Capstone Pharmacy Review

Edited by

Barb Mason, PharmD, FASHP
Professor of Pharmacy Practice
College of Pharmacy
Idaho State University
Ambulatory Care Clinician
Boise Veteran Affairs Medical Center
Boise, Idaho

Debra Parker, PharmD, BCPS
Chair and Associate Professor
College of Pharmacy
The University of Findlay
Findlay, Ohio

Rex S. Lott, PharmD, BCPP
Professor of Pharmacy Practice
College of Pharmacy
Idaho State University
Mental Health Clinical Pharmacist
Boise Veteran Affairs Medical Center
Clinical Associate Professor
Department of Psychiatry and Behavioral Sciences
School of Medicine
University of Washington
Boise, Idaho

JONES & BARTLETT
LEARNING

World Headquarters
Jones & Bartlett Learning
5 Wall Street
Burlington, MA 01803
978-443-5000
info@jblearning.com
www.jblearning.com

Jones & Bartlett Learning books and products are available through most bookstores and online booksellers. To contact Jones & Bartlett Learning directly, call 800-832-0034, fax 978-443-8000, or visit our website, www.jblearning.com.

Substantial discounts on bulk quantities of Jones & Bartlett Learning publications are available to corporations, professional associations, and other qualified organizations. For details and specific discount information, contact the special sales department at Jones & Bartlett Learning via the above contact information or send an email to specialsales@jblearning.com.

Production Credits
Publisher: William Brottmiller
Senior Acquisitions Editor: Katey Birtcher
Editorial Assistant: Kayla Dos Santos
Editorial Assistant: Sean Fabery
Associate Production Editor: Jill Morton
Marketing Manager: Grace Richards
Manufacturing and Inventory Control Supervisor: Amy Bacus
Composition: Laserwords Private Limited, Chennai, India
Cover Design: Scott Moden
Cover Images: (Background) © Morgan Lane Photography/ShutterStock, Inc.,
(left) Courtesy of Rhoda Baer/National Cancer Institute,
(middle) © Paul Morley/ShutterStock, Inc.,
(right) © 18percentgrey/ShutterStock, Inc.
Chapter Opener Image: © Evgeny Karandaev/ShutterStock, Inc.
Printing and Binding: Courier Companies
Cover Printing: Courier Companies

To order this product, use ISBN: 978-1-2840-3155-3

Library of Congress Cataloging-in-Publication Data

Capstone pharmacy review / edited by Barb Mason, Debra Parker, and Rex S. Lott.
p. ; cm.
Includes bibliographical references and index.
ISBN 978-0-7637-8442-3 – ISBN 0-7637-8442-7
I. Kennedy, Barb J. II. Parker, Debra. III. Lott, Rex S.
[DNLM: 1. Pharmacological Phenomena–Outlines. 2. Drug Therapy–methods–Outlines. QV 18.2]

615.5–dc23

2012031185

6048

Printed in the United States of America
17 16 15 14 13 10 9 8 7 6 5 4 3 2 1

Dedication

To my parents, Charlie and Evelyn, who gave me roots and wings, and my husband, Jim, and daughter, Stacia, who keep me grounded, yet let me soar, thanks to their support and love.

—Barb Mason, PharmD, FASHP

With appreciation to my family, especially Devin, Olivia, Sophia, and Reese, for their constant love and support.

—Debra Parker, PharmD, BCPS

My thanks and recognition go to my colleagues and mentors who provided me opportunities, support, and encouragement over the years. Special thanks go to Melvin R. Gibson, Allen I. White, Philip Hansten, Peter Penna, and Lloyd Young. I also want to recognize the students and colleagues who, over the years, never hesitated to question me or stimulate me to think harder. Finally, I'd like to thank my children, David and Joann, and my wife, Mary, for their support.

—Rex S. Lott, PharmD, BCPP

Brief Contents

Contents

Preface

HOW TO USE THIS BOOK

As you have already successfully reached the pinnacle of pharmacy education through graduation, you might think it a little insulting that we would include a section on "How to use this book." There is no doubt that how individual NAPLEX candidates study for exams differs, and how they use the various study tools differs as well. The format and platform with which to access the study material can be just as much of a factor in exam success as the quality of the information presented. Some learners demand already-printed content at their fingers, whereas others prefer online access and mobile applications. When the editors conceived the idea for *Capstone Pharmacy Review* (CPR), it was based on our idea for a study system stemming from a collective 70 years of pharmacy practice and teaching. We welcome your ideas and feedback on your successes and the elements that worked best for your NAPLEX study, as we continuously work on new and improved future editions.

The title says it all: *Capstone Pharmacy Review*. What you have just purchased is more than just a review book. Rather, it is a system designed to meet the needs of all levels of students studying for the NAPLEX exam. Students differ tremendously in how much they study for the NAPLEX exam, but all uniformly agree that the ideal amount of time invested in studying should be no more or no less than what it takes to pass the exam. Trying to figure out that threshold is the key to knowing when you are ready for the test.

Throughout your pharmacy curriculum, your course work was guided by competencies—that theme will follow you throughout your career. This system is the one and only NAPLEX review offering that emphasizes the three competencies on which the NAPLEX is based. It enables individuals to readily focus on their weak areas and direct their study time accordingly. If you are strong in Competency Area 1, which accounts for 56% of the test, but less so in Competency Area 2, which represents 33% of the test, then you know where your emphasis should be. Both the topic section content and the exam questions can be sorted to focus on those areas of study in which you need the most help.

The book content begins with a Foundational Pharmacy Review to address those concepts presented early in your pharmacy curriculum. Not all students will need to start with this section. Like most things in pharmacy, competencies are not black and white. There is a good chance that information you study for Competency 1 will overlap with the material needed for Competency 2. We consider it a healthy approach to not silo information, but rather integrate it as we are required to do every day in pharmacy practice. Most readers would expect a logical flow from Competency 1 to 2 to 3, but the editors intentionally started the Competency portion of the book with Competency 2. The Foundational Pharmacy Review precedes the Competency 2 section and consists of a concise review of common therapeutic agents jointly written by a pharmacologist and a medicinal chemist. Additional topics in the Foundational Pharmacy Review include a review of chemical pharmacologic classes of therapeutic agents, biopharmaceutics, pharmacokinetics/therapeutic drug monitoring, basic principles of drug interactions, and pharmacoeconomic principles. Because pharmacoeconomics for the first time has been incorporated into the recently released NAPLEX Competency Blueprint, we include a brief review of this area in the Foundational Pharmacy Review. For many readers, this first section will form a firm study foundation before you move on to Competency 2; it will also boost your confidence, which is extremely important in exam preparation. Other readers may opt to skip the Foundational Pharmacy Review section and return to only those topics in that section they later identify as weak after taking the practice exam. Regardless of which section or chapter is reviewed, whether in printed format or online, the material stands alone and does not require a sequenced approach; instead, it lends itself well to "jumping around."

A multitude of pharmacists from diverse practices, backgrounds, and walks of life contributed to this book. PharmD students also assisted in the review of the book. They are able to provide you with a perspective beyond what your academic alma mater could do alone. The academic professor-writers in the group were quick to agree that not all PharmDs are created equal; thus some NAPLEX candidates will need more prep time regarding certain sections and certain topics than others.

The comprehensive inclusion of topics beyond what is available in all competing NAPLEX review offerings ensures that student needs will be met for content review. Self-care topics are emphasized in this CPR Board prep system. This focus reflects the statistics showing that the majority of graduates enter into retail pharmacy as well as similar statistics showing inconsistent curricular offerings on over-the-counter drugs. Topics that have significant OTC and prescription elements are intentionally separated and provided as distinct sections. While this material may appear repetitive to some extent, it was an intentional approach by the editors to reinforce that content. If you are not one of those students who needs study time for a certain section, then the editors suggest you skip that section and move on to the next.

The format is intended to be consistent throughout so you become familiar with the text's style and do not have to deal with the classroom challenges many of you have encountered with team-taught courses and the need to "read the minds" of your professors. The heading format for Competency 1 directly follows the information in the NAPLEX Blueprint. Not all of these headings are applicable to every therapeutic topic, so any deviation in the format should not be viewed as an omission. The section content is rich in tables that include information such as drug indications, mechanisms of action, common doses, generic names, trade names, and dosage form availability. These tables lend themselves well to flash card and print-and-review study.

The Tips Worth Tweeting feature is a nod to the social networking offerings so vital to this generation of learners; it represents a more contemporary version of the highlighted or bulleted lists of key information. CPR's lack of extensive content on pathophysiology, which is so prevalent in pharmacotherapy courses throughout PharmD curricula, is consistent with the NAPLEX competencies.

This CPR Board review system complements other NAPLEX review systems on the market and can easily be used side by side with them in study sessions. Some students like to jump to a practice exam first to determine the areas in which they are weak and go from there. Reviewing answers with explanations to exam questions is a sure-fire way to retain information learned. For additional content, students can then go to those texts that have topic content reviews. Not all NAPLEX review books have content review elements, however, so some students find themselves going to their old class notes and becoming overwhelmed with content for what is an entry-level exam. This CPR Board review system is meant to serve as a "happy medium"—offering content and practice exams for students who prefer to set aside a specified study time, while still enabling those students on the fly to take advantage of the online mobile applications through which they can pick up threads of information and study intermittently.

The NAPLEX Competency Statements

The NAPLEX Competency Statements provide a blueprint of the topics covered on the examination. They offer important information about the knowledge, judgment, and skills you are expected to demonstrate as an entry-level pharmacist. A strong understanding of the Competency Statements will aid in your preparation to take the examination.

AREA 1: ASSESS PHARMACOTHERAPY TO ASSURE SAFE AND EFFECTIVE THERAPEUTIC OUTCOMES (APPROXIMATELY 56% OF TEST)

1.1.0 Identify, interpret, and evaluate patient information to determine the presence of a disease or medical condition, assess the need for treatment and/or referral, and identify patient-specific factors that affect health, pharmacotherapy, and/or disease management.

- 1.1.1 Identify and assess patient information including medication, laboratory, and disease state histories.
- 1.1.2 Identify patient-specific assessment and diagnostic methods, instruments, and techniques and interpret their results.
- 1.1.3 Identify and define the etiology, terminology, signs, and symptoms associated with diseases and medical conditions and their causes and determine if medical referral is necessary.
- 1.1.4 Identify and evaluate patient genetic, and biosocial factors, and concurrent drug therapy, relevant to the maintenance of wellness and the prevention or treatment of a disease or medical condition.

1.2.0 Evaluate information about pharmacoeconomic factors, dosing regimen, dosage forms, delivery systems, and routes of administration to identify and select optimal pharmacotherapeutic agents for patients.

- 1.2.1 Identify specific uses and indications for drug products and recommend drugs of choice for specific diseases or medical conditions.
- 1.2.2 Identify the chemical/pharmacologic classes of therapeutic agents and describe their known or postulated sites and mechanisms of action.
- 1.2.3 Evaluate drug therapy for the presence of pharmacotherapeutic duplications and interactions with other drugs, food, and diagnostic tests.
- 1.2.4 Identify and evaluate potential contraindications and provide information about warnings and precautions associated with a drug product's active and inactive ingredients.
- 1.2.5 Identify physicochemical properties of drug substances that affect their solubility, pharmacodynamic and pharmacokinetic properties, pharmacologic actions, and stability.
- 1.2.6 Evaluate and interpret pharmacodynamic and pharmacokinetic principles to calculate and determine appropriate drug dosing regimens.
- 1.2.7 Identify appropriate routes of administration, dosage forms, and pharmaceutical characteristics of drug dosage forms and delivery systems, to assure bioavailability and enhance therapeutic efficacy.

Note: This blueprint took effect on March 1, 2010.

1.3.0 Evaluate and manage drug regimens by monitoring and assessing the patient and/or patient information, collaborating with other healthcare professionals, and providing patient education to enhance safe, effective, and economic patient outcomes.

1.3.1 Identify pharmacotherapeutic outcomes and endpoints.

1.3.2 Evaluate patient signs and symptoms, and the findings of monitoring tests and procedures to determine the safety and effectiveness of pharmacotherapy. Recommend needed follow-up evaluations or tests when appropriate.

1.3.3 Identify, describe, and provide information regarding the mechanism of adverse reactions, allergies, side effects, iatrogenic, and drug-induced illness, including their management and prevention.

1.3.4 Identify, prevent, and address methods to remedy medication nonadherence, misuse, or abuse.

1.3.5 Evaluate current drug regimens and recommend pharmacotherapeutic alternatives or modifications.

AREA 2: ASSESS SAFE AND ACCURATE PREPARATION AND DISPENSING OF MEDICATIONS (APPROXIMATELY 33% OF TEST)

2.1.0 Demonstrate the ability to perform calculations required to compound, dispense, and administer medication.

2.1.1 Calculate the quantity of medication to be compounded or dispensed; reduce and enlarge formulation quantities; and calculate the quantity or ingredients needed to compound the proper amount of the preparation.

2.1.2 Calculate nutritional needs and the caloric content of nutrient sources.

2.1.3 Calculate the rate of drug administration.

2.1.4 Calculate or convert drug concentrations, ratio strengths, and/or extent of ionization.

2.2.0 Demonstrate the ability to select and dispense medications in a manner that promotes safe and effective use.

2.2.1 Identify drug products by their generic, brand, and/or common names.

2.2.2 Identify whether a particular drug dosage strength or dosage form is commercially available and whether it is available on a nonprescription basis.

2.2.3 Identify commercially available drug products by their characteristic physical attributes.

2.2.4 Assess pharmacokinetic parameters and quality assurance data to determine equivalence among manufactured drug products, and identify products for which documented evidence of inequivalence exists.

2.2.5 Identify and provide information regarding appropriate packaging, storage, handling, administration, and disposal of medications.

2.2.6 Identify and provide information regarding the appropriate use of equipment and apparatus required to administer medications.

2.3.0 Demonstrate the knowledge to prepare and compound extemporaneous preparations and sterile products.

2.3.1 Identify techniques, procedures, and equipment related to drug preparation, compounding, and quality assurance.

2.3.2 Identify the important physicochemical properties of a preparation's active and inactive ingredients.

2.3.3 Identify the mechanism of and evidence for the incompatibility or degradation of a product or preparation and methods for achieving its stability.

AREA 3: ASSESS, RECOMMEND, AND PROVIDE HEALTHCARE INFORMATION THAT PROMOTES PUBLIC HEALTH (APPROXIMATELY 11% OF TEST)

3.1.0 Identify, evaluate, and apply information to promote optimal health care.

3.1.1 Identify the typical content of specific sources of drug and health information for both healthcare providers and consumers, and recommend appropriate resources to address questions or needs.

3.1.2 Evaluate the suitability, accuracy, and reliability of clinical and pharmacoeconomic data by analyzing experimental design, statistical tests, interpreting results, and formulating conclusions.

3.2.0 Recommend and provide information to educate the public and healthcare professionals regarding medical conditions, wellness, dietary supplements, and medical devices.

3.2.1 Recommend and provide healthcare information regarding the prevention and treatment of diseases and medical conditions, including emergency patient care and vaccinations.

3.2.2 Recommend and provide healthcare information regarding nutrition, lifestyle, and other nondrug measures that promote health or prevent the progression of a disease or medical condition.

3.2.3 Recommend and provide information regarding the documented uses, adverse effects, and toxicities of dietary supplements.

3.2.4 Recommend and provide information regarding the selection, use, and care of medical/surgical appliances and devices, self-care products, and durable medical equipment, as well as products and techniques for self-monitoring of health status and medical conditions.

About the Editors

Barb Mason, PharmD, FASHP, started her career at South Dakota State University, developing a geriatric curriculum and initiating ambulatory care pharmacy services at the Sioux Falls Veterans Administration (VA). The 9-month teaching position allowed her to do summer itinerate pharmacy work with the Indian Health Service and serve as a relief pharmacist for community pharmacies across the state. This experience was followed by a director of pharmacy education position at the University of Arkansas Medical Sciences AHEC-El Dorado. In her current position with Idaho State University and the Boise VA, Dr. Mason has been active in state pharmacy organizations and pharmacy residency education. She has been recognized during her career as Most Influential Professor, Teacher of the Year, and Pharmacist of the Year. Through her experiences, she has been party to the evolution of a network of colleagues who were instrumental in the origination, creation, and completion of this book. The breadth of their experiences, contributions, feedback, and support is the foundation of this project.

Debra Parker, PharmD, BCPS, received her doctorate of pharmacy degree from Ohio Northern University, and began her professional practice with a residency in pharmacy practice at Riverside Methodist Hospital in Columbus, Ohio. Throughout her career, she has gained experience in drug information, independent pharmacy, and collaborative private practice, where she has directed multiple ambulatory care clinics. Dr. Parker now serves as an associate professor and chair of the department of pharmacy practice at The University of Findlay College of Pharmacy. She is a board-certified pharmacotherapy specialist as well as a certified anticoagulation provider, a clinical lipid specialist, and a certified diabetes educator, and enjoys teaching these topics as part of The University of Findlay curriculum. In addition to her academic responsibilities, Dr. Parker continues to maintain a clinical practice with St. Rita's Health Management Group in Lima, Ohio. Past recognitions include Ohio Northern University Preceptor of the Year, The University of Findlay Teacher of the Year, and the Ohio Pharmacists Association Innovative Pharmacy Practice Award.

Rex S. Lott, PharmD, BCPP, is a professor in the department of practice and administrative sciences at Idaho State University's College of Pharmacy. He has practiced and taught psychiatric and neurologic pharmacy for more than 35 years. He earned a bachelor of pharmacy degree from Washington State University in 1972 and a doctor of pharmacy degree from the University of Minnesota in 1977. Dr. Lott was an assistant professor of clinical pharmacy at Washington State University from 1972 until 1978. He has been a psychiatric clinical pharmacist in Minnesota's state hospital system and was also a clinical assistant professor at the University of Minnesota College of Pharmacy. From 1985 to 1997, Dr. Lott served as director of pharmacy in two institutions for developmentally disabled adults in Washington State. During that time, he also worked as a long-term care consultant pharmacist and maintained a private practice as a pharmacotherapy consultant. From 1994 until 1997, he was also a clinical associate professor with the University of Washington School of Pharmacy. In 1997, Dr. Lott returned to academia as a full-time faculty member at Idaho State University with a practice in psychiatric pharmacy at the Boise, Idaho, Veterans Administration Medical Center. In 2008, he was also appointed as a clinical associate professor in the department of psychiatry and behavioral sciences at the University of Washington's School of Medicine. He precepts students from Idaho State University, and, since 2008, has taught third- and fourth-year residents in the University of Washington's Idaho Track Psychiatry Residency.

Section Coordinators

James R. Clem, PharmD
Professor and Department Head of Pharmacy Practice
College of Pharmacy
South Dakota State University
Sioux Falls, SD

Larry Dent, BS Pharm, PharmD, BCPS, RPh
Associate Professor of Pharmacy Practice
Skaggs School of Pharmacy
University of Montana
Missoula, MT
Clinical Account Manager, Rx Services
Government Healthcare Solutions
Xerox State Healthcare, LLC
Anchorage, AK

Teresa K. Hoffmann, PharmD, CDE, CLS, BCPS
Ambulatory Care Residency Program Director
Health Management Group
St. Rita's Medical Center
Lima, OH

Sandra Hrometz, BS Pharm, PhD
Associate Professor of Pharmacology
College of Pharmacy
Ohio Northern University
Ada, OH

Michael Klepser, PharmD, BCPS
Professor of Pharmacy Practice
College of Pharmacy
Ferris State University
Kalamazoo, MI

Catherine M. Oliphant, PharmD
Associate Professor of Pharmacy
College of Pharmacy
Idaho State University
Pocatello, ID

Katherine Kelly Orr, PharmD
Clinical Associate Professor
College of Pharmacy
University of Rhode Island
Charleston, RI

Tracy K. Pettinger, PharmD, BCPS
Clinical Assistant Professor
College of Pharmacy
Idaho State University
Pocatello, ID

Jennifer D. Smith, PharmD, CPP, BC-ADM, CDE
Associate Professor of Pharmacy
Campbell University College of Pharmacy and Health Sciences
Wilson, NC

Contributors List

John Arross, BS, RPh
Wyoming Medical Center
Casper, WY

Nathan R. Ash, PharmD, CACP
St. Rita's Medical Center
Lima, OH

Alberto Augsten, PharmD
Memorial Regional Hospital
Hollywood, FL

Katie Hinkle-Axford, PharmD, BCPS
College of Pharmacy
Ferris State University
Big Rapids, MI

Matt Beachnau, PharmD
Munson Medical Center
Traverse City, MI

Scott J. Bergman, PharmD, BCPS
Edwardsville School of Pharmacy
Southern Illinois University
Springfield, IL

Amy C. Bower, PharmD
Borgess Medical Center
Kalamazoo, MI

Sherril Brown, DVM, PharmD, BCPS
Skaggs School of Pharmacy
University of Montana
Missoula, MT

Katherine A. Campbell-Petkewicz, PharmD
VA Hospital
Hines, IL

Glenda Carr, PharmD
College of Pharmacy
Idaho State University
Meridian, ID

Jaclynn Chin, PharmD
South Dakota State University
Brookings, SD

James R. Clem, PharmD
South Dakota State University
Sioux Falls, SD

Kevin W. Cleveland, PharmD
College of Pharmacy
Idaho State University
Pocatello, ID

Curtis D. Collins, PharmD, MS
University Michigan Health System Hospital
Ann Arbor, MI

Emily H. Collins-Lucey, PharmD
Mercy Hospital
St. Louis, MO

Halley Connor-Hustedde, PharmD
Edwardsville School of Pharmacy
Southern Illinois University
Chatham, IL

Jill. A. Covyeou, PharmD
College of Pharmacy
Ferris State University
Essexville, MI

Kendall M. Crane, PharmD, BCPS
Boise VA Medical Center
Boise, ID

Christopher W. Crank, PharmD, MHSM, BCPS
Rush University Medical Center
Chicago, IL

Robyn Cruz, PharmD, BCPS, BCPP
Sioux Falls VA Health Care System
Sioux Falls, SD

Jean E. Cunningham, BSPS, PharmD, BCPS
College of Pharmacy
The University of Findlay
Findlay, OH

Gina Davis, PharmD
College of Pharmacy
Idaho State University
Pocatello, ID

Larry Dent, BS Pharm, PharmD, BCPS, RPh
Skaggs School of Pharmacy
University of Montana
Missoula, MT

Michaela M. Doss, PharmD, BCPS
OSF Saint Francis Medical Center
Peoria, IL

Richard Dudley, RPh, PhD
College of Pharmacy
The University of Findlay
Findlay, OH

Sandra Earle, PharmD
College of Pharmacy
The University of Findlay
Findlay, OH

Lori J. Ernsthausen, PharmD, BCPS
College of Pharmacy
The University of Findlay
Findlay, OH

John Erramouspe, PharmD, MS
College of Pharmacy
Idaho State University
Pocatello, ID

Nathan Everson, PharmD
Henry Ford Hospital
St. Ignace, MI

Debra K. Farver, PharmD
Avera Sacred Heart Hospital
Yankton, SD

Danielle P. Fennema, PharmD
Health Management Group St. Rita's
Medical Center
Lima, OH

Debra K. Gardner, PharmD
The Ohio State University Medical Center
Columbus, OH

Teddie Gould, BS, MS, PharmD, BCPS
College of Pharmacy
Idaho State University
Pocatello, ID

Randi Lynn Griffiths, PharmD, BCPS
VA Medical Center
Boise, ID

Payal K. Gurnani, PharmD, BCPS
Rush University Medical Center
at Rush Medical College
Chicago, IL

Jennifer K. Hagerman, PharmD
College of Pharmacy
Ferris State University
Grand Rapids, MI

Katherine S. Hale, PharmD, BCPS
Skaggs School of Pharmacy
University of Montana
Missoula, MT

Greg Hall, PharmD

Shannon Hartke, PharmD candidate
College of Pharmacy
The University of Findlay
Findlay, OH

Jennifer Hawkey, PharmD candidate
College of Pharmacy
The University of Findlay
Findlay, OH

Thaddaus R. Hellwig, PharmD, BCPS
Sanford Medical Center
Sioux Falls, SD

Tanner W. Higgenbothom, PharmD
College of Pharmacy
Idaho State University
Chubbuck, ID

Teresa K. Hoffmann, PharmD, CDE, CLS, BCPS
Health Management Group St. Rita's
Medical Center
Lima, OH

Sandra L. Hrometz, BS Pharm, PhD
College of Pharmacy
Ohio Northern University
Ada, OH

Jolie Jantz, PharmD, BCPS
College of Pharmacy/Kootenai Medical Center
Idaho State University
Coeur d'Alene, ID

Mindy Jock, PharmD
Munson Medical Center
Traverse City, MI

Annette M. Johnson, PharmD
College of Pharmacy
South Dakota State University
Sioux Falls, SD

Karen L. Kier, BS, MSC, PhD, BCPS
College of Pharmacy
Ohio Northern University
Ada, OH

Michael Klepser, PharmD, FCCP
College of Pharmacy
Ferris State University
Kalamazoo, MI

Jamie Ridley Klucken, PharmD, MBA
Bernard J. Dunn School of Pharmacy
Shenandoah University
Winchester, VA

H. Stephen Lee, PharmD
College of Pharmacy
Ferris State University
Big Rapids, MI

Jean C. Lee, PharmD, BCPS, AAHIVE
Saint Mary's Health Care
Grand Rapids, MI

Joy K. Lehman, PharmD, BCNSP
The Ohio State University Medical Center
Columbus, OH

Terri L. Levien, PharmD
College of Pharmacy
Washington State University
Spokane, WA

B. Shane Martin, PharmD
VA Medical Center
Chillicothe, OH

Suzanne Lifer, PharmD candidate
College of Pharmacy
The University of Findlay
Findlay, OH

Srikumaran Melethil, PhD, JD
Law and Science Consulting
The University of Findlay
Findlay, OH

Kimberly Messerschmidt, BS Pharm, PharmD
Sanford Medical Center
Sioux Falls, SD

Michael M. Milks, BS Pharm, PhD
College of Pharmacy
Ohio Northern University
Ada, OH

Nicole Murdock, PharmD, BCPS
College of Pharmacy
Idaho State University
Pocatello, ID

Michelle R. Musser, PharmD
Blanchard Valley Medical Associates
Findlay, OH

Jerod L. Nagel, PharmD, BCPS
University of Michigan Hospitals and Health Centers
Ann Arbor, MI

Amber Norris, PharmD
Leonidas, MI

Kelley Oehlke, PharmD
South Dakota State University
Sioux Falls, SD

Mark E. Olah, PhD
College of Pharmacy
Ohio Northern University
Ada, OH

Catherine M. Oliphant, PharmD
College of Pharmacy
Idaho State University
Meridian, ID

Katherine Kelly Orr, PharmD
College of Pharmacy
University of Rhode Island
Charleston, RI

Christopher T. Owens, PharmD, BCPS
College of Pharmacy
Idaho State University
Pocatello, ID

Vinita B. Pai, PharmD, MS
The Ohio State University Medical Center
Columbus, OH

Laura Perry, PharmD, BCPS
College of Pharmacy
The University of Findlay
Findlay, OH

Stacy J. Peters, PharmD
South Dakota State University
Sioux Falls, SD

Tracy K. Pettinger, PharmD, BCPS
College of Pharmacy
Idaho State University
Pocatello, ID

Sarah J. Popish, PharmD, BCPP
US Department of Veterans Affairs
Sierra Pacific Network
Martinez, CA

Adam D. Porath, PharmD, BCPS
Renown Regional Medical Center
Reno, NV

Kendra Procacci, PharmD, BCPS, AE-C
Skaggs School of Pharmacy
University of Montana
Missoula, MT

Brooke Pugmire, PharmD, BCPS
College of Pharmacy
Idaho State University
Pocatello, ID

Anna Ratka, PharmD, PhD
Texas A&M Health Science Center
Irma Lerma Rangel College of Pharmacy
Kingsville, TX

Kristin McCray-Sampson, PharmD, BCPS
VA Medical Center
Boise, VA

M. Chandra Sekar, PhD
College of Pharmacy
The University of Findlay
Findlay, OH

Bradley W. Shinn, BS, PharmD
College of Pharmacy
The University of Findlay
Findlay, OH

Jennifer D. Smith, PharmD, CPP, BC-ADM, CDE
Campbell University College of Pharmacy and Health Sciences
Wilson, NC

Lindsay R. Snyder, BSPS, PharmD, BCPS
Saint Joseph Regional Medical Center
South Bend, IN

Kenneth R. Speidel, BS Pharm, PharmD
College of Pharmacy
The University of Findlay
Findlay, OH

Michelle L. Steed, PharmD, CDE
College of Pharmacy/Kootenai Medical Center
Idaho State University
Coeur d'Alene, ID

Seth Thomas, PharmD
St. Luke's Regional Medical Center
Boise, ID

Jeffrey M. Tingen, PharmD, MBA
University of Michigan
Ann Arbor, MI

Mary Ann Tucker, PharmD, BCPS
Blanchard Valley Medical Associates
Findlay, OH

Connie Valente, PharmD

Heather L. VandenBussche, PharmD
Ferris State University
Kalamazoo, MI

Thomas G. Wadsworth, PharmD, BCPS
Idaho State University
Meridian, ID

Courtenay Gilmore Wilson, PharmD, BCPS
Mountain Area Health Education Center
Family Health Center
Asheville, NC

Reviewers

John S. Clark, PharmD, MS, BCPS
Associate Director of Pharmacy
University of Michigan Hospitals and Health Centers
Clinical Assistant Professor
College of Pharmacy
University of Michigan
Ann Arbor, MI

Flora G. Estes, PharmD
Assistant Dean for Practice Programs
Assistant Professor of Pharmacy Practice
College of Pharmacy and Health Sciences
Texas Southern University
Houston, TX

Kylee Funk
Pharmacy Student
University of Michigan
Ann Arbor, MI

Reza Karimi, RPh, PhD
Associate Dean for Academic Affairs and Assessment
Pacific University
Forest Grove, OR

Laurie Mauro, PharmD
Professor of Clinical Pharmacy
College of Pharmacy
The University of Toledo
Toledo, OH

Vincent F. Mauro, PharmD, FCCP
Professor of Clinical Pharmacy
College of Pharmacy
The University of Toledo
Toledo, OH

Foundational Pharmacy Review

SECTION

1

Chemical/Pharmacological Classes of Therapeutic Agents

CHAPTER 1

Contributors: Mark E. Olah and Richard Dudley

THERAPEUTIC AGENTS FOR RESPIRATORY DISORDERS

Asthma

Asthma is a chronic inflammatory disease of the pulmonary airways that results in substantial bronchoconstriction. Thus the major drug classes used in the treatment of asthma are anti-inflammatory agents and direct-acting bronchodilators. Drugs in both groups are available for oral administration or inhalation.

Bronchodilators intended for asthma therapy are fairly selective agonists of the **beta$_2$-adrenergic receptor** located on bronchial smooth muscle. These agonists include albuterol and long-acting agents such as salmeterol and formoterol. Activation of the beta$_2$-adrenergic receptor results in activation of adenylyl cyclase and generation of cAMP, with a resulting relaxation of bronchial smooth muscle.

Theophylline also produces bronchodilation in people with asthma. This effect likely occurs due to an increase in cAMP. Additional proposed mechanisms of action include activation of bronchial adenosine receptors and inhibition of the phosphodiesterases responsible for cAMP degradation.

Most anti-inflammatory drugs used to treat asthma are administered chronically. **Corticosteroids** are commonly used for treatment of asthma; agents employed include beclomethasone and fluticasone, both of which are administered via inhalation—a method that reduces the likelihood of systemic effects. These corticosteroids generally act by stimulating glucocorticoid receptors, with subsequent transcriptional regulation of pro- and anti-inflammatory mediators. The activity of various inflammatory cell types, such as eosinophils and leukocytes, is also modified.

Cromolyn also produces anti-inflammatory effects by inhibiting the release of histamine and other inflammatory mediators from mast cells. Cromolyn appears to stabilize mast cell membranes and prevent release of these mediators.

Cysteinyl leukotrienes also play a role in asthma. These compounds are bronchoconstrictors but also have pro-inflammatory effects. **Zileutin** is a competitive inhibitor of 5-lipoxygenase, the enzyme responsible for the generation of cysteinyl leukotrienes from arachadonic acid. Thus zileutin blocks the biosynthesis of cysteinyl leukotrienes. **Zafirlukast** and **montelukast** block a leukotriene receptor, the CysLT1 receptor, and inhibit the actions of cysteinyl leukotrienes. Through their interference with leukotriene-mediated activity, zileutin, zafirlukast and montelukast promote bronchodilation and, to a lesser extent, have an anti-inflammatory effect.

Chronic Obstructive Pulmonary Disease

Chronic obstructive pulmonary disease (COPD), like asthma, is characterized by both bronchoconstriction and airway inflammation. Thus many of the drugs used for asthma may also be employed in COPD.

Muscarinic receptor antagonists (ipratropium, tiotropium) may be useful in

COPD. These agents are nonselective antagonists at all five muscarinic receptors, although their beneficial effect of bronchodilation is most likely due to blockade of the M3 muscarinic receptor on bronchial smooth muscle.

THERAPEUTIC AGENTS FOR CARDIOVASCULAR DISORDERS

Hyperlipidemia

The **HMG-CoA reductase inhibitors ("statins")** are competitive inhibitors of the rate-limiting enzyme in cholesterol biosynthesis. Reduction in cholesterol synthesis by these agents promotes increased expression of hepatic LDL receptors that are responsible for LDL-cholesterol uptake. The cumulative result of these actions is a significant reduction in plasma levels of LDL-cholesterol. Statins may produce a slight increase in HDL-cholesterol in individuals with low HDL levels and lower triglycerides in hypertriglyceridemic individuals.

A major safety concern with statins is the potential for development of skeletal muscle myopathy, which may progress to rhabdomyolysis and eventual renal failure. Multiple mechanisms secondary to HMG-CoA reductase inhibition may account for the skeletal muscle damage. Hepatotoxicity has also been associated with statin administration.

Ezetimibe is an inhibitor of the Niemann-Pick C disease-like protein (NPC1L1), which is found on enterocytes of the small intestine. Blockade of NPC1L1 reduces intestinal absorption of dietary cholesterol with no direct effects on cholesterol biosynthesis. However, secondary to the reduction of LDL-cholesterol, cholesterol biosynthesis may be increased. Thus ezetimibe is often used in combination with a statin to counteract this reflex increase.

Bile acid sequestrants, such as cholestyramine, colestipol, and colesevelam, are positively charged resins. After oral administration, these agents are not systemically absorbed, but rather act in the intestine to bind bile acids. The bile acids then cannot be reabsorbed and are excreted. In response to the reduction of the recycling of bile acids, the liver increases LDL-receptor expression and directs cholesterol toward bile acid synthesis with a reduction in plasma LDL-cholesterol levels. Adverse drug reactions are restricted to the GI system (dyspepsia, bloating, constipation). Bile acid sequestrants may interfere with the absorption of many drugs, so concomitant administration with other agents should be avoided.

Niacin (nicotinic acid) has a very widespread beneficial effect on the lipid profile. Effects include reduction of LDL-cholesterol and triglyceride levels and increased HDL-cholesterol level. Niacin may also decrease lipoprotein a (Lp[a]) levels. These effects occur via multiple mechanisms. Triglycerides and LDL-cholesterol may be lowered secondary to niacin-mediated inhibition of hormone-sensitive lipase in adipose tissue, which results in a decrease in free fatty acid transportation to the liver. This effect may occur due to the activation of a G-protein–coupled receptor on adipocytes. Niacin decreases hepatic clearance of Apo A-1, a precursor of HDL. The end result is an increase in mature HDL levels. Niacin frequently causes a transient dermal flushing reaction owing to an increase in prostaglandin levels with subsequent vasodilation. The flushing reaction is more common with immediate-release forms of niacin. Sustained-release preparations of niacin may cause hepatoxicity with flu-like syndrome and elevated liver enzymes.

Fibrates (clofibrate, gemfibrozil, fenofibrate) promote a decrease in triglyceride levels with moderate and variable effects on other lipoproteins. Fibrates activate peroxisome proliferator-activated receptor a (PPARa) on hepatocytes, which produces several effects that promote fatty acid oxidation and, therefore, decreased synthesis of triglycerides. Gemfibrozil may increase the occurrence of myopathy in patients who are also receiving a statin.

Thromboembolic Disorders

Most available anticoagulant drugs produce their effects by binding to and enhancing the activity of the endogenous anticoagulant protein antithrombin. Antithrombin primarily inhibits thrombin and Factor Xa via a suicide inhibition. **Unfractionated heparin** (UFH), **low-molecular-weight heparin** (LMWH), and synthetic **fondaparinux** all possess the critical pentasaccharide sequence necessary for antithrombin binding and activation. LMWH and fondaparinux primarily direct antithrombin activity against Factor Xa.

Direct thrombin inhibitors, including lepirudin, bivalirudin, argatroban, and dabigatrin, bind directly to the active site of thrombin to produce their anticoagulant effects. Direct thrombin inhibitors do not require interaction with antithrombin to produce an effect.

With all of the previously mentioned agents, the major adverse effect is undesired bleeding or hemorrhage. Heparin-induced thrombocytopenia is a concern with UFH, but the incidence of this event is much lower with LMWH and fondaparinux.

Warfarin inhibits vitamin K epoxide reductase, the enzyme responsible for generation of the reduced form of vitamin K. The reduced form of vitamin K is a necessary cofactor for the post-translational carboxylation of prothrombin, Factor VII, Factor IX, and Factor X. As a result of warfarin administration, the active forms of these clotting factors are not released and their plasma levels decline. As is true for the parenteral anticoagulants, the major adverse effect associated with warfarin is hemorrhage. Because of the risk of warfarin-induced birth defects, warfarin administration is avoided in pregnant women.

The majority of **antiplatelet drugs** act via an inhibition of platelet activator signaling or through blockade of glycoprotein IIb-IIIa (GP IIb-IIIa), which is the final mediator of platelet aggregation.

Aspirin inhibits cyclooxygenase-1 (COX-1) and disrupts formation of thromboxane A_2, a mediator of platelet activation. **Clopidogrel** and **prasugrel** are both prodrugs whose active metabolites are irreversible antagonists of the P2Y12 purinergic receptor on platelets. Blockade of the P2Y12 purinergic receptor prevents its activation by ADP, a potent platelet activator.

Abciximab, a chimeric antibody, and **tirofiban**, a nonpeptide antagonist, bind to extracellular regions of GP IIb-IIIa and inhibit activity of this key mediator of platelet aggregation.

Dipyridamole is an inhibitor of the adenosine transporter and blocks phosphodiesterase. Both of these actions ultimately result in increased intracellular cAMP within the platelets, which produces antiplatelet effects.

Most **thrombolytic** drugs act by mimicking the actions of the endogenous fibrinolytic protein, tissue plasminogen activator (t-PA). Human t-PA is available as recombinant protein. **Reteplase** and **tenecteplase** are variants of t-PA that have been genetically engineered to increase their plasma half-lives.

Hypertension

Most drugs used to treat hypertension lower blood pressure by either reducing cardiac output or decreasing peripheral vascular resistance by promoting vasodilation. Many, but not all, of these agents act to regulate the sympathetic nervous system and its role in controlling both cardiac and vascular function.

Antihypertensive drugs that target the sympathetic nervous system are often collectively referred to as **sympatholytics**. This group includes **beta-adrenergic receptor antagonists (beta blockers)**, **alpha-adrenergic receptor antagonists (alpha blockers)**, and **centrally acting sympatholytics**. Beta blockers, through antagonism of cardiac beta-adrenergic receptors, decrease heart rate and contractility. Blockade of renal b_1-adrenergic receptors decreases release of renin and subsequent production of angiotensin II, a potent vasoconstrictor. Beta blockers also promote vasodilation through an unknown mechanism. Alpha blockers such as prazosin promote vasodilation and decrease peripheral vascular resistance through their actions on vascular receptors. Centrally acting α_2-adrenergic receptor agonists such as clonidine and methyldopa decrease sympathetic outflow, thereby decreasing both cardiac output and peripheral vascular resistance.

Diuretics, particularly thiazide diuretics, are useful in treating hypertension. These drugs decrease intravascular volume through their diuretic effects. Additionally, through an unknown mechanism, thiazide diuretics eventually promote vasodilation, which also promotes lowering of blood pressure.

Vasodilation that results in a decrease in peripheral vascular resistance may also be produced by drugs that do not directly regulate the sympathetic nervous system. All classes of **calcium-channel blockers** decrease the influx of calcium necessary for vascular contraction and produce vasodilation. The dihydropyridine calcium-channel blockers such as nifedipine have few direct cardiac effects; as a consequence, reflex tachycardia subsequent to vasodilation may be significant. Conversely, other calcium-channel blockers such as verapamil and diltiazem antagonize cardiac calcium channels, so they cause less reflex tachycardia.

Angiotensin-converting enzyme (ACE) inhibitors and **angiotensin receptor blockers (ARBs)** have different mechanisms and sites of action, yet both classes of drugs ultimately act to inhibit the blood pressure–elevating effects of angiotensin II. Angiotensin II is a direct-acting vasoconstrictor (increases peripheral vascular resistance); it also promotes the release of aldosterone, which causes sodium and water retention and, therefore, increases blood volume. ACE inhibitors interfere with the biosynthesis of angiotensin II by preventing the conversion of angiotensin I to angiotensin II. ARBs block the ability of angiotensin II to activate its receptor, known as the AT1 angiotensin receptor.

Heart Failure

The development of heart failure typically occurs as a result of the body's compensatory response to ischemic cardiac damage or some other pathological event such as chronic hypertension. Initially, multiple interrelated reflex mechanisms serve to compensate for impaired cardiac function. However, these compensatory responses eventually become detrimental and pathologic changes such as cardiac remodeling and hypertrophy occur. In concert with other related events such as fluid retention and changes in vascular tone, heart failure develops. Many of the first-line agents employed in patients with heart failure are directed at inhibiting components of these reflex mechanisms. The major components of these neuroendocrine mechanisms that may be therapeutically targeted in heart failure are the sympathetic nervous system and the renin–angiotensin–aldosterone system. Additional drugs used in heart failure include positive inotropic agents and vasodilators.

Selective beta blockers have been shown to be beneficial in heart failure. These agents include **metoprolol**, **bisoprolol**, and **carvedilol**. Through blockade of primarily peripheral β_1-adrenergic receptors and decreased CNS sympathetic outflow, these agents antagonize the effects of enhanced sympathetic drive, including tachycardia, vasoconstriction, increased renin release, and cardiac remodeling and hypertrophy. In addition, the antiarrhythmic effects of such medications may be beneficial in heart failure patients. Carvedilol may have additional beneficial effects through blockade of β_2- and alpha-adrenergic receptors.

Several drugs used in the treatment of heart failure inhibit components of the renin–angiotensin–aldosterone system—for example, **ACE inhibitors**, **ARBs**, and **aldosterone antagonists**. By blocking the activity of angiotensin-converting enzyme and thereby ultimately decreasing production of angiotensin II, ACE inhibitors may counteract the detrimental effects of angiotensin II, including vasoconstriction, cardiac hypertrophy and remodeling, and aldosterone secretion. ACE inhibitors may also increase plasma levels of bradykinin, which may have beneficial effects in heart failure. ARBs, by acting as competitive antagonists at the angiotensin AT1 receptor, produce beneficial effects similar to those following ACE inhibitor use in patients with heart failure. Aldosterone antagonists, which are also referred to as mineralocorticoid receptor antagonists, include spironolactone and eplerenone. Aldosterone may promote many responses—such as sodium and water retention, cardiac remodeling, and alterations in sympathetic and parasympathetic tone—that have negative effects in heart failure. Thus blockade of aldosterone receptors in various tissues may trigger a beneficial response in heart failure.

Other drugs for heart failure include **positive inotropic agents**, which increase the force of cardiac contraction. Digoxin produces positive inotropic effects through blockade of the cardiac plasma membrane Na^+,K^+-ATPase. Blockade of this ion pump decreases the efflux of intracellular Na^+. The resulting increase in intracellular Na^+ ultimately results in an increase in intracellular Ca^{++} content via alterations in the equilibrium of the cardiac Na^+-Ca^{++} exchanger. Na^+ efflux in exchange for Ca^{++} influx is increased, and Ca^{++} efflux is decreased. The end result is an increase in intracellular Ca^{++} available for cardiomyocyte contraction. Digoxin may also produce beneficial effects in heart failure by regulating autonomic nervous system activity. Specifically, digoxin may increase parasympathetic tone and decrease sympathetic tone—both actions that are beneficial in heart failure.

Additional positive inotropic agents that are used in heart failure include dobutamine, which is an agonist at β_1- and β_2-adrenergic receptors. Inamrinone and milrinone both inhibit a cAMP phosphodiesterase; the resulting increase in intracellular levels of cAMP leads to enhanced cardiac contraction. These drugs may also promote vasodilation.

Vasodilators may be useful in heart failure patients as well. Nitrates (nitroglycerin, sodium nitroprusside) serve as intracellular nitric oxide donors. Nitric oxide activates soluble guanylyl cyclase, which produces cGMP that may produce vasorelaxation in both venous and arterial beds. Nitrate-induced venous relaxation increases venous capacitance and decreases preload. Arterial vasodilation decreases afterload. Hydralazine produces primarily arteriolar vasodilation, and, therefore decreases afterload. Nesiritide is a recombinant version of human brain natriuretic peptide (BNP). Like endogenous BNP, it activates a membrane-spanning guanylyl cyclase and promotes cGMP production. The beneficial effects of nesiritide occur partly as a result of vasodilation and partly due to its diuretic activity.

Angina

Angina occurs when the cardiac blood supply provided by the coronary vasculature does not match the metabolic demands of the heart. Major determinants of cardiac metabolic requirements are heart rate, force of contraction, and systolic wall stress. The most common form of angina is chronic stable angina, also known as classic or exertional angina. The pathology underlying chronic stable angina is narrowing or stenosis of coronary arteries, typically as a result of atherosclerotic plaque development that results in impaired coronary blood flow. A second, less common form of angina is variant angina, also referred to as vasospastic angina or Prinzmetal angina. In variant angina, impaired coronary blood flow occurs as a result of a contraction or spasm of the coronary artery. This spasm may occur in either an atherosclerotic or nonatherosclerotic coronary vessel. The pharmacologic goal in the treatment of angina is to lessen the imbalance between cardiac supply and cardiac demand. In chronic stable angina, this goal is primarily accomplished by lowering cardiac demand. In variant angina, increasing coronary supply is often therapeutically beneficial.

Calcium-channel blockers (CCBs) inhibit the influx of calcium through L-type voltage-dependent calcium channels. All CCBs are active at the calcium channel of vascular smooth muscle and, therefore, promote vasodilation. Dihyropyridine CCBs such as nifedipine have little activity at cardiac calcium channels, whereas nondihydropyridine CCBs such as verapmil and diltiazem are effective in blocking cardiac calcium channels and, therefore, in decreasing heart rate and force of contraction. CCBs are effective in angina because they decrease cardiac demand. These agents promote vasodilation and decrease peripheral vascular resistance, thereby decreasing cardiac wall stress. Verapamil and diltiazem also decrease cardiac demand by decreasing heart rate and cardiac contractility. The ability of CCBs to dilate coronary arteries is beneficial in variant angina.

Beta blockers are beneficial in angina as a result of their ability to decrease myocardial oxygen demand. This reduction is accomplished primarily by direct blockade of cardiac β_1-adrenergic receptors, with an end result of decreased heart rate and contractility. Beta blockers, through a decrease in heart rate, may also increase diastolic perfusion time, which in turn improves coronary blood flow and myocardial perfusion.

Organic nitrates such as nitroglycerin produce vasodilation by generating nitric oxide in vascular smooth muscle. Nitric oxide activates soluble guanylyl cyclase, which produces cGMP that may produce vasorelaxation in both venous and arterial beds. At therapeutic doses of nitrates, venous dilation results in lessened blood return to the heart and, in tandem, a decrease in preload. Decreased preload is beneficial in angina, as ventricular end diastolic pressure and volume are reduced and, in turn, myocardial oxygen demand is reduced. Higher doses of nitrates cause arterial dilation, with a decrease in cardiac afterload and a concomitant decrease in myocardial demand.

THERAPEUTIC AGENTS FOR ENDOCRINE DISORDERS

Female Reproductive Hormones (Estrogen and Progesterone)

The ovary is the principal site for estrogen and progesterone synthesis, while the adrenal gland (zona reticularis) makes a minimal contribution to the synthesis/production of these two hormones. The structures of both estrogen and progesterone are built on a general steroid scaffold, so they are quite similar. However, differences in three-dimensional shape and hydrogen binding characteristics allow for their respective receptors to discriminate between both hormones.

The most potent form of estrogen in the female is estradiol (often abbreviated E2), followed by estrone (E1) and estriol (E3). The number following E represents the number of hydroxyl (—OH) groups in the hormone. Like other steroid agents and hormones, E2 binds its receptor, causing conformational changes that lead to the formation of a homodimer (it binds with another estrogen receptor). This complex targets a hormone response element upstream of a gene of interest and either initiates or suppresses its transcription. Progesterone, also a steroid hormone, follows a similar pattern of binding and DNA transcription regulation.

Both estrogen and progesterone are critical in the development and maintenance of secondary female sex characteristics. Estradiol is involved in many aspects of metabolism (lipid regulation, protein synthesis, metabolic rate), skeletal structure, and fluid balance, and it even contributes to the coagulation process indirectly. The menstrual cycle and ovulation are also under the control of estrogen and progesterone. All of these effects can be considered the mechanisms of action for estradiol. Mechanisms of action for progesterone include induction of changes in the uterine lining, converting it from a proliferative tissue to a secretory tissue; maintenance of pregnancy after conception; and when used therapeutically, encouraging implantation of an embryo.

Therapeutic uses of estrogens and progestins (synthetic progesterone analogs) include contraception, hormone replacement therapy, and regulation of the menstrual cycle (amenorrhea or dysmenorrhea). Estradiol specifically has been used to treat vasomotor symptoms associated with menopause, in prophylaxis against osteoporosis, and in the treatment of vaginal or vulvar atrophy.

The most common use of estrogens/progestins is in the form of oral contraceptives. Combined oral contraceptives, when used appropriately, can suppress the release of follicle-stimulating hormone (FSH) and luteinizing hormone (LH) from the anterior pituitary. Mechanistically, through a negative feedback loop, constant stimulation of receptors on the hypothalamus and anterior pituitary prevents the release of FSH and LH, which will subsequently prevent follicle development and Graafian follicle rupture, or ovulation.

Antidiabetic Agents

Insulin is a polypeptide hormone synthesized by beta cells in the pancreas. Insulin is released into the system secondary to increased plasma glucose concentration or incretin stimulation of beta cells. The binding of insulin to its receptor causes phosphorylation of the receptor, and the subsequent phosphorylation of insulin-receptor substrates in the cytosol of target tissue. The net result of insulin binding is a translocation of glucose transporters (GLUT-4) from the cytosol to the cell surface, where glucose can then bind and be transported into the cell.

Many analogs of insulin are currently available. These medications display the same biological activity as native human insulin. However, their onset of action or duration of action is modulated through alterations in the amino acid sequence of the A chain or the B chain of insulin.

Lispro (Humalog), **aspart** (Novolog), and **glulisine** (Apidra) are rapid-acting analogs with a general onset of action of less than 30 minutes. This rapid action is due to minor alterations (reverse order, additions, or deletions) in amino acid sequence. These changes discourage insulin hexamer formation, or hasten insulin dissociation into monomers, which allows for absorption into the circulation.

Detemir (Levemir) and **glargine** (Lantus) are long-acting analogs of human insulin. Detimir has been modified on the B chain with a saturated fatty acid (myristic acid). The addition of this fatty acid allows for plasma protein binding. The rate of dissociation from plasma proteins occurs over a 10- to 12-hour period, allowing for twice-daily dosing. Glargine has several modifications to the parent hormone that result in this analog precipitating in tissue upon subcutaneous administration (the pH of glargine in the vial is approximately 4; upon injection of this medication into an area of pH 7.4, microprecipitates form). These precipitates slowly dissolve and are absorbed into the circulation. One noteworthy point is that glargine lacks a peak effect and instead mimics the body's basal insulin release.

NPH insulin, also known as N (Humulin N or Novolin N), is an intermediate-acting insulin that is formulated with zinc and the basic protein protamine. The combination of zinc and protamine leads to insulin aggregate formation and results in a suspension. Upon subcutaneous administration, these aggregates disassociate and are absorbed.

The **sulfonylurea** class of insulin-secreting agents includes glimepride, glyburide, and glipizide. Older agents with less favorable pharmacokinetic profiles exist but are sparingly used. These medications include acetohexamide, chlorpropamide, and tolazimide. Insulin secretion is dependent upon beta-cell depolarization secondary to closure of a specific potassium channel (K_{ATP}) expressed on the beta cell's surface. In nondiabetic patients, glucose will be metabolized, resulting in generation of ATP, which then causes closure of the potassium channels. The membrane potential becomes positive and depolarization occurs as a result of potassium accumulation. This results in exocytosis of insulin-containing granules. Sulfonylureas have as their targets the K_{ATP} channel. They bind to the channel, causing closure and subsequent depolarization. This is followed by the secretion of insulin. Sulfonylureas are used only when the patient has the ability to synthesize and secrete insulin.

Meglitinides such as repaglinide and nateglinide are also classified as secretagouges. Administration of these agents will stimulate insulin secretion in a similar manner as described for the sulfonylureas. One difference seen with the meglitinides is their relatively short duration of action and rapid onset of action. Their ability to stimulate insulin secretion is dependent on the presence of glucose. They are much less likely to cause hypoglycemia than are sulfonylureas.

Thiazolidinediones (TZDs) include pioglitazone (Actos) and rosiglitazone (Avandia). These drugs are considered insulin-sensitizing agents and improve peripheral utilization of glucose. The molecular target of the TZDs is a nuclear receptor called peroxisome proliferator activated receptor γ (PPAR-γ). Upon binding, the ligand–receptor complex will dimerize with a second receptor (such as vitamin D or retinoic acid) and target response elements located upstream of target genes involved in metabolism. The increased turnover of these metabolic genes has been shown to improve glucose utilization.

Metformin (Glucophage) is a biguanide derivative that has also been shown to improve peripheral utilization of glucose. Target tissues for metformin include the liver and skeletal muscle. Gluconeogenesis—that is, new sugar production—is inhibited by metformin administration. Notably, metformin does not cause hypoglycemia.

Sitagliptin (Januvia) and **saxagliptin** (Onglyza) are small-molecule inhibitors of an enzyme called dipeptidyl peptidase IV (DPP IV). The DPP IV enzyme is a protease responsible for inactivating incretin hormones. Prolonging the duration of action of incretin hormones has been shown to have beneficial effects in diabetic patients. In addition to stimulating insulin secretion secondary to the presence of nutrition in the GI tract, incretins have been suggested to be insulinotropic. They are capable of stimulating beta cell growth.

Exenatide (Byetta) is an incretin analog derived from natural sources. Native incretins such as GLP-1 are released from L cells in the small intestine due to the presence of food in the GI tract. Once bound to their receptors on pancreatic beta cells, they stimulate the secretion of insulin. The duration of action, however, is very short (approximately 2–3 minutes), as incretins are quickly metabolized by soluble and membrane-bound DPP IV. Exenatide is an incretin analog with a longer duration of action (2–4 hours).

Thyroid Hormones

Levothyroxine (T_4) and liothyronine (T_3) are the principal thyroid hormones. These iodine-containing molecules are synthesized and stored in the thyroid gland and released secondary to stimulation by the anterior pituitary hormone known as thyroid-stimulating hormone (TSH). Once released into the circulation, thyroid hormones quickly become bound to plasma proteins (thyroid-binding globulin, transthyretin, and, to a lesser extent, albumin). Upon dissociation from the plasma protein, T_4 can cross a cell membrane and undergo a de-iodination reaction to generate the more potent hormone T_3. Triiodothyronine (T_3) binds tightly to its receptor (thyroid hormone receptor) and the ligand–receptor complex will form a dimer with a second receptor (a steroid receptor such as vitamin D or vitamin A). This heterodimer will then bind hormone response elements in DNA upstream of a gene of interest and modulate its transcription. The thyroid hormones are heavily involved in regulating many aspects of metabolism, including normal growth and development, controlling basal metabolic rate, and protein synthesis at many levels.

Synthetic levothyroxine (Synthroid, Levoxyl) is the mainstay of therapy for treating hypothyroid patients, and its mechanism of action is virtually identical to that of naturally produced T_4. Similar to naturally occurring T_4, synthetic T_4 will bind plasma proteins, and upon dissociation will be converted to the active form T_3.

Antithyroid Agents

Graves' disease—the most common form of hyperthyroidism—results from the production of antibodies capable of stimulating the release of thyroid hormones. The resulting increase in thyroid hormone concentration leads to the symptoms associated with the disease: increased metabolic rate, weight loss, increased heart rate, and intolerance to heat. Treatment for hyperthyroidism is centered on reducing thyroid hormone synthesis and secretion and is accomplished with two drugs, methimazole (Tapazole) and propylthiouracil (PTU). The mechanism of action for these drugs can be described as inhibition of critical enzymes required in the synthesis of T_4 and T_3—specifically, thyroperoxidase (TPO). When this enzyme is inhibited, the thyroid gland becomes unable to oxidize and incorporate iodine into tyrosine residues in thyroglobulin. Also, inhibition of TPO prevents the formation of thyronine, a prerequisite for T_4 synthesis.

THERAPEUTIC AGENTS FOR GASTROINTESTINAL DISORDERS

Histamine-2 Receptor Antagonists

Gastric acid secretion can be stimulated through several receptor-mediated pathways. Gastrin can bind its receptor on the parietal cell surface and increase acid secretion. Also, cholinergic stimulation can cause acid secretion through muscarinic receptor activation on gastric parietal cells. The histamine 2 (H2) receptor on parietal cells, once activated by histamine, can also stimulate the secretion of gastric acid. Antagonizing any of these receptors is a rational approach to suppressing acid secretion. However, to date, only antagonists to the H2 receptor have been successfully developed and marketed. Cimetidine (Tagamet), ranitidine (Zantac), famotidine (Pepcid), and nizatidine (Axid) are all agents described as H2 receptor antagonists. Mechanistically, these drugs are competitive inhibitors of the H2 receptor located on gastric parietal cells. Preventing the binding and stimulation of these receptors decreases gastric acid secretion, and raises intra-gastric pH. This increase in pH allows for the healing of ulcers, and alleviates the symptoms of gastroesophageal reflux disease (GERD) and gastritis.

Proton Pump Inhibitors

The final step in gastric acid secretion involves the expulsion of a proton (H^+) from the parietal cell. This is accomplished by the H^+/K^+ ATPase pump following stimulation of the parietal cell by histamine, gastrin, or acetylcholine. Proton pump inhibitors (PPIs), such as omeprazole (Prilosec), pantoprazole (Protonix), lansoprazole (Prevacid), and rabeprazole (Aciphex), suppress acid secretion by inhibiting the H^+/K^+ ATPase pump. After acid-catalyzed activation, the PPI will covalently bind to a cysteine residue(s) on the pump, locking it into a conformation that is no longer capable of pumping protons. As seen with H2 receptor antagonists, gastric pH increases and healing of ulcers is supported. Also, relief of GERD and symptomatic gastritis will occur.

Antiemetics

Nausea and vomiting have diverse underlying causes. Infection, motion sickness, cancer chemotherapy, and pregnancy can all contribute to nausea and vomiting. Apart from chemotherapy, many other drugs can cause nausea as well. The chemoreceptor trigger zone (CTZ) is weakly protected by the blood–brain barrier and is susceptible to activation by drugs and many neurotransmitters. Receptors expressed on the CTZ include histaminic, dopaminergic, serotonergic, muscarinic, and substance P/neurokinin 1 receptors. Antagonizing any of these receptors is a rational approach to the treatment/prevention of nausea.

Classical **antihistamines** such as diphenhydramine (Benadryl) can block histamine receptor activation on the CTZ and prevent nausea/vomiting. Promethazine (Phenergan), although chemically classified as a phenothiazine, blocks histamine receptors to alleviate nausea/vomiting. Unlike other phenothiazines used clinically, it is a weak antagonist at dopamine receptors.

Phenothiazines were initially marketed as antipsychotics. They block dopamine receptors throughout the CNS, and were observed to alleviate nausea and vomiting. Today, however, prochlorperazine (Compazine) is perhaps the only phenothiazine used clinically for nausea and vomiting. Promethazine has greater affinity for the histamine receptor.

Serotonin receptors are ubiquitous, and the 5-HT_3 receptor subtype is heavily involved in nausea. This receptor is expressed on the CTZ and throughout the GI tract. Activation of this receptor will lead to emesis. The **5-HT_3 receptor antagonists** have proved useful in the treatment and prevention of nausea secondary to chemotherapy and anesthesia. These agents, which include ondansetron (Zofran), granisetron (Kytril), dolasetron (Anzemet), and palonosetron (Aloxi), prevent serotonin from binding and activating receptors that will subsequently activate the vomiting center in the CNS. These agents are routinely used in the hospital and the outpatient setting.

The substance P/neurokinin 1 receptor is expressed on the CTZ as well. A relatively newer agent, aprepitant (Emend), has been developed as an antagonist of this receptor. Aprepitant is indicated for chemotherapy-induced nausea and vomiting as well as postoperative nausea and vomiting.

Agents for Inflammatory Bowel Disease

Inflammatory bowel disease (IBD) includes disorders such as ulcerative colitis and Crohn's disease. These two conditions differ slightly by location and lesion severity, but both involve the GI tract. The cause of IBD is unknown, but environmental and genetic factors have been implicated in its etiology. Bacterial infections have also been suggested as initiating IBD. The inflammation seen with IBD is typically localized at the mucosal layer in the small and large intestines. Secondary to a precipitating event, a local inflammation occurs. The severity of this inflammation correlates with levels of discomfort. Therapy is often aimed at suppressing the host immune response, which is the major contributor to inflammation. Several agents are used clinically to suppress the immune system, including derivatives of 5-aminosalicylic acid as well as corticosteroids.

Several agents that consist of, or evolve from, **5-aminosalicyclic acid** are in clinical use—for example, sulfasalazine (Azulfidine), mesalamine (Asacol and Pentasa), osalazine (Dipentum), and balsalazide (Colazal). These agents suppress the production of substances that potentiate the immune response in the GI tract. The precise mechanism by which they act remains unknown, although decreased production of tumor necrosis factor alpha (TNF-α) and inhibition of the production of arachidonic acid (a precursor to prostaglandins) at the mucosal level has been suggested.

THERAPEUTIC AGENTS FOR INFECTIOUS DISEASES

Antiviral Agents

Many viruses exist and are infectious to humans. Only a handful of viral infections, however, can be treated with the currently available antiviral agents. Herpesvirus, influenza, and human immunodeficiency virus (HIV) represent the major viruses for which drug therapy is prescribed. Targets of antiviral therapy include viral polymerase enzymes that elongate the DNA strand; neuraminidase enzymes for influenza; and for HIV, reverse transcriptase, HIV protease, HIV integrase, and HIV entry inhibitors.

The herpesvirus is a double-stranded DNA virus responsible for infections including oral herpes (HSV-1), genital herpes (HSV-2), chickenpox, shingles, Epstein-Barr virus infection, and mononucleosis. Nearly all medications used to treat herpesvirus act to inhibit viral DNA polymerase. Agents include the nucleoside analogs acyclovir (Zovirax), famciclovir (Famvir), and valcyclovir (Valtrex). All three agents are prodrugs, and must be metabolized by a viral kinase enzyme (viral thymidine kinase [TK]) to the monophosphate nucleotide. Subsequent kinase reactions will convert this monophosphate into the diphosphate and triphosphate. For example, acyclovir will be taken up into a virally infected cell and become phosphorylated by viral TK to acyclovir monophosphate. Cellular kinases will then convert the acyclovir monophosphate to acyclovir triphosphate. This triphosphate then serves as a substrate for viral DNA synthesis. In fact, viral DNA polymerase will incorporate acyclovir into the growing strand of viral DNA. Once inserted, acyclovir will cause DNA chain termination, as it lacks an equivalent 3'-hydroxyl group as seen in deoxyribose. Notably, mammalian DNA polymerase does not use nucleoside analogs in DNA synthesis. Also, both famcyclovir and valcyclovir must be processed via a hydrolysis reaction prior to being phosphorylated. The presence of additional groups in the structures of valcyclovir and famcyclovir increase their bioavailability.

The influenza virus contains a segmented, negative-strand RNA genome packaged in an envelope. Humans are typically infected with three different versions of the virus—H1N1, H2N2, and H3N2 (where H = hemagglutinin and N = neuraminidase). Transmission occurs via inhalation of aerosolized droplets, yet the virus can persist on inanimate objects (fomite contamination) for days. The respiratory tract is the primary site of infection. The influenza virus will spread from an infected cell through a process known as budding.

As newly formed virus particles form at the cell surface, the hemagglutinin protein remains attached to the cell. However, an enzyme called neuraminidase will cleave a bond connecting the hemagglutinin to the cell surface receptor. Therefore, inhibition of the neuraminidase enzyme can prevent the spread of the infection and shorten the duration of illness. Neuraminidase inhibitors such as zanamivir (Relenza) and oseltamivir (Tamiflu) work in this capacity; they inhibit influenza neuraminadase by serving as transition-state mimetics.

The HIV virus contains two strands of negative-polarity RNA packaged in a virion along with several enzymes: reverse transcriptase (RT), protease, and integrase. All three of these enzymes are targets of currently available anti-HIV agents. The first class of antiretroviral agents made available to treat HIV comprised the **reverse transcriptase inhibitors**. The prototypical agent was zidovudine (Retrovir), a nucleoside analog of the pyrimidine thymidine. The key structural difference between these molecules (zidovudine and thymidine) that leads to activity against HIV virus occurs at the 3'-hydroxyl group on the deoxyribose ring. In thymidine, the hydroxyl group is maintained and its presence allows for viral DNA chain elongation. In contrast, in zidovudine and all other nucleoside reverse transcriptase inhibitors, this hydroxyl group is absent, or is replaced with a functional group that disallows viral DNA elongation. The net result of incorporation of a nucleoside analog into the growing viral DNA strand is chain termination. Many agents are available in this class, including lamivudine (Epivir), zalcitibine (Hivid), and didanosine (Videx). Newer agents include emtricitabine (Emtriva) and tenofovir (Viread). Much like the agents discussed for herpesvirus infections, the RT inhibitors must be activated via kinase enzymes as well. The formation of a diphosphate and a triphosphate is obligatory for activity.

In addition to the nucleoside RT inhibitors, a second class of RT inhibitors is available. These agents are dubbed the **non-nucleoside reverse transcriptase inhibitors (NNRTIs)**. Unlike the nucleoside agents, they do not compete for binding with natural substrates, and do not require activation via phosphorylation. Instead, they are noncompetitive inhibitors that bind to an allosteric site on the HIV reverse transcriptase enzyme. Essentially, a small lipophilic pocket exists on the enzyme into which these drugs can bind. Doing so causes a conformational change in the enzyme that prevents viral DNA synthesis. Agents in this class include nevirapine (Viramune), efavirenz (Sustiva), and delavirdine (Rescriptor). The most recently marketed agent is etravirine (Intelence).

The HIV protease enzyme is critical in the life cycle of HIV and is the target of **protease inhibitors**. A brief review of the flow of genetic material reveals its importance. The entire HIV genome, once inserted in the host genome, is transcribed by host cells' polymerase enzymes to generate a long primary transcript. This transcript is translated into a large protein that lacks function until processed by the protease enzyme. This dimeric enzyme will cleave the protein at specific sites to generate small proteins and enzymes necessary for subsequent viral replication and budding. Thus, inhibition of the protease enzyme will disrupt the HIV life cycle and inhibit replication. Saquinavir (Invirase or Fortovase) was the first protease inhibitor to be marketed; other agents include indinavir (Crixivan), lopinavir/ritonavir (Kaletra), and nelfinavir (Viracept). Fosamprenavir (Lexiva) and darunavir (Prezista) are newer protease inhibitors. These compounds are also transition-state mimetics that occupy the active site of the protease enzyme to cause the inhibition.

Protease inhibitors, when combined with reverse transcriptase inhibitors, afford the patient a potent cocktail of drugs that has proved able to prevent the inevitable progression of HIV into acquired immunodeficiency syndrome (AIDS). Today, HIV is considered a chronic disease, and patients are said to die *with* HIV, not *from* HIV. This change in the disease's status is largely due to the administration of highly active, antiretroviral therapy (HAART).

In addition to the previously mentioned medications used to treat HIV, several relatively newer medications have become available. These agents include entry inhibitors such as enfuvirtide (Fuzeon) and maraviroc (Selzentry), and an integrase inhibitor called raltegravir (Isentress).

A coreceptor for entry is required for HIV to infect CD4+ T cells. The CD4 protein/receptor is the primary attachment molecule, but a second receptor called CCR5 or CXCR4 is also required. CCR5, a G-protein–coupled receptor, is a chemokine receptor located on the surface of T cells. To date, its function or necessity in normal physiology has not been elucidated. Its role in HIV entry is significant enough that antagonizing the receptor with a small molecule prevents viral entry and infection. During the entry process, the virion glycoprotein gp120 also binds to CD4, causing a conformation change in the virion that reveals a second glycoprotein, gp41. Acting like a harpoon, gp41 extends into the plasma membrane of the T cell, and then attempts to fold the gp41 proteins back upon themselves. This folding brings the HIV virion membrane within fusion distance of the T cell's membrane. Once the membranes fuse, the virus slips into the host cell and begins its life cycle. Enfuvirtide (Fuzeon) is a peptide drug containing a sequence of amino acids that has a strong interaction with the extended form of gp41. Once interaction has occurred, the gp41 is unable to fold back upon itself, such that fusion and entry are inhibited.

Antifungal Agents

It is possible to exploit the differences in metabolism between fungi and humans for the development of selectively toxic antifungal agents. Several classes of antifungals exist, but have very different indications. These classes include **polyene antifungals** (amphotericin B and nystatin), **azole antifungals** (fluconazole, voriconazole, itraconazole), **squalene epoxidase inhibitors** (terbinafine), and one fungal **cytosine deaminase inhibitor** (flucytosine). The final class of antifungals is the **echinocandins**, a group of relatively new antifungal agents with a unique molecular target, fungal beta-1,3-glucan synthase.

Polyene antifungals, such as amphotericin B, are available in a conventional form (Fungizone), and in a complex with lipids, liposomes, or cholesteryl sulfate (Abelcet, Ambisome, Amphotec). Mechanistically, amphotericin has affinity for the fungal sterol ergosterol found in the fungal plasma membrane. Amphotericin B binds to ergosterol and forms pores in the plasma membrane, thereby causing nutrient and ion loss. This ultimately leads to fungal cell death. As therapy with amphotericin B continues, the risk for renal dysfunction increases, especially with conventional amphotericin. The risk is diminished with lipid formulations, however. Amphotericin B is administered intravenously.

The most commonly used azole antifungal agents are available in both oral and parenteral formulations, and include fluconazole (Diflucan) and voriconazole (Vfend). The molecular target of these drugs is the fungal cytochrome enzyme CYP51 (14α-demethylase). This enzyme is critical for the synthesis of the fungal sterol ergosterol. Ergosterol provides structure and support for fungal cells and is not present in humans. Selectively inhibiting its synthesis proves to be fatal for fungi. While humans also have a similar enzyme, the human isoform is not inhibited at clinical concentrations. However, other enzymes, including drug metabolizing enzymes in the liver, are inhibited secondary to azole antifungal administration. Cytochrome-P450 3A4, 2C19, and 2C9 are inhibited and will have diminished capacity to metabolize other drug substrates.

Terbinafine (Lamisil) is an allylamine derivative capable of inhibiting the fungal enzyme squalene epoxidase. This enzyme is critical in the synthesis of ergosterol as well. Upon its administration, fungal cells are unable to synthesize intermediates leading to the formation of ergosterol and, as occurs with azole antifungals, cell death ensues. Terbinafine represents the only oral version of allylamine, but several topical agents are available, including butenafine (Mentax) and naftifine (Naftin).

Echinocandins are inhibitors of the fungal enzyme beta-(1,3)-glucan synthase. This enzyme is responsible for the formation of glucan polymers that contribute to a portion of the fungal cell. Humans do not need such polymer in their cells; thus echinocandins are selectively toxic to fungi. Upon administration of these agents, polymers of glucan are not synthesized, and the cell wall becomes weak and compromised—a state that is ultimately toxic to fungal cells. Caspofungin (Cancidas) was the first approved echinocandin, followed by micafungin (Mycamine) and anidulafungin (Eraxis). These agents are available for parenteral use only.

Antibacterial Drugs (Antibiotics)

Antibacterial or antimicrobial agents may be either bactericidal or bacteriostatic. Many of these drugs produce their effects by selectively targeting processes in bacteria while sparing mammalian (host) cells. This includes inhibition of bacterial cell-wall synthesis, targeting of the bacterial ribosome to inhibit protein translation, and targeting of other bacteria–specific processes.

Agents acting to **disrupt bacterial cell-wall synthesis** are typically bactericidal, as loss of cell–wall integrity results in cell lysis.

Penicillins bind to a group of bacterial proteins known as penicillin binding proteins (PBPs). This group includes transpeptidase, which is the enzyme responsible for cross-linking of the cell–wall. Penicillin-induced inhibition of transpeptidase is a major mechanism of its bactericidal effect. Additionally, penicillins may regulate other PBPs—for example, promoting the activation of autolysins, which act to break down the existing cell membrane.

Similar to penicillins, **cephalosporins** contain a β-lactam ring and promote destruction of the cell wall through mechanisms similar to those described for the penicillins. Cephalosporins are typically classified by generation, which generally also represents their spectrum of antibacterial activity. This may in part reflect differential sensitivity of individual cephalosporins to β-lactamases that may inactivate these drugs.

Members of the **carbapenem** class of antibiotics also contain a β-lactam ring and cause bacterial cell-wall destruction and cell lysis.

Several other antibacterial drugs produce their effects through inhibition of cell-wall synthesis by varying mechanisms, as shown in Table 1-1.

The cell membrane of bacteria may also be targeted by antibiotic drugs. Insertion of **daptomycin** results in pore formation with loss of intracellular potassium. **Polymyxin B** and **colistin** bind predominantly to the lipopolysaccharide component of the cell membrane of gram-negative organisms.

Table 1-1 Antibacterial Drugs That Inhibit Cell-Wall Synthesis

Drug	Mechanism
Bacitracin	Inhibits the dephosphorylation of bactoprenol, which is the lipid transporter of cell wall precursors. The inability of bactoprenol to be dephosphorylated results in loss of precursor shuttling.
Fosfomycin	Inhibits the initial step in formation of bacterial cell wall precursors.
Vancomycin	Binds to peptide precursors of the cell wall that terminate in D-alanine–D-alanine, and inhibits transglycosylase and transpeptidase reactions necessary for cell-wall synthesis.

Many antibiotics produce their effects through inhibition of bacterial protein translation, specifically through binding to and inhibition of the bacterial ribosome. The bacterial ribosome is composed of a 30S and 50S subunit with a key protein translation site—the peptidyl transferase center. For most antibiotics that act as protein synthesis inhibitors, binding interactions occur between the drug and specific nucleotides of ribosomal RNA. As shown in Table 1-2, these drugs may be classified by binding to the 30S or 50S ribosomal subunit.

In addition to disruption of bacterial cell walls and inhibition of protein translation, several antibiotics use various other mechanisms of action to produce their antibacterial effects. These agents are listed in Table 1-3.

Table 1-2 Protein Synthesis Inhibitors: Binding Sites

Drug	Binding Site
Chloramphenicol	50S
Clindamycin	50S
Dalfopristin/quinipristin	50S (individual agents bind to partially overlapping but distinct sites; binding of dalfopristin enhances the binding affinity of 50S and quinipristin)
Linezolid	50S
Macrolides (including erythromycin, clarithromycin, azithromycin, and ketolides)	50S
Aminoglycosides	30S
Tetracyclines	30S
Retapamulin	30S (binding target may be a ribosomal protein)

Table 1-3 Other Antibiotics: Mechanisms of Action

Drug	Mechanism
Fluoroquinolones	Depending on the specific organism, inhibits DNA gyrase or topoisomerase IV
Metronidazole	Undergoes activation to a reactive compound that damages bacterial DNA and possibly proteins
Nitrofurantoin	Undergoes reduction to generate reactive compounds that damage bacterial DNA
Methenamine	Generates formaldehyde in the urinary bladder
Rifampin	Inhibits DNA-dependent RNA polymerase, thereby preventing RNA synthesis
Mupirocin	Disrupts protein synthesis by inhibiting isoleucyl tRNA synthetase
Sulfonamide/ trimethoprim	Disrupt biosynthesis of tetrahydrofolic acid by bacteria at two successive steps in the pathway

THERAPEUTIC AGENTS FOR ARTHRITIC DISORDERS AND OSTEOPOROSIS

Osteoarthritis

Osteoarthritis is an inflammatory condition characterized by joint swelling and pain. Common sites of inflammation include the knees, back, and wrists. The exact cause of osteoarthritis is unknown, but a decrease in cushioning cartilage in the joints is a contributory factor. Treatment is aimed at reducing inflammation and pain relief. This may be accomplished with **acetaminophen (Tylenol)**, as well as with one of the many **nonsteroidal anti-inflammatory drugs (NSAIDs)**. While acetaminophen has been shown to block central prostaglandin (PG) synthesis and inhibit peripheral pain neurotransmission, the NSAIDs attack inflammation by inhibiting peripheral prostaglandin production. Because prostaglandins mediate inflammation, suppressing their formation is a reasonable approach to treating osteoarthritis.

Classical NSAIDs include indomethacin (Indocin), ibuprofen (Motrin), and naproxen (Naprosyn). There are certainly more agents available, and all NSAIDs share a common mechanism of action: inhibition of cyclooxygenase-1 and -2 (COX-1 and -2). COX-1 is constitutively active, and is required for maintenance of protective barriers in the stomach and ensuring renal blood flow. COX-2 is an inducible enzyme, which will be turned on secondary to injury. When COX enzymes are inhibited, precursors to prostaglandins are not readily synthesized and inflammatory prostaglandins are not produced. Older

NSAIDs are relatively nonselective in their action and will inhibit both COX-1 and COX-2. The disadvantage to this approach is a reduction in the prostaglandins responsible for cytoprotective effects in the stomach and a decrease in vasodilating prostaglandins required for adequate perfusion of the kidney. **Selective COX-2 inhibitors** such as celecoxib (Celebrex) are associated with a decreased incidence of GI bleed and acute renal failure.

Gout

Gout is a result of elevated uric acid levels. Once a threshold level of solubility for uric acid in the plasma is reached, this purine metabolite will start to precipitate out of plasma. The most common site for uric acid crystals to deposit is in the joints of the great toe. Most individuals with elevated uric acid have a diminished capacity to excrete the by-product. Treatment is aimed at decreasing production or inhibiting renal tubular reabsorption. Decreased production is accomplished with chronic administration of **inhibitors of the enzyme xanthine oxidase**. Purines are oxidized to hypoxanthine, xanthine, and then uric acid, with the latter two substances being formed by xanthine oxidase. Inhibition of this enzyme—the mechanism of action for drugs such as allopurinol (Zyloprim) and febuxostat (Uloric)—prevents the formation of uric acid and increases the formation of xanthine, which is more water soluble relative to uric acid. **Uricosuric agents**, such as probenecid, prevent reabsorption of uric acid by inhibiting anionic transporters in the renal tubule.

Osteoporosis

Osteoporosis is characterized by a loss in bone mass. Postmenopausal women are at greatest risk for this condition, although elderly men may be affected as well. Fracture is the major complication from osteoporosis. As women age, estrogen production decreases. The loss of endogenous estrogen also means loss of positive bone-forming effects in women. As a result, bone breakdown outpaces bone formation. In the past, estrogen replacement therapy was considered the mainstay of therapy. **Estrogens**, such as conjugated equine estrogens (Premarin), and other forms of estrogen have differing effects on tissues. For instance, in bone, estrogen stimulates protein synthesis and bone formation, perhaps by inhibiting osteoclast activity. Estrogens also stimulate tissue proliferation in uterine and breast tissue. These effects increase the risk of cancers; for this reason, estrogens have fallen out of favor for treatment and prevention of osteoporosis.

Selective estrogen receptor modulators (SERMs) have proved to be useful agents for the treatment and prevention of osteoporosis. Remarkably, SERMs such as raloxifene (Evista) are able to positively modulate estrogen receptors in bone tissue and antagonize estrogen receptors in other tissues such as breast tissue. This dual action decreases the risk of cancers seen with estrogen administration.

The **bisphosphonate** class includes drugs such as alendronate (Fosamax), ibandronate (Boniva), and risedronate (Actonel). These agents are useful for treating osteoporosis, as they indirectly increase bone density by inhibiting the actions of osteoclasts and osteoclast precursors. As such, new bone formation will outpace bone resorption, leading to an increase in bone mass.

Rheumatoid Arthritis

Rheumatoid arthritis (RA) is typically characterized by joint inflammation, but may involve other tissues and organs systems. A genetic predisposition and environmental exposure seem to be required for development of the disease. Treatment for RA is aimed at decreasing proliferation of joint tissue and suppressing inflammation and activation of the immune system. Agents in clinical use include nonsteroidal anti-inflammatory agents (NSAIDs), steroids, agents that target tumor necrosis factor alpha (TNF-α), and a constellation of drugs referred to as disease-modifying antirheumatic drugs (DMARDs).

NSAIDs were previously discussed in the osteoarthritis section. The reader is referred there for a review of their mechanism of action and rationale for use.

Corticosteroids have been shown to improve the symptoms associated with RA, specifically decreasing inflammation. However, long-term administration of these agents produces undesirable effects (Cushing's syndrome, glucose abnormalities, and osteoporosis). Mechanistically, steroids such as prednisone and methylprednisolone reduce inflammation by altering the activity of phospholipase A_2, an enzyme responsible for liberating arachidonic acid from plasma membranes. The decreased amount of arachidonic acid corresponds to a decrease in prostaglandin production. Other mechanisms suggested for the anti-inflammatory effects of corticosteroids include inhibition of leukocyte infiltration into inflamed areas and modification of protein synthesis. Both corticosteroids and NSAIDs are useful for the initial symptomatic treatment of RA, but overall these drugs do little to alter the progression of the disease.

Disease-modifying antirheumatic drugs (DMARDs) are a collection of drugs used to prevent the progression of rheumatoid arthritis. Included in this class are methotrexate, leflunomide (Arava), hydroxychloroquine (Plaquenil), cyclosporine (Sandimmune), and azathioprine (Imuran). The rationale for the use of these agents is their ability to suppress proliferation of immune cells that might otherwise contribute to the inflammation of affected joints in the RA patient. A brief description of the mechanism of action for each agent is provided here.

Methotrexate (Rheumatrex) is a dihydrofolate reductase inhibitor. Administration of methotrexate will prevent the synthesis of thymidine from uridine. Proliferation of white cells, which is common in RA patients, requires a steady supply of DNA precursor substrates. Administration of methotrexate induces thymidine starvation, thereby suppressing white cell proliferation.

Leflunomide (Arava) is a prodrug that requires metabolic activation to an active metabolite prior to exerting any effect. The active metabolite, teriflunomide, is a dihydroorotate dehydrogenase inhibitor. Inhibition of this enzyme prevents de novo pyrimidine synthesis. The end result is a decrease in the production of DNA precursor substrates similar to that described for methotrexate.

Hydroxychloroquine (Plaquenil) has been suggested to inhibit immune cell migration, thereby preventing infiltration of joints with leukocytes.

Cyclosporine (Sandimmune) is a calcineurin inhibitor. Upon binding to its intracellular receptor, cyclosporine prevents the production of gene products responsible for the activation and proliferation of T cells. Specifically, cyclosporine has been shown to down-regulate the expression of interleukin (IL)-2, IL-3, and IL-4 as well as TNF-α. As such, T cells remain in a dormant phase and do not progress from the G_0 to G_1 phase of the cell cycle.

Azathioprine (Imuran), after metabolism, generates the antimetabolite 6-mercaptopurine (6-MP). This metabolite has been shown to suppress purine synthesis and has been suggested to inhibit DNA, RNA, and protein synthesis.

Tumor necrosis factor alpha (TNF-α) is involved in the pathology of rheumatoid arthritis, and is present in high levels in RA patients. Antagonizing the effects of TNF-α at the receptor level or quenching soluble TNF-α has been shown to slow the progression of RA. Many biological agents have been developed to treat RA, as well as other diseases associated with increased levels of TNF-α. **Monoclonal antibodies**, by binding to TNF-α, decrease the production of pro-inflammatory cytokines (various interleukins), leukocyte mobilization, and eosinophil and neutrophil activation. Included in the armamentarium of monoclonal antibodies for RA are infliximab (Remicade), adalimumab (Humira), golimumab (Simponi), and certolizumab pegol (Cimzia). These monoclonal antibodies are either chimeric (mouse and human: infliximab), fully human (adalimumab and golimumab), or Fab fragments (certolizumab). Certolizumab pegol is a pegylated Fab fragment of a humanized monoclonal antibody directed against TNF-α. Pegylation affords this biological agent a longer half-life by decreasing the rate of elimination.

In addition to monoclonal antibodies, soluble fusion proteins are available that contain the receptor for TNF-α conjugated to the Fc portion of human IgG. Etanercept (Enbrel) binds circulating TNF-α, thereby diminishing the inflammatory response.

OPIOID ANALGESICS

Opioids are widely used in both hospital and ambulatory settings. Many diseases and acute conditions require the administration of opioids. Severe cases of arthritis, cancer pain, surgical pain, and traumatic injury, for example, may all necessitate prescription of a potent opioid. The prototypical opioids, morphine and codeine, are derived from natural sources. Derivatives of morphine and codeine have been synthesized and include hydromorphone, hydrocodone, and oxycodone. Some opioids are combined with acetaminophen in a single dosage form as well. Still other opioid analgesics are completely synthetic. Fentanyl, meperidine, and tramadol are all considered synthetic opioids, for example. Potency varies among these agents and is usually expressed in relation to the potency of morphine.

The opioid analgesics can be described as agonists of the opioid receptor. There are currently three known opioid receptors: mu, kappa, and delta. The mu receptor is associated with most opioid binding, and activation decreases the ascending pain signaling pathway. The perception and the response to pain are altered in patients who are administered opioids.

THERAPEUTIC AGENTS FOR PSYCHIATRIC AND NEUROLOGIC DISORDERS

Antidepressants

The exact cause of depression remains elusive, and the disease manifests as a complex series of symptoms. While much progress has been made in determining the etiology of depression, the most likely cause remains an imbalance in the complicated regulation of neurotransmitters including norepinephrine (NE) and serotonin (5-HT). Support for this mechanism was provided by the administration of reserpine, an alkaloid that depleted biogenic amines. Early experiments showed that laboratory animals given reserpine developed depression symptoms. It has been suggested that a deficiency in either NE or 5-HT exists in the depressed patient and contributes to depression. This notion is further complemented by the observation that administration of agents capable of inhibiting the reuptake of NE or 5-HT, or both, dramatically improves the course of the disease. Today, treatment of depressive disorders is focused on agents that increase the synaptic concentration of norepinephrine, serotonin, or both.

Tricyclic antidepressants (TCAs) were among the first agents used to treat depression. Included in this class are amitriptyline (Elavil), nortriptyline (Pamelor), imipramine (Tofranil), and desipramine (Norpramin). Amitriptyline and imipramine are tertiary amines that are metabolized to active secondary amine compounds (nortriptyline and desipramine, respectively). These active metabolites are also used as antidepressants. The primary mechanism of action for TCAs is inhibition of norepinephrine reuptake into the presynaptic terminal. A specific norepinephrine transporter exists on these terminals, and TCAs bind to and inhibit its normal function. The net result is an increased concentration of norepinephrine in the synapse and a more robust postsynaptic receptor activation. TCAs have variable effects on the reuptake of serotonin.

Selective serotonin reuptake inhibitors (SSRIs) increase synaptic concentrations of serotonin. Through a similar mechanism of action as described for TCAs, these drugs inhibit serotonin transport back into a presynaptic terminal. This effect increases the serotonin signaling on a postsynaptic receptor. The prototypical agent in this class is fluoxetine (Prozac). Also included in this class are paroxetine (Paxil), sertraline (Zoloft), citalopram (Celexa), and escitalopram (Lexapro; the active S-enantiomer of citalopram). Clomipramine (Anafranil) is also an SSRI pharmacologically, although chemically it is a member of the TCA class.

An additional class of antidepressants is the **serotonin-norepinephrine reuptake inhibitors (SNRIs)**. TCAs and SSRIs have the capacity to block the reuptake of both NE and 5-HT. However, the predominant neurotransmitter affected by TCAs is NE, and SSRIs have significantly more preference for 5-HT reuptake. The SNRIs, which include duloxetine (Cymbalta) and venlafaxine/desvenlafaxine (Effexor/Pristiq), inhibit both NE and 5-HT reuptake. It has been suggested that this combined mechanism produces a more rapid clinical effect compared to NE or 5-HT reuptake alone.

Dopamine has also been implicated in the pathogenesis of depression. One specific agent, bupropion (Wellbutrin), inhibits dopamine reuptake and produces an antidepressant effect. Bupropion, or its active metabolite, may have a weak reuptake inhibitory effect on norepinephrine as well. This small molecule exerts a similar effect as described for the other agents acting on the dopamine reuptake transporter, increasing synaptic dopamine concentrations.

Antiepileptic Agents

Epilepsy and other seizure disorders are highly variable in their classification and etiology. The medications used to treat seizure disorders typically target an ion channel (sodium, calcium, and possibly potassium), either suppressing neuronal depolarization or causing neuronal hyperpolarization (chloride channels). Many antiepileptic agents exist, and it is difficult to group them into classes. Following is a list of miscellaneous agents and a brief description of their proposed mechanisms of action. This mechanism is unknown for several agents.

Carbamazepine, **oxcarbazepine**, and **phenytoin** all exert their antiepileptic effects by inhibiting Na^+ ion influx. This inhibition prevents depolarization of neuronal membranes, stabilizes the neuronal membrane, and prevents the spread of seizures across the CNS.

Gabapentin (Neurontin) and **pregabalin (Lyrica)** probably exert their effects through blockade of voltage-gated Ca^{2+} channels. Blocking such channels prevents the release of neurotransmitters thought to be involved in epilepsy.

The exact mechanism of action for **levetiracetam (Keppra)** is unknown, but research suggest that this agent is capable of inhibiting Ca^{2+} channels in a similar manner to that described for gabapentin. Also, levetiracetam has been suggested to augment gamma-aminobutyric acid (GABA) activity, which contributes to suppressing seizures.

Lamotrigine (Lamictal) has been shown to inhibit the release of the excitatory amino acid glutamate. Lamotrigine may also exert an inhibitory effect on Na^+ channels, thereby stabilizing the neuronal membrane.

Vigabatrin (Sabril) is an irreversible inhibitor of GABA transaminase, an enzyme responsible for the metabolism of GABA. Its administration prolongs the inhibitory effects of GABA.

Tiagabine (Gabatril) seems to augment GABA activity by inhibiting GABA reuptake into presynaptic neurons.

Topiramate (Topamax) has several suggested mechanisms: inhibiting Na^+ channels, enhancing GABA activity, and also blockade of glutamate receptors.

Zonisamide (Zonegran), through an unknown mechanism, has been shown to stabilize neuronal membranes.

Valproic acid/sodium valproate (Depakene/Depakote) has several suggested mechanisms of action. It appears that valproic acid increases CNS concentrations of GABA, possibly by inhibiting GABA metabolism or preventing its reuptake. Valproic acid may also exert an inhibitory effect on voltage-gated Na^+ channels.

Anxiolytics

Anxiety has a broad definition that incorporates both psychological and physiological aspects. Characteristic symptoms of anxiety include uneasiness and unnecessary worrying. Stress often brings on anxious feelings, yet this is regarded as a normal response. When anxiety dominates an individual's life such that daily performance or routine behaviors are impaired, an anxiety diagnosis can often be made. Counseling is often the best approach to treating anxiety, but when counseling fails, drug therapy can be initiated. Drugs used to treat anxiety disorders include the benzodiazepines, the SSRIs, and buspirone.

All **benzodiazepines** can alleviate the symptoms of anxiety. While some of these agents are marketed as sedative/hypnotics rather than as antianxiety agents, their effects do not differ. Benzodiazepines with longer half-life (e.g., diazepam [Valium] and flurazepam [Dalmane]), when used as sedative/hypnotics, may produce a "hangover" effect. Benzodiazepines with shorter half-lives, such as alprazolam (Xanax), lorazepam (Ativan), and clonazepam (Klonopin), are often used for anxiety and tend to not produce a comparable hangover effect. The mechanism of action for benzodiazepines capitalizes on their ability to bind the benzodiazepine receptor located on $GABA_A$ ion channels. Upon binding, the benzodiazepine–receptor complex will cause a conformation change to the receptor, increasing the affinity for the natural ligand GABA. The net effect of this drug–receptor interaction is more frequent neuronal hyperpolarization and suppressed neurotransmission. When neurons in the CNS involved in the management of stress/anxiety are hyperpolarized, they are unable to fire and a calming effect is noted.

Selective serotonin reuptake inhibitors are used as first-line agents in the treatment of anxiety disorders when chronic treatment is indicated. Unfortunately, the SSRIs, as is true with their administration for depression, take time to achieve a maximal effect. The mechanism of action for treatment of anxiety is probably identical to that for depression.

Buspirone (Buspar) is neither a benzodiazepine nor a SSRI. This stand-alone agent acts as a partial agonist for the particular serotonin receptors believed to be involved in anxiety (the $5\text{-}HT_{1A}$ receptor). As with SSRIs, the maximal effect is seen only after 2–3 weeks of therapy, and this drug must be taken on a regular basis.

Migraine-Abortive Agents

Migraine headaches are painful and debilitating, such that prompt termination of the headache is desirable. Some patients may be able to quickly terminate a migraine attack with NSAIDs, aspirin, or acetaminophen. For those who do not respond to traditional analgesics, rapid relief of migraine can be achieved with the **serotonin agonist ("triptan")** class of antimigraine agents. Mechanistically, the triptans act as agonists of serotonin receptors located in several key areas of the CNS. Activation of these receptors ($5\text{-}HT_{1B/1D}$) leads to intracranial vasoconstriction, suppression of pain neurotransmission through the trigeminal nerve tracts, and inhibition of presynaptic release of inflammatory mediators/vasodilators. Also included in this class of agents are rizatriptan (Maxalt), naratriptan (Amerge), eletriptan (Relpax), and zolmitriptan (Zomig).

Sedatives/Hypnotics

Disorders of initiating and maintaining sleep (DIMS) and insomnia affect a large portion of the population. Causes of insomnia are most often behavioral. When lifestyle modifications fail to treat the disorder, sedatives/hypnotics can be used. These agents include benzodiazepines; the nonbenzodiazepines ("Z" drugs), zolpidem (Ambien), zaleplon (Sonata), and eszopiclone (Lunesta); and a melatonin analog, ramelteon (Rozerem).

Benzodiazepines used for insomnia include temazepam (Restoril), triazolam (Halcion), and (rarely) flurazepam (Dalmane). These agents have an identical mechanism of action as described for their use in anxiety. They bind to benzodiazepine receptors on $GABA_A$ channels, increasing GABA affinity and resulting in chloride ion influx and hyperpolarization of neuronal membranes. The benzodiazepines produce clinically relevant anxiolytic effects and sedation. However, the Z drugs, such as zolpidem, have an increased specificity for $GABA_A$ receptors found on neurons primarily involved in sedation/wakefulness; these agents have far less activity as antianxiety agents. When zolpidem (and other Z drugs) binds to receptors, GABA affinity for its binding site is increased and hyperpolarization ensues. The net effect is a decrease in sleep latency, or the time required to fall asleep.

Melatonin, an endogenous neurohormone made by the pineal gland, has also been used to treat insomnia. Ramelteon (Rozerem), a conformationally constrained melatonin analog, has been approved for insomnia. Mechanistically, ramelteon can be described as an agonist of the melatonin-1 and -2 receptors (MT_1 and MT_2). The MT_1 receptor is believed to be involved in the sleep–wake cycle.

ANNOTATED BIBLIOGRAPHY

Abraham D, *Burger's Medicinal Chemistry and Drug Discovery Online.* Hoboken, NJ: John Wiley and Sons; 2009.

Foye WO, Lemke TL, Williams DA, eds. *Principles of Medicinal Chemistry.* 6th ed. Philadelphia: Lippincott Williams & Wilkins; 2007.

Hardman JG, Limbird LE, Goodman Gilman, A eds. *Goodman & Gilman's The Pharmacological Basis of Therapeutics.* 10th ed. New York: McGraw-Hill; 2007.

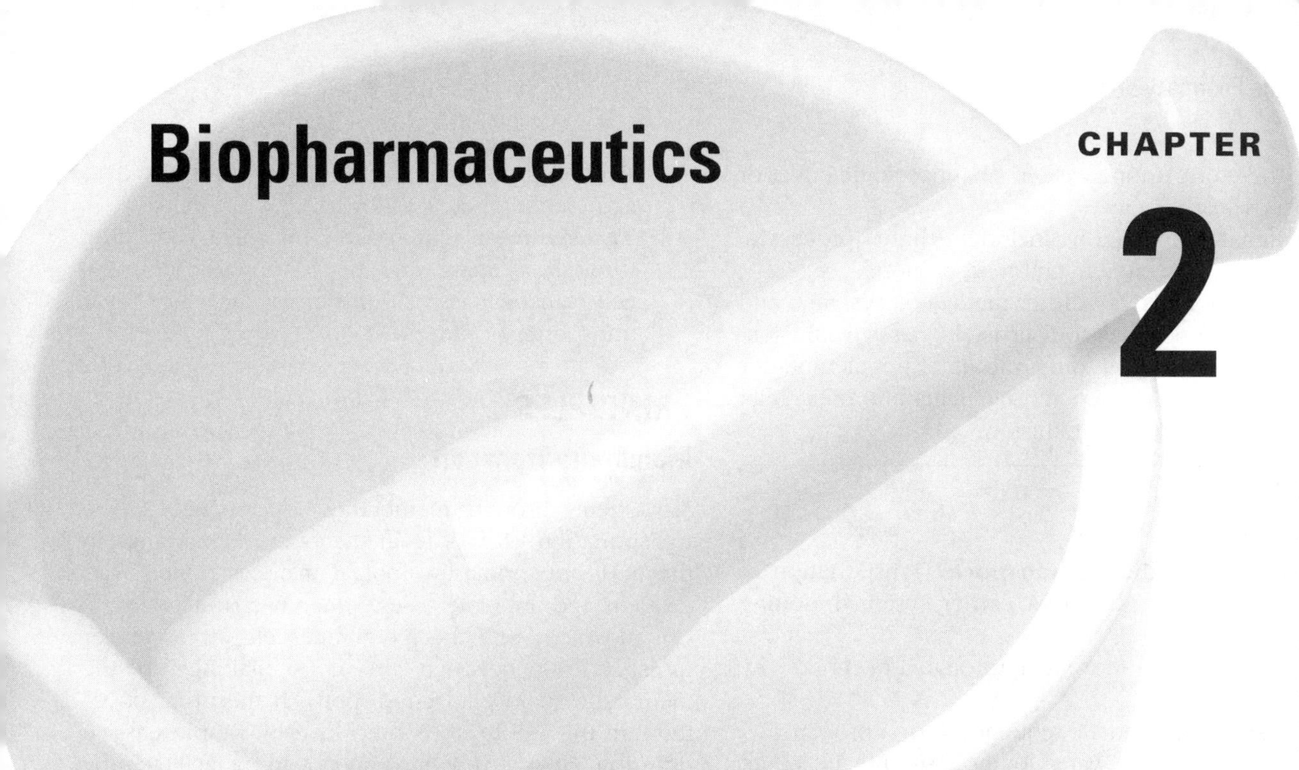

Biopharmaceutics

CHAPTER

2

Contributor: Sandra Earle

The physiochemical properties of drugs determine how they will move and interact with the body. By understanding a few principles, predictions about how and where a drug will move in the body can be accurately made. These principles can then be applied to the processes that a drug undergoes as it moves through the body.

Tips Worth Tweeting

- A drug must be sufficiently small and lipophilic, and must be uncharged (un-ionized), to undergo passive diffusion.
- Passive diffusion does not require energy—just a concentration gradient.
- Active transport requires a carrier, attraction to the carrier, and energy.
- Any fixed-capacity system can follow Michaelis-Menten kinetics and be nonlinear.
- Michaelis-Menten kinetics are determined by the system's capacity and affinity.
- If the drug concentration is much less than the concentration where half the carriers are occupied (K_m), the system will be concentration–independent.
- Genetic polymorphisms can dictate how much enzyme capacity or transporter capacity an individual patient possesses.
- A drug must be dissolved to be absorbed.
- Consumption of food slows drug absorption, but may not change the amount of drug ultimately absorbed.
- Drugs can be metabolized by enzymes in the gut wall before reaching the systemic circulation.
- Drugs can be pumped out of the gut wall and back into the gut lumen after being absorbed.
- Efflux pumps can be up-regulated and down-regulated by drugs.
- Gut enzymes can be either induced or inhibited by drugs and food.
- Drugs can be metabolized in the liver before reaching the systemic circulation.
- The more highly protein bound a drug is, the more important binding displacement becomes.
- Only non-protein-bound drug (free drug) can move between membranes and interact with receptors or drug-metabolizing enzymes.
- Polar drugs can be excreted in the urine. Nonpolar drugs must be metabolized to make them more polar for excretion by the kidneys.
- The CYP450 family of enzymes is responsible for most drug metabolism.
- Drugs can be substrates, inducers, and inhibitors of specific isoenzymes in the CYP450 family.
- Enzyme induction will likely cause a decrease in drug concentration and therefore cause a possible decrease in or loss of therapeutic efficacy.
- Enzyme inhibition will likely cause an increase in drug concentration and,

therefore, an increase in pharmacologic effect or possible toxicity.

- Renal elimination includes three processes: filtration, secretion, and reabsorption.
- Secretion is a carrier-mediated system, and reabsorption is accomplished by passive diffusion.
- Movement of a drug through the membranes between a woman and her fetus and breastmilk occurs by passive diffusion.

Key Terms

Carrier-mediated transport: Transportation of a drug molecule via a carrier system requiring energy.
Endocytosis: Movement through a membrane by engulfment.
Genotype: Genetic sequencing for a protein.
Hydrophilic: "Water loving"; soluble in water, insoluble in nonpolar lipids. Similar to lipophobic ("lipid fearing").
Lipophilic: "Lipid loving"; soluble in nonpolar lipids, insoluble in aqueous solutions. Similar to hydrophobic ("water fearing"). The higher the partition coefficient (PC), the more lipophilic the compound.
Michaelis-Menten kinetics: Description of a nonlinear rate of a reaction that can be applied to many processes.
Paracellular transport: Movement of a drug through a membrane by passing between cells.
Partition coefficient (PC): Ratio of drug concentrations at equilibrium between n-octanol (mimics lipophilic membranes) and water. The higher the PC, the more lipophilic the compound.
P-glycoprotein (P-gp): An important efflux pump found on the gut wall, blood–brain barrier, hepatocytes, and renal tubular cells.
Phenotype: How a genotype expresses itself.
Polymorphism: When at least two different phenotypes (1 wild + 1 or more mutations) occur in a population.
Prodrug: A drug that must be metabolized to acquire therapeutic efficacy.
Transcellular transport: Movement of a drug through a membrane by passing through the cell; can be passive diffusion or facilitated by a transporter or pump.

PRINCIPLES

Membrane Transport

Movement through membranes is essential to the transportation of a drug in the body. Membranes in the body are primarily lipoidal matrices dotted with proteins and, in some cases, aqueous channels. Drugs can move through the membrane cells (transcellular transport) or between the cells making up the membrane (paracellular transport). If the drug moves through the cell itself, it can move by simple passive diffusion; alternatively, movement can be facilitated by a transport system. Drugs can also cross membranes by endocytosis (i.e., a large molecule may be engulfed by the cell).

Passive Diffusion

Drugs move by passive diffusion by naturally following a concentration gradient. Because the movement is due to the energy of the molecules, no energy is required for the transport. The rate of transport is based on Fick's first law of diffusion:

$$\text{Rate of transport} = \frac{\text{Permeability} \times \text{Surface area} \times \text{Concentration difference}}{\text{Membrane thickness}} \quad (2\text{-}1)$$

Carrier-Mediated Transport

Many drugs are transported via carrier systems rather than by passive diffusion. This method does not require the concentration gradient or permeability characteristics needed for passive diffusion, but a transporter and energy are required to move the drug. The number of transport sites will be limited, so competition for these sites may occur. Up- or down-regulation of

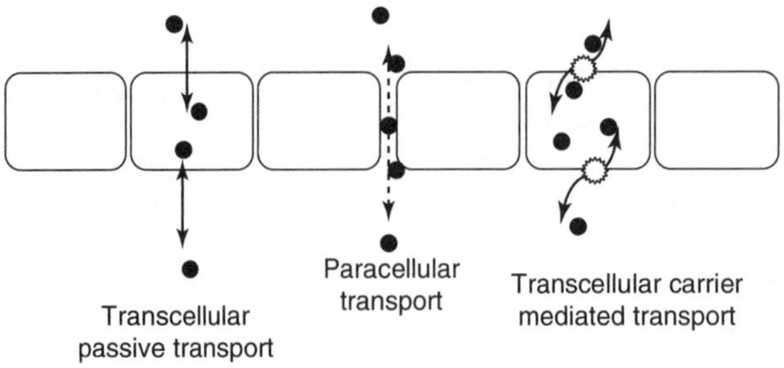

Figure 2-1 Forms of Drug Molecule Transport

Table 2-1 Factors That Enhance Drug Transport

Membrane Properties That Enhance Transport by Passive Diffusion	
Membrane thickness	Very thin membranes, like those in blood capillaries, facilitate very rapid transport of even large, polar, charged molecules; the thicker the membrane, the more important the permeability characteristics of the drug.
Available surface area	Larger surface areas offer greater opportunity for transport; the small intestine is most important site of drug absorption because of its large surface area.
Drug Properties That Enhance Transport by Passive Diffusion	
Small size	Molecular weight of less than 300 g/mol increases the likelihood of passive diffusion. Protein-bound drugs not small enough.
Charge	Ionized drugs less likely to be transported. Use the Henderson-Hasselbalch equation to estimate the degree of ionization.
Lipophilic	Nonpolar/lipophilic drugs more likely to be transported; a higher oil:water partition coefficient (PC) predicts more rapid transport.
Large concentration gradient	A larger difference between concentrations on opposite sides of the membrane predicts faster transport to the less concentrated side.

the number of transporters may occur. The direction of the transport can be either into the cell (influx) or out of the cell (efflux). Some transporters are listed in Table 2-2.

P-glycoprotein (P-gp) is the best studied member of a family of efflux transporters called the multidrug resistance proteins (MRPs). It plays a major role in moving drugs from the intestinal wall back into the gut lumen. P-gp is also found in the liver (moves drugs from hepatocytes back into the blood), in the kidneys (moves drugs from tubular cells back into the urine), and as part of the blood–brain barrier (moves drugs from brain epithelial cells back into the blood). Its discovery on tumor cells that were resistant to anticancer drugs greatly increased awareness of this transporter.

Table 2-2 Drug Transporters

Influx Transporters	Efflux Transporters
OAT (organic anion transporter)	P-gp (P-glycoprotein)
OCT (organic cation transporter)	BCRP (breast cancer resistance protein)
	BSEP (bile salt export pump)
	MRP (multidrug resistance proteins)

Many drugs are substrates, inducers, and inhibitors of P-gp. These drugs are also commonly substrates of CYP3A4. P-gp may act as a "gatekeeper" to regulate exposure of drugs to CYP450 enzymes in the gut wall. P-gp can be up- and down-regulated by some drugs and foods—an important source of drug and disease interactions. Additionally, genetic variants of P-gp may be more or less effective than the wild type. As more is learned about this polymorphism, patient-specific information may become useful to determine individual dosing regimens based on P-gp phenotype.

Michaelis-Menten Kinetics and Drug Transport

Any transport system that has a fixed capacity (i.e., carrier-mediated transport) is saturable at some point. When this occurs, the rate or extent of the process can no longer increase proportionally to the dose or concentration; that is, it is no longer a linear relationship. In this case, the process will follow Michaelis-Menten kinetics. The Michaelis-Menten relationship is shown in Equation 2-2. Hepatic metabolism, plasma protein binding, and facilitated (carrier-mediated) transport all follow this principle:

$$Rate\ of\ Reaction = \frac{V_{max} \cdot C}{K_m + C} \qquad (2\text{-}2)$$

where

V_{max} = maximal rate of the reaction (capacity)
K_m = concentration at which $\frac{1}{2}V_{max}$ is reached (affinity)
C = concentration.

Metabolism

In the case of drug metabolism by hepatic enzymes, hepatic intrinsic clearance (CL_{int}) is governed by Michaelis-Menten kinetics:

$$CL_{int} = \frac{Rate\ of\ Reaction}{C} = \frac{V_{max}}{K_m + C}. \qquad (2\text{-}3)$$

The maximal rate of metabolism (V_{max}) is determined by the number of enzymes available, or the capacity of the enzyme system. The number of enzymes (and, therefore, V_{max}) can be increased by the addition of an enzyme inducer. The drug concentration where 50% of V_{max} is achieved is K_m and serves as a measure of the affinity of the system. The lower the value of K_m, the higher the affinity between drug and enzyme. Knowledge of relative K_m (which are often referred to as K_i in the literature) between two drugs could predict which drug would be preferentially metabolized and suggest which drug–drug interactions might occur.

In most cases, metabolism is linear because drug concentrations achieved in the therapeutic range are much smaller than the K_m value of the system. In such a scenario, concentration is unimportant in the denominator of Equation 2-3 and, therefore, is unimportant in the determination of CL_{int}. CL_{int} would then be linear and determined only by the relative capacity (number of enzymes available or V_{max}) and affinity (how attracted the drug is to the enzyme or K_m) of the drug–enzyme system. This will result in concentration-independent, linear clearance of the drug (Figure 2-2):

$$CL_{int} = \frac{V_{max}}{K_m + C} \approx \frac{V_{max}}{K_m}. \qquad (2\text{-}4)$$

However, if K_m is not much smaller than the concentrations seen, then drug concentration becomes a determinant of the enzyme activity (CL_{int}) and the clearance of the drug. This happens with phenytoin in the therapeutic range. In this case, CL_{int} and therefore the *CL* of phenytoin are partly determined by the concentration (as in Equation 2-3) and will be saturable. As concentration increases, CL_{int} will decrease, causing concentration-dependent or nonlinear metabolism and clearance (Figure 2-3).

Nonlinear metabolism makes dosing a challenge. Small changes in doses produce disproportionately large changes in concentrations. Also, because *CL* is constantly changing, there is no true $t_{1/2}$.

Protein Binding and Carrier-Mediated Transport

Plasma protein binding and active, carrier-mediated transport are also saturable systems that exhibit nonlinearity. Again, each system will have a capacity (V_{max}) and affinity (K_m). In the case of plasma protein binding, the capacity will be determined by the number of binding sites available. The K_m or affinity measure is termed K_d in the case of binding and is the concentration producing half saturation of binding sites. If K_d is much greater than the concentrations achieved, binding will be concentration–independent and linear. Most drugs exhibit linear binding in the therapeutic range, although valproic acid and disopyramide demonstrate nonlinear binding in their therapeutic ranges. For these drugs, free fraction increases as concentration increases, making interpretation of total drug concentrations difficult.

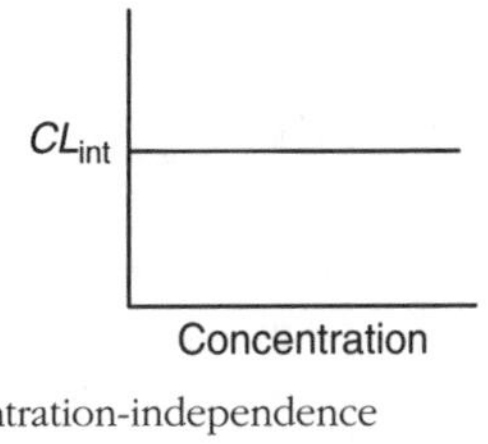

Figure 2-2 Concentration-independence

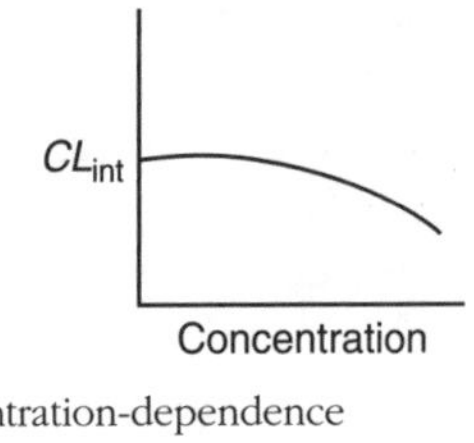

Figure 2-3 Concentration-dependence

Analogously, the capacity of carrier-mediated transport will be the number of carrier systems available; K_m is called K_T in this case. If K_T is much greater than the concentration, transport will be linear. If the concentration approaches K_T, transport will be concentration–dependent and will slow with increasing concentration.

Pharmacogenomics

Genetic differences in individuals can affect drug movement and drug response. By understanding these

Table 2-3 Sources of Polymorphism

	Enzyme/Gene	Ethnic Frequency of Poor Metabolizers
Phase I enzymes	CYP 2D6	Approximately 10% of all Caucasians
	CYP 2C9	Approximately 3% of all Caucasians
	CYP 2C19	Approximately 20% of all Asians Approximately 3% of all African Americans and Caucasians
	Dihydropyrimidine dehydrogenase	Approximately 1% of the total population
Phase II enzymes	*N*-acetyltransferase	52% of all Caucasians 25% of all Asians
	Uridine diphosphate-glycuronosyl-transferase	Approximately 10% of all Caucasians Approximately 3% of all Asians
	Thiopurine *S*-methyltransferase	1 in 300 Caucasians 1 in 2,500 Asians
	COMT	25% of all Caucasians
Pharmacologic receptors	Angiotensin-converting enzyme	
	β_2 receptors	
	Bradykinin receptors	
	Estrogen receptor-α	
	Glycoprotein IIIa	
	Serotonin	

possible differences, predictions can be made about an individual's response to a given drug, and an optimal therapeutic plan can be developed.

Genetic differences in metabolizing enzymes and transport systems have been identified and can sometimes be used to optimize therapy. Genetic differences in pharmacologic receptors may be important in choice of therapy. "Polymorphism" is said to exist when there is a significant subpopulation with a specific variant gene expression. Some important sources of polymorphism are identified in Table 2-3.

A DRUG'S TRIP THROUGH THE BODY

Bioavailability

The bioavailability of a drug (F) is determined by many factors, including the route of administration, dosage form, physiological status of the patient, and properties of the drug itself. If given orally, the drug must first be absorbed (f_a). Then it must cross the gut wall without being metabolized or pumped back into the intestine by an efflux pump (f_g). Finally the drug must circulate through the liver without undergoing metabolism (f_{fp}) before reaching the systemic circulation, where it can act on receptors:

$$F = f_a \times f_g \times f_{fp}. \qquad (2\text{-}5)$$

Absorption (f_a)

Most absorption in the gut occurs in the small intestine because of the great amount of surface area available there; this absorption usually results from passive diffusion. Before reaching the site of absorption, a drug must first be liberated from its dosage form. Then it must survive exposure to the acidic environment in the stomach without being destroyed and reach the absorption site without being adsorbed (bound) or complexed by food or another drug. Once it reaches the site of absorption, the drug will be absorbed either by passive diffusion or by active transport; this amount accounts for the fraction of drug absorbed (f_a).

Liberation

A drug must be dissolved to be absorbed. Most drugs are given as tablets, capsules, or solutions. A drug in a solution form is already dissolved and does not need to be liberated. In contrast, capsules must dissolve and release their contents containing the active drug, which must then dissolve to be available for absorption. Compressed tablets must also disintegrate into smaller particles before a drug can undergo dissolution. The smaller the particle size in the formulation, the more quickly the drug will dissolve and be ready for absorption.

Gastric Effects

Gastric emptying time is often the rate-limiting step in absorption. Gastric emptying is slowed by consumption of food (especially fat). This relationship explains why it is recommended that many drugs be taken on an empty stomach. Drugs such as anticholinergics and diseases such as diabetes can also slow gastric emptying time, thereby slowing the absorption rate. The stomach is very acidic, and some drugs may be destroyed when exposed to the very low pH in this organ.

Adsorption and Complexing

A drug may be adsorbed (bound) or complexed in the gastrointestinal lumen, in which case it will be found in the feces in the bound or complexed form. Adsorption occurs when a drug is attracted to and clings to another entity. Adsorption with charcoal, for example, is commonly used to prevent drugs from being absorbed in cases of overdose. Drugs can also complex with compounds to make them incapable of being absorbed. Calcium and iron supplements are common ions that will complex with drugs (e.g., tetracycline antibiotics or levothyroxine), making them too big for absorption.

Gut Wall Metabolism and Efflux

Once the drug is absorbed into the gut wall (f_a), efflux pumps (e.g., P-gp) in gut wall cells can propel the drug back into the gut lumen. Enzymes in the gut wall also may metabolize the drug. Cytochrome P450 (CYP450) 3A enzymes are found in high concentrations in the small intestinal wall. There is great potential for inducers and inhibitors of these systems to alter the fraction of drug escaping gut metabolism (f_g). For example, grapefruit juice is an inhibitor of CYP450 3A and may significantly increase f_g for substrates of this enzyme (Figure 2-4).

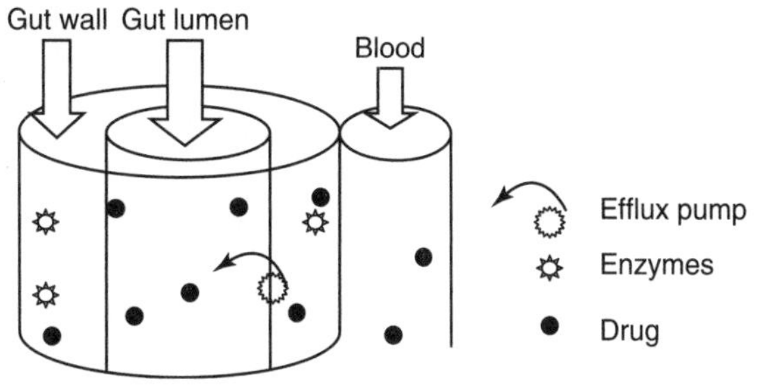

Figure 2-4 Drug Metabolization in the Gut

First Pass Through the Liver

Once the drug has been absorbed (f_a) and escapes metabolism or efflux from the gut wall (f_g), it is then taken by the portal vein to the liver, which is the major organ responsible for clearance of drugs by metabolism. The liver is rich in enzymes for both Phase I and Phase II metabolism reactions. A fraction of the absorbed drug (f_{fp}) may escape first-pass metabolism by the liver before reaching the systemic circulation. Drugs extensively metabolized by hepatic enzymes in the liver will often have a very low bioavailability if given by the oral route because much of the drug is metabolized in the first pass. For this reason, these drugs may need to be administered by a non-oral route to attain sufficient concentrations at receptor sites. Examples of routes that avoid first-pass metabolism are topical (e.g., patches) and parenteral.

Biliary Clearance and Enterohepatic Cycling

Drugs may also undergo biliary elimination or enterohepatic cycling. In this case, after the drug is absorbed and delivered via the portal vein to the liver; a portion may be secreted—by active, carrier-mediated transport—into the bile and stored in the gallbladder. The drug in the bile will then be transported back into the intestine and possibly reabsorbed to complete what is called an enterohepatic cycle. Alternatively, the drug may not be reabsorbed and will be eliminated in the feces. Biliary transport of drugs can be competitively inhibited. Drugs that have high biliary clearance are often polar, ionized molecules with molecular weights greater than 250 g/mol. Metabolites of drugs are often eliminated via biliary secretion (Figure 2-5).

Distribution and Protein Binding

Once the drug reaches the systemic circulation, it is distributed throughout the body. The extent of this distribution is measured as volume of distribution and is an important determinant of how and where the drug may act and how long it stays in the body. When the drug reaches the circulation, it may become bound to a protein in the plasma. Only unbound drug can move to other tissues, where it may also be bound to tissue proteins. Because of the size of proteins, only free or unbound drug can pass through membranes from the plasma to and from the tissue and interact with pharmacologic receptors. The extent of protein binding is a major determinant of volume of distribution of a drug. Volume of distribution is important because it affects the elimination rate constant and half-life and must be considered in some dosing calculations.

Distribution

Three different volumes of distribution may be utilized in pharmacokinetics: central volume of distribution (V_c), volume of distribution at steady state (V_{ss}), and apparent volume of distribution ($V_{dapparent}$). The first two are physiologic volumes, and the third is a calculated value.

Central Volume of Distribution

Initially, the drug will become distributed in the plasma and highly perfused organs. This is generally called the

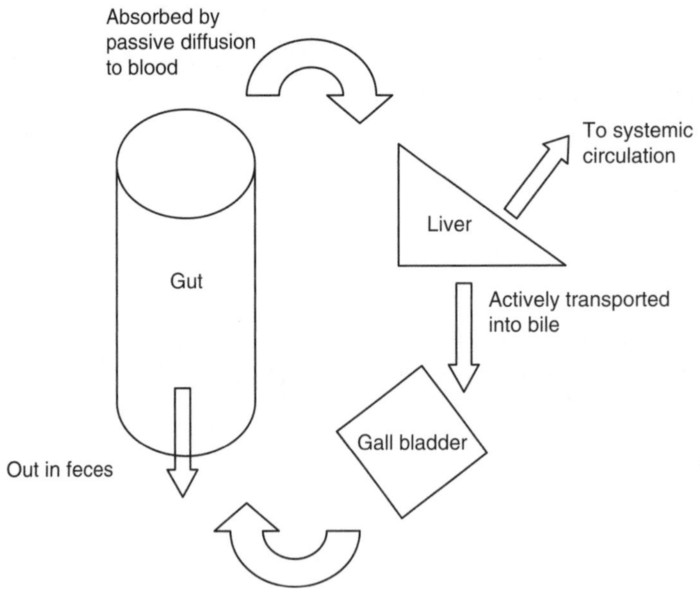

Figure 2-5 Enterohepatic Cycling

central volume of distribution and is used to calculate loading doses.

Steady-State Volume of Distribution

As a drug reaches its steady state, it moves into other tissues in the body. In an average 70-kg patient, the plasma volume (V_p) is approximately 3 L (0.04 L/kg) and the tissue volume (V_T) is approximately 39 L (0.56 L/kg). Distribution of a drug depends on how highly it is bound in the plasma compartment in relation to the tissue compartment. Because only free or unbound drug can move between plasma and tissue compartments, drug molecules that are bound to plasma proteins are "stuck" in the smaller plasma compartment and cannot move to the tissue compartment; therefore, such a drug will have a smaller volume of distribution. The opposite case can also be true: if a drug is more highly bound in the larger tissue compartment, it will have a relatively large volume of distribution. This relationship is described in Equation 2-6 and Figure 2-6:

$$V_{ss} = V_p + \left(V_T \cdot \frac{f_{up}}{f_{ut}} \right), \tag{2-6}$$

where

f_{up} = fraction unbound in plasma
f_{ut} = fraction unbound in tissues.

Apparent Volume of Distribution

The apparent volume of distribution is the calculated volume necessary to account for the resulting concentration when a known amount of drug is given. This is not a physiologic volume but is often considered to be similar to V_{ss}:

$$C = \frac{Dose}{V}. \tag{2-7}$$

The size and lipophilicity of drugs also determine where they are distributed. Large molecules will not be able to leave the plasma compartment and will have a volume of distribution roughly equal to the V_p. (V_p is the smallest possible volume for a drug.) Relatively small, but polar drugs will not be able to traverse lipophilic cell membranes and, therefore, will be able to reach only the plasma and interstitial volumes (approximately 0.17 L/kg). Small, lipophilic drug molecules will be able to move throughout all the available spaces.

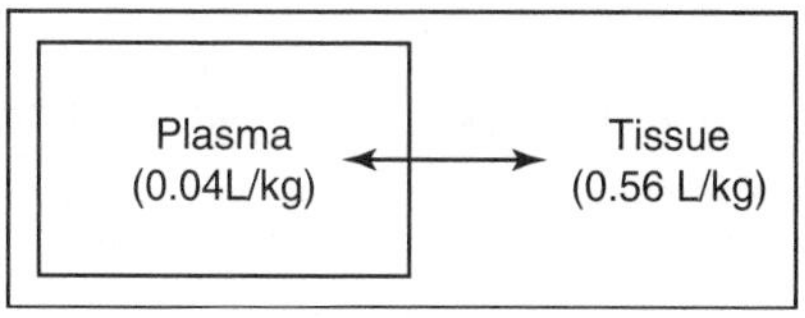

Figure 2-6 Size and Lipophilicity of Drugs Determines Distribution

Protein Binding

Protein binding is important for many reasons. Only free drug is active and able to move through membranes and interact with receptors, so protein binding is important in determining active concentrations and volumes. Also, in many cases, only free drug can be cleared; therefore, clearance may be dependent upon the unbound fraction in plasma (f_{up}). Drugs are bound to proteins in a reversible fashion. The fraction bound is determined by the capacity (amount of protein available) and the affinity of the drug for the binding site (see the earlier discussion of Michaelis-Menten pharmacokinetics).

$$Drug + Protein \leftrightarrow Drug - Protein\ Complex$$

Significance of Protein Binding

In clinical practice, total concentrations (both free and bound) of drugs are measured. To determine the free concentration of a drug, the total concentration should be multiplied by the fraction unbound (free fraction) in the plasma (f_{up}):

$$C_{free} + C_{tot} \cdot f_{up}. \tag{2-8}$$

Equation 2-8 illustrates the importance of knowing whether plasma protein binding has changed. Protein binding changes are significant only if the drug is highly bound to begin with. The more highly bound, the more significant binding changes will be.

Plasma protein binding also is a determinant of the hepatic clearance of low extraction (i.e., non-first-pass drugs) (Equation 2-9) and glomerular filtration clearance in the kidney (Equation 2-10). In both of these cases, only free drug is available for clearance:

$$CL_{H,Low\ E} \approx CL_{int} \times f_{up} \tag{2-9}$$

$$CL_{gf} = GFR \times f_{up}. \tag{2-10}$$

Changes in protein binding can occur as a result of changes in the amount of plasma proteins available (capacity) or competitive inhibition of binding (relative affinity) through binding displacement.

Binding Proteins

Drugs are bound in the plasma primarily to albumin, α_1-acid glycoprotein (AAG): and lipoproteins. The quantity of each of these proteins can be altered by disease states (Table 2-4).

Competition between drugs for AAG and/or albumin binding sites may result in displacement of the drug with lower affinity for the site ($\uparrow K_d$). This will cause the f_{up} to increase for that drug. Competitive displacement does not occur with lipoproteins.

Table 2-4 Protein Binding

Binding Protein	Drugs to Which the Protein Preferentially Binds	Disease States That Alter Proteins
Albumin	Weak acids	Renal failure, Cirrhosis, Burns } ↓alb Pregnancy Surgery
AAG	Weak bases and neutral	Crohn's disease, Cancer, Rheumatoid arthritis } ↑AAG AMI Trauma
Lipoproteins	Weak bases and neutral	Changes in cholesterol levels

Consequences

If the f_{up} of a drug increases due to a decrease in the number of binding protein sites available or competitive displacement, an increase in the free concentration of the drug will occur (Equation 2-8). This increase will likely be temporary, because the clearance rate is often also dependent upon the f_{up} of the drug (Equations 2-9 and 2-10). This is the case for low-extraction drugs. An increase in the f_{up} of such a drug results in an increase in clearance. After SS is reestablished, there will be no change in the free concentration (and, therefore, no change in pharmacologic effect), but the total concentration will be decreased. In practice, lower plasma concentrations of drugs that are observed under these circumstances may be misinterpreted as an indication of a need for dosage increase.

Metabolism

After a drug has been absorbed and distributed, it will be eliminated by being metabolized or by being excreted, or by a combination of the two. Polar drugs are more easily excreted in the urine. More lipophilic drugs may need to be metabolized into a new, more polar form to make them suitable for renal elimination.

Metabolism primarily occurs in the liver, but any tissue with metabolizing enzymes (e.g., the gut wall) can be a site of biotransformation. Two major classes of reactions result in metabolism: Phase I reactions and Phase II reactions. Drugs may undergo metabolism by any combination of these reactions.

Phase I

Phase I reactions make compounds more polar with simple, nonsynthetic oxidation, reduction, and hydrolysis reactions. The CYP450 family of enzymes is most responsible for drug metabolism. This large group of enzymes can be broken down into several isoenzyme subfamilies. A drug may be a substrate, an inducer, or an inhibitor of any of these subfamilies. Some drugs induce or inhibit their own metabolism. Genetic polymorphisms seen in 2D6, 2C9, and 2C19 (Table 2-5) may be sources of many drug interactions and toxicities.

Phase II

Phase II reactions are conjugation reactions that generally attach a group to the drug molecule that makes the molecule more polar. Glucuronidation, sulfation, acetylation, and methylation are all examples of Phase

Table 2-5 Selected Examples of CYP Isoenzyme Substrates, Inducers, and Inhibitors

CYP Isoenzyme	Substrates	Inducers	Inhibitors
1A2	Theophylline Caffeine	Charbroiled food Smoking Phenytoin St. John's wort	Erythromycin Ketoconazole Omeprazole Oral contraceptives
2C9	S-warfarin Phenytoin Fluvastatin Glipizide Glyburide	Phenobarbital Phenytoin Rifampin Carbamazepine	Cimetidine Fluconazole Fluoxetine Fluvastatin Sertraline
2C19	Omeprazole Lansoprazole Diazepam	Phenobarbital Phenytoin Rifampin Carbamazepine	Fluconazole Fluoxetine Fluvastatin Sertraline
2D6	β-blockers Codeine Dextromethorphan Fluoxetine TCA	St. John's wort Ritonavir Phenobarbital Phenytoin Rifampin Carbamazepine	Cocaine Ritonavir Paroxetine Fluoxetine Bupropion
3A4	Cyclosporine Saquinavir Ritonavir Lovastatin Tacrolimus Tamoxifen Nifedipine Verapamil Zolpidem	St. John's wort Ritonavir Phenobarbital Phenytoin Rifampin Carbamazepine	Erythromycin Fluconazole Fluoxetine Grapefruit juice Saquinavir Zileuton Clarithromycin St. John's wort

II reactions. Genetic polymorphisms also play a role in Phase II enzymes. (Table 2-3) The enzymes responsible for Phase II reactions can be induced or inhibited by drugs in the same fashion as the CYP450 enzymes.

Alteration in Enzymes

Hepatic clearance of a drug is highly dependent upon the activity of the enzyme(s) responsible for its metabolism (hepatic intrinsic clearance or CL_{int}). It is also dependent upon the rate of introduction of the drug to the liver (liver blood flow, Q) and the fraction of drug unbound to plasma proteins (f_{up}). If, however, the drug has a high affinity for the enzymes and the CL_{int} is very large in comparison to Q, liver blood flow will be the rate-limiting step and will determine hepatic clearance. Such an agent is called a high-extraction or high-first-pass drug:

$$CL_{high\,E} \approx Q. \tag{2-11}$$

If the drug does not have a high affinity for the enzyme and Q is much greater than CL_{int}, CL_{int} and the unbound drug fraction become the rate-limiting step and, therefore, the determinant of the clearance of these drugs. Agents that exhibit this property are called low-extraction drugs:

$$CL_{low\,E} \approx CL_{int} \cdot f_{up}. \tag{2-12}$$

Changes in enzyme activity will alter the clearance of only low-extraction drugs. However, CL_{int} is a determinant of the fraction that escapes the first-pass effect (f_{fp}) for high-extraction drugs:

$$f_{fp} \approx \frac{Q}{CL_{int} \cdot f_{up}}. \tag{2-13}$$

Enzyme Induction

Hepatic enzymes may be induced by drugs, or a patient may have more enzyme available because of genetic predisposition. Occasionally, drugs may induce the enzymes responsible for their own clearance (i.e., carbamazepine). When enzymes are induced, V_{max} (the capacity of the system) is increased. This change generally happens slowly because new enzymes must be synthesized to increase the number available.

Enzyme induction results in an increase in clearance of low-extraction drugs and a decrease in f_{fp} of orally administered, high-extraction drugs. In both cases, drug concentrations will be decreased. This could result in a lack of efficacy of the drug. In both cases, an increase in dose rate may be necessary:

$$\downarrow C_{ss,low\,E} = \frac{F \cdot DR}{CL} \approx \frac{F \cdot DR}{\uparrow CL_{int} \cdot f_{up}}.$$

$$\downarrow C_{ss,high\,E} = \frac{F \cdot DR}{CL} \approx \frac{f_a \cdot f_g \cdot \frac{Q}{\uparrow CL_{int} \cdot f_{up}} DR}{Q}.$$

Induction of metabolism may increase transformation of a prodrug (the inactive parent compound) to the active metabolite. Enzyme induction may also result in problems if the metabolite formed is toxic.

When an inducer is discontinued, enzyme activity (CL_{int}) will return to normal over time. This will result in the opposite effect seen from the induction. The net effect will be similar to that following addition of an enzyme inhibitor (discussed in this next section), and may result in unexpected drug interactions.

Enzyme Inhibition

Hepatic enzymes can be competitively or noncompetitively inhibited, or a reduced number of enzymes may be genetically predetermined (Table 2-5). Two drugs metabolized by the same enzyme may compete for that enzyme's active site. The drug with the higher affinity for the enzyme (lower K_m) would be preferentially metabolized; such drugs are called competitive inhibitors. Compounds with imidazole, pyridine, or quinolone groups have a high propensity for causing enzyme inhibition. Some drugs can inhibit the enzymes needed for their own metabolism; they are called auto-inhibitors (e.g., clarithromycin). Enzyme inhibition happens relatively quickly. The onset of potential increased effects or toxicity is only dependent upon the half-lives of the inhibitor and the substrate.

Enzyme inhibition may decrease the clearance of low-extraction drugs and increase the f_{fp} of orally administered, high-extraction drugs. In both cases, concentrations will be increased and toxicity or concentration-related side effects may occur. A decrease in dosage may be necessary:

$$\uparrow C_{ss,low\,E} = \frac{F \cdot DR}{CL} \approx \frac{F \cdot DR}{\downarrow CL_{int} \cdot f_{up}}.$$

$$\uparrow C_{ss,high\,E} = \frac{F \times DR}{CL} \approx \frac{f_a \cdot f_g \cdot \frac{Q}{\downarrow CL_{int} \cdot f_{up}} DR}{Q}.$$

Inhibition of enzymes that metabolize a prodrug may result in lack of efficacy due to decreased conversion to the active metabolite form. Decreased enzyme activity may have a positive effect if the metabolite formed is toxic.

When an inhibitor is discontinued, enzyme activity (CL_{int}) will increase to normal levels fairly quickly in cases of competitive inhibition. This will result in the opposite effect seen with enzyme inhibition.

Excretion

Excretion results in elimination of a drug from the body without changes being made in the drug molecule. If a drug is more polar, it is more likely to be excreted unchanged by the kidneys. A drug that is more lipophilic will need to be metabolized before it is suitable for excretion. The kidney is the primary site of excretion, but drugs may also be excreted through bile, saliva, breastmilk, placenta, and lungs.

Renal Excretion

Three processes are involved in renal clearance: filtration, secretion, and reabsorption. Filtration and secretion add drug to the glomerular filtrate for elimination, while reabsorption removes drug from the glomerular filtrate and returns it to the blood (Figure 2-7).

- **Filtration.** Only free drug can be filtered because bound drug is too large. Therefore filtration clearance (glomerular filtration rate, GFR) is determined by blood flow to the glomerulus and the fraction of unbound drug (f_{up}); see Equation 2-10.
- **Secretion.** Tubular secretion occurs in the proximal tubule. It is a carrier-mediated transport process requiring energy. The carriers moving a drug are specific for either acids or bases. Drugs that compete for these carriers may cause drug interactions; that is, acids will compete with acids and bases with bases. The drug with the higher affinity (lower K_T) will be preferentially transported from the blood into the renal tubules for excretion.
- **Reabsorption.** Drugs can be reabsorbed back into the blood in the distal tubule. While some drugs (e.g., lithium) and nutrients undergo active reabsorption, most drugs are subject to simple passive diffusion (driven by a concentration gradient) for this process. Drugs must be lipophilic and non-ionized to be reabsorbed. Therefore alterations in urine pH or concentration gradient can alter reabsorption. For example, if the urine is alkalinized by sodium bicarbonate, weak acids would be more ionized, decreasing reabsorption; weak bases would be less ionized, favoring reabsorption. Conversely, if the urine were acidified by taking large doses of vitamin C, weak acids would be less ionized, favoring reabsorption, and weak bases would be more ionized, decreasing reabsorption.

Analyzing the net effect of these three processes allows prediction of drug interactions. If renal clearance is less than filtration clearance, the predominant process must be reabsorption. If renal clearance is greater than filtration clearance, secretion must be the predominant process.

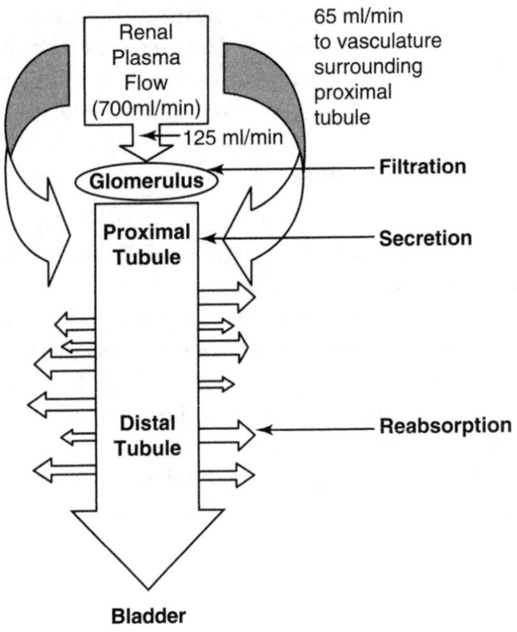

Figure 2-7 Representation of Renal Clearance in Kidney

Breastmilk

Excretion of drugs into breastmilk is of great concern to nursing mothers. Most drug excretion in human milk occurs through passive diffusion. As a consequence, the drug must be small enough (low molecular weight and/or unbound), lipophilic enough, and un-ionized to pass into breastmilk. There must also be a concentration gradient. The choice of a drug that is unlikely to diffuse through a membrane would be prudent in nursing mothers.

- **Concentration gradient.** A concentration gradient arises if any drug is present in the blood; therefore, nursing when blood concentrations are at their lowest would decrease this gradient. It is good practice to suggest breastfeeding a child just before taking the medication.
- **Size.** Drugs with a molecular weight less than 300 daltons will be small enough to diffuse into breastmilk, but those with a molecular weight greater than 6,000 daltons will be too large.
- **Ionic character.** Breastmilk has a pH of approximately 7.1, making it slightly more acidic than blood (pH 7.4). Drugs that are weak bases will become more highly ionized when moving to the more acidic milk side of the membrane. Ionization will inhibit such a drug from being able to move back into the blood, so weak bases will become trapped in breastmilk—a phenomenon called "ion trapping." Therefore weak bases are often less desirable for use by nursing mothers.
- **Lipophilicity.** A very low partition coefficient (low lipophilicity) helps minimize transport of drug from blood to milk.

Placenta

Predicting the movement of a drug from the mother's blood to the placenta and on to the fetus is important to pregnant women. Most placental transport occurs via passive diffusion, so the principles involved in breast-milk transfer of drugs also apply to placental transfer. Drugs with a pK_a in the range of 4.3–8.5 are likely to be transferred across the placenta. Fetal plasma and amniotic fluid are more acidic than maternal blood; therefore, ion trapping of weak bases on the baby's side of the placenta can occur. Drugs with a molecular weight less than 600 daltons are more likely to be transferred.

CONCLUSION

By applying the principles of biopharmaceutics, patient care can be improved by the pharmacist. Knowing the physiochemical properties of a drug can help the healthcare team as a whole make better drug therapy choices and anticipate drug interactions.

Pharmacokinetics

CHAPTER

3

Contributor: Sandra Earle

Tips Worth Tweeting

- k is determined by $\frac{CL}{V}$. k does not determine CL or V.
- The value e^{-kt}) determines the fraction of drug remaining at time t.
- The value $(1 - e^{-kt})$ determines the fraction of the steady state (SS) achieved at time t.
- The accumulation factor $\left(\frac{1}{1-e^{-k\tau}}\right)$ can "fast forward" any concentration from the first-dose concentration-time curve to SS.
- The multiple dosing factor $\left(\frac{1-e^{-nk\tau}}{1-e^{-k\tau}}\right)$ can "fast forward" any concentration from the first-dose concentration-time curve to n doses.
- Area under the concentration-time curve (AUC) is an important measure of drug exposure and can be used to calculate the clearance rate.
- The clearance rate is important because it is a determinant of drug exposure (AUC, $C_{SS,avg}$) and influences how long the drug remains in the body ($t_{1/2}$, k).
- Volume of distribution is important because it is a determinant of C_{max} if given by IV bolus and influences how long the drug remains in the body ($t_{1/2}$, k).
- Bioavailability is important because it is a determinant of drug exposure (AUC, $C_{SS,avg}$).
- The elimination rate constant (k) and half-life are important because they are measures of how long a drug remains in the body and how long it takes to reach SS.
- High-first-pass drugs have high extraction ratios and low bioavailability; their clearance depends on hepatic blood flow.
- Hepatic intrinsic clearance (enzyme activity), plasma protein binding, and renal tubular secretion all follow Michealis-Menten kinetics.
- Only free drug can pass through membranes and interact with systemic receptor sites.
- Total drug concentrations will reflect free concentrations as long as plasma protein binding remains constant.
- Drug and disease interactions should be anticipated when drugs or diseases are added *and* when they are removed or resolved.

Pharmacokinetics (PK) utilizes mathematics to study the relationship between drug dosage regimens and the resulting drug concentrations in the body. When drug concentrations can be correlated with drug effects, PK can be used to target given effects of the drug, to predict drug and disease interactions, and to optimize the response to drugs.

As soon as a drug is taken or administered, it goes on a journey through the body. PK paramenters guide this journey. If it is taken orally, the drug must travel from the gastrointestinal tract to the systemic circulation; it will then be distributed throughout the body and be eliminated. At any step in this process, the drug may encounter receptors where it can exert its pharmacologic effects (either therapeutic or adverse). Where the drug becomes distributed depends on its physiochemical properties. Elimination of the parent drug is accomplished primarily by either metabolism or the removal of the parent drug from the body via the kidneys or bile.

The details of a drug's journey through the body are presented in the Biopharmaceutics chapter, in this text. This journey involves bioavailability, absorption, distribution, metabolism, and excretion or elimination (ADME) processes. Still other concepts or processes are important to the characterization of a drug's pharmacokinetic behavior; these processes are discussed in this chapter.

CLEARANCE

Clearance is a measure of the efficiency of drug removal from the body. The two major organs of clearance in the body are the kidneys and the liver. Total body clearance is the sum total of all of the organ clearances. The fraction of administered, bioavailable drug that is recovered unchanged (not metabolized) in the urine (f_e), is the fraction of drug eliminated by the kidneys. Any drug not recovered unchanged in the urine must have been eliminated by another organ of clearance.

The relationships among volume of distribution, clearance, elimination rate constant (k), and half-life are important in determining the biopharmaceutics of any agent. The volume of distribution (V) is an important determinant of how long a drug remains in the body. Both the half-life ($t_{½}$) of a drug (Equation 3-1) and the elimination rate constant (k) (Equation 3-2) are determined by the volume of distribution and the clearance (CL) of a drug. Neither half-life nor k determines CL or V, however. The half-life not only dictates how long a drug remains in the body, but also determines how long it takes to reach a steady state (SS):

$$t_{½} = \frac{0.693 \cdot V}{CL} \quad (3\text{-}1)$$

$$k = \frac{CL}{V}. \quad (3\text{-}2)$$

Clearance is also important because it is a determinant of the average amount of drug in the body after steady state has been achieved:

$$C_{ss,avg} = \frac{F \cdot DR}{CL}. \quad (3\text{-}3)$$

Hepatic clearance (CL_H) is discussed in the Biopharmaceutics chapter. To briefly review, hepatic clearance is determined by hepatic blood flow (Q_H), hepatic enzyme activity or intrinsic hepatic clearance (CL_{int}), and plasma protein binding (i.e., the unbound fraction of drug in plasma, f_{up}). Hepatically cleared drugs that are highly extracted by liver enzymes are considered high-first-pass drugs; they will have a relatively low F because only a small fraction (f_{fp}) survives the first pass through the liver. Doses will likely be different depending on the route by which the drug is administered. For such drugs, Q_H is the most important determinant of CL_H, and alterations in Q_H (e.g., owing to congestive heart failure or arrhythmias) will change their clearance. Hepatically cleared drugs with low extraction efficiency will not have a high first-pass effect. Their clearance correlates with the product of CL_{int} and f_{up}. If either of these values is altered by disease or drug interactions, clearance will be altered.

Renal clearance is also discussed in the Biopharmaceutics chapter.

THERAPEUTIC DRUG MONITORING

Most drugs do not require determination of plasma or tissue concentrations—that is, therapeutic drug monitoring (TDM)—for optimization of therapy. If a standard dosage regimen produces the wanted effect in all or most patients, there is no reason to measure drug concentrations. TDM is useful only if the following criteria apply:

- Absence of a well-defined dose–response relationship
- Presence of a well-defined concentration–response relationship (pharmacodyamics)
- A relatively narrow therapeutic range
- Interpatient variability in the dose regimen–concentration relationship (pharmacokinetics)
- Accurate drug assays available

In addition to serving as a guide for dosage adjustment, drug concentrations may be used to assess patient adherence.

For appropriate interpretation of measured drug concentrations, the following information should be either known or obtained:

- Which condition is being treated?
- Is the patient suffering from any dose-related toxicities or signs of lack of efficacy?
- Is the patient at steady state?
- Were all doses given at the appropriate time? If not, when were they given?
- When was (were) the sample(s) drawn in relation to the dose given?
- Are there any patient-specific factors that might influence pharmacokinetic parameters (e.g., volume status, albumin concentrations)?

If it is determined that targeting concentrations of a drug will improve patient outcomes, utilizing pharmacokinetics will be an important tool for dosage regimen design and monitoring.

BASIC CALCULATIONS TO DETERMINE PHARMACOKINETIC PARAMETERS

Characterization of the Concentration-Time Curve

To determine the initial pharmacokinetic parameters of a given drug in a patient, concentrations of drug in plasma will be measured over time after drug administration. If a drug is given as a bolus intravenous injection, bioavailability and rate of administration do not have to be considered. The resulting concentration-time curve would look something like Figure 3-1.

The maximum concentration (C_{max}) will be achieved immediately after the drug is given at time 0; the drug will subsequently be distributed and cleared from the body. Because a known amount of drug was introduced into the body, if C_{max} is measured, the initial volume of distribution (V_c) can be calculated (Equation 3-4). The concentration at any time after the drug has been administered can be

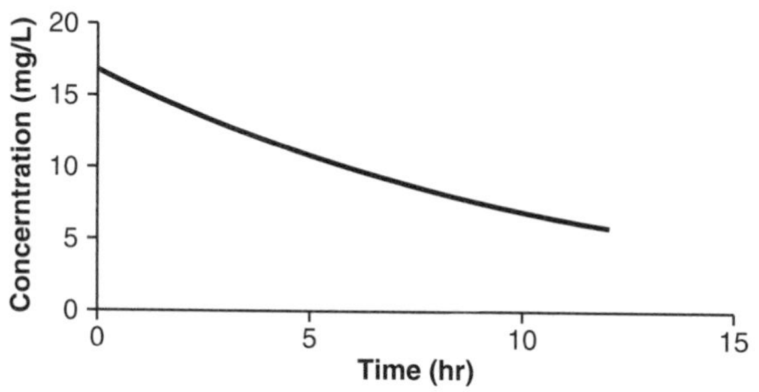

Figure 3-1 Plasma Concentration vs. Time Curve After Bolus Intravenous Drug Administration

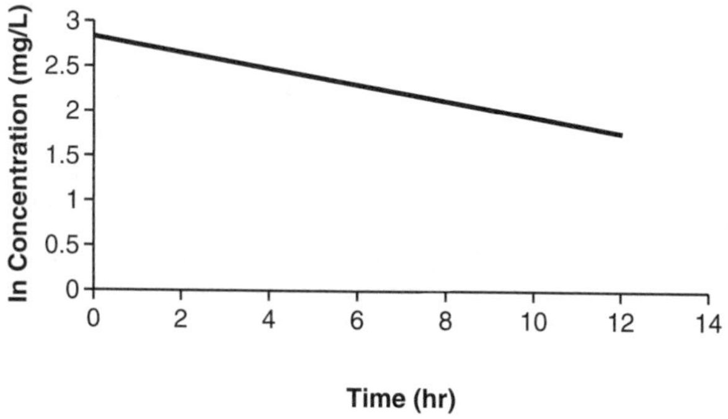

Figure 3-2 ln Plasma Concentration vs. Time Curve After Bolus Intravenous Drug Administration

determined by multiplying C_{max} or C_0 by the fraction of drug remaining at time t (e^{-kt}); see Equation 3-5:

$$C = \frac{Dose}{V_c} \tag{3-4}$$

$$C_t = C_0 e^{-kt}. \tag{3-5}$$

The drug is eliminated from the body in a log-linear manner. Therefore, if the ln concentration-time curve were plotted, it would form a straight line, as in Figure 3-2. The slope of this line is k and the y-intercept is ln C_{max}.

To determine the rate of elimination from the body (k), plasma concentrations are collected and measured at two or more different time points after administration. From these concentrations, the slope of the line describing the elimination of the drug can be determined using Equation 3-6, which is a rearrangement of Equation 3-5:

$$k = \frac{(\ln C_2 - \ln C_1)}{t_2 - t_1}. \tag{3-6}$$

Notice that Equation 3-6 is a simple "rise over run" calculation. Memorization is not necessary if you understand the basic principle. This number will be negative because the slope of the line is negative. However, the elimination rate constant is not negative; it is the fraction of drug removed per time, so it cannot be negative. The $t_{½}$ and time to steady state (approximately $5t_{½}$) can be determined once the value of k is established:

$$t_{½} = \frac{0.693}{k}. \tag{3-7}$$

Once the elimination rate constant and one other concentration on the concentration-time curve are known, any concentration at any time point can be determined (Equation 3-5). The elimination rate constant is an important pharmacokinetic variable, because it indicates how long the drug stays in the body. This rate is determined by clearance and volume, as shown in Equation 3-2. Again, it is important to note that k is the dependent variable in this relationship. The elimination rate constant does not *determine* clearance or volume; however, the relationship between these parameters may be used to *calculate CL* or *V* if the other two variables are known.

Multiple Compartments

The simplistic example given in the previous subsection is helpful when trying to grasp the basic concepts

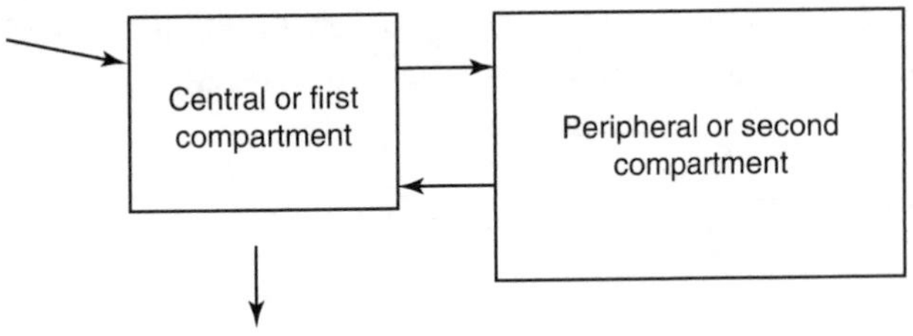

Figure 3-3 Diagram of Two-compartment Model

underlying the concentration-time curve and the information that can be gathered from it. In reality, drugs are rarely given by IV bolus and rarely, if ever, have instantaneous distribution. Instead, most drugs are distributed into several groups of tissues—compartments—at different rates. Most drugs enter into at least two compartments; many become distributed into even more. Most of the calculations presented here assume that a drug follows a one-compartment pharmacokinetic model, for the sake of simplicity. In most cases, assuming one compartment results in a small but acceptable margin of error.

A two-compartment model is often represented schematically as shown in Figure 3-3. In a typical two-compartment model, the first compartment is called the central compartment. It represents the tissues where the drug is administered, and from which the drug is distributed and eliminated. It is physiologically envisioned as the blood and highly perfused organs. The second compartment is called the peripheral compartment; it represents the group of tissues into which the drug becomes distributed more slowly. The drug must also move back out of the tissues of the peripheral compartment and return to the central compartment to be eliminated. If a concentration-time curve of a two-compartment-model drug were characterized, the line depicting the log concentration versus time would not be straight (Figure 3-4).

The concentration-time curve for a two-compartment model features an initially steeper decline, representing drug distribution. The second phase of the line is flatter, depicting the slower elimination of the drug. This second phase is called the terminal phase for a two-compartment model; its slope is used to determine

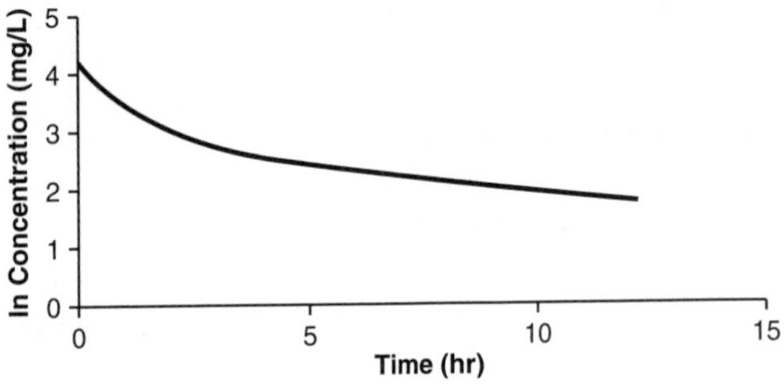

Figure 3-4 ln Plasma Concentration vs. Time Curve for Two-Compartment Model After Bolus Intravenous Drug Administration

k and $t_{½}$. The biexponential line formed by these data can be analyzed to characterize both compartments, with each having a slope (k) and y-intercept (C_{max}) to describe them. When the two compartmental lines are added, the equation to describe the concentration at any time can be determined:

$$C_t = C_1 e^{-k_1 t} + C_2 e^{-k_2 t}. \quad (3\text{-}8)$$

As more compartments are added, the pertinent equations and models become increasingly more complex. Most calculations become too cumbersome without the help of a computer for a model that assumes more than two compartments. For these reasons, the remainder of the discussion will assume a one-compartment model.

Area Under the Curve

The area under the concentration-time curve (AUC) is a model-independent parameter that measures drug exposure. It is commonly used to correlate with goals for both efficacy and toxicity. AUC can also be used to determine CL, V, $C_{SS,avg}$, and F:

$$AUC_{0\to\infty} = \frac{Dose_{IV}}{CL} = \frac{F \cdot Dose_{PO}}{CL} \quad (3\text{-}9)$$

$$AUC_{0\to\infty} = \frac{Dose_{IV}}{V \cdot k} = \frac{F \cdot Dose_{PO}}{V \cdot k} \quad (3\text{-}10)$$

$$C_{ss,avg} = \frac{AUC_{ss,0\to\tau}}{\tau} \quad (3\text{-}11)$$

$$F = \frac{Dose_{IV}}{AUC_{IV}} \cdot \frac{AUC_{PO}}{Dose_{PO}}. \quad (3\text{-}12)$$

AUC can be determined in several ways. The most commonly used method is the trapezoidal rule, in which the sum of the areas of rectangles formed between each successive concentration–time point is determined. In this method, the areas between successive concentrations are treated as rectangles. The height of each rectangle is the average of the two observed points, and the width of the rectangle is the difference between the two time points (Figure 3-5). The area between the last observed time point and infinity is a triangle that assumes a log-linear decline. It is based on the quotient of the last time point observed and the elimination rate constant (k). The sum of these rectangles and the triangle gives a good estimate of AUC.

Nonlinearities

Many pharmacokinetic processes demonstrate Michealis-Menten kinetic relationships, in that they have a saturable or fixed capacity and an affinity or dissociation

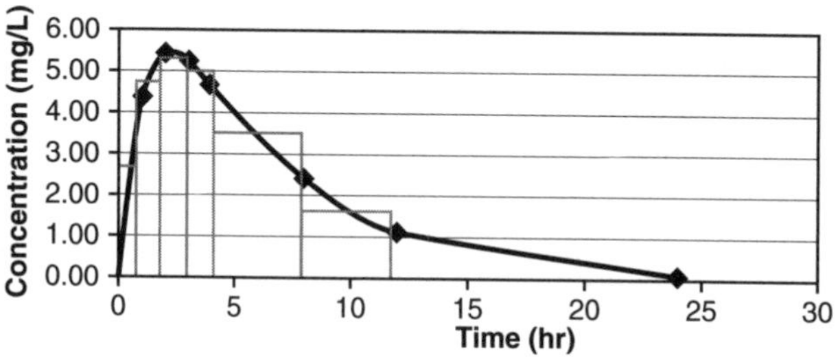

Figure 3-5 Trapezoidal Rule for Estimation of AUC

constant that describes the relationship between the drug and binding or metabolic sites. These processes include pharmacodynamics, plasma protein binding, hepatic intrinsic clearance, and renal tubular secretion. These processes are discussed at length in the Biopharmaceutics chapter.

Protein Binding

Only free drug can pass easily through membranes and interact with pharmacodynamic receptors to cause therapeutic or possibly toxic effects. Therefore, free drug concentrations correlate more closely with pharmacologic effect. While free or unbound concentrations of drugs should be of the highest interest, most pharmacokinetic equations calculate total concentrations, rather than unbound or free concentrations. Additionally, most laboratories report total concentrations—not free concentrations—of drugs, and most therapeutic ranges are listed as total concentrations. It is much easier (and much less expensive) for laboratories to measure total drug concentration rather than just the free drug concentration. As long as the free fraction of drug in the plasma (f_{up}) remains constant, total concentration will be proportional to free concentration, and total concentrations can be used to effectively determine what is happening with the free concentration. As soon as f_{up} changes, however, this will no longer be true. It is almost always acceptable to look at total concentrations and feel confident that they are proportional to the free concentration, unless f_{up} is thought to be altered by drugs or disease or is changing with concentration. This consideration is especially important when interpreting total concentrations of low-extraction drugs cleared by the liver. Protein binding relationships and interactions are discussed thoroughly in the Biopharmaceutics chapter.

DOSAGE REGIMEN DESIGN

The pharmacist can easily control dosage regimens given to patients to optimize the outcomes of their therapy. If a drug's target effect can be correlated with a concentration or range of concentrations, a regimen should be designed to target this concentration range. Drugs are commonly given as IV boluses, constant IV infusions, IV short infusions, and orally. Each of these methods is discussed here.

IV Bolus

An IV bolus is given to achieve a target concentration immediately. It does not have to take into consideration how the drug will be removed. As a consequence, giving an IV bolus is much like adding an amount of instant coffee to a coffee cup. To get the appropriate amount of coffee in the water, the amount of water (volume) and desired concentration of coffee (C_{target}) must be known. If the drug is already present in the patient's body (C_{obs}), or if the drug is given as a salt form, that fact needs to be taken into consideration when determining the dose:

$$Dose = \frac{(C_{target} - C_{obs}) \cdot V_c}{S}. \qquad (3\text{-}13)$$

Conversely, if the volume of distribution and dose given are known, the resulting concentration, which would be C_{max}, can be determined by rearranging Equation 3-13:

$$C_{max} = \frac{S \cdot Dose}{V_C}. \qquad (3\text{-}14)$$

After an IV bolus dose is administered, the concentration will fall in a log-linear fashion, as seen in Figure 3-6 and described by Equation 3-5. By combining Equation 3-5 and Equation 3-14, any concentration at any time t can be determined:

$$C_t = \overbrace{\frac{S \cdot Dose}{V_C}}^{C_{max}} \times \overbrace{e^{-kt}}^{\text{Fraction of drug remaining at time } t}. \qquad (3\text{-}15)$$

This example demonstrates how pharmacokinetic equations are built by combining equations to get the result needed. In this case, by using the equation to calculate the value of C_{max} after an IV bolus with the

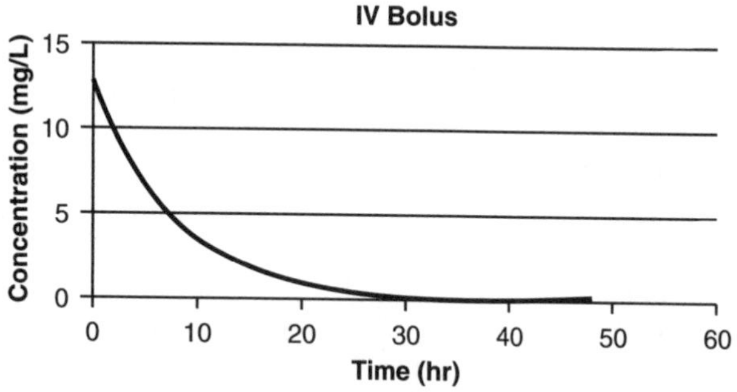

Figure 3-6 Plasma Concentration vs. Time Curve for Two-compartment Model After Bolus Intravenous Drug Administration

equation that describes the log-linear decay of drugs after administration, the concentration at any time after the administration of the IV bolus can be determined (Equation 3-15).

Repeat IV Bolus (Multiple Dosing)

If an IV bolus dose is repeated in a regular pattern (e.g., 500 mg IV bolus every 12 hours), the drug concentration will continue to increase until it reaches steady state (SS) at approximately five half-lives. It takes one half-life to achieve 50% of the eventual steady state. It takes two half-lives to achieve 75% of SS, three half-lives to achieve 87.5% of SS, four half-lives to achieve 93.8% of SS and five half-lives to reach approximately 97% of SS. The steady state will theoretically never be reached, but after three to five half-lives the patient is considered to have reached a clinical SS. To determine the fraction of SS achieved at any time, Equation 3-16 can be used:

$$1 - e^{-kt} = \text{fraction of SS achieved at time } t. \qquad (3\text{-}16)$$

Any concentration at a specific time after the first dose is given can be used to determine the corresponding concentration at SS, by utilizing the accumulation factor (Equation 3-17). The accumulation factor uses the elimination rate constant (k) and the dosing interval (τ):

$$\frac{1}{1 - e^{-k\tau}} = \textit{Accumulation Factor}. \qquad (3\text{-}17)$$

Therefore, C_{max} at SS can be predicted by utilizing C_{max} after the first bolus dose (Equation 3-18). By combining C_{max} from the first dose and multiplying it by the accumulation factor, C_{max} at SS can be determined:

$$C_{max,ss} = C_{max,1st\ dose}\left(\frac{1}{1 - e^{-k\tau}}\right). \qquad (3\text{-}18)$$

In fact, any concentration at any time t after the IV bolus dose is administered can be determined at SS by combining Equation 3-15, which determines the concentration at any time t after the dose is given, and the accumulation factor (Equation 3-17), which "fast forwards" results to SS:

$$C_{t,ss} = \overbrace{\frac{S\ Dose}{V_C}}^{C_{max}\text{ first dose}} \times \underbrace{e^{-kt}}_{\text{Fraction remaining at time } t} \times \overbrace{\frac{1}{1 - e^{-k\tau}}}^{\text{Accumulation factor}}. \qquad (3\text{-}19)$$

If SS is not reached, this same concept can be used to "fast forward" to the corresponding concentration at any time t after the dose was given, after n doses, by using the multiple dosing function (MDF; Equation 3-20). Note as n gets larger, the numerator will approach 1, so that the equation can be simplified into the accumulation factor (Equation 3-17):

$$MDF = \frac{1 - e^{-nk\tau}}{1 - e^{-k\tau}}. \qquad (3\text{-}20)$$

As an example, C_{max} on the third dose ($n = 3$) would be determined by "fast forwarding" the first dose C_{max} to the third dose by combining the equation for C_{max} (Equation 3-14) and the MDF for the third dose (Equation 3-20):

$$C_{max,\ third\ dose} = \overbrace{\frac{S \cdot Dose}{V}}^{C_{max},\text{ first dose}} \times \overbrace{\frac{1 - e^{-3k\tau}}{1 - e^{-k\tau}}}^{\text{MDF, third dose}}.$$

This expression could also be used to find a concentration at any time t after any dose before steady state. For example, if you wanted to know the concentration 4 hours after the dose was given of the second dose, the calculation would start with finding C_{max} for the first dose (Equation 3-14). The concentration 4 hours later would then be determined by identifying the fraction of drug left in 4 hours (Equation 3-15). Finally, to "fast forward" to the second dose, the MDF for the second dose would be used (Equation 3-20):

$$C_{4hr\ post,\ 2nd\ dose} = \overbrace{\frac{S \cdot Dose}{V}}^{C_{max},\text{ first dose}} \times \underbrace{e^{-k(4hr)}}_{\text{Fraction of drug remaining after 4 hours}} \times \overbrace{\frac{1 - e^{-2k\tau}}{1 - e^{-k\tau}}}^{\text{MDF, second dose}}.$$

These concepts can be utilized for any multiple dosing regimen, including repeated short infusions and oral dosing. The equations presented here are very powerful in predicting concentrations with a given dosage regimen or in determining doses when target concentrations are given.

Constant IV Infusions

When giving a constant IV infusion, the targeted concentration may not be reached until SS. Instead, a drug given by constant IV infusion is often combined with an IV bolus to achieve the targeted concentration immediately; then, as the IV bolus decays, the continuous infusion builds to the targeted concentration at SS. The two dosage regimens together allow the target concentration to be reached immediately (Figure 3-7).

The value of C_{SS} is dependent only upon the infusion rate ("drug in" or K_0) and "drug out" (CL) (Figure 3-8). The salt form would be taken into consideration if needed:

$$C_{SS} = \frac{S \cdot K_0}{CL}. \qquad (3\text{-}21)$$

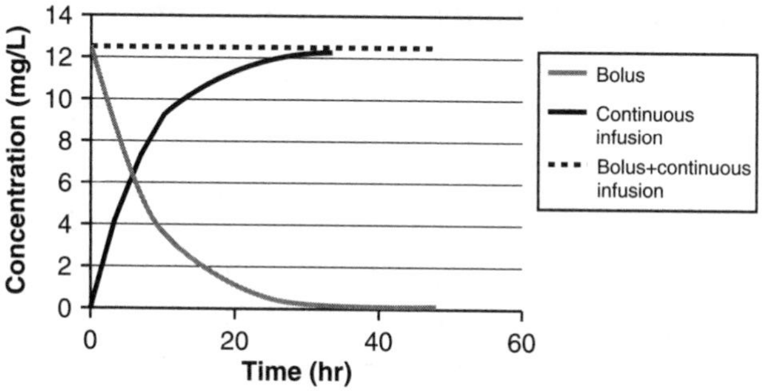

Figure 3-7 Bolus Plus Constant Infusion Drug Administration

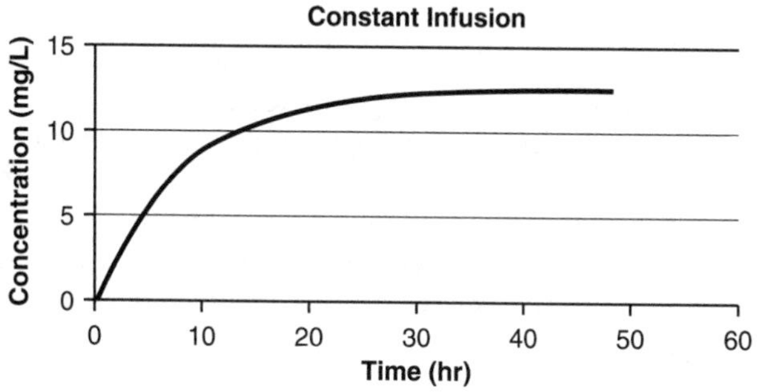

Figure 3-8 Constant Intravenous Infusion to Achieve Steady State

If the constant infusion is stopped before reaching SS, the SS equation is multiplied by $(1 - e^{-kt})$, which represents the fraction of SS achieved at time t (Equation 3-16). Equation 3-22 describes the concentration at any time t after starting a constant infusion:

$$C_t = \overbrace{\frac{S \cdot K_0}{CL}}^{C_{SS}} \overbrace{\left(1 - e^{-kt}\right)}^{\text{Fraction of SS achieved at time } t}. \tag{3-22}$$

When the constant infusion is stopped, Equation 3-22 can be utilized to determine the concentration when the infusion is stopped at time t (t = time of infusion). This would be the highest concentration achieved—that is, C_{max}. The concentration at any later time could be determined by utilizing the log-linear decline of a linear one-compartment model, as described in Equation 3-5.

$$C_t = \overbrace{\overbrace{\frac{S \cdot K_0}{CL}}^{C_{SS}} \overbrace{\left(1 - e^{-kt_{infusion}}\right)}^{\text{Fraction of SS achieved at end of infusion}}}^{C_{max}\text{ (when infusion stopped at } t_{infusion}\text{)}} \times \underbrace{e^{-kt}}_{\text{Fraction remaining at time "t" after infusion is stopped}} \tag{3-23}$$

This will determine the concentration at any time t after a constant infusion is stopped. Equation 3-23 is a combination of Equations 3-5 and 3-22. Thus this example again illustrates how pharmacokinetic equations are built to calculate the concentration you would like to determine.

Short IV Infusions

Many drugs are given as short IV infusions. These doses are treated as constant infusions that are stopped at the end of the infusion time. Therefore, if the dose is given over 1 hour, the concentration at the end of this "constant infusion" can be determined by using Equation 3-22. This calculation combines the determinants of C_{SS} for a constant infusion (Equation 3-21) and the fraction of SS achieved at the end of the infusion—in this case, 1 hour (Equation 3-16):

$$C_t = \frac{S \cdot K_0}{CL}\left(1 - e^{-kt-kt_{infusion}}\right). \tag{3-24}$$

When the constant infusion stops, that will be the highest concentration; that is, it will be C_{max} (Figure 3-9).

The concentration at any time after the short infusion is stopped can be determined by the product of C_{max} from Equation 3-22 and the fraction of drug remaining at time t after the end of the infusion. For example, if the short infusion is given once every 24 hours (τ), the minimum concentration (C_{min}) could be determined by the following expression:

$$C_t = \frac{S \cdot K_0}{CL}\left(1 - e^{-kt_{infusion}}\right) \times e^{-k(\tau - t_{infusion})}. \tag{3-25}$$

These equations can be "fast forwarded" to SS by using the accumulation factor (Equation 3-17). Therefore $C_{SS,max}$ and $C_{SS,min}$ can be calculated by multiplying Equations 3-24 and 3-25, respectively, by the accumulation factor (Table 3-1). They could also be "fast forwarded" to any dose before reaching SS in the same manner by using the MDF (Equation 3-20).

It is sometimes difficult to find population estimates of drug clearance. Indeed, it is often easier to find estimates of volumes of distribution and elimination rate

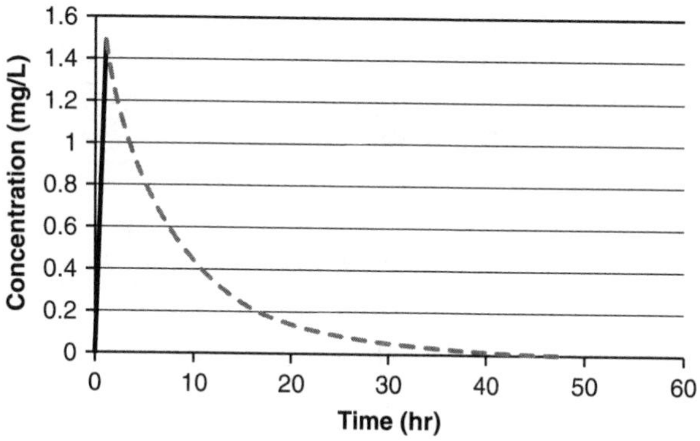

Figure 3-9 Decay of Plasma Concentration from C_{max} Following Discontinuation of Constant Intravenous Infusion

Table 3-1 Calculation of Minimum and Maximum Short IV Infusion Concentrations

	C_{max}	C_{min}
At SS	$\frac{S \cdot K_0}{CL}\left(1-e^{-kt_{infusion}}\right) \times \left(\frac{1}{1-e^{-k\tau}}\right)$	$\frac{S \cdot K_0}{CL}\left(1-e^{-kt_{infusion}}\right) \times e^{-k(\tau - t_{infusion})}\left(\frac{1}{1-e^{-k\tau}}\right)$
At *n* doses	$\frac{S \cdot K_0}{CL}\left(1-e^{-kt_{infusion}}\right) \times \left(\frac{1-e^{-nk\tau}}{1-e^{-k\tau}}\right)$	$\frac{S \cdot K_0}{CL}\left(1-e^{-kt_{infusion}}\right) \cdot e^{-k(\tau - t_{infusion})} \times \left(\frac{1-e^{-nk\tau}}{1-e^{-k\tau}}\right)$

constants in the literature. The relationship in Equation 3-2 can be used to calculate a clearance based on this relationship ($CL = kV$) as long as it is clearly understood that clearance is not determined by the elimination rate constant and volume.

Oral Dosing

Most drugs are given orally, and the concepts discussed previously can also be applied to oral dosing. The challenging aspect of oral dosing is determining the point at which C_{max} occurs. C_{max} occurs at t_{max} when the rate of drug absorption is equivalent to the rate of drug elimination. The absorption rate constant (k_a) is the fraction of drug absorbed per unit of time. The value of t_{max} is calculated as follows:

$$t_{max} = \frac{ln \frac{k_a}{k}}{k_a - k}. \quad (3\text{-}26)$$

The concentration at any time t after an oral dose is administered is the sum of the two factors of absorption and elimination working in opposition and is described by the following equation:

$$C_t = \left(\frac{F \cdot Dose}{V}\right) \times \left(\frac{k_a}{k_a - k}\right) \times \left(e^{-kt} - e^{-k_a t}\right). \quad (3\text{-}27)$$

The value of C_{max} can be calculated using the value of t_{max} determined in Equation 3-27. Likewise, the value of C_{min} can be determined by substituting the τ time as the value for t in the same equation. These equations can be "fast forwarded" to SS or a dose before SS is reached by using the accumulation factor (Equation 3-17) and MDF (Equation 3-20), respectively:

$$C_{t.ss} = \left(\frac{F \cdot Dose}{V}\right) \times \left(\frac{k_a}{k_a - k}\right) \times \left(e^{-kt} - e^{-k_a t}\right) \times \left(\frac{1}{1-e^{-k\tau}}\right)$$

$$C_{t.dose\text{“}n\text{”}} = \left(\frac{F \cdot Dose}{V}\right) \times \left(\frac{k_a}{k_a - k}\right) \times \left(e^{-kt} - e^{-k_a t}\right) \times \left(\frac{1-e^{nk\tau}}{1-e^{-k\tau}}\right).$$

Utilization of Equations

The equations described in this section may be rearranged as necessary to calculate drug concentrations when dosing regimens and pharmacokinetic parameters are known (or guessed) using population information. These same equations can be rearranged to determine dosing regimens when pharmacokinetic parameters are known (or guessed) to achieve targeted concentrations. Finally, if known concentrations result from a given dosage regimen in a patient, individual pharmacokinetic parameters can be calculated by these equations.

DOSAGE REGIMENS

Pharmacists can design dosing regimens to ensure that patients are achieving adequate but not toxic concentrations of needed medications. While it is easy to adjust how much drug is given (the dose rate) and how often (the dose interval), it is much more difficult to alter pharmacokinetic parameters such as bioavailability, distribution, and clearance of drug in a patient. The dosing regimen is made up of two components: the dose rate (*DR*) and the dose interval (τ).

The dose rate is the amount of drug the patient is receiving per unit of time. A constant infusion is an easy example. If a patient is receiving a 2 mg/min drip of lidocaine, his dose rate is 2 mg/min. If, however, a patient is receiving 1 g of cefotaxime every 8 hours, the dose rate is 125 mg/hr or 3 g/day.

The dose interval is how often the patient is receiving the drug. In the preceding example, the cefotaxime dose interval is every 8 hours.

The dose rate and dose interval work together to determine the dose. Do not confuse dose with dose rate, however. If the patient who was receiving 1 g of cefotaxime every 8 hours developed renal impairment, less drug should be given and thus the *DR* should be decreased. His τ may also be increased, causing the dose to remain unchanged.

Average Concentration at Steady State

The two factors targeted when trying to maximize efficacy and minimize toxicity are the average concentration at steady state ($C_{SS,avg}$) and the peak-to-trough ratio ($P:T$). $C_{SS,avg}$ is an overall average concentration seen during a dosing interval at steady state. Consequently, the determinants of $C_{SS,avg}$ are very important. They are a balance of the drug coming in—bioavailability (F) and dose rate (DR)—and the drug going out—clearance (CL):

$$C_{ss,avg} = \frac{F \cdot DR}{CL}. \quad (3\text{-}28)$$

Therefore, if there is a change in CL, F, or DR, $C_{SS,avg}$ will also change. Such a change may result in a toxic or subtherapeutic concentration. By altering the dose rate to accommodate that change, the pharmacist can avoid such a problem. For example, if a patient goes into acute renal failure while taking a drug that is cleared by the kidneys, the clearance rate will decrease. The result will be an increase in $C_{SS,avg}$ and possible toxicity. The pharmacist will therefore recommend a decrease in the dose rate for the drug that the patient is receiving. This will result in the necessary decrease in the $C_{SS,avg}$.

Peak-to-Trough Ratio

The ratio of the C_{max} to the C_{min} or peak-to-trough ratio ($P:T$) is also important in determining a safe, effective dosing regimen. These ratios determine the variability of drug concentration within a dosing interval. If a drug is not given often enough, it may have a very large, possibly unacceptable $P:T$ ratio. For example, if a drug is given once a day compared to three times daily, and the dose rate or total daily dose is the same, the peak concentration will be relatively high and the trough concentration relatively low (Figure 3-10). This could result in toxic peak concentrations and subtherapeutic trough concentrations.

The more often a drug is dosed or the smaller the individual doses into which the daily dose is divided,

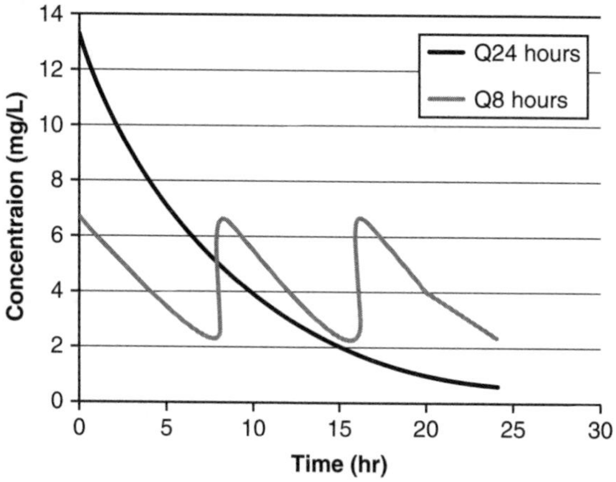

Figure 3-10 Peak:trough Comparisons for Once Daily vs. Three Times Daily Administration of the Same Drug Dose

the less variation there will be between the peak and trough concentrations. This smoothing out of the concentrations may be desirable, but it should be weighed carefully with the ability of patients to comply with difficult dosing regimens. In addition, it is not always desirable to have a small $P:T$ ratio. For example, it is advantageous for aminoglycosides to have a large peak-to-trough ratio. High peak concentrations of aminoglycosides are associated with better bacterial kill, and low trough concentrations may decrease the risk for nephrotoxicity. The elimination rate constant (k) and dosing interval (τ) determine the peak-to-trough ratio:

$$P:T = \frac{1}{e^{-k\tau}}. \quad (3\text{-}29)$$

Recall that k is determined by CL and V. Thus, if there is a change in CL, V_d, or dosing interval (τ), there will be a change in the peak-to-trough ratio.

It is helpful to realize that for every half-life of the drug given, the peak-to-trough ratio will be 2. Therefore, the peak concentration will be twice the trough concentration. If dosing is more frequent, there will be less variation between the peak and trough concentrations; if dosing is more frequent, there will be a greater deviation between peak and trough concentrations.

Initial Doses

When a drug is given to a patient for the first time, population averages are employed as the patient's pharmacokinetic parameters. Depending on the therapeutic concentration goals, a loading dose (LD) may or may not be needed. An LD is needed when it will take too long to achieve therapeutic concentrations using just a maintenance dosing regimen. This often occurs for drugs with a long half-life. The LD is based on the target concentration and the V_c. Also a miniload may be necessary to increase a patient's drug concentration quickly. The equation for loading dose is as follows (Equation 3-13):

$$Dose = \frac{\left(C_{\text{target}} - C_{\text{obs}}\right) \cdot V_c}{S}.$$

Initial maintenance dosage regimens are determined by choosing a target $C_{SS,max}$, $C_{SS,min}$, $C_{SS,avg}$, or C_{SS} (constant infusion) and target $P:T$.

If dosing is based upon a target $C_{SS,avg}$, the DR can be determined first, utilizing population CL ($V \times$ k) and F estimates. The DR will be given as an amount per unit of time, rather than as a dose (Equation 3-28):

$$C_{ss,\,avg} = \frac{F \cdot DR}{CL}.$$

This is followed by choosing an appropriate dose interval (τ) to allow for acceptable fluctuations within the dosing interval. Dosing once every half-life is a good rule of thumb, but the $P{:}T$ ratio can be targeted with a population k. The dose can be determined by combining the dose rate and dose interval.

If the maintenance dosage regimen is based upon a $C_{SS,max}$ and/or a $C_{SS,min}$, an optimal τ will need to be chosen first:

$$\tau = \left| -\frac{1}{k}\left[ln\frac{C_{min,target}}{C_{max,target}} \right] \right| + t_i. \tag{3-30}$$

After an optimal τ is chosen, the dose can be determined by rearranging the appropriate $C_{SS,max}$ and/or a $C_{SS,min}$ equations for the administration method chosen. For example, if short infusions are being given, the $C_{SS,max}$ equation in Table 3-1 can be rearranged to calculate the optimal dose to achieve the targeted $C_{SS,max}$:

$$K_0 = \left(\frac{C_{ss,max,target} \cdot CL}{1 - e^{-kt_{infusion}}} \right) \times \left(1 - e^{-k\tau}\right). \tag{3-31}$$

The K_0 value is an infusion rate and is given as an amount per unit of time. Thus, to determine the dose, K_0 is multiplied by the time of infusion. The initial dosing regimen recommendation should include the approximate concentrations predicted, any monitoring that should be done, and the times at which serum concentrations should be drawn to monitor the drug therapy.

Sampling Times

As a general rule, the trough concentration (C_{min}) is usually monitored. If C_{min} is within therapeutic range, the patient is likely not suffering from lack of efficacy due to inadequate serum concentrations. Nevertheless, this finding does not ensure that the patient's $C_{SS,avg}$ and $C_{SS,max}$ will be appropriate. Because the time to C_{max} can vary significantly for orally administered drugs, it is difficult to determine when to draw a concentration to capture the C_{max}. If any two concentrations are drawn during the elimination phase, the values of k, $t_{½}$, V, and CL can be determined along with C_{max}, C_{min}, and any other concentration. There are drugs for which both the trough and the peak concentrations may be monitored (e.g., aminoglycosides). If trying to determine k when giving a short infusion, be sure to allow sufficient time after giving a drug for initial distribution. A good rule of thumb is to wait 1 hour after giving a 0.5-hour infusion and to wait 0.5 hour if giving an infusion over 1 hour.

It is important to ensure that the blood sample drawn will have a concentration that will be higher than the minimum detection limit of your lab. The pharmacist should predict what the concentration will be before it is drawn, to ensure it is within the detectable range. A C_{min} measurement may be too low. If a concentration-related toxicity is suspected, a serum concentration sample should be drawn as soon as possible to determine the toxicity range for that patient.

Modification of Dosing Regimens

After starting a patient on a dosage regimen based on population information, optimization of the individual patient's drug therapy must be verified. The most important monitoring includes clinical evaluation of the patient. Drug concentrations are simply one tool in evaluating therapy. Evaluating the patient's clinical status in light of his or her drug concentrations will help to determine if a change in dosing regimen is necessary.

To evaluate SS concentrations ($C_{SS,avg}$, $C_{SS,max}$, $C_{SS,min}$, or C_{SS}), the patient must have reached a steady state. It is often appropriate to measure concentrations before reaching SS to avoid toxicity or lack of efficacy. If the patient is at SS, the pharmacist should determine if the C_{SS} concentrations observed in the serum sample(s) is(are) appropriate for the patient. If the C_{SS} concentrations are elevated, the patient's drug exposure may be too high, putting him or her at risk for concentration-related toxicity; in such a scenario, the dose rate should be decreased. If the C_{SS} concentrations are too low, the opposite would be true and the dose rate should be increased.

What would cause a change in C_{SS} concentrations? The determinants of $C_{SS,avg}$ are "drug in" (F X DR) and "drug out" (CL):

$$C_{ss,avg} = \frac{F \cdot DR}{CL} = \frac{Drug\ In}{Drug\ Out}.$$

If CL or F is altered, there will be a resulting change in $C_{SS,avg}$, possibly necessitating a change in DR. If there is a possible change in plasma protein binding, it will be important to consider $C_{SS,avg,free}$ rather than just $C_{SS,avg}$. If a change in DR is deemed necessary and the patient is at SS, as long as there is no reason to think there might be a nonlinearity or change in CL or F, $C_{SS,avg}$ becomes proportional to DR. Therefore the adjustment in DR can be made using a simple proportion:

$$\frac{DR_1}{C_{ss,avg_1}} = \frac{DR_2}{C_{ss,ss,avg_2}}.$$

It is often important to consider the variability in the C_{max} and C_{min} concentrations ($P{:}T$). If C_{max} is too high and C_{min} is too low (large $P{:}T$), the dosing interval may be too long, so the dosing interval should be shortened, with the patient taking the drug more often during the day. It is rare (with the exception of aminoglycosides) that C_{max} would be too low and C_{min} too high (too small $P:T$). In this case, the τ should be increased, which would allow for greater change between C_{max} and C_{min}. What would cause a change in this variability ($P:T$)? Changes in V or CL will cause a change in k and, therefore, change the $P:T$ ratio.

PREDICTING DRUG AND DISEASE INTERACTIONS

Drugs administered concurrently and diseases that patients might have can alter PK parameters. This factor may result in changes in steady-state concentrations or $P:T$ ratios that could cause concentration-related toxicity or lack of efficacy. To predict these changes, the determinants of F, V, and CL should be examined. Many potential changes in these parameters are discussed thoroughly in the Biopharmaceutics chapter. Some important examples are briefly mentioned here.

Altered Bioavailability

A change in F can occur due to a change in f_a, f_g, or f_{fp}. Examples would include changes in formulation or addition of drug that adsorbs the first drug. Adding an agent that inhibits CYP P450 3A4 in the gut wall (e.g., grapefruit juice), for instance, will increase f_g, thereby increasing F and $C_{SS,avg}$. It also must be remembered that when these interacting drugs are removed, F will also be affected. Changes in bioavailability affect only $C_{SS,avg}$, so altering the dose rate appropriately should alleviate the problems caused by the bioavailability changes.

Altered Volume of Distribution

Changes in plasma or tissue protein binding or changes in the volumes of tissue will alter the volume of distribution of drugs. If a drug is highly bound to albumin and the patient has hypoalbuminemia, f_{up} will be elevated and V will be increased, resulting in a longer half-life and longer time required to achieve a steady state. This would allow for the dose interval to be increased because the $P:T$ ratio will be decreased. If a drug is highly bound to AAG, and the amount of AAG is increased (e.g., after an acute myocardial infarction), f_{up} would decrease, V would decrease, and an increase in the $P:T$ ratio, a shorter half-life, and a shorter time to SS would occur. In this case, a shorter dose interval may be helpful.

Altered Clearance

The determinants of the clearance rate are complex, as many organs may be involved. If a CYP P450 2D6 inhibitor is added to a regimen containing a low-extraction drug that is hepatically cleared and is a 2D6 substrate, there would be a decrease in the clearance rate of the first drug. This would cause an increase in $C_{SS,avg}$, possibly resulting in concentration-dependent toxicity. In this scenario, the dose rate should be decreased to avoid toxicity. This change would also decrease the $P:T$ ratio. Although this effect may not be clinically important, it may be possible to increase the dose interval, making the dosing regimen easier for the patient. Remember that the dose rate should probably be increased and the dose interval decreased after discontinuation of the 2D6 inhibitor. A good resource for updated CYP P450 data is http://medicine.iupui.edu/flockhart/table.htm.

Renal clearance is dependent upon filtration, secretion, and reabsorption. If a drug is a highly secreted (renal clearance is greater than filtration clearance), weak base, and a second drug is added that is a highly secreted, weak base, it is likely that the two agents will compete for the same secretion sites. This competition would drive down the clearance of the first drug, which is dependent upon secretion for its clearance, and would result in an increase in $C_{SS,avg}$ and a decrease in the $P:T$ ratio. The dose rate should be decreased before the patient would possibly suffer from a toxicity. Also, while clinically unimportant, it may be possible to increase the dose interval, making the dosing regimen easier for the patient. Remember that the dose rate should probably be increased and the dose interval decreased when the secreted drug is discontinued.

These are just a few examples of how PK concepts can be applied to predict and avoid drug–drug and drug-disease interactions. By taking advantage of the various mathematical and physiologic models describing drugs' sojourn through the body, pharmacists can predict and avoid drug interactions and tailor dosage regimens to result in the best outcome for patients.

Key Terms

Apparent volume of distribution (V_d): Calculated volume that would be necessary to account for all the drug or the concentration of drug in the body. It is calculated by: $V_d = \frac{Dose}{C}$ or by relating clearance and k: $V_d = \frac{CL}{K}$.

Area under the concentration-time curve (AUC): $Units = \frac{amount \times time}{vol}$. The area measured under the concentration-time curve that results after administration of the drug. It assesses patient exposure to a drug better than just a concentration at a point in time. In some cases, it may be helpful in determining the efficacy and/or toxicity of a given drug. It is determined by the dose given, F, if given other than intravenously, and by the clearance rate.

Average concentration at steady state ($C_{SS,avg}$): $Units=\frac{Amount}{Volume}$. The drug concentration representing the average concentration achieved during a steady-state dosing interval. It is similar to, but not determined by, the average of $C_{SS,max}$ and $C_{SS,min}$. It is often the target concentration when determining which dose rate to administer.

Bioavailability (F): The fraction of the administered dose that is available to the systemic circulation. Determined by f_a, f_g, and f_{fp}. Bioavailability is important in determining the dose rate needed to achieve a certain targeted $C_{SS,avg}$ if a drug is given by other than the intravenous route.

Central volume of distribution (V_c): Hypothetical volume into which a drug is initially distributed. It includes blood and highly perfused tissues. It is important for determining loading doses.

Clearance (CL): $Units=\frac{Volume}{Time}$. The volume of serum, plasma, or blood that has all of the drug removed per unit of time by the eliminating organ. Total body clearance is the sum of the clearances of all the eliminating organs. It is also the rate of elimination with respect to the given plasma concentration ($CL=\frac{k}{C}$). Clearance of any organ is determined by the blood flow to that organ (Q) and the extraction efficiency of that organ (E): $CL = Q \times E$.

Dose interval (τ): *Units = time.* The frequency of intermittent drug administration; it is important in determining the variance between the $C_{SS,max}$ and $C_{min,SS}$ or P:T. One of the factors that pharmacists can control. As a rule of thumb, drugs can be given once every half-life.

Dose rate (DR): $Units=\frac{Amount}{Time}$. The amount of drug administered per unit of time; may be thought of as the daily dose. It is important in determining $C_{SS,avg}$ and is one of the factors that pharmacists can control.

Elimination rate constant (k): $Units=Time^{-1}$. The fraction of drug removed in a given time. It is determined by measuring the slope of the terminal portion of the line formed by log serum concentrations versus time. This constant is important for determining how often to dose a drug and how long it will take to achieve a steady state. It is determined by total body clearance (CL) and volume of distribution (V), and is inversely related to half-life ($t_{½}$).

First-order (linear) elimination: The rate of a drug's elimination is directly proportional to the concentration of the drug in the serum.

Fraction absorbed (f_a): The fraction of the drug given that is able to be absorbed into the circulation.

Fraction that escapes first-pass effect (f_{fp}): The fraction of the drug that escapes metabolism in the liver as the blood passes through the liver before reaching the systemic circulation. f_{fp} is related to the hepatic extraction ratio of a drug (E): $f_{fp} = 1 - E$.

Fraction that escapes gut metabolism (f_g): The fraction of the drug absorbed that is able to escape metabolism in the gut and escape the efflux pumps located in the gut wall (e.g., P-glycoprotein).

Half-life ($t_{½}$): *Units = time.* The time required for half of the drug to be removed from the body if the drug is subject to first-order elimination. It is important for determining how often to dose a drug and how long it will take to achieve steady state. The half-life is determined by total body clearance (CL) and volume of distribution (V), and it is inversely related to the elimination rate constant (k).

Hepatic extraction ratio (E): The fraction of the absorbed dose metabolized during each pass through the liver. It is determined by Q_H, CL_{intH}, and f_{up} and is an important determinant of CL_H.

Maximum concentration at steady state ($C_{max,SS}$): $Units=\frac{Amount}{Volume}$. The highest concentration achieved after intermittent dosage administration at steady state. $C_{max,SS}$ will remain constant from dose to dose; it may be correlated with dose-related toxicity problems.

Michaelis-Menten (nonlinear) elimination: The rate of a drug's elimination does not change in proportion to the concentration of that drug in the serum. Instead, as serum drug concentrations rise, the rate of elimination increases less than proportionally. This effect occurs when there is a capacity-limited elimination process. Examples are hepatic enzymes and transport sites for renal tubular secretion. When all available or nearly all available enzymes are in use, the process reaches a saturation point, which results in the rate of elimination becoming fixed. $CL=\frac{Vmax}{Km+C}$

Minimum concentration at steady state ($C_{min,SS}$): $Units=\frac{Amount}{Volume}$ The lowest concentration within a steady-state dosing interval. $C_{min,SS}$ will remain constant from dose to dose; it may be correlated with dose-related lack of efficacy.

Peak-to-trough ratio (P:T): A comparison of C_{max} to C_{min}; important for understanding how much variation there is between the C_{max} and C_{min} concentrations within a dosing interval.

Steady state (SS): The point in therapy when the amount of drug administered exactly replaces the amount of drug removed. SS is technically never achieved, but for clinical purposes five half-lives (97% of SS) is considered to be at SS.

Therapeutic range (*TR*): A statistical range of desirable drug concentrations, for which the *majority* of patients show an effective therapeutic response with minimal drug-related side effects—*not* an absolute for every patient. Individual patients can have good therapeutic response with "subtherapeutic" drug concentrations or can experience toxicity with "therapeutic" drug concentrations. Therapeutic ranges are often indication specific.

Volume of distribution (*V*): Where the drug becomes distributed in the body. It is important for determining how long the drug stays in the body (determinant of half-life) and whether a drug will be removed by hemodialysis (larger volumes will not be removed significantly). *V* is primarily determined by binding of the drug to plasma and tissue binding sites as well as lipophilicity.

Volume of distribution at steady state (V_{SS}): Actual blood and tissue volumes into which a drug becomes distributed. This value can be used to estimate the amount of drug in the body:

$$\text{Amount of drug in body} = V_{ss} \times C_{ss,avg}.$$

DRUGS COMMONLY SUBJECT TO THERAPEUTIC DOSE MONITORING

Aminoglycosides (Gentamicin and Tobramycin)

Use: parenteral antibiotics, gram-negative infections

TR: Extended-interval dosing: peak 20 mg/L; trough too low to measure

Traditional dosing: peak 5–10 mg/L; trough < 2 mg/L

CL: renal; approximated by GFR

V_d : 0.25 L/kg; adjust for obesity and/or alterations in extracellular fluid status

$t_{½}$: 2–3 hr

Concentration-related side effects: nephro- and ototoxicity[2–5]

Aminoglycoside dosage regimens are determined in an unusual way because peak and trough levels rather than $C_{SS,avg}$ are targeted. Dosing goals are also unconventional because high peak concentrations are the best predictors of efficacy, and low trough concentrations are necessary to avoid toxicity. Therefore, a relatively new dosing method has been used: extended-interval or "once-daily" dosing.[1] To improve the likelihood of high peak and low trough concentrations during a dosage interval, a longer dose interval is desirable. Thus, rather than using conventional dosing schedules (every 8 or 12 hours), longer schedules (every 24 hours) have been used. This method has been tested in many patient groups with good success.

Clinical Insights

1. Serum concentrations should be monitored if aminoglycoside therapy is expected to continue for more than a few days. Determination of two serum concentrations allows determination of the patient's pharmacokinetic parameters and optimization of the dosage regimen. Nomograms for extended-interval dosing allow for only one midpoint concentration to be drawn.[1]
2. Although the disposition of aminoglycosides is better described by a two- or three-compartment model, no clinically significant difference is seen in predicted trough concentrations using a one-compartment model versus a two-compartment model.[6] Be sure to wait for 0.5–1 hour after the end of infusion to ensure the distribution phase has ended before drawing a "peak" sample.
3. Serum creatinine lags behind changes in renal function by at least 24 hours. Therefore, urine output, if available, should be used in conjunction with the serum creatinine to monitor aminoglycoside therapy.
4. Nephrotoxicity induced by aminoglycosides is usually reversible on discontinuation of the drug. Although high trough concentrations have been associated with renal toxicity, such concentrations may also be the result—and not the cause—of renal dysfunction. In fact, elevated trough concentrations are an early indicator of renal damage.[3,7]

Carbamazepine

Use: antiepileptic, focal and some generalized seizures; bipolar disorder

TR: 4–12 mg/L

CL: hepatic 3A4; epoxide active metabolite; auto-induction

V_d: 1.4 L/kg

$t_{½}$: initial, 15 hr; after induction, 10 hr

Concentration-related side effects: CNS (nystagmus, ataxia, blurred vision, and drowsiness). *Not* concentration-related: dermatological and hematological effects, the most serious of which is the rare, but potentially fatal, aplastic anemia.[8–10]

Carbamazepine undergoes auto-induction; it induces enzymes responsible for its own clearance and

Table 3-2 Pharmacokinetic Equations

	Equations	When to Use	When Not to Use
Area under the concentration-time curve (AUC) Units: (amount/volume) × time	$AUC_{0-\infty} = \left[\frac{(C_1 + C_2)}{2} \times (t_2 - t_1)\right]$ $\left[\frac{(C_2 + C_3)}{2} \times (t_3 - t_2)\right] + \ldots + \frac{C_{last}}{k}$ 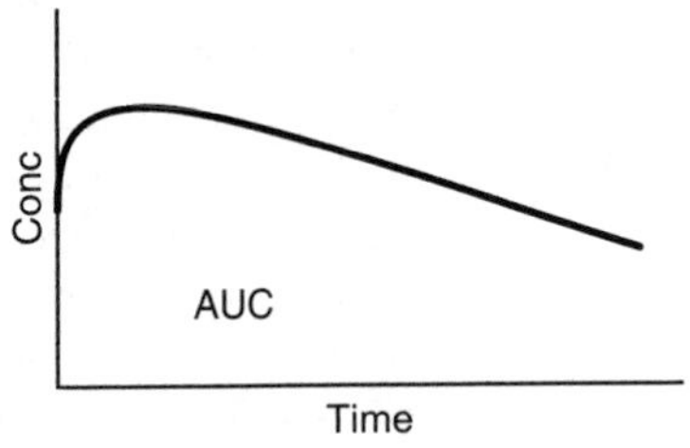 **Figure 3-11** AUC for Oral concentration vs. Time Curve	To determine $AUC_{0-\infty}$ given concentration time data after administration of drug	If only want to measure to end of τ
	$AUC_{0-t} = \left[\frac{(C_1 + C_2)}{2} \times (t_2 - t_1)\right] + \left[\frac{(C_2 + C_3)}{2} \times (t_3 - t_2)\right] + \ldots + \left[\frac{(C_{nexttolast} + C_{last})}{2} \times (t_{nexttolast} - t_{last})\right]$	To determine AUC_{0-t} given concentration time data after administration of drug	If want to measure to ∞
	$AUC_{0-\infty} = \frac{Dose_{IV}}{CL}$	Determine AUC or *CL* from AUC if dose given IV	If given by other than IV
	$AUC_{0-\infty} = \frac{F \times Dose_{PO}}{CL}$	Determine AUC or *CL* from AUC if dose given other than IV	
Bioavailability (*F*) Units: (fraction)	$F = fa \times fg \times f_{fp}$	Determine F, f_a, f_g, or f_{fp} given the others	
	$f_{fp} = \frac{Q_H}{Q_H + (CL_{int} \times f_{up})}$ Low-hepatic-extraction drug: $f_{fp} \sim 1$ High-hepatic-extraction drug: $f_{fp} \sim \frac{Q}{CL_{int} \times f_{up}}$	Determine f_{fp} Assume the "well-stirred jar" model	Assume parallel tube model
	$F = \frac{AUC_{nonIV}}{AUC_{IV}}$	Used to determine *F* when the same dose is given by IV and non-IV routes	If different doses given
	$F = \frac{AUC_{nonIV}}{AUC_{IV}} \times \frac{Dose_{IV}}{Dose_{nonIV}}$	To determine *F* when comparing differing doses	
Total body clearance (*CL*) Units: volume/time	$CL = CL_H + CL_R + \ldots$	To determine total body clearance, all organ clearances must be summed	
Hepatic $CL(CL_H)$ Units: volume/time	$CL_H = Q_H \times E_H$ Low extraction: $CL_H \cong CL_{int} \times f_{up}$ High extraction: $CL_H \cong Q_H$	• To determine what will alter hepatic clearance • Low-extraction drugs: the rate limitation to clearance is the enzyme activity (CL_{int}) and fraction unbound in plasma (f_{up}).	

Table 3-2 (*continued*)

	Equations	When to Use	When Not to Use
Hepatic $CL(CL_H)$ Units: volume/time		• High-extraction drugs: rate limitation to clearance is liver blood flow (Q)	
Hepatic extraction efficiency (E_H) Units: none	$E_H = \dfrac{CL_{int} \times f_{up}}{Q_H + (CL_{int} \times f_{up})}$	According to the "well-stirred jar" model	
Hepatic intrinsic clearance = enzyme activity (CL_{int}) Units: volume/time	$CL_{int} = \dfrac{V_{max}}{K_m + C}$	Michaelis-Menten V_{max}: maximum rate of metabolism; capacity of the system or number of enzymes available K_m: concentration at which $\frac{1}{2}V_{max}$ is reached; measure of affinity	
Renal clearance (CL_R) Units: volume/time	$CL_R = (CL_{gf} + CL_{TS})(1 - E_{TR})$	CL_{gf} = filtration clearance CL_{ts} = tubular secretion clearance E_{TR} = efficiency of tubular reabsorption	
Elimination rate constant (k) Units: time^{-1}	$k = \dfrac{\ln C_2 - \ln C_1}{t_2 - t_1}$ 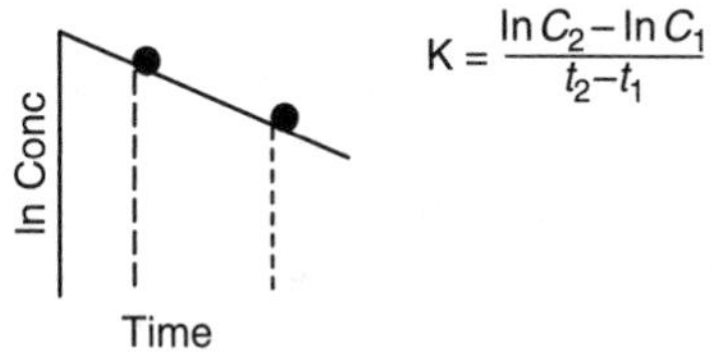 **Figure 3-12** Determination of k from ln Concentration vs. Time Curve	To determine k when given 2 concentration-time points during the decay phase of a drug considered to be linear, and gathered during a time that is considered to be reflecting only one compartment	If the concentrations given are not gathered during the decay phase of a drug that is considered to be linear and within one compartment
	$k = \dfrac{CL}{V}$	• To determine how changes in V and/or CL might alter k • To determine k if given CL and V • To determine CL if given k and V • To determine V if given K and CL	
Half-life ($t_{½}$) Units: time	$t_{½} = \dfrac{0.693}{k}$	To determine $t_{½}$ from k, or vice versa	
	$t_{½} = \dfrac{0.693 \times V}{CL}$	To determine how changes in V and/or CL might alter $t_{½}$	
Central volume of distribution (V_c) Units: volume	$Vc = \dfrac{Dose\ (injected\ instanteneously)}{C_0}$	To determine V_c or dose to achieve a target C_0	

(continues)

Table 3-2 (*continued*)

	Equations	When to Use	When Not to Use
Apparent volume of distribution (V) Units: volume	$V = \frac{Dose}{C}$ $k = \frac{CL}{V}$		
Volume of distribution at steady state (V_{SS}) Units: volume	$V_{ss} = V_p + \left[V_T \times \frac{f_{up}}{f_{ut}} \right]$ Given: $V_p = 0.07$ L/kg $V_T = 0.53$ L/kg	Determine V_{SS}, f_{ut}, or f_{up}, given the other parameters	

Table 3-3 Dosing Equations

	Equations	When to Use	When Not to Use
Model of decay of one compartment, first-order elimination	$C_t = C_0 e^{-kt}$ 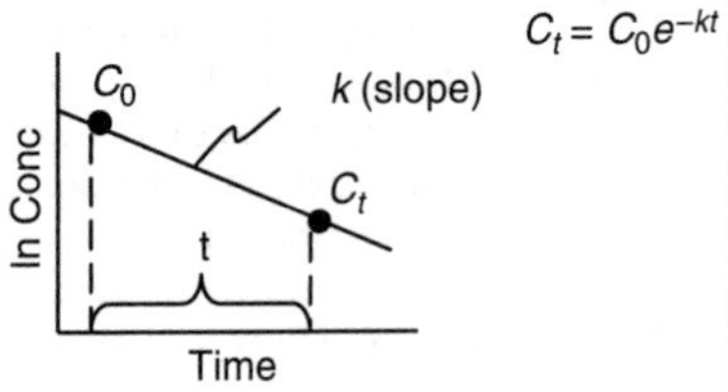 **Figure 3-13** ln Concentration vs. Time Curve for One Compartment First-order Drug Elimination	• To determine concentration at any time (C_t) during decay of a drug following one-compartment, linear kinetics when given k, an earlier concentration (C_0), and the time between C_0 and C_t (t) • To determine concentration from an earlier concentration (C_0) when all of the above conditions are met • To determine time (t) between two given concentrations (C_0 and C_t) when all of the above conditions are met • To determine elimination rate constant (k) when all of the above conditions are met	• Multiple compartments • Nonlinear clearance
Model of decay, two compartments, linear Units: amount/volume	$C_t = C_1 e^{-k_1 t} + C_2 e^{-k_2 t}$	To determine concentration at any time t during the decay of the drug if a two-compartment model	Nonlinear
Concentration at time t after oral dose Units: amount/volume	$C_t = \left(\frac{F \cdot Dose}{V} \right) \times \left(\frac{k_a}{k_a - k} \right) \times \left(e^{-kt} - e^{-k_a t} \right)$	To determine concentration at any time t after PO administration	Flip flop (when $k_a < k$)
Time of maximal concentration after PO dose (t_{max}) Units: time	$t_{max} = \frac{\ln \frac{k_a}{k}}{k_a - k}$	Determine time when C_{max} occurs after a PO dose	Flip flop (when $k_a < k$)
Loading dose (LD) Units: amount	$LD = \frac{V_c \cdot (C_{target} - C_{observed})}{S}$	Determine LD when V_c, target concentration, and any drug already in the body is known	

Table 3-3 (*continued*)

	Equations	When to Use	When Not to Use
Concentration at steady state Units: amount/volume	$C_{ss} = \frac{DR}{CL}$ or $= \frac{k_0}{CL}$	• To determine the plasma concentration at steady state (C_{SS}) when a constant infusion is given at a certain dose rate (*DR*) and *CL* • To determine *DR* if given a target C_{SS} and *CL* • To determine *CL* if given *DR* and the resulting C_{SS}	If not at steady state If nonlinear *CL*
	$C_{SS,avg} = \frac{S \cdot F \cdot DR}{CL}$	• To determine average concentration during a dosing interval at steady state • To determine how changes in *DR*, *CL*, and *F* will affect $C_{SS,avg}$	
	$C_{SS,avg} = \frac{AUC_{SS,0-\tau}}{\tau}$	• To determine $C_{SS,avg}$ given AUC_{SS} and τ	
Concentration before steady state, constant infusion Units: amount/volume	$C_t = \frac{DR}{CL}\left(1 - e^{-kt}\right)$	To determine plasma concentration at time *t* prior to reaching steady state if given a constant infusion and *DR*, *CL*, and *k* are known	
Multiple dosing function (MDF) Units: none	$MDF = \frac{1 - e^{-nk\tau}}{1 - e^{-k\tau}}$ C_t at dose n = C_t at first dose × MDF	Use to multiply any known concentration after the first dose by any concentration at that same time on subsequent doses (*n*)	
Accumulation factor Units: none	$Accumulation\ Factor = \frac{1}{1 - e^{-k\tau}}$ C_t at SS = C_t at first dose × AF	Use to multiply any known concentration after the first dose by any concentration at that same time at SS	
Calculating new *DR* if known $C_{SS,avg}$ at *DR*	$DR_{new} = \frac{DR_{given} \times C_{ss,target}}{C_{ss,observed}}$	Determine new *DR* when measured concentration at SS; assumes *CL* and *F* remain constant	Nonlinear *CL* or Nonlinear *F* $C_{observed}$ not at SS
Calculating new dose regimen based on $C_{SS,avg}$	Determine *DR* $DR = \frac{C_{target} \times CL}{F}$	Determine *DR* if *CL* and *F* are known at SS	Must be linear clearance and bioavailability
	Determine τ, dose q $t_{½}$ $t_{½} = \frac{0.693 \times V}{CL}$ **or** base on known target peak and trough as below	Determine τ if can dose every $t_{½}$	
Calculating new dose regimen based on target C_{max} and C_{min} (e.g., aminoglycosides)	Determine optimal τ $\tau = \left\| -\frac{1}{k}\left[ln\frac{C_{min,target}}{C_{max,target}}\right] \right\| + t_i$ t_i = time of infusion	Determine optimal dosing interval given target peak and trough; *k* must have been determined at SS	Multicompartmental Not at SS
	Determine optimal dose (using optimal τ from above) $K_0 = V \times k \times C_{max,target}\left(\frac{1 - e^{-k\tau}}{1 - e^{-kti}}\right)$ K_0 is in terms of amount/time—*not* dose	Determine optimal dose using optimal τ and target C_{max}; *V* and *k* must have been determined at SS	

(continues)

Table 3-3 (*continued*)

	Equations	When to Use	When Not to Use
Calculating new dose regimen based on target C_{max} and C_{min} (e.g., aminoglycosides)	Determine what $C_{SS,max}$ would be expected using a given dosing regimen $C_{max} = \frac{K_0}{V \times k}\left(\frac{1-e^{-kti}}{1-e^{-k\tau}}\right)$	Determine $C_{SS,max}$ when given a defined dosing regimen	
	Determine what $C_{SS,min}$ would be expected using a given dosing regimen $C_{min} = C_{max}e^{-k(\tau - ti)}$	Determine $C_{SS,min}$ when given a defined dosing regimen	
Adjustment of total phenytoin concentrations when protein binding displacement	In hypoalbuminemia: $C_{normal} = \frac{C_{observed}}{[(0.2)(Alb)+(0.1)]}$	Determine what would have been the observed concentration if normal binding; Alb is given in g/dL	
	In renal failure: $C_{normal} = \frac{C_{observed}}{[(0.1)(Alb)+(0.1)]}$	Determine what would have been the observed concentration if normal binding; Alb is given in g/dL	

the clearance of other drugs (e.g., other antiepileptic agents). Clearance increases with time of exposure. It takes 3–4 weeks for full induction. Therefore, as clearance increases, concentrations and half-life decrease. For this reason, the dose rate should increase and the dose interval should decrease over the first month of administration.

Cyclosporine

Use: immunosuppression
TR: depends upon assay
CL: hepatic; P-gp substrate; 3A4 substrate
V_d: 4-5 L/kg
$t_{½}$: 6–12 hr
f_{ut} < 0.1 (bound to lipoproteins)
Concentration-related side effects: renal vasoconstriction (renal impairment), neurotoxicity (headache, tremor, parasthesias, seizures) and hypertension

Cyclosporine is at risk for many interactions because it is a CYP 3A4 and P-glycoprotein substrate; many drugs and diseases can affect these enzymes, causing changes in *CL* and *F*. Cyclosporine is also highly plasma protein bound, making binding displacement situations significant. The result of subtherapeutic concentrations is very serious. Many cases of organ rejection result from drug–drug or drug–disease interactions that alter cyclosporine's *CL*, *F*, or *V*.

Digoxin

Use: CHF and atrial fibrillation
TR: CHF 0.5–1 µg/L; atrial fibrillation 1.5–2.5 µg/L
CL: renal (primarily) + hepatic; P-gp substrate; CHF decreases CL_H; CL_R approximated by GFR
V_d: 3.8 (weight kg) + (3.1 × CrCl); dosed on IBW; decreased in renal failure
$t_{½}$: 36–48 hr
Concentration-related side effects: decreased heart rate, arrhythmias, vision changes

Digoxin has a relatively large volume of distribution and a long half-life. Its volume and clearance are affected by many diseases and drugs.

Clinical Insights[11–13]

1. Interpretation of serum digoxin concentrations for optimal dosing design should ideally be made after a steady state is attained.
2. Blood sampling for determination of any digoxin serum concentrations must take into account the drug's prolonged distribution phase. Clinicians should wait at least 6 hours after an intravenous dose and 8 hours after an oral dose to obtain blood samples. Therefore, a standard collection time (preferably as a trough concentration before administration of the patient's daily dose) should be instituted.

3. For rapid control of ventricular rate in the acute management of atrial fibrillation, digoxin loading doses generally are divided into three or four doses (e.g., one-half, one-quarter, one-quarter given every 6 hours) to assess the clinical effect of each dose before administration of the next dose. In this clinical setting, determination of digoxin concentrations in between dosing is probably of minimal benefit and is not cost-effective.
4. Determination of digoxin concentrations is appropriate for patients with significant renal impairment, for patients with clinical deterioration after initial good response, when toxicity or drug interaction (e.g., with quinidine) is suspected, and for evaluating noncompliance and/or the need for continued therapy.
5. Some medical conditions (e.g., hypokalemia, hyperthyroidism, hypothyroidism) can change the sensitivity of the patient to pharmacologic effects of digoxin independent of any change in concentration. Therefore, in addition to renal function and concurrent therapy, electrolytes (especially potassium) and thyroid status should be assessed.

Ethosuximide

Use: antiepileptic (absence seizures)
TR: 40–100 mg/L[14–18]
CL: hepatic; 3A4 (subject to induction and inhibition)
V_d: 0.7 L/kg
$t_{½}$: 50 hr

Clinical Insights

Ethosuximide may exhibit nonlinear kinetics in higher concentrations.[19,20] Therefore, caution needs to be exercised with dosage increments at the upper end of the therapeutic range.

Lidocaine

Use: local anesthetic, antiarrhythmic
TR: 2–5 mg/L[21–25]
CL: hepatic; high extraction, so it is a high-first-pass drug; CHF and cirrhosis (↓Q) decrease *CL*; active metabolites: MEGX and GX
V_1: 0.5 L/kg
V_2 1.3 L/kg
$t_{½}$: 100 min
f_{ut}: 0.3 (AAG)
Concentration-related side effects: CNS side effects (e.g., dizziness, mental confusion, blurred vision); seizures are usually associated with concentrations exceeding 9 mg/L[21–25]

Lidocaine is highly extracted by the liver, which results in a very low oral bioavailability. Its pharmacokinetic profile follows a two-compartment model. To maintain lidocaine concentrations within the therapeutic range, it is necessary to administer "minibolus" doses (half of original loading dose) every 8–10 minutes.

Clinical Insights

1. Concurrent medical conditions, such as congestive heart failure and liver disease, can decrease the clearance of lidocaine and the expected therapeutic responses with the usual doses. Therefore, a reduction of dose by as much as 40% may be necessary for these patients.
2. MEGX is primarily eliminated by the liver, whereas GX is eliminated by both the liver and the kidneys. Therefore, in patients with liver and/or renal disease, accumulation of lidocaine metabolites may contribute to CNS toxicity.
3. AAG is an acute-phase reactant; as such, its concentration can increase with stress or pathophysiologic conditions such as acute myocardial infarction (especially during the first week after infarction). An increase in serum concentrations of AAG decreases the free fraction of lidocaine temporarily due to increased protein binding. The increase and subsequent decrease in AAG concentration can further complicate interpretation of lidocaine kinetics and effects in patients. Careful clinical monitoring and interpretation of plasma concentrations are required.
4. Because lidocaine is rapidly distributed to the brain and the heart, intravenous bolus doses should be administered at a rate not faster than 50 mg/min, so that the patient is not exposed to transient but toxic concentrations of lidocaine, especially in the brain. Seizures and arrhythmias may occur and may not always be preceded by other toxic signs (e.g., confusion, dizziness).
5. Lidocaine clearance decreases with continuous dosing.[25,26] Therefore, infusions lasting longer than 24 hours require diligent monitoring of concentrations and clinical responses. If necessary, doses should be reduced.

Lithium

Use: bipolar disorder
TR: 0.5–1.5 mEq/L
CL: renal; treated like sodium; actively reabsorbed; 0.25 × CrCl
V: 0.7 L/kg
$t_{½}$: 20 hr

Concentration-related side effects: gastrointestinal (i.e., nausea, vomiting, anorexia, epigastric bloating, abdominal pain) and CNS (i.e., lethargy, fatigue, muscle weakness, tremor)[27–29]

Clinical Insights

1. Administering lithium preparations with meals will decrease the rate of absorption and achievable peak concentrations. Meals, therefore, may help minimize the incidence of some adverse effects (e.g., tremor, gastrointestinal upset, polyuria). Side effects may also be minimized in some patients through use of slow-release lithium dosage formulations.
2. The daily dose of lithium should usually be divided into two or more doses, and trough concentrations should be obtained 12 hours after the last dose.
3. Lithium reabsorption follows sodium reabsorption in the proximal tubule. Therefore, patients with precipitous changes in fluid balance or electrolytes due to drug therapy (e.g., thiazide diuretics) that result in increased sodium (and lithium) reabsorption are at increased risk of toxicity.

Phenobarbital

Use: antiepileptic
TR: 15–40 mg/L[30,31]
CL: hepatic (primary) + renal; low extraction; enzyme inducer
V: 0.7 L/kg
$t_{½}$: 5 days
f_{ut}: 0.5
Concentration-related side effects: sedation and ataxia[31]

Clinical Insights

1. For treatment of status epilepticus, a loading dose of 15 mg/kg can be administered intravenously, usually in three divided doses of 5 mg/kg.
2. Because phenobarbital is distributed to fatty tissue, loading doses for morbidly obese patients should be based on total body weight.[32]

Phenytoin

Use: antiepileptic
TR: 10–20 mg/L; free: 1–2 mg/L
CL: hepatic; nonlinear; substrate for 2C9/2C19; enzyme inducer 3A4; subject to induction and inhibition
V: 0.65 L/kg
$t_{½}$: undefined because of the nonlinear clearance rate
f_{ut}: 0.1 (albumin)
Concentration-related side effects: nystagmus, ataxia, and confusion[33]; gingival hyperplasia, folate deficiency, and peripheral neuropathy are not related to concentration

Phenytoin has nonlinear clearance in its therapeutic range; this factor, accompanied by its high plasma protein binding, may make dosing very difficult. Phenytoin metabolism is saturable. Therefore, modest changes in the dose rate can result in disproportionate changes in steady-state plasma concentrations. The high protein binding presents a challenge in the interpretation of phenytoin concentrations in patients with altered protein binding (e.g., patients with renal failure or hypoalbuminemia, and patients taking drugs that displace phenytoin from binding sites).

Clinical Insights

1. Oral bioavailability of phenytoin can be reduced significantly by concomitant oral nutrition supplements (e.g., Osmolite) administered as nasogastric (NG) feedings. The most practical way of circumventing this problem is to administer phenytoin intravenously. If that is not possible, then stop NG feeding 2 hours before dose administration, flush the NG tube with 60 mL of water after dose administration, and then wait 2 hours before resuming NG feeding.
2. Only phenytoin extended-release capsules should be dosed once daily. As is true for many extended-release formulations, the capsules should not be crushed.
3. Hypotension may occur with intravenous phenytoin administration due to the propylene glycol diluent.[34] Therefore, the rate of phenytoin infusion should not exceed 50 mg/min. Fosphenytoin, a prodrug of phenytoin, is available for parenteral use. The addition of a phosphate group to the chemical structure of phenytoin results in a more soluble chemical entity; therefore, there is no need for propylene glycol as a diluent for fosphenytoin.
4. Fosphenytoin dosing should be expressed in terms of "phenytoin equivalent" (PE)—the molecular weight of fosphenytoin is 1.5 times that of phenytoin.
5. Protein binding displacement makes interpretation of a total phenytoin concentration difficult.[35–37] When protein binding displacement occurs, the total concentration of phenytoin is usually lower after a steady state is reestablished. However, the unbound (pharmacologically active) concentration remains the same. Dose regimen adjustment is usually not necessary in patients with altered binding only.

6. Equations to "equate" the measured total phenytoin concentration to that which would be observed under normal binding conditions should be used so that inappropriate dosage adjustments can be avoided.[38,39]

Procainamide[40–45]

Use: antiarrhythmic
TR: 4–8 mg/L (may need much higher concentrations in some patients)
CL: hepatic and renal; CL_H by acetylation (acetylation phenotype: slow and fast acetylators); active metabolite: NAPA (renal clearance)
V: 2 L/kg
$t_{½}$: 3 hr
Concentration-related side effects: gastrointestinal disturbances, weakness, mild hypotension, and ECG changes (10–30% prolongation of the PR, QT, or QRS intervals)

Clinical Insights

1. Hypotension may occur if intravenous procainamide is administered too quickly. The rate of infusion should not be faster than 25 mg/min.
2. The short plasma half-life of procainamide dictates use of 3- to 4-hour dosing intervals for the rapid-release products and every-6-hours intervals for the sustained-release formulations.
3. Wax matrix carcasses or "skeletons" of the sustained-release tablets may appear intact in the stool. Such an event is not of concern because the drug is absorbed despite the recovery of the wax matrix.
4. Most clinical laboratories report the concentrations of both procainamide and NAPA (the active metabolite of procainamide). The electrophysiologic activity of NAPA is different from that of procainamide, and monitoring of NAPA concentrations is not necessary to evaluate efficacy. However, assessment of NAPA concentrations may be appropriate in some patients[61] (e.g., those with diminished renal function) because NAPA is primarily eliminated by the kidneys and accumulates to a much greater extent than procainamide.
5. In addition to concentration monitoring, baseline ECG and QT interval should be assessed, if possible, before initiation of therapy or before dosage increase. Prolongation of QT interval > 25–50% of the baseline value necessitates at least the consideration of dosage reduction.

Valproic Acid/Divalproex[46–51]

Use: antiepileptic
TR: 50–100 mg/L (nonlinear protein binding at upper ranges)
CL: hepatic; nonlinear clearance due to nonlinear protein binding; 3A4 substrate; can induce (rarely) and inhibit (commonly) metabolism of other drugs
V: 0.14 L/kg
f_{ut}: 0.05–0.2 (albumin); nonlinear in upper end of therapeutic range
$t_{½}$: 10–12 hr
Concentration-related side effects: gastrointestinal disturbances, sedation, drowsiness, and hepatoxicity (toxic metabolite). *Not* concentration-related: alopecia, a benign essential tremor, and thrombocytopenia.

Clinical Insights

1. Although the rate of absorption from the use of enteric-coated tablets may be slower, this formulation may minimize gastrointestinal side effects.
2. Diurnal variation in valproic acid clearance has been reported, such that concentrations of valproic acid are lower in the afternoon or evening than in the morning. Therefore, it is important to standardize blood sampling times (e.g., morning trough concentration) for therapeutic drug monitoring.
3. Valproic acid can inhibit the metabolism of a number of other drugs, such as phenobarbital and phenytoin. In addition, it can displace highly protein-bound drugs, such as phenytoin, from their albumin binding sites. Potential drug–drug interactions should be considered when adding or deleting medications within patients' regimens.
4. Although valproic-acid–induced hepatotoxicity is rare, it is a serious complication of therapy and should be considered in any patient with elevated liver enzymes. Unfortunately, the predictive value of laboratory monitoring for occurrence of hepatotoxicity induced by valproic acid is low.

Vancomycin[52–63]

Use: antibiotic for gram-positive infections
TR: peak < 40–50 mg/L; trough ~ 10 mg/L
CL: renal; approximated by CrCl
V: 0.7 L/kg *or* 0.17 × (age) + (0.22 × TBW in kg) + 15
f_{ut}: 0.5
$t_{½}$: 6–7 hr

Concentration-related side effects: nephrotoxicity when combined with other nephrotoxins; rarely otoxicity

Clinical Insights

1. "Red man syndrome" (characterized by flushing, tachycardia, and hypotension) is associated with histamine release. Its incidence is higher with rapid infusion rates. To minimize its occurrence, vancomycin should be infused slowly (e.g., 1 g over at least 60 minutes). Despite this rate of infusion, some patients will experience flushing and tachycardia. The syndrome may also be managed by premedication with an antihistamine.
2. Efficacy is related to maintaining adequate concentrations of drug. Therefore achieving a "therapeutic trough" is very important.

ANNOTATED BIBLIOGRAPHY

1. Nicolau D, et al. Experience with a once-daily aminoglycoside dosing program administered to 2,184 adult patients. *Antimicrob Agents Chemother* 1995;39:650–655.
2. Jackson GG, Arcieri G. Ototoxicity of gentamicin in man: a survey and controlled analysis of clinical experience in the United States. *J Infect Dis* 1971;124(suppl):130.
3. Schentag JJ, et al. Clinical and pharmacokinetic characteristics of aminoglycoside nephrotoxicity in 201 critically ill patients. *Antimicrob Agents Chemother* 1982;5:721.
4. Wilfret JN, et al. Renal insufficiency associated with gentamicin therapy. *J Infect Dis* 1971;124(suppl):148.
5. Federspil P, et al. Pharmacokinetics and ototoxicity of gentamicin, tobramycin, and amikacin. *J Infect Dis* 1976;134(suppl):200.
6. Hatton RC, Massey KL, Russell WL. Comparison of the predictions of one- and two-compartment microcomputer programs for long-term tobramycin therapy. *Ther Drug Monit* 1984;6:432–437.
7. Goodman EL, et al. Prospective comparative study of variable dosage and variable frequency regimens for administrations of gentamicin. *Antimicrob Agents Chemother* 1975;8:434.
8. So EL, et al. Seizure exacerbation and status epilepticus related to carbamazepine-10,11 epoxide. *Ann Neurol* 1994;35:743–746
9. Rane A, Hojer B, Wilson JT. Kinetics of carbamazepine and its 10.11-epoxide metabolite in children. *Clin Pharmacol Ther* 1976;19:276–283.
10. Bertilsson L. Clinical pharmacokinetics of carbamazepine. *Clin Pharmacokinet* 1978;3:128.
11. Smith TW. Digitalis toxicity: epidemiology and clinical use of serum concentration measurements. *Am J Med* 1975;58:470.
12. Smith TW, Harber E. Digoxin intoxication: the relationship of clinical presentation to serum digoxin concentration. *J Clin Invest* 1970;49:2377.
13. Aronson JK, Hardman M. ABC of monitoring drug therapy: digoxin. *Br J Med* 1992;305:1149–1152.
14. Browne TR, et al. Ethosuximide in the treatment of absence seizures. *Neurology* 1975;25:515.
15. Sherwin AL, et al. Improved control of epilepsy by monitoring plasma ethosuximide. *Arch Neuro.* 1973;27:178.
16. Penry JK, et al. Ethosuximide: relation of plasma levels to clinical control. In: Woodbury DM, Penry JK, Schmidt RP, eds. *Anti-epileptic Drugs.* New York, NY: Raven Press; 1972:431–441.
17. Sherwin AL, Robb JP. Ethosuximide: relation of plasma levels to clinical control. In: Woodbury DM, Penry JK, Schmidt RP, eds. *Anti-epileptic Drugs.* New York, NY: Raven Press; 1972:443–448.
18. Sherwin AL, et al. Plasma ethosuximide levels: a new aid in the management of epilepsy. *Ann Royal Coll Surg Can* 1971;14:48.
19. Bauer LA, et al. Ethosuximide kinetics: possible interactions with valproic acid. *Clin Pharmacol Ther* 1982;31:741–745.
20. Smith GA, et al. Factors influencing plasma concentrations of ethosuximide. *Clin Pharmacokinet* 1979;4:38–52.
21. Gianelly R, et al. Effect of lidocaine on ventricular arrhythmias in patients with coronary heart disease. *N Engl J Med* 1967;277:1215.
22. Jewett DE, et al. Lidocaine in the management of arrhythmias after acute myocardial infarction. *Lancet* 1968;1:266.
23. Seldon R, Sasahara AA. Central nervous system toxicity induced by lidocaine. *JAMA* 1967;202:908.
24. Thompson PD. Lidocaine pharmacokinetics in advanced heart failure, liver disease, and renal failure in humans. *Ann Intern Med* 1973;78:499.
25. LeLorier J, et al. Pharmacokinetics of lidocaine after prolonged intravenous administrations in uncomplicated myocardial infarction. *Ann Intern Med* 1977;87:700–702.
26. Davidson R, Parker M, Atkinson A. Excessive serum lidocaine levels during maintenance infusions: mechanisms and prevention. *Am Heart J* 1982;104:203–208.
27. Elizur A, et al. Intra:extracellular lithium ratios and clinical course in affective states. *Clin Pharm Ther* 1972;13:947.
28. Salem RB. A pharmacist's guide to monitoring lithium drug–drug interactions. *Drug Intell Clin Pharm* 1982;16:745.

29. Amdisen A. Lithium. In: Evans WE, Schentag JJ, Jusko WJ, eds. *Applied Pharmacokinetics: Principles of Therapeutic Drug Monitoring*. 2nd ed. Vancouver: Applied Therapeutics; 1986:978–1002.
30. Buchthal F, et al. Relation of EEG and seizures to phenobarbital in serum. *Arch Neurol* 1968;19: 567.
31. Plass GL, Hine CH. Hydantoin and barbiturate blood levels observed in epileptics. *Arch Int Pharmacodyn Ther* 1960;128:375.
32. Wilkes L, Danziger LH, Rodvold KA. Phenobarbital pharmacokinetics in obesity: a case report. *Clin Pharmacokinet* 1992;22:481–484.
33. Kutt H, et al. Diphenylhydantoin metabolism, blood levels and toxicity. *Arch Neurol* 1964;11: 642.34.
34. Louis S, et al. The cardiocirculatory changes caused by intravenous dilantin and its solvent. *Am Heart J* 1967;74:523.
35. Lund L. Effects of phenytoin in patients with epilepsy in relation to its concentration in plasma. In: David DS, Prichard NBC, eds. *Biological Effects of Drugs in Relation to Their Concentration in Plasma*. Baltimore, MD: University Park Press; 1972:227.
36. Lascelles PT, et al. The distribution of plasma phenytoin levels in epileptic patients. *J Neurol Neurosurg Psychiatry* 1970;33:501.
37. Reidenberg MM. The binding of drugs to plasma proteins and the interpretation of measurements of plasma concentrations of drugs in patients with poor renal function. *Am J Med* 1977;62: 466.
38. Winter M. *Basic Clinical Pharmacokinetics*. 3rd ed. Vancouver: Applied Therapeutics; 1994:312–316.
39. Liponi DL, et al. Renal function and therapeutic concentrations of phenytoin. *Neurology* 1984;34:395.
40. Koch-Weser J. Pharmacokinetics of procainamide in man. *Ann N Y Acad Sci* 1971;169:370.
41. Koch-Weser J, Klein SW. Procainamide dosage schedules, plasma concentrations and clinical effects. *JAMA* 1971;215:1454.
42. Engel TR, et al. Modification of ventricular tachycardia by procainamide in patients with coronary artery disease. *Am J Cardiol* 1980;46:1033.
43. Giardina EV, et al. Efficacy, plasma concentrations and adverse effects of a new sustained release procainamide preparation. *Am J Cardiol* 1980;46:855.
44. Greenspan AM, et al. Large dose procainamide therapy for ventricular tachyarrhythmia. *Am J Cardiol* 1980;46:453.
45. Vlasses PH, et al. Lethal accumulations of procainamide metabolite in renal insufficiency [abstract]. *Drug Intell Clin Pharm* 1984;18:493.
46. Kodama Y, et al. Binding parameters of valproic acid to serum protein in healthy adults at steady-state. *Ther Drug Monit* 1992;14:55–60.
47. Pinder RM, et al. Sodium valproate: a review of its pharmacological properties in therapeutic efficacy in epilepsy. *Drugs* 1977;13:81.
48. Graham L, et al. Sodium valproate, serum level, and critical effect in epilepsy: a controlled study. *Epilepsia* 1979;20:303.
49. Sherard ES, et al. Treatment of childhood epilepsy with valproic acid: result of the first 100 patients in a 6-month trial. *Neurology* 1980:30:31.
50. Suchy FJ, et al. Acute hepatic failure associated with the use of sodium valproate. *N Engl J Med* 1979;300:962.
51. Donalt JT, et al. Valproic acid and fatal hepatitis. *Neurology* 1979;29:273.
52. Alexander MB. A review of vancomycin. *Drug Intell Clin Pharm* 1974;8:520.
53. Kirby WMM, et al. Treatment of staphylococcal septicemia with vancomycin. *N Engl J Med* 1960;262:49.
54. Banner WN Jr, Ray CG. Vancomycin in perspective. *Am J Dis Child* 1984;183:14.
55. Cunha BA, Ristuccia AM. Clinical usefulness of vancomycin. *Clin Pharm* 1982;2:417.
56. Rotschafer JC, et al. Pharmacokinetics of vancomycin: observations in 28 patients and dosage recommendations. *Antimicrob Agents Chemother* 1982;22:391.
57. Blouin RA, et al. Vancomycin pharmacokinetics in normal and morbidly obese subjects. *Antimicrob Agents Chemother* 1982;21:575.
58. Mollering RC, et al. Vancomycin therapy in patients with impaired renal function: a nomogram for dosage. *Ann Intern Med* 1981;94:343.
59. Farber BF, Mollering RC Jr. Retrospective study of the toxicity of preparations of vancomycin from 1974 to 1981. *Antimicrob Agents Chemother* 1983;23:138.
60. Ryback MJ, et al. Nephrotoxicity of vancomycin, alone and with an aminoglycoside. *J Antimicrob Chemother* 1990;25:679–687.
61. Newfield P, Roizen MF. Hazards of rapid administration of vancomycin. *Ann Intern Med* 1979; 91:581.
62. Cook FV, Farrar WE. Vancomycin revisited. *Ann Intern Med* 1978;88:813.
63. Lanese DM et al. Markedly increased clearance of vancomycin during hemodialysis using polysulfone dialyzers. *Kidney Int* 1989;35:1409.

Principles of Drug Interactions

CHAPTER

4

Contributor: Rex S. Lott

INTRODUCTION

The possibility that one drug may alter the action of another is a primary monitoring concern for pharmacists. While drugs may interact in a way that produces positive or improved patient outcomes, drug–drug interactions are usually of concern because of the potential for harmful results. This chapter reviews basic principles and mechanisms of drug interactions with the goal of reinforcing skills of assessment and evaluation. The focus will be on drug interactions with potentially negative consequences or outcomes.

Key Terms

- **Precipitant drug:** A drug (or sometimes a nutrient) that causes a change in the effect of another drug.
- **Object drug:** A drug whose activity is altered by a drug interaction.
- **Pharmacokinetic (ADME) interactions:** Drug interactions resulting from a change in the plasma concentration versus time profile of the object drug. ADME is an acronym:
  - **A**bsorption
  - **D**istribution
  - **M**etabolism
  - **E**limination or **E**xcretion of active (unchanged) drug
- **Pharmacodynamic interactions:** Drug interactions resulting from additive or antagonistic pharmacologic effects of the interacting drugs. When pharmacodynamic interactions occur, there is often a less clearly identifiable precipitant or object drug.

Much of the terminology regarding drug interactions is also discussed in the chapters on biopharmaceutics, pharmacokinetics, and chemical and pharmacological classes of therapeutic agents.

MECHANISMS OF DRUG–DRUG INTERACTIONS

Pharmacodynamic Mechanisms and Examples

Many pharmacodynamic interactions are easily recognized if one maintains awareness of the mechanisms of the pharmacological effect of the interacting drugs and/or the clinical results of the pharmacologic effect of the interacting drugs. The following list is not meant to be complete, but presents some well-documented potential interactions.

Antagonism

Drugs may adversely interact when one drug antagonizes the pharmacologic action of the other.

- **Mirtazapine + clonidine or guanfacine:** Clonidine and guanfacine exert their antihypertensive action by stimulating alpha$_2$-adrenergic receptors in the central nervous system. Mirtazapine is an antagonist at $alpha_2$-adrenergic receptors, and this effect is believed to result in increased serotonergic and adrenergic transmission and an antidepressant response. Mirtazapine will reduce or eliminate the antihypertensive response to clonidine or guanfacine.

- **Beta-adrenergic blockers (nonselective) + adrenergic bronchodilators:** The effects of these drugs are directly antagonistic. Nonselective beta blockers such as propranolol are highly likely to reduce or eliminate the bronchodilating actions of agents such as albuterol and salmeterol.
- **Noncardioselective beta-adrenergic blockers + epinephrine:** This under-recognized drug interaction may have serious consequences. Epinephrine causes both alpha-adrenergic stimulation (vasoconstriction) and beta-adrenergic stimulation (vasodilation and cardiac stimulation). Patients receiving noncardioselective beta blockers such as propranolol may exhibit dramatically elevated blood pressure when they are given epinephrine because the beta-adrenergic effects of epinephrine are blocked and the alpha-adrenergic effects are left unopposed. This can occur even with infiltration of lidocaine plus epinephrine during surgery.

Additive Pharmacologic Activity

Drugs may increase each other's effect because they act through similar or identical mechanisms. Interactions may also occur because each drug's pharmacologic activity results in similar or increased clinical manifestations—even though the drugs may cause the manifestations via different pharmacologic actions.

- **Diphenhydramine + olanzapine:** Each of these drugs has potent antihistamine properties. Their combined administration may increase the risk that a patient will develop increased antihistaminic side effects (e.g., sedation).
- **Thioridazine + disopyramide:** Both of these drugs act to prolong the QTc interval. Their combined administration puts patients at increased risk of ventricular arrhythmia.
- **Diphenhydramine + diazepam:** Each of these drugs is sedating, although sedation occurs from different mechanisms. Nonetheless, their combined use may cause an increased risk of sedative side effects.
- **Lamotrigine + carbamazepine:** Combined use of these drugs may produce symptoms suggestive of carbamazepine intoxication (double vision, ataxia, sedation). Some references attribute this outcome to an effect of lamotrigine in increasing concentrations of carbamazepine's active epoxide metabolite, but this mechanism has largely been ruled out. The interaction appears to be a pharmacodynamic one.

Pharmacokinetic Mechanisms and Examples

The majority of drug interactions probably occur through pharmacokinetic mechanisms. Typically, the precipitant drug alters some aspect of the pharmacokinetics of the object drug, causing either an increase or a decrease in serum concentrations and, therefore, the pharmacologic effect of the object drug. These effects can occur at a number of stages.

Absorption

Interference with the absorption of one drug by another is a well-documented cause of drug interactions. Changes in absorption can also be caused by dietary substances.

- **Decreased absorption:** Antacids (especially those containing polyvalent cations such as aluminum and magnesium) can bind a number of drugs and decrease or prevent their absorption. Tetracyclines, quinolone antibiotics, some azole antifungals (itraconazole and ketoconazole), and levothyroxine are examples. In the case of tetracyclines, the increased pH caused by antacids can also interfere with dissolution of tetracyclines and further impair their absorption.
- **Increased absorption:** Many drugs are susceptible to extensive first-pass metabolism by CYP 3A4 in the gut wall. Grapefruit juice contains a substance that inhibits intestinal (but not hepatic) CYP3A4. When this enzyme is inhibited, first-pass metabolism is reduced and the amount of drug absorbed into the systemic circulation is increased. The net result may be significantly increased effect of the drug. Examples of drugs susceptible to this interaction are: alprazolam, triazolam, felodipine, cyclosporine, simvastatin, and lovastatin.

Distribution

Drug interactions involving altered distribution most commonly involve changes in binding to serum proteins (especially albumin). Pharmacokinetic aspects of serum protein binding are thoroughly discussed in the Pharmacokinetics chapter of this text, and they are briefly summarized here.

For many highly protein-bound drugs, hepatic metabolic clearance is dependent upon the *free fraction (% unbound)*. If these drugs are displaced from serum protein binding, only a transient increase in their *free concentration* will occur, so their pharmacologic effect will increase for only the amount of time required for the free concentration to return to its pre-displacement value. Therefore, for many highly protein-bound drugs, displacement from protein binding will have only a transient effect on their pharmacologic activity. However, if the displacing drug also inhibits the metabolism of the displaced drug, there may be a persistent increase in the free concentration and pharmacologic effect of the displaced drug.

- **Warfarin:** Warfarin is a highly bound drug whose clearance depends on the free fraction. Warfarin may be displaced from albumin binding by other highly bound drugs (e.g., trichloracetic acid, the metabolite of chloral hydrate and triclofos). Because warfarin's free fraction is increased, its hepatic clearance is also increased. A transient (approximately 1 week) increase in the anticoagulant effect of warfarin is well documented after this displacement. Temporary dosage adjustment may be warranted. However, after increased clearance returns unbound concentrations to baseline, the previous dose of warfarin will again be appropriate.
- **Phenytoin:** Phenytoin is highly bound to albumin. Phenytoin follows Michaelis-Menten pharmacokinetics, and, as a result, hepatic enzymes involved in phenytoin clearance are near their maximum capacity. Therefore, it may not be possible for phenytoin clearance to increase in proportion to the free fraction. In turn, displacement of phenytoin from albumin binding sites may result in persistent increases in free serum concentration and clinical effect. This outcome may be particularly likely to occur when phenytoin is displaced by valproate, because valproate also inhibits the hepatic enzymes responsible for phenytoin metabolism.

Metabolism

The vast majority of pharmacokinetic drug interactions probably involve alterations in the metabolism of object drugs by precipitant drugs. In recent years, understanding of the role of CYP450 enzymes in drug metabolism has increased significantly. An increasing amount of information is also becoming available about other drug-metabolizing enzymes such as UGT. The various isoforms of CYP450 are discussed in the chapters on biopharmaceutics and pharmacokinetics. Basic concepts are summarized here.

In terms of hepatic metabolism by CYP450 and UGT, drugs fall into three groups:

- **Substrates:** A drug may be a substrate for one or more metabolic enzymes. This means that those enzymes are responsible for either the oxidative metabolism (CYP450) or glucuronidation (UGT) of the drug. These processes convert lipid-soluble molecules into more water-soluble molecules that are more easily excreted in urine or bile. Some drugs are metabolized by UGT without being metabolized first by CYP450; lamotrigine is an example of this type of drug.
- **Inducers:** Inducers stimulate the liver to synthesize more drug-metabolizing enzymes. Many drugs are narrow-spectrum inducers and stimulate increased synthesis of only a limited number of enzymes. For example, omeprazole is a narrow-spectrum inducer; it induces CYP1A2. Phenobarbital induces a number of enzymes: CYP1A2, CYP2B6, CYP2C9/10/19, CYP3A3/4, and UGT.
- **Inhibitors:** Drugs may be either narrow- or broad-spectrum inhibitors of either CYP450 isoforms or UGT. Inhibition may be competitive, in which case the drug binds strongly with an enzyme's active site and prevents other drugs from being bound and metabolized. Inhibition may also be allosteric; in that situation, the inhibitor binds to the enzyme in such a way that it alters the ability of the enzyme to bind other drugs that may be substrates. For example, valproate is an inhibitor of several CYP450 enzymes as well as UGT.

Knowledge of those enzymes that are either inhibited or induced by specific drugs as well as knowledge of the drugs that are metabolized by specific enzymes can allow prediction of potentially significant drug interactions.

Elimination or Excretion of Active (Unchanged) Drug

Drug interactions involving elimination or excretion of unchanged drug most commonly occur in the kidneys. These drug interactions may occur through several mechanistic processes:

- **Altered glomerular filtration:** Changes in glomerular filtration may occur because of altered filtration pressure (e.g., through lowered blood pressure or through altered vascular tone in the glomerulus). Reduced glomerular filtration may also occur as a result of administration of nephrotoxic drugs. Highly protein-bound drugs are not significantly filtered at the glomerulus.
- **Altered tubular secretion:** Renal tubular secretion is usually an active process. Secretion, along with filtration, contributes to renal drug clearance. The active processes involve transport proteins that tend to be specific for either cationic (basic) drugs or anionic (acidic) drugs. Interactions may occur between drugs that compete for these transport proteins. The interaction between

probenecid and penicillins is an example of a therapeutically useful interaction of this type. Probenecid competes with penicillins for renal tubular secretion, which results in increased serum concentrations of penicillins for a longer time period. Probenecid can also decrease tubular secretion of other agents such as methotrexate. This interaction can be potentially harmful if not recognized. Inhibition of P-glycoprotein–mediated renal tubular secretion of digoxin by agents such as quinidine and erythromycin represents another well-recognized drug–drug interaction involving this mechanism.

- **Altered tubular reabsorption:** Reabsorption of drugs from renal tubular fluid is often passive, although it may be an active process. Passive reabsorption often depends on the degree of ionization and the lipid solubility of the drug in the tubular fluid. The degree of ionization is usually dependent upon both the pK_a of the drug and urine pH. Weakly acidic drugs will be more likely to be ionized at high pH and, therefore, will be less likely to be reabsorbed. Drugs that are weak bases will tend to be non-ionized at high pH and may be more likely to be reabsorbed. As an example, urine alkalinization can increase renal reabsorption of amphetamine and prolong the action of this drug.
- Tubular reabsorption of some drugs may also be an active process and can sometimes be indirectly affected. This process results in the accumulation of lithium in patients who take thiazide diuretics, for example. Thiazide diuretics do not increase renal lithium excretion. They do cause a compensatory increase in proximal tubular sodium reabsorption, however, and this process also increases lithium reabsorption. The result can be significantly increased lithium serum concentrations when thiazide diuretics are added to lithium therapy.

Additional mechanistic considerations in monitoring and evaluating drug interactions involve recognition of several other factors:

1. Discontinuation of a precipitant drug may cause significant changes in the effect of an object drug. These situations can be considered "inverse drug interactions." Withdrawal of a metabolic enzyme inhibitor from stable therapy will result in decreased serum concentrations and clinical effects of substrates of that enzyme. For example, if a patient was stabilized on chronic therapy with cimetidine and nifedipine, and cimetidine was then discontinued, the loss of metabolic inhibition would likely result in a decreased effect of nifedipine. Conversely, discontinuation of a metabolic enzyme inducer may cause increased serum concentrations and clinical effects of drugs that are substrates of the induced enzyme.
2. Inhibition of metabolism of object drugs that are prodrugs may result in decreased therapeutic response rather than increased therapeutic response to these medications. Several examples of this type of interaction are clinically important:

   a. Drugs that inhibit CYP2D6 prevent metabolic conversion of codeine to morphine. This may significantly reduce the analgesic effect of codeine.
   b. CYP2D6 inhibition prevents conversion of tamoxifen to its active metabolite and may reduce the effectiveness of tamoxifen.
   c. CYP2C19 inhibitors such as omeprazole may interfere with conversion of clopidogrel to its active metabolite, thereby reducing the antiplatelet effect of clopidogrel.

3. Genetic factors may play a significant role in determining the actual clinical outcomes associated with administration of interacting combinations of drugs. Genetic polymorphisms result in patients' phenotypes differing with respect to their CYP450 metabolizing capacity.

   a. Approximately 5–10% of Caucasians and 8% of African Americans are poor metabolizers (PMs) with respect to CYP2D6.
   b. Approximately 1% of Caucasians and African Americans are ultra-rapid metabolizers with respect to CYP2D6.
   c. Only approximately 1% of Asians are PMs for CYP2D6.
   d. Approximately 2–4% of Caucasians, 4–7% of African Americans, and 18–20% of Asians are PMs with respect to CYP2C19.

Administration of inhibitors of these CYP enzymes to PMs will have little additional effect on metabolism of substrates for these enzymes. As a result, no apparent drug interaction will occur when patients receive these inhibitors. Conversely, administration of inhibitors to normal or ultra-rapid metabolizers may result in profound changes in drug response.

EVALUATION, ASSESSMENT, AND MONITORING OF POTENTIAL DRUG INTERACTIONS

Practicing pharmacists generally are not able to memorize every potential drug interaction. Most pharmacists will be familiar with interactions that are serious, common, or of particular interest owing to their area of expertise. Therefore, pharmacists often must rely on electronic drug interaction monitoring systems that are a part of computerized dispensing systems ("clinical decision support" [CDS] systems). Depending on the particular system in use and the settings applied, pharmacists may be faced with multiple alerts regarding potential drug interactions. Evaluating these alerts and assessing the possible risks to patients and the potential need for intervention require awareness and application of evaluation principles. Beyond that step, some consideration needs to be given to appropriate monitoring strategies. Some of the principles and concepts important to assessing the significance of alerts regarding possible drug interactions are highlighted here.

Route of Administration

Actual occurrence of drug interactions may depend on the route of administration.

- **Example:** Antacids containing calcium, aluminum, or magnesium bind tetracycline antibiotics and decrease their absorption. Both the antacid and the antibiotic must be administered orally for this interaction to be significant.
- **Example:** Grapefruit juice can significantly increase serum concentrations of drugs that undergo significant first-pass metabolism in the gut wall by CYP34A. Orally administered felodipine would be expected to interact in this way; intravenously administered felodipine would not.

Dose

Many drug interactions are dose dependent. The larger the baseline dose or serum concentration of the object drug, the more likely a change in its metabolism is to cause significant change in its effect. Likewise, higher doses of precipitant drugs are usually more likely to exert an effect on the object drug.

- **Example:** A patient receiving carbamazepine with a serum concentration of 4 mcg/mL who is given a drug that inhibits CYP3A4 may experience a doubling of the carbamazepine concentration. This is far less likely to cause clinically significant adverse effects than if the baseline serum concentration were 9 mcg/mL.

Order of Administration

Addition of an object drug (especially when the dose of this drug will be titrated to clinical response) to existing therapy with a precipitant drug is less likely to cause negative outcomes than if the precipitant drug is added to stabilized therapy with the object drug.

- **Example:** Quinidine reduces digoxin clearance by inhibiting P-glycoprotein. Initiation of digoxin therapy and titration of its dose and serum concentrations in a patient who is already receiving quinidine is less likely to result in harm than addition of quinidine to the regimen of a patient who is stabilized on digoxin.

Individual Drugs Versus Therapeutic or Pharmacologic Class

Drug interaction warnings are often generalized to all members of a specific therapeutic or pharmacologic class. Depending on the mechanism of the interaction, members of a class may interact very differently.

- **Example:** Some, but not all, quinolone antibiotics inhibit CYP1A2. Enoxacin is a potent inhibitor, whereas ciprofloxacin is only moderately potent. Levofloxacin and ofloxacin have only minimal inhibitory activity.
- **Example:** Cimetidine, at full therapeutic doses, is a potent inhibitor of several CYP450 enzymes. Other H2 antagonists lack this effect.
- **Example:** Of the selective serotonin reuptake inhibitor (SSRI) antidepressants, only fluoxetine and paroxetine significantly inhibit CYP2D6. Other SSRIs (e.g., citalopram, fluvoxamine, sertraline) have mild or no inhibitory activity at that enzyme, although they may have effects on other CYP450 enzymes.

Time Course of Drug Interactions

Estimating the probable time course of a drug interaction can be an important aspect of assessing the interaction's potential significance and developing appropriate strategies for monitoring possible manifestations of an interaction. Some drug interactions may be manifested quickly, while others may not cause changes in patients' status for weeks. A number of characteristics of the drugs involved that will determine the probable time course of a particular interaction:

Half-lives of Precipitant and Object Drugs

The shorter the half-life of either the precipitant drug or the object drug, the more rapidly accumulation to new steady-state concentrations will occur, and the more rapidly manifestations of a drug interaction are likely to appear. Likewise, a longer half-life for either drug may delay the appearance of the drug interaction. In situations where manifestations are delayed, the drug interaction may not be identified as responsible for the change in the patient's status.

Precipitant drugs with long half-lives may not reach the concentrations required for interaction effects for several days to weeks. For example, if diazepam were added to treatment with another medication that had prominent sedative side effects, the full effect of the additive sedation might not be detectable for approximately 10 days because diazepam's active metabolite (desmethyldiazepam) has a half-life of approximately 48 hours.

Object drugs with long half-lives (especially if the half-life is increased by the drug interaction) may require an extended time before the full effects of the interaction are seen. For example, valproate inhibits the hepatic metabolism of phenobarbital. If valproate is added to a stable phenobarbital regimen, 1–2 weeks of therapy may be required for the full effect of the interaction to become apparent—either as symptoms exhibited by the patient or as increased phenobarbital serum concentrations. This is the case because phenobarbital's usual half-life is approximately 2–4 days and will be increased by inhibition of its metabolism.

Dosage

As noted earlier, dosage of either drug may influence the likelihood of an interaction's occurrence. Dosage may also influence the speed of onset of the interaction. If an object drug is being administered at high dosage and its metabolism or elimination is decreased, it will reach potentially toxic concentrations relatively quickly. Larger doses of a precipitant drug would also be expected to result in a more rapid onset of an interaction.

Interaction Mechanism

Along with factors mentioned previously, the mechanism of the interaction may dramatically influence the time course.

- **Absorption:** These interactions essentially amount to a change in the dose of the object drug (decreased absorption is essentially the same as decreasing the dose; increased absorption is essentially the same as increasing the dose). When one of these interactions occurs, serum concentrations of the object drug will start to change immediately, but the rate of change in the concentration and the time required to achieve a new steady state will depend on the object drug's half-life.
- **Protein binding:** The increased pharmacologic effect of the object drug in these interactions is likely to be a transient one because clearance of that drug is increased. For object drugs with long half-lives, free concentrations will take longer to return to baseline, and clinical manifestations of these increased concentrations are more likely to be observed. The likelihood of manifestations resulting from protein-binding displacement also depends on the mechanism of pharmacologic effect of the object drug. As an example, displacement of a sulfonylurea such as tolbutamide might quickly produce a brief decrease in blood glucose. Displacement of an anticoagulant such as warfarin might result in a temporary change in INR, but several days would be required for this to be observable.
- **Enzyme induction:** Enzyme induction is a relatively slow process; CYP450 enzymes that are subject to induction generally "turn over" every approximately 1–6 days. The initial effects of an enzyme inducer may be detectable in 1–2 days, but usually at least 1–2 weeks is required for full enzyme induction. The onset of full enzyme induction will also be influenced by the half-life of the inducer. For example, rifampin is a potent enzyme inducer with a half-life of approximately 5 hours. When rifampin therapy is initiated, its serum concentrations reach steady state in less than 2 days, and one would expect to see its enzyme-inducing effects much more quickly than with a drug such as phenobarbital which has a very long half-life. When enzyme inducers are discontinued, the loss of enzyme induction will depend on the turnover rate for the enzyme as well as the half-life of the inducer.
- **Enzyme inhibition:** The onset of significant enzyme inhibition is often quite rapid (less than 1–2 days), although maximal inhibition may be delayed until the inhibitor has accumulated to its final steady-state concentrations. The time course of appearance of clinical manifestations of the interaction may be delayed if the object drug has a long half-life. It is important to consider that the object drug will have a new, longer half-life under these circumstances
- **Renal excretion:** These interactions will follow a time course similar to that seen with interactions resulting from enzyme inhibition.

In individual patient situations, evaluating the potential time course of a possible drug interaction can help determine an appropriate monitoring strategy for detecting adverse outcomes and prevent unnecessary, expensive testing and evaluation.

MANAGEMENT OF DRUG INTERACTIONS

Appropriate management of actual or potential drug interactions depends on a thorough, accurate assessment of the significance of the specific interaction and the risks of harm to the patient receiving the medications. As noted previously, the first step when dealing with a potential interaction is to assess whether factors such as order of administration, dose, and so on predict that an adverse outcome is likely. Depending on this assessment, several options may be available:

1. **Avoid administering the interacting drugs.** Often, it may be possible to replace either the precipitant or the object drug with another agent that is less likely to engage in an adverse interaction. For example, it may be possible to replace propranolol with metoprolol in a patient with asthma who is using an albuterol inhaler. While monitoring and patient education are still very important, use of these drugs may be less likely to result in adverse outcomes.
2. **Administer the potentially interacting drugs with close monitoring and/or extensive patient education.** This approach may be necessary when both drugs are needed to treat a specific patient's conditions. Careful monitoring and educating the patient regarding the possible negative effects of the interaction may allow early intervention in situations where an adverse interaction does occur.
3. **Adjust the dosage of the object drug.** This approach is often practical and successful in situations involving well-known pharmacokinetic interactions. As an example, if addition of a thiazide diuretic is necessary in a patient stabilized on lithium, lithium dosage can be reduced by 25–35% to compensate for the effect of the diuretic. Further monitoring will be needed to ensure that the dosage adjustment was appropriate.

ANNOTATED BIBLIOGRAPHY

DeVane CL. Clinical significance of drug binding, protein binding, and binding displacement drug interactions. *Psychopharmacol Bull* 2002;36:5–21.

Hansten PD, Horn JR. *Drug Interactions: Analysis and Management*. St Louis, MO: Facts and Comparisons Publishing Group, Wolters Kluwer Health; 2011.

Horn JR, Hansten PD, Chan L-N. Proposal for a new tool to evaluate drug interaction cases. *Ann Pharmacother* 2007;41:674–680.

Principles of Pharmacoeconomics

CHAPTER

5

Contributor: Barb Mason

CURRICULUM AND COMPETENCIES

Tips Worth Tweeting

- Pharmacoeconomics measures costs and consequences in drug treatment.
- Perspectives of the patient, provider, payer, and society are included in pharmacoeconomic measurement.
- Pharmacoeconomics includes clinical, economic, and humanistic aspects of outcomes.
- There are four basic types of pharmacoeconomic research: cost-minimization analysis (CMA), cost-benefit analysis (CBA), cost-utility analysis (CUA), and cost-effectiveness analysis (CEA).

Patient Care Scenario: Community Setting

A 53-year-old male presents to your pharmacy with a combination antihypertensive drug. The medication is not covered by his insurance plan. The pharmacist checks with the insurance formulary, and then calls the physician and requests an alternative. Use of this medication will require the patient to undergo periodic lab draws, and the patient lives in a rural setting without ready lab access. The physician, pharmacist, and patient discuss a different class of medication that may be used that may be more cost-effective.

Pharmacoeconomics is incorporated in the pharmacy curriculum in individual courses or as a stand-alone course following the guidelines established by the Accreditation Council for Pharmacy Education. The Naplex Competency Blueprint for the first time has incorporated the topic of pharmacoeconomics in the following three statements:

Competency 1: Safe and Effective Therapeutic Outcomes

1.2.0 Evaluate information about pharmacoeconomic factors, dosage regimen, dosage forms, delivery systems, and routes of administration to identify and select optimal pharmacotherapeutic agents for patients.

1.3.0 Evaluate and manage drug regimens by monitoring and assessing the patient and/or patient information, collaborating with other healthcare professionals, and providing patient education to enhance safe, effective, and economic patient outcomes.

Competency 3: Health Care Information That Promotes Public Health

3.1.2 Evaluate the suitability, accuracy, and reliability of clinical and pharmacoeconomic data by analyzing experimental design, statistical test, interpreting results, and formulating conclusions.

Pharmacy graduates and Naplex candidates need to have the knowledge and skills to understand and apply pharmacoeconomic research in pharmacy practice decision making. Pharmacoeconomics is one type of outcomes research.

PHARMACOECONOMIC MEASUREMENTS

Pharmacoeconomics measures costs and consequences in drug treatment. The most basic pharmacoeconomic equation compares the costs associated with providing a pharmacy product or service to the outcome of the product or service. The value of pharmacy products and services is determined by applying specific pharmacoeconomic methods to compare costs, assess consequences, and make decisions. Perspectives of the patient, provider, payer, and society are all included in the measurement.

PHARMACOECONOMIC APPLICATIONS

Pharmacoeconomics can be applied to the examination of drugs, medical devices, diagnostics, biotechnology, surgery, and disease prevention/wellness. Pharmacoeconomic evaluation is used to assist with formulary decisions, clinical practice guideline development, evaluation of the pharmacists' contribution to healthcare teams, and a variety of healthcare decisions. By definition, pharmacoeconomics includes clinical, economic, and humanistic aspects of outcomes. Outcomes can be patient reported, caregiver reported, or clinician reported. Economic comparisons must also take into consideration social, legal, ethical, and political aspects when decisions are made.

TYPES OF PHARMACOECONOMIC RESEARCH

Four basic types of pharmacoeconomic research are undertaken: cost-minimization analysis (CMA), cost-benefit analysis (CBA), cost-utility analysis (CUA), and cost-effectiveness analysis (CEA). Each differs in the method used to measure outcomes. More than one type of analysis may be used in one study, and the differences are less distinct than they may seem.

Key Terms

Cost analysis: the measurement and comparison of costs of various options without the measurement of outcomes.

Cost-benefit analysis (CBA): evaluates both costs and benefits in monetary terms so decisions can be made about benefits of programs versus cost of implementation. CBA can address different effectiveness measures. Outcomes or benefits and all inputs are converted to a dollar value, realizing that it is difficult to place a monetary value on health outcomes.

Cost-consequence analysis (CCA): an analysis in which costs and outcomes are included but are not used in direct calculations or direct comparisons.

Cost-effectiveness analysis (CEA): answers the questions of whether a new drug with increased efficacy is worth a higher price. CEA requires the same effectiveness measures as other types of pharmacoeconomic analysis, and compares total cost of therapy to the consequences when the outcomes for the alternative are not equal. CEA is reported as the cost per unit of clinical outcome measures. CEA research is some of the most commonly published pharmacoeconomic analysis. Outcomes are measured in natural units with which clinicians are familiar and routinely monitor, such as cholesterol or glucose levels. A monetary value is not assigned to the clinical outcome in this analysis, leaving this judgment for the clinician and patient.

Cost-effectiveness ratio (CER): the costs of an intervention divided by the units of effectiveness of the intervention.

Cost-minimization analysis (CMA): answers the question of how costs compare for drugs that are therapeutically equivalent. It compares the total cost difference between treatment alternatives that produce the same patient outcomes (i.e., generic versus brand-name equivalent). CMA is considered the easiest pharmacoeconomic research to conduct because the outcomes are assumed to be equal. Comparing different classes of medications using CMA would not be appropriate if different outcomes existed.

Cost-of-illness (COI): assesses the actual direct or indirect costs associated with a given disease state, economic burden, or society.

Cost-utility analysis (CUA): answers the question of what value is placed on a new drug that improves quality of life. CUA considers both quantity and quality of life and offers a societal perspective. Patient length of life (quantity) does not take into consideration the quality or utility of life. CUA measures outcomes based on years of life adjusted by utility weights that incorporate patient and societal factors.

Decision analysis models: tools to analyze cost and outcomes data in pharmacoeconomic analysis. They are usually presented in graphical format or as decision trees.

Direct costs: the most obvious costs associated with providing treatment or prevention. Costs are defined by transaction or monetary exchange, such as drug, hospitalization, and laboratory costs.

Direct nonmedical costs would include items such as transportation and ancillary costs such as food or lodging expenses incurred because of illness or health care.

Discounting: the adjustment of costs and consequences when comparisons cannot be made at one point in time.

ECHO model: a model that organizes outcomes of medical care with the dimensions of economic, clinical, and humanistic outcomes.

Effectiveness: real-world outcomes measured in routine clinical practice.

Efficacy: the optimal effect of a drug under carefully controlled conditions, such as a clinical trial used as evidence in a new drug application submitted to the Food and Drug Administration (FDA).

External validity: when the study results are valid in a population external to the specific study population.

Health-related quality of life: the functional effect of an illness and the consequent therapy on a patient as perceived by the patient.

Incremental costs: the difference in estimated costs between two or more interventions. It may include the extra cost of an intervention over an alternative, taking into account the additional effect, benefit, or outcome the intervention provides.

Incremental cost-effectiveness ratio (ICER): the ratio of the difference in costs divided by the difference in outcomes.

Indirect benefits: the increases in productivity or earnings that occur because of an intervention.

Indirect costs: the cost of lost productivity to patients secondary to a disease, condition, or illness.

Intangible benefits: benefits caused by a decrease in intangible costs.

Intangible costs: the costs of pain, suffering, or fatigue and the anxiety that occurs due to an illness or its treatment. These costs are difficult to measure or place a monetary value on.

Internal validity: when the study results are valid in the specific study population studied.

Opportunity costs: the economic benefit forgone when using one therapy instead of the next best alternative therapy.

Perspective: whose costs are relevant based on the study purpose (i.e., the payer, patient, institution, or provider).

Pharmacoeconomics: economic assessment that evaluates the value of pharmaceutical products, services, or programs through clinical, economic, and humanistic outcomes in the prevention, diagnosis, treatment, and management of disease.

Quality-adjusted life-year (QUALY): life years gained in an outcome, adjusted by patient preferences for health states.

Quality of life: a person's overall well-being, which may be related to health factors or nonhealth factors, such as environmental, economic, or political factors.

Societal costs: costs to all sectors such as the insurance company and patient.

ANNOTATED BIBLIOGRAPHY

Bootman JL. Pharmacoeconomics and outcomes research. *Am J Health Syst Pharm* 1995;52(suppl 3): S16–S19.

NAPLEX Competency 2—Safe and Accurate Preparation and Dispensing of Medications

SECTION

2

The Basics of Pharmaceutical Calculations

CHAPTER

6

Contributors: *Courtenay Gilmore Wilson and Jamie Ridley Klucken*

SETTING UP CALCULATIONS

The first step to being able to perform pharmaceutical calculations appropriately is to set up the calculations properly.

Proportional Calculations

Proportional calculations involve using a *known* ratio to determine an *unknown* value in a similar ratio. They are commonly used to determine simple drug dosing problems. In the following example, we solve for *x* by multiplying *a* and *d* and dividing by *b*

$$\frac{a}{b} = \frac{x}{d} \quad \Rightarrow \quad x = \frac{(a \cdot d)}{b}.$$

Example

What is the volume of a 250 mg/5 mL suspension required to give a dose of 300 mg?

$$\frac{250\,\text{mg}}{5\,\text{ml}} = \frac{300\,\text{mg}}{x\,\text{mL}}.$$

Change to:

$$\frac{x\,\text{ml}}{300\,\text{mg}} = \frac{5\,\text{mL}}{250\,\text{mg}}.$$

Solve:

$$x\,\text{mL} = \frac{(5\text{ mL} \cdot 300\text{ mg})}{250\text{ mg}}$$

$$x\,\text{mL} = 6\,\text{mL}.$$

Dimensional Analysis

Dimensional analysis is a method of checking an equation or solution for validity by setting up dimensions (units of measurement). This method is important in pharmaceutical calculations because it is a way to ensure the patient gets the right dose of medication.

Both sides of the equation should have the same dimensions for the equation to be correct.

Example

$$\cancel{\text{kg}} \cdot \frac{\cancel{\text{mg}}}{\cancel{\text{kg}}} \cdot \frac{\text{mL}}{\cancel{\text{mg}}} = \text{mL}.$$

If the dimensions on each side of the equation are not equal, the equation has been set up incorrectly.

Dimensional analysis is simple if you follow these steps:

1. **Write the desired final units** (right-hand side).
2. **List all available data pertinent to the question *and* any necessary conversion factors** (left-hand side). Include units for all numbers. Include drug names for all units, if dealing with more than one drug.

3. **Invert dimensions** so that all possible units cross out, leaving you with the desired units in the numerator position.
4. **Perform calculations.** Cancel units out, leaving only the desired final units.

Example

Calculate the appropriate dose (mL) of medication for a 180-lb individual. The suspension is 250 mg/mL with a dosing recommendation of 15 mg/kg.

Step 1: = ____________mL

Step 2:

Data:			Conversion Factors:
180 lb	$\frac{250\text{ mg}}{\text{mL}}$	$\frac{15\text{ mg}}{\text{kg}}$	$\frac{2.2\text{ lb}}{1\text{ kg}}$

Step 3: $180\text{ lb}\cdot\frac{1\text{ kg}}{2.2\text{ lb}}\cdot\frac{15\text{ mg}}{\text{kg}}\cdot\frac{\text{mL}}{250\text{ mg}}=x\text{ mL}$

Step 4: $180\,\cancel{\text{lb}}\cdot\frac{1\,\cancel{\text{kg}}}{2.2\,\cancel{\text{lb}}}\cdot\frac{15\,\cancel{\text{mg}}}{\cancel{\text{kg}}}\cdot\frac{\text{mL}}{250\,\cancel{\text{mg}}}=4.9\text{ mL}$

Example

ProAir HFA metered-dose inhalers (MDIs) contain 20 mg of albuterol each. How many doses are in each MDI if each actuation delivers 90 mcg of albuterol?

$$\frac{1\text{ dose}}{90\text{ mcg}}\cdot\frac{1{,}000\text{ mcg}}{1\text{ mg}}\cdot\frac{20\text{ mg}}{1\text{ MDI}}=\frac{x\text{ doses}}{\text{MDI}}$$

$$x=\frac{222\text{ doses}}{\text{MDI}}.$$

If the prescription reads, "2 puffs q 4 hr for SOB," how many MDIs should you dispense for a 90-day supply?

$$\frac{1\text{ MDI}}{222\text{ doses}}\cdot\frac{2\text{ doses}}{4\text{ hrs}}\cdot\frac{24\text{ hrs}}{1\text{ day}}\cdot 90\text{ days}=x\text{ MDI}$$

$$x\text{ MDI}=4.86\text{ MDIs (or 5 MDIs)}.$$

Example

JK is a 10-year-old boy (Ht 4'4", Wt 76 lb) whose mother brings a prescription to you that reads:

Amoxicillin 400 mg/5mL
Give 90 mg/kg/day po tid for 10 days

How many milliliters of suspension are in each dose?

$$76\text{ lb}\cdot\frac{1\text{ kg}}{2.2\text{ lb}}\cdot\frac{90\text{ mg}}{1\text{ kg}\cdot\text{day}}\cdot\frac{1\text{ day}}{3\text{ doses}}\cdot\frac{5\text{ mL}}{400\text{ mg}}=\frac{x\text{ mL}}{\text{dose}}$$

$$\frac{x\text{ mL}}{\text{dose}}=\frac{12.95\text{ mL}}{\text{dose}}\left(\text{or }\frac{13\text{ mL}}{\text{dose}}\right).$$

How many milliliters total should you dispense?

$$\frac{13\text{ mL}}{\text{dose}}\cdot\frac{3\text{ doses}}{1\text{ day}}\cdot 10\text{ days}=x\text{ mL}$$

$$x\text{ mL}=390\text{ mL}.$$

If the suspension comes in bottles of 250 mL, how many bottles should you dispense?

$$\frac{1\text{ bottle}}{250\text{ mL}}\cdot 390\text{ mL}=x\text{ bottles}$$

$$x\text{ bottles}=1.56\text{ bottles (or 2 bottles)}.$$

Example

SE presents the following prescription for her insulin:

Insulin aspart
Sig: Inject 20 units SQ tid ac
Disp: 90-day supply

How many vials of aspart do you need to dispense to accurately fill this prescription?

$$\frac{1\text{ vial}}{10\text{ mL}}\cdot\frac{1\text{ mL}}{100\text{ units}}\cdot\frac{20\text{ units}}{\text{dose}}\cdot\frac{3\text{ doses}}{1\text{ day}}\cdot 90\text{ days}=x\text{ vials}$$

$$x\text{ vials}=5.4\text{ vials (or 6 vials)}$$

UNITS OF MEASURE

Now that we understand how to set up calculations, we need to understand the various conversion factors we will be using in these calculations.

Metric System

The basic units used in the metric system are the gram (measure of weight), liter (measure of volume) and meter (measure of length). Prefixes are used to express quantities that are much greater or much less than these

Prefix	Symbol	Conversion
mega-	m	10^6
kilo-	k	10^3
deca-	da	10^1
base		—
deci-	d	10^{-1}
centi-	c	10^{-2}
milli-	m	10^{-3}
micro-	μ or mc	10^{-6}
nano-	n	10^{-9}
pico-	p	10^{-12}

basic units. It is important to understand how to convert between these various measures.

Examples

Convert the following:

1. 180 mcg to mg:

$$180 \text{ mcg} \cdot \frac{1 \text{ mg}}{1,000 \text{ mcg}} = 0.18 \text{ mg}$$

2. 6.9 g to mg:

$$6.9 \text{ g} \cdot \frac{1,000 \text{ mg}}{1 \text{ g}} = 6,900 \text{ mg}$$

3. 2,800 g to kg:

$$2,800 \text{ g} \cdot \frac{1 \text{ kg}}{1,000 \text{ g}} = 2.8 \text{ kg}$$

Conversion Factors

It is also important to understand how to convert between different systems of measure. Some of the most commonly used conversion factors are listed below. Many of these conversion factors should be memorized, as they are commonly used in pharmacy (as denoted by *).

It is common to round the following:

*1 tsp = 5 mL

*1 tbsp = 15 mL

*1 fl oz = 30 mL

*1 gr = 65 mg

Unit		SI
	Length	
*1 inch		2.54 centimeter (cm)
	Volume	
1 teaspoon (tsp)		4.928 milliliter (mL)
1 tablespoon (tbsp)	3 tsp	14.786 mL
1 fluid ounce (fl oz)	2 tbsp	29.573 mL
1 cup (cp)	8 fl oz	236.588 mL
1 pint (pt)	2 cp	473.176 mL
1 quart (qt)	2 pt	946 mL
1 gallon (gal)	4 qt	3,785 mL
	Mass	
1 grain (gr)		64.789 milligrams (mg)
1 dram (dr)		1.771 grams (g)
1 ounce (oz)		28.349 g
1 pound (lb)		453.592 g
*2.2 lb		1 kilogram (kg)

Examples

Convert the following:

1. 65 inches to cm

$$65 \text{ in} \cdot \frac{2.54 \text{ cm}}{1 \text{ in}} = 165.1 \text{ cm}$$

2. 8 mL to tsp

$$8 \text{ mL} \cdot \frac{1 \text{ tsp}}{5 \text{ mL}} = 1.6 \text{ tsp}$$

3. 180 mL to fl oz

$$180 \text{ mL} \cdot \frac{1 \text{ fl oz}}{30 \text{ mL}} = 6 \text{ fl oz}$$

4. 180 lb to kg

$$180 \text{ lb} \cdot \frac{1 \text{ kg}}{2.2 \text{ lb}} = 81.8 \text{ kg}$$

Specific Gravity and Density

Density is the measure of an object's weight divided by its volume. Specific gravity (SpGr) is a unitless measure that represents the ratio between the density of one material and the density of a standard material at a specific temperature. In particular, for liquids, water is the standard material. Because water has a density of 1g/mL, the volume of water is the same as the weight of water. Thus the specific gravity of liquids may be determined by calculating the weight of the liquid divided by the weight of the same volume of water. Both specific gravity and density are used to convert between the volume and weight of an object or liquid

$$\text{Density} = \frac{\text{Weight}}{\text{Volume}}$$

$$\text{SpGr} = \frac{\text{Weight of } x \text{ mL of a material}}{\text{Weight of } x \text{ mL of a standard}}.$$

Example

What is the weight of 200 mL of boric acid (specific gravity 1.44)?

$$1.44 = \frac{x \text{ g of 200 mL of boric acid}}{200 \text{ mL of water} (1 \frac{\text{g}}{\text{mL}})}$$

$$x = 288 \text{ g of boric acid.}$$

Temperature

It's very important for pharmacists to understand the relationship between the Fahrenheit and Celsius temperature scales. This is a common conversion with which you must be comfortable. The following equations provide a way to convert between the two measures of temperature:

$$9°C = 5°F - 160$$

$$x°C = \frac{5}{9}°F - 17.778$$

$$x°F = \frac{9}{5}°C + 32.$$

It is also imperative to understand what a normal body temperature is as well as when a fever is considered medically significant.

Example:

Normal body temperature is considered 98.6°F. What is this temperature in Celsius?

$$x°C = \frac{5}{9}(98.6) - 17.778$$

$$x = 37°C.$$

A fever is considered medically significant when the body temperature greater than 38°C. What is this temperature in Fahrenheit?

$$x°F = \frac{9}{5}(38) + 32$$

$$x = 100.4°F.$$

Additionally, it is important to understand the difference between temperatures taken by various routes. Oral temperature is normally used for individuals aged 5 and older. Rectal temperature is normally used for individuals younger than age 5 years. It is important to note that rectal temperature is 1°F (0.5°C) *higher* than oral temperature and that axillary temperature is 1°F (0.5°C) *lower* than oral temperature. Ear thermometers are used commonly as well; they will be set to read at either an oral or rectal setting

$$\text{Rectal } -1°F \text{ (or } -0.5°C) = \text{Oral Temperature}$$

$$\text{Axillary } +1°F \text{ (or } +0.5°C) = \text{Oral Temperature.}$$

Example

JD, a dad who uses your pharmacy, comes to the store asking for some help. His daughter has been fighting a cold, and her pediatrician instructed JD to call if she develops a fever greater than 39°C. JD has a thermometer and states that his daughter has been running an oral temperature of 100.8°F. Should JD call the pediatrician?

$$x°C = \frac{5}{9}(100.8°F) - 17.778$$

$$x = 38.2°C.$$

JD should not call the pediatrician yet. When should you instruct JD to call the pediatrician?

$$x°F = \frac{9}{5}(39°C) + 32$$

$$x = 102.2°F.$$

JD should call the pediatrician when his daughter's temperature is greater than 102.2°F.

PATIENT-SPECIFIC DOSING

An integral role of the pharmacist, whether in the community or a clinical setting, is to ensure the proper dosing regimen based on the patient's specific characteristics. This often means adjusting the dose based on body weight, body mass index (BMI), body surface area (BSA), and creatinine clearance (CrCl). This section elucidates the various ways these calculations may be done in practice.

Body Weight

Several different measures of body weight, including total body weight (TBW), ideal body weight (IBW), and adjusted body weight (ABW), are used in various calculations. The TBW is merely how much the individual weighs. Recall how to convert between pounds (lb) and kilograms (kg):

$$\text{wt in lb} \cdot \frac{1\,\text{kg}}{2.2\,\text{lb}} = \text{wt in kg.}$$

The IBW is a measure of how much a person should weigh based on gender and height, otherwise known as lean body mass. This calculation is important because many medications are dosed based on the IBW—specifically, medications that do not distribute well into fat. Two IBW formulas are available, based on gender (assuming that females have less muscle mass than males). The formulas for IBW (in kilograms) are as follows:

$$\text{Male: } IBW = 50 + 2.3(\text{height in inches} - 60)$$

$$\text{Female: } IBW = 45.5 + 2.3(\text{height in inches} - 60).$$

Example

JR is a 57-year-old male who weighs 119 kg and is 69 inches tall. What is his IBW?

Male: $IBW = 50 + 2.3(\text{height in inches} - 60)$

$$IBW = 50 + 2.3(69 - 60)$$

$$IBW\ (kg) = 70.7.$$

Example

AR is prescribed a medication that should be dosed 4 mg/kg (in IBW) po divided twice daily. AR is female, weighs 150 lb, and is 5 feet, 2 inches tall. What dose of this medication should she receive?

Female: $IBW = 45.5 + 2.3(\text{height in inches} - 60)$

$$IBW = 45.5 + 2.3(62 - 60)$$

$$IBW\ (kg) = 50.1.$$

Daily dose calculation:

$$\frac{x\text{ mg}}{\text{day}} = \frac{4\text{mg}}{\text{kg}}(\text{IBW in kg}) = \frac{4\text{mg}}{\text{kg}}(50.1\text{ kg})$$

$$= 200.4\left(\text{or } 200\,\frac{\text{mg}}{\text{day}}\right)$$

Individual dose calculation:

$$\frac{200\text{ mg}}{1\text{ day}} \cdot \frac{1\text{ day}}{2\text{ dose}} = \frac{100\text{ mg}}{\text{dose}}$$

The ABW is an adjusted version of the IBW. This calculation assumes that overweight individuals have more muscle mass compared to individuals at IBW. It is often used when the individual's TBW is 30% greater than his or her calculated IBW. The formula for ABW (in kilograms) is as follows:

$$ABW\ (\text{kg}) = \text{IBW} + 0.4(\text{TBW} - \text{IBW})$$

Example

CR is a 55-year-old female who weighs 100 kg and is 62 inches tall. What is her ABW?

Female: $IBW = 45.5 + 2.3(\text{height in inches} - 60)$

$$IBW = 45.5 + 2.3(62 - 60)$$

$$IBW = 49.6\text{ kg}.$$

Use ABW because CR's current weight is more than 30% greater than her calculated IBW.

$$ABW\,(\text{kg}) = \text{IBW} + 0.4(\text{TBW} - \text{IBW})$$

$$ABW(\text{kg}) = 49.6\text{kg} + 0.4(100\text{ kg} - 49.6\text{ kg})$$

$$ABW(\text{kg}) = 69.76\text{ kg}.$$

Body Surface Area

Some medications—especially chemotherapeutic agents—are dosed according to a patient's body surface area. The BSA (expressed in square meters, m^2) is calculated using the following formula:

$$BSA = \sqrt{\frac{(\text{height in cm})(\text{weight in kg})}{3,600}}.$$

Example

RD is to be started on carboplatin for treatment of her ovarian cancer. The dose should be 360 mg/m^2. RD weighs 140 lb and is 63 inches tall. What should her dose be?

$$Height\ in\ cm = 63\text{ in} \cdot \frac{2.54\text{ cm}}{1\text{ in}} = 160.02\text{ cm}$$

$$Weight\ in\ kg = 140\text{ lb} \cdot \frac{1\text{ kg}}{2.2\text{ lb}} = 63.63\text{ kg}$$

$$BSA = \sqrt{\frac{(160.02)(63.63)}{3,600}} = \sqrt{2.83} = 1.68\text{ m}^2$$

$$Dose = 360\frac{\text{mg}}{\text{m}^2} \cdot 1.68\text{ m}^2 = 604.8\text{ mg}.$$

Oftentimes, the dose for a child is determined from the dose for the adult and the average adult BSA, which is 1.73 m^2. The following proportion will help determine the child's dose:

$$\frac{\text{Adult dose}}{\text{Average adult BSA}} = \frac{\text{Child's dose}}{\text{Child's BSA}}.$$

Example

Sam (Wt 25 kg, Ht 53 inches) is a 5-year-old child who must receive a dose of a medication. The adult dose is 300 mg. What dose should Sam be given?

$$BSA = \sqrt{\frac{(53\text{ in})\frac{2.54\text{ cm}}{\text{in}}(25\text{ kg})}{3,600}} = 0.9669\text{ m}^2.$$

$$Child's\ dose = \frac{(\text{Adult dose})(\text{Child's BSA})}{\text{Average adult BSA}}$$

$$Child's\ dose = \frac{(300\ \text{mg})(0.9669\ \text{m}^2)}{1.73\ \text{m}^2} = 167.67\ \text{mg}.$$

Creatinine Clearance

Many medications are dosed according to a patient's renal function. Creatinine clearance (CrCl) is a measure of a patient's renal function based on age, gender, body weight, and serum creatinine (SCr). Although the MDRD equation is commonly used for staging kidney disease, the Cockroft-Gault equation should be used for drug dosing.

$$CrCl = \frac{(140 - \text{Age})(\text{Actual Body Wt in kg})(0.85\ \text{if female})}{(72)(\text{SCr in mg/dL})}.$$

Note: Some clinicians prefer using IBW in this calculation. Although the original formula was derived using actual body weight (TBW), it excluded people weighing more than 130% of IBW.

Example

JL is a 68-year-old female with a complicated UTI that is sensitive to ciprofloxacin. Ciprofloxacin dosage must be corrected for renal function when CrCl is less than 50 mL/min. JL's vital signs are as follows: weight 145 lb, height 66 inches, BP 134/82, P 72, T 39°C. Her lab results are as follows: Na 142 mg/dL, K 4.2 mg/dL, SCr 1.5 mg/dL, Cl 95 mg/dL, Glu 139 mg/dL. What is JL's CrCl? Should her dose be adjusted?

$$CrCl = \frac{(140 - 68)\left(145\ \text{lb} \cdot \frac{\text{kg}}{2.2\ \text{lb}}\right)(0.85)}{(72)(1.5)} = 37.35\ \text{mL/min}.$$

Because the CrCl is less than 50 mL/min, JL's dose should be adjusted.

Example

BR is a 72-year-old male (Ht 74 inches, Wt 224 lb) with newly diagnosed diabetes. His primary care provider (PCP) calls to ask if glyburide is an appropriate choice for BR. He informs you that BR's SCr is 1.4 mg/dL. Glyburide should not be used in patients if the CrCl is less than 50 mL/min. What should you tell BR's PCP?

$$CrCl = \frac{(140 - 72)\left(224\ \text{lb} \cdot \frac{\text{kg}}{2.2\ \text{lb}}\right)}{(72)(1.4)} = 68.69\ \text{mL/min}.$$

The CrCl is greater than 50 mL/min, so glyburide would be appropriate in this patient.

IV Infusions

It is essential that pharmacists be able to determine appropriate infusion rates and doses for intravenous preparations. In fact, pharmacists working in an inpatient setting perform these calculations daily.

Example

You receive an order for vancomycin 1,000 mg IV q 12 hours in 200 mL D_5W, which should be infused over 90 minutes. At what rate (mg/min) should the infusion be set?

$$x\frac{\text{mg}}{\text{min}} = \frac{1{,}000\ \text{mg}}{90\ \text{min}} = 11.11\frac{\text{mg}}{\text{min}}.$$

Example

You receive a call from the floor nurse asking to clarify the parameters of a patient's infusion pump. The patient is supposed to receive 25 mg/hr of a particular medication, which comes in premade bags of 500 mg in 200 mL. At what flow rate (mL/hr) should the infusion pump be set?

$$x\frac{\text{mL}}{\text{hr}} = \frac{200\ \text{mL}}{500\ \text{mg}} \cdot \frac{25\ \text{mg}}{1\ \text{hr}} = 10\frac{\text{mL}}{\text{hr}}.$$

CONCENTRATIONS

Percentage Strength

Concentrations may be expressed as percentage strength. Percentage signifies the number of units of drug (numerator) per 100 units of total drug product (denominator). Drug concentrations can be calculated in several ways.

Percent weight-in-weight (% w/w) is grams of ingredient in 100 grams of product (mixture). It is expressed in g/100 g.

Example

What is the concentration of a preparation containing 20 mg of drug in 400 mg of product?

Convert mg to grams:

$$20\ \text{mg} \cdot \frac{1\ \text{g}}{1{,}000\ \text{mg}} = 0.020\ \text{g}$$

$$400\ \text{mg} \cdot \frac{1\ \text{g}}{1{,}000\ \text{mg}} = 0.400\ \text{g}.$$

Determine the concentration (% w/w = g/100 g):

$$\frac{x\ \text{g}}{100\ \text{g}} = \frac{0.020\ \text{g}}{0.400\ \text{g}} \rightarrow x\ \text{g} = \frac{(0.020\ \text{g} \cdot 100\ \text{g})}{0.400\ \text{g}} \rightarrow$$

$$x = \frac{5\ \text{g ingredient}}{100\ \text{g product}} = 5\%\ \text{w/w}.$$

Percent volume-in-volume (% v/v) is milliliters of ingredient in 100 milliliters of product (solution). It is expressed in mL/100 mL.

Example

What is the concentration of a solution containing 15 mL of drug in 60 mL of solution?

Determine the concentration (% v/v = mL/100 mL):

$$\frac{x\,\text{mL}}{100\,\text{mL}} = \frac{15\,\text{mL}}{60\,\text{mL}} \rightarrow x\,\text{mL} = \frac{(15\,\text{mL} \cdot 100\,\text{mL})}{60\,\text{mL}} \rightarrow$$

$$x = \frac{25\,\text{mL ingredient}}{100\,\text{mL product}} = 25\%\ \text{v/v}.$$

Percent weight-in-volume (% w/v) is grams of ingredient in 100 milliliters of product (solution). It is expressed in g/100 mL.

Example

What is the concentration of a solution containing 50 mg of drug in 50 mL of solution?

Convert mg to grams:

$$50\,\text{mg} \cdot \frac{1\,\text{g}}{1{,}000\,\text{mg}} = 0.050\,\text{g}.$$

Determine concentration (% w/v = g/100 mL):

$$\frac{x\,\text{g}}{100\,\text{mL}} = \frac{0.050\,\text{g}}{50\,\text{mL}} \rightarrow x\,\text{mL} = \frac{(0.050\,\text{g} \cdot 100\,\text{mL})}{50\,\text{mL}} \rightarrow$$

$$x = \frac{0.1\,\text{g ingredient}}{100\,\text{mL product}} = 0.1\%\ \text{w/v}.$$

Ratio Strength

Concentrations may be expressed as ratio strength (parts) when the ingredient is highly diluted. To solve these problems we use proportional calculations.

Percent weight-in-weight, or % (w/w), is the grams of ingredient in 100 grams of product (mixture). It is expressed in g/100 g.

Example

What is the concentration in (w/w) of a preparation with a ratio strength of 1:5,000?

Known: 1 g ingredient in 5,000 g product
Unknown: x g ingredient in 100 g product

Determine the concentration (% w/w = parts/100 g):

$$\frac{x\,\text{g}}{100\,\text{g}} = \frac{1\,\text{g}}{5{,}000\,\text{g}} \rightarrow x\,\text{g} = \frac{(1\,\text{g} \cdot 100\,\text{g})}{5{,}000\,\text{g}} \rightarrow$$

$$x = \frac{0.02\,\text{g ingredient}}{100\,\text{g product}} = 0.02\%\ \text{w/w}.$$

Percent volume-in-volume, or % (v/v), is milliliters of ingredient in 100 milliliters of product (solution). It is expressed in mL/100 mL.

Example

What is the concentration in (v/v) of a solution with a ratio strength of 1:2,000?

Known: 1 mL ingredient per 2,000 mL product
Unknown: x mL ingredient per 100 mL product

Determine the concentration (% v/v = parts/100 mL):

$$\frac{x\,\text{mL}}{100\,\text{mL}} = \frac{1\,\text{mL}}{2{,}000\,\text{mL}} \rightarrow x\,\text{mL} = \frac{(1\,\text{mL} \cdot 100\,\text{mL})}{2{,}000\,\text{mL}} \rightarrow$$

$$x = \frac{0.05\,\text{mL ingredient}}{100\,\text{mL product}} = 0.05\%\ \text{v/v}.$$

Percent weight-in-volume is grams of ingredient in 100 milliliters of product (solution). It is expressed in g/100 mL.

Example:

What is the concentration in (w/v) of a solution with a ratio strength of 1:4,000?

Known: 1 g ingredient per 4,000 mL product
Unknown: x g ingredient per 100 mL product

Determine the concentration (% w/v = parts/100 mL):

$$\frac{x\ \text{g}}{100\ \text{mL}} = \frac{1\ \text{g}}{4{,}000\ \text{mL}} \rightarrow x\ \text{g} = \frac{(1\text{g} \cdot 100\ \text{mL})}{4{,}000\ \text{mL}} \rightarrow$$

$$x = \frac{0.025\ \text{g ingredient}}{100\ \text{mL product}} = 0.025\%\ \text{w/v}.$$

Parts

Parts are used to indicate the relative amounts of each ingredient when compounding medications. Parts are unitless until the compounder decides the units to assign to each ingredient. It is important to note that once assigned, the units must be the same for each ingredient (i.e., grams for solids and milliliters for liquids).

Example

Compounding instructions: Make a 400 g supply of the following:

Calcium carbonate: magnesium oxide: sodium bicarbonate 5:2:3

Translation:

$$5\ \text{parts}\ CaCO_3 + 2\ \text{parts}\ MgO + 3\ \text{parts}\ NaHCO_3 = 10\ \text{parts total}.$$

Calculation for compounding:

$$\frac{5 \text{ parts } CaCO_3}{10 \text{ parts total}} = \frac{x \text{ g}}{400 \text{ g}} \rightarrow x \text{ g} = \frac{(5 \text{ parts } CaCO_3)\cdot(400 \text{ g})}{10 \text{ parts total}}$$
$$\rightarrow x = 200 \text{ g } CaCO_3$$

$$\frac{2 \text{ parts MgO}}{10 \text{ parts total}} = \frac{x \text{ g}}{400 \text{ g}} \rightarrow x \text{ g} = \frac{(2 \text{ parts MgO})\cdot(400 \text{ g})}{10 \text{ parts total}}$$
$$\rightarrow x = 80 \text{ g MgO}$$

$$\frac{3 \text{ parts } NaHCO_3}{10 \text{ parts total}} = \frac{x \text{ g}}{400 \text{ g}}$$
$$\rightarrow x \text{ g} = \frac{(3 \text{ parts } NaHCO_3)\cdot(400 \text{ g})}{10 \text{ parts total}}$$
$$\rightarrow x = 120 \text{ g } NaHCO_3.$$

As a final check, note that the total weight of all ingredients in this product is 400 g.

Parts per Million

Parts per million (ppm) indicates the amount of trace substances in water. It is expressed in terms of grams of substance per 1,000,000 mL of water.

Example

If the standard dilution of fluoride is 1 ppm, calculate the ppm for the following and interpret it: A water supply is determined to have 0.8 g fluoride for every 350,000 mL water.

$$\frac{0.8 \text{ g fluoride}}{350{,}000 \text{ mL } H_2O} = \frac{\text{x g fluoride}}{1{,}000{,}000 \text{ mL } H_2O}$$
$$\rightarrow x = \frac{(0.8 \text{ g})(1{,}000{,}000 \text{ mL})}{350{,}000 \text{ mL}} = (\text{or } 2.3 \text{ ppm}).$$

Interpretation: 2.3 ppm exceeds the standard dilution of fluoride.

Molarity

We have previously discussed concentration in metric form (g/L), but will now discuss concentration in molar form (moles/L). Molarity is commonly used outside of the United States in reporting laboratory values. Thus it is commonly seen in medical journals that are not printed in the United States.

$$\text{Molarity} = \frac{\text{Moles of solute}}{\text{Liter of solution}}$$

$$\text{Millimolarity} = \frac{\text{millimoles of solute}}{\text{Liter of solution}}.$$

A mole is equal to the molecular weight in grams (GMW), and a millimole is the molecular weight in milligrams.

Mole: molecular weight in grams (GMW)

- $\text{GMW} = \frac{\text{grams}}{\text{mole}}.$

Millimole: molecular weight in milligrams (mGMW)

- $\text{mGMW} = \frac{\text{millligrams}}{\text{millimole}}.$

Osmolarity

Osmotic pressure is determined by the number of particles in a given amount of solution. This measurement of concentration is important in terms of the rate and the extent to which particles diffuse across a membrane, especially if the solution is given intravenously or intraocularly.

It is important to be able to convert between milliosmoles in a solution and the molar concentration of that solution. To do so, we must first understand how to calculate milliosmoles.

Calculating Milliosmoles

Determine into how many particles a given substance will dissociate.

- **Covalent substances** will not dissociate. An example of a covalent substance is glucose.

  Milliosmoles = millimoles

- **Ionic bonds dissociate readily into species. An example of an ionic bond is MgO.**

  Milliosmoles = # of particles.

Example

Millimole	Species	Milliosmole
1 millimole dextrose	1 dextrose (covalent bond)	1 milliosmole dextrose
1 millimole NaCl	1 Na^+ + 1 Cl^-	2 milliosmoles NaCl
1 millimole $CaCl_2$	1 Ca^{++} + 2 Cl^-	3 milliosmoles $CaCl_2$
1 millimole $NaC_2H_3O_2$	1 Na^+ + 1 $C_2H_3O_2^-$ (covalent bond)	2 milliosmoles $NaC_2H_3O_2$

If 1 L of solution contains 9 g of NaCl, calculate the number of milliosmoles per liter. NaCl has a molecular weight of 58.5 mg/mmol.

1 millimole NaCl dissociates into two species (1 Na^+ and 1 Cl) => 2 milliosmoles NaCl per mmol

$$\frac{9 \text{ g}}{\text{L}} \cdot \frac{1{,}000 \text{ mg}}{\text{g}} \cdot \frac{1 \text{ mmol}}{58.5 \text{ mg}} \cdot \frac{2 \text{ mOsmol}}{\text{mmol}} = 308 \frac{\text{mOsmol}}{\text{L}}.$$

Milliequivalents

Ionic equivalency conveys the electrical activity of ions in the body. Equivalence defines the weight of a substance that can *replace* or *combine with* 1 g of hydrogen. Every ion with a single charge is considered equivalent to one hydrogen ion (because hydrogen has a single charge). If an ion has a + 2 charge, it is considered the equivalent of two hydrogen ions. Of note: Only the positive *or* negative charges should be counted, not both.

Ion	Equivalency
+1 charge	1 equivalent
Single bonded ion	1 equivalent
+2 charge	2 equivalents

Because the concentration of a drug in the human body is usually so small, we generally use milliequivalents rather than equivalents. With the following formulas, we are able to convert between amounts of drugs (mg) and milliequivalents (mEq).

$$\text{Equivalent weight (Eq)} = \frac{\text{MW in g}}{\text{Valence}}$$

$$\text{MilliEquivalent weight (mEq)} = \frac{\text{MW in mg}}{\text{Valence}}.$$

MW: molecular weight (g or mg)
Valence: electrons that can participate in a chemical bond (electrons in outer shell)

Note: Do not add valence electrons in molecules.

Examples

Na^+	Cl^-	NaCl	Ca^{++}
MW: 23 mg	MW: 35.5 mg	MW: 58 mg	MW: 40 mg
Valence: 1	Valence: 1	Valence: 1	Valence: 2

Examples

How many milligrams of NaCl are in each milliequivalent of NaCl?

$$1\text{mEq NaCl} \cdot \frac{(23 \text{ mg Na}) + (35.5 \text{ mg CL})}{1} = 58.5 \text{ mg NaCl}$$

How many milligrams of $CaCO_3$ are in each milliequivalent of $CaCO_3$?

$$1\text{mEq } CaCO_3 \cdot \frac{(40 \text{ mg Ca}) + (60 \text{ mg } CO_3)}{2} = 50 \text{ mg } CaCO_3$$

How many milligrams of Ca^{++} are in each milliequivalent of $CaCO_3$?

$$1\text{mEq } CaCO_3 \cdot \frac{(40 \text{ mg Ca})}{2} = 20 \text{ mg Ca}.$$

How many milligrams of CO_3 are in each milliequivalent of $CaCO_3$?

$$1\text{mEq } CaCO_3 \cdot \frac{(60 \text{ mg } CO_3)}{2} = 30 \text{ mg } CO_3 \text{ per mEq of } CaCO_3.$$

COMPOUNDING

Compounding is a unique responsibility entrusted to the profession of pharmacy. To maintain this trust, all pharmacists must be able to compound high-quality medications that meet specific standards.

Batch Preparation

Formulas for compounded products include the specific proportions of the various ingredients needed to make the product. When compounding, it is often necessary to use this formula to determine the amount of each ingredient that is required to make a predetermined amount of finished product.

Example

How much diphenydramine would you need to compound 500 mL of the following solution?

Diphenydramine HCl: 250 mg
Glycerin: 5 mL
Syrup for sweetening: 30 mL
Distilled water: qs to 100 mL

$$\frac{x \text{ mg diphenhydramine}}{500\text{mL}} = \frac{250\text{mg diphenhydramine}}{100\text{mL}}$$

$$x\text{mg diphenhydramine} = \frac{(250 \text{ mg}) \cdot (500 \text{ mL})}{100 \text{ mL}}$$
$$= 1,250 \text{ mg diphenhydramine}.$$

Dilutions

Dilutions are used commonly in pharmacy when the desired concentration of a product is not available and, therefore, must be made from a stronger concentration of the same product. This may be done using a simple proportion:

$$(\text{Quantity}_1) \cdot (\text{Concentration}_1) = (\text{Quantity}_2) \cdot (\text{Concentration}_2).$$

Examples

If 500 mL of a solution that is 20% v/v is diluted to 1,000 mL, what is the new percentage strength?

$$(500 \text{ mL}) \cdot (20\%) = (1,000 \text{ mL}) \cdot (x\%) \rightarrow x\%$$
$$= \frac{(500 \text{ mL}) \cdot (20\%)}{1,000 \text{ mL}} \rightarrow 10\%.$$

How much distilled water must be added to 500 mL of a 6% w/v solution to make a new solution with a concentration of 2%?

$$(500\,\text{mL})\cdot(6\%) = (500\,\text{mL} + x)\cdot(2\%) \rightarrow x\text{mL} = \left(\frac{(500\,\text{mL})\cdot(6\%)}{2\%}\right) - 500\,\text{mL}$$

$$x = 1{,}000\text{mL}.$$

Percentage Error

Percentage error (PE) is a variable used to indicate the sensitivity of a balance; it describes to what degree a scale may be inaccurate. The formula for PE is as follows:

$$\%\ \text{error} = \frac{|(\text{Actual weight}) - (\text{Measured weight})|}{\text{Quantity desired}}.$$

Example

A scale has a PE of 2%. If you intend to measure 5 g of a powder, how much powder could you have actually measured?

$$0.02 = \frac{|(x) - (5\ g)|}{5\ g} \rightarrow x\text{vg} = ((5\ \text{g})\cdot(0.02)) + 5\ \text{g} \rightarrow x = 5.1\ \text{g}.$$

Example

Your pharmacy has recently upgraded to a brand-new scale to be used for all of your compounding. You wish to compare the two scales to see if the older scale was still measuring accurately. For your test, you weigh out 2.50 g of sugar on your old balance. You then weigh this same amount of sugar on your new scale, which reads 2.28 g. What is the PE of the old scale?

$$x = \frac{|(2.28\ \text{g}) - (2.50\ \text{g})|}{2.50\ \text{g}} = \frac{0.22}{2.5} = 0.088 = 8.8\%.$$

Minimum Measurable

As discussed in the preceding subsection, percentage error (PE) indicates by what degree a balance may be inaccurate. Balances also have a defined sensitivity requirement (SR), which indicates the smallest amount of weight that the balance can detect. The PE and SR are used to determine the minimum measurable amount of a balance.

$$\text{Minimum measurable quantity} = \frac{(\text{Sensitivity requirement})\cdot 100\%}{\text{Percentage error}}.$$

Example

USP requires that balances used in compounding have a PE of no more than 5%. The SR for Class A prescription balances is 6 mg. What is the minimum measurable quantity for these balances?

$$x\,\text{mg} = \frac{(6\ \text{mg})\cdot 100\%}{5\%} = 6\ \text{mg}\cdot 20 = 120\ \text{mg}.$$

Alligations

Alligations are used when the pharmacist must compound a new concentration from two different concentrations—one stronger and one weaker than the desired concentration. This situation often arises when certain concentrations are not available from the manufacturer. To calculate how much of each of the existing concentrations are needed, follow these steps ([] denotes concentration):

1. Determine the number of parts needed of the strongest concentration (Parts [S]) from the strength of the desired concentration (Strength [D]) and the strength of the weakest concentration (Strength [W]):

   Parts [S] = (Strength [D]) – (Strength [W]).

2. Determine the number of parts needed of the weakest concentration (Parts [W]) from the strength of the strongest concentration (Strength [S]):

   Parts [W] = (Strength [S]) – (Strength[D]).

The following graphic will help you determine how much of the two existing concentrations are needed to make the new concentration.

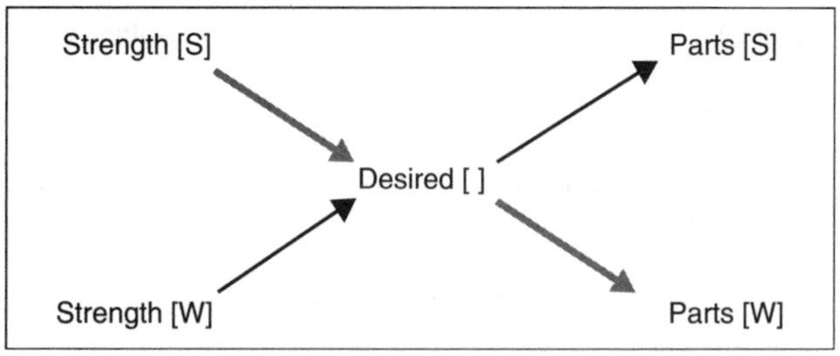

3. Parts [S] + Parts [W] = Total # of parts in solution
4. Use the desired volume of the final solution to set up equations based on the particular quantity you are trying to calculate:

$$\frac{x\,\text{mL concentration of interest}}{\text{Total mL}} = \frac{\text{Parts concentration of interest}}{\text{Total parts}}.$$

Example

You receive notice from your supplier that 3% NaCl is unavailable; however, you are able to order plenty of 20% NaCl and 0.9% NaCl. Because it is imperative that you have 3% NaCl in stock for urgent cases of hyponatremia, you decide to compound a small supply.

How much of the 20% NaCl would you need to compound 1,000 mL of the 3% concentration?

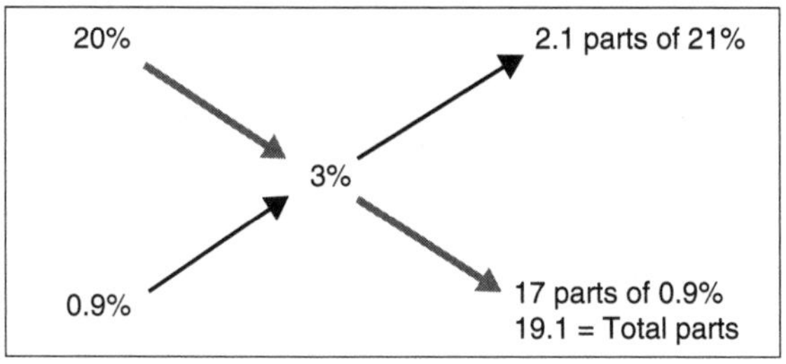

$$\frac{x\,\text{mL } 20\%}{1{,}000\text{ mL}} = \frac{2.1\text{ Parts } 20\%}{19.1} \rightarrow x\,\text{ml } 20\%$$

$$= \frac{(2.1)\cdot(1{,}000\text{ mL})}{19.1} = 109.94\text{ mL.}$$

How much of the 0.9% NaCl would you need to compound 1,000 mL of the 3% concentration?

$$x\text{ mL of } 0.9\% = (\text{Total mL}) - (\text{mL of } 20\%)$$
$$= 1{,}000\text{-}109.94 = 890.06\text{ mL.}$$

Or

$$\frac{x\,\text{mL } 0.9\%}{1{,}000\text{ mL}} = \frac{17\text{ Parts } 0.9\%}{19.1} \rightarrow x\,\text{ml } 0.9\%$$

$$= \frac{(17)\cdot(1{,}000\text{ mL})}{19.1} = 890.05\text{ mL.}$$

ANNOTATED BIBLIOGRAPHY

1. Ansel HC. *Pharmaceutical Calculations.* 13th ed. Philadelphia: Lippincott Williams & Wilkins; 2010.
2. Khan MA, Reddy IK. *Pharmaceutical and Clinical Calculations.* 2nd ed. Lancaster, PA: Technomic; 2000.
3. O'Sullivan TA. *Understanding Pharmacy Calculations.* Washington, DC: American Pharmaceutical Association; 2002.
4. *USP Pharmacists' Pharmacopeia.* 2nd ed. Rockville, MD: U.S. Pharmacopeial Convention; 2008.

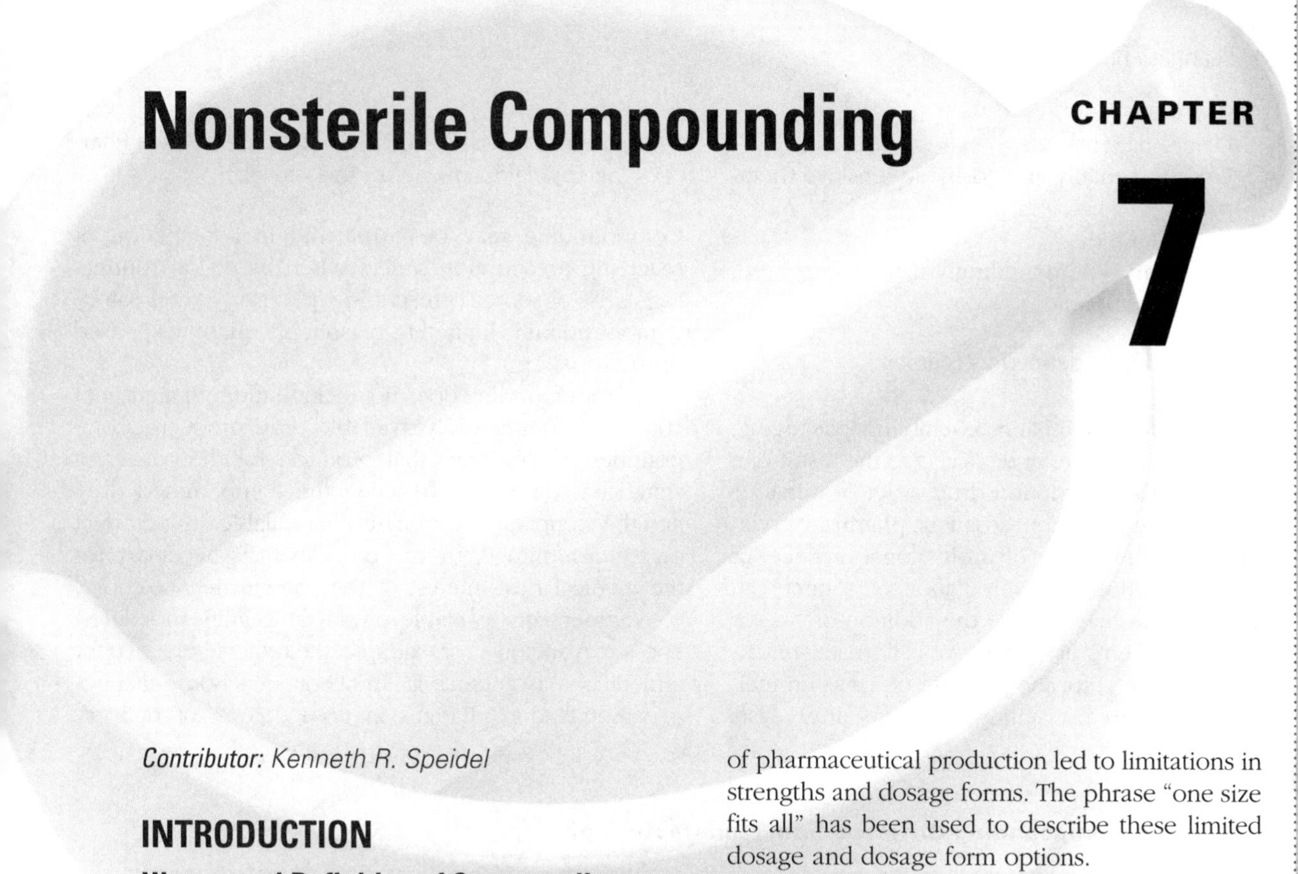

Nonsterile Compounding

CHAPTER 7

Contributor: *Kenneth R. Speidel*

INTRODUCTION

History and Definition of Compounding

Prior to a discussion on what pharmaceutical compounding is, it is necessary to understand where the practice came from. The history of pharmacy is the history of compounding. Prior to the 1820s, drug manufacturing did not exist; thus any medication that was needed was compounded. These compounds were prepared by the pharmacists of the day, known as the alchemists. Indeed, the practice of compounding dates back to the physician priests of ancient Egypt, who were divided into two groups. The first group included the healers who actually went and attended to the sick; the second group stayed back and prepared the medicine for the sick. This bifurcation in roles also marked the start of the separation between physician and pharmacist.

Pharmacy is unique in that it is the only profession that has the training and knowledge to be able to make formulations for specific patient populations. In the United States in the nineteenth century, most towns had a compounding pharmacist. In 1820, early pharmacists and physicians combined their efforts and issued the *National Formulary*. During the early twentieth century, almost all prescriptions dispensed were compounded. The 1900s, however, soon saw the introduction of commercially prepared pharmaceuticals. Many strengths and dosage forms were made available, although over time the economics of pharmaceutical production led to limitations in strengths and dosage forms. The phrase "one size fits all" has been used to describe these limited dosage and dosage form options.

By the 1980s, most schools and colleges of pharmacy did not include compounding in their curriculum. However, in the late 1980s, pharmacists and practitioners realized the need for revisiting compounding as a part of pharmacy practice. Today, compounding has become a common component of the pharmacy practice.

Reasons for the Growth of Pharmacy Compounding

- Limited dosage forms and/or strengths
- Limited strengths
- A recognized need to have a combination of medications administered within the same dosage form
- A greater number of patients being treated at home for complex and sometimes terminal conditions (e.g., hospice)
- Manufacturer shortages or discontinuation of medications
- The growing complexity of veterinary pharmacotherapy
- Orphan drugs
- New therapeutic approaches
- The need to create individualized support for patients in special populations
    - Pediatrics
    - Geriatrics
    - Bio-identical hormone replacement therapy
    - Pain management

- Dental patients
- Environmentally and cosmetic sensitive therapies
- Sports injuries
- Veterinary compounding: small, large, herd, exotic, companion

Compounding is defined as follows:

[T]he preparation, mixing, assembling, packaging, or labeling of a drug or device 1) as the result of a practitioner's prescription drug order or initiative based on the practitioner/patient/pharmacist relationship in the course of professional practice, or 2) reconstitution or manipulation of commercial products that may require the addition of one or more ingredients as a result of a licensed practitioner's order 3) for the purpose of, or as an incident to, research, teaching, or chemical analysis and not for sale or dispensing (United States Pharmacopeial Convention, Inc., 2005b).

Compounding may be conducted in anticipation of receiving prescription orders when based on routine, regularly observed prescribing patterns. Anticipatory compounding is limited to reasonable quantities, based on such patterns.

Compounding does not include the preparation of copies of commercially available drug products. Compounded preparations that produce, for the patient, a significant difference between the compounded drug and the comparable commercially available drug product or are determined, by the prescriber, as necessary for the medical best interest of the patient are not copies of commercially available products. "Significant" differences may include, for example, the removal of a dye for a medical reason (such as an allergic reaction), changes in strength, and changes in dosage form or delivery

Table 7-1 How Is Compounding Different from Manufacturing?

Manufacturing	Compounding
Most drug products are prepared in finished dosage form from bulk materials and mass distributed for resale.	Compounding dosage forms utilize bulk drug materials and/or manufactured drug products.
Use large-scale production in manufacturing plants.	Uses small-size equipment in small pharmacy areas in state-licensed pharmacies.
Regulations require new drug applications (NDAs) or abbreviated new drug applications (ANDAs) before a drug can be brought to market.	Requires a prescription. Compounded prescriptions are exempt from NDAs. While the FDA says that NDAs are legally necessary, the agency has not required them.
The sources of bulk drugs used for compounding are subject to FDA inspection and inspection by State Boards of Pharmacy.	The sources of bulk drugs used for compounding are subject to FDA inspection and inspection by State Boards of Pharmacy.
All distribution points and storage facilities for manufactured drug products are subject to FDA inspection.	The only distribution point and storage facility (i.e., the pharmacy) is subject to State Boards of Pharmacy inspection. (May also include nursing homes and nursing stations in hospitals.)
Manufacturers have extended patent protection in the form of chemical patents, process patents, and use patents.	Pharmacists generally have no patent protection.
Physicians prescribe manufactured products when they believe they are the best therapy for the patient. When a prescription is written by a physician, State Boards of Pharmacy direct that it must be filled with manufactured products unless such products are unavailable or a physician specifically directs it to be compounded.	Physicians prescribe compounded products when they believe they are the best therapy for the patient.
Manufactured products are designed to meet the vast majority of patient needs (97–99%).	Compounding meets unique needs (often critical) for very small patient populations (1–3%). Compounding accounts for approximately 11% of prescriptions when reconstituted products are included.
Manufacturers make claims about safety and efficiency and may promote their products for labeled uses.	Pharmacists make no claims about safety and efficiency and may not promote particular uses of compounded medications.
Two centuries old.	Fifty centuries old.
The FDA is the expert in regulating manufacturing.	State Boards of Pharmacy are the experts in regulating the practice of pharmacy, including compounding.

mechanism. Price differences are not considered to be a "significant" difference that justifies compounding.

Standards also note that a pharmacy may advertise or otherwise promote that it provides prescription drug compounding services. Such advertising should include only those claims, assertions, or inference of professional superiority in the compounding of drug products that can be independently and scientifically substantiated.

Compounding is a part of the practice of pharmacy that is subject to regulation and oversight from the State Boards of Pharmacy. Although state rules and regulations on the practice of compounding vary, many of the same tenets can be found as underlying precepts. It is universally accepted in all states that a pharmacist cannot manufacture medications under the guise of performing compounding. This point often suggests that in each case of compounding, there is most often a patient, prescriber, and pharmacist relationship that is initiated and maintained. Nevertheless, it is important to recognize that some states allow for compounding for licensed prescriber "office use," although most often this does not include prescribers reselling compounded medications.

CATEGORIES OF COMPOUNDING

1. Nonsterile: simple
2. Nonsterile: complex
3. Sterile: low risk
4. Sterile: moderate risk
5. Sterile: high risk
6. Nuclear pharmacy
7. Veterinary compounding

Categories are based upon the following characteristics:

- Degree of difficulty
- Stability information and warnings
- Packaging and storage requirements
- Dosage forms
- Complexity of calculations
- Local versus systemic effect
- Level of risk to the compounder
- Potential for risk or harm to the patient

Nonsterile Compounding

- Simple: Mixing two or more commercial products to form a new compounded preparation; simple activities not requiring advanced calculations, dilutions, or working with hazardous materials
- Complex: Special training, equipment, environment, facilities, and procedures required; specialized dosage forms. Includes compounding using bulk chemicals; compounded preparations requiring complex calculations; compounded preparations requiring aliquots, dilutions, or other forms; compounding using hazardous materials

Sterile Compounding

- Low Risk: International Organization for Standardization (ISO) Class 5 working conditions; sterile ingredients, products, components, and devices; limited manipulations; simple transfer; single transfers from ampules, bottles, bags, and vials using sterile syringes with sterile needles, and other means; manually measuring and mixing up to three products to compound a drug admixture or nutritional solution
- Moderate Risk: Multiple individual or small doses combined or pooled for multiple patients or for one patient on multiple occasions; complex aseptic manipulations; long compounding process; no bacteriostatic agents; medications administered over several days; total parenteral nutrition (TPN) solutions; filling reservoirs with multiple drug products; filling reservoirs for administration over several days and transfer from multiple ampules/vials into a single, final sterile container
- High Risk: Nonsterile ingredients or a nonsterile device is employed before terminal sterilization; sterile ingredients, components, devices, or mixtures are exposed to air quality inferior to ISO Class 5; nonsterile preparations are exposed for at least 6 hours before being sterilized; assumption that the chemical purity and content strength of ingredients meet the original or compendial strength specifications

Compounding of Radiopharmaceuticals (Nuclear)

- Preparation of radiopharmaceuticals
- Complex due to handling, packaging, and regulatory agency requirements

Veterinary Compounding

- Preparation of veterinary pharmaceuticals
- Complex due to the uniqueness of patients and/or different regulations

STANDARDS OF PRACTICE

United States Pharmacopeia (USP)

- Has set official standards for drugs in the United States since 1906

- *Pharmacists' Pharmacopeia* introduced in 1820
- USP developed for pharmacy in 1900
- 1900s: USP became more oriented toward manufacturing
- 2000s: USP must meet the needs of both pharmacists and manufacturers
- January 2004: *USP: Pharmacists Edition* was created

U.S. Pharmacopeia Activities (2000–2010)

- Almost 200 official monographs related to compounding
- More monographs being prepared
- Chapters relating to compounding
  - USP <795> Pharmaceutical Compounding Nonsterile
  - USP <797> Pharmaceutical Compounding Sterile
  - USP <1160> Pharmaceutical Calculations
  - USP <1163> Quality Assurance in Pharmaceutical Compounding

USP is an independent organization. USP regulations, numerically greater than 1,000, are generally not recognized as enforceable but rather are considered informational. In contrast, USP standards, numerically less than 1,000, are generally enforceable and are considered requirements. The USP <795> nonsterile standard, for example, was created in 1996 and made enforceable in 1997. This standard is intended to protect both patient and pharmacist. It contains information on responsibility, facilities and equipment, stability, ingredient selection, and the compounding process based on dosage form, records, and documentation. Some areas noted in USP <795> include the following:

1. Responsibility of the compounding pharmacist
   a. Assurance of quality
   b. Controlled processes
   c. Error prevention and documentation
2. Environment and equipment
   a. Must have adequate space
   b. Appropriate conditions
   c. Lighting, temperature, ventilation, and storage
   d. Potable water
   e. Purified water for all compounds
   f. Equipment must be rinsed and cleaned each time it is used
   g. Clean and sanitary conditions
   h. Cleaning is necessary in the environment to reduce cross-contamination
   i. Working surface must be nonreactive with each product used
   j. Must be able to accurately measure products and have all equipment to do so
3. The stability of compounded drugs is the responsibility of the compounder. An appropriate beyond-use date (BUD) must be established for each compound. USP has established the following guidelines for BUD:
   a. Solids and nonaqueous liquids prepared from commercially available dosage forms: 25% of the remaining ingredient expiration *or* 6 months
   b. Solids and nonaqueous liquids prepared from bulk ingredients: 6 months
   c. Water-containing formulations (prepared from ingredients in solid form): 14 days when refrigerated
   d. All other formulations: 30 days *or* the intended duration of therapy, whichever is earlier
4. Ingredient selection
   a. Use USP- and NF-grade ingredients if available
   b. If not available, use high-quality ingredients from a reliable source; use Certificates of Analysis (C of A) to establish the quality of the ingredients used
   c. Always check the FDA's "do not compound" list
5. Acceptable strength, quality, and purity suggested checklist questions:
   a. Have the physical, chemical, medicinal, dietary, and pharmaceutical uses of the drug substance been reviewed?
   b. Are the quantity and quality of each active ingredient identifiable?
   c. Will the active ingredient be effectively absorbed, locally or systemically according to the prescribed purpose, from the preparation and route of administration?
   d. Are there added substances, either confirmed or potentially present from manufactured products, that might be expected to cause an allergic reaction, irritation, toxicity, or undesirable organoleptic response from the patient? Are there added substances, confirmed or potentially present, that may be unfavorable?
   e. Were all calculations and measurements confirmed to ensure that the preparation will be compounded accurately?
6. The compounding process: 13 steps to minimize and maximize the prescriber's intent
7. Quality control
8. Patient counseling

Pharmacy Compounding Accreditation Board (PCAB)

The Pharmacy Compounding Accreditation Board is an organization that was founded by eight of the nation's leading pharmacy organizations, which joined together to create a voluntary system of standard compliance for compounding pharmacies.

The mission of PCAB is to enhance the public good by serving pharmacists, patients, and prescribers through organizing and carrying out a comprehensive program of voluntary accreditation in the practice of pharmacy compounding. The organization seeks to promote, develop, and maintain principles, policies, and standards for the practice of pharmacy compounding in the public interest, and by applying these principles, policies, and standards in the accreditation of pharmacies that offer pharmacy compounding, to improve the quality and safety of pharmacy compounding provided to the general public. PCAB accreditation enables both the public and prescribers to identify those pharmacies that satisfy the organization's criteria. PCAB also provides a public forum that supplies information on the practice of pharmacy compounding to educate the public on the importance of pharmacy compounding.

The PCAB standards cover the following general areas:

- Regulatory compliance
- Personnel
- Facilities and equipment
- Chemicals, components, and completed compounded preparations
- Compounding process standard
- Beyond-use dating, stability, and sterility
- Completed compounded preparations
- Practitioner and patient education
- Quality assurance plan
- Self-assessment

PHARMACY COMPOUNDING REGULATIONS

Pharmacy State Boards

State Boards of Pharmacy are the agencies responsible for regulating pharmacy practices, including compounding, in their respective state. There exists some diversity in pharmacy compounding requirements from state to state, with some being very active in the practice area and others not. Supporting these state boards is the National Association of Boards of Pharmacy (NABP), an independent association that assists its member state boards and jurisdictions in developing, implementing, and enforcing uniform standards, including those dealing with compounding, for the purpose of protecting the public health.

Food and Drug Administration

In 1997, as part of the Food and Drug Administration Modernization Act (FDAMA), the Food, Drug and Cosmetic Act (FDCA) of 1938 was amended to clarify the status of pharmacy compounding under federal laws. According to the FDA, this act creates a special exemption to ensure continued availability of compounded drug products prepared by pharmacists, thereby providing patients with individualized therapies not available commercially. The law, however, seeks to prevent manufacturing under the guise of compounding by establishing parameters within which the practice is appropriate and lawful. The 1997 amendment, however, was legally challenged on the grounds of impermissible regulation of commercial speech and was invalidated by the U.S. Supreme Court in 2002. Subsequent to the Supreme Court decision, the FDA issued a guidance document suggesting areas in which it will exercise enforcement activities against compounding pharmacies. Broadly stated, the FDA will defer to state boards regarding less significant violations of the FDCA unless the pharmacy's activities raise concerns similar to those associated with a drug manufacturer.

Of additional importance to pharmacists, the FDA publishes a list of drugs that cannot be compounded (except under specific conditions mentioned). The "List of Drug Products That Have Been Withdrawn or Removed from the Market for Reasons of Safety or Effectiveness" was originally published in the *Federal Register,* Volume 64, Number 44. A listing is available at http://www.fda.gov/ohrms/dockets/98fr/100898b.txt. A few examples from this list are provided here:

- Camphorated oil: all drug products containing camphorated oil
- Chlorhexidine gluconate: all tinctures of chlorhexidine gluconate formulated for use as a patient preoperative skin preparation
- Chloroform: all drug products containing chloroform
- Diethylstilbestrol: all oral and parenteral drug products containing 25 mg or more of diethylstilbestrol per unit dose
- Dipyrone: all drug products containing dipyrone
- Fenfluramine hydrochloride: all drug products containing fenfluramine hydrochloride
- Gonadotropin chorionic: all drug products containing chorionic gonadotropins of animal origin
- Nitrofurazone: all drug products containing nitrofurazone (except topical drug products formulated for dermatologic application)

- Phenformin hydrochloride: all drug products containing phenformin hydrochloride
- Potassium chloride: all solid oral dosage form drug products containing potassium chloride that supply 100 mg or more of potassium per dosage unit (except for controlled-release dosage forms and those products formulated for preparation of solution prior to ingestion)
- Sulfathiazole: all drug products containing sulfathiazole (except those formulated for vaginal use)
- Tetracycline: all liquid oral drug products formulated for pediatric use containing tetracycline in a concentration greater than 25 mg/mL

Drug Enforcement Agency

Compounding pharmacy is not an easy venue in which to process and manage controlled substances, owing to the limited capacity of some pharmacy computer systems to track quantities received, utilized, and dispensed; unlike many retail systems, pharmacy computer systems may not support point-of-sale updating of quantities on hand. Complicating the process further is the need to inventory many of the controlled substances in the form of bulk powders and liquids—a factor that makes inventory control much more complex than simply counting tablets or capsules as part of an organization's scheduled manual audits.

The Drug Enforcement Agency (DEA) website provides additional information on the Controlled Substances Act: www.usdoj.gov/dea/pubs/csa.html. It is important for all pertinent pharmacy personnel to be familiar with the various scheduled controlled substances. In some cases, a compounding pharmacy may purchase a controlled substance under one class, but once the compound is formulated, the prescription dispensed may be classified within another category. For example, hydrocodone powder is a Class II substance; however, if combined with a common co-ingredient such as acetaminophen, it then becomes a Class III scheduled compound. If the compound's only active ingredient is hydrocodone, then the rules and regulations for dispensing a Class II substance would apply; if it is a Class III substance, then those rules and regulations apply, which will make refills and reordering an easier process.

Miscellaneous Regulatory Agencies

Healthcare workers who prepare or administer hazardous drugs or work in areas where they are used may be exposed to those substances through a variety of avenues, including air, work surfaces, and contaminated clothing. Workplace exposure has been shown to be associated with health effects such as skin rashes, decreased fertility, spontaneous abortions, congenital malformations, and possibly leukemia and other cancers. Additionally, the handling, transporting, shipping, and destruction of hazardous chemicals can contaminate nonemployees and the general public. The level of health risk corresponds to the extent of exposure and the potency of the hazardous drug. Potential adverse effects can be minimized or eliminated through proper handling and use of protective equipment, as well as the proper containment and disposal.

In addition to the State Boards of Pharmacy, several federal agencies have oversight in the area of hazardous chemicals:

Occupational and Safety Health Administration

The Occupational and Safety Health Administration (OSHA) was founded in 1970 as an agency for the U.S. Department of Labor. Its main mission is to prevent the occurrence of workplace illness, injury, or death by establishing safety and health guidelines and regulations that all businesses, including pharmacies, must follow. Failure to follow the guidelines set up by OSHA may result in fines and potentially the closure of the pharmacy.

OSHA has established standards for electrical hazards, fire, hazardous materials, personal protection, violence, and other areas. These guidelines are intended to promote safety in the workplace by encouraging employees to follow all safety precautions when working with everything from heavy machinery to hazardous chemicals. If there is an incident or a report, OSHA is likely to investigate the event and determine whether it involved human error or equipment malfunction.

OSHA defines a hazardous chemical in its Federal Hazard Communication Standard (HCS) as "any chemical that is a physical or health hazard." A health hazard is defined as a chemical for which statistically significant evidence supports the contention that acute or chronic health effects may occur in exposed employees. Such chemicals include carcinogens, toxic and highly toxic agents, reproductive toxins, irritants, corrosives, sensitizers, and agents that produce target organ effects.

National Institute for Occupational Safety and Health

The National Institute for Occupational Safety and Health (NIOSH) develops and establishes occupational health and safety standards, conducts research to develop new criteria for improving health and safety standards, and makes recommendations on those standards. This agency was created by the Occupational Safety and Health Act of 1970. It is part of the Centers for Disease Control and Prevention (CDC) in the Department of Health and Human Services.

Some activities that NIOSH agents may undertake include the investigation of hazardous working conditions, evaluation of workplace hazards, development of scientifically valid recommendations for worker protection after conducting research in relevant areas, and education and training for individuals working or preparing to work in the field of occupational safety or health. Whereas OSHA is responsible for investigation and fines after workplace injuries, NIOSH is responsible for researching and developing policies to prevent workplace injuries before they happen.

Key Terms

NIOSH Hazardous Drug Alert: A chemical or drug that exerts one or of the following activities: genotoxicity, carcinogenicity, teratogenicity/ development toxicity, reproductive toxicity, organ toxicity at low dose, and structure/toxicity profile for a new drug that mimics the structure/toxicity profile of existing hazardous drugs.

Environmental Protection Agency

The Environmental Protection Agency (EPA) implements federal laws designed to promote public health by protecting the United States' air, water, and soil from harmful pollution. In the event of an incident of a reported exposure through the air, water, or soil due to a chemical from a pharmacy, the EPA may have jurisdiction.

COMPOUNDING FACILITIES

Many facility designs are possible for areas where nonsterile preparations are compounded. As contrasted with sterile facilities, a smaller degree of specificity exists. When a facility is designed, it is important that it is designed to ensure a safe work environment for laboratory employees and that the resulting preparation is not contaminated. Several considerations for facility design are in this section.

Countertops

Countertops come in many different materials, surfaces, and styles. To select the countertop that suits an organization's needs, it must consider how the countertop will be used and which materials, chemicals, and temperatures it will come in contact with; in addition, the countertop's quality, design, and cost must be taken into account.

Lighting

Adequate, glare-free lighting is necessary throughout the laboratory facility. Unshielded lighting, the presence of harsh shadows and annoying reflections, and insufficient illumination are to be avoided in the design of the laboratory. Shielded fluorescent lights are particularly effective in providing sufficient lighting without direct glare. Placement of workstations facing windows or reflective walls tends to produce visual fatigue.

Floors

Floors should be as durable and maintenance free as possible. They should be kept dry and free from accumulated debris. Finishes should be antislip. Mats should be in good condition.

Carpeting is not recommended for laboratory areas.

Ventilation, Heating, Cooling, and Indoor Air Quality

While specific sources of chemical-related emissions are generally controlled, such as with powder containment hoods, fume hoods, and local exhaust ventilation, general room and building ventilation have a considerable effect on the air quality in the laboratory and associated areas.

In design of the ventilation system, air intakes and exhausts should be located so as to avoid reentry of contaminated air. Powder containment or fume hoods and biological safety cabinets should be located in low-traffic areas and away from air supply locations. Additional general ventilation may be required for stockroom and storerooms in the facility.

Closely related to the ventilation requirements is the need for proper heating and cooling of room air in the pharmacy. Suitable room temperature throughout the year provides comfort to the employees in the facility, thereby encouraging their efficiency and productivity. Winter heating that yields a temperature in the range of 68°F to 74°F and summer cooling to 75°F to 78°F, with appropriate relative humidity, seems to provide the optimal indoor environment. Specific requirements of certain types of analytical equipment and computer operations may require different room conditions and separate systems may be indicated. Some chemicals can have characteristics that can be affected by environmental conditions such as hygroscopic (water gaining) or efflorescence (water loss) traits.

Sanitation Facilities and Lunch and Break Areas

Eating, drinking, smoking, and applying cosmetics are not permitted in areas where hazardous materials are stored or used, or where the potential for occupational exposure to blood or other potentially infectious materials is present. Cross-contamination between food items and hazardous materials is an obvious hazard and should be avoided.

Lunchrooms or break rooms and sanitation facilities, such as restrooms, must be distinctly separated from the main laboratory areas. Employees must, as a matter of routine, be responsible for washing, cleaning, and any other decontamination required when passing from the laboratory to other areas. Any laboratory coats, gloves, or other protective equipment must be removed prior to leaving the laboratory.

COMPOUNDING TECHNIQUES

In the compounding process, the pharmacist must be sure of the purity and stability of the ingredients. The technician is limited to measuring, mixing, molding, and packaging. Each of these steps must then be checked by the pharmacist. The finished product must be stable for its intended use. Some of the procedures used in compounding are outlined in this section.

Geometric Dilution

Definition: A process used to mix two materials evenly to create a homogeneous mixture.

Purpose of geometric dilution: If an even distribution is not obtained in a compounded product, then many quality issues can arise. Failure to utilize the concept of geometric dilution can result in loose powders not being mixed into a base, gritty consistency of the product, or unreliable drug concentrations in each dose. Imbalanced distribution of the active ingredient in the base will result in an inconsistent concentration of the active ingredient throughout the mixture. As a consequence, the patient will receive different doses of medication with each use, and perhaps varying therapeutic effects. In addition, it is possible for the patient to suffer adverse reactions due to this discrepancy.

Procedure for geometric dilution: The smallest quantity of the active ingredient is first placed into the mixing surface (i.e., mixing slab, mortar). An equal amount of base or diluent is then added and mixed thoroughly. Next, amounts of base or diluents equal to the amount of mixture on the mixing surface are added in stages, with the preparation being mixed thoroughly with each new addition. This is repeated until the entire base or diluent is added to the mixture and smoothly distributed.

Trituration

Definition: Can be a compounding process as well as a dilution that results in the formation of an aliquot.

Procedure for trituration: A powder is ground to a finer state in a mortar using a pestle. Trituration is also used to blend several powders together while reducing particle size at the same time.

Dilution

Definition: Mixture of a potent drug powder with an inert diluent powder, usually lactose, in a definite proportion by weight. A weighable portion (i.e., an aliquot) of the mixture containing the desired quantity of substance may then be used to maintain an acceptable range of accuracy.

Procedure for dilution: Using ratio and proportion, the weight of drug and lactose required to make the trituration can be determined, as well as the weight of the aliquot to be used to fill the prescription.

$$\frac{\text{Weight of drug in trituration}}{\text{Weight of trituration}} = \frac{\text{Weight of drug in aliquot}}{\text{Weight of aliquot}}$$

Levigation

Definition: Triturating a powdered drug in a mortar or spatulating it on an ointment slab with a solvent in which it is insoluble, with the goal of reducing the drug's particle size.

EQUIPMENT

The main pieces of equipment used to compound nonsterile medications are identified in this section.

Balance

The balance is perhaps the single-most important piece of equipment in nonsterile compounding. The most popular form is the torsion balance. The main accessories are weighing papers, or weighing boats, and weights.

Class A Prescription Balance

- Two-pan torsion balance
- Internal and external weights
- Capacity: minimum, 120 mg; maximum, 60 g
- Sensitivity: usually 6 mg

Electronic (Digital) or Analytical Balance

- Various sizes and shapes
- Often used to weigh quantities smaller than 120 mg
- Sensitivities vary: usually ≤ 1 mg

Weighing

It is generally agreed that pharmaceutical products should be prepared with a low percentage of error. The official compendia allow a tolerance of ± 5% for most formulas, although greater accuracy may be required for very potent drugs with greater toxicity potential. This same degree of accuracy is expected in all extemporaneously compounded products. Most pharmaceutical products allow for a tolerance of only **5% error**.

$$\% \text{ error} = \frac{\text{error of measurment}}{\text{quantity desired}} \times 100\%$$

If the sensitivity of the balance is known, we can calculate the percentage of possible error when any amount of the substance is weighed.

$$\% \text{ error} = \frac{\text{sensitivity}}{\text{quantity desired}} \times 100\%$$

As an example, the Class A prescription balance has a sensitivity of 6 mg. What percentage of error would result from weighing 50 mg of a drug on the balance?

$$\% \text{ error} = \frac{6 \text{ mg}}{50 \text{ mg}} \times 100\% = 12\%$$

Similarly, we can calculate the smallest quantity that can be weighed, on a balance of known sensitivity, to maintain a desired level of accuracy. This weight is referred to as the **least weighable quantity (LWQ)**.

$$\text{LWQ} = \frac{\text{sensitivity}}{\% \text{ error tolerated}} \times 100\%$$

As an example, consider the least weighable quantity that will result in an error of 5% or less on a Class A prescription balance:

$$\text{LWQ} = \frac{6 \text{ mg}}{5\%} \times 100\% = 120 \text{ mg}$$

When a prescription formula calls for the incorporation of a component weighing less than 120 mg, special methods must be employed to obtain that weight of the component. When the component must be incorporated as a solid into powders, tablets, capsules, or pastes, the *trituration method* is used.

The balance is used to measure solids, but there are several options for measuring volumes. Common volumetric vessels include pipets, cylindrical and conical graduates, burets, syringes, and volumetric flasks. Always use the smallest device that will accommodate the desired volume of liquid. Use a graduated pipet or syringe to measure volumes less than 1 mL. Oily and viscous liquids are difficult to remove from graduates and pipettes; in these cases, syringes may be a better choice.

Liquids develop a meniscus when they are poured into containers; that is, the surface of the liquid curves downward toward the center. To compensate for this effect, hold the graduate at eye level and read the mark at the bottom of the meniscus.

Droppers are also used to deliver small doses of liquid medication. The dropper must be calibrated by dropping the formulation slowly into a small graduate and counting the number of drops need to make several milliliters in the graduate; using these data, calculate the number of drops per milliliter.

Syringes are also used for liquid measure. Their sizes range from 0.5 mL to 60 mL. They are easy to use and especially good choices for viscous liquids.

Other Equipment

Hot plates with or without a magnetic stirrer, blenders, and electric ointment mills are used to reduce particle size and homogenize mixtures. Electronic mortars and pestles, manual capsule machines, and tube sealing presses are also used in nonsterile compounding.

Other essential items needed for compounding include a mortar (the vessel) and pestle (grinds materials in the mortar), ointment slab or papers, spatula, molds (e.g., suppository or troche), and other equipment for specialized compounding.

FORMS OF COMPOUNDED MEDICATIONS

Capsules

Definition: Solid dosage forms often intended for oral administrations that contain one or more active pharmaceutical ingredients (APIs) in a gelatin capsule that consists of a body and a cap. There are 8 sizes of capsules, ranging from #000 to #5. Size 5 holds 60–130 mg, and size #000 holds 616–1,370 mg. Gelatin capsules are derived from animal sources; cellulose capsules are available for those patients desiring preparations derived from nonanimal sources. Pharmacies preparing capsule formulations often use manual 100- or 300-count capsule machines or use the hand-fill or punch method.

Oral Liquids

Suspensions

Definition: Mixture of two substances resulting in two phases, where one is finely divided and dispersed (or suspended) in the other. The particles in a suspension are visible under a microscope and can be seen by the naked eye; and precipitate if allowed to stand undisturbed (e.g., milk of magnesia).

Common suspending agents: It is important to pick the appropriate suspending agent/solvent for the drug, as the viscosity of the suspending agents affects the settling rate. The following options are available:

- Xanthan gum
- Polysorbate-80
- Simple syrup
- Methylcellulose
- Ora-Sweet SF

Solutions

Definition: A homogeneous mixture of two or more substances, where the solute(s) is (are) dissolved in a solvent.

Types (noninclusive):

- Syrups: A syrup is a concentrated or nearly saturated solution of sucrose in water. Syrups with flavoring agents are called flavoring syrups (e.g., cherry syrup). Medical syrups contain medication, whereas simple syrup (syrup USP) is 850 g of sucrose in 450 mL of water.
- Elixirs: Elixirs contain alcohol and water. Alcohol serves as the solvent for a drug. The amount of alcohol will vary with the amount of drug to be dissolved. Elixirs should be avoided with selected patient populations.

Emulsions

Definition: Unstable system consisting of at least two immiscible liquids. Very useful to mask taste and improve palatability of orally administered formulations.

Types:

- Oil in water (o/w) oil dispersed in an aqueous phase
- Water in oil (w/o) water dispersed in an oil phase

A lower hydrophilic–lipophilic balance (HLB) value (1–9) favors a water in oil (w/o) emulsion; a higher HLB value (≥ 10) favors an oil in water emulsion (o/w) emulsion.

Flavoring agents should be compatible and incorporated into the dominant (external) phase of an emulsion if intended for oral administration.

An emulsifying agent (i.e., an emulsifier) is a stabilizing agent in emulsions to prevent separation. Emulsifying agents include the following options, among others:

- Acacia is a gum that is a natural polysaccharide derived from the sap of the African acacia tree.
- Tween (polysorbate) is a hydrophilic, nonionic surfactant and emulsifier derived from polyethoxylated sorbitan and oleic acid.
- Span is a lipophilic agent produced from sorbitol and lauric acid, a normal fatty acid from vegetable or animal origin.

Semisolid Dosage Forms

Creams

Definition: An emulsion of oil and water components often combined with an active pharmaceutical ingredient that demonstrates a fluid-like consistency when applied to the skin.

Lotions

Definition: An aqueous preparation easily absorbed by the skin, generally consisting of a fine, insoluble powder permanently suspended in the preparation. Lotions are useful when a thin layer of medication is needed over a large area. The formulation can be oil-in-water (e.g., Keri Lotion) or water-in-oil (e.g., Lubriderm Lotion). Most lotions are oil-in-water formulations.

Emulsifying agents, such as cetearyl alcohol, are often used to keep the emulsion together in a lotion. The emulsifying agent prevents the oil and aqueous phases from separating by reducing the surface tension.

The difference between lotions and creams is usually recognized as being that lotions are thinner than creams and less oily than ointments. Lotions usually contain more alcohol (to emulsify the ingredients) than creams do—a factor that can actually lead to drying of the skin.

Gels

Definition: A colloidal dispersion composed of small inorganic particles or large organic molecules in which the particles restrict movement of the dispersed medium. Gels are fine dispersions of 5–10 microns.

Types:

- Carbomers: An often-used brand name, Carbopol, is a polymer that forms an acid aqueous solution (pH of approximately 3.0). The gel thickens as a pH increase occurs upon the addition of a pH enhancer such as sodium hydroxide or triethanoloamine.

- Cellulose derivatives: Methylcellulose, hydroxyethylcellulose, hydroxypropyl cellulose, hrdroxypropyl methylcellulose, and hydroxypropyl cellulose are commonly used derivatives.
- Poloxamers: These copolymers of polyoxyethylene and polyoxypropylene form reverse thermal gels, which exist as gels at room or body temperature and as liquids at cool temperatures, in concentrations from 15% to 50%. Pluronic F-127 is often combined with a lecithin and isopropyl palmitate solution (LIPS) to prepare a PLO gel (pluronic lecithin organogel). The pluronic poloxamer is often the dominant phase in which water-soluble active pharmaceutical ingredients are dissolved. The LIPS is the phase into which oil-soluble APIs are dissolved. The two phases are combined under shear stress, which forms a microemulsion with the API that can be used as a delivery vehicle, allowing for the transcutaneous administration of the API.

Ointments

Definition: A viscous or semisolid substance used on the skin as a protective, cosmetic, emollient, or medicament. Ointments remain on the skin for an extended time, which allows for the retention of cutaneous-derived moisture and aids in the retention and contact time of APIs contained within the ointment.

Types (noninclusive):

- Water in oil (w/o): cold cream
- Oil in water (w/o): emollient cream

Pastes

Definition: A substance that contains more solid material than an ointment and often consists of more than 20% solids, making its consistency much stiffer and causing more difficulty in spreading. Pastes generally are not formulated to allow the penetration of an API into the skin but more so for their ability and intended use to absorb serous discharges or for their protective ability (e.g., zinc oxide.)

Suppositories

Definition: A semisolid dosage form intended for insertion into the rectum, vagina, or urethra, thereby providing either localized or systemic therapy.

- Rectal route: A viable route when nausea and vomiting prevent the effective administration of a medication through the oral route. Hepatic first-pass metabolism is not completely avoided due to some absorption via the superior hemorrhoidal vein, which terminates into the hepatoportal vein. Drugs intended for systemic activity often demonstrate an erratic absorption profile. The maximum amount of a solid material contained in a suppository should be less than 30% of the base volume. Excess suppository volume introduced into the rectum can result in defecation—an important consideration for the compounder of a suppository.
- Vaginal route: Often used to attain a local effect in or near the vaginal tract. Systemic absorption can occur and must be considered when selecting APIs.
- Urethral route: Often used for local effects such as anesthetization or antimicrobial activities of the urethra. Some dosage forms are used for erectile dysfunction in males. The female urethral suppository can be 25–70 mm in length; the male version is 50–125 mm in length.

Suppository bases: Suppository bases should be nonirritating, and should melt at body temperature and in the presence of mucous secretions.

- Oleaginous bases: Include cocoa butter (theobroma oil). Newer synthetic triglyceride bases (e.g., MBK, FattiBase) are associated with formulation issues than the traditional cocoa butter.
- Water-soluble/water-miscible bases: Melt in mucosal fluids. Melting does not depend on body temperature alone, which affords an advantage during storage and handling relative to oleaginous bases. Water-soluble/water-miscible bases are often used for vaginal and urethral administration. Glycerinated gelatin is often used for vaginal suppositories. Polyethylene glycol (PEG) bases offer the advantage of being water soluble and can be formulated in different hardness and melting points based on type or combination of PEG used.

Lozenges and Troches

Definition: semisolid preparations formulated to dissolve in the mouth for local effect (lozenge) or systemic use (troche). These dosage forms can be hard or soft ("gummy") depending on the type of base used. Typical bases include sugars, polyethylene glycol (PEG), or gelatin to form a "chewy" dosage form.

Medicated Sticks

Definition: A semisolid dosage form often used to administer medications for topical activity. Can be applied to the skin and lips and can contain anesthetic APIs, antibiotics, antivirals, emollient agents, and sunscreens.

ANNOTATED BIBLIOGRAPHY

Allen LV Jr. *The Art, Science and Technology of Pharmaceutical Compounding,* 2nd ed. Washington, DC: American Pharmaceutical Association; 2002.

American Society of Health-System Pharmacists. ASHP guidelines: minimum standards for pharmacies in hospitals. *Am J Health Syst Pharm* 1995;52: 2711–2717.

Bormel G, Valentino JG, Williams RL, McElhiney LF. Application of USP-NF standards to pharmacy compounding international. *J Pharm Compounding* 2009;7:361–363.

Food and Drug Administration Modernization Act of 1997. Application of federal law to practice of pharmacy compounding [Page 111 STAT. 2296]. Public Law 105-115 105th Congress. Updated June 18, 2009; cited October 14, 2009. Available at: http://www.fda.gov/Drugs/GuidanceCompliance RegulatoryInformation/PharmacyCompounding /ucm155666.htm.

McElhiney LF. An overview of United States Pharmacopeia Chapter <795> and American Society of Health-System Pharmacists guidelines for nonsterile compounding. *Int J Pharm Compounding* 2009;13:525–530.

National Association of Boards of Pharmacy. Model State Pharmacy Act and model rules of the National Association of Boards of Pharmacy, 2007. Available at: http://www.nabp.net/ftpfiles/nabp01 /lelreport2007.pdf. Accessed March 4, 2010.

Pharmacy Compounding Accreditation Board. Standards with compliance indicators. Available at: http://www.pcab.info/standards.shtml.

Shrewsbury R. *Applied Pharmaceutics in Contemporary Compounding,* 2nd ed. Englewood, CO: Morton; 2008.

United States Pharmacopeial Convention, Inc. *USP Drug Information, Vol. III: Approved Drug Products and Legal Requirements.* Taunton, MA: Quebecor World; 1998.

United States Pharmacopeial Convention, Inc. *USP-Pharmacists' Pharmacopeia.* Rockville, MD: Author; 2005a;408–413.

United States Pharmacopeial Convention, Inc. *<795> Pharmaceutical Compounding—Nonsterile Preparations: The United States Pharmacopeia 29/ National Formulary 25.* Rockville, MD: Author; 2005b:2731–2735.

http://www.fda.gov/ohrms/dockets/98fr/100898b.txt

http://www.usdoj.gov/dea/pubs/csa.html

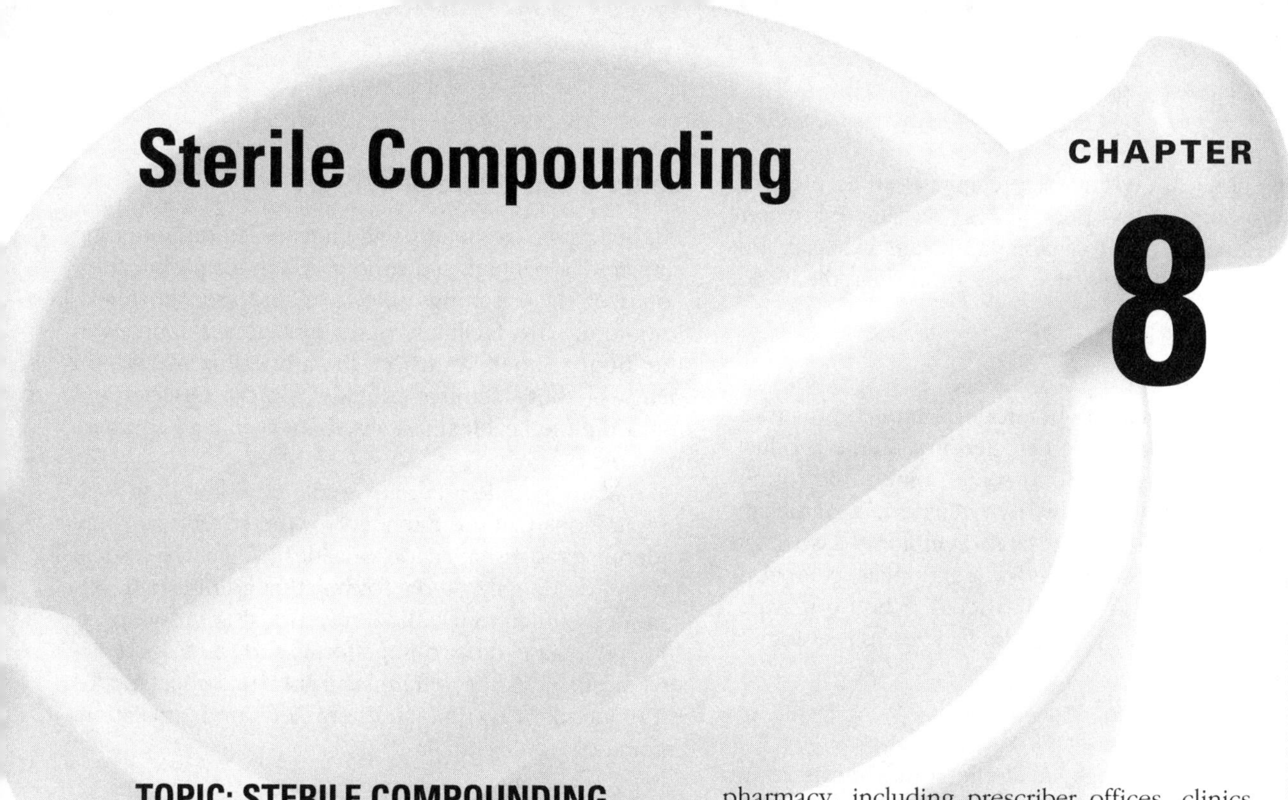

Sterile Compounding

CHAPTER

8

TOPIC: STERILE COMPOUNDING

Contributor: Kenneth R. Speidel

Introduction

Definition of Compounding

Compounding is defined as the preparation, mixing, assembling, packaging, or labeling of a drug or device (1) as the result of a practitioner's prescription drug order or initiated based on the practitioner–patient–pharmacist relationship in the course of professional practice; (2) through reconstitution or manipulation of commercial products that may require the addition of one or more ingredients, as a result of a licensed practitioner's order; or (3) for the purpose of, or incident to, research, teaching, or chemical analysis, and not for sale or dispensing.

Compounding may be conducted in anticipation of receiving prescription orders when based on routine, regularly observed prescribing patterns. Anticipatory compounding is limited to reasonable quantities, based on such patterns.

There often exist misperceptions and misunderstandings that the term "compounding" refers only to nonsterile preparations, does not include activities within a hospital pharmacy, and pertains only to the profession of pharmacy. Compounding of sterile dosage forms within U.S. hospitals has been a common and acceptable practice for many decades. Additionally, USP <797> includes guidelines for compounded sterile products (CSPs) that are prepared and handled in a variety of settings outside of a pharmacy, including prescriber offices, clinics, and other healthcare facilities.

It is important for pharmacists to be competent in the subject of sterile product preparation due to the common utilization of sterile formulations in many healthcare settings. This chapter provides basic knowledge of the definitions, regulations, standards of practice, and other considerations to enable the pharmacist to advance toward competency in safely handling CSPs.

Critical Requirements of Final Preparations of Compounded Sterile Products

Personnel preparing CSPs must be aware of critical aspects of final preparations:

- Sterility
- Particulate material solutions
- Endotoxin/pyrogen-free
- Potency
- pH
- Osmotic pressure

Sterility

Sterility is the freedom from bacteria and other microorganisms. Formulations must be sterile.

Particulate-free

Particulate-free solutions must be maintained in the final preparation. The pharmacist performing compounding must consider various means, such as a light box and visual inspection, plus final filtration, to ensure these particles are not present. Particulates can consist of rubber stopper cores, chemical crystals, or precipitates (e.g., metal or glass, to name a few possibilities). Sterile suspensions and ointments may contain particulate material, but these are usually the active drug or an ingredient, not contaminants.

Pyrogen-free

Pyrogens are metabolic by-products of living microorganisms. If pyrogens are detected in a sterile product, bacteria have proliferated at some point in the formulation process. In humans, pyrogens cause significant discomfort but are rarely fatal. Symptoms associated with their presence include fever and chills, cutaneous vasoconstriction, increased arterial blood pressure, increased heart workload, and other physiological manifestations.

Potency

The potency of drugs in sterile formulations is an important consideration. In the past, CSPs were often prepared just prior to administration. Today, with increased demands on time, home infusion therapy, central filling of orders to compound CSPs, and enhanced evidence-based stability data, longer "beyond use" dates (BUDs) have been utilized. The USP has developed BUD guidelines for CSPs for which BUDs are not available.

pH

Physiological pH is approximately 7.4. When injected into human tissue, a product with this pH is optimal for tissue comfort. Many commercially available products, because of the nature of the chemicals within them, do not exist at physiological pH and are known to cause discomfort upon administration. CSPs as close to possible to physiologic pH will improve tolerance.

Osmotic Pressure

Osmotic pressure is a characteristic of any solution that results from the number of dissolved particles in the solution. Blood has an osmolarity of approximately 300 milliosmoles per liter (mOsmol/L). Ideally, any sterile solution will be formulated to have this osmolarity. The most commonly used large volume parenteral solutions have osmolarities similar to that of blood (e.g. 0.9% sodium chloride solution –308 mOsmol/L) and 5% dextrose solution –252 mOsmol/L).

Intravenous solutions that have higher osmolarity values (hypertonic) or lower osmolarity values (hypotonic) may cause damage to red blood cells, pain, and tissue irritation. Nevertheless, in some therapeutic situations, it may be necessary to administer hypertonic or hypotonic solutions. In these cases, the solutions are usually given slowly through large veins to minimize reactions.

Settings and Routes of Delivery

Pharmacists have been providing sterile compounding services for patients in a variety of settings for decades. Some of these settings include acute care hospitals, long-term care facilities, outpatient clinics, and even the home (home infusion therapy). Pharmacists in many of these settings provide clinical services and assist the medical team to assess and manage complex therapies.

Many people associate sterile compounding with preparations that are intended for the parenteral route (administered by injection outside the gastrointestinal tract). Additionally, sterile formulation administration is further assumed to use the intravenous (IV) route only. In reality, many other dosage forms and routes of delivery exist, including intramuscular (IM), subcutaneous (SQ), intradermal (ID), intrathecal, epidural, inhalation, intranasal, and ophthalmic.

Routes of Delivery of Compounded Sterile Preparations

Intravenous (IV) Route

Drugs delivered by the IV route have a rapid onset of action. Solutions are administered directly into a vein and, therefore, directly into the blood supply. Most solutions are water based (aqueous), but glycols, alcohols, and nonaqueous solvents are also possible.

Intramuscular (IM) Route

Solutions or suspensions administered via the IM route are injected deep into the muscle fibers under the subcutaneous layer of skin. Needles are generally 19 to 22 gauge and 1 inch to 1.5 inches long, depending on the intended size and location of the muscle. Principal IM sites are the gluteal (buttock), deltoid (upper arm), and vastus lateralis (thigh) muscles. Injection sites must be rotated when multiple injections are required. Use of the IM route is limited by volume: only 2 mL (deltoid) to 5 mL (gluteus) of solution can be injected. This route generally results in lower but longer-lasting blood concentrations (depot). Usually an IM injection is more painful than other routes. A "Z-tract" is a technique used for IM administration of medications that stain the skin (e.g., iron preparations).

Subcutaneous (SQ, SC) Route

With the SQ or SC route, solutions or suspensions are administered beneath the surface of the skin. This approach can be used for both short-term and long-term therapies. The choice of site allows for the implantation of a cannula or needle beneath the surface of the skin, thereby allowing the drug to be infused slowly over a longer period of time. Frequently used sites include the lower abdomen, anterior aspect of the thigh, upper back, and posterior upper arm. Injection sites must be rotated to prevent irritation. The maximum amount injected is usually 2 mL or less. Needles are generally $^3/_8$ to 1 inch in length and 24 to 28 gauge.

Intradermal (ID) Route

With the ID route, the drug is administered into the very top layer of the skin (usually in the forearm) and usually a small amount of solution (approximately 0.1 mL) is delivered. This approach is often used for diagnostic reasons, desensitization, or immunization. Adverse effects are generally local. Intradermal injections may create a wheal (i.e., a raised blister-like area). Needles are generally $^3/_8$ inch long and 23 to 26 gauge.

Intra-arterial Route

With the intra-arterial route, the drug is administered directly into an artery. This technique delivers a high concentration of a drug to the site of action. This route is generally used for radiopaque materials and some antineoplastic agents.

Ophthalmic (OS, OD, OU) Route

Drugs are administered to the eye for local treatment of various eye conditions and for anesthesia. Eye products or preparations must be sterile in the final container, and their pH must be carefully controlled. The eye can retain approximately 7 to 10 microliters of medication. Some systemic absorption can occur. Ophthalmic formulations occur as eye drops (suspensions or solutions) and ointments.

Intranasal Route

The surface of the nasal cavity is very large, has a rich blood supply, and can hold about 20 mL. Most intranasal formulations are used for their decongestant activity on the nasal mucosa. More recently, intranasal preparations have been used for immunization and migraine headaches. Intranasal absorption of some drugs could result in blood concentrations close to IV administration. Intranasal formulations include solutions, suspensions, sprays, aerosols, and inhalers.

Inhalation Route

The inhalation route is used to deliver drugs to the pulmonary system (lungs). The drugs administered in this way affect lung function—for example, bronchodilators, steroids, antiallergy medications. Most of the inhalation dosage forms are aerosols that depend on the power of compressed or liquefied gas to expel the drug from the container. Particle size is critical (1–10 microns); if the particles are too large, the drug is swallowed.

Intrathecal Route

The intrathecal route involves administration of solutions into the lumbar spine. Local anesthetics and analgesics are commonly administered via this route. Solutions must be preservative free.

Categories of Compounding: A Review

1. Nonsterile simple
2. Nonsterile complex
3. Sterile-low risk
4. Sterile-moderate risk
5. Sterile-high risk
6. Nuclear pharmacy
7. Veterinary compounding

Categories of compounding are based on the following characteristics:

- Degree of difficulty
- Stability information and warnings
- Packaging and storage requirements
- Dosage forms
- Complexity of calculations
- Local versus systemic effect
- Level of risk to the compounder
- Potential for risk of harm to patient

Sterile Compounding

Low Risk

- International Organization for Standardization (ISO) Class 5 working conditions
- Sterile ingredients, products, components, and devices
- Limited manipulations
- Simple transfers
- Single transfers from ampules, bottles, bags, and vials using sterile syringes with sterile needles
- Manually measuring and mixing up to three products to compound a drug admixture or nutritional solution

Moderate Risk

- Multiple individual or small doses combined or pooled for multiple patients or to one patient on multiple occasions
- Complex aseptic manipulations
- Long compounding process
- No bacteriostatic agents or medications that are administered over several days
- Total parenteral nutrition (TPN) solutions
- Filling reservoirs with multiple drug products
- Filling reservoirs for administration over several days
- Transfer from multiple ampules/vials into single, final sterile container

High Risk

- Nonsterile ingredients or a nonsterile device is employed before terminal sterilization
- Sterile ingredients, components, devices, or mixtures that are exposed to air quality inferior to ISO Class 5
- Nonsterile preparations that are exposed for at least 6 hours before being sterilized
- Assumption that the chemical purity and content strength of the ingredients meets the original or compendial strength specifications

Standards of Practice

The USP

The U.S. Pharmacopeial Convention (USP) is an independent organization. USP regulations numerically greater than 1,000 are generally not recognized as enforceable and, therefore, are considered informational; conversely, USP standards numerically less than 1,000 are generally enforceable and are considered requirements. USP 797 Pharmaceutical Compounding: Sterile Preparations was revised in June 2008 and covers the following areas pertaining to compounding sterile preparations:

- Responsibility of compounding personnel
- CSP microbial contamination risk levels
- Personnel training and evaluation in aseptic manipulation skills
- Immediate-use CSPs (compounded sterile preparations)
- Single-dose and multiple-dose containers
- Hazardous drugs as CSPs
- Radiopharmaceuticals as CSPs
- Allergen extracts as CSPs
- Verification of compounding accuracy and sterility
- Environmental quality and control
- Suggested standard operating procedures (SOPs)
- Elements of Quality Control
- Verification of automated compounding devices for parenteral nutrition compounding
- Finished preparation release checks and tests
- Storage and beyond-use dating
- Maintaining sterility, purity, and stability of dispensed and distributed CSPs
- Patient or caregiver training
- Patient monitoring and adverse events reporting
- Quality assurance program

The criteria for the various CSP risk levels are identified in Table 8-1.

USP guidelines establish minimum allowable standards for compounding. These guidelines were developed as a comprehensive approach to compounding. Training protocols, staffing, strict SOPs encompassing every activity, and strictly controlled processes are at the heart of these standards. Environmental standards are the same for each "risk" level—low, medium, and high. An important aspect of these environmental standards is that they depend on all of the other standards embedded within USP guidelines.

State Boards of Pharmacy

State-to-state variability is observed regarding regulations pertaining to compounding sterile preparations (CSPs). Many states require a separate distinction within the licensure of a pharmacy; others do not. Various states incorporate requirements that the pharmacy preparing CSPs be compliant with standards such as USP <797>. Some states have promulgated their own requirements for sterile preparations. The practicing pharmacist must be aware of the requirements for compounding sterile preparations in the state in which the pharmacy is located as well as any states in which the pharmacy provides CSPs to patients and practitioners (if permitted in the respective state).

CSP Work Environment

The expectation is that the compounding environment will be within a building with fixed support systems. The obtaining of materials, packaging, the compounding process, and the output is also expected to be well controlled. It is recognized that mistakes happen when any aspect of this comprehensive and controlled environment is subject to excessive stress.

Several design methods for clean rooms have been developed. One of the most basic relies on "dependent" air. The conditioned and filtered air poured into one room is first vented into the next room to provide clean air and then vented to the next room; this air is dependent on the prior room to provide the necessary clean air. An accident in a room upstream can affect the downstream rooms, however, so this is not a very robust or adaptable system.

Other designs take advantage of classic architecture, most often using a central HVAC and HEPA filtration system. This central filtration unit would house ducts to transfer clean air to the vents of a clean room. Unfortunately, the materials utilized in the ceiling and walls are often coated materials that can be easily damaged. Thus, this design is often inefficient and meets only the minimum air exchange and filtration coverage requirements. Anterooms are often tiny and materials introduction an afterthought in such designs, and occupational exposure issues typically have not been considered.

Table 8-1 CSP Risk-Level Criteria

Criteria	Low-Risk Level	Medium-Risk Level	High-Risk Level
Compounding conditions	• Compounded entirely under ISO Class 5 (Class 100) conditions • Compounding involves only transfer, measuring, and mixing manipulations, with closed or sealed packaging systems, that are performed promptly and attentively • Manipulations are limited to aseptically opening ampules, penetrating sterile stoppers on vials with sterile needles and syringes, and transferring sterile liquids in sterile syringes to sterile administration devices and packages of other sterile products	• Conditions listed under low risk level • Multiple individual or small doses of sterile products are combined or pooled to prepare a CSP that will be administered either to multiple patients or to one patient on multiple conditions • The compounding process includes complex aseptic manipulations other than the single-volume transfer • The compounding process has an unusually long duration • The sterile CSPs do not contain broad-spectrum bacteriostatic agents, and are administered over several days	• Nonsterile ingredients are incorporated, or a nonsterile device is employed before terminal sterilization • Sterile ingredients, components, devices, and mixtures are exposed to air quality inferior to ISO Class 5 (Class 100) • Nonsterile preparations are exposed for no more than 6 hours before being sterilized • Nonsterile preparations are terminally sterilized, but are not tested for bacterial endotoxins • It is assumed that the chemical purity and content strength of ingredients meet their original or compendial specifications in unopened or in opened packages of bulk ingredients
QA program	• Formalized in writing • Describes specific monitoring and evaluation activities • Describes reporting and evaluation of results • Identifies follow-up activities when thresholds are exceeded • Delineates individual responsibilities for each aspect of the program	• Formalized in writing • Describes specific monitoring and evaluation activities • Describes reporting and evaluation of results • Identifies follow-up activities when thresholds are exceeded • Delineates individual responsibilities for each aspect of the program	• Formalized in writing • Describes specific monitoring and evaluation activities • Describes reporting and evaluation of results • Identifies follow-up activities when thresholds are exceeded • Delineates individual responsibilities for each aspect of the program
QA practices	• Routine disinfection and quality testing of direct compounding environment • Visual confirmation of personnel processes regarding gowning and other measures • Review of orders and packages of ingredients to ensure correct identity and amounts of ingredients • Visual inspection of CSP • Media-fill test procedure performed at least annually	• Routine disinfection and quality testing of direct compounding environment • Visual confirmation of personnel processes regarding gowning and other measures • Review of orders and packages of ingredients to ensure correct identity and amounts of ingredients • Visual inspection of CSP • Media-fill test procedure performed at least annually	• Routine disinfection and quality testing of direct compounding environment • Visual confirmation of personnel processes regarding gowning and other measures • Review of orders and packages of ingredients to ensure correct identity and amounts of ingredients • Visual inspection of CSP • Media-fill test procedure performed at least semi-annually
Outcome monitoring	Yes	Yes	Yes
Reports/ documents	• Written policies and procedures • Adverse event reporting • Complaint procedures • Periodic review of quality control documents	• Written policies and procedures • Adverse event reporting • Complaint procedures • Periodic review of quality control documents	• Written policies and procedures • Adverse event reporting • Complaint procedures • Periodic review of quality control documents

(*continues*)

Table 8-1 (*continued*)

Criteria	Low-Risk Level	Medium-Risk Level	High-Risk Level
Patient and caregiver training	• Formalized program that includes: ○ Understanding of the therapy provided ○ Handling and storage of the CSP ○ Appropriate administration techniques ○ Use and maintenance of any infusion device involved ○ Use of printed material ○ Appropriate follow-up	• Formalized program that includes: ○ Understanding of the therapy provided ○ Handling and storage of the CSP ○ Appropriate administration techniques ○ Use and maintenance of any infusion device involved ○ Use of printed material ○ Appropriate follow-up	• Formalized program that includes: ○ Understanding of the therapy provided ○ Handling and storage of the CSP ○ Appropriate administration techniques ○ Use and maintenance of any infusion device involved ○ Use of printed material ○ Appropriate follow-up
Maintaining product quality and control once the CSP leaves the pharmacy (both institutional based and NICPs)	• Packaging, handling, and transport ○ Written policies and procedures including the packaging, handling, and transport of chemotoxic/hazardous CSPs • Use and storage ○ Written policies and procedures • Administration ○ Written policies and procedures dealing with such issues as hand washing, aseptic technique, site care, and so on • Education/training ○ Written policies and procedures dealing with proper education of patients and caregivers ensuring all of the above	• Packaging, handling, and transport ○ Written policies and procedures including the packaging, handling, and transport of chemotoxic/hazardous CSPs • Use and storage ○ Written policies and procedures • Administration ○ Written policies and procedures dealing with such issues as hand washing, aseptic technique, site care and so on • Education/training ○ Written policies and procedures dealing with proper education of patients and caregivers ensuring all of the above	• Packaging, handling, and transport ○ Written policies and procedures including the packaging, handling, and transport of chemotoxic/hazardous CSPs • Use and storage ○ Written policies and procedures • Administration ○ Written policies and procedures dealing with such issues as hand washing, aseptic technique, site care and so on • Education/training ○ Written policies and procedures dealing with proper education of patients and caregivers ensuring all of the above
Storage and beyond-use dating	• Specific labeling requirements • Specific beyond-use dating policies, procedures, and requirements • Policies regarding storage	• Specific labeling requirements • Specific beyond-use dating policies, procedures, and requirements • Policies regarding storage	• Specific labeling requirements • Specific beyond-use dating policies, procedures, and requirements • Policies regarding storage
Storage conditions and beyond-use dating for completed CSP	In the absence of sterility testing, storage periods (before administration) shall not exceed the following: • Room temperature ≤ 48 hours • 2–8° C≤ 15 days • ≤ 20°C ≤ 45 days	In the absence of sterility testing, storage periods (before administration) shall not exceed the following: • Room temperature ≤ 30 hours • 2–8°C ≤ 7 days • ≤ 20°C ≤ 45 days	In the absence of sterility testing, storage periods (before administration) shall not exceed the following: • Room temperature ≤ 24 hours • 2–8°C ≤ 3 days • ≤ 20°C ≤ 45 days

Table 8-1 (*continued*)

Criteria	Low-Risk Level	Medium-Risk Level	High-Risk Level
Finished product release checks and tests	• Written policies and procedures that address: ○ Physical inspections ○ Compounding accuracy checks ○ Sterility testing ○ Pyrogen testing ○ Potency testing	• Written policies and procedures that address: ○ Physical inspections ○ Compounding accuracy checks ○ Sterility testing ○ Pyrogen testing ○ Potency testing	• Written policies and procedures that address: ○ Physical inspections ○ Compounding accuracy checks ○ Sterility testing ○ Pyrogen testing ○ Potency testing
CSP work environment	• Appropriate solid surfaces • Limited (but necessary) furniture, fixtures, and so on • Ante area • Buffer zone	• Appropriate solid surfaces • Limited (but necessary) furniture, fixtures, and so on • Ante area • Buffer zone	• Appropriate solid surfaces • Limited (but necessary) furniture, fixtures, and so on • Ante area • Buffer zone
Equipment	• Written policies and procedures that address calibration, routine maintenance, and personnel training	• Written policies and procedures that address calibration, routine maintenance, and personnel training	• Written policies and procedures that address calibration, routine maintenance, and personnel training
Components	• Written policies and procedures that address: ○ Sterile components ○ Nonsterile components	• Written policies and procedures that address: ○ Sterile components ○ Nonsterile components	• Nonsterile drug components must meet the compendial standards if available • Written policies and procedures that address: ○ Sterile components ○ Nonsterile components
Processing: aseptic technique	• Written policies and procedures that address specific training and performance evaluation • Critical operations are carried out in an sterile compounding environment	• Written policies and procedures that address specific training and performance evaluation • Critical operations are carried out in an sterile compounding environment	• Written policies and procedures that address specific training and performance evaluation • Critical operations are carried out in an sterile compounding environment
Environmental control and monitoring program	• Policies and procedures that address: ○ Cleaning and sanitizing the workspaces (Direct and Contiguous Compounding Area, DCCA) ○ Personnel and gowning ○ Standard operating procedures	• Policies and procedures that address: ○ Cleaning and sanitizing the workspaces (Direct and Contiguous Compounding Area, DCCA) ○ Personnel and gowning ○ Standard operating procedures	• Policies and procedures that address: ○ Cleaning and sanitizing the workspaces (Direct and Contiguous Compounding Area, DCCA) ○ Personnel and gowning ○ Standard operating procedures
Verification procedures: sterility testing	No	No	Yes

(*continues*)

Table 8-1 (*continued*)

Criteria	Low-Risk Level	Medium-Risk Level	High-Risk Level
Validation procedures: environmental control/ monitoring	• Certification of LAFW and barrier isolates every 6 months • Certification of the buffer room/zone and anteroom/ zone every 6 months • Bacterial monitoring using an appropriate manner at least monthly	• Certification of LAFW and barrier isolates every 6 months • Certification of the buffer room/ zone and anteroom/zone every 6 months • Bacterial monitoring using an appropriate manner at least monthly	• Certification of LAFW and barrier isolates every 6 months • Certification of the buffer room/ zone and anteroom/zone every 6 months • Bacterial monitoring using an appropriate manner at least weakly
Validation procedures: personnel training and evaluation	Initially and annually thereafter: • Didactic review • Written testing • Media-fill testing	Initially and annually thereafter: • Didactic review • Written testing • Media-fill testing	Initially and annually thereafter: • Didactic review • Written testing • Media-fill testing

Dependent Rooms with Contained Workstations

In a dependent room design, the cleanest room receives filtered air directly from the source. Air flows from this room into other, less clean rooms. The environment in each room is dependent on the quality and quantity of air arriving from the upstream side of the air flow. If a problem occurs upstream, it affects the rest of the downstream facility. Often, the cleanest room will not have a laminar air flow workstation (LAFW), but the less clean areas of the facility will have one or more LAFWs in them as a workspace. Some designs also depend on the air flow from these LAFWs to maintain required air exchanges.

Independent Rooms with Contained Workstations

Another classic design is the independent system. In this design, the required air flow in each of the rooms is such that the room operates without needing assistance from other rooms. Within these rooms, LAFWs are usually placed and used as a direct and contiguous compounding area (DCCA) or aseptic workspace.

Open Architecture

An open architecture system is where filtered air is supplied directly over workspaces without the use of LAFWs. Filter arrays are designed such that they are directly over the DCCA and critical work area, providing this area with 100% filtration coverage. Air returns are located near the floor, thereby providing a flow of air down and away from the workspace. Wall-mounted arrays are seen in nonpharmaceutical applications. In pharmaceutical practice, having a clean air supply reach the face of personnel before it reaches the active biological agents will decrease the chance of occupational exposure. Movable stainless steel, solid shelf tables are utilized as workspaces. Storage carts are also movable, and any shelving on the wall is removable and off the floor. This setup facilitates cleaning and the sanitization of the entire facility; it also provides for a high degree of adaptability and ease of use. By adding arrays of filtered air in strategic places throughout the facility, it becomes possible to create workspaces throughout the facility.

Anterooms

Just prior to entering the anteroom, particle-producing agents such as makeup or jewelry should be removed. Anterooms serve as the first line of defense against particulate and microbial contamination. A clean room without this vital component starts out with many difficult obstacles to overcome. The anteroom is the barrier to dirty air currents. When the external door is open, the internal door should remain closed to prevent the entry of particles. The positive pressure of the anteroom will also inhibit the influx of particulates and their attendant microbes.

The anteroom should be the place where personnel wash their hands to the elbow and cover their particle-producing clothing and body with gloves, gowning materials, shoe covers, and head covers. This process should be started on the least clean side of the line of demarcation. When the shoe covers are placed over the feet, they should be placed on the cleaner side of the line of demarcation. Once shoe covers are placed on the feet, they should never cross over to the least clean side of the line of demarcation. This "de-particle-ization" of the employees is a key component of operating a successful clean room.

Another key attribute of the anteroom is the processing of reusable and disposable devices and depyrogenated glassware. These steps focus on the removal of particulates and microbes. As reusable and disposable devices and depyrogenated glassware are transported through the anteroom, they are wiped down with sterile isopropyl alcohol. Cardboard should never be taken into the anteroom, as it is a major source of particles as well as a source of microbes. Equipment, devices, and steri-wrapped items should be unboxed in the room prior to the anteroom. The carts and conveyances used on the exterior can be brought into the anteroom, but only to the line of demarcation. At this point, equipment, devices, and steri-wrapped items should be wiped and placed in a conveyance that is used only on the cleaner side of the line of demarcation. Steri-wrapped items can be opened over the line of demarcation into a clean conveyance on the cleaner side of the line of demarcation.

Without an anteroom to perform these tasks, the incursion of particulates and the attendant microbes into the clean room is a certainty, increasing the risk of infection to the patient.

Buffer Rooms and Zones

Buffer rooms are, in effect, the clean areas of the clean room. These areas should be controlled environments with a positive pressure to the anteroom and the exterior of the clean room facility. Without this pressure differential to discourage the incursion of particulates and the attendant microbes, the likelihood of contamination of preparations increases. Several variables need to be controlled in the buffer room or zone.

- The temperature and humidity should be controlled to allow for the appropriate filtration of air into the facility not only for the protection of the CSP, but also for the comfort of personnel. This type of control also keeps personnel within the clean room from perspiring outside their garments. If personnel do perspire to the outer side of a garment, that perspiration facilitates the transport of microbes across the garments, thus creating the potential for microbial contamination of a CSP.
- Another aspect of control is the cleaning and sanitization required within a buffer room. This is a two-step process in which cleaning removes dirt and residues (particle reduction) while sanitation decreases microbial counts. The two processes need to be done thoroughly and regularly according to guidelines.
- Particulate counting and microbial monitoring are also means of environmental control. They allow a buffer room operator to notice trends in clean room procedures that run counter to a safe working environment. Once it is understood which behaviors are undesirable, procedures can be changed and more appropriate behavior implemented.
- Quality control of air entering a room as well as the air return system will enhance the cleanliness of the buffer room. By maintaining a higher pressure with sufficiently clean air within the buffer room, the particulate and attendant microbes can be kept within required levels.

The control of the personnel, equipment, and devices entering the buffer room is one of the most important elements of control for a sterile compounding facility. Cleaning and sanitizing to reduce or eliminate particulate and microbial presence is of extreme importance. These tedious but important aspects of clean room operations may have the greatest impact on maintaining quality control over the CSP.

Air Quality Relative to Particle Counts

The USP has established standards for room and or DCA classification, as shown in Table 8-2.

Particulate counts are utilized as a method of approximating viable microbial particles in the air. Viable microbial particles are often associated physically with particulate matter. The size of particles measured and counted depends on the classification desired. Most counters will measure the 0.3- and 0.5-micron particles needed for classification under ISO 5 (Class 100), which is the standard for sterile compounding. Environments whose requirements exceed ISO Class 5 will also measure 5-micron particles. For anything under ISO 4 (Class 10) conditions, it would be necessary to measure the 0.1-micron particles. The "not to exceed" numbers in Table 8-2 apply to a single cubic foot of air. If any of the numbers in the environment exceed the listed levels, the area tested does not meet standards for classification. It is important to note that it is not the average number but rather a consistent number that is considered. A clean room is a controlled environment in which particulate counts are maintained below those listed levels at all times. Measuring

Table 8-2 Particulate Counts per Cubic Foot for ISO Classifications

Clean Room Class	Class Limits "Not To Exceed" Particle per Cubic Foot for Particle Sizes Shown				
	0.1 Micron	0.2 Micron	0.3 Micron	0.5 Micron	5 Micron
ISO 3	35.0	7.50	3.0	1.0	—
ISO 4	350	75.0	30.0	10.0	—
ISO 5	—	750	300	100	—
ISO 6	—	—	—	1,000	7.0
ISO 7	—	—	—	10,000	70.0
ISO 8	—	—	—	100,000	700

the levels on a continuous basis gives the best view of the facility's ability to maintain this control. If intermittent measurement is used instead, it is important to measure at a time of peak use or a time most likely to produce problematic results.

A clean room is a controlled environment that is able to attain and maintain the standards necessary to produce a sterile CSP. It is an environment shielded from contaminated air currents, whether they come from unfiltered air ducts or from open entrances. The clean air flow of most laminar air flow systems can easily be disrupted by movement from traffic, air conditioning, or open entrance air currents. A person walking creates a plume of disturbed air approximately 30 feet behind his or her body. This disturbed air picks up contaminants from the floor and raises them to higher levels in the room. It takes roughly 8 minutes for a 0.5-micron particle to settle to the floor through Brownian motion from a height of 5 feet.

Personnel Preparation to Enter a Controlled Environment

While sterile compounding areas may seem to be designed to maintain a controlled environment, the reality is that the most problematic sources of contamination are overlooked. The most problematic issue, by far, is the human body. The human body produces enormous amounts of particles. While sitting, a person produces 100,000 particles/ft^3/min; while walking, he or she produces 10 million particles/ft^3/min.

The human body sheds particles from the skin; these particles are usually impregnated with bacteria. This shedding can be enhanced by makeup, perfume, cologne, poor personal hygiene, or conditions such as eczema or dandruff. If an odor can be detected, then particles are being produced. It is essential that personnel receive training in proper use of barrier controls to prevent end-product contamination. Some common barrier controls are outlined here:

- Hair cover (also applies to bald heads): Skin sloughs; a hair cover provides product and personnel protection
- Face mask: Do not compound with a cold or other upper respiratory infection; a face mask provides product protection
- Gown: Provides product, personnel, and environmental protection
- Gloves: Provides product and personnel protection
- Goggles: Provides personnel protection
- Shoe covers: Provides product, personnel, and environmental protection

It is important for personnel performing aseptic manipulations to avoid introducing objects that shed particles into the anteroom or buffer room; these include pencils, cardboard cartons, paper towels, and cotton items. Only lint-free paper-related products (e.g., boxes, work records) may be brought into the anteroom or clean room. Compounding personnel must remove personal outer garments; cosmetics; artificial nails; hand, wrist, and body jewelry that can interfere with the fit of gowns and gloves; and visible body piercing above the neck. The wearing of artificial nails or extenders is prohibited while working in the sterile compounding environment. Natural nails must be kept neat and trimmed.

The following garbing techniques must be performed in the following order after entrance into an anteroom:

1. Don shoe covers.
2. Put on a sterile head cap/facial hair cover.
3. Put on a sterile mask/eye protection.
4. Perform hand hygiene procedure.
5. Don a sterile disposable gown.
6. Perform antiseptic hand cleansing and don sterile gloves.
7. Wash sterile gloves with 70% isopropyl alcohol or foaming sterile alcohol.

Aprons

Acid aprons worn over a bunny suit will provide better protection than the bunny suit alone, and can be removed much more quickly. They are recommended when working with large volumes of chemicals or whenever highly corrosive or toxic materials are being used. Be especially careful to wear proper protection when heating and mixing chemicals. Remove aprons carefully to prevent any chemicals on them from contaminating other areas.

Gloves

Gloves may be made of a number of different materials with varying resistances. Sometimes double gloving (in which a second pair of gloves is worn over the initial gloves) will suffice for adequate extra protection. When working with mixtures, choose gloves that are suitable for all of the chemicals in the mixture. If one component in the mixture can penetrate the gloves, it may carry the other components with it, exposing you to all the chemical hazards in the mixture. Gloves should be removed when leaving the clean room to prevent harmful chemicals from being transported to other areas.

Eyewear

Safety glasses should be worn in the clean room at all times. They provide protection against flying objects and some chemical splashes. When working with chemicals, especially when heating or mixing chemicals, goggles that seal around the face will provide better protection and prevent injury. Face shields should be worn whenever working with corrosive chemicals.

High-Risk Operations

High-risk operations require attention to minimizing the risk of contamination on lab coats, bunny suits, and other garb to be worn in the anteroom or clean area. Preferably, fresh, clean garb should be donned upon each entry into the anteroom or clean room area to avoid liberating contaminants from previously worn garb. Alternatively, garb that has been worn may be removed with the intention of regarbing for reentry into the anteroom or clean area and stored during the interim under proper control and protection in the anteroom area. Garb worn or taken outside the confines of the anteroom area cannot be worn in the clean room area.

Direct Compounding Area

The direct compounding area (DCA) is required to be, at a minimum, an ISO 5 environment. Thus each cubic foot is allowed to contain a maximum of 3,520 particles of 0.5 micron or greater size, which may or may not be associated with microbes. Under controlled and nonstressed circumstances, this would lead to a level of assurance that the preparations compounded would be sterile. Several designs for DCAs exist, with the most common being the use of a laminar flow workbench (hood). Aseptic biological cabinets and aseptic isolators are also used. In addition, some facilities use an open architecture design, creating a DCA without the use of a hood in an ISO 5 room.

Laminar Flow Hoods (Horizontal and Vertical)

- The hood controls airborne contamination of sterile products.
- Laminar flow hoods used in sterile compounding **must** be at least an ISO 5/Class 100 (less than 100 particles of 0.05 micron size per cubic foot).
- Room air is filtered through a high-efficiency particulate air (HEPA) filter, which removes 99.97% of all particles 0.3 micron or larger.
- Parallel air streams bathe the work area with a velocity sufficient to keep the area free of particles and microorganisms.
- The direction of air flow may be horizontal or vertical.
- Horizontal flow hoods are most commonly used, with the more costly vertical flow hoods being reserved for agents that might produce an environmental hazard (e.g., cytotoxic agents, radioactive agents, antimicrobial agents).

Laminar flow hoods are effective only when they are properly used by trained personnel. Operators need to be well aware that any interruption of the air flow will interfere with the effectiveness of the hood, and that

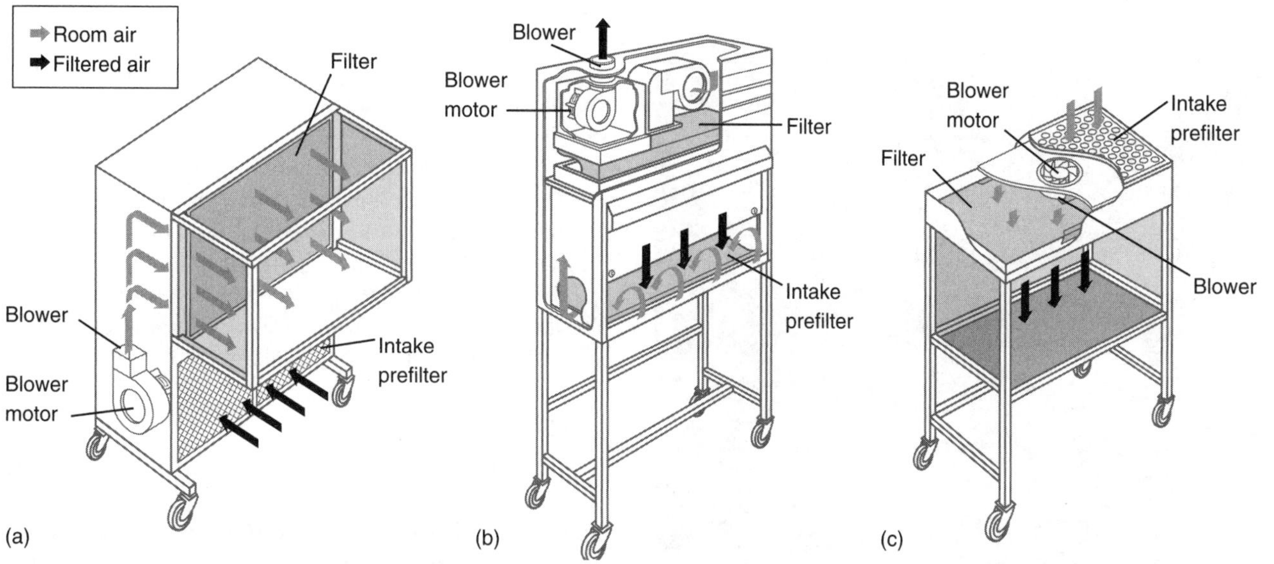

Figure 8-1 Laminar Flow Hoods: (a) Horizontal Flow Hood, (b) Vertical Flow BSC, (c) Vertical Flow Hood

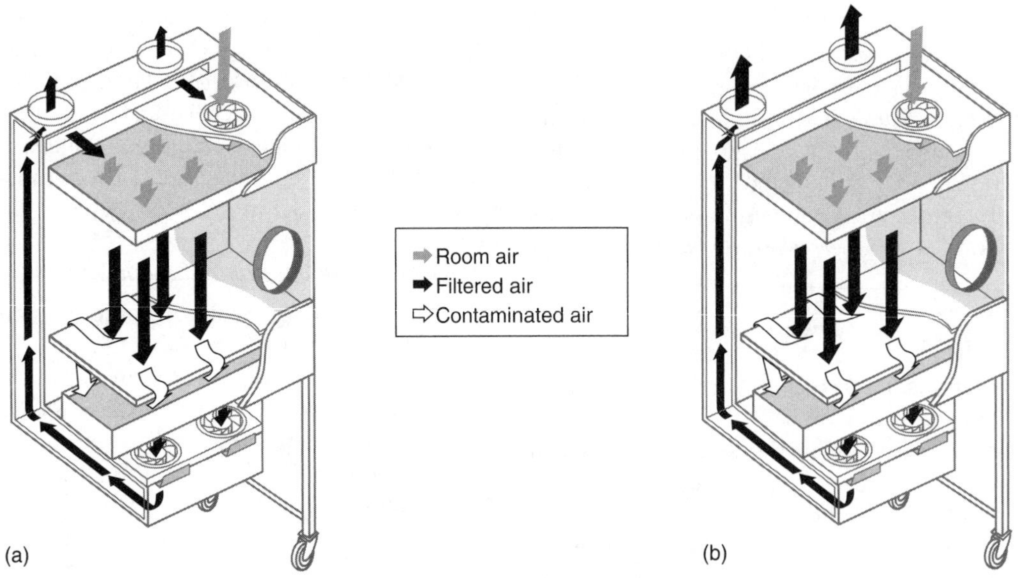

Figure 8-2 Compounding Aseptic Isolators

downstream contamination occurs when any object comes between the HEPA filter and the sterile product, interrupting the parallel flow and creating dead space. Cross-stream contamination may occur due to rapid movements of the operator in the hood. Backward contamination may be caused when turbulence is created by objects being placed in the hood, by fast traffic passing the hood, or by coughing, sneezing, and other actions of the operator.

A laminar flow hood does not produce sterilization, but merely prevents contaminants from settling onto the surface of the sterile product. Any movement of greater velocity and different direction than that of the hood's air flow will create turbulence that reduces the hood's effectiveness. Contamination may be minimized by working at a smooth, steady pace at least 6 inches into the hood.

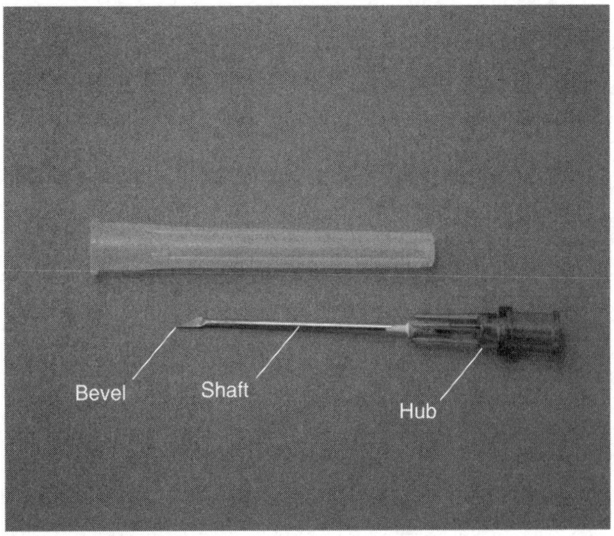

Figure 8-3 Needle

Needles and Syringes

Needles

A needle has three parts: the hub, the shaft, and the bevel. The hub is located at one end of the needle and is the part that attaches to the syringe. The shaft is the long, slender stem of the needle that is beveled at one end to form a point. The hollow bore of the needle shaft is known as the lumen. Disposable needles should always be used when preparing admixtures, as they are presterilized and individually wrapped to maintain sterility.

Needle size is designated by length and gauge. The length of a needle is measured in inches from the juncture of the hub and the shaft to the tip of the point. Needle lengths range from $^3/_8$ inch to 3½ inches; some special-use needles are even longer. The gauge of a needle, which designates the size of the lumen, ranges from 27 (the finest) to 13 (the largest).

Syringes

The basic parts of a syringe are the barrel, plunger, and tip. The barrel is a tube that is open at one end and tapers into a hollow tip at the other end. The plunger is a piston-type rod with a slightly cone-shaped top that passes inside the barrel of the syringe. The tip

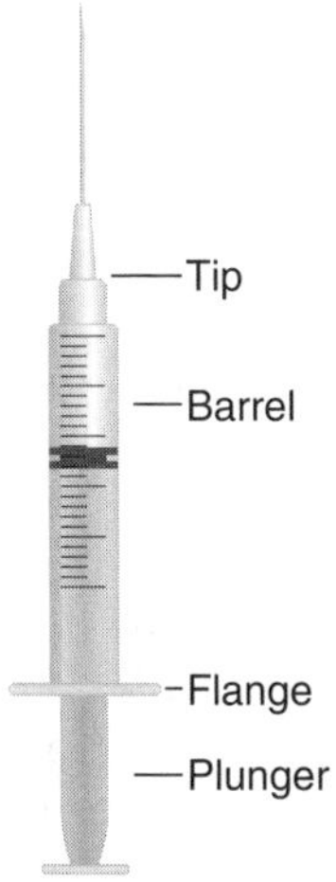

Figure 8-4 Syringe

of the syringe provides the point of attachment for a needle. The volume of solution inside a syringe is indicated by graduation lines on the barrel; these lines may be in milliliters or fractions of a milliliter, depending on the capacity of the syringe. The larger the capacity, the larger the interval between graduation lines.

Three types of syringe tips are commonly used: Slip-Tip, Luer-Lok, and eccentric. Slip-Tips allow the needle to be held on the syringe by friction. The needle is reasonably secure, but it may come off if not properly attached or if considerable pressure is used. Luer-Lok tips incorporate a collar with grooves that lock the needle in place. Eccentric tips, which are off-center, are used when the needle must be parallel to the plane of injection, such as in an intradermal injection.

Syringes come in a variety of sizes, ranging from 1 to 60 mL. As a rule, you should select a syringe whose capacity is the next size larger than the volume to be measured. For example, a 3 mL syringe should be selected to measure 2.3 mL, or a 5 mL syringe to measure 3.8 mL. With this approach, the graduation marks on the syringe will be in the smallest possible increments for the volume measured. Syringes should not be filled to capacity because the plunger can be easily dislodged.

Aseptic Techniques

Aseptic techniques are defined as the sum total of methods and manipulations required to minimize the contamination of sterile compounded formulations. The following are considered minimum requirements for good aseptic technique:

- Conduct all manipulations inside a properly maintained and certified laminar flow hood. Allow the laminar flow hood to operate for at least 30 minutes before use to produce a particle-free environment. Maintain a designated "clean" area around the hood.
- Remove all jewelry, and scrub hands and arms to the elbows with a suitable antibacterial agent. Sterile gloves are worn in addition to scrubbing.
- Wear lint-free clothing or clothing covers, head and facial hair covers, and a mask.
- Clean all flat surfaces of the hood with sterile 70% isopropyl alcohol, or another antibacterial scrub such as benzalkonium chloride solution, working first from top to bottom, then from back to front.
- Assemble all necessary supplies in the hood, checking each for packaging damage, expiration dates, and particulate material. Use only presterilized needles, syringes, and tubing for medication transfers.
- Remove the dust covering from supplies before placing them in the hood.
- Make sure there are no objects between the HEPA filter and the sterile surfaces, and that there is adequate space between objects. Place the smaller supplies closer to the HEPA filter and the larger supplies farther away from the filter.
- Swab all surfaces that require entry (puncture) with 70% isopropyl alcohol. Avoid excess alcohol or lint that might be carried into the solution.
- Pay close attention to hand position and the direction of air flow over injection ports or objects being manipulated. Minimize hand movements within the hood.
- To assemble needles and syringes, peel back the protective coverings and attach the needle and syringe, twisting them to lock them in place. When handling syringes and needles, be sure not to touch any surface that will come in contact with the sterile solution. Only the exterior of the syringe barrel, plunger tip, and needle cap or sheath may be safely handled.
- Perform all manipulations at least 6 inches inside the outer edge of the LAFW or 4 inches inside a BSC.
    - The 6-inch rule (horizontal hoods): In a horizontal hood, air moves from the back to the front. The flow rate of the hood air prevents an inward flow of room air. It is important not to position critical sites downstream of objects at any time (shielding them from sterile air). All critical operations should be performed at least 6 inches into the hood (to ensure an environment of sterile air).

- The 4-inch rule (vertical hoods): In a vertical hood, air moves from top to bottom. As the air moves to the work surface and toward the front or rear vents, there is potential for pickup of surface contamination. Therefore, critical operations should not be carried out directly over any vent and manipulations must be performed above the level of the work surface, preferably 4 inches above the work surface.
- Do not remove the hands from the hood until the compounding procedure is complete and the final inspection of the formulation has been made.
- Examine all formulations before removing them from the hood.
- Place all syringes and needles in puncture-proof containers and dispose of them according to proper procedures.

Aseptically Transferring a Drug from a Vial

Two types of parenteral vials are used in making admixtures:

- A vial that already has the drug in solution
- A vial that requires a lyophilized powder to be dissolved in a diluent to make a solution

In either case, a needle will be used to penetrate the rubber closure on the vial.

If the drug is already in solution, then the aseptic transfer technique is as follows:

1. Draw into the syringe a volume of air equal to the volume of drug solution to be withdrawn.
2. Place the vial on the work area surface, and penetrate the vial without coring.
3. Invert the vial. Use one hand to hold the vial and the barrel of the syringe, and the other hand to hold the syringe barrel.
4. Inject the air into the vial and withdraw the drug solution. It may be necessary to use successive small injections and withdrawals to exchange the air in the syringe with the solution in the vial.
5. Fill the syringe to a slight excess of the drug solution. Remove all air bubbles from the syringe by tapping the syringe. Once air bubbles have been removed, fill the syringe to the correct volume.
6. Withdraw the needle from the vial.
7. Transfer the solution in the syringe into a final container, again minimizing coring.

If the drug is a lyophilized powder in a vial, it will need to be reconstituted before it can be withdrawn.

1. Determine the correct volume of suitable diluent to use.
2. Perform steps as described previously for drugs in solution to draw the correct volume of diluent into a syringe.
3. Transfer the diluent into the vial containing the lyophilized powder.
4. Once the diluent is added, remove a volume of air into the syringe equal to slightly more than the volume of diluent added. This will create a negative pressure in the vial and decrease the likelihood that aerosol droplets will be sprayed when the needle is withdrawn.
5. Withdraw the needle.
6. Swirl the vial until the drug is dissolved.
7. Using a new needle and syringe, perform steps 1–6 again to withdraw the correct volume of reconstituted drug solution into the syringe.
8. Transfer the reconstituted drug solution in the syringe into a final container, again minimizing coring.

Aseptically Transferring a Drug from a Glass Ampule

Ampules have a colored stripe around the neck if they are pre-scored; the stripe indicates the neck has been weakened by the manufacturer to facilitate opening. Some ampules are not pre-scored by the manufacturer, so the neck must first be weakened (scored) with a fine file. The ampule should always be opened by breaking it at the neck.

1. Hold the ampule upright and tap the top to remove solution from the head space.
2. Swab the neck of the ampule with an alcohol swab.
3. Wrap the neck with an alcohol pad or gauze, and grasp the top with the thumb and index finger of one hand. With the other hand, grasp the bottom of the ampule.
4. Quickly snap the ampule, moving your hands away and out from you. Do not open the ampule toward the HEPA filter or any other sterile supplies in the hood. If the ampule does not snap easily, rotate it slightly and try again.
5. Inspect the opened ampule for any particles of glass that might have fallen inside.
6. Hold the ampule at a 20-degree downward angle.
7. Insert a needle or straw into the ampule, taking care not to touch the ampule neck where it is broken.
8. Position the needle in the shoulder area of the ampule, with the beveled edge down. This will avoid pulling glass particles into the syringe.

9. Withdraw the solution, keeping the needle submerged to avoid withdrawing air into the syringe.
10. Withdraw the needle from the ampule and remove all air bubbles from the syringe.
11. Transfer the solution to the final container using a filter needle or membrane filter.

Aseptically Adding Drug Solution to Large-Volume Parenteral Solutions and Small-Volume Parenteral Solutions

Large-volume parenteral (LVP) solutions are used as primary or continuous infusion solutions by administering them at a slow infusion rate. Drug additives can then be introduced directly into the LVP with a syringe and needle. Drug additives are also put in minibags and used as a piggyback on the LVP.

All of these scenarios require a syringe and needle to transfer the drug additive solution into a plastic bag or administration set injection port. The needle must be at least ½ inch long and not less than 19 gauge to ensure that the inner diaphragm of the port will be penetrated and that the protective rubber cover will reseal.

1. Remove the protective covering from the injection port.
2. Assemble the needle and syringe, and aseptically withdraw the necessary drug additive volume.
3. Swab the injection port with an alcohol swab.
4. Hold the injection port with one hand and insert the needle into the port with the other hand. Hold the port in such a way that the fingers are out of the way in case the needle punctures through the port. The injection port should be fully extended to minimize the chance of punctures through the port.
5. Inject the drug additive solution.
6. Remove the needle.
7. Mix and inspect the admixture.

CSP Sterilization

The sterilization process is intended to eliminate from the CSP any bacteria and other microorganisms that could result in a negative patient outcome. Methods commonly used in pharmacy compounding include filtration, moist-heat sterilization (autoclave), and dry-heat sterilization (convection oven).

Filtration

Filtration is used to remove particles—either particulate matter or microorganisms—from solutions. The choice of the filter will determine which particulates are the greatest cause of concern. Filtration is used for materials that are chemically or physically unstable if sterilized by heat, gas, or radiation. It is important to validate the integrity of the filter by conducting a bubble-point test. After a filter is used, its integrity can be determined by exposing the wetted filter to a high pressure. If the filter is intact, the appearance of bubbles on the filter surface should occur when the pressure is in the range of 50–55 psi. Conversely, if the filter integrity has been compromised, the bubble-point pressure will be much lower.

Moist-Heat Sterilization (Autoclave)

Moist heat sterilization is a commonly used method in which sterilization occurs through the application of high-pressure steam. When steam contacts the object to be sterilized, the moisture condenses and loses heat to the object. It is important to ensure that the chemical(s) to be sterilized can sustain temperatures of 120°C or greater.

Dry-Heat Sterilization (Convection Oven)

The dry-heat sterilization technique is useful to depyrogenate equipment and for oil and powder sterilization. This method takes longer than moist-heat sterilization. As with the autoclave, it is important to ensure any chemicals intended for sterilization can tolerate temperatures of more than 160°C.

Inspections and End Product Evaluations

The compounded formulation should be inspected for the following:

- Container integrity or leaks
- Particulate material properties such as color, odor, fill volume, and consistency

Preparations in flexible containers should be squeezed to ensure the absence of unintended holes and slits. Glass bottles should be examined for cracks and leaking stoppers.

Visual inspection will show two of the six characteristics of parenteral solutions: (1) particulate material and (2) stability, if such stability is physically characterized by precipitation or crystallization. The presence (or absence) of particulate material is best determined when the parenteral is held against an illuminated light/dark background.

Stability

Compounded sterile preparation stability refers to physical, chemical, and microbial stability. Anything not intended for immediate use must have a defined beyond-use date. Stability needs to be confirmed prior to the administration of the CSPs.

Compatibility

Components within a CSP can exhibit physiochemical effects such as acid–base reactions or solubility issues resulting in a physical change in the CSP that, in turn, could lead to a precipitate or inactivity of the active pharmaceutical ingredient (API). These changes can render the CSP incompatible for administration to a patient. The compatibility of two or more CSPs that come in contact with each other must be considered prior to and during their administration. It is not uncommon to combine two or more CSPs into one syringe or container (e.g., IV bag, eyedrops) to improve compliance and ease of administration. Additionally, the simultaneous administration of multiple CSPs into administration tubing (Y-site) or single-lumen catheters provides the opportunity for the CSPs to contact each other, which could result in an incompatibility. Pharmacists providing CSPs must have access to references that will enable them to determine the compatibility of multiple CSPs or their respective components.

Compatibility and Stability

- The National Coordinating Committee on Large Volume Parenterals (NCCLVP) defines instability as "a phenomenon which occurs when an LVP or LVP drug product (IV admixture) is modified due to storage conditions (e.g., time, light, temperature, sorption)." An unsuitable product may be formed under conditions of instability.
- Incompatibility is defined as "a phenomenon which occurs when a drug is mixed with others and produces an unsuitable product by some physiochemical means." The new product may be unsuitable for administration either because the "active" drug has been modified (e.g., increase in toxicity) or because some physical change (e.g., solubility) has occurred.
- If the stability or incompatibility of a given formulation is not known, the pharmacist should anticipate the likelihood of these problems.

Special Considerations and Precautions

Certain pharmaceutical preparations require special precautions in their preparation to minimize product contamination or environmental hazards. The following information may serve as a helpful guideline for a few of these classes of drugs.

Parenteral Nutrition Solutions

Because of their high risk for bacterial growth and their vast potential for drug incompatibilities, parenteral nutrition products require special attention. Strict adherence to aseptic technique and frequent sterility testing are essential. Whenever feasible, it is desirable to maintain a separate hood for nutrition solutions to avoid cross-contamination with other medicinal agents.

Table 8-3 Storage Conditions and Beyond-Use Dating for Completed CSPs per USP <797>

Low-Risk CSPs	Medium-Risk CSPs	High-Risk CSPs
In the absence of sterility testing, storage periods (before administration) shall not exceed the following: • Room temperature ≤ 48 hours • 2–8°C ≤ 15 days • ≤ 20°C ≤ 45 days	In the absence of sterility testing, storage periods (before administration) shall not exceed the following: • Room temperature ≤ 30 hours • 2–8°C ≤ 7 days • ≤ 20°C ≤ 45 days	In the absence of sterility testing, storage periods (before administration) shall not exceed the following: • Room temperature ≤ 24 hours • 2–8°C ≤ 3 days • ≤ 20°C ≤ 45 days

Cytotoxic Agents (Cancer Chemotherapy Agents)

Cytotoxic agents present an environmental hazard. It is now known that prolonged exposure to these agents may lead to the development of cancers. For this reason, special precautions must be taken to minimize the exposure of pharmacy personnel to these medications. These agents should be prepared in a shielded vertical flow hood, so that materials are not blown into the operator's face. When possible, it is best to have the responsibility for preparing these agents rotated among pharmacy personnel to minimize any one individual's exposure. It is desirable that pregnant women be exempted from preparation of these agents.

Radiopharmaceuticals

Radiopharmaceutical agents also represent an environmental hazard and must be handled carefully. In addition to adhering to the guidelines set forth for cytotoxic agents, pharmacists may further reduce exposure to these agents by working with them in protective lead vial shields. Special storage and disposal of these agents is required.

Antibiotics

Due to the allergenicity of the penicillins, it is desirable to work with these agents in a shielded vertical flow hood to avoid environmental contamination. When working with any antibiotics, it is important to remember that prolonged exposure may lead to infections of exposed areas by nonsusceptible bacteria and fungi. Pharmacists who must prepare large numbers of antibiotic doses should wash their hands frequently to avoid infections of the hands and nail beds.

Disposal Precautions

Discarded gloves, needles, syringes, ampules, vials, and prefilled syringes used in preparing sterile formulations represent a potential source of contamination and should be disposed of properly. Receptacles that are leak proof, puncture proof, sealable, and easily identifiable should be used for this purpose. Needles and syringes should be placed in "sharps" containers. They should not be clipped or recapped so as to prevent aerosolization or accidental needle sticks. Excess solutions should be returned to their original vial, an empty vial, or some other suitable closed container.

ANNOTATED BIBLIOGRAPHY

Anderson L, Higby GJ. *The Spirit of Voluntarism, a Legacy of Commitment and Contribution: United States Pharmacopeia, 1820–1995.* Rockville, MD: US Pharmacopeial Convention; 1995:14–29, 41–294.

Applied microbiology products: Steritest Sterility Testing System. Millipore Corporation. Available at: www.millipore.com/appmicro/products.nsf/docs/steritest/#Liquid. Accessed May 23, 2004.

Bormel G, Valentino JG, Williams RL. Application of USP-NF standards to pharmacy compounding. *IJPC* 2003;7(5):361–363.

Code of Federal Regulations, Title 21 § 808, 812 and 820 (1996). Available at: www.gmp1st. com/mdreg.htm. Accessed April 1, 2004.

Joint Commission on Accreditation of Healthcare Organizations. Joint Commission to survey compliance with new USP-NF chapter on compounding sterile preparations. *Joint Commission Perspectives* 2004;24(4):4–5.

Kawamura K, Abe H. Consideration of media fill tests for evaluation and control of aseptic processes: A statistical approach to quality criteria. *PDA J Pharm Sci Tech* 2002;56(5):235–241.

Leake M. PostScription. *IJPC* 2002;6(6):480.

Limited FDA survey of compounded drug products. U.S. Food and Drug Administration. Available at: www.fda.gov/cder/pharmcomp/survey.htm. Accessed March 4, 2004.

Lyman RA, Urdang G. Preface. In: Lyman RA, ed. *Pharmaceutical Compounding and Dispensing.* Philadelphia, PA: JB Lippincott, 1949:v.

Morris AM, Schneider PJ, Pedersen CA, et al. National survey of quality assurance activities for pharmacy-compounded sterile preparations. *Am J Health Syst Pharm* 2003;60(24):2567–2576.

National Institute of Occupational Safety and Health. Preventing occupational exposures to antineoplastic and other hazardous drugs in healthcare systems. NIOSH alert. March 2004. Available at: www.cdc.gov/niosh/docs/2004-HazDrugAct. Accessed May 21, 2004.

Newton DW, Trissel LA. A Primer on *USP* Chapter <797> "Pharmaceutical Compounding—Sterile Preparations," and USP Process for Drug and Practice Standards. *IJPC* 2004;8(4):251–263.

Rahe H. Overview of USP Chapter <797> "Pharmaceutical Compounding—Sterile Preparations: The Potential Impact for Compounding Pharmacies." *IJPC* 2004;8(2):89–94.

Rich DS. *USP-NF—Chapter 797 Legal and JCAHO Implications: Practical Application of USP to Pharmaceutical Compounding, Packaging and Dispensing.* Presentation at a seminar sponsored by the United States Pharmacopeia, Gaithersburg, MD, August 6–7, 2004.

Spencer J, Mathews AW. As druggists mix customized brews, FDA raises alarm. "Compounders" often meet special needs, but industry falls in regulatory gap. Rare fungus in the steroids. *Wall Street Journal* (February 27, 2004): A1, A6.

Talley CR. Sterile compounding in hospital pharmacies. *Am J Health Syst Pharm* 2003;60(24):2563.

Thompson CA. USP publishes enforceable chapter on sterile compounding. *Am J Health Syst Pharm* 2003;60(18):1814, 1817–1818, 1822.

Trissel LA. *Handbook on Injectable Drugs.* 12th ed. Bethesda, MD: American Society of Health-System Pharmacists; 2003.

U.S. Food and Drug Administration: FDA history. Available at: www.fda.gov/oc/history/default.htm Accessed January 30, 2003.

U.S. Food and Drug Administration. *Guidelines on General Principle for Process Validation.* Rockville, MD: Author; 1987.

U.S. Food and Drug Administration. *Human Drug Current Good Manufacturing Practice Notes.* Rockville, MD: Author; 1999:7(2).

U.S. Pharmacopeial Convention, Inc. Available at: www.usp.org. Accessed January 30, 2004.

U.S. Pharmacopeial Convention, Inc. *<795> Pharmaceutical Compounding—Nonsterile Preparations. United States Pharmacopeia 29—National Formulary 25.* Rockville, MD: Author; 2005:2731–2735.

U.S. Pharmacopeial Convention, Inc. *Chapter <1116> Microbiological Evaluation of Cleanrooms and Other Controlled Environments. United States Pharmacopeia 2—National Formulary 22.* Available at: www.uspnf.com. Accessed January 19, 2004.

U.S. Pharmacopeial Convention, Inc. *Chapter <1211>, Sterilization and Sterility Assurance of Compendial Articles. United States Pharmacopeia*

27—National Formulary 22. Rockville, MD: Author; 2004:2616–2620.

U.S. Pharmacopeial Convention, Inc. General chapters: an official in-process revision announcement. *Pharmacopeial Forum* 2003;29(6):1825.

U.S. Pharmacopeial Convention, Inc. *United States Pharmacopeia 25—National Formulary 20*. Rockville, MD: Author; 2001:2053–2057.

U.S. Pharmacopeial Convention, Inc. *United States Pharmacopeia 26—National Formulary 21*. Rockville, MD: Author; 2003.

U.S. Pharmacopeial Convention, Inc. *United States Pharmacopeia 27. Chapter <797> "Pharmaceutical Compounding—Sterile Preparations."* Rockville, MD: Author; 2004:2350–2370.

U.S. Pharmacopeial Convention, Inc. *United States Pharmacopeia 27—National Formulary 22*. Rockville, MD: Author; 2004:2350–2370.

U.S. Pharmacopeial Convention, Inc. *United States Pharmacopeia 27, Supplement 1. Chapter <797> "Pharmaceutical Compounding—Sterile Preparations."* Rockville, MD: Author; 2004:3121–3138.

NAPLEX Competency 1—Safe and Effective Therapeutic Outcomes

SECTION

3

Chemotherapeutic Principles and Agents

CHAPTER

9

Contributor: Teddie Gould

Tips Worth Tweeting

- Antineoplastic agents make up one of the largest groups of drugs.
- Because chemotherapy affects cell functioning and cell division, these agents have numerous toxicities, and some carry "black box" warnings.
- Myelosuppression is the most common dose-limiting toxicity of cytotoxic chemotherapy.
- Many agents cause significant nausea and vomiting, requiring patients to have proper antiemetic therapy.
- All cytotoxic agents should be considered "hazardous drugs." Safe handling procedures should be implemented due to the risks of carcinogenicity, mutagenicity, and teratogenicity associated with these agents.
- Chemotherapy drugs may be dosed in units of mg/m^2 rather than mg/kg.
- Many of these drugs require refrigeration and have special preparation and administration requirements.
- Breast and prostate cancers are the most frequently occurring cancers in women and men, respectively.
- Hormonal therapy has a different side-effect profile and is much better tolerated than chemotherapy.
- Because most advanced cancers cannot be cured, use of screening for early detection is important.
- Although very few agents used to treat cancer are in the top 200 drugs, errors associated with their dispensing and use have the potential to inflict great harm.

Patient Care Scenario: Ambulatory Setting

62 y/o F, white, 172 lbs, BMI 28.6, NKA, (–) alcohol and smoking
PMH: stage II breast cancer diagnosed 12/08, hypertension, osteoarthritis, depression
Laboratory: potassium 4.6 mEq/dL, Cr 1.1 mg/dL, BUN 15 mg/dL, calcium 9.2 mEq/dL, WBC 5,400 cells/mm^3, hemoglobin 12.8 g/dL, platelet count 195,000 cells/mm^3, liver function tests normal

Date	Physician	Drug	Quantity	Sig	Refills
6/10	Buchin	Paroxetine 20 mg	60	One po daily	4 refills
6/10	Buchin	Lisinopril 40 mg	60	One po daily	6 refills
6/10	Buchin	Naproxen 500 mg	120	One po bid	6 refills
8/20	Porter	Tamoxifen 20 mg	60	One po daily	4 refills

Notes: Patient is s/p lumpectomy, radiation therapy, and 6 months of chemotherapy with doxorubicin, cyclophosphamide, and paclitaxel. She takes the following OTCs and herbals: calcium 600 mg twice daily, vitamin D 800 units daily, and glucosamine/chondroitin twice daily.

1.1.0 Patient Information

Before dispensing chemotherapy in an institutional setting, the following information should always be updated and used to assess the appropriateness of drug dosing: patient height, weight, renal function, hepatic function, and CBC. In a retail setting, chemotherapy agents should not be dispensed without verifying the indication.

Medication information to be collected should include a current list of OTC and herbal medications and any medications the patient may be obtaining from outside sources. With regard to herbal medications, look for St. John's Wort, which can increase the metabolism of some antineoplastic agents. For patients on cytotoxic chemotherapy, look for OTC or herbal products with antiplatelet effects; they will increase the risk of bleeding if the patient becomes thrombocytopenic. For patients with breast cancer, find out whether they are taking any estrogen-containing medications or any herbal products with estrogenic properties. Growth of most breast cancers is hormonally driven, so estrogens are contraindicated in patients with a history of breast cancer, even if they appear to have been cured.

Laboratory information applicable to cancer and cancer treatment is all-encompassing. The cancer itself can affect any body organ and, therefore, almost any laboratory test. Also, many cancer treatments have toxic effects that are monitored using common laboratory tests (CBC, sCr). Given this fact, you should at least be familiar with the normal values for the CBC and standard chemistry panel. One common test for prostate cancer is the prostate-specific antigen (PSA) test. While it is not specific for cancer, it is used to screen, predict prognosis, assess treatment effect, and monitor for recurrence. A normal PSA level is usually in the range of 0–4 ng/mL. (Note that finasteride, dutasteride, and saw palmetto can interfere with PSA interpretation by lowering PSA levels.) Tests commonly used for determining prognosis and treatment of breast cancer assess for estrogen and progesterone receptor levels in tumor tissue, along with over-expression of human epidermal growth factor receptor 2 (HER2). Hormone receptor-positive patients have the option of being treated with hormonal therapy. HER2-positive patients are candidates for treatment with trastuzumab.

Signs and Symptoms

The ACS uses the following acronyms to help everyone remember the general signs and symptoms of cancer.

Seven Warning Signs of Cancer in Adults

Change in bowel or bladder habits
A sore that does not heal
Unusual bleeding or discharge
Thickening or lump in breast or elsewhere
Indigestion or difficulty swallowing
Obvious change in wart or mole
Nagging cough or hoarseness

Seven Warning Signs of Cancer in Children

Continued, unexplained weight loss
Headaches with vomiting in the morning
Increased swelling or persistent pain in bones or joints
Lump or mass in abdomen, neck, or elsewhere
Development of whitish appearance in the pupil of the eye
Recurrent fevers not caused by infections
Excessive bruising or bleeding
Noticeable paleness or prolonged tiredness

Wellness, Prevention, and Genetic Factors

Antineoplastic agents that are affected by pharmacogenomics include tamoxifen, irinotecan, mercaptopurine, thioguanine, fluorouracil, and capecitabine. See supplemental information for more details.

1.2.0 Pharmacotherapy

General Principles

- Traditional antineoplastic agents (cytotoxic agents) target rapidly proliferating cells, employing various mechanisms to interfere with cell growth. They tend to be toxic to normal cells as well. Most of these agents work by damaging DNA, interfering with DNA synthesis, or interrupting other steps in cell division.
- Several different methods are used for classifying anticancer agents; thus agents may be classified differently depending on the reference used. Classification is commonly based on mechanism of action, chemical structure, or source of origin.
- The higher the dose of chemotherapy, the greater the proportion of tumor cells killed.
- When attempting to achieve cure, the rule is to give the maximum tolerated dose. Most cytotoxic agents have a particular dose-limiting toxicity that prevents a higher dose from being given. Two common dose-limiting toxicities are bone marrow suppression (myelosuppression) and mucositis.
- Decreasing the dose intensity decreases the cure rate.
- Because of their side effects on rapidly growing cells, chemotherapy regimens are often given in pulsed-dose fashion, which allows normal cells to recover between cycles. Most treatment cycles are repeated every 3 to 4 weeks, which is the amount of time it normally takes the bone marrow to recover. Some agents cause delayed bone marrow toxicity and require a longer interval between cycles; other regimens may be administered at shorter intervals.

Table 9-1 Key Terms

ACS	American Cancer Society.
Adjuvant therapy	Therapy given in addition to primary therapy to eradicate micrometastases and prevent recurrence. Adjuvant therapy is commonly used in breast and colorectal cancer.
Alopecia	Hair loss.
ANC	Absolute neutrophil count. Number of neutrophils/mm^3. An ANC of less than 500 puts the patient at very high risk of infection. ANC = total WBC × (% of segmented + band neutrophils).
Angiogenesis	Growth of new blood vessels.
Antiemetic	Agent used to prevent or treat nausea and vomiting.
Antineoplastic	For the purposes of this chapter, this term applies to any agent used to treat cancer, including cytotoxic agents, targeted agents, and hormonal agents. Synonymous with "anticancer."
Carcinogen	Agent that leads to the development of cancer.
Chemoprotective agent	Agent given prior to chemotherapy to prevent toxicity. Examples are dexrazoxane, amifostine, and mesna.
Chemotherapy	For the purposes of this chapter, this term applies to any antineoplastic agent other than a hormonal agent.
Cytotoxic agent	For the purposes of this chapter, this term applies to any antineoplastic agent interfering with cell division and having toxic effects on rapidly growing cells.
Extravasation	Leaking of chemotherapy into the tissue surrounding an intravascular injection site.
Hand–foot syndrome	Palmar–plantar erythrodysesthesia. Tender erythema of the hands and soles of the feet followed by desquamation. It is a side effect of some chemotherapy agents.
HER2	Human epidermal growth factor receptor 2.
Histologic grade	Measure of how well tumor cells are differentiated. The higher the grade, the less differentiated and the poorer the prognosis.
Hormonal therapy	For the purposes of this chapter, this term applies to any antineoplastic agent with a hormonal mechanism.
Intrathecal	Into the spinal canal.
Leukopenia	Low white blood cell count.
Malignancy	Characterized by uncontrolled growth.
Metastases	Tumor spread to distant sites. Singular: metastasis.
Mucositis	Side effect of chemotherapy caused by injury to rapidly growing cells lining the gastrointestinal tract.
Myelosuppression	Suppression of blood cell formation in the bone marrow.
Nadir	Lowest point. In chemotherapy, it refers to the point in time when blood cell counts are at their lowest level.
Neoadjuvant therapy	Treatment used to reduce local tumor size before performing surgery or radiation therapy.
Neutropenia	Low neutrophil count.
Palliation	Therapy delivered with the goal of making a patient comfortable and providing the best quality of life.
Pancytopenia	Decrease in WBC, RBC, and platelet counts.
Primary therapy	Therapy used to treat a localized tumor with curative intent (surgery or radiation therapy).
Stomatitis	Mucositis specifically involving the oral mucosa.
Thrombocytopenia	Low platelet count.
TNM staging	Assessment of tumor size, lymph node involvement, and presence of metastases, used in determining the degree of solid tumor spread.
Tumor stage	Solid tumors are often staged as I–IV. Stage I = localized; Stage II–III = local/regional; Stage IV = distant metastases.
Vesicant	Agent that causes blistering or ulceration of tissue when extravasated.
Xerostomia	Dry mouth; lack of saliva production.

Table 9-2 Cancer Prevention

Cancer Type	Prevention	Comments
Lung cancer	Avoid smoking/smoking cessation.	Smoking is the number one cause of lung cancer. Smokers should be identified at each contact within the healthcare system, assessed for their readiness to quit, and assisted in whatever way possible. Tobacco use also increases the risk of oral cancer.
Skin cancer	Limit UV exposure, wear protective clothing, use sunscreen (SPF ≥ 15), avoid sunburn. Topical fluorouracil can be used to treat actinic keratoses, which are considered to be premalignant lesions.	Risk of nonmelanoma skin cancers (basal cell and squamous) is related to cumulative sun exposure. Risk of melanoma is related to history of sunburn and sun exposure early in life.
Cervical cancer	Human papillomavirus vaccine: • Gardasil 0.5 mL IM; three doses given at the following intervals: 0, 2, and 6 months • Cervarix 0.5 mL IM; three doses given at the following intervals: 0, 1, and 6 months	Human papillomavirus (HPV) causes most cases of cervical cancer. Guidelines for the use of HPV vaccine to prevent cervical cancer were published in 2007. The current ACS recommendation is routine vaccination, primarily for females aged 11–12 years, but also for females aged 13–18 years to "catch up" if the opportunity for vaccination was previously missed.
Breast cancer	Tamoxifen 20 mg daily Raloxifene 60 mg daily	Both agents are FDA approved for breast cancer prevention in high-risk women. The recommended duration of therapy is 5 years.
Prostate cancer	Finasteride 5 mg daily	Shown to reduce the incidence of prostate cancer, but not FDA approved for this indication.

- Because cancer cells are heterogeneous, use of a combination of agents with differing mechanisms of action is usually preferred. Regimens are also designed to include agents with nonoverlapping toxicities.
- Chemotherapy protocols are very specific with regard to agents used, dose, timing, and route of administration. Regimens are often referred to by acronyms (e.g., FOLFOX, BEP, CMF).
- Many newer agents target particular antigens on cancer cells or specific receptors, or pathways involved in tumor cell growth (e.g., monoclonal antibodies, tyrosine kinase inhibitors, and epidermal growth factor receptors). These agents, which are referred to as targeted therapies, have a somewhat different side-effect profile than traditional chemotherapy agents.
- Some cancers, such as prostate and breast cancer, are under hormonal control and, therefore, are best treated with hormonal agents.

More than 100 different drugs are used in the treatment of cancer. While knowing the correct dose of these medications is crucial, doses for any given agent will vary with the regimen employed. The best strategy is to determine which regimen the patient is receiving and calculate the patient's dose based on that.

Agents in Table 9-5 are used in the treatment of breast and prostate cancer. Some of these agents (GnRH agonists) have additional indications beyond their use in cancer treatment.

Routes of Administration

Antineoplastics are given by a variety of routes. Most of the cytotoxic and targeted agents are given intravenously either by bolus, short-term infusion, or prolonged infusion (over 24 hours or longer). Many of these agents are vesicants or irritants if allowed to leak outside of the vein. For this reason, they are sometimes administered via a central line into a large blood vessel with rapid flow. Other less common routes of administration include intravesicular (bladder instillation for bladder cancer), intrapleural (for malignant pleural effusions), intraperitoneal (for ovarian cancer), intra-arterial (via hepatic artery for liver metastases), and topical (see the discussion of fluorouracil). Many chemotherapy agents do not penetrate the CNS—a system that can be a site of cancer metastases as well as a primary site of occurrence. For this reason, methotrexate and cytarabine are sometimes given intrathecally. Note that only a few agents can be given this way. *Never* give vinca alkaloids or anthracyclines intrathecally.

Drug and Food Interactions

For notes on drug and food interactions occurring with cytotoxic drugs, see the comments sections for individual agents in Tables 9-3, 9-4, and 9-5. There is surprisingly little information regarding drug interactions with the cytotoxic agents. Obviously, many of the drugs have pharmacodynamic interactions manifested as additive side effects (e.g., additive bone marrow

Table 9-3 Selected Oral Chemotherapy Agents[2]

Drug	Brand Name	Pharmacologic Class	Comments
Capecitabine	Xeloda 150 and 500 mg tablets	Antimetabolite, oral prodrug of 5FU, pyrimidine analog	For colorectal and breast cancer. Given in 3-week cycles: 2 weeks on, 1 week off. 2,500 mg/m^2 total daily dose divided into two doses. Give with food. Reduce dose in patients with renal dysfunction. Side effects: hand–foot syndrome, diarrhea, ↓ bone marrow. Significant DDI with warfarin.
Erlotinib	Tarceva 25, 100, and 150 mg tablets	Tyrosine kinase inhibitor that affects epidermal growth factor signaling	For non-small-cell lung cancer and pancreatic cancer. Take on an empty stomach (food increases absorption and toxicity). Metabolized by CYP 3A4; watch for DDI. Do not take with antacids. Do not drink grapefruit juice. Side effects: severe rash, diarrhea. Numerous other warnings and precautions (pulmonary, hepatic).
Etoposide	VePesid 50 mg capsules Also available as an injection	Epipodophyllotoxin	Oral etoposide is indicated for small-cell lung cancer. The oral dose is twice the IV dose. Take with or without food. Reduce dose in renal and hepatic dysfunction. Refrigerate. Side effects: ↓ bone marrow.
Gefitinib	Iressa 250 mg tablets	Tyrosine kinase inhibitor that affects epidermal growth factor signaling	For non-small-cell lung cancer. Take with or without food. Metabolized by CYP 3A4. Side effects: rash, diarrhea. Warning for pulmonary toxicity.
Imatinib	Gleevec 100 and 400 mg tablets	Tyrosine kinase inhibitor	Primary indication is chronic myelogenous leukemia. Usual maximum dose is 600 mg/day. Take with food. Avoid grapefruit juice. Reduce dose in hepatic dysfunction. Metabolized by CYP 3A4 and inhibits 3A4 and 2D6; watch for DDI (warfarin). Side effects: rash, fluid retention, ↓ bone marrow, hepatoxicity, muscle cramps.
Mercaptopurine (6-MP)	Purinethol 50 mg tablets	Antimetabolite, purine analog	For acute lymphocytic leukemia (maintenance therapy). 1.5–2.5 mg/kg/day. Take on an empty stomach. Major DDI with allopurinol; inhibits 6-MP metabolism. Dose *must* be reduced to one-third to one-fourth of the usual dose. Side effects: ↓ bone marrow, hepatotoxicity.
Methotrexate	2.5, 5, 7.5, 10, and 15 mg tablets Rheumatrex and Trexall are brand names for tablets	Antimetabolite, folic acid antagonist	In addition to treating malignancy, methotrexate is used orally for conditions such as rheumatoid arthritis and psoriasis. May be taken with or without food. See Table 9-4 for more information.
Thalidomide	Thalimid 50, 100, and 200 mg capsules	Immunomodulator	For multiple myeloma. Providers and pharmacists must be registered with the manufacturer's S.T.E.P.S. program for the drug to be obtained. Females of reproductive age must have a current pregnancy test that is negative. Take shortly before bedtime to avoid sedation. Side effects: teratogenicity, rash, VTE, sedation, peripheral neuropathy.

DDI = drug–drug interaction; S.T.E.P.S = System for Thalidomide Education and Prescribing Safety; VTE = venous thromboembolism.

suppression). For patients receiving agents that cause thrombocytopenia and bleeding, avoid drugs with antiplatelet effects and do not give drugs by the IM route. The very significant drug interaction between mercaptopurine and allopurinol requires a substantial dose reduction for mercaptopurine. NSAIDs should not be administered with methotrexate, as these agents block its renal tubular secretion and lead to increased toxicity. Among the newer agents, tyrosine kinase inhibitors (e.g., imatinib) have significant interactions with the cytochrome P450 enzyme system. All of these drugs are metabolized by CYP 3A4 and may also affect substrates of 3A4 and other CYP enzymes. With several of these agents, including imatinib, it is recommended that

Table 9-4 Common Parenteral Chemotherapy Agents[2]

Drug	Brand Name	Pharmacologic Class	Comments
Bevacizumab	Avastin 25 mg/mL in 4 and 16 mL vials	Monoclonal antibody against vascular endothelial growth factor (VEGF); inhibits angiogenesis	Approved for breast, colorectal, renal, and non-small-cell lung cancers and glioblastoma. Side effects: hypertension, GI perforation, hemorrhage, wound healing complications.
Bleomycin	Blenoxane 15 and 30 unit vials for reconstitution	Antitumor antibiotic	Approved for lymphoma, testicular, and head and neck cancers. Reduce dose in patients with renal dysfunction. Side effects: hypersensitivity, give 1–2 unit test dose in lymphoma. Dose-limiting side effect is pulmonary fibrosis, avoid a cumulative dose of more than 400 U.
Carboplatin	Paraplatin Powder and solution for injection in various sizes	Platinum compound/ alkylating agent	Approved for ovarian cancer. Dosed in units of mg/m^2 and also by AUC using the Calvert formula. Reduce dose in patients with renal dysfunction. Side effects: ↓ bone marrow, N/V (including delayed), hypersensitivity, peripheral neuropathy, ototoxicity.
Cisplatin (CDDP)	Platinol, Platinol-AQ 1 mg/mL in various vial sizes	Platinum compound/ alkylating agent	Broad-spectrum agent. Usual dose range is 20–100 mg/m^2 per cycle. Verify all orders for more than 100 mg/m^2 per cycle. Use with caution in patients with renal dysfunction. Side effects: nephrotoxicity (dose limiting), N/V (including delayed), hypersensitivity, peripheral neuropathy, ototoxicity, ↓ bone marrow. Hydrate pre- and post-infusion.
Cyclophosphamide	Cytoxan, Neosar 500 mg, 1 g, and 2 g powder for injection 25 and 50 mg tablets	Alkylating agent	Broad-spectrum agent. Prodrug. Dosed in units of both mg/kg and mg/m^2. Side effects: ↓ bone marrow, N/V, hemorrhagic cystitis. Hydrate pre- and post-infusion.
Cytarabine	Ara-C, Cytosine arabinoside, Cytosar Powder and solution for injection Depo-Cyt (liposomal for intrathecal use)	Antimetabolite, pyrimidine	Used for acute leukemias. DepoCyt is a liposomal formulation for q 14 day intrathecal use. Side effects: ↓ bone marrow, stomatitis.
Dacarbazine	DTIC-Dome Powder for injection; 100 and 200 mg vials	Alkylating agent	Approved for melanoma and Hodgkin's disease. Side effects: ↓ bone marrow, N/V.
Docetaxel	Taxotere Solution for injection containing Polysorbate 80	Taxane/antimitotic	Approved for breast, lung, and prostate cancer. Pretreat all patients with dexamethasone starting one day before to prevent both fluid retention and hypersensitivity. Metabolized by 3A4. Avoid in hepatic dysfunction. Side effects: ↓ bone marrow, hypersensitivity, peripheral neuropathy, fluid retention.
Doxorubicin	Adriamycin Powder and solution for injection Doxil (pegylated liposomal)	Anthracycline/DNA intercalating agent	Broad-spectrum agent. Reduce dose in patients with hepatic dysfunction. Side effects: ↓ bone marrow, cardiac toxicity (cumulative dose limiting), vesicant, infusion reactions with liposomal. Turns urine red.

Table 9-4 (*continued*)

Drug	Brand Name	Pharmacologic Class	Comments
Fluorouracil (5-FU)	Adrucil 50 mg/mL in various vial sizes Topical cream 0.5%, 1%, and 5% Solution 2% and 5% (Efudex, Carac, Fluoroplex)	Antimetabolite, pyrimidine	Broad-spectrum agent. Used with leucovorin in colon cancer. Leucovorin enhances binding to thymidylate synthase. Side effects: stomatitis (dose limiting for prolonged IV infusions), ↓ bone marrow (dose limiting for IV bolus and short-term infusion), diarrhea. 5% topical strength used for superficial basal cell carcinomas.
Gemcitabine	Gemzar Injection	Antimetabolite, pyrimidine	Approved for breast, lung, ovarian, and pancreatic cancers. Side effects: ↓ bone marrow, rash.
Ifosfamide	Ifex Powder for injection, 1 and 3 g vials	Alkylating agent	Approved for testicular cancer. Reduce dose in patients with renal dysfunction. Side effects: ↓ bone marrow, hemorrhagic cystitis. Hydrate patient and give with mesna (Mesnex) to prevent bladder toxicity.
Irinotecan	Camptosar 20 mg/mL in 2 and 5 mL vials	Camptothecin/ topoisomerase inhibitor	Approved for colorectal cancer. Given IV only. Side effects: ↓ bone marrow, diarrhea (dose limiting), N/V. Use atropine for early diarrhea, and loperamide (high dose) for late diarrhea.
Methotrexate (MTX)	Vials for injection both with and without preservative Also available as tablets	Antimetabolite, folic acid antagonist	Broad-spectrum agent. Reduce dose in patients with renal dysfunction. Antidote is leucovorin. Side effects: ↓ bone marrow (dose limiting), stomatitis, pulmonary fibrosis, hepatoxicity, nephrotoxicity in large doses. Hydrate and alkalinize urine to prevent nephrotoxicity.
Oxaliplatin	Eloxatin Powder and solution for injection in various sizes	Platinum compound/ alkylating agent	Approved for colorectal cancer. Side effects: peripheral neuropathy, N/V (including delayed), hypersensitivity.
Paclitaxel	Taxol Onxol 6 mg/mL solution containing Cremophor EL and absolute alcohol as diluents Abraxane Albumin-bound paclitaxel injection	Taxane/antimitotic	Approved for ovarian, breast, and lung cancer. With Taxol, pretreat all patients with corticosteroids, diphenhydramine, and H_2 blockers to prevent hypersensitivity. Abraxane does not require pretreatment. Metabolized by CYP 2C8 and 3A4. Side effects: ↓ bone marrow, hypersensitivity, peripheral neuropathy.
Rituximab	Rituxan 10 mg/mL in 10 and 50 mL vials	Monoclonal antibody against CD20 (cell surface antigen found on normal and malignant B lymphocytes)	Approved for B-cell non-Hodgkin's lymphoma. Side effects: hypersensitivity reactions (pretreat with acetaminophen and antihistamine), ↓ bone marrow.
Trastuzumab	Herceptin Powder for injection 440 mg	Monoclonal antibody to HER2 receptor, an epidermal growth factor receptor found in approximately 20% of women with breast cancer.	Approved for breast cancer. Side effects: hypersensitivity reactions, cardiotoxicity.

(*continues*)

Table 9-4 (*continued*)

Drug	Brand Name	Pharmacologic Class	Comments
Vincristine	Oncovin Vincasar PFS 1 mg/mL in a variety of vial sizes	Vinca alkaloid, antimitotic	Approved for acute leukemia and some lymphomas. Dose: 1.4 mg/m^2 or 2 mg/week limit. Reduce dose in patients with hepatic impairment. Side effects: neurotoxicity (dose limiting), vesicant.
Vinblastine	Velban Powder for injection and solution	Vinca alkaloid, antimitotic	Broad-spectrum agent. Reduce dose in patients with hepatic dysfunction. Side effects: ↓ bone marrow (dose limiting), vesicant.

N/V = nausea and vomiting.

Table 9-5 Hormonal Agents[2]

Drug	Brand Name/Dose Form	Pharmacologic Class	Comments
Anastrozole	Arimidex Oral tablet, 1 mg	Aromatase inhibitor, selective, nonsteroidal, competitive	Approved for adjunctive therapy and treatment of advanced breast cancer in postmenopausal women. Dose is 1 mg daily. Side effects: estrogen deprivation, hot flashes, fatigue, osteoporosis.
Bicalutamide	Casodex Oral tablet 50 mg	Antiandrogen	Used for treatment of prostate cancer in combination with a GnRH agonist (or orchiectomy). Use may be short term to block the flare in symptoms caused at start of GnRH agonist or continued in combination. Dose is 50 mg daily. Side effects: hepatotoxicity, hot flashes, loss of libido, gynecomastia, osteoporosis.
Exemestane	Aromasin Oral tablet 25 mg	Aromatase inhibitor, selective, steroidal, irreversible	Approved for the treatment of advanced breast cancer in postmenopausal women who have failed on tamoxifen. Dose is 25 mg daily with food. Side effects: similar to anastrozole.
Flutamide	Eulexin Oral capsules 125 mg	Antiandrogen	Used for prostate cancer in the same manner as bicalutamide. Dose is 250 mg tid. Side effects: hepatotoxicity, hot flashes, loss of libido, gynecomastia, osteoporosis.
Goserelin	Zoladex Injectable implants: • 3.6 mg: 1 month • 10.8 mg: 3 month	GnRH (LHRH) agonist	Approved for prostate cancer and breast cancer. May be used as monotherapy or in combination with an antiandrogen. Given SC. Side effects: hormone deprivation, hot flashes, loss of libido, osteoporosis, temporary disease flare.
Fulvestrant	Faslodex Injection 50 mg/mL	Pure antiestrogen	Only approved for metastatic breast cancer in postmenopausal women after failing on antiestrogen. Similar side effects as noted with tamoxifen.
Histrelin	Vantas, Supprelin LA 12-month injectable implant, 50 mg	GnRH (LHRH) agonist	Approved for advanced prostate cancer. Given SC. Side effects: similar to those of goserelin. Refrigerate.
Letrozole	Femara Oral tablets 2.5 mg	Aromatase inhibitor, selective, nonsteroidal, competitive	Approved for adjunctive therapy, extended adjuvant therapy (after 5 years of tamoxifen), and treatment of advanced breast cancer in postmenopausal women. Dose is 2.5 mg daily. Side effects: estrogen deprivation, hot flashes, fatigue, osteoporosis.

Table 9-5 (*continued*)

Drug	Brand Name/Dose Form	Pharmacologic Class	Comments
Leuprolide	Lupron, Eligard Injections available: Daily use (1 mg/0.2 mL), 1-month(7.5 mg), 3-month(22.5 mg), 4-month(30 mg), and 6-month(45 mg)	GnRH (LHRH) agonist	Approved for prostate cancer. Administered IM or SC depending on the product. See goserelin for additional information.
Nilutamide	Nilandron Oral tablets 150 mg	Antiandrogen	Used for prostate cancer in the same manner as bicalutamide. Dose is 150 mg daily. Side effects: hot flashes, loss of libido, gynecomastia, osteoporosis, interstitial pneumonitis, delayed visual adaptation to the dark, alcohol intolerance.
Tamoxifen	Nolvadex Oral tablets 10 mg and 20 mg Soltamox Oral solution 10 mg/5 mL	Some sources refer to tamoxifen as an antiestrogen, others as a SERM	Approved for premenopausal and postmenopausal women for breast cancer prevention, as adjuvant therapy in early-stage disease, and as palliative therapy in advanced disease. Usual dose is 20 mg qd. Metabolized to active metabolites by CYP 2D6; watch for DDI. Side effects: estrogen deprivation, hot flashes, endometrial cancer, VTE. Potential for initial flare reaction with or without hypercalcemia when used for *metastatic* breast cancer.
Toremifene	Fareston 60 mg tablet	Some sources refer to toremifene as an antiestrogen, others as a SERM	Approved only for metastatic breast cancer in postmenopausal women. Similar side effects as noted with tamoxifen.
Triptorelin	Trelstar Depot Injection 3.75 mg monthly depot Trelstar LA 11.25 mg 84-day depot	GnRH (LHRH) agonist	Given IM. Approved for prostate cancer. See goserelin for additional information.

GnRH = gonadotropin hormone-releasing hormone; LHRH = luteinizing hormone-releasing hormone; SERM = selective estrogen receptor modulator; VTE = venous thromboembolism.

patients avoid grapefruit juice. Avoid inhibitors of CYP 2D6 in patients on tamoxifen, as these agents decrease the formation of active metabolites.

Contraindications, Warnings, and Precautions

As a whole, cytotoxic drugs represent a highly toxic group of agents with numerous warnings and precautions. Labeling for the vast majority includes "black box" warnings.

Physiochemical Properties Affecting Solubility, Pharmacodynamics, Pharmacokinetics, and Stability

Several of the chemotherapy agents have solubility issues that require them to be formulated with agents such as absolute alcohol (carmustine), Polysorbate 80 (docetaxel), and Cremophor EL (paclitaxel). In the case of docetaxel and paclitaxel, these vehicles may be responsible for hypersensitivity reactions. They may also cause leaching of DEHP plasticizer from IV tubing. For this reason, non-PVC tubing and containers should be used to administer these agents. Platinum compounds can precipitate on contact with aluminum, so it is important to avoid the use of aluminum needles in the preparation of cisplatin, carboplatin, and oxaliplatin.

Some drugs have been developed in different formulations to decrease side effects. Examples include pegylated liposomal doxorubicin, which is used to decrease cardiac toxicity, and albumin-bound paclitaxel, which is used to decrease the risk of hypersensitivity reactions. These formulations are not generically equivalent and cannot be used interchangeably with the drug's conventional formulation. Given the large number of agents being discussed and the potential for IV incompatibilities, appropriate references should be consulted before mixing any of these drugs. Many of these drugs require storage under refrigeration.

1.3.0 Safety, Monitoring, and Patient Education

Pharmacotherapeutic Outcomes

Goals of therapy and monitoring parameters will depend on the patient, type of cancer, and stage of disease. The goal of therapy will be either cure (in early-stage cancers) or palliation (in advanced-stage and metastatic cancers).

Safety

In general, chemotherapy agents are highly toxic and cause a wide range of side effects. One method of classifying these side effects is shown in Table 9-6. Toxicities are sometimes graded on a universal scale of 0–4, depending on the degree of severity. Grade 4 is the most severe and considered life threatening. Hormonal agents have a completely different set of toxicities related to hormone deprivation (see Table 9-5).

Table 9-6 Classification of Chemotherapy Side Effects

Category	Side Effect
Acute effects on rapidly growing cells	Bone marrow suppression
	Mucositis, stomatitis, diarrhea
	Alopecia
Other acute effects	Nausea and vomiting
	Extravasation reactions
	Hypersensitivity reactions
	Hyperuricemia
Organ system toxicity	Cardiac
	Renal
	Bladder
	Neurologic
	Pulmonary
	Dermatologic
	Hepatic
	Ocular
	Reproductive
Long term	Carcinogenicity/second malignancies
	Teratogenicity

Pharmacists play an important role in the prevention and management of antineoplastic side effects.

Acute Effects on Rapidly Growing Cells

Bone Marrow Suppression

Bone marrow suppression is the most common dose-limiting toxicity of the cytotoxic agents. In fact, it is so common that it is easier to remember the drugs that do not cause bone marrow suppression than the ones that do. Of the agents listed in Tables 9-3 and 9-4, only bleomycin, bevacizumab, trastuzumab, and vincristine are bone marrow sparing. WBCs are most sensitive to these agents, followed by platelets and finally RBCs. The usual time course for WBC effects is as follows: onset, 7–10 days; nadir, 10–14 days; recovery, 21–28 days. This time course is important in determining treatment intervals. Symptoms include infection, bleeding, and fatigue.

Patients are at greatest risk of infection and febrile neutropenia when their ANC is less than 500 cells/mm^3. For regimens associated with a 20% or greater risk of febrile neutropenia, prophylaxis with WBC growth factors (colony-stimulating factors [CSFs]) is indicated. Anemia occurs less commonly and can be due to the cancer itself or to chemotherapy. Use of erythropoiesis-stimulating agents (ESAs) such as epogen or darbepoetin may be indicated for some patients.

Patients should be counseled on good hygiene and hand washing. They should avoid crowds and sick people during the neutropenic period. They should also report any signs of infection, including temperature of 100.5°F or greater or sore throat. Marrow suppressive chemotherapy should be held for an ANC less than 1,500 and a platelet count less than 100,000.

Another agent used specifically with high-dose methotrexate to prevent bone marrow and other toxicity is leucovorin calcium. It is given either IV or orally every 6 hours starting 12 to 24 hours after completion of the methotrexate therapy. The duration of therapy depends on the blood levels of methotrexate. See the supplemental material for information on the mechanism of action. Note that other names for leucovorin are citrovorum factor and folinic acid, *not* folic acid. A similar product, levoleucovorin (Fusilev), is given IV at half the dose of racemic leucovorin. Leucovorin is also used in some chemotherapy regimens to potentiate the effects of fluorouracil.

Effects on Cells Lining the GI Tract: Mucositis/Stomatitis

The side effects of mucosistis and stomatitis are most common with cell cycle phase-specific agents. Common causes mentioned earlier include bleomycin, cytarabine, docetaxel, doxorubicin, fluorouracil, methotrexate, and vinblastine. The time course over which

Table 9-7 White Blood Cell Growth Factors[2]

Agent	Brand Name/ Synonym	Adult Dose	Timing	Comments
Filgrastim	Neupogen, G-CSF Available in 300 mcg and 480 mcg vials and prefilled syringes	5 mcg/kg SC or IV daily	Initiate 24–72 hours after chemotherapy; continue until ANC is at least 2,000	Primary indication is prophylaxis, but may be used for high-risk patients in whom neutropenia has already developed. Most common side effect: bone pain. Refrigerate
Pegfilgrastim	Neulasta, G-CSF Available in 6 mg/0.6 mL single-use, prefilled syringe	6 mg SC each cycle	Initiate 24–72 hours after chemotherapy	Same as filgrastim. Pegylation extends the drug's half-life, allowing a dosing interval of once per cycle. Refrigerate.

Sargramostim (Leukine, Prokine, GM-CSF) is another agent for the prevention of neutropenia, but tends to be used more often in specialty practice.

Table 9-8 Erythropoiesis-Stimulating Agents Used for Anemia of Cancer and Chemotherapy-Induced Anemia

Agent	Brand Name/ Synonym	Adult Dose	Comments
Epogen	Procrit Injection	40,000 units SC weekly; increase to 60,000 units if no response in 4 weeks	Only indicated for hemoglobin levels less than 10 g/dL or hematocrit less than 30%. If hemoglobin does not rise at least 1 g/dL within 8 weeks of initiation, discontinue. "Black box" warning indicates this agent carries an increased risk of mortality and possible tumor promotion. Maintain adequate iron stores. Monitor CBC weekly. Goal is a hemoglobin level of 10–12 g/dL and to avoid transfusions. ESAs must now be prescribed under a REMS (risk evaluation and mitigation strategy) program. Medication guides are required for patients, and healthcare providers must undergo training.
Darbepoetin	Aranesp Injection	2.25 mcg/kg/week SC or 200 mcg SC every 2 weeks; increase to 300 mcg if no response in 4 weeks	Same as epogen.

these side effects develop parallels WBC suppression. Monitor patients for erythema of the mouth, oral ulceration, bleeding, pain, and difficulty chewing or swallowing. Patients should be counseled to see a dentist before starting chemotherapy and to maintain good oral hygiene so as to decrease the risk of mucositis. Other than that, treatment is symptomatic and supportive.

Patient counseling tips include the following recommendations:

- Avoid acidic, salty, spicy, or sharp-textured foods that could irritate the mouth.
- Avoid tobacco and caffeine.
- Avoid alcohol-containing products.
- Use warm saline mouthwashes, including $NaHCO_3$.
- Try cold substances such as ice pops or ice chips to reduce pain.
- Eat soft or pureed foods.
- Use a soft-bristle toothbrush or foam swab for mouth hygiene, along with proper flossing.

The following topical agents are sometimes used to relieve pain in mucositis:

- Viscous lidocaine
- Dyclonine spray
- Benzocaine in Orabase
- Diphenhydramine mouthwash (avoid elixir)
- Maalox and diphenhydramine mouthwash
- Gelclair—bioadherent gel/protective barrier

In some cases, opiates may be needed for pain control.

Watch for oral candida and herpes infections and treat them as needed, using clotrimazole troches, nystatin suspension, or systemic therapy. These agents may also be used prophylactically in high-risk patients.

Other GI side effects include xerostomia, diarrhea, and constipation. Irinotecan, in particular, causes dose-limiting diarrhea. Manage late-onset diarrhea with high-dose loperamide (Imodium). *In this case it is acceptable to exceed the usual dose limit of 16 mg/day.*

Alopecia

Many chemotherapy agents cause alopecia due to their effects on rapidly dividing hair cells. While not dose limiting, this side effect is highly concerning to patients. Scalp hair is most susceptible, but eyebrows, eyelashes, facial hair, pubic hair, and axillary hair can also be affected. Patients should be counseled in advance to expect alopecia. Hair loss often begins 7 to 14 days after treatment starts and becomes prominent at 1 to 2 months. Hair growth generally resumes 1 to 2 months after chemotherapy is completed. Common culprits that cause this side effect include bleomycin, cyclophosphamide, docetaxel, doxorubicin, fluorouracil, ifosphamide, irinotecan, and paclitaxel.

Other Acute Side Effects

Chemotherapy-Induced Nausea and Vomiting

Chemotherapy-induced nausea and vomiting (CINV) is a common—and the most dreaded—side effect of chemotherapy. If not controlled, it may affect patient compliance with chemotherapy. The risk of this side effect depends on the agent as well as the dose and individual patient factors.

Chemotherapy agents are classified according to their emetogenic potential, sometimes using the Hesketh classification. Cisplatin is considered the most emetogenic and the "gold standard" for testing antiemetic agents. Other commonly used agents with high emetogenic potential are high-dose cyclophosphamide, dacarbazine, cytarabine, doxorubicin, carboplatin, and oxaliplatin. Combinations of agents also increase the risk of CINV.

Nausea and vomiting can be separated into subtypes based on their time course and underlying cause. Each type responds differently to treatment.

Principles of therapy are as follows:

- The goal is to completely prevent nausea and vomiting.
- It is easier to prevent CINV than to treat it. Prevention is best done by using *scheduled* around-the-clock dosing, starting 30 to 60 minutes *before* chemotherapy and *continuing* for a minimum of 24 hours after chemotherapy is complete.
- Patients should also receive prn antiemetics for breakthrough symptoms.
- A combination of agents often gives the best results.
- For agents causing delayed nausea, treat the patient for at least 3 to 5 days.
- A combination of aprepitant, a $5HT_3$ receptor blocker, and a corticosteroid is the most effective regimen.
- For short-acting serotonin$_3$ ($5HT_3$) receptor blockers, the oral route is as effective as the IV route and is less expensive. All three $5HT_3$ agents are considered equally effective.
- Corticosteroids enhance the effectiveness of $5HT_3$ receptor blockers, so these agents should be given in combination.
- Palonosetron and aprepitant are the most effective agents for preventing delayed nausea and vomiting.

See the supplemental materials for information on the neurotransmitters involved in vomiting and the mechanism of action of antiemetics.

Patient counseling should include the following points:

- Avoid large meals; eat small meals instead. Avoid consuming solid food for 8 to 12 hours before chemotherapy.
- Avoid the kitchen during meal preparation, as food smells can worsen CINV.
- Eat foods that are at room temperature, rather than very hot or very cold foods.
- Limit fluid intake at meal times so as not to fill up.
- Avoid sweets and fatty foods.

Table 9-9 Classification of Nausea and Vomiting

Type	Onset	Comments
Acute	Usual onset 1–2 hours, peak at 5–6 hours, subsides in 24 hours	Easiest to control. For highly emetogenic regimens, use a combination of aprepitant, a $5HT_3$ antagonist, and a corticosteroid with or without benzodiazepine.
Delayed	Onset after 24 hours, peak at 2–3 days, can persist for 6–7 days	Most difficult to control. Frequent causes: cisplatin, carboplatin, high-dose cyclophosphamide, doxorubicin. Palonosetron and aprepitant are the most effective agents for preventing delayed nausea and vomiting. Corticosteroids are the most effective for treatment of this side effect.
Anticipatory	Before chemotherapy is given	Conditioned response that occurs as a result of prior bad experiences. Giving a benzodiazepine (lorazepam) beforehand can help prevent it.
Breakthrough	Occurs despite prophylaxis	Try prochlorperazine, metoclopramide, or lorazepam prn.

Table 9-10 Antiemetic Agents for the Prevention and Treatment of CINV[2]

Drug Class	Agent	Brand Name	Adult Dose/Comments
$5HT_3$ receptor blocker	Dolasetron	Anzemet Tablets and injection	Single daily dose of 100 mg or 1.8 mg/kg, IV or po.
	Granisetron	Kytril Tablets, oral solution, injection Sancuso Transdermal patch	Oral: single daily dose of 2 mg or 1 mg bid. IV: single daily dose of 1 mg or 10 mcg/kg. Apply the patch 24–48 hours before chemotherapy and leave on for at least 24 hours after chemotherapy; it may be left on for as long as 7 days.
	Ondansetron	Zofran Tablets, ODT, oral solution, injection	Oral: single daily dose of 24 mg or 8 mg given bid-tid. IV: single dose of 32 mg or 0.15 mg/kg at 8-hr intervals × 3. Doses may vary depending on the emetogenicity of the chemotherapy.
	Palonosetron	Aloxi Capsules and injection	Longest half-life and higher binding affinity compared to other $5HT_3$ receptor blockers. Single dose of 0.25 mg IV or 0.5 mg oral, not to be repeated for 7 days.
NK_1 inhibitor	Aprepitant	Emend 40, 80, and 125 mg capsules	Given as a 3-day regimen for moderately to highly emetogenic chemotherapy in combination with a $5HT_3$ receptor blocker and a corticosteroid. Day 1, 125 mg; days 2 and 3, 80 mg. Good for prevention of delayed CINV. Inhibits CYP 3A4, induces 2C9, and is metabolized by 3A4. Potentially significant interaction with warfarin (increased INR), oral contraceptives (decreased effect), and dexamethasone (need to reduce the dose of dexamethasone by 40–50%).
	Fosaprepitant	Emend Injection	Metabolized to aprepitant. May give 115 mg IV on day 1 in place of oral aprepitant. Follow with oral aprepitant 80 mg on days 2 and 3.
Benzamide analog	Metoclopramide	Reglan 10 mg tablets and injection	May be helpful for delayed CINV and prn use for breakthrough nausea and vomiting. Dose: 40–60 mg po q 4–6 hr. Can give as much as 1–2 mg/kg IV q 3–4 hr. High doses can cause extrapyramidal side effects, in which case diphenhydramine should be added.
Phenothiazines Dopamine$_2$ (D_2) receptor blocker	Prochlorperazine and others	Compazine Oral tablet and spansule, injection, and suppository	Best for preventing mild to moderate CINV, prn use for breakthrough nausea and vomiting, and (possibly) preventing delayed nausea. Dose: 10 mg po or IV q 4–6 hr, 15 mg spansule q 8–12 hr, 25 mg prn q 12 hr.
Butyrophenones D_2 receptor blockers	Droperidol Haloperidol	Inapsine Injection Haldol	"Black box" warning for QT-interval prolongation with droperidol. Less sedating alternative to phenothiazines.
Benzodiazepines	Lorazepam and others	Ativan Tablets, oral solution, injection	Useful for patients with an anxiety component in CINV and for preventing anticipatory nausea and vomiting. Dose: 0.5–2 mg po/IV/SL q 4–6 hr. For anticipatory CINV: 0.5–2 mg q 8 hr starting the night before chemotherapy.
Cannabinoid	Dronabinol	Marinol 2.5 mg, 5 mg, and 10 mg capsules	Dose: 5 mg tid-qid starting 1–3 hours before chemotherapy. C-III. Second- or third-line agent for mild to moderately emetogenic regimens. Common side effects: sedation, other CNS effects.
	Nabilone	Cesamet 1 mg capsules	Dose: 1–2 mg, bid-tid starting 1–3 hours before chemotherapy. C-II. Second- or third-line agent for mild to moderately emetogenic regimens. Common side effects: sedation, other CNS effects.
Corticosteroid	Dexamethasone	Decadron Tablets and injection	Dose: 4–20 mg orally or IV. Enhances the effectiveness of $5HT_3$ receptor blockers. Useful for delayed CINV. Minimal side effects when used short term, but watch for glucose intolerance in diabetics. For delayed CINV: 8 mg daily or bid.
	Methylpredniso-lone	Solu-Medrol Injection Medrol Tablets	Dose: 40–125 mg IV. Other than dose, same comments as for dexamethasone.

NK = neurokinin; ODT = orally disintegrating tablet.

Histamine$_2$ blockers or proton pump inhibitors can also be added.

- Eat slowly and chew food well.
- Dry foods such as crackers or toast may help to settle the stomach.
- Lie down or rest.

Extravasation Reactions

Many chemotherapy agents are irritants or vesicants if allowed to leak into soft tissues. Of these, anthracyclines are the most notorious vesicants and cause the most damage. Other vesicants include vincristine and vinblastine. Some drugs create problems only if extravasated in large quantities or if highly concentrated. Examples of irritants include cisplatin, epipodophyllotoxins, and taxanes.

Patients should be told to report any pain, burning, tingling, or itching either during or after IV chemotherapy administration. The best method of preventing or minimizing these reactions is to have guidelines in place for safe administration, to use central venous catheters for delivering chemotherapy when possible, and to have established procedures for the management of extravasation. Antidotes should be readily available, if needed. All occurrences should be documented in the patient's medical record.

Hypersensitivity Reactions

Signs and symptoms of hypersensitivity reactions include anaphylaxis, bronchospasm, hypotension, fever, chills, pruritis, and rash. In some cases, these reactions may be caused by the delivery vehicle (e.g., Cremophor EL, Polysorbate 80) rather than the active ingredient. Premedication with diphenhydramine, acetaminophen, and corticosteroids (either alone or in combination) is recommended for some of these agents. Slowing the infusion rate may help in some cases. Have epinephrine, diphenhydramine, and corticosteroids on hand when agents with potential for hypersensitivity reactions are administered.

Table 9-12 Commonly Used Agents with "Black Box" Warnings for Hypersensitivity Reactions[2]

Bleomycin	Oxaliplatin
Carboplatin	Paclitaxel
Cisplatin	Rituximab
Docetaxel	Trastuzumab
Doxorubicin, conventional and liposomal	

Hyperuricemia/Tumor Lysis Syndrome

Hyperuricemia and tumor lysis syndrome are caused by the release of uric acid during cell lysis. These side effects are related more to the type of cancer being treated than to the specific chemotherapy agents being used. Cancers with large cell burdens, such as acute leukemias and lymphomas, are most likely to cause hyperuricemia and tumor lysis syndrome. Pretreat the patient with allopurinol or rasburicase in addition to ensuring hydration and alkalinization of the urine.

Organ System Toxicity

See Table 9-13.

Long-Term Toxicities

Chemotherapy agents are associated with many additional side effects, including infertility (temporary or permanent), hepatotoxicity, ocular toxicity, and a variety of other dermatologic effects. Hormonal agents tend to have a completely different side-effect profile including hot flashes, loss of libido, gynecomastia, disease flare, thrombosis, and osteoporosis.

2.1.0 Dosage Calculations

Medication errors are a concern with any drug, but are particularly acute with antineoplastic agents. Errors

Table 9-11 Antidotes Used for Extravasation Reactions[3]

Agent	Use	Comments
Dexrazoxane (Totect)	Anthracyclines	The Totect brand of dexrazoxane is FDA approved for this use. Start it within 6 hours of extravasation, and give it as an IV infusion once daily for 3 days. Also apply cold compresses to the site of extravasation and elevate it if possible.
Dimethyl sulfoxide (DMSO) 99% (weight/volume)	Anthracyclines, mitomycin	Apply 1–2 mL topically every 6 hours × 14 days; do not cover. Also apply cold compresses to the site of extravasation and elevate it if possible.
Hyaluronidase (Amphadase, Hylenex, Vitrase)	Vinca alkaloids, etoposide, teniposide, taxanes	Enzyme used to aid local dispersion. Inject 150 units locally using the "pin cushion" technique. Also apply warm compresses. For taxanes, use cold compresses.
Sodium thiosulfate	Mechlorethamine, cisplatin, oxaliplatin	1/6 M solution (prepare using 4 mL of 10% solution for injection mixed with 6 mL of sterile water for injection). Inject locally using the "pin cushion" technique.

Table 9-13 Organ System Toxicities of Commonly Used Chemotherapy Agents

Toxicity	Causative Agents	Manifestations/Monitoring	Comments
Cardiac	Anthracyclines/ doxorubicin	Can cause acute symptoms (arrhythmia, pericarditis), but the greatest concern is irreversible heart failure. Perform a baseline ejection fraction and serial follow-up.	Dose limiting, related to the total cumulative dose. Dexrazoxane (Zinecard) is a chemoprotective agent that can be used for prophylaxis. Pegylated liposomal doxorubicin was developed to decrease cardiac toxicity.
	Trastuzumab	Signs and symptoms of chronic heart failure.	Not dose limiting. Not recommended in combination with anthracyclines due to the increased risk of cardiac toxicity.
Nephrotoxicity	Cisplatin	Decreased GFR, increased sCr, hypomagnesemia, hypokalemia. Monitor sCr and clCr before each dose.	Dose limiting. The risk is cumulative. Prevent this toxicity with hydration. Mannitol and/or furosemide can also be used. Administer in a saline vehicle.* Amifostine (Ethyol) is approved for preventing nephrotoxicity due to cisplatin. Carboplatin is less nephrotoxic.
	Methotrexate	Acute renal failure due to precipitation of methotrexate in the renal tubules.	Can be seen with high-dose methotrexate. Alkalinize the urine and hydrate.
Hemorrhagic cystitis	Ifosfamide	Microscopic and gross hematuria, dysuria, frequency, urgency. Monitor signs and symptoms and perform urinalysis.	Caused by formation of the acrolein metabolite, which concentrates in the bladder. All doses *must* be given with mesna to prevent hemorrhagic cystitis (mesna is a chemoprotective agent). Give the first dose IV immediately before ifosfamide, followed by 2 more doses that may be either IV or oral.
	Cyclophos-phamide	Same as for ifosfamide.	Prevent hemorrhagic cystitis with hydration and frequent voiding. Option: use mesna with high doses.
Neurotoxicity	Vincristine	Peripheral: "stocking-glove" paresthesias, loss of DTR, motor weakness. Autonomic: primarily constipation. Monitor symptoms and DTR.	Peripheral neuropathy is dose limiting and cumulative. Use prophylactic stool softeners and laxatives. Never give intrathecally.
	Cisplatin	Peripheral sensory neuropathy: paresthesias, tingling, numbness in hands and feet. May lead to sensory ataxia. Also ototoxicity, tinnitus. Monitor symptoms.	Related to cumulative dose.
	Oxaliplatin	Peripheral sensory neuropathy: hand, foot, and perioral paresthesia, exacerbated by cold. Monitor symptoms.	Dose limiting, cumulative, progressive.
	Taxanes	Numbness, pain, tingling in "stocking glove" distribution. Impairment of fine motor skills. Monitor symptoms and DTR.	Linked to paclitaxel more than docetaxel. Can be dose limiting.
Pulmonary	Bleomycin	Dyspnea, tachypnea, fever, nonproductive cough. Monitor symptoms; perform a chest x-ray if needed.	Causes both hypersensitivity pneumonitis and pulmonary fibrosis. Dose limiting, related to the cumulative dose.
Hand–foot syndrome	Fluorouracil Capecitabine	Tender erythema of the palms of the hands and the soles of the feet. Can start with tingling or burning, progress to erythema and swelling, and then lead to blistering and desquamation.	Patients should be counseled on this side effect and told to report any early symptoms to their physician. Capecitabine has been reported to cause photosensitivity.
Rash	Imatinib	Erythematous macules and papules on the face, arms, and trunk.	
	Erlotinib	Acneiform/pustular rash, dry skin, fissuring. Occurs in a high percentage of patients.	Generally indicates the drug is working. Treat with topical agents and supportive care. Avoid sun exposure.

DTR = deep tendon reflexes.

* Chloride keeps cisplatin in nonaquated form, which is less toxic. The aquated form has higher protein and tissue binding.

involving this group of drugs have the potential to cause extreme harm or may even be fatal. Among other things, always check and double-check the dose and route of administration.

Anticancer agents are dosed in a variety of ways: fixed dose (mg), body weight (mg/kg), or body surface area (mg/m^2, g/m^2). In the process of verifying correct doses, make sure you know which dosing method is being used. There is a big difference in a dose calculated in mg/kg as compared with one calculated in mg/m^2! Cancer drugs, in particular, are sometimes dosed based on body surface area (BSA). Some evidence indicates that drug clearance correlates better with BSA than with weight alone. BSA can be calculated using an equation or from various nomograms based on the patient's height and weight. Pharmacists should perform their own BSA and dose calculations independent of the prescriber as a double-check system.

Mosteller method:

$$\text{BSA in m}^2 = \text{square root of } \frac{(\text{height in cm} \times \text{weight in kg})}{3{,}600}$$

Du Bois method:

$$\text{BSA in m}^2 = 0.007184 \times \text{height in cm}^{0.725} \times \text{weight in kg}^{0.425}$$

See the appendix for an adult BSA nomogram.

In addition, the area under the curve (AUC) is sometimes used for dosing carboplatin. In this case, the Calvert formula can be used to determine the patient's dose:

$$\text{Total dose (mg)} = (\text{target AUC}) \times (\text{GFR} + 25)$$

The usual AUC for IV carboplatin is in the range of 4–7.5. A modified Calvert formula is used in children. If you do not have this text handy when you are out in practice, you can find the needed equation in either *Facts & Comparisons* or *AHFS Drug Information* under the "carboplatin" entry.

2.2.0 Dispensing

Be aware when you are dispensing cytotoxic agents that some of the parenteral agents are available in more than one formulation. For example:

- Doxorubicin: conventional and liposomal
- Cytarabine: conventional (with and without preservative) and liposomal for intrathecal use
- Methotrexate: with and without preservative
- Paclitaxel: conventional (formulated with Cremophor EL) and albumin-bound
- GnRH analogs: slow-release formulations dosed at varying intervals

Proper Storage

A number of chemotherapeutic products require refrigeration. See the comments sections of Tables 9-3 and 9-15.

Proper Handling and Disposal

Cytotoxic agents are considered hazardous and should be handled and disposed of accordingly. Hazardous drugs are defined as any drug causing cancer, teratogenic effects, reproductive toxicity, organ toxicity, or genotoxicity at low doses.

When preparing parenteral agents, personal protective equipment should be worn and drugs prepared either in a Class II contained vertical-flow biological safety cabinet (BSC) using closed-system drug transfer devices (e.g., PhaSeal system) or in a Class III BSC. For dispensing, all such agents should be placed inside a sealed plastic bag and clearly labeled: "Chemotherapy. Handle with Gloves. Dispose of Properly." This bag should be placed inside of a second sealed plastic bag for further transfer.

For oral cytotoxic agents, gloves should be worn when handling them. Use only a designated counting tray, and do not use an automatic counting machine.

Table 9-14 Long-Term Toxicities

Toxicity	Causative Agents	Manifestations/ Monitoring	Comments
Carcinogenicity	Alkylating agents Anthracyclines Epipodophyllotoxins	Development of leukemias and second malignancies	Median time to development after chemotherapy is 15 years.
Teratogenicity	Concern with all of the chemotherapy agents		Most agents are classified into pregnancy categories D and X. Birth control should be considered for any patient at risk of becoming pregnant. Use special precautions when handling cytotoxic agents.

Proper Preparation and Administration

Platinum compounds interact with aluminum, so they should not be mixed with or administered using aluminum needles. Some agents should not be administered via PVC tubing or containers due to the potential for leaching DEHP plasticizer. An inline filter should be used during paclitaxel administration. Depending on the agent, chemotherapy may be administered by many methods: intravenous, intramuscular, subcutaneous, intrathecal, intraperitoneal, intrapleural, intra-arterial, intravesicular, oral, topical, or even intracranial implant. Only cytarabine and methotrexate should be given by the intrathecal route. Always use preservative-free formulations when preparing injections for delivery via this route.

Table 9-15 Storage and Administration[2]

Drug	IV	IM	SC	IP	IT	Refrigerate*	Comments
Bevacizumab	√					√	Infuse over 60–90 minutes. Do not use dextrose-containing solutions.
Bleomycin	√	√	√			√	Can also be given intrapleurally. Do not use dextrose-containing solutions.
Carboplatin	√			√			Reacts with aluminum.
Cisplatin	√			√			Infuse over 6–8 hours. Dilute in saline-containing solution. Reacts with aluminum. Compatible with mannitol in the same admixture. Y-site compatibility with furosemide. If not used within 6 hours, protect the diluted solution from light.
Cyclophosphamide	√						Also available in tablet form.
Cytarabine	√		√		√	√ for DepoCyt only	DepoCyt (liposomal form) is for intrathecal use only.
Dacarbazine	√					√	
Docetaxel	√						Avoid PVC tubing and containers; a Polysorbate 80 vehicle leaches plasticizer.
Doxorubicin	√					√ solution for injection and liposomal	Store powder for injection at room temperature.
Fluorouracil	√						Can be given intra-arterially via the hepatic artery for hepatic metastases.
Gemcitabine	√						
Ifosfamide	√						Must be administered with mesna.
Irinotecan	√						Infuse over 90 minutes.
Methotrexate	√	√			√		Also available in tablet form, but the primary route of delivery for malignancy is IV. Use preservative-free vials for intrathecal injections.
Oxaliplatin	√						Do not mix in sodium chloride-containing solutions. Reacts with aluminum.
Paclitaxel	√						Conventional formulation: infuse over 3 hours. Avoid PVC tubing and containers (Cremophor EL vehicle leaches plasticizer). Use 0.22-mcm inline filter for administration. Do not filter the albumin-bound formulation; PVC tubing can be used with this formulation.
Rituximab	√					√	Administer as IV infusion only.
Trastuzumab	√					√	Give as IV infusion: first dose over 90 minutes, subsequent doses over 30–60 minutes. Do not use dextrose-containing solutions.
Vinblastine	√					√	Fatal if given intrathecally.
Vincristine	√					√	Fatal if given intrathecally.

IV = intravenous; IM = intramuscular; SC = subcutaneous; IP = intraperitoneal; IT = intrathecal.

* Store in a refrigerated site prior to reconstitution or mixing.

Table 9-16 Summary of American Cancer Society Cancer Screening Guidelines

Guidelines for Asymptomatic Persons of Average Risk with Negative Screening Results[1]			
Cancer Site	**Population**	**Test or Procedure**	**Frequency**
Breast	Women, aged 20 years and older	Mammography	Annually, beginning at age 40
		Clinical breast exam	Recommended as part of a periodic health exam, at a minimum every 3 years for ages 20–39, and annually thereafter.
		Breast self-examination	Beginning in the early 20s, educate women on the importance of breast self-awareness and to report any changes.
Colorectal	Men and women, aged 50 years and older	Colonoscopy **or**	Every 10 years
		Flexible sigmoidoscopy **or**	Every 5 years
		Barium enema **or**	Every 5 years
		CT colonography **or**	Every 5 years
		Stool tests for blood: fecal occult blood test **or** fecal immunochemical test	Annually
		Stool DNA test	Uncertain
Cervical	Women, aged 18 years and older	Papanicolaou (Pap) test (test for cervical cytology) Human papillomavirus DNA testing: optional	Screening should begin approximately 3 years after beginning sexual intercourse, but no later than 21 years of age. Frequency of screening depends on the type of test. For conventional Pap tests, the recommended frequency is annually. There is an option to decrease the frequency of testing if previous exams have been normal.
Prostate	Men, aged 50 years and older	PSE and DRE	Discuss the pros and cons of screening. Offer these options to the patient.

3.1.0 Quality Information Sources on Cancer Topics

- American Cancer Society (ACS)
- American Society of Clinical Oncologists (ASCO)
- National Cancer Institute (NCI)
- National Comprehensive Cancer Network (NCCN)

Information for patients is available at www.chemocare.com.

3.2.0 Cancer Screening

Cancer screening plays an important role in the early detection of some cancers and has been shown to save lives, particularly in patients with cervical cancer, breast cancer, and colorectal cancer. For other cancers (e.g., lung, ovarian), there is no adequate method of routine screening available. Finally, screening for some cancers, such as prostate cancer, is highly controversial. With prostate cancer, effects of screening on mortality are equivocal while exposing patients to the risks of overtreatment.

Recommendations for cancer screening are available from several organizations and do not always agree. Guidelines from the American Cancer Society and the United States Preventive Services Task Force are the most widely publicized. Pharmacists can play an important role in educating the public regarding the benefits of cancer screening and providing current recommendations.

Table 9-17 Comprehensive Listing of Antineoplastic Agents by Chemical Classification/Mechanism of Action

Alkylating Agents				
Chemical Class	**Agent**	**Synonym/Brand Name**	**Major Toxicity**	**Comments**
Bis-chloroethylamines (Nitrogen mustards)	Nitrogen mustard Injection	meclorethamine, Mustargen	Bone marrow ↓, vesicant, N/V	Use in 15" of reconstitution, rapid decomposition Neutralize with sodium thiosulfate
	Cyclophosphamide Oral and injection	Cytoxan, Neosar	Bone marrow ↓, N/V, hemorrhagic cystitis	Hydrate patient, prodrug that needs to be activated Also causes SIADH and alopecia
	Ifosfamide Injection	Ifex	Bone marrow ↓, hemorrhagic cystitis	Hydrate patient and give with mesna (Mesnex) to prevent bladder toxicity
	Melphalan (2 mg) Oral and injection	L-PAM, Alkeran, l-phenylalanine mustard	Bone marrow ↓	Refrigerate. Take on an empty stomach. Used for multiple myeloma
	Chlorambucil (2 mg) Oral	Leukeran	Bone marrow ↓	Good oral bioavailability, used in CLL
	Estramustine Oral	Emcyt (140 mg cap)	Bone marrow ↓, estrogenic SE	Combination of estrogen and nitrogen mustard. Take on empty stomach. Refrigerate. Used in metastatic prostate cancer
Nitrosoureas	Carmustine Injection and implant	BCNU, BiCNU Gliadel Wafer	Delayed bone marrow ↓, N/V, pulmonary fibrosis	Refrigerate, absolute alcohol diluent, absorbs to PVC, use glass container. Infuse over 1–2 hr. Irritant if extravasated. Crosses BBB. Gliadel wafers for intracranial implantation.
	Lomustine Oral	CCNU, CeeNu	Delayed bone marrow ↓, N/V	Take on empty stomach
	Streptozocin Injection	Zanosar	Renal, N/V, delayed BM ↓	Refrigerate, light sensitive, hydrate to prevent nephrotoxicity. Monitor renal function, proteinuria, avoid extravasation
Alkyl sulfonate	Busulfan Oral and injection	Myleran (2 mg tab) Busulfex injection	Bone marrow ↓, pulmonary fibrosis	Delayed/prolonged BM suppression, used in CML
Ethylenimine (Aziridine)	Thiotepa Injection	triethylenethiophos-phoramide, Thioplex	Bone marrow ↓	Refrigerate, intravesicular administration for bladder cancer
Triazine	Dacarbazine Injection	DTIC-Dome	Bone marrow ↓, N/V	Refrigerate. Used for melanoma and Hodgkin's disease
	Temozolomide Oral and injection	Temodar	Bone marrow ↓	For glioblastoma. Prodrug of an active metabolite of dacarbazine. Take capsules on an empty stomach. Refrigerate injection

(continues)

Table 9-17 (*continued*)

Chemical Class	Agent	Synonym/Brand Name	Major Toxicity	Comments
Metals (**Platinum complexes**)	Cisplatin Injection	CDDP, Platinol, Platinol-AQ	Nephrotoxicity, N/V, peripheral neuropathy	Hydrate. Reacts with aluminum Black box warning re: hypersensitivity rxns
	Carboplatin Injection	Paraplatin	Bone marrow ↓, N/V, hypersensitivity	Reacts with aluminum. Black box warning re: hypersensitivity rxns
	Oxaliplatin Injection	Eloxati	Peripheral neuropathy, N/V	Reacts with aluminum. Black box warning re: hypersensitivity rxns
Other	Procarbazine (50 mg) Oral	Matulane	Bone marrow ↓, CNS	Weak MAOI, flushing with alcohol. Part of MOPP regimen for Hodgkin's disease
	Altretamine (50 mg) Oral	hexamethylmelamine Hexalen	Bone marrow ↓, N/V, paresthesias	Used for ovarian CA. 260 mg/m^2 in 4 divided doses after meals and bedtime. Take for 14-21 days out of 28.
	Bendamustine Injection	Treanda	Bone marrow ↓, skin reactions	Used for CLL, non-Hodgkin's lymphoma. Watch for DDI with CYP 1A2 inhibitors (will ↓ formation of active metabs)

Antimetabolites				
Category	**Agent**	**Synonym/Brand Name**	**Major Toxicity**	**Comments**
Folic acid antagonists	Methotrexate Oral and injection Vials for injection both with and without preservative	MTX	Bone marrow ↓, stomatitis	Leucovorin antidote, pulmonary fibrosis, nephrotoxicity in large doses, extensive renal excretion. Use preservative-free vials for intrathecal injections
	Pemetrexed Injection	Alimta	Bone marrow ↓, stomatitis, rash	Pretreat w/ corticosteroid to decrease incidence and severity of rash. Supplement with B12 & folate. For mesothelioma
	Pralatrexate Injection	Folotyn	Bone marrow ↓, stomatitis	Refrigerate. Supplement with B12 & folate.
Pyrimidine analogs	Cytarabine Injection (IV and intrathecal)	Ara-C, Cytosine arabinoside, Cytosar DepoCyt intrathecal	Bone marrow ↓, stomatitis	Used for acute leukemias DepoCyt is liposomal formulation for q 14 day intrathecal use, refrigerate DepoCyt only
	Fluorouracil Injection	5-FU, Adrucil	Stomatitis, bone marrow ↓, diarrhea	Broad spectrum, used w/ leucovorin in colon cancer. Leucovorin enhances binding to thymidylate synthase
	Capecitabine Oral 150 and 500 mg tablets	Xeloda	Diarrhea, bone marrow ↓	Oral prodrug of 5FU. Hand-foot syndrome. Significant DDI w/ warfarin. For colorectal and breast cancer. Given in 3 week cycles, 2 weeks on, one week off. Give with food

	Floxuridine Injection	FUDR	Stomatitis, bone marrow ↓, hepatotox	Intra-arterial for liver metastases in colon cancer
	Gemcitabine Injection	Gemzar	Bone marrow ↓, rash	For breast, lung, ovarian, and pancreatic cancers
	Azacitidine Injection	Vidaza	Bone marrow ↓	Indicated for myelodysplastic syndrome
	Decitabine Injection	Dacogen	Bone marrow ↓	Indicated for myelodysplastic syndrome
	Nelarabine Injection	Arranon	Bone marrow ↓, CNS and peripheral neuropathy	For leukemia/lymphoma.
Purine analogs	Thioguanine (40 mg) Oral	6-TG, Tabloid	Bone marrow ↓	For acute leukemia. Give on empty stomach
	Mercaptopurine (50 mg) Oral	6-MP, Purinethol	Bone marrow ↓, hepatotoxicity	Take on empty stomach. For leukemia. **Major DDI with allopurinol, inhibits 6-MP metabolism**
	Fludarabine Injection and oral	Fludara injection Oforta tablets	Bone marrow ↓	Refrigerate injection. Tablets should not be crushed
	Clofarabine Injection	Clolar	Bone marrow ↓	For acute lymphoblasitc leukemia
Adenosine analogs	Pentostatin Injection	2-deoxycoformycin, Nipent	Bone marrow, N/V Nephrotoxicity, rash	Refrigerate. Used for hairy cell leukemia
	Cladribine Injection	Leustatin	Bone marrow ↓	Refrigerate. Used for hairy cell leukemia
Other	Hydroxyurea Oral 200, 300, 400, 500 mg caps	Hydrea	Bone marrow ↓, mucositis	For CML, thrombocytosis, polycythemia vera. Can take with food to decrease GI upset

Antitumor Antibiotics and Other Natural Products

Category	Agent	Synonym/Brand Name	Major Toxicity	Comments
Anthracyclines	Doxorubicin Injection	Adriamycin Doxil (liposomal)	Bone marrow ↓, cardiac, vesicant, infusion reactions with liposomal	Store powder at room temperature, refrigerate solution and liposomal. Turns urine red, reduce dose in hepatic dysfunction. Broad spectrum agent.
	Daunorubicin Injection	Cerubidine DaunoXome (liposomal)	Bone marrow ↓, vesicant, N/V, cardiac	Refrigerate. Turns urine red, reduce dose in hepatic dysfunction. Used for leukemia
	Idarubicin Injection	Idamycin	Bone marrow ↓, N/V, cardiac, vesicant	Refrigerate. Turns urine red, reduce dose in hepatic dysfunction
	Epirubicin Injection	Ellence	Bone marrow ↓, cardiac, vesicant	Refrigerate. Turns urine red, reduce dose in hepatic dysfunction
	Valrubicin Injection for bladder instillation	Valstar	Bladder irritation	Refrigerate. Intravescicular administration only, retain x 2 hr, avoid PVC tubing. Solution is red.

(*continues*)

Table 9-17 (*continued*)

Category	Agent	Synonym/Brand Name	Major Toxicity	Comments
Anthracycline-related (anthracendione)	Mitoxantrone Injection	Novantrone	Bone marrow ↓, N/V, stomatitis, vesicant	Blue-green urine, less cardiac toxicity than anthracyclines
Other antitumor antibiotics	Dactinomycin Injection	Actinomycin-D, Cosmegen	Bone marrow ↓, N/V, vesicant	Bone marrow toxicity is delayed and cumulative
	Mitomycin Injection	Mutamycin	Bone marrow ↓, N/V	Bone marrow ↓ is cumulative
	Bleomycin Injection	Blenoxane	Hypersensitivity, pulmonary	Avoid cumulative dose >400U, refrigerate, give test dose in lymphoma. Reduce dose in renal dysfunction. Can be given IV, IM, SC, intrapleural
Camptothecins	Topotecan Injection and oral	Hycamtin	Bone marrow ↓, diarrhea	Approved for small-cell lung cancer. Refrigerate. Do not crush, chew or break capsules.
	Irinotecan Injection	Camptosar	Bone marrow ↓, diarrhea	Atropine for early diarrhea, loperamide for late diarrhea. For colorectal cancer.
Enzymes	Asparaginase, Pegaspargase (PEG) Injection	l-asparaginase, Elspar, Oncaspar	Hypersensitivity	Test dose recommended by manufacturer. Conjugation of asparaginase with PEG to ↓ hypersensitivity. Refrigerate, don't shake. For acute leukemia.
Epothilones	Ixabepilone Injection	Ixempra	Bone marrow ↓, peripheral neuropathy	Cremophor EL vehicle, premedicate for hypersensitivity rxns, DDI with CYP 3A4. Avoid PVC containing infusion bags or sets as plasticizer may leach. Refrigerate. Requires inline filter. Used for metastatic breast cancer.

Plant Alkaloids

Category	Agent	Synonym/Brand Name	Major Toxicity	Comments
Vinca alkaloids	Vincristine Injection	VCR, Oncovin Vincasar PFS	Neurotoxicity, vesicant	Refrigerate, 1.4 mg/m^2 or 2 mg /wk limit, SIADH, hepatic metabolism. Fatal if given intrathecally
	Vinblastine Injection	VBL, Velban	Bone marrow ↓, vesicant	Refrigerate. Fatal if given intrathecally
	Vinorelbine Injection	Navelbine	Bone marrow ↓, vesicant,	Refrigerate.
Epipodophyllotoxin	Etoposide Oral and injection	VePesid, VP-16, Etopophos, Toposar	Bone marrow ↓	Refrigerate capsules. Hypotension if given too fast, absolute alcohol diluent, avoid PVC tubing. Used for small-cell lung cancer.
	Teniposide Injection	VM-23, Vumon	Bone marrow ↓, hypersensitivity, mucositis	Cremophor EL/absolute alcohol diluent. Avoid PVC tubing. Refrigerate, slow IV to avoid ↓BP
Taxanes	Paclitaxel Injection Albumin bound paclitaxel Injection	Taxol Abraxane	Bone marrow ↓, hypersensitivity, peripheral neuropathy	Taxol: Cremophor EL/absolute alcohol diluent, avoid PVC tubing, infuse over 3 hr, use 0.22 mcm filter, pretreat all patients with corticosteroids, diphenhydramine and H_2 blockers to prevent hypersensitivity. Abraxane: does not require pretreatment, filtering, or avoidance of PVC. Metabolized by CYP 2C8, 3A4
	Docetaxel Injection	Taxotere	Bone marrow ↓, hypersensitivity, peripheral neuropathy, fluid retention	Pretreat all patients with dexamethasone starting 3 days before to prevent both fluid retention and hypersensitivity. Avoid PVC tubing. Metabolized by 3A4. Contains polysorbate 80.

Monoclonal Antibodies			
Category	**Agent**	**Synonym/ Brand Name**	**Comments—SE hypersensitivity, give as IV infusion, not IV bolus**
Monoclonal antibodies	Alemtuzumab Injection	Campath	MAB to CD52, cell surface antigen on all B and T lymphocytes and some other hematopoietic cells. Used in B-cell CLL for patients that have failed alkylating agents and fludarabine. SE: bone marrow ↓, infusion reactions. Give as 2 hr infusion. Refrigerate.
	Bevicizumab Injection	Avastin	Blocks binding of VEGF to its receptors. Infuse over 60-90 min. SE: hypertension, GI perforation, wound healing complications. Refrigerate.
	Cetuximab Injection	Erbitux	MAB that binds to EGFR and blocks effects for EGF. For colorectal, head and neck cancer. SE: infusion reactions, skin rash, photosensitivity. Infuse over 1-2 hr. Use 0.22 mcm in-line filter. Refrigerate.
	Gemtuzumab ozogamicin Injection	Mylotarg	MAB for patients with CD-33 positive AML. SE: hypersensitivity, hepatoxicity, bone marrow ↓, premedicate, infuse over 2 hr, use UV protective bag over IV bag during infusion, use in-line filter. Refrigerate.
	Ibritumomab tiuxetan Injection	Zevalin	Radiopharmaceutical given in conjunction w/ rituximab, for non-Hodgkin's lymphoma. SE: hypersensitivity, skin rxn, bone marrow ↓. Premedicate. Use in-line filter. Refrigerate.
	Ofatumumab Injection	Arzerra	Used for CLL, binds to portion of CD20 antigen on B-lymphocytes. SE: Infusion reactions, bone marrow ↓. Give by infusion only. Premedicate. Use in-line filter. Refrigerate.
	Panitumomab Injection	Vectibix	MAB to EGFR and blocks effects of EGF. Used for colorectal cancer. SE: hypersensitivity, skin reactions. Give as 60-90 minute infusion. Use in-line filter. Refrigerate.
	Rituximab Injection	Rituxan	MAB against CD20 (cell surface antigen found on normal and malignant B-lymphocytes). Used for B-cell non-Hodgkin's lymphoma. Hypersensitivity rxns (pretreat with acetaminophen and antihistamine), bone marrow ↓
	Tositumomab Injection	Bexxar	Iodine containing radiopharmaceutical. For non-Hodgkin's lymphoma. SE: hypersensitivity reactions, bone marrow ↓. Thyroid protective agents must be given 24 hr before. Infuse over 60 minutes, premedicate, use in-line filter. Refrigerate.
	Trastuzumab Injection	Herceptin	MAB to HER-2 receptor, an epidermal growth factor receptor found in ~20% of women with breast cancer. SE: hypersensitivity rxns, cardiotoxicity. Give as 30–90 minute infusion. Refrigerate

Newer Agents and Miscellaneous			
Category	**Agent**	**Synonym/Brand Name**	**Comments—watch CYP450 drug interactions with tyrosine kinase inhibitors**
Tyrosine kinase inhibitors	Sorafenib Oral	Nexavar	Multikinase inhibitor. Skin rash, hand foot syndrome, metabolized by CYP3A4, inhibits 2C9. Take on empty stomach.
	Dasatinib Oral	Sprycel	Bone marrow suppression, fluid retention, QT >, used for CML
	Imatinib Oral	Gleevec	Used for CML. Metabolized by CYP 3A4, inhibits 3A4 and 2D6, watch for DDI. Avoid grapefruit juice. SE rash, fluid retention, bone marrow ↓, hepatoxicity, take with food
	Lapatinib Oral	Tykerb	QT>, ↓LVEF , diarrhea, avoid grapefruit juice, black box warning for hepatoxicity
	Nilotinib Oral	Tasigna	Bone marrow, > QT, used for CML, watch DDI with CYP3A4

(*continues*)

Table 9-17 (*continued*)

Category	Agent	Synonym/Brand Name	Comments—watch CYP450 drug interactions with tyrosine kinase inhibitors
	Pazopanib Oral	Votrient	QT>, black box warning for hepatoxicity
	Sunitinib Oral	Supent	↓LVEF. Metabolized by 3A4
mTOR inhibitors	Temsirolimus Injection	Torisel	Premedicate for hypersensitivity rx, DDI with CYP3A4, metabolite is sirolimus, immunosuppression, increased infection, hyperglycemia. Avoid PVC containing infusion bags or sets as plasticizer may leach. For advanced renal cell carcinoma
	Everolimus Oral	Afinitor	For advanced renal cell carcinoma
Proteosome inhibitors	Bortezomib Injection	Velcade	For lymphoma, multiple myeloma. SE: peripheral neuropathy, bone marrow ↓, hypotension. Metabolized by CYP 3A4, 2C19, 1A2, watch DDI. Give as IV bolus.
Histone deacetylase inhibitors	Vorinostat Oral	Zolinza	QT >
	Romidepsin Injection	Istodax	Metabolized by CYP3A.
Epidermal growth factor receptor inhibitors	Erlotinib Oral	Tarceva	Metabolized by CYP 3A4. Interstitial lung disease, rash, diarrhea. Take on an empty stomach.
	Gefitinib Oral	Irresa	Metabolized by CYP 3A4. Interstitial lung disease, diarrhea, rash
Biological response modifiers	Denileukin diftitox Injection	Ontak	Diphtheria toxin combined with protein that binds to IL-2 receptor found on activated T-lymphocytes and macrophages. Used for cutaneous T-cell lymphoma. Store frozen. SE hypersensitivity, vascular leak syndrome
	Aldesleukin Injection	Proleukin IL-2; interleukin-2	Used for renal cell carcinoma, melanoma. SE: capillary leak syndrome, nephrotoxicity, hypotension, flu-like sx, impaired neutrophil function/infection. Pretreat with NSAID. Give as IV infusion over 15 minutes, continuous IV infusion or SC. Do not use bacteriostatic water or sodium chloride to reconstitute, dilute with D5W. Refrigerate.
	Interferon-α Injection	Intron-A	For some leukemias, lymphomas, melanoma. Give IM, SQ, or IV. SE: depression, fatigue, fever, chills, malaise, myalgias. Refrigerate.
Miscellaneous	Mitotane Oral	Lysodren	Used for adrenal cortical tumors
	Porfimer sodium Injection	Photofrin	Component of photodynamic therapy involving drug administration followed by laser treatment. SE: photosensitivity
	Tretinoin Oral, 10 mg capsule	Vesanoid, all-trans-retinoic acid (ATRA)	Retinoid , used for acute promyelocytic leukemia. SE: hyperlipidemia, hypothyroidism, APL syndrome (fever, respiratory distress, edema). Take with food. Do not crush or chew capsules.
	Bexarotene Oral and topical gel	Targretin	Retinoid for cutaneous lymphoma. SE: hyperlipidemia, hypothyroidism, photosensitivity. Take with food. Metabolized by CYP 3A4.
	Arsenic trioxide Injection	Trisenox	Used for APL (acute promyelocytic leukemia). SE QT>, APL syndrome, bone marrow
	Thalidomide	Thalomid	Birth control should be used with all chemotherapy agents, but absolute must for thalidomide. Can only be supplied by pharmacists in the S.T.E.P.S. restricted distribution program. Side effect include peripheral neuropathy and VTE (in some situations prophylaxis with warfarin or LMWH is recommended). Approved for use in multiple myeloma.

	Lenalidomide Oral capsules	Revlimid	Used for myelodysplastic syndrome, multiple myeloma. SE: bone marrow ↓, VTE, skin rxns. Birth control should be used with all chemotherapy agents, but absolute must for lenalidomide. Only available through restricted distribution program (RevAssist). Do not break, chew or open capsules.

Hormonal Agents

Category	Agent	Synonym/Brand Name	Comments
Selective estrogen receptor modulators (SERMs)	Tamoxifen (Oral) 10 mg, 20 mg tablets Solution 10 mg/5 ml	Nolvadex	Usual dose is 20 mg daily. SE: hot flashes, endometrial cancer, thromboembolism. Potential for initial flare reaction with or without hypercalcemia when used for **metastatic** breast cancer. Indicated for breast cancer prevention, adjuvant therapy in early stage disease, and as palliative therapy in advanced disease
	Toremifene (Oral)	Fareston	Treatment of advanced breast cancer
	Raloxifene (Oral)	Evista	Approved for breast cancer prevention, not used for treatment
Pure antiestrogen	Fulvestrant (Injection)	Faslodex	Refrigerate
Aromatase inhibitors (selective)	Anastrozole (Oral) 1 mg	Arimidex	**Only for use in postmenopausal women.** SE: estrogen deprivation, hot flashes, fatigue, osteoporosis
	Exemestane (Oral) 25 mg	Aromasin	**Only for use in postmenopausal women.** SE: estrogen deprivation, hot flashes, fatigue, osteoporosis. Take after meals to increase absorption.
	Letrozole (Oral) 2.5 mg	Femara	**Only for use in postmenopausal women.** SE: estrogen deprivation, hot flashes, fatigue, osteoporosis
Antiandrogens	Flutamide (Oral)	Eulexin	TID dosing. SE: hepatotoxic, hot flashes, loss of libido, osteoporosis
	Bicalutamide (Oral)	Casodex	SE: hot flashes, loss of libido, osteoporosis
	Nilutamide (Oral)	Nilandron	SE: hot flashes, loss of libido, osteoporosis. Black box warning for pulmonary fibrosis. Delayed dark adaptation.
LHRH agonists	Leuprolide (Injection)	Lupron, Eligard	SE: flare reactions. Available in daily, 1-month, 3-month, 4-month and 6-month dose forms
	Goserelin (Injection)	Zoladex	SE: flare reactions. Available in 1- and 3-month implants
	Triptorelin (Injection)	Trelstar Depot Trelstar LA	Trelstar Depot given every month, Trelstar LA every 3 months
	Histrelin (Injection)	Vantas, Supprelin LA	12-month implant. Refrigerate.
Progestins	Megestrol acetate (Oral)	Megace	Third and fourth line agents for advanced breast cancer
	Medroxyprogesterone acetate (Oral and Injection)	Provera Depo-Provera	

Key to abbreviations: AML = acute myelocytic leukemia; APL = acute promyelocytic leukemia; BBB = blood brain barrier; CA = cancer; CLL = chronic lymphocytic leukemia; CML = chronic myelogenous leukemia; CNS = central nervous system; CYP = cytochrome P450; DDI = drug-drug interaction; EGFR = epidermal growth factor receptor; HER-2 = human epidermal growth factor receptor 2; IM = intramuscular; IV = intravenous; LHRH = luteinizing hormone releasing hormone; LMWH = low molecular weight heparin; LVEF = left ventricular ejection fraction; MAB = monoclonal antibody; MAOI = monoamine oxidase inhibitor; Mcm = micrometer; Rxn = reaction; SC = subcutaneous; N/V = nausea and vomiting; PEG = polyethylene glycol; PVC = polyvinyl chloride; SE = side effects; SIADH = syndrome of inappropriate antidiuretic hormone; VEGF = vascular endothelial growth factor; VTE = venous thromboembolism

ANNOTATED BIBLIOGRAPHY

1. Smith RA, et al. Cancer screening in the United States, 2009: a review of current American Cancer Society guidelines and issues in cancer screening. *CA Cancer J Clin* 2009;59:27–41.
2. Facts & Comparisons. Available at: http://onlinefactsandcomparisons.com. Accessed April 9, 2010.
3. Seung AH. Adverse effects of chemotherapy and targeted agents. In: Koda-Kimble MA, Young LY, Alldredge BK, Corelli RL, Guglielmo BJ, Kradjan, Williams BR, eds. *Applied Therapeutics: The Clinical Use of Drugs*. 9th ed. Philadelphia, PA: Lippincott, Williams & Wilkins; 2009:89-1–89-40.
4. Antineoplastic agents. In: McEvoy GK, ed. *AHFS: Drug Information*. Bethesda, MD: American Society of Health-System Pharmacists; 2010. Available at: http://online.statref.com. Accessed April 9, 2010.
5. Micromedex Healthcare Series. Available at: http://www.thomsonhc.com. Accessed April 9, 2010.
6. DiPiro JT, Talbert RL, Yee GR, Matzke GR, Wells BG, Posey LM. *Pharmacotherapy: A Pathophysiologic Approach*. 7th ed. New York, NY: McGraw-Hill; 2008.

Cardiovascular

CHAPTER

10

TOPIC: ANGINA

Section Coordinator: Teresa K. Hoffmann
Contributor: Teresa K. Hoffmann

Angina Overview

The proper treatment of angina requires an understanding of the different types of angina as well as the underlying cause. Pharmacists have a role in treating each specific type of angina with the most appropriate drugs and monitoring for side effects as well as drug interactions.

Tips Worth Tweeting

- Angina is chest pain that occurs due to increased myocardial oxygen demand.
- It is very important to determine whether a patient has stable or unstable angina.
- Consider pain type, quality, radiation, severity, and timing when addressing angina.
- Stable angina is caused by a fixed obstruction, whereas unstable angina could be a sign of plaque rupture.
- Patients can develop nitrate tolerance after prolonged use.
- Make sure patients on sustained-release nitrates have a nitrate-free interval.
- IV nitroglycerin binds to PVC bags, tubing, and filters.
- Consider other chronic conditions before starting prophylactic angina therapy.
- Calcium-channel blockers are the first choice in treatment of Prinzmetal's angina.

1.1.0 Patient Information

Medication-Induced Causes of Angina

- Vasodilators
- Excessive thyroid replacement
- Vasoconstrictors
- Beta blockers (Prinzmetal's angina)

Laboratory Values

- Complete blood count (CBC): rule out anemia
- Troponin I: rule out unstable angina/acute myocardial infarction (MI)

Disease States Associated with Angina

- Anemia
- Coronary artery disease (CAD)
- Hyperthyroidism
- Valvular heart disease
- Uncontrolled hypertension
- Hypoxemia

Instruments and Techniques Related to Patient Assessment

The description of chest pain follows the mnemonic PQRST:

- Provokes: aggravating and alleviating factors
- Quality: burning, crushing, or stabbing

Table 10-1 Classification of Angina

Terminology	Aggravated by	Alleviated by	Location
Stable angina	Effort or emotion	Rest Nitroglycerin (NTG)	Substernal with radiation
Unstable angina	Spontaneous, can occur at rest (nocturnal)	NTG	Substernal with radiation
Prinzmetal's angina (unstable)	Spontaneous Hyperventilation Stress Exposure to cold May be cyclical	NTG	Substernal with radiation

- Radiation
- Severity
- Timing

Wellness and Prevention

Because stable angina is often due to a fixed obstruction in one of the coronary arteries, prevention focuses on preventing and treating CAD. It is recommended that patients maintain a healthy body weight, exercise at least 30 minutes per day on at least 4 days per week, and limit saturated fats while eliminating trans-fats in the diet. Patients are further advised to increase their consumption of fresh fruits and vegetables, polyunsaturated fats (e.g., almonds, olive oil, canola oil) and fatty fish, such as salmon, mackerel, and tuna.

Other important issues to address include smoking cessation, proper management of blood pressure and lipids, appropriate treatment of diabetes mellitus, and the avoidance of triggers such as over-the-counter decongestants, energy supplements/drinks, and large amounts of caffeine.

Table 10-2 Signs and Symptoms of Angina

Symptom	Stable Angina	Unstable Angina
Midsternal chest pain	Present	Present
Chest "tightness"	Present	Present
Radiation to left shoulder/ arm/hand, neck, jaw, or back	Present	Present
Nausea	Not present	Present
Shortness of breath (SOB)	Present	Present
Sweating	Not present	Present
Improves with rest	Yes	No
Improves within 10 minutes	Yes	No

1.2.0 Pharmacotherapy

Mechanism of Action by Class

Nitrates

- Produce vasodilation of cardiac arteries and collateral vessels, thereby increasing oxygen supply
- Decrease preload by venodilation

Beta Blockers

- Decrease inotropy and heart rate, leading to decreased oxygen demand

Calcium-Channel Blockers

- Decrease coronary vascular resistance, thereby increasing coronary circulation
- Negative inotropy and decreased heart rate (especially verapamil/diltiazem)

Ranolazine

- Inhibits myocardial fatty acid oxidation, which increases glucose oxidation

Table 10-3 Angina Medications: Drugs, Indications, and Routes of Administration

Drug	Approved Indications	Routes of Administration
Nitrates		
Amyl nitrite	Acute relief	Nasal inhalation
Isosorbide dinitrate	Prophylaxis	Oral
Isosorbide mononitrate	Prophylaxis	Oral
Nitroglycerin	Acute relief Prophylaxis	IV, sublingual tablets, lingual spray Topical, oral, sublingual tablets, lingual spray
Beta Blockers		
Nadolol	Prophylaxis	Oral
Propranolol		Oral
Atenolol		Oral
Metoprolol		Oral, IV
Calcium-Channel Blockers		
Nifedipine	Prophylaxis	Oral
Nicardipine	Prophylaxis	Oral, IV
Amlodipine	Prophylaxis	Oral
Verapamil	Acute relief, prophylaxis	Oral, IV
Diltiazem	Prophylaxis	Oral, IV
Miscellaneous		
Ranolazine	Prophylaxis	Oral

- Helps the myocardium use oxygen more efficiently

Interaction of Drugs with Foods and Laboratory Tests

Nitrates

- Contraindication: Phosphodiesterase inhibitors
- Precautions: Pancuronium, alteplase, antihypertensives, alcohol

Beta Blockers

- Precautions: Sulfonylureas, antihypertensives, negative inotropes, epinephrine

Calcium-Channel Blockers

- Non-dihydropyridine (non-DHP): CYP 450 3A4 substrates/inhibitors
  - Precautions: Amiodarone, barbiturates, itraconazole, cyclosporine, cimetidine, rifampin, anesthetics, statins, antihypertensives, negative inotropes, dofetilide, buspirone, carbamazepine, digoxin, alcohol, phenytoin, imipramine, moricizine, ranolazine, sirolimus, tacrolimus, quinidine, grapefruit juice
- Dihydropyridine (DHP): CYP 450 3A4 substrates
  - Precautions: "Azole" antifungals, barbiturates, carbamazepine, cimetidine, phenytoin, rifampin, anesthetics

Ranolazine

- P-glycoprotein substrate
- CYP 450 3A substrate
- CYP 450 3A, 2D6 inhibitor
- Additive prolongation of QT interval
  - Contraindications: Barbiturates, carbamazepine, cisapride, macrolides, dronedarone, efavirenz, griseofulvin, itraconazole, ketoconazole, lopinavir/ritonavir, modafinil, nelfinavir, nevirapine, phenytoin, rifampin, ritonavir, voriconazole
  - Precautions: Aprepitant, cyclosporine, diltiazem, paroxetine, QT-interval-prolonging drugs, verapamil, digoxin, simvastatin

Contraindications, Warnings, and Precautions

Contraindications

- Nitrates: Phosphodiesterase inhibitors due to profound hypotension
- NTG patches: History of adhesive allergy
- Beta blockers: Class IV heart failure, sick sinus syndrome (SSS), second- or third-degree heart block, hypotension (SBP < 90), ventricular tachycardia (VT), cardiogenic shock
- All calcium-channel blockers: SSS, second- or third-degree heart block, hypotension (SBP < 90)
- Non-DHP: Left ventricular dysfunction, Wolff-Parkinson-White (WPW) syndrome, ventricular tachycardia (VT), acute MI, cardiogenic shock, recent IV beta blocker use
- Ranolazine: Patients taking strong CYP 3A inducers or inhibitors, clinically significant hepatic disease

Table 10-4 Physiochemical Properties, Solubility, Pharmacodynamics, and Pharmacokinetic Properties

Drug	Onset	Peak
NTG Oral ER	20–45 min	90 min
NTG Sublingual	1–3 min	5–15 min
NTG Ointment	30–60 min	3–4 hours
NTG Patch	30–60 min	
NTG Spray	2 min	
NTG IV	1–5 min	

Table 10-5 Biopharmaceutical Principles and Pharmaceutical Characteristics of Dosage Forms

Drug	Dosage Form	Bioavailability
Nitrates		
Isosorbide dinitrate	Oral ER	22%
	Oral IR	58%
Isosorbide mononitrate	Oral ER	80–100%
	Oral IR	93–100%
Nitroglycerin	SL tablet	38.5%
	Patch	75%
Beta Blockers		
Nadolol	Oral tablet	20–40%
Propranolol	Oral	30–70%
Atenolol	Oral	46–60%
Metoprolol	Oral IR	50%
	Oral ER	65–70%
Calcium-Channel Blockers		
Nifedipine	Oral IR and modified release	30–60%
	Oral sustained release	30–50%
Nicardipine	Oral capsule	35%
Amlodipine	Oral tablet	60–65%
Verapamil	Oral IR/ER/CR	20–35%
Diltiazem	Oral IR/CD/SR/XT	35–40%
Miscellaneous		
Ranolazine	Extended-release tablet	55%

Table 10-6 Angina Medications: Generic Names, Brand Names, and Dosage Form Availability

Generic	Brand Name	Strengths Available
Nitroglycerin SL	Nitrostat	0.3, 0.4, 0.6 mg
Nitroglycerin spray	Nitrolingual, Nitromist	0.4 mg
Nitroglycerin ER capsules	Nitro-time	2.5, 6.5, 9 mg
Nitroglycerin patch	Minitran, Nitro-Dur, Nitrek	0.1, 0.2, 0.3, 0.4, 0.6 mg/hr
Nitroglycerin patch	Nitro-Dur	0.8 mg/hr
Nitroglycerin ointment	Nitro-Bid	2%
Nitroglycerin solution		5 mg/mL
Nitroglycerin in 5% dextrose		100, 200, 400 mcg/mL
Nadolol	Corgard	20, 40, 60, 80, 120, 160 mg
Propranolol IR tablets	Inderal	10, 20, 40, 60, 80, 90 mg
Propranolol ER capsules	Inderal LA	60, 80, 120, 160 mg
Propranolol ER capsules	InnoPran XL	80, 120 mg
Propranolol intensol oral solution	Inderal	80 mg/mL
Propranolol IV	Tenormin	1 mg/mL
Atenolol	Lopressor	25, 50, 100 mg
Metoprolol tartrate tablets	Toprol XL	25, 50, 100 mg
Metoprolol succinate tablets	Lopressor	25, 50, 100, 200 mg
Metoprolol IV		1 mg/mL
Nifedipine IR capsules	Procardia	10, 20 mg
Nifedipine ER tablets	Adalat CC, Procardia XL, Afeditab CR, Nifedical XL, Nifediac CC	60, 90 mg
Nicardipine IR capsules		20, 30 mg
Nicardipine ER tablets	Cardene SR	20, 45, 60 mg
Nicardipine IV	Cardene IV	0.1, 0.2 mg/mL
Amlodipine tablets	Norvasc	2.5, 5, 10 mg
Verapamil IR tablets	Calan	40, 80, 120 mg
Verapamil ER tablets	Calan ER, Isoptin SR	120, 180, 240 mg
	Covera HS	180, 240 mg
Verapamil ER capsules	Verelan PM	100, 120, 180, 200, 240, 300, 360 mg
Verapamil for injection		2.5 mg/mL
Diltiazem IR tablets	Cardizem	30, 60, 90, 120 mg
Diltiazem LA tablets	Cardizem LA	120, 180, 240, 300, 360, 420 mg
Diltiazem ER capsules	Cardizem CD, Cartia XT, Dilacor XR, Dilt CD, Dilt XR, Diltia XT, Diltzac, Taztia XT, Tiazac	120, 240 mg
	Cardizem CD, Cartia XT, Dilt CD, Diltzac, Taztia XT, Tiazac	300 mg
	Cardizem CD, Diltzac, Taztia XT, Tiazac	360 mg
	Tiazac	
	Cardizem	420 mg
Diltiazem for injection	Cardizem	5 mg/mL
Diltiazem powder for injection		25 mg
Ranolazine ER tablets	Ranexa	500, 1,000 mg

Warnings and Precautions

- Nitrates: IV NTG binds to PVC plastics in IV bags, tubing, and filters; may aggravate angina caused by hypertrophic cardiomyopathy; tolerance can develop after prolonged use; include 10- to 12-hour nitrate-free interval
- NTG patches: Do not defibrillate over patch
- Amyl nitrite: Extremely flammable
- Beta blockers: Diabetes mellitus, reactive airway disease, sinus bradycardia, WPW, peripheral vascular disease, Prinzmetal's angina, emphysema, chronic obstructive pulmonary disease (COPD), hypotension
- All calcium-channel blockers: Edema, sinus bradycardia, hypotension
- Ranolazine: Prolonged QT syndrome
- Atenolol
  - Half-life increased to 28 hr in renal patients
  - Food decreases AUC by 20%
- Propranolol: Food increases absorption by 53%
- Verapamil: Grapefruit juice increases bioavailability by 30%

1.3.0 Monitoring

Pharmacotherapeutic Outcomes

The goals of therapy are to reduce symptoms of angina, increase physical function, and improve quality of life.

Safety and Efficacy Monitoring and Patient Education

Nitrates

- Use SL tabs and spray for immediate relief of angina.
- Store SL tabs in the original glass bottle.
- SL tabs may be used until the expiration date on the bottle.
- Call 911 if chest pain does not resolve after the first tablet or spray.
- Patients may take up to two additional tablets at 5-minute intervals until an ambulance arrives.
- Replace the product if tablets are powdery.
- Sit or lie down before use.
- Do not use in the presence of recent use of tadalafil, vardenafil, or sildenafil.
- Sustained-release products may cause headache, which can be treated with acetaminophen. Sometimes loss of headache can mean loss of effectiveness due to tolerance.
- If using a patch, remove it for 12 hours daily.
- At least an 8-hour, nitrate-free interval is needed to reduce tolerance.

Calcium-Channel Blockers

- Ideally, use long-acting DHP and NDHP
- Preferred in Prinzmetal's angina

Beta Blockers

- Do not abruptly discontinue these medications due to risks of acute angina or even myocardial infarction.

Ranolazine

- Do not crush or chew
- No clinical effect on heart rate or blood pressure

Adverse Drug Reactions

- Nitrates: Headache (50%), dizziness, postural hypotension, flushing, reflex tachycardia, coronary steal
- Beta blockers: Bradycardia, hypotension, fatigue, nightmares, erectile dysfunction, worsening blood glucose control
- Calcium-channel blockers: Edema, dizziness, reflex tachycardia (DHP), fatigue hypotension, bradycardia (NDHP), headache, constipation (esp. verapamil)
- Ranolazine: Dizziness, headache, constipation, nausea

ANNOTATED BIBLIOGRAPHY

Drug Facts and Comparisons. Wolters Kluwer Health, Inc. Updated periodically.

Micromedex Healthcare Series. Greenwood Village, CO: Thomson Reuters (Healthcare) Inc. Updated periodically.

Talbert RL. Ischemic heart disease. In DiPiro JT, Talbert RL, Yee GC, Matzke GR, Wells BG, Posey LM, eds. *Pharmacotherapy: A Pathophysiologic Approach*. 7th ed. Available at: http://0-www.accesspharmacy.com.polar.onu.edu/content.aspx?aID=3180000.

TOPIC: ACUTE CORONARY SYNDROME

Section Coordinator: Teresa K. Hoffmann
Contributor: Michelle R. Musser

Acute Coronary Syndrome Overview

Acute coronary syndrome can lead to significant morbidity and mortality. Appropriate management of this condition is multifaceted and requires careful diagnosis, risk assessment, treatment selection, and medication management. Pharmacists have a large role to play in both the acute and chronic care of patients with acute coronary syndrome.

Tips Worth Tweeting

- Acute coronary syndrome causes significant morbidity and mortality.
- Acute coronary syndrome is caused by the rupture of atherosclerotic plaques and subsequent thrombosis formation, leading to a decrease in myocardial oxygen supply and possible myocardial cell death.
- Acute coronary syndromes consist of three distinct conditions: unstable angina (UA), non-ST-segment elevation myocardial infarction (NSTEMI), and ST-segment elevation myocardial infarction (STEMI).
- Classification of acute coronary syndrome and risk stratification is important to ensure appropriate management.
- Early treatment of patients with UA/NSTEMI and STEMI should include aspirin (ASA), clopidogrel, beta blocker therapy, and angiotensin-converting enzyme inhibitor (ACEI) therapy as well as analgesic, nitrate, and oxygen use.
- Long-term treatment should include use of ASA, beta blockers, ACEI therapy, and clopidogrel, along with use of a hydroxymethylglutaryl-CoA (HMG-CoA) reductase inhibitor (statin) as a lipid-lowering agent.
- The cornerstone of treatment for STEMI patients is reperfusion therapy, through either the use of fibrinolytic agents or percutaneous intervention (PCI).
- PCI is the preferred reperfusion therapy in hospitals with proper facilities and experienced staff.
- The use of fibrinolytic therapy requires careful consideration of the patient's condition and past medical history.
- The treatment of UA/NSTEMI patients is based on risk stratification; it includes angiography and PCI in high-risk and some moderate-risk patients, and conservative medical management in most low-risk patients.
- Important agents in the acute management of acute coronary syndrome patients include antiplatelet agents, anticoagulant agents, and anti-ischemic agents.
- Treatment of acute coronary syndrome includes long- term risk factor modification for all patients, including lipid-lowering therapy, blood pressure control, blood glucose control, and smoking cessation.

Epidemiology of Acute Coronary Syndrome

- Cardiovascular disease is the leading cause of death in the United States.
- Each year more than 1.5 million American experience an acute coronary syndrome (ACS).
- Approximately 220,000 people will die of a myocardial infarction (MI) each year.
- Coronary heart disease (CHD) is the leading cause of premature chronic disability in the United States.
- The cost of CHD, including both direct and indirect costs, was estimated at $151.6 billion in 2007.

Pathophysiology

- The underlying cause of ACS is the formation of atherosclerotic plaques.
- The primary cause of ACS is atherosclerotic plaque rupture, followed by clot or thrombus formation over the ruptured plaque.
- Plaque rupture leads to the release of vasoactive substances, including adenosine diphosphate (ADP) and thromboxane A_2; these substances induce platelet adhesion and activation as well as vasoconstriction.
- Conformation of glycoprotein IIb/IIIa (GP IIb/IIIa) surface receptors leads to formation of fibrin bridges.
- Blood components exposed to the endothelium activate the extrinsic coagulation cascade, leading to the production of thrombin and the production of fibrin from fibrinogen.
- A thrombus containing more platelets than fibrin usually produces an incomplete occlusion of a coronary vessel, whereas a thrombus containing more fibrin relative to platelets is more likely to completely occlude a coronary vessel.
- Narrowing or occlusion of a coronary artery leads to reduced myocardial perfusion, leading to an imbalance between myocardial oxygen supply and demand. This imbalance can lead to eventual myocardial ischemia and cell death.

Classification of Acute Coronary Syndromes

Acute coronary syndromes consist of three distinct conditions: unstable angina (UA), non-ST-segment elevation myocardial infarction (NSTEMI), and ST-segment elevation myocardial infarction (STEMI). Distinguishing between these three conditions is essential in the proper management of patients with ACS.

1.1.0 Patient Information

Signs and Symptoms

- Symptoms
  - Midline anterior anginal chest pain at least 20 minutes in duration; may radiate to the shoulder, down the left arm, to the back, or to the jaw

Table 10-7 Comparison of ACS Conditions

ACS	ECG Changes	Biochemical Markers	Symptoms	Occlusion	Myocardial Damage
UA	• None (or transient)	Negative	• Rest angina • New onset (< 2 months) angina • Angina that increases in frequency, duration, or intensity	• Incomplete • Platelet rich	• Ischemia
NSTEMI	• ST segment changes: ST depression • T wave inversion	Positive	• More prolonged or intense rest angina	• Incomplete • Platelet rich	• Less extensive • May cause necrosis
STEMI	• ST segment changes: ST elevation	Positive	• Unremitting chest discomfort	• Complete • Fibrin rich	• More extensive and persistent • Leads to myocardial necrosis

  - Associated symptoms include nausea, vomiting, diaphoresis, and shortness of breath
- ECG
  - Essential to classification of ACS and proper treatment
  - Should be obtained and interpreted within 10 minutes of presentation
- Biochemical markers
  - Indicate myocardial cell death
  - Troponin and creatinine kinase (CK-MB) rise following myocardial cell death
  - Routine practice is to obtain troponin and CK-MB levels upon presentation and then twice more over the next 12–24 hours
  - Both markers appear in the blood within 6 hours of infarction; troponins remain elevated for up to 10 days, while CK-MB levels return to normal within 2 days
  - Positive biochemical markers include one troponin level above the laboratory-specific decision limit or two CK-MB levels above the laboratory-specific decision limit

Management of Acute Coronary Syndromes

Goals of Therapy

- Restoration of blood flow through the affected coronary artery
- Relief of ischemic chest pain
- Prevention of complications
- Prevention of death

Risk Stratification

- Factors
  - Symptoms
  - ECG findings
  - Medical history
  - Troponin or CK-MB levels
- STEMI patients are at the highest risk of death, so timely reperfusion therapy is essential in eligible STEMI patients
  - Initiate fibrinolytic therapy within 30 minutes of presentation
  - Perform primary percutaneous intervention within 90 minutes of presentation
- Stratification for NSTEMI patients is more complex due to varied outcomes in this group
  - Thrombolysis in myocardial infarction (TIMI) risk score
    - One point is given for each TIMI risk score criterion and the points are totaled
    - The patient is assigned the corresponding risk

Table 10-8 TIMI Risk Score Criteria for NSTEMI Patients

Past Medical History	Clinical Presentation
Age ≥ 65 years old	ST-segment depression (≥ 0.5 mm)
Use of aspirin in the past seven days	Positive biochemical marker for infarction
Known CAD (≥ 50% stenosis of coronary artery)	2 or more episodes of chest discomfort in the past 24 hours
3 or more risk factors for coronary artery disease (CAD) • Hyperlipidemia • Hypertension • Smoking • Family history of premature CHD • Diabetes mellitus	

Table 10-9 Classification and Recommendations in the ACC/AHA Guidelines for the Management of UA/NSTEMI and STEMI Patients

Classification	Interpretation
Class I	• Treatment or procedure should be performed or given • Procedure or treatment is useful or effective
Class IIa	• It is reasonable to perform or administer treatment • Recommendation in favor of treatment or procedure being useful or effective
Class IIb	• Procedure or treatment may be considered • Recommendation has less well-established usefulness or effectiveness
Class III	• Procedure or treatment should not be performed or administered • Recommendation that treatment is not useful or effective and may be harmful

- High risk: TIMI risk score of 5–7 points
- Moderate risk: TIMI risk score of 3–4 points
- Low risk: TIMI risk score of 0–2 points

Additional findings indicating high risk (alone or in combination):

- ST-segment depression
- Positive biochemical marker for infarction
- Deep symmetric T-wave inversion (> 2 mm)
- Acute heart failure
- Diabetes mellitus
- Chronic kidney disease
- Refractory chest discomfort
- Recent MI (within the past 2 weeks)

Low-risk patients should undergo a noninvasive stress test:

- Negative stress test: Indicates noncardiac chest pain
- Positive stress test: Patient may undergo angiography with revascularization

Moderate-risk patients with positive biochemical markers should undergo angiography with revascularization. Moderate-risk patients with negative biochemical markers may either undergo angiography with revascularization or a noninvasive stress test.

High-risk patients should undergo angiography with revascularization.

The following sections discussing the management of UA/NSTEMI and STEMI patients are adapted from the American College of Cardiologists (ACC) and American Heart Association (AHA) guidelines. The classification system for the recommendations in these guidelines is described in Table 10-9.

Management of UA/NSTEMI Patients

Table 10-10 Anti-ischemic and Analgesic Therapy in UA/NSTEMI Patients

Class I	Supplemental oxygen in patients with arterial saturation less than 90% or in patients in respiratory distress
	Sublingual nitroglycerin for patients with ongoing chest pain
	Intravenous nitroglycerin indicated in first 48 hours for persistent ischemia, heart failure, or hypertension
	Oral beta blocker therapy should be initiated within first 24 hours
	Oral non-dihydropyridine calcium-channel blockers (non-DHP CCB) should be used in patients with contraindications for beta blocker therapy
	ACEI therapy should be initiated within the first 24 hours of presentation in patients with pulmonary congestion or left ventricular ejection fraction (LVEF) ≤ 40%
	An angiotensin receptor blocker (ARB) should be used in patients who are intolerant of ACEI
	Nonsteroidal anti-inflammatory drugs (NSAIDs) should be discontinued
Class IIa	May administer supplemental oxygen to all patients during first 6 hours after presentation
	Intravenous morphine sulfate may be used for patients with uncontrolled chest pain despite nitroglycerin
	Intravenous beta blockers may be used for hypertension
	Oral long-acting non-DHP CCBs may be used for patients with recurrent ischemia if beta blockers and nitrates have been used fully
	ACEI therapy may be useful in all patients
Class IIb	May use long-acting non-DHP CCB instead of beta blocker therapy
	May use immediate-release DHP CCB with beta blocker therapy in patients with ongoing symptoms
Class III	Nitrates should be avoided in patients recently using a phosphodiesterase inhibitor for erectile dysfunction
	Immediate-release DHP CCBs should not be used with beta blocker therapy
	Avoid intravenous ACEI therapy within the first 24 hours of presentation

Table 10-11 Antiplatelet Therapy in UA/NSTEMI Patients

Class I	ASA should be administered to all patients as soon as possible and continued indefinitely
	Clopidogrel should be given to patients who are unable to take aspirin
	For patients with a history of gastrointestinal (GI) bleeding who will receive clopidogrel or ASA, drugs to minimize recurrent GI bleeding should be used concomitantly
	For patients selected for an initial invasive strategy, ASA with clopidogrel or an intravenous GP IIb/IIIa inhibitor (eptifibatide or tirofiban preferred) should be initiated prior to angiography • Abciximab is preferred only if PCI is likely and there will be no appreciable delay to angiography
	For patients selected for initial conservative approach, clopidogrel should be added to ASA and anticoagulant therapy as soon as possible and continued for at least 1 month and ideally up to 1 year
Class IIa	For patients selected for an initial conservative approach, a GP IIb/IIIa inhibitor can be added to clopidogrel, ASA, and anticoagulant therapy if there is ongoing ischemic discomfort before angiography
	For patients selected for an initial invasive approach, antiplatelet therapy with clopidogrel and a GP IIb/IIIa inhibitor may be used
	For patients selected for an initial invasive approach, GP IIb/IIIa inhibitor administration prior to angiography may be omitted if bivalirudin is selected as the anticoagulant and at least 300 mg of clopidogrel was administered at least 6 hours prior to planned catheterization
Class IIb	For patients selected for an initial conservative approach, eptifibatide or tirofiban may be added to anticoagulant and antiplatelet therapy
Class III	Abciximab should only be used if PCI is planned

Table 10-12 Anticoagulant Therapy in UA/NSTEMI Patients

Class I	Anticoagulant therapy should be initiated as soon as possible after presentation
	For patients selected for an initial invasive approach, regimens include enoxaparin or unfractionated heparin (UFH) • Fondaparinux or bivalirudin are possible regimens with a lower level of established efficacy
	For patients selected for an initial conservative approach, regimens include enoxaparin or unfractionated heparin (UFH) • Fondaparinux is a treatment regimen with a lower level of established efficacy, but it is preferred for patients with an increased risk of bleeding
Class IIa	For patients selected for an initial conservative approach, enoxaparin or fondaparinux is preferred unless coronary artery bypass surgery (CABG) is planned within 24 hours

Table 10-13 Additional Antiplatelet and Anticoagulant Therapy Considerations in UA/NSTEMI Patients

Class I	For patients classified as low risk and managed conservatively with no angiography performed • Continue ASA indefinitely • Continue clopidogrel at least 1 month, and ideally up to 1 year • Discontinue GP IIb/IIIa inhibitors if started • Continue UFH for 48 hours or administer enoxaparin or fondaparinux for the duration of hospitalization, up to 8 days, and then discontinue
	For patients where CABG is selected after angiography • Continue ASA • Continue UFH • Discontinue other antiplatelets and anticoagulants at appropriate intervals prior to CABG
	For patients where PCI is selected after angiography • Continue ASA • Give clopidogrel loading dose if not given • Administer a GP IIb/IIIa inhibitor (abciximab, eptifibatide, or tirofiban) if not already started • Discontinue anticoagulant therapy after PCI for uncomplicated cases

(*continues*)

Table 10-13 (*continued*)

Class I (cont'd)	For patients managed medically after angiography with no CAD found • Antiplatelet and anticoagulant therapy is given at the clinician's discretion • Patients with atherosclerosis should receive long-term ASA and other secondary prevention measures
	For patients managed medically after angiography identifies the presence of CAD • Continue ASA • Administer a clopidogrel loading dose if not already given • Discontinue GP IIb/IIIa inhibitors if started • Continue UFH, enoxaparin, or fondaparinux therapy for the duration of hospitalization
	For patients selected for an initial conservative approach not undergoing stress testing or angiography • Continue ASA indefinitely • Continue clopidogrel at least 1 month, and ideally up to 1 year • Discontinue GP IIb/IIIa inhibitors if started • Continue heparin for 48 hours or enoxaparin or fondaparinux for the duration of hospitalization and then discontinue anticoagulant therapy
Class IIa	If PCI is selected after angiography, GP IIb/IIIa inhibitor administration prior to angiography may be omitted if bivalirudin is selected as the anticoagulant and at least 300 mg of clopidogrel was administered at least 6 hours prior to planned catheterization
Class IIb	If PCI is selected after angiography, GP IIb/IIIa inhibitor administration prior to angiography may be omitted if not started prior to angiography in certain patients
Class III	Intravenous fibrinolytic therapy is not indicated for patients without acute ST-segment elevation, true posterior MI, or presumed new left bundle branch block

Table 10-14 Long-Term Medical Management in UA/NSTEMI Patients

Class I	Continue ASA indefinitely • 75–162 mg daily in patients without stenting • 162–325 mg daily for 1 month, then 75–162 mg daily indefinitely after bare-metal stent implantation • 162–325 mg daily for 3 months after sirolimus drug-eluting stent implantation or 6 months after paclitaxel drug-eluting stent placement, then 75–162 mg daily indefinitely • Use clopidogrel in patients who are allergic to ASA
	Continue clopidogrel 75 mg daily • At least 1 month and ideally up to 1 year in patients without stenting or in patients after bare-metal stent implantation • At least 12 months to all patients after drug-eluting stent placement
	Continue beta blockers
	Continue ACEIs in patients with heart failure, LVEF < 40%, hypertension, or diabetes mellitus (use ARBs for patients intolerant of ARBs or in combination regimens in patients with persistent symptomatic heart failure and LVEF < 40%)
	Give nitroglycerin to treat ischemic symptoms
	Assess lipids within 24 hours of admission
	Give HMG-CoA reductase inhibitors to all UA/NSTEMI patients
	LDL goal of < 100 mg/dL (goal of < 70 mg/dL is also acceptable)
	Blood pressure control
	Blood glucose control
	Smoking cessation
	Weight management
	Physical activity

Table 10-14 (*continued*)

Class IIa	ACEI therapy is reasonable in all post-UA/NSTEMI patients (use ARBs in patients intolerant of ACEIs)
	May use ASA 75–162 mg daily after PCI if bleeding is a concern
Class IIb	Encourage consumption of omega-3 fatty acids
Class III	Dipyridamole is not recommended in post UA/NSTEMI patients

Management of STEMI Patients

Table 10-15 Routine Measures in STEMI Patients

Class I	Supplemental oxygen for patients with arterial saturation < 90%
	Sublingual nitroglycerin for patients with ongoing chest pain
	Intravenous nitroglycerin is indicated for persistent ischemia, heart failure, or hypertension
	Morphine sulfate is the analgesic of choice
	Aspirin 162–325 mg should be chewed upon presentation, if not taken already
	Oral beta blocker therapy should be given promptly
Class IIa	Give oxygen to all patients during the first 6 hours after presentation
Class III	Nitrates should be avoided in patients who recently used a phosphodiesterase inhibitor for erectile dysfunction

Table 10-16 Fibrinolytic Reperfusion in STEMI Patients

Class I	All STEMI patients should undergo rapid evaluation for reperfusion therapy and have reperfusion strategy implemented promptly • If primary PCI within 90 minutes of first medical contact is not possible, patients should undergo fibrinolytic therapy unless contraindicated
	Fibrinolytic therapy is indicated for STEMI patients with symptom onset within the prior 12 hours and ST elevation > 0.1 mV in at least two contiguous precordial leads or at least two adjacent limb leads or with new left bundle branch block
	Patients should be assessed for neurologic contraindications for fibrinolytic therapy • Patients with substantial risk of intracranial hemorrhage (ICH) should be treated with PCI
	Any change in neurological status during or after reperfusion therapy should be considered to be ICH until proven otherwise • Discontinue fibrinolytic, anticoagulant, and antiplatelet therapies until imaging rules out ICH
Class IIa	Fibrinolytic therapy is indicated for STEMI patients with symptom onset within the prior 12 hours and a 12-lead ECG consistent with true posterior MI
	Fibrinolytic therapy is indicated for STEMI patients with symptom onset within the prior 12–24 hours with continued ischemic symptoms and ST elevation > 0.1 mV in at least two contiguous precordial leads or at least two adjacent limb leads or with new left bundle branch block
Class III	Fibrinolytic therapy should not be used in patients with initial symptoms beginning more than 24 hours earlier
	Fibrinolytic therapy should not be used in patients with ST-segment depression unless true posterior MI is expected

Table 10-17 PCI Reperfusion in STEMI Patients

Class I	All STEMI patients should undergo rapid evaluation for reperfusion therapy and have reperfusion strategy implemented promptly
	Diagnostic angiography should be performed for all candidates for primary PCI
	If immediately available, PCI should be performed for STEMI patients by persons skilled in the procedure
	PCI is preferred if symptom duration exceeds 3 hours
	PCI is preferred if symptom duration is within 3 hours and the expected door-to-balloon time minus the expected door-to-needle time is within 1 hour • If this interval is more than 1 hour, fibrinolytic therapy is preferred
	PCI should be performed within 12 hours of symptom onset in fibrinolytic-ineligible patients
Class IIa	PCI can be performed with symptom onset in the prior 12–24 hours with severe heart failure, hemodynamic instability, or persistent ischemic symptoms
	PCI can be performed within 12–24 hours of symptom onset in fibrinolytic-ineligible patients with severe heart failure, hemodynamic instability, or persistent ischemic symptoms
Class III	PCI should not be performed for asymptomatic, hemodynamically stable patients more than 12 hours after STEMI onset

Table 10-18 Ancillary Therapy to Reperfusion Therapy in STEMI Patients

Class I	UFH for patients undergoing PCI or surgical revascularization or reperfusion with alteplase, reteplase, or tenecteplase
	UFH for patients undergoing reperfusion with streptokinase or urokinase who are at high risk for systemic emboli
	Aspirin 75–162 mg daily should be continued indefinitely after STEMI, with an initial dose of 162–325 mg daily
	Patients undergoing PCI should receive clopidogrel for at least 1 month after bare-metal stent implantation, for 3 months with sirolimus drug-eluting stent implantation, for 6 months with paclitaxel drug-eluting stent implantation, and up to 1 year for patients not at high risk for bleeding
Class IIa	Clopidogrel is indicated for patients receiving fibrinolytic therapy who are unable to take ASA
	Begin abciximab therapy as early as possible prior to PCI
Class IIb	May use UFH for patients undergoing reperfusion with streptokinase
	Low-molecular-weight heparin (LMWH) may be used as an acceptable alternative to UFH in patients younger than age 75 who are receiving fibrinolytic therapy • Enoxaparin with full-dose tenecteplase is most extensively studied combination
	Treatment with tirofiban or eptifibatide may be considered prior to PCI
Class III	LMWH should not used as an alternative to UFH in patients older than age 75 who are receiving fibrinolytic therapy
	LMWH is not an acceptable alternative to UFH for patients younger than age 75 who are receiving fibrinolytic therapy but have significant renal dysfunction (serum creatinine > 2.5 mg/dL in men and > 2.0 mg/dL in women)

Table 10-19 Other Pharmacological Measures in STEMI Patients

Class I	ACEIs should be given orally within the first 24 hours of STEMI in patients with an anterior infarction, pulmonary congestion, or LVEF < 40% • ACEIs should be given during convalescence from STEMI and continued on a long-term basis
	Valsartan and candesartan should be used for patients who are intolerant of ACEIs, have signs of heart failure, or have LVEF < 40%
	Verapamil or diltiazem may be used to relieve ongoing ischemia if beta blockers are ineffective or for patients who are unable to take beta blockers
	Oral beta blocker therapy should continue if received within the first 24 hours of STEMI with no adverse effects, or should be started if not received earlier
	Nitroglycerin may be used beyond the first 48 hours following STEMI for recurrent angina or persistent heart failure

Table 10-19 (*continued*)

	ASA should be continued indefinitely Clopidogrel should be used in patients who are unable to take ASA Clopidogrel should be continued for patients who are undergoing stent implantation
	Oxygen may be continued beyond the first 6 hours for STEMI patients with arterial oxygen desaturation or overt pulmonary congestion
Class IIa	ACEIs may be useful given orally within the first 24 hours of STEMI in all patients without relevant contraindications (although the expected benefits are less for these patients than for patients with LVD)
	Verapamil or diltiazem may be used to relieve ongoing ischemia if beta blockers are ineffective or in patients who are unable to take beta blockers
	Valsartan and candesartan may be used as an alternative to an ACEI in patients with signs of heart failure or LVEF < 40%
	Patients who are not undergoing reperfusion should receive subcutaneous UFH or LMWH for at least 48 hours or until they are ambulatory
Class IIb	Continuing nitrate use beyond the first 24–48 hours in the absence of recurrent angina or heart failure may be helpful (although this benefit is not well established)
	Deep vein thrombosis (DVT) prophylaxis with LMWH or subcutaneous UFH until the patient is ambulatory may be useful (although its effectiveness is not well established)
Class III	Avoid intravenous ACEI within the first 24 hours of STEMI
	Verapamil and diltiazem are contraindicated for patients with STEMI and LVD heart failure
	Nifedipine is contraindicated for STEMI patients

Table 10-20 Long-Term Medical Management in STEMI Patients

Class I	ASA 75–162 mg daily should be given indefinitely
	Use clopidogrel in patients who are allergic to ASA or warfarin, with a target INR of 2.5–3.5 for patients younger than age 75 with a low risk of bleeding
	ACEI should be prescribed at discharge
	Valsartan or candesartan may be used as alternative therapy for patients who are intolerant of ACEIs and for patients with signs of heart failure and LVEF < 40%
	Beta blocker therapy should be continued for all patients except for low-risk patients
	Blood pressure control
	Blood glucose control
	Assess lipid profile within 24 hours of admission
	Target LDL is less than 100 mg/dL
	HMG-CoA reductase inhibitor agents are the preferred choice to manage lipids
	Weight management
	Smoking cessation
	Physical activity
Class IIa	May add niacin or fibrate therapy to raise HDL levels for patients with LDL < 100 mg/dL
	Valsartan or candesartan may be used as an alternative to ACEIs for patients with signs of heart failure and LVEF < 40%
	May give beta blocker therapy to low-risk patients
Class IIb	Combination of an ACEI and an ARB may be considered for patients with persistent symptomatic heart failure and LVEF < 40%
Class III	Avoid the use of ibuprofen
	Avoid the use of short-acting DHP CCBs

1.2.0 Safe and Accurate Preparation and Dispensing of Medications

Pharmacology of Acute Coronary Syndrome Agents

Table 10-21 Antiplatelet Agents

Drug	Mechanism of Action	Contraindications	Warnings	Dosing	Adverse Effects	Monitoring
Aspirin	Inhibition of prostaglandin (PG) synthesis and platelet aggregation via inhibition of cyclooxygenase	• Hypersensitivity to NSAID • Active bleeding or severe bleeding risk	• Bleeding disorders • Alcohol use of 3 or more drinks per day • GI symptoms including peptic ulcer disease • Renal failure • Severe hepatic insufficiency	• Initial dose of 162–325 mg daily • 75–162 mg daily indefinitely for patients not receiving stent implantation • Initial doses continued for 30 days in patients receiving a bare-metal stent implantation, for 3 months for patients receiving a sirolimus drug-eluting stent, and for 6 months for patients receiving a paclitaxel drug-eluting stent, followed by 75–162 mg daily indefinitely	• Bleeding • GI symptoms	• Signs of bleeding • GI symptoms • Complete blood count (CBC)

Clopidogrel (Plavix)	Selective and irreversible inhibition of ADP binding to platelet receptors and subsequent activation of ADP-mediated GP IIb/IIIa complex	• Active bleeding or severe bleeding risk
		• Hypersensitivity
			• Concomitant use with CYP2C19 inhibitors should be avoided
			• Impaired CYP2C19 function, including genetic variation; may reduce clopidogrel efficacy
			• Concomitant use with drugs that may induce bleeding of preexisting GI lesion
			• History of GI lesions with a tendency to bleed, such as ulcers
			• Severe liver disease
			• Severe renal impairment
			• Premature discontinuation of therapy for PCI patients may increase the risk of stent thrombosis, MI, and death
			• Risk of increased bleeding from trauma, surgery, or other pathological condition
			• Discontinue use 5 days prior to the procedure if an antiplatelet effect is not desired, including in patients planning to undergo CABG
				• 300–600 mg (Class IIa recommendation in NSTEMI patients) loading dose
				  ○ May omit the loading dose in patients older than age 75 when given fibrinolytics
				• 75 mg daily maintenance dose
				  ○ Use indefinitely in patients with ASA allergy
				  ○ Use at least 1 month and ideally up to 1 year for NSTEMI patients without stenting or for NSTEMI patients after bare-metal stent implantation
				  ○ Use at least 12 months for NSTEMI patients after drug-eluting stent placement
				  ○ Patients undergoing PCI should receive clopidogrel for at least 1 month after bare-metal stent implantation, for 3 months with sirolimus drug-eluting stent implantation, for 6 months with paclitaxel drug-eluting stent implantation, and up to 1 year for patients not at high risk for bleeding
					• Bleeding
					• GI symptoms
					• Rash
					• Thrombotic thrombocytopenic purpura (TTP)
						• Signs of bleeding
						• GI symptoms
						• CBC

Ticlopidine (Ticlid)	Same as clopidogrel	• Hypersensitivity
		• Active bleeding
		• Neutropenia
			• **Black box warning**
			  ○ Can cause life-threatening hematologic adverse reactions, including neutropenia, agranulocytosis, TTP, and aplastic anemia
			  ○ Hematologic adverse reactions cannot be reliably predicted by any identified demographic or clinical characteristics
				• 250 mg twice daily following PCI stent implantation
				• Rarely used due to side effects		

		• Thrombocy-Topenia • Severe liver impairment	○ During the first 3 months of treatment, patients receiving ticlopidine must be hematologically and clinically monitored for evidence of neutropenia or TTP ○ If any such evidence is seen, ticlopidine should be immediately discontinued • Predisposition to bleeding, including gastric or duodenal ulcers • Underlying hematologic disorders • Liver disease • Discontinue 10 to 14 days prior to surgery • Discontinue if absolute neutrophil count (ANC) is less than 1,200/mm^3 or if platelet count is less than 80,000/mm^3 • May elevate serum cholesterol and triglyceride levels		• Rash • GI symptoms • Hematolo-gical disturbances • TTP	• CBC with differential, including absolute neutrophil and platelet counts • Hepatic function testing • Signs of bleeding • Signs of infection
Prasu-grel (Effient)	• Inhibition of platelet activation and aggregation via irreversible inhibition of the platelet ADP receptor	• Active pathological bleeding • History of transient ischemic attack or stroke	• Increased risk of subsequent cardiovascular events if prasugrel is discontinued in the first few weeks after use • Significant bleeding has occurred with risks such as propensity to bleed, body weight less than 60 kg, and concomitant use of medications that increase risk • Concomitant use of medications that increase bleeding risk is not recommended • Not recommended for patients older than age 75, except for patients with diabetes or history of myocardial infarction • Recent or recurrent GI bleeding • Severe hepatic impairment • Do not start for patients who are likely to undergo urgent CABG • Increased risk of stent thrombosis, myocardial infarction, and death with premature discontinuation following stent implantation • Discontinue at least 7 days prior to elective surgery • TTP reported with other thienopyridines after exposure of less than 2 weeks • Risk of bleeding increased with recent trauma or surgery	• 60 mg loading dose for patients undergoing PCI • 10 mg daily maintenance dose taken with ASA 75–325 mg daily ○ Consider 5 mg daily for patient under 60 kg ○ Use at least 12 months for patients receiving stent implantation ○ May continue beyond 15 months in patients receiving drug-eluting stents	• Hypertension • Hyperlipide-mia • Bleeding • Headache	• CBC with platelet count • Signs of bleeding • Lipid panel

Table 10-22 Anticoagulant Agents

Drug	Mechanism of Action	Contraindications	Warnings	Dosing	Adverse Effects	Monitoring
UFH	• Combination with antithrombin III blocks thrombosis through inactivation of Factor Xa and inhibition of prothrombin (Factor II) conversion to thrombin (Factor IIa) • Prevents fibrin formation from fibrinogen during active thrombosis	• Active, uncontrollable bleeding except when due to disseminated intravascular coagulation (DIC) • Instances in which blood coagulation tests cannot be performed at necessary intervals • Severe thrombocytopenia	• Increased risk of hemorrhage for patients with bleeding disorders • Discontinue if testing shows that coagulation is excessively prolonged or if hemorrhage occurs • Increased risk of hemorrhage with gastrointestinal ulceration, hepatic disease with impaired hemostasis, or hypertension • Heparin-induced thrombocytopenia (HIT) and thrombocytopenia and thrombosis (HITT) may occur up to several weeks after discontinuing therapy • Thrombocytopenia may occur; discontinue therapy if recurrent thrombosis develops or if the platelet count falls below 100,000/mm^3	• In STEMI patients, administer 60 units/kg IV bolus (maximum: 4,000 units), followed by a constant IV infusion at 12 units/kg/hr (maximum 1,000 units/hr) • In NSTEMI patients, administer 60–70 units/kg IV bolus (maximum: 5,000 units), followed by a constant IV infusion at 12–15 units/kg/hr (maximum: 1,000 units/hr) • Titrated to maintain an activated partial thromboplastin time (aPTT) of 1.5–2.5 times control for NSTEMI patients and 50–70 seconds for STEMI patients • The first aPTT level should be measured at 4–6 hours for NSTEMI and STEMI in patients not treated with fibrinolytics • The first aPTT level should be measured at 3 hours in patients with STEMI who are treated with fibrinolytics • Continue for at least 48 hours or until the end of PCI	• Bleeding • HIT	• Signs of bleeding • CBC with platelet count • aPTT
LMWH: enoxaparin (Lovenox)	Activity against Factor Xa and antithrombin (anti-Factor IIa)	• Active major bleeding • Hypersensitivity to enoxaparin or heparin • Thrombocytopenia associated with a positive test for antiplatelet antibody in the presence of enoxaparin sodium	• Increased risk of epidural or spinal hematoma with concomitant use of enoxaparin and neuraxial anesthesia or spinal puncture, presence of an indwelling epidural catheter, concomitant use of drugs affecting hemostasis, or traumatic or repeated epidural or spinal puncture; increased risk of epidural or spinal hematoma • Increased risk of bleeding in patients with bleeding disorders, in elderly patients, and in low-weight patients • Enoxaparin is not interchangeable with heparin or another LMWH on a unit-for-unit basis • Recent history of GI ulceration or hemorrhage	• 1 mg/kg subcutaneous (SC) every 12 hours for patients with NSTEMI (CrCl ≥ 30 mL/min) • 1 mg/kg SC every 24 hours (CrCl 15–29 mL/min) for NSTEMI or STEMI • For patients undergoing PCI following initiation of SC enoxaparin for NSTEMI, a supplemental 0.3 mg/kg IV dose of enoxaparin should be administered at the time of PCI if the last dose of SC enoxaparin was given 8–12 hours prior to PCI • Administer enoxaparin 30 mg IV bolus followed immediately by 1 mg/kg SC every 12 hours (first two doses, administer a maximum of 100 mg for patients weighing more than 100 kg who are younger than age 75	• Bleeding • HIT	• Signs of bleeding • CBC with platelet count • aPTT • Serum creatinine

			• Use with extreme caution in patients with a history of HIT • Increased risk of bleeding in patients with renal impairment; dose adjustment is necessary in patients with severe renal impairment (creatinine clearance [CrCl] < 30 mL/min) • Thrombocytopenia may occur; discontinue therapy if the platelet count falls below 100,000/mm^3	• Administer enoxaparin 0.75 mg/kg SC every 12 hours (first two doses, administer a maximum of 75 mg for patients weighing more than 75 kg who are 75 years or older and have STEMI • Continue throughout hospitalization or up to 8 days for STEMI • Continue for the duration of the hospital stay or until the end of PCI for NSTEMI • Avoid enoxaparin if CrCl < 15 mL/min • Avoid use for patients undergoing CABG		
Fondaparinux (Arixtra)	Selectively binds to ATIII and potentiates the neutralization of Factor Xa, causing disruption of the blood coagulation cascade and inhibition of thrombin formation and thrombus development	• Active major bleeding • Bacterial endocarditis • Severe renal impairment (CrCl < 30 mL/min) • Thrombocytopenia associated with positive in vitro test for antiplatelet antibody in the presence of fondaparinux sodium	• Same warnings as for LMWH in regard to the risk of epidural or spinal hematoma • Increased risk of bleeding in patients with bleeding disorders, diabetic retinopathy, and patients 65 years or older • Discontinue concomitant use of agents that increase the risk of hemorrhage prior to initiation of fondaparinux sodium, or monitor the patient closely if coadministration is necessary • Discontinue in case of hemorrhage or unexpected changes in coagulation parameters • May cause an allergic reaction due to the latex in the needle guard of the prefilled fondaparinux syringe for patients with latex allergies • Increased risk of bleeding for patients with moderate renal impairment (CrCl of 30–50 mL/min) • Discontinue therapy if severe renal impairment (CrCl < 30 mL/min) occurs while on fondaparinux therapy	• 2.5 mg IV bolus followed by 2.5 mg SC once daily starting on hospital day 2 in STEMI patients • 2.5 mg SC once daily in NSTEMI patients • Continue until hospital discharge	• Bleeding	• Signs of bleeding • CBC with platelet count • aPTT • Serum creatinine

(*continues*)

Table 10-22 (*continued*)

Drug	Mechanism of Action	Contraindications	Warnings	Dosing	Adverse Effects	Monitoring
			• Moderate and severe thrombocytopenia has been reported; discontinue therapy if the platelet count falls below 100,000/mm^3			
Bivalirudin (Angiomax)	Directly inhibits thrombin by specifically binding to the catalytic site and to the anion-binding exosite of circulating and clot-bound thrombin, leading to inhibition of thrombogenic activity	• Active major bleeding • Hypersensitivity	• Preexisting disease states associated with increased risk of bleeding • Increased risk of bleeding in elderly patients • Intravenous injection and infusion administration only • Renal impairment may require dose adjustment	• Administer 0.1 mg/kg IV bolus, followed by 0.25 mg/kg/hr infusion in NSTEMI patients • Administer a second bolus of 0.5 mg/kg IV and increase the infusion rate to 1.75 mg/kg/hr in patients who undergo PCI • Discontinue at the end of PCI or continue for up to 4 hours	• Bleeding	• Signs of bleeding • CBC with platelet count • Serum creatinine • aPTT
GP IIb/IIIa inhibitors	• Inhibit platelet aggregation by specifically binding to the GP IIb/IIIa receptor, the major surface receptor involved in the final common pathway for platelet aggregation • Inhibition of platelet aggregation occurs in a dose-dependent manner • Tirofiban is a nonpeptide platelet glycoprotein (GP) antagonist • Abciximab is a chimeric human–murine monoclonal antibody Fab (fragment antigen-binding) fragment	• Hypersensitivity • Uncontrolled hypertension • Prior stroke • Active bleeding • Recent abnormal bleeding • History of bleeding diathesis • Recent major surgery or trauma • Thrombocytopenia • Dependence on renal dialysis (eptifibatide)		• Abciximab (Reopro): ○ 0.25 mg/kg IV bolus, followed by 0.125 mcg/kg/min (maximum: 10 mcg/min) for 12 hours for PCI ○ Not recommended in NSTEMI patients ○ No dose adjustment required for patients with renal insufficiency • Eptifibatide (Integrilin): ○ 180 mcg/kg IV bolus × 2, 10 minutes apart, with an infusion of 2 mcg/kg/min for 18–24 hours for PCI ○ 180 mcg/kg IV bolus, followed by an infusion of 2 mcg/kg/min for 18–24 hours in NSTEMI patients ○ Dose adjustments are needed for patients with renal insufficiency • Tirofiban (Aggrastat): ○ Not approved for PCI use ○ 0.4 mg/kg IV bolus administered over 30 minutes, followed by an infusion of 0.1 mcg/kg/min for 18–24 hours for NSTEMI patients without PCI ○ Dose adjustments are needed in patients with renal insufficiency	• Bleeding • Acute thrombocytopenia	• Signs of bleeding • CBC with platelet count

Table 10-23 Fibrinolytic Agents

Mechanism of Action	Contraindications	Dosing	Adverse Effects	Monitoring
• Streptokinase initiates activation of the endogenous fibrinolytic system upon binding to plasminogen, producing a complex that accelerates the transformation of plasminogen into proteolytic and fibrinolytic plasmin • Alteplase is a recombinant tissue plasminogen activator that binds to fibrin and enhances the conversion of plasminogen to plasmin, initiating fibrinolysis with limited systemic proteolysis • Tenecteplase and reteplase have mechanism of action similar to that of alteplase	• Absolute: ○ Active internal bleeding ○ Any previous ICH ○ Ischemic stroke within 3 months ○ Known intracranial neoplasm ○ Known structural vascular lesion ○ Suspected aortic dissection ○ Significant closed head or facial trauma within 3 months • Relative: ○ Severe, uncontrolled hypertension (> 180/100 mmHg) ○ History of ischemic stroke for more than 3 months ○ Dementia or known intracranial pathology not covered in the absolute contraindications ○ Current use of anticoagulants ○ Known bleeding diathesis ○ Traumatic or prolonged (> 10 minutes) cardiopulmonary resuscitation (CPR) ○ Major surgery less than 3 weeks prior to presentation ○ Noncompressible vascular puncture ○ Recent internal bleeding (within 2–4 weeks) ○ Previous streptokinase use or prior allergic reaction (streptokinase only) ○ Pregnancy ○ Active peptic ulcer ○ History of severe, chronic, poorly controlled hypertension	• Streptokinase (Streptase): 1.5 million units IV over 60 minutes • Alteplase (Activase): 15-mg IV bolus, followed by 0.75 mg/kg IV over 30 minutes (maximum 50 mg) followed by 0.5 mg/kg (maximum 35 mg) over 60 minutes (maximum dose: 100 mg) • Reteplase (Retavase): 10 units IV × 2 doses, with each dose separated by 30 minutes • Tenecteplase (TNKase): ○ Weight < 60 kg: 30 mg IV bolus ○ Weight 60–69.9 kg: 35 mg IV bolus ○ Weight 70–79.9 kg: 40 mg IV bolus	• Bleeding (including ICH)	• Signs of bleeding • CBC with platelet count • aPTT • Mental status

ANNOTATED BIBLIOGRAPHY

ACC/AHA 2007 guidelines for the management of patients with unstable angina/non ST-elevation myocardial infarction: executive summary: a report of the American College of Cardiology/American Heart Association Task Force on Practice Guidelines (Writing Committee to Revise the 1999 Guidelines for the Management of Patients with Acute Myocardial Infarction). *Circulation* 2007;116: 803–877.

ACC/AHA guidelines for the management of patients with ST-elevation myocardial infarction: executive summary: a report of the American College of Cardiology/American Heart Association Task Force on Practice Guidelines (Writing Committee to Revise the 1999 Guidelines for the Management of Patients with Acute Myocardial Infarction). *Circulation* 2004;110:588–636.

DiPiro JT, Talbert RL, Yee GC, Matzke GR, Wells BG, Posey LM, eds. *Pharmacotherapy: A Pathophysiologic Approach*. 6th ed. New York: McGraw-Hill; 2005.

Micromedex Healthcare Series. Greenwood Village, CO: Thomson Reuters (Healthcare) Inc. Updated periodically.

TOPIC: ARRHYTHMIAS

Section Coordinator: *Teresa K. Hoffmann*
Contributor: *Mary Ann Tucker*

Arrhythmias Overview

Arrhythmias can originate in both the atria and the ventricles of the heart. To treat each type of arrhythmia properly, pharmacists must understand the differences in arrhythmias and be knowledgeable about the various classes of antiarrhythmic medications to ensure their safe and appropriate use.

Tips Worth Tweeting

- Antiarrhythmic medications are not always the first choice in treating arrhythmias, as major trials have shown increased mortality with their use in several clinical situations; nondrug therapies such as ablation and use of an internal cardioverter-defibrillator (ICD) may be more effective treatment options.
- Proarrhythmia is a major side effect of all arrhythmias; the risk of this adverse reaction requires routine monitoring of EKG, blood pressure, and pulse.
- Amiodarone is the most commonly prescribed antiarrhythmic medication. It is FDA indicated for the treatment of ventricular arrhythmias, but is often used off-label to treat supraventricular arrhythmias. Amiodarone is efficacious in terminating arrhythmias, but side effects are frequent and may be serious; therefore, its use requires prudent monitoring.
- Almost all antiarrhythmic medications can cause new-onset heart failure or worsen it if already present. Amiodarone does not have a negative inotropic effect on heart muscle, so it may be used for patients with left ventricular dysfunction.
- Rate control with beta blockers, calcium-channel blockers, or digoxin, along with prevention of thromboembolism with aspirin or warfarin, is as effective as rhythm control for arrhythmias and has the ability to prevent thromboembolism. Rate control offers the advantage of fewer adverse reactions and less need for monitoring compared to rhythm control. Rhythm control should be reserved for those patients who remain symptomatic despite rate control.
- Monitoring with most antiarrhythmic medications should focus on EKG (QT prolongation), blood pressure, pulse, electrolytes (potassium and magnesium), liver and renal function, and drug interactions.

Patient Care Scenario: Ambulatory Setting

CC: "I feel my heart beating fast, and I'm short of breath."
HPI: BH is a 68-year-old female with a history of hypertension. She presents to her internist today complaining of a 1-week history of palpitations and dyspnea on exertion (DOE).
ROS: Negative
P/E: Normal except cardiovascular: Heart rate 104, irregular.
BP: 132/76; wt: 134 lbs; ht: 65 inches

Diagnostic Tests:

- 2D Echocardiogram: Mild left ventricular hypertrophy with ejection fraction of 35%, normal valve function
- EKG: Atrial fibrillation with a ventricular rate of 110

Current Medications:

- Hydrochlorothiazide 25 mg daily
- Calcium carbonate 500 mg twice a day
- Aspirin 81 mg daily

Drug Allergies: Penicillin (rash)

1.1.0 Patient Information

Normal and Abnormal Cardiac Conduction

Normal electrical activity within the heart is initiated by the sinoatrial (SA) node and moves through cardiac tissue as a wavefront, eventually gaining access to the ventricle through the atrioventricular (AV) node and a large bundle of conducting tissue referred to as the bundle of His. From the bundle of His, the cardiac conduction system splits into three bundle branches—one right bundle branch and two left bundle branches. All three of these branches eventually become the Purkinje system.

This conduction system as a whole innervates the mechanical myocardium and initiates the contractile process. Electrical stimulation of the myocardial cells results in changes in membrane potential over time, also known as an action potential curve, owing to the movement of specific ions across the cell membrane. The most notable ions responsible for this change in membrane potential are sodium, potassium, and calcium; most antiarrhythmic medications target at least one of these ions. After a cell group within the heart is electrically stimulated, a brief period of time follows in which those cells cannot be excited again; this is known as the refractory period.

Abnormal conduction leading to tachyarrhythmias is divided into two general categories: arrhythmias resulting from an abnormality in impulse generation (autonomic tachycardias such as sinus tachycardia and junctional tachycardias) and arrhythmias resulting from an abnormality in impulse conduction (reentrant tachycardias such as atrial flutter, atrial fibrillation, AV nodal reentry, and recurrent ventricular tachycardia).

Key Terms

Atrial fibrillation and atrial flutter:

- The most common supraventricular tachycardias.
- Overall prevalence: 0.4%. The prevalence increases with age, as more than 6% of all patients older than age 80 have been diagnosed with this arrhythmia.
- **Atrial fibrillation:** *irregularly irregular* supraventricular rhythm with no discernible p waves (atrial activity). Ventricular response is generally 120–180 beats per minute, and the pulse feels irregular.
- Atrial fibrillation is the result of multiple atrial reentrant loops.
- **Atrial flutter:** *regular* supraventricular rhythm with characteristic flutter waves ("sawtooth" waves) due to a single, dominant reentrant substrate. Ventricular rate is usually measured in factors of 300 beats per minute (150, 100, or 75 beats per minute).
- Several forms of heart and pulmonary disease can cause atrial distention leading to atrial fibrillation and atrial flutter, including ischemia and infarction, hypertension, valvular disorders, dilated or hypertrophic cardiomyopathy, acute pulmonary embolus, and pulmonary hypertension. Atrial fibrillation may also occur in association with states of high adrenergic tone such as thyrotoxicosis, alcohol withdrawal, sepsis, and excessive physical exertion.

Paroxysmal supraventricular tachycardia (PSVT):

- Reentry regular tachycardia with a rate of 160–240 beats per minute that is abrupt in onset and termination.
- Cause can be idiopathic, fever, drug-induced (beta agonists, anticholinergics, sympathomimetics).

Nonsustained ventricular tachycardia (NSVT):

- Three or more beats originating from the ventricles, more than 100 beats per minute, terminating spontaneously in less than 30 seconds.
- Wide QRS pattern.

Torsades de pointes:

- Ventricular tachycardia with a prolonged QT interval and EKG characterized by twisting of the peaks of the QRS complexes around the isoelectric line during the arrhythmia.

Sustained ventricular tachycardia (SVT)/pulseless ventricular tachycardia/ventricular fibrillation (VF):

- **Sustained ventriculation tachycardia:** ventricular tachycardia greater than 30 seconds in duration and/or requiring termination due to hemodynamic compromise.
- **Ventricular fibrillation:** rapid (more than 300 beats per minute), grossly irregular ventricular rhythm with marked variability in QRS cycle length, morphology, and amplitude.
- No recognizable P waves, QRS complexes, or T waves.
- Results in hemodynamic instability—absent pulse and blood pressure.

Signs and Symptoms

Table 10-24 Signs and Symptoms of Arrhythmias

Arrhythmia	Atrial fibrillation/ atrial flutter	Paroxysmal supraventricular tachycardia	Ventricular arrhythmias
Symptoms	• Palpitations • Shortness of breath • Fatigue • Edema • Chest discomfort	• Palpitations • Weakness • Shortness of breath • Lightheadedness • Chest pressure • Anxiety	• Chest discomfort • Syncope • Palpitations • Rapid or absent pulse • Low or absent blood pressure • Loss of consciousness
Complications	• Embolism leading to ischemic stroke • Increased risk of stroke if in the presence of heart failure, hypertension, age greater than 75 years, diabetes, or previous stroke/TIA	• Increased risk of heart failure	• Sudden cardiac death

Treatment Goals of Arrhythmias

Atrial Fibrillation/Atrial Flutter Treatment

- Restore and maintain sinus rhythm by electrical cardioversion and/or administration of antiarrhythmic drugs.
    - Also known as *rhythm control.*
    - Historically, antiarrhythmic drugs were used to restore and maintain sinus rhythm, as this approach approximately doubles the chances of a patient remaining in sinus rhythm.
    - Rhythm control exposes patients to adverse events from antiarrhythmic drugs.
    - Rhythm control has been thought to lessen symptoms, lower risk of stroke, increase quality of life, and reduce mortality, but these benefits have never been demonstrated in clinical trials.

OR

- Control ventricular rate with digoxin, beta blockers (e.g., metoprolol, atenolol, carvedilol), or non-dihydropyridine calcium-channel blockers (e.g., verapamil, diltiazem).
    - Also known as *rate control.*
    - Rate control is generally preferred over rhythm control as a treatment approach due to the better side-effect profiles of the medications and the lack of an apparent advantage for rhythm control over rate control in large randomized clinical trials.

AND

- Prevent thromboembolism.
    - Aspirin 325 mg daily:
        - Age younger than 65 years and no risk factors (risk factors include heart failure, hypertension, diabetes, and previous stroke/TIA).
        - Age younger than 65 years and coronary artery disease but no risk factors.
        - Age 65–76 years but no risk factors (warfarin is also acceptable in this group).
    - Warfarin (goal INR of 2–3): Indicated for any patient who does not meet criteria for aspirin therapy.

Paroxysmal Supraventricular Tachycardia Treatment

- Synchronized direct current cardioversion if the patient is severely symptomatic and/or hemodynamically unstable
- Non-drug therapy to increase vagal tone:
    - Carotid sinus massage
    - Valsalva maneuver
    - Squatting
    - Deep breathing

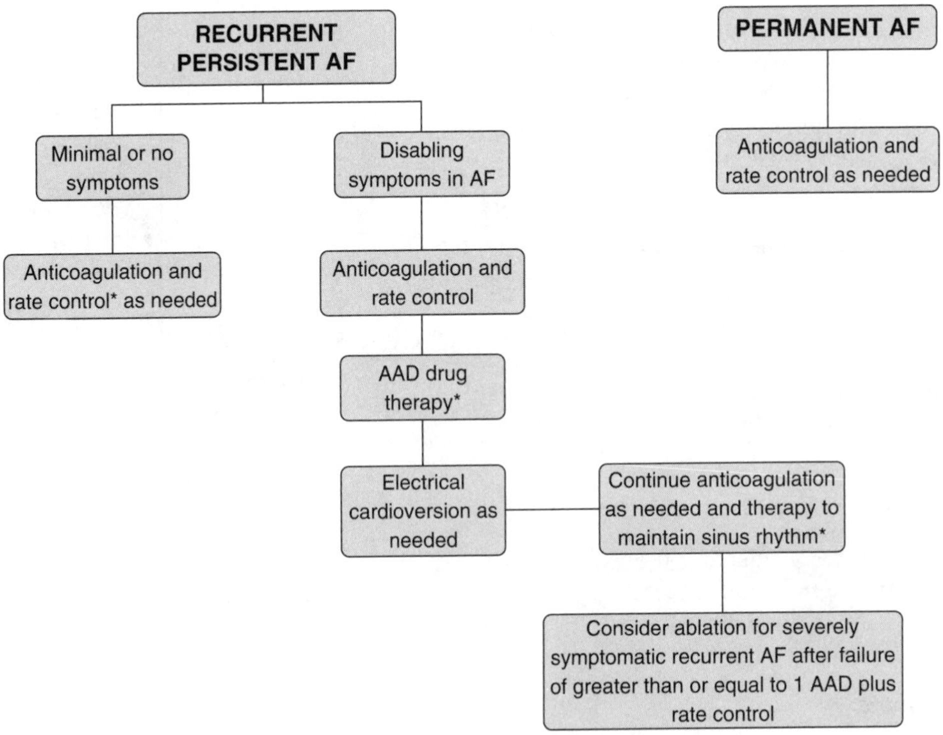

Figure 10-1 Rate vs. Rhythm Control for Atrial Fibrillation

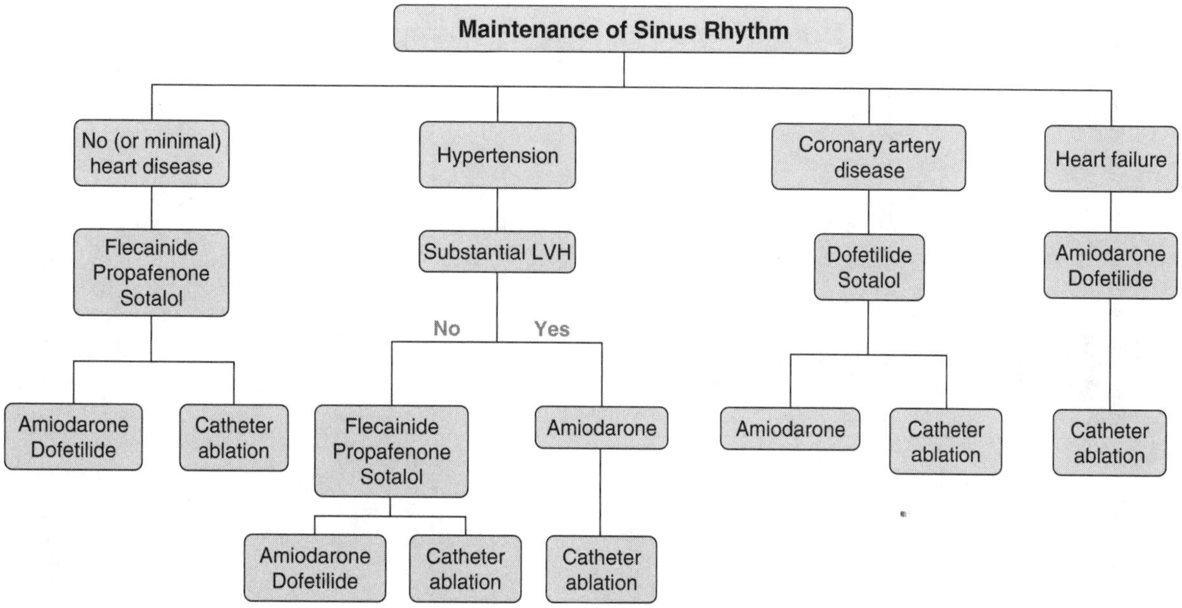

Figure 10-2 Antiarrhythmic Drug (AAD) Therapy for Atrial Fibrillation

- AV-nodal blocking agents:
  - Adenosine
  - Digoxin
  - Beta blockers
  - Calcium-channel blockers
  - Combination of the above medications
- Type Ic antiarrhythmic medications
  - Flecainide
  - Propafenone
- Prevention: Ablation with radiofrequency current

Nonsustained Ventricular Tachycardia Treatment

- Electrophysiologic studies
  - If no inducible sustained VT/VF, then do not use any antiarrhythmic drug on a chronic basis except beta blockers for palpitation control
  - If sustained VT/VF, consider an ICD or empiric amiodarone

Torsades de Pointes Treatment

- Direct-current cardioversion (DCC)
- Magnesium sulfate 2 g IV over 2–60 minutes, then infusion
- Discontinue all agents that prolong the QT interval
- Correct exacerbating factors such as hypokalemia or hypomagnesemia

Sustained Ventricular Tachycardia/Pulseless Ventricular Tachycardia/Ventricular Fibrillation Treatment:

- DCC
- Cardiopulmonary resuscitation (CPR)
- Epinephrine 1 mg IV/IO, repeat every 3–5 minutes

Table 10-25 Classification and Mechanism of Action of Antiarrhythmic Medications

Type	Drug	Conduction	Refractory	Automaticity	Mechanism of Action: Ion Blocked
Ia	Quinidine Procainamide Disopyramide	Decrease	Increase	Decrease	Sodium (intermediate)
Ib	Lidocaine Mexilitine	Neutral/ Decrease	Decrease	Decrease	Sodium (fast)
Ic	Flecainide Propafenone Moricizine	Decrease	Neutral	Decrease	Sodium (slow)
II	Beta blockers	Decrease	Increase	Decrease	Potassium
III	Amiodarone Dronedarone Dofetilide Sotalol Ibutilide	Neutral	Increase	Neutral	Potassium
IV	Verapamil Diltiazem	Decrease	Increase	Decrease	Calcium

Table 10-26 Antiarrhythmic Medications: Drug Indications, Dosing Regimens, Routes of Administration, and Pharmacodynamic/ Pharmacokinetic Properties

Drug	FDA Indications	Dosage Forms	Loading Dose	Maintenance Dose	Pharmacodynamic/Pharmacokinetic Properties
Quinidine (Quinidex, Quinaglute, Quinalan)	• Atrial fibrillation • Atrial flutter • Life-threatening ventricular arrhythmias	• 80 mg/mL • 324 mg extended-release tab	• 200 mg po every 2–3 hours for 5–8 doses	• 328–648 mg po every 8–12 hours	• Hepatic metabolism • Strong inhibitor of CYP 3A4 and 2D6
Procainamide (Pronestyl)	• Life-threatening ventricular arrhythmias	• 100 mg/mL • 500 mg/mL • 250 mg cap • 500 mg cap	• 20 mg/min IV	• 2–6 mg/min IV	• CYP 2D6 substrate • 50% renally excreted unchanged • 50% hepatically metabolized to *N*-acetylprocainamide (NAPA)
Disopyramide (Norpace, Norpace CR)	• Life-threatening ventricular arrhythmias	• 100 mg cap • 150 mg cap • 100 mg CR cap • 150 mg CR cap	• 200–300 mg po	• 400–800 mg/day po divided every 6 hours (immediate release) or every 12 hours (controlled release)	• CYP 3A4 substrate • 20% renally excreted as metabolite (mono-*N*-dealkylated)
Lidocaine	• Ventricular arrhythmias • Ventricular fibrillation	• 0.2 % • 0.4 % • 0.5 % • (in D_5W)	• 50–100 mg IV over 2–3 minutes; may repeat every 5 minutes up to 300 mg per 1-hour period	• 1–4 mg/min IV	• Hepatic metabolism • CYP 3A4 and 2D6 substrate • CYP 1A2 inhibitor (strong), 2D6, and 3A4 inhibitor (moderate) • Active metabolites: mono-ethylglycinexylidide (MEGX) and glycinexylidide (GX)
Mexiletine (Mexitil)	• Life-threatening ventricular arrhythmias	• 150 mg cap • 200 mg cap • 250 mg cap	• 400 mg po, then 200 mg po 8 hours later	• 200–300 mg po every 8 hours	• CYP 1A2 and 2D6 substrate • CYP 1A2 inhibitor • Urinary alkalinizers (antacids, sodium bicarbonate, acetazolamide) increase levels • Urinary acidifiers (cimetidine) decrease levels
Flecainide (Tambocor)	• Atrial fibrillation • Atrial flutter • PSVT • Ventricular tachycardia	• 50 mg tab • 100 mg tab • 150 mg tab	• 50 mg po every 12 hours	• 300–400 mg every 12 hours	• CYP 1A2 and 2D6 substrate • CYP 2D6 inhibitor • Urinary alkalinizers increase levels
Propafenone (Rythmol, Rythmol SR)	• Atrial fibrillation • Atrial flutter • PSVT	• 150 mg IR tab • 225 mg IR tab • 300 mg IR tab	• 150 mg every 8 hours • 225 mg every 12 hours	• 225–300 mg every 8 hours • 325–425 mg every 12 hours	• CYP 2D6, 3A4, and 1A2 substrate • CYP 1A2 and 2D6 inhibitor • Reduce digoxin dose by 25% to decrease digoxin toxicity

	• Ventricular arrhythmias	• 225 mg SR cap • 325 SR cap • 425 SR cap			• Reduce warfarin dose, as this combination increases INR
Moricizine (Ethmozine)	• Life threatening ventricular arrhythmias		• 200–300 mg every 8 hours	• Increase by 15 mg/day every 3 days	• Extensive first-pass hepatic metabolism
Amiodarone (Pacerone, Cordarone)	• Ventricular fibrillation • Ventricular tachycardia • Often used off-label for atrial fibrillation and atrial flutter	• 100 mg tab • 200 mg tab • 400 mg tab • 50 mg/mL	• 15 mg/min IV for 10 minutes (150 mg), then 1 mg/min IV for 6 hours (360 mg), then 0.5 mg/min IV for 18 hours (540 mg)	• 200–800 mg po daily	• CYP 2C8 and 2C9 major substrate • CYP 1A2, 2C8, 2C9, 2D6, and 3A4 inhibitor • Reduce warfarin, digoxin, quinidine, and procainamide by 30–50% to prevent toxicities • Elimination half-life: 40–55 days
Dronedarone (Multaq)	• Atrial fibrillation • Atrial flutter	• 400 mg tab	• 400 mg po every 12 hours	• 400 mg po every 12 hours	• Hepatic metabolism, mostly CPY 3A4 • Elimination half-life: 13–19 hours
Dofetilide (Tikosyn)	• Atrial fibrillation • Atrial flutter	• 0.125 mg cap • 0.25 mg cap • 0.5 mg cap	• 0.5 mg po every 12 hours (adjust in patients with renal dysfunction)	• 0.25–0.5 mg po every 12 hours	• Hepatic metabolism • CYP 3A4 substrate • Renal excretion: 80% unchanged
Sotalol (Betapace, Betapace AF, Sorine)	• Atrial fibrillation • Atrial flutter • Life-threatening ventricular arrhythmias	• 80 mg tab • 120 mg tab • 160 mg tab • 240 mg tab	• 80 mg po every 12 hours (adjust in patients with renal dysfunction)	• 160–360 mg po daily depending on renal function	• Not metabolized • Renal excretion as unchanged drug by glomerular filtration and tubular secretion • Contraindicated in patients with CrCl < 40 mL/min • Dialyzable through hemodialysis
Ibutilide (Corvert)	• Atrial fibrillation (recent onset) • Atrial flutter (recent onset)	• 0.1 mg/mL	• Weight > 60 kg: 1 mg over 10 minutes • Weight < 60 kg: 0.01 mg/mL over 10 minutes	• Cardioversion only	• Renal excretion: 82% as active metabolite • Fecal excretion: 19% • Elimination half-life: 6 hours
Verapamil (Calan, Calan SR, Covera-HS, Isoptin SR, Verelan, Verelan PM)	• Atrial arrhythmias • PSVT	• 2.5 mg/mL • 40 mg tab • 80 mg tab • 120 mg tab • 100 mg ER cap • 120 mg ER cap • 180 mg ER cap • 200 mg ER cap	• 80–160 mg po every 8 hours • 5–10 mg IV over 2–3 minutes, may repeat × 1 in 30 minutes	• 80–160 mg po every 8 hours	• CYP 3A4 substrate • CYP 3A4 moderate inhibitor

(*continues*)

Table 10-26 (*continued*)

Drug	FDA Indications	Dosage Forms	Loading Dose	Maintenance Dose	Pharmacodynamic/Pharmacokinetic Properties
Verapamil (Calan, Calan SR, Covera-HS, Isoptin SR, Verelan, Verelan PM) *(continued)*		• 240 mg ER cap • 300 mg ER cap • 360 mg ER cap • 120 mg ER tab • 180 mg ER tab • 240 mg ER tab			
Diltiazem (Cardizem, Cardizem CD, Cartia XT, Dilacor XR, Tiazac, Dilt-CD, Dilt-XR, Ditia XT)	• Atrial arrhythmias • PSVT	• 5 mg/mL • 30 mg tab • 60 mg tab • 90 mg tab • 120 mg tab • 120 mg ER cap • 180 mg ER cap • 240 mg ER cap • 420 mg ER cap • 60 mg 12-hour ER cap • 90 mg 12-hour ER cap • 120 mg 12-hour ER cap • 120 mg 24-hour ER cap • 180 mg 24-hour ER cap • 240 mg 24-hour ER cap • 300 mg 24-hour ER cap • 360 mg 24-hour ER cap • 420 mg 24-hour ER cap	• 0.25 mg/kg IV over 2 minutes; if no response after 15 minutes, may give second bolus of 0.35 mg/kg IV over 2 minutes	• 15 mg/hr IV infusion	• CYP 3A4 substrate • CYP 3A4 moderate inhibitor

Table 10-27 Antiarrhythmic Medications: Contraindications, Warnings, Precautions, Side Effects, and Monitoring

Drug	Contraindications	Warnings	Precautions	Side Effects	Monitoring
Quinidine	• Cisapride • Dronedarone • Itraconazole • Nelfinavir • Ritonavir • Saquinavir • Sparfloxacin • Voriconazole • Ziprasidone	• Doses are *not* interchangeable: 267 mg quinidine gluconate = 200 mg quinidine sulfate • Decrease digoxin dose by half • Can increase INR • Antacids, sodium bicarbonate, and acetazolamide alkalinize the urine and increase quinidine levels • Beta blockers, verapamil, amiodarone, diltiazem, cimetidine, and erythromycin increase quinidine levels	• Rheumatic fever • Thyrotoxicosis • Bradycardia • Use of digoxin • Heart failure • Hypokalemia • Hypomagnesemia • Hypotension • Liver disease • Structural heart disease (increased mortality) • Renal impairment	• QT prolongation • Torsades de pointes • Nausea/vomiting/ diarrhea • Photosensitivity • Dermatitis • Tinnitus • Deafness • Bitter taste • Flushing	• Symptomatic improvement • CBC • EKG • Blood pressure • Liver function tests within first few weeks of therapy
Procainamide	• Cisapride • Dronedarone • Sparfloxacin • Thioridazine • Ziprasidone	• Prolonged use of procainamide often leads to a positive ANA test, with or without symptoms of SLE • Discontinue procainamide if blood dyscrasias are identified	• Ischemic heart disease • Blood dyscrasias • Cardiomyopathy • Heart failure • Digoxin • First-degree heart block • Liver disease • Myasthenia gravis • Renal impairment	• Systemic lupus erythematosus (SLE) • QT prolongation • Torsades de pointes • Hypotension • GI disturbance • Flushing/rash	• ANA titer • Blood pressure • Pulse • CBC: weekly for the first 3 months and frequently thereafter • Renal function • Plasma concentration: 4–12 mcg/mL
Disopyramide	• Cisapride • Dronedarone • Sparfloxacin • Thioridazine • Ziprasidone	• Should be used only for life-threatening arrhythmias	• Heart failure • Geriatrics • Hypokalemia • Hyperkalemia • Glaucoma • Hypoglycemia • Liver disease • Renal impairment • Sick sinus syndrome • Wolff-Parkinson-White syndrome • BPH	• QT prolongation • Torsades de pointes • Constipation • Urinary retention/ delay in passing urine • Impotence • Hypoglycemia	• Signs and symptoms of heart failure • EKG • Blood pressure • Pulse • Liver and renal function • Blood glucose

(*continues*)

Table 10-27 (*continued*)

Drug	Contraindications	Warnings	Precautions	Side Effects	Monitoring
Lidocaine	• Dihydroergotamine	• Cimetidine, propranolol, ciprofloxacin, diltiazem, verapamil, grapefruit juice, digoxin, erythromycin, ketoconazale: increased lidocaine levels	• Bradycardia • Mexilitine or Class III antiarrhythmic • Hepatic disease	• Hypotension • Dizziness • Numbness • Blurred vision	• Therapeutic range: 1.5–5 mcg/mL
Mexiletine	• Levomethadyl	• Should be used only for life-threatening arrhythmias	• Heart failure • Hypokalemia • Hypotension • Blood dyscrasias • Liver disease • Parkinson's disease (causes tremor) • Seizure disorder	• Lightheadedness • Palpitations • Ataxia • Confusion • Dizziness • Blurred vision • GI distress • Tremor	• EKG • CBC • Liver function
Flecainide	• Cisapride • Ritonavir • Saquinavir • Thioridazine • Ziprasidone	• Withdrawal of therapy should be done in the hospital setting	• Atrial fibrillation • Heart failure • Hypokalemia • Hyperkalemia • Geriatrics • Liver disease • Renal impairment • Sick sinus syndrome	• Dizziness • Blurred vision • Photopsia • Dyspnea • Cardiac dysrhythmia	• EKG • Pulse • Liver and renal function • Trough plasma level (adults): 0.2–1 mcg/mL
Propafenone	• Cisapride • Ritonavir • Saquinavir • Thioridazine • Ziprasidone	• Considerable risk in patients with structural heart disease • Should be used only for life-threatening arrhythmias	• Heart failure • Elevated ANA titers • Hematologic disorders • Impaired spermatogenesis	• Atrioventricular block • CHF • Chest pain • Agranulocytosis • Angina • Dizziness • Headache	• EKG • Pulse • Signs and symptoms of heart failure • ANA titer • Liver function
Moricizine	• Cisapride • Sparfloxacin	• Should be used only for life-threatening arrhythmias • Withdrawal of therapy should be done in the hospital setting	• Heart failure • Hypokalemia • Geriatrics • Liver disease • Renal impairment • Sick sinus syndrome	• Decompensated heart failure • Dizziness • Headache • Dysrhythmia	• EKG • Blood pressure • Pulse • Liver and renal function • Signs and symptoms of heart failure

Amiodarone	• Cisapride • Dronedarone • Indinavir • Ritonavir • Saquinavir • Sparfloxacin • Thioridazine • Ziprasidone	• Amiodarone has several potentially fatal toxicities, the most important of which is pulmonary toxicity • Liver injury is common, but is usually mild and evidenced only by abnormal liver enzymes; overt liver disease can occur, however, and has been fatal in a few cases • Amiodarone can exacerbate the arrhythmia—for example, by making the arrhythmia less well tolerated or more difficult to reverse	• Pulmonary toxicity • Hepatic disease • Acute MI, especially with IV administration • Bradycardia • Concomitant use with CYP 3A4 inhibitors and QT-prolonging drugs • Hypokalemia • Hypomagnesemia • Hypotension, especially with IV administration • Thyroid abnormalities	• Elevated liver enzymes • Corneal deposits • Hypothyroidism • Hyperthyroidism • QT prolongation • Hypotension • Photosensitivity • Blue-gray discoloration of skin • Movement disorder • GI disturbances	• EKG for efficacy and QT prolongation • Liver enzymes • Thyroid function • Chest x-ray • Pulmonary function tests with diffusion capacity • Ophthalmic examinations including fundoscopy and slit-lamp examinations • Pacing and defibrillation thresholds
Dronedarone	• Amiodarone • Cisapride • Clarithromycin • Cyclosporine • Disopyramide • Dofetilide • Gatifloxacin • Ibutilide • Indinavir • Itraconazole • Ketoconazole • Levofloxacin • Mefloquine • Methadone • Moxifloxacin • Mefazodone • Melfinavir • Paliperidone • Procainamide • Quinidine • Quinine • Ritonavir • Saquinavir	• Contraindicated in patients with NYHA Class IV heart failure or NYHA Class II–III heart failure with a recent decompensation; these patients have a more than twofold increase in mortality when given dronedarone • Strong CYP 3A4 inhibitors (ketoconazole) and Class I or III antiarrhythmics must be discontinued prior to initiation of dronedarone	• CYP 3A4 inducers (e.g., carbamazepine, phenobarbital, phenytoin, St. John's wort) should be avoided • Grapefruit juice should be avoided • Heart failure (new-onset or worsening) has been reported • Avoid in pregnancy • QT prolongation may occur	• QT prolongation • Abdominal pain • Diarrhea • Indigestion • Nausea • Vomiting • Asthenia • Increased serum creatinine • Heart failure	• EKG • Signs and symptoms of heart failure

(*continues*)

Table 10-27 (*continued*)

Drug	Contraindications	Warnings	Precautions	Side Effects	Monitoring
Dronedarone *(continued)*	• Sotalol • Thioridazine • Vardenafil • Voriconazole • Ziprasidone				
Dofetilide	• Cimetidine • Cisapride • Dronedarone • Hydrochlorothi-azide • Itraconazole • Ketoconazole • Megestrol • Prochlorperazine • Sparfloxacin • Sulfamethoxazole • Thioridazine • Trimethoprim • Verapamil • Ziprasidone	• Initiation should be done in a hospital for a minimum of 3 days with continuous EKG monitoring and creatinine clearance calculations	• AV block • Bradycardia • QT-prolonging drugs • Hypokalemia • Hypomagnesemia • Liver disease • Moderate QT prolongation prior to therapy • Potassium-depleting diuretics • Renal impairment	• Chest pain • QT prolongation • Torsades de pointes • Atrioventricular block • Diarrhea • Dizziness • Headache • Dyspnea	• EKG • Blood pressure • Pulse • Renal function at baseline and every 3 months thereafter
Sotalol	• Cisapride • Dronedarone • Sparfloxacin • Thioridazine • Ziprasidone	• Initiation should be done in a hospital with continuous cardiac monitoring • Betapace AF is indicated for patients in NSR to prevent symptomatic atrial fibrillation/atrial flutter • Betapace is *not* approved for the atrial fibrillation/atrial flutter indication and should not be substituted for Betapace AF due to significant differences in the drug's labeling	• Avoid abrupt withdrawal • Bronchospastic disease • QT interval–prolonging drugs • Heart failure • Diabetes • Hypokalemia • Hypomagnesemia • Hyperthyroidism • Peripheral vascular disease • Renal impairment • Recent MI • Sick sinus syndrome	• Chest pain • CHF • Edema • QT prolongation • Torsades de pointes • Palpitations • Hypotension	• EKG • Blood pressure • Pulse • Signs and symptoms of heart failure • Renal function • Serum potassium and magnesium

Ibutilide	• Cisapride • Dronedarone • Sparfloxacin • Thioridazine • Ziprasidone	• Can cause fatal arrhythmias such as torsades de pointes, with and without QT-interval prolongation • Must be administered in a facility due to the need for continuous EKG monitoring • Patients with atrial fibrillation/atrial flutter must be anticoagulated	• Bradycardia • Heart failure • Hypokalemia • Hypomagnesemia • Liver disease • Other antiarrhythmics should not be given within 4 hours of ibutilide infusion • Recent MI • QT interval prolongation prior to treatment	• Bradyarrhythmia • Hypertension • Hypotension • QT prolongation • Torsades de pointes • Palpitations • Ventricular arrhythmias	• EKG • Blood pressure • Pulse
Verapamil	• Dofetilide	• Do not use in Wolff-Parkinson-White syndrome, Lown-Ganong-Levine syndrome, or sick sinus syndrome • Contraindicated when SBP < 90 mm Hg • Contraindicated in left ventricular dysfunction • Drug interactions: 3A4 inhibitors	• Heart failure may occur • Elevated liver enzymes • Implement dose reduction if any type of AV block occurs • Hypotension • Dizziness • Pulmonary edema • Renal function impairment	• Edema • Hypotension • Dizziness • Headache • Constipation • Nausea	• EKG • Pulse • Renal function • Liver function • Signs and symptoms of heart failure
Diltiazem	• Cisapride	• Contraindicated in acute MI with pulmonary congestion • Do not administer IV beta blockers within a few hours of IV diltiazem • Contraindicated when SBP < 90 mm Hg • Do not use IV diltiazem in ventricular tachycardia • Drug interactions: 3A4 inhibitors	• Concomitant use of beta blockers or digoxin • Dermatologic reactions • Hepatic impairment • Hypotension • Renal impairment • Supraventricular arrhythmias with hemodynamic compromise • Left ventricular dysfunction	• Atrioventricular block • Congestive heart failure exacerbation • Edema • Bradyarrhythmia • Gingival hyperplasia • Dizziness • Headache	• Angina • EKG • Blood pressure • Pulse • Signs and symptoms of heart failure • Liver function

- Vasopressin 40 U IV/IO to replace the first or second dose of epinephrine
- Amiodarone 300 mg IV/IO once, then consider additional 150 mg IV/IO
- Lidocaine 1–1.5 mg/kg first dose, then 0.5–0.75 mg/kg IV/IO; maximum 3 doses or 3 mg/kg

ANNOTATED BIBLIOGRAPHY

ACC/AHA/ESC 2006 guidelines for the management of patients with atrial fibrillation: a report of the American College of Cardiology/American Heart Association Task Force on Practice Guidelines and the European Society of Cardiology Committee for Practice Guidelines. *J Am Coll Cardiol* 2006;48:e149–e246.

ACC/AHA/ESC 2006 guidelines for management of patients with ventricular arrhythmias and the prevention of sudden cardiac death: a report of the American College of Cardiology/American Heart Association Task Force and the European Society of Cardiology Committee for Practice Guidelines. *J Am Coll Cardiol* 2006;48:e247–e246.

DiPiro JT, Talbert RL, Yee GC, Matzke GR, Wells BG, Posey LM, eds. *Pharmacotherapy: A Pathophysiologic Approach*. 6th ed. New York: McGraw-Hill; 2005.

Handbook of Emergency Cardiovascular Care for Healthcare Providers. American Heart Association; 2008.

Micromedex Healthcare Series. Greenwood Village, CO: Thomson Reuters (Healthcare) Inc. Updated periodically.

TOPIC: SHOCK

Section Coordinator: Teresa K. Hoffmann
Contributor: Teresa K. Hoffmann

Shock Overview

Successful treatment of shock involves the proper choice of vasopressors and inotropes and the treatment of the underlying cause. Pharmacists play a critical role in choosing the correct drug for the patient and making the drug quickly available in medical emergencies.

Tips Worth Tweeting

- Shock is defined as hypotension (SBP < 90 mm Hg or drop in BP > 40 mm Hg from baseline) with clinical signs of end-organ failure that is unresponsive to initial therapy.
- Aggressive fluid replacement (within first 6 hours) improves mortality.
- Mortality rates for shock are in the range of 30% to 50%.
- Shock results from profound pump failure and the activation of compensatory mechanisms.
- Start vasopressors and inotropes at low doses and titrate to the desired effect.
- Wean the patient off pressors/inotropes as soon as clinically possible while constantly monitoring hemodynamic parameters.
- Vasopressors carry a "black box" warning regarding extravasation.

1.1.0 Patient Information

Classification of Shock

- Cardiogenic: due to "pump" failure
- Septic: due to vascular resistance failure (caused by capillary leak)
- Hypovolemic: due to rapid loss of vascular volume

Signs and Symptoms

See Table 10-28 and Table 10-29.

Wellness and Prevention

Unfortunately, shock cannot always be prevented. Focus on preventing or treating the cause. Causes may include MI, infection, blood loss, dehydration, aortic/mitral stenosis, third-spacing fluid, and pericardial effusion.

1.2.0 Pharmacotherapy

Mechanism of Action by Class

Vasopressors (Increase BP)

- Dopamine: Precursor of norepinephrine (NE) that stimulates three types of receptors
  - D_1 receptors (0.5–3 mcg/kg/min), producing increased perfusion

Table 10-28 Symptoms of Shock

Oliguric renal failure
Mental status changes
Hypotension
Lactic acidosis
Organ failure (liver, stomach, brain, kidneys)
Tachycardia
Pulmonary edema
Tachypnea
Dyspnea
Decreased oxygenation

Table 10-29 Signs of Shock

Sign/Parameter	Normal Range
Blood pressure (BP)	120–140/80–90 mm Hg
Heart rate (HR)	60–100 bpm
Cardiac output (CO)	5–8 L/min
Central venous pressure (CVP)	2–6 mm Hg
Mean arterial pressure (MAP)	80–100 mm Hg
Mean pulmonary artery pressure (MPAP)	12–15 mm Hg
Pulmonary artery pressure (PAP)	20–30/8–12 mm Hg
Pulmonary capillary wedge pressure (PCWP)	5–12 mm Hg
Cardiac index (CI)	2.5–4.2 L/min/m^2
Perfusion pressure (PP)	> 50 mm Hg
Stroke volume (SV)	60–130 mL/beat
Stroke volume index (SVI)	30–75 mL/beat/m^2
Systemic vascular resistance (SVR)	800–1,440 dynes/sec/cm^{-5}
Systemic vascular resistance index (SVRI)	1,300–2,100 dynes/sec/cm^{-5}
Mixed venous oxygen saturation (SvO_2)	70–75%

- Beta$_1$ receptors (3–10 mcg/kg/min), producing positive inotropy
- Alpha$_1$ receptors (10–20 mcg/kg/min), producing vasoconstriction and positive chronotropy, which leads to increased myocardial oxygen demand (ischemia)

- Epinephrine: Potent alpha- and beta-receptor agonist
  - Low dose (0.01–0.05 mcg/kg/min): $\beta > \alpha$
  - High dose ($\geq$ 0.1 mcg/kg/min): $\alpha > \beta$
- Norepinephrine
  - Greater alpha than beta agonist activity
  - Produces profound vasoconstriction
  - Phenylephrine: Pure alpha agonist

Inotropes (Increase CO)

- Dobutamine: Primarily beta$_1$ agonist, producing inotropy with some vasodilation
- Milrinone: Phosphodiesterase inhibitor, producing vasodilation and decreased afterload

Interaction of Drugs with Foods and Laboratory Tests

Vasopressors

- Contraindication: Topical cocaine
- Precautions: Ergot alkaloids, linezolid, phenytoin, tricyclic antidepressants, atomoxetine, beta blockers, nonselective alpha blockers, beta$_2$ agonists, monoamine oxidase inhibitors (MAOIs)

Table 10-30 Shock Medications: Drugs, Indications, and Routes of Administration

Drug	Approved Indications	Routes of Administration
Vasopressors		
Dopamine	Shock (after adequate fluid replacement)	IV
Epinephrine	Anaphylactic shock	IV, IM
Norephinephrine	Shock (after adequate fluid replacement)	IV
Phenylephrine	Shock (after adequate fluid replacement)	IV
Inotropes		
Dobutamine	Short-term management of patients with cardiac decompensation	IV
Milrinone	Short-term therapy for acutely decompensated heart failure	IV

Dobutamine

- Contraindication: Topical cocaine
- Precautions: Ergot alkaloids, linezolid, phenytoin, tricyclic antidepressants, atomoxetine, betablockers, nonselective alpha blockers, beta$_2$ agonists

Milrinone

- Precautions: Anagrelide

Contraindications, Warnings, and Precautions

Contraindications

- Dopamine: Sulfite hypersensitivity, pheochromocytoma, VF
- Epinephrine: Narrow-angle glaucoma, organic brain damage, local anesthesia of the digits, active childbirth labor
- Norepinephrine: Severe volume depletion except as an emergency measure to maintain perfusion until volume is replaced, vascular thrombosis, cyclopropane anesthesia, halothane anesthesia, profound hypoxia, sulfite sensitivity
- Phenylephrine: VT
- Dobutamine: Sulfite hypersensitivity, idiopathic hypertrophic subaortic stenosis
- Milrinone: Hypersensitivity to milrinone or inamrinone

Warnings and Precautions

- Dopamine: Avoid extravasation by infusing into a large vein, cardiovascular disease, post-MI

Table 10-31 Shock Medications: Physiochemical Properties, Solubility, Pharmacodynamics, and Pharmacokinetic Properties

Drug	Onset (min)	Duration (min)
Dopamine	5	< 10
Epinephrine	5–10	< 60
Norepinephrine	1–2	1–2
Phenylephrine	10–15	15–30
Dobutamine	1–10	10 1 week if multidose
Milrinone	90	3–5 hours (lengthened in renal failure)

- Epinephrine: Cardiovascular disease, cerebrovascular disease, diabetes, Parkinson's disease, thyroid disease
- Norepinephrine: Avoid extravasation by infusing into a large vein
- Phenylephrine: Avoid extravasation by infusing into a large vein, hyperthyroidism, partial heart block, bradycardia, severe CAD, hypertension
- Dobutamine: Aortic stenosis, atrial fibrillation, hypovolemia, post-MI
- Milrinone: Arrhythmias, liver dysfunction, severe hypotension due to hypovolemia, hypokalemia, hypomagnesemia, acute MI, renal dysfunction

1.3.0 Monitoring

Pharmacotherapeutic Outcomes

Stabilize the patient and treat the underlying cause.

Safety and Efficacy Monitoring and Patient Education

Treatment goals are as follows:

- MAP ≥ 65 mm Hg
- SvO_2 ≥ 70%
- CI ≥ 3 L/min/m^2
- paO_2 ≥ 80 mm Hg
- SBP > 90 mm Hg

Adverse Drug Reactions

- Dopamine: Ectopic beats, tachycardia, palpitation, vasoconstriction, headache
- Epinephrine: Chest pain, flushing, hypertension, tachycardia, vasoconstriction, ventricular ectopy, anxiety headache, xerostomia
- Norepinephrine: Arrhythmias, bradycardia, peripheral ischemia, headache, anxiety, dyspnea

Table 10-32 Shock Medications: Generic Names, Brand Names, and Dosage Forms Available

Generic	Brand Name	Strengths Available
Dopamine	Inotropin	Premixed infusion in D_5W: 0.8, 1.6, 3.2 mg/mL Injection solution: 40, 80, 160 mg/mL
Epinephrine	Adrenalin	0.1, 1 mg/mL
Norepinephrine	Levophed	1 mg/mL
Phenylephrine	Neo-Synephrine	10 mg/mL
Dobutamine	Dobutrex	Premixed infusion in dextrose: 1, 2, 4 mg/mL Injection solution: 12.5 mg/mL
Milrinone	Primacor	Premixed infusion in D_5W: 200 mcg/mL Injection solution: 1 mg/mL

- Phenylephrine: Decreased CO, hypertension, reflex bradycardia, severe peripheral and visceral vasoconstriction, anxiety, insomnia, metabolic acidosis, extravasation, decreased renal perfusion, hypersensitivity reactions
- Dobutamine: Tachycardia, hypertension, ventricular ectopy, premature ventricular contractions (dose related), fever, headache
- Milrinone: Ventricular ectopy, nonsustained ventricular tachycardia, supraventricular arrhythmia, hypotension, chest pain, headache

2.2.0 Select and Dispense Medications in a Manner That Promotes Safe and Effective Use

See Table 10-32.

ANNOTATED BIBLIOGRAPHY

Drug Facts and Comparisons. Wolters Kluwer Health, Inc. Updated periodically.

Lexi-Drugs. Lexi-Comp, Inc.; February 28, 2010.

Maclaren R, Rudis MI, Dasta JF. Use of vasopressors and inotropes in the pharmacotherapy of shock. In DiPiro JT, Talbert RL, Yee GC, Matzke GR, Wells BG, Posey LM, eds. *Pharmacotherapy: A Pathophysiologic Approach*. 7th ed. Available at: http://0-www.accesspharmacy.com.polar.onu.edu/content.aspx?aID=3191927.

Micromedex Healthcare Series. Greenwood Village, CO: Thomson Reuters (Healthcare) Inc. Updated periodically.

TOPIC: HEART FAILURE

Section Coordinator: Teresa K. Hoffmann
Contributor: Danielle P. Fennema

Heart Failure Overview

Heart failure is an ongoing public health problem that affects more than 5 million Americans. It accounts for at least 20% of all hospitalizations, with the estimated annual costs in the United States for this disorder totaling more than $30 billion. Heart failure is a complex clinical symptom that can result from structural and/or functional cardiac impairment, leading to decreased ability of the ventricle to fill with or eject blood. Thus, heart failure is defined as the inability of the heart to provide sufficient blood supply to meet the body's metabolic demands. It may be the underlying cause in nearly every form of cardiac disease, including coronary atherosclerosis, myocardial infarction, valvular disease, hypertension, congenital heart disease, and cardiomyopathies. This disorder is becoming more prevalent due to the aging of the population and increases in risk factors such as hypertension, diabetes, and consumption of a high-fat diet.

Tips Worth Tweeting

- Heart failure is classified using two methods: (1) New York Heart Association (NYHA) functional classes, which categorize patients based on symptoms alone, and (2) American College of Cardiology/American Heart Association (ACC/AHA) stages, which categorize patients based on symptoms and cardiac structural damage.
- Lifestyle modifications play a major role in managing heart failure.
- Not all medications in each class have an indication for heart failure (e.g., beta blockers).
- Every patient with heart failure should be taking an ACE inhibitor and a beta blocker (unless there is a contraindication).
- Patients with renal disease will typically require higher doses of loop diuretics to produce adequate diuresis.
- Aldosterone antagonists reduce morbidity and mortality in patients with heart failure.
- Although thiazide diuretics have an FDA indication for edema as adjunct therapy, clinically they are minimally effective.
- Digoxin does not reduce morbidity and mortality but may improve symptoms of heart failure.

Key Terms

Cardiac output is the volume of blood being pumped by the heart, in particular by the ventricle per minute. For normal individuals, it is the amount of blood needed to meet the body's total metabolic needs; patients with heart failure, however, are unable to meet these metabolic demands. The metabolic needs of the body include supplying enough blood, oxygen, and nutrients to organs. Cardiac output (CO), the volume of blood ejected from the ventricle per minute, is a product of stroke volume (SV) and heart rate (HR):

$$CO = SV \times HR$$

Stroke volume is the volume of blood ejected with each contraction. It is influenced by three major factors: preload, afterload, and myocardial contraction. **Preload** is the amount of myocardial stretch at the end of diastole (i.e., just prior to contraction), which reflects end-diastolic volume (EDV) or end-diastolic pressure (EDP). Preload has a direct effect on stroke volume. **Afterload** is the resistance that the ventricle must overcome to empty during contraction, which reflects arterial or systolic ventricular pressure; it has an inverse effect on stroke volume. **Myocardial contractility**, or inotropic state, accounts for changes in the force generated by the myocardium independent of preload and afterload. It also has a direct relationship with stroke volume.

↑ Preload = ↑ SV
↓ Afterload = ↑ SV
↑ Contractility = ↑ SV

Systolic heart failure is the inability of the ventricle to contract normally. **Diastolic heart failure** is the inability of the ventricle to relax (diastole) normally, resulting in a filling defect (low end-diastolic volume).

Causes of Heart Failure

Common causes of heart failure include cardiac events such as myocardial infarction, coronary artery disease, valvular heart disease, arrhythmias, cardiomyopathy, and uncontrolled hypertension. Other causes are as follows:

- Diabetes mellitus
- Hyperlipidemia
- Smoking
- Alcoholism
- Obesity
- Rheumatic fever
- Pheochromocytoma
- Severe anemia
- Amyloidosis
- Emphysema
- Collagen vascular disease
- Thyroid disorder
- Cardiotoxic medications (e.g., doxorubicin, daunorubicin, cyclophosphamide)

The following medications, among others, exacerbate heart failure symptoms:

- Nonsteroidal anti-inflammatory drugs (NSAIDS)
- Cyclooxygenase-2 (COX-2) inhibitors
- Glucocorticoids
- Androgens
- Estrogens
- Salicylates at high doses
- Thiazolidinediones

Diagnosis

Heart failure is usually diagnosed based on symptoms and then confirmed with a physical exam and a complete medical history.

Physical Findings

- Weak, rapid pulse
- Hypotension
- Abnormal heart sounds
- Pulmonary, abdominal, or extremity edema
- Cardiomegaly
- Jugular venous distention
- Hepatomegaly

Laboratory Testing

CBC, BNP, BUN, SCr, and electrolytes are all tested in case of heart failure.

Other Diagnostic Tests

- Chest x-ray
- Electrocardiogram
- Electrocardiography
- Tests used to measure EF, such as cardiac catheterization, multiple gated acquisition (MUGA) scan, magnetic resonance imaging (MRI), or computerized tomography

Classifications of Heart Failure

The NYHA functional classes focus on symptomatic heart failure based on the clinician's subjective evaluation. These classes do not address preventive measures or the progression of heart failure. The NYHA functional classes consider clinical diagnosis of heart failure starting at Class II, which is based only on symptoms.

- Class I: Patients without symptoms and no limitations with normal physical activity, but symptomatic with strenuous exercise.
- Class II: Patients with symptoms with normal activity or moderate exertion.
- Class III: Patients with symptoms with minimal exertion; marked limitations in physical activity, including activities of daily life.
- Class IV: Patients symptomatic at rest, requiring hospitalization, or intravenous inotropic support.

The ACC/AHA guidelines subdivide heart failure into four stages, but these stages do not directly correlate with the NYHA functional classes.

- Stage A: Patients who are at high risk of developing heart failure due to comorbid conditions, such as diabetes mellitus or hypertension, with no structural heart disease detectable.
- Stage B: Patients who are asymptomatic, but have detectable structural heart disease (e.g., left ventricular dysfunction, fibrosis).
- Stage C: Patients with structural heart disease and current or history of heart failure symptoms.
- Stage D: Patients with end-stage refractory heart failure, with symptoms of heart failure at rest despite all possible therapies.

Nonpharmalogic Therapy

The key to preventing heart failure is to eliminate as many risk factors for heart failure as possible. Lifestyle modifications can often help relieve signs and symptoms of heart failure and even prevent the disease from worsening.

- Smoking cessation: Smoking damages the blood vessels, and causes hypoxia and tachycardia.
- Sodium restriction: Excess sodium induces water retention, which makes the heart work harder and causes shortness of breath and peripheral edema. Patients with heart failure should be restricted to less than 2,000 mg of sodium daily.
- Daily weight: Recording daily weight assists in detecting fluid accumulation in the body. A gain of more than 3 pounds per day is significant and requires evaluation by a physician.
- Exercise: Exercise was once forbidden for heart failure patients, but it has been proved to maintain the health of the rest of the body; moreover, conditioning reduces the demands on the heart muscle.
- Stress reduction: Anxiety may cause tachycardia and tachypnea, which can exacerbate heart failure.
- Sleep improvement: Elevate the head of the bed, propping it up at a 45-degree angle to decrease shortness of breath.
- Alcohol restriction: Excessive alcohol is a direct cardiotoxin, and can weaken the heart muscle and increase the risk of arrhythmias, which could exacerbate heart failure.

Table 10-33 ACC/AHA Heart Failure Goals of Therapy

Heart Failure Classes	Goals of Therapy
Stage A: High-risk patients, without structural heart disease	Treat underlying disease states: • Control hypertension, diabetes, obesity, metabolic syndrome, and hyperlipidemia • Encourage regular exercise • Discourage alcohol, tobacco, and illicit drug use Medications: • ACEI/ARB for diabetic or vascular patients*
Stage B: Asymptomatic patients, with structural heart disease	All treatments from Stage A Medications: • ACEI/ARB for diabetic or vascular patients* • Beta blocker for appropriate patients
Stage C: Symptomatic patients, with structural heart disease	All treatments from Stages A and B Medications: • ACEI/ARB for diabetic or vascular patients* • Beta blocker for appropriate patients • Diuretics for fluid retention • Aldosterone antagonists • ARB added to standard therapy • Digitalis • Hydralazine/nitrates Medical devices: • Biventricular pacing • Implantable defibrillator
Stage D: Refractory, end stage, with symptoms at rest despite maximal medical therapy	All treatments for Stages A, B, and C End-of-life care/hospice Other treatments: • Transplant • Chronic inotropes • Mechanical support • Experimental drugs or surgery

* ARB to be used if the patient is ACEI intolerant.

Acute Decompensated Heart Failure

Acute decompensated heart failure (ADHF) is sudden-onset worsening of chronic heart failure and/or a new cardiac event such as myocardial infarction, atrial fibrillation, or fluid overload.

Table 10-34 Common Symptoms and Physical Signs of Heart Failure

Left Ventricular Heart Failure	Right Ventricular Heart Failure
Tachypnea	Constipation
Diaphoresis	Peripheral edema
Orthopnea	Bloating
Pulmonary rales	Jugular venous distention
Dyspnea on exertion	Right upper quadrant pain
Pulmonary edema	Hepatomegaly
Paroxysmal nocturnal dyspnea	Ascites
Cheyne-Stokes respirations	Hepatojugular reflux
Hemoptysis	Anorexia
Loud P_2	Nausea
Cough	
S_3 gallop ($\pm$ S_4)	

Hemodynamic Classifications

1. Normal: warm and dry
   - CI (cardiac index) > 2.2 L/min, PCWP (pulmonary capillary wedge pressure) < 18 mm Hg
   - Goal PCWP 15–18 mm Hg
2. Pulmonary congestion: warm and wet
   - CI > 2.2 L/min, PCWP > 18 mm Hg
3. Hypoperfusion: cold and dry
   - CI < 2.2 L/min, PCWP < 18 mm Hg
4. Pulmonary congestion and hypoperfusion: cold and wet
   - CI < 2.2 L/min, PCWP > 18 mm Hg

Table 10-35 Signs and Symptoms of ADHF

Congestion (Elevated PCWP)	Hypoperfusion (Decreased CO)
Dyspnea on exertion or at rest	Fatigue
Orthopnea, paroxysmal nocturnal dyspnea	Altered mental status
Peripheral edema	Sleepiness
Rales	Cold extremities
Early satiety, nausea/vomiting	Worsening renal function
Ascites	Narrow pulse pressure
Hepatomegaly, splenomegaly	Hypotension
Jugular venous distention	Hyponatremia
Hepatojugular reflux	

1.2.0 Pharmacotherapy

Mechanism of Action by Class

- Potassium-sparing diuretics: Aldosterone receptor antagonist; work in the distal renal tubules, causing Na^+ and H_2O excretion while holding onto K^+ and H^+
- Loop diuretics: Inhibit reabsorption of Na^+ and Cl^- in the ascending loop of Henle and distal renal tubules, interfering with the Cl^- binding co-transport system, thereby causing excretion of H_2O, Na^+, Cl^-, Mg^+, and Ca^{++}
- Thiazide diuretics:
    - Inhibit Na^+ reabsorption in the distal renal tubules, resulting in excretion of Na^+, H_2O, K^+, and H^+
    - Thiazide diuretics are used for hypertension but, with the exception of metolazone, are only minimally effective in the treatment of edema
- Angiotensin-converting enzyme inhibitors (ACEIs): Block the conversion of angiotensin I to angiotensin II, thereby blocking vasoconstriction and aldosterone release
- Angiotensin receptor blockers (ARBs):
    - Block angiotensin II from binding to the AT 1 receptor
    - Block smooth muscle contraction and aldosterone release
- Beta blockers:
    - Decrease inotropy and heart rate, leading to decreased oxygen demand
    - Nonselective alpha- and beta-adrenergic receptor antagonists lead to vasodilation, decreased peripheral vascular resistance, heart rate, and cardiac output
- Vasodilators: Cause direct arterial vasodilatation, decreasing systemic resistance
- Cardiac glycosides:
    - Inhibit Na/K^+ ATPase pump, increase intracellular Ca^{2+}, and increase contractility (positive inotrope) and CO
    - Prolong the refractory period by enhancing vagal tone and suppressing the AV node
- Nesiritide: B-type natriuretic peptide that binds to guanylate cyclase receptors on vascular smooth muscle and endothelial cells, leading to increased cGMP, smooth muscle relaxation, and reduction in systemic arterial pressure
- Positive inotropes:
    - $Beta_1$ agonists: Stimulate adenylate cyclase to convert ATP into cAMP, leading to increased cardiac output and slight peripheral vasodilation
    - PDE inhibitors: Inhibit cAMP breakdown in the heart to increase cardiac output and in the vascular smooth muscle to decrease systemic vascular resistance

Table 10-36 Indications for Heart Failure Drugs

Drug	Approved Indications	Routes of Administration
K^+-Sparing Diuretics		
Spironolactone Triamterene Amiloride	HF/edema	Oral
Eplerenone	HF/HTN	Oral
Loop Diuretics		
Furosemide	HF/edema	Oral, IV, IM
Torsemide		Oral, IV
Bumetanide		Oral, IV
Thiazide Diuretics		
Hydrochlorothiazide Metolazone Chlorthalidone	HF/edema	Oral
ACEIs		
Enalapril Fosinopril Lisinopril Quinapril Captopril	HF	Oral
ARBs		
Candesartan Valsartan	HF	Oral
Beta Blockers		
Bisoprolol Carvedilol Metoprolol succinate	HF	Oral
Vasodilators		
Nitroprusside	ADHF	IV
Nitroglycerin	ADHF	IV
Isosorbide dinitrate/ hydralazine	HF	Oral
B-Type Natriuretic Peptides/Vasodilators		
Nesiritide	ADHF	IV
Cardiac Glycosides		
Digoxin	HF	Oral, IV
Inotropic Therapy		
Dobutamine	ADHF	IV
Milrinone	ADHF	IV

Interaction of Drugs with Foods and Laboratory Tests

- Thiazide diuretics: Antihypertensives, anesthetics, anticoagulants, antigout agents, lithium, probenecid, NSAIDs, antidiabetic agents, corticosteroids, corticotropin, amphotericin B, alcohol
- K^+-sparing diuretics: Digoxin, potassium preparations, ACEIs/ARBs, NSAIDs
- Loop diuretics: Antihypertensives, NSAIDs, digoxin, lithium, cisplatinum, aminoglycosides, probenecid, theophylline
- ACEIs: Antihypertensives, potassium preparations, sulfonylureas, NSAIDs, allopurinol, tetracycline
- ARBs: Antihypertensives, NSAIDs, potassium preparations
- Beta blockers: Antihypertensives, sulfonylureas, negative inotropes, epinephrine, barbiturates, carbamazepine, rifamipin, sulfasalazine, phenobarbitol
- Vasodilators: Antihypertensives, NSAIDs
- Nesiritide: Antihypertensives
- Cardiac glycosides: Minor CYP 3A4 substrate; antihypertensives, amiodarone, quinidine, verapamil, erythromycin, clarithromycin, azole antifungals, cyclosporine, propafenone, spironolactone, cholestyramine, metoclopramide; hypokalemia may enhance effects
- Inotropic therapy: Antihypertensives, tricyclic antidepressants

Contraindications, Warnings, and Precautions

Contraindications

- Thiazide diuretics: Persistent anuria/oliguria
- K^+-sparing diuretics: Anuria, pregnancy, hyperkalemia ($K^+ > 5.5$ mEq/L), acute renal insufficiency (SCr > 2 mg/mL)
- Loop diuretics: Sulfa allergy (except for ethacrynic acid), anuria, hepatic coma, severe renal impairment
- ACEIs: Angioedema, pregnancy, bilateral renal artery stenosis
- ARBs: Angioedema, pregnancy, bilateral renal artery stenosis
- Beta blockers: Second- and third-degree heart block, sinus bradycardia, sinus node dysfunction, sick sinus syndrome, cardiogenic shock, Class IV heart failure, ventricular tachycardia
- Vasodilators: Dissecting aortic aneurysm; nitroglycerin: anemia, severe early myocardial infarction, increased ICP (sublingual), concurrent use of phosphodiesterase inhibitors such as sildenafil or vardenafil (increased hypotensive effect), constrictive pericarditis, pericardial tamponade, restrictive cardiomyopathy (intravenous)
- Cardiac glycosides: VT
- Nesiritide: Cardiogenic shock, systolic BP < 90 mm Hg, pregnancy
- Dobutamine: Idiopathic hypertrophic subaortic stenosis

Warnings and Precautions

- Thiazide diuretics: Caution in patients with sulfa allergy, diabetes, gout, renal failure (CrCl < 30 mL/min), dyslipidemia, photosensitivity, electrolyte imbalances; hypokalemia, hypochloremic alkalosis, hyponatremia, hypomagnesemia, hypercalcemia
- K^+-sparing diuretics: Caution with potassium intake/supplements, fluid/electrolyte loss, hypotension
- Loop diuretics: Caution with potassium intake/supplements, fluid/electrolyte loss, hypotension, hyperuricemia, ototoxicity with rapid IV administration, photosensitivity, cirrhosis
- ACEIs: Caution with hyperkalemia, orthostatic hypotension, rash, hepatotoxicity, pancreatitis, cholestatic jaundice, renal impairment, development of cough
- ARBs: Caution with hyperkalemia, orthostatic hypotension, renal impairment
- Beta blockers: Caution in patients with diabetes mellitus, hypotension, peripheral vascular disease, reactive airway disease, sinus bradycardia, WPW syndrome, Prinzmetal's angina, emphysema, chronic obstructive pulmonary disease (COPD)
- Vasodilators: Caution with fluid retention, tachycardia, aggravation of angina, fluid/sodium retention; hydralazine: mitral valve rheumatic heart disease, reflex tachycardia, lupus-like syndrome, dizziness, headache; minoxidil: acute MI, hirsuitism, pericardial effusion
- Cardiac glycosides: Caution with second- and third-degree heart block, VT, WPW syndrome
- Dobutamine: Caution with concomitant MAOI use

Pharmacodynamic and Pharmacokinetic Properties

- Hydrochlorothiazide: Ineffective when CrCl < 30 mg/dL
- Amiloride and triamterene: Onset within 2 hours
- Spironolactone: Onset within 24–48 hours
- Oral loop diuretics: Onset in 1–2 hours, while IV loops take action within minutes
  - Loop diuretic equivalent oral dosages: furosemide 40 mg = bumetanide 1 mg = torsemide 10 mg
  - Equivalent IV dose of a loop diuretic is generally half that of the oral dose

- Beta blockers: Mask the signs of hypoglycemia except for sweating and hunger
- Nesiritide serum: $t_{1/2}$ = 2 minutes (initial); 18 minutes (terminal)
- Digoxin
  - Improves short-term signs and symptoms, exercise tolerance, and quality of life; decreases hospital stay; does *not* decrease morbidity or mortality
  - The therapeutic range for HF (0.5–1 ng/mL) is lower than that for arrhythmias.
  - When changing from oral digoxin (tablets or liquid) or IM to IV therapy, reduce dosage by 20% to 25%

1.3.0 Monitoring

Pharmacotherapeutic Outcomes

The goals of therapy are to decrease signs and symptoms of heart failure, to improve quality of life, and to decrease morbidity and mortality.

Safety and Efficacy Monitoring and Patient Education

Thiazide Diuretics

- Take as directed, with meals, early in the day to avoid nocturia.

K^+-Sparing Diuretics

- Monitor potassium intake and avoid salt substitutes.
- Take after meals to decrease GI upset.

Loop Diuretics

- Take early in the day to avoid nocturia.
- Monitor potassium intake and avoid salt substitutes.

ACEIs

- Monitor potassium intake and avoid salt substitutes.
- Report any swelling of the lips, mouth, or face. Also report any bothersome, dry cough.
- Take all doses on an empty stomach, 1 hour before or 2 hours after meals.
- Do not take if you become pregnant.

ARBs

- Monitor potassium intake and avoid salt substitutes.
- May be taken with or without food.
- Do not take if you become pregnant.

Table 10-37 Heart Failure Medications: Biopharmaceutical Principles and Pharmaceutical Characteristics of Dosage Forms

Drug	Dosage Forms	Bioavailability
Thiazide Diuretics		
Chlorthalidone	Oral	65–75%
Hydrochlorothiazide		60–80%
Metolazone		40–65%
K^+-Sparing Diuretics		
Spironolactone	Oral	> 90%
Amiloride		15–25%
Triamterene		30–70%
Eplerenone		69%
Loop Diuretics		
Furosemide	Oral, IV, IM	60–64%
Torsemide	Oral, IV	80%
Bumetanide	Oral, IV	80–95%
ACEIs		
Enalapril	Oral	60%
Fosinopril		36%
Lisinopril		Decreased with NYHA Class II–IV heart failure
Quinapril		28% (ramipril, active drug)
Ramipril		44% (ramiprilat, prodrug)
Captopril		70–75%
ARBs		
Candesartan	Oral	15%
Valsartan		25%
Beta Blockers		
Bisoprolol	Oral	80%
Carvedilol		25–35%
Metoprolol succinate		85%
Vasodilators		
Isosorbide/hydralazine	Oral	Isosorbide ER: 22%; IR 58% Hydralazine 38–50%—
Nitroglycerin	IV	100% (IV)—
Sodium nitroprusside	IV	100% (IV)—
B-Type Natriuretic Peptides		
Nesiritide	IV	100% (IV)—
Cardiac Glycosides		
Digoxin	Oral, IV	80%
Inotropic Therapy		
Dobutamine	IV	100% (IV)—
Milrinone	IV	100% (IV)

Beta Blockers

- Do not suddenly stop taking these medications, as it could worsen the condition.
- Mask the signs of hypoglycemia (except for sweating and hunger).

Vasodilators

- Do not drink alcohol.

Nesiritide

- Monitor BP, hemodynamic responses, BUN, creatinine, and urine output.
- The patient should remain in bed while receiving infusion until instructed otherwise.

Cardiac Glycosides

- Digoxin toxicity can occur with serum levels greater than 0.8–2.2 ng/mL and/or with symptoms of severe nausea/vomiting, visual disturbances (green halos), and CNS effects.
- Trough levels should be obtained just prior to administering the next dose.

Inotropic Therapy

- Monitor BP, hemodynamic response, and arrhythmias.

Adverse Drug Reactions

Thiazide Diuretics

- Hypokalemia, hypercalcemia, hyponatremia, hypomagnesemia, hyperuricemia, hypercholesterolemia, hypertriglyceridemia, photosensitivity, skin rash, sexual dysfunction, pancreatitis

K^+-Sparing Diuretics

- Hyperkalemia, hyponatremia, GI disturbances, rash, sexual dysfunction, nephrolithiasis, hyperchloremic metabolic acidosis
- Spironolactone: Gynecomastia, hair loss, menstrual irregularities

Loop Diuretics

- Hypernatremia, hyperuricemia, hyperglycemia, hypokalemia, hypocalcemia, hypomagnesemia, hypochloremia, first-dose orthostatic hypotension (especially with furosemide and torsemide), ototoxicity, blood dyscrasias, metabolic alkalosis, photosensitivity

ACEIs

- Cough, rash, increased SCr, hyperkalemia, first-dose orthostatic hypotension, taste changes, angioedema, fetal abnormalities, hepatotoxicity, pancreatitis, proteinuria

ARBs

- Increased SCr, hyperkalemia, angioedema, hypotension, fetal abnormalities

Beta blockers

- Fatigue, depression, bradycardia, sexual dysfunction, hypertriglyceridemia, dyslipidemia, orthostatic hypotension, bronchospasm, glucose intolerance, vivid dreams

Vasodilators

- Hydralazine: Reflex tachycardia, lupus-like syndrome, fluid retention, dizziness, headache, aggravation of angina
- Nitroglycerin: Headache, dizziness, nausea/vomiting, flushing, postural hypotension, reflex tachycardia, coronary steal
- Sodium nitroprusside: Hypotension, cyanide or thiocyanate toxicity

Nesiritide

- Hypotension, headache, abdominal pain, insomnia, anxiety, confusion, tachycardia

Cardiac Glycosides

- Visual disturbances (e.g., scotomas, yellow/green halos), CNS effects (e..g, hallucinations, delirium, confusion), gynecomastia, nausea/vomiting, abdominal pain, bradycardia, arrhythmias

Inotropic Therapy

- Dobutamine: Proarrhythmic, tachycardia, hypokalemia, myocardial ischemia, tachyphylaxis, possible increase in mortality with long-term use
- Milrinone: Proarrhythmic, hypotension (avoid bolus), tachycardia, thrombocytopenia (less than 1%), possible increase in mortality with long-term use

2.2.0 Select and Dispense Medications in a Manner That Promotes Safety and Efficacy

Table 10-38 Thiazide Diuretics

Drug	Brand Name	Available Strengths
Chlorthalidone	Thalitone	15, 25, 50, 100 mg
Hydrochlorothiazide	Microzide	12.5 mg
	HydroDiuril	25 mg
	Hydro-Par	50 mg
		100 mg
Metolazone	Zaroxolyn	2.5, 5, 10 mg

Table 10-39 K⁺-Sparing Diuretics

Drug	Brand Name	Available Strengths
Spironolactone	Aldactone	25, 50, 100 mg
Amiloride	Midamor	5 mg
Triamterene	Dyrenium	50, 100 mg
Eplerenone	Inspra	25, 50 mg

Table 10-40 Loop Diuretics

Drug	Brand Name	Available Strengths
Furosemide Furosemide oral solution Furosmide IV	Lasix	20, 40, 80 mg 10 mg/mL, 40 mg/5 mL 10 mg/mL
Torsemide	Demadex	5, 10, 20, 100 mg
Bumetanide Bumetanide IV	Bumex	0.5, 1, 2 mg 0.25 mg/mL

Table 10-41 Angiotensin-Converting Enzyme Inhibitors

Drug	Brand Name	Available Strengths
Captopril	Capoten	12.5, 25, 50, 100 mg
Enalapril Enalaprilat IV	Vasotec	2.5, 5, 10, 20 mg 1.25 mg/mL
Fosinopril	Monopril	10, 20, 40 mg
Lisinopril	Zestril, Prinivil	2.5, 5, 10, 20, 30, 40 mg
Quinapril	Accupril	5, 10, 20, 40 mg

Table 10-42 Angiotensin Receptor Blockers

Drug	Brand Name	Available Strengths
Candesartan	Atacand	4, 8, 16, 32 mg
Valsartan	Diovan	40, 80, 160, 320 mg

Table 10-43 Beta Blockers

Drug	Brand Name	Available Strengths
Bisoprolol	Zebeta	5, 10 mg
Metoprolol tartrate Metoprolol succinate Metoprolol IV	Lopressor Toprol XL Lopressor	25, 50, 100 mg 25, 50, 100, 200 mg 1 mg/mL
Carvedilol Carvedilol ER	Coreg Coreg CR	3.125, 6.25, 12.5, 25 mg 10, 20, 40, 80 mg

Table 10-44 Vasodilators

Drug	Brand Name	Available Strengths
Isosorbide dinitrate/ hydralazine	Bidil	20 mg/37.5 mg
Hydralazine	Apresoline	10, 25,50, 100 mg
Sodium nitroprusside IV	Nitropress	50 mg
Nitroglycerin for injection Nitroglycerin in 5% dextrose		5 mg/mL 100, 200, 400 mcg/ mL

Table 10-45 B-Type Natriuretic Peptide

Drug	Brand Name	Available Strengths
Nesiritide	Natrecor	1.5 mg powder for IV

Table 10-46 Cardiac Glycosides

Drug	Brand Name	Available Strengths
Digoxin Digoxin liquid caps Digoxin IV	Lanoxin Lanoxicaps	0.125, 0.25, 0.5 mg; 0.05 mg/mL 0.05, 0.1, 0.2 mg 0.1 mg/mL, 0.25 mg/mL

Table 10-47 Inotropic Therapy

Drug	Brand Name	Available Strengths
Dobutamine IV Dobutamine in 5% dextrose	Dobutrex	12.5 mg/mL 1 mg/mL, 2 mg/mL, 4 mg/mL
Milrinone IV	Primacor	1 mg/mL

ANNOTATED BIBLIOGRAPHY

American Heart Association. *Heart Disease and Stroke Facts, 2009 Update.* Dallas, TX: Author; 2009.

DiPiro JT, Talbert RL, Yee GC, et al. *Pharmacotherapy: A Pathophysiologic Approach.* 6th ed. New York: McGraw-Hill; 2005.

Drug Facts and Comparisons. Wolters Kluwer Health, Inc. Updated periodically.

Frankel SK, Fifer MA. Pathophysiology of heart failure. In: Braunwald E, ed. *Heart Disease: A Textbook of Cardiovascular Medicine.* Philadelphia: W. B. Saunders; 1997:189–215.

Hunt SA, Abraham WT, Chin MH, et al. ACC/AHA 2005 guideline for the diagnosis and management of chronic heart failure in the adult—summary article: a report of the American College of Cardiology/American Heart Association Task Force on Practice Guidelines (writing committee to update the 2001 guidelines for the evaluation and management of heart failure). *J Am Coll Cardiol* 2005;46:1116–1143.

Micromedex Healthcare Series. Greenwood Village, CO: Thomson Reuters (Healthcare) Inc. Updated periodically.

TOPIC: HYPERTENSION/HYPERTENSIVE EMERGENCY

Section Coordinator: Teresa K. Hoffmann
Contributor: Danielle P. Fennema

Hypertension Overview

Hypertension affects approximately 50 million people in the United States, or nearly 25% of the population. Of those patients taking antihypertensive medications, it is estimated that only one in three has controlled blood pressure (less than 140/90 mm Hg). Uncontrolled high blood pressure can lead to hypertension, hypertensive urgency, or even hypertensive emergency leading to end-organ damage. Adequately controlling blood pressure reduces the risk of complications such as ischemic heart disease, heart failure, nephropathy, chronic kidney disease, cardiovascular disease, myocardial infarction, hypertensive urgencies/emergencies, retinopathy, transient ischemic attack, and stroke. The Seventh Report of the Joint National Committee (JNC VII) established national guidelines to classify and treat hypertension.

Tips Worth Tweeting

- Guidelines per JNC VII call for a blood pressure of less than 140/90 mm Hg or less than 130/80 mm Hg for patients with diabetes mellitus and/or chronic kidney disease.
- All patients with hypertension should be encouraged to adopt lifestyle modifications, including the DASH diet, reduction of sodium and alcohol intake, weight loss, and increased physical activity.
- Although treatment of hypertension should be individualized, medications include, but are not limited to, thiazide diuretics, beta blockers, angiotensin-converting enzyme inhibitors (ACEIs), and angiotensin receptor blockers (ARBs). Many other classes of medications can be used to lower blood pressure as well.
- Most patients with hypertension will require two or more drugs to achieve their BP goals.

1.1.0 Patient Information

Causes of Hypertension

- Idiopathic
- Sleep apnea
- Chronic kidney disease
- Renovascular disease
- Cushing's syndrome or steroid therapy
- Pheochromocytoma
- Thyroid/parathyroid disease
- Coarctation of aorta
- Primary aldosteronism
- Drug-induced

Medication-Induced Causes of Hypertension

- Corticosteroids
- NSAIDs
- Decongestants
- Amphetamines
- Appetite suppressants
- Caffeine
- Alcohol
- Cyclosporine
- Estrogens
- Oral contraceptives
- Thyroid hormone
- Venlafaxine

Laboratory Testing and Diagnostic Workup

- History and physical (including a review of possible risk factors and causes)
- Blood pressure
- Heart rate
- Laboratory tests including urinalysis, blood glucose, hematocrit, lipid panel, potassium, creatinine, and calcium

Table 10-48 Classifications of Hypertension per JNC V-II

BP Classification*	Systolic BP (mm Hg)	Diastolic BP (mm Hg)
Normal	< 120	< 80
Pre-HTN	120–139	80–89
Stage 1 HTN	140–159	90–99
Stage 2 HTN	≥ 160	≥ 100

*Determined by the highest BP category.

Note: Target blood pressure for patients with CKD or DM: < 130/80 mm Hg.

Table 10-49 Comparison of Hypertensive Urgency and Hypertensive Emergency

Hypertensive Urgency	Hypertensive Emergency
Not life threatening	Potentially life threatening
BP elevated to a level that could be harmful if sustained; without end-organ damage (EOD).	BP elevated with EOD, also known as target-organ damage (TOD), such as intracranial hemorrhage, encephalopathy, unstable angina, AMI, and acute left ventricular failure with pulmonary edema.
Treatment: Onset of action for drugs within 15–30 minutes; peak effect in 2–3 hours. Monitor BP every 15–30 minutes and reduce BP gradually over 24–48 hours.	Treatment: Initial goal is to reduce MAP ≤ 25% within 30–60 minutes, and to reach 160/100 mm Hg within 2–6 hours. Measure BP every 5–10 minutes until MAP is achieved. Maintain goal BP for 1–2 days; attempt further BP reduction over several weeks.
Oral treatment or slower-acting parenteral drugs over several hours or days.	IV treatment preferred and requires immediate pressure reduction.

Table 10-50 Effects of Lifestyle Modifications on Blood Pressure

Lifestyle Modification	Approximate Systolic BP Reduction
Weight reduction: Maintain/attain a BMI < 25 kg/m^2	5–20 mm Hg per 10 kg weight lost
Dietary Approaches to Stop HTN (DASH) eating plan: Diet high in fruits, vegetables, and low-fat dairy products, with reduced saturated and total fat	8–14 mm Hg
Dietary Na^+ reduction: Reduce Na^+ intake to ≤ 2.4 g of Na^+ per day	2–8 mm Hg
Physical activity: Engage in regular aerobic physical activity such as brisk walking (at least 30 minutes per day, most days of the week)	4–9 mm Hg
Moderate consumption of alcohol • Men: 2 drinks per day • Women: 1 drink per day	2–4 mm Hg

Signs and Symptoms of End-Organ/Target-Organ Damage

- Fundoscopic: Papilledema, hemorrhage
- Neurologic: Confusion, seizures, coma, visual deficits
- Cardiac: S_4 gallop, ischemic changes on ECG, pulmonary edema, chest pain
- Renal: Oliguria, progressive azotemia, hematuria, proteinuria

Wellness and Prevention

Encourage lifestyle modifications for all patients.

Other important issues include routine blood pressure monitoring, smoking cessation, and proper management of comorbidities and complications.

1.2.0 Pharmacotherapy

Mechanism of Action by Class

Thiazide Diuretics

- Inhibit Na^+ reabsorption in the distal renal tubules, resulting in excretion of Na^+, H_2O, K^+, and H^+

Potassium-Sparing Diuretics

- Aldosterone receptor antagonists; cause Na^+ and H_2O excretion in the distal renal tubules, but spare K^+ and H^+ loss

Loop Diuretics

- Inhibit reabsorption of Na^+ and Cl^- in the ascending loop of Henle and distal renal tubules, interfering with the Cl^- binding cotransport system and causing excretion of H_2O, Na^+, Cl–, Mg^+, and Ca^{++}

Angiotensin-Converting Enzyme Inhibitors

- Block the conversion of angiotensin I to angiotensin II, thus blocking vasoconstriction and aldosterone release

Angiotensin Receptor Blockers

- Block angiotensin II from binding to AT 1 receptors
- Block smooth muscle contraction and aldosterone release

Beta Blockers

- Decrease inotropy and heart rate, leading to decreased oxygen demand

Combined Alpha-Beta Blockers

- Nonselective alpha- and beta-adrenergic receptor antagonists cause vasodilation and decreased peripheral vascular resistance, heart rate, and cardiac output

Alpha Blockers

- Block alpha-adrenergic receptors, leading to vasodilation, decreased total peripheral vascular resistance, and decreased blood pressure

Calcium-Channel Blockers

- Decrease coronary vascular resistance, thereby increasing coronary circulation

Table 10-51 Antihypertensive Medications: Indications and Routes of Administration

Drug	Approved Indications	Routes of Administration
Thiazide Diuretics		
Chlorothiazide Chlorthalidone Hydrochlorothiazide Indapamide Metolazone	HTN	Oral
K^+-Sparing Diuretics		
Spironolactone	HTN	Oral
Amiloride Eplerenone Triamterene	Not-FDA-labeled for HTN	Oral
Loop Diuretics		
Furosemide	HTN	Oral, IV, IM
Torsemide		Oral, IV
Ethacrynic acid	Not-FDA-labeled for HTN	Oral, IV
ACEIs		
Benazepril Enalapril Fosinopril Lisinopril Moexipril Perindopril Quinapril Ramipril Trandolapril	HTN	Oral
Captopril	HTN, HTN urgency	Oral
Enalaprilat	HTN, HTN emergency	IV
ARBs		
Candesartan Eprosartan Irbesartan Losartan Olmesartan Telmisartan Valsartan	HTN	Oral
Beta Blockers		
Acebutolol Betaxolol Bisoprolol Carteolol Metoprolol succinate Nadolol	HTN	Oral

Table 10-51 (*continued*)

Drug	Approved Indications	Routes of Administration
Nebivolol Penbutolol Pindolol Timolol		
Atenolol Metoprolol tartrate Propranolol		Oral, IV
Esmolol	HTN emergency	IV
Alpha/Beta Blockers		
Carvedilol	HTN	Oral
Labetalol	HTN, HTN urgency/ emergency	Oral, IV
Alpha Blockers		
Doxazosin Prazosin Terazosin	HTN	Oral
Phentolamine	HTN emergency	IV, IM
Calcium-Channel Blockers		
Diltiazem Verapamil	HTN	Oral, IV
Nicardipine	HTN, HTN emergency	Oral, IV
Amlodipine Felodipine Isradipine Nifedipine Nisoldipine	HTN	Oral
$Alpha_2$ Agonists		
Clonidine	HTN, HTN urgency	Oral, transdermal
Guanabenz Guanfacine	HTN	Oral
Methyldopa	HTN	Oral, IV
Adrenergic Antagonists		
Reserpine	HTN	Oral
Guanethidine	Adjunct HTN, renal HTN	Oral
Vasodilators		
Hydralazine	HTN	Oral, IV
Minoxidil		Oral
Sodium nitroprusside Nitroglycerin Diazoxide	HTN emergency	IV
Dopamine Agonists		
Fenoldopam	HTN emergency	IV

- Negative inotropic and chronotropic cardiac effects (especially verapamil and diltiazem)

Centrally Acting Alpha$_2$-Adrenergic Agonists

- Decrease norepinephrine release, leading to decreased sympathetic outflow and deceased blood pressure

Peripheral Adrenergic Antagonists

- Decrease catecholamine and 5-HT levels, leading to decreased peripheral resistance and increased plasma volume and, in turn, decreased cardiac output
- Positive inotropic and chronotropic effects on heart muscle and vasodilator effects on vascular smooth muscle

Vasodilators

- Direct arterial vasodilatation; decrease systemic resistance

Dopamine Agonists

- Bind to alpha$_2$ adrenoreceptors
- Act rapidly as vasodilators and increase renal blood flow

Interaction of Drugs with Foods and Laboratory Tests

Thiazide Diuretics

- Antihypertensives, anesthetics, anticoagulants, antigout agents, lithium, probenecid, NSAIDs, antidiabetic agents, corticosteroids, corticotropin, amphotericin B, alcohol

K^+-Sparing Diuretics

- Digoxin, potassium preparations, ACEIs/ARBs, NSAIDs
- Eplerenone: CYP 450 3A4 substrate/inhibitors

Loop Diuretics

- Antihypertensives, NSAIDs, digoxin, lithium, cisplatinum, aminoglycosides, probenecid, theophylline

ACEIs

- Antihypertensives, potassium preparations, sulfonylureas, NSAIDs, allopurinol, tetracycline

ARBs

- Antihypertensives, NSAIDs, potassium preparations

Beta Blockers

- Antihypertensives, sulfonylureas, negative inotropes, epinephrine

Alpha/Beta Blockers

- Antihypertensives, sulfonylureas, negative inotropes, epinephrine

Alpha Blockers

- Antihypertensives, NSAIDs, tricyclic antidepressants, indomethacin, MAOIs, phosphodiesterase inhibitors

Calcium-Channel Blockers

- Non-dihydropyridine (non-DHP): CYP 450 3A4 substrates/inhibitors; amiodarone, barbiturates, itraconazole, cyclosporine, cimetidine, rifampin, anesthetics, statins, antihypertensives, negative inotropes, dofetilide, buspirone, carbamazepine, digoxin, alcohol, phenytoin, imipramine, moricizine, ranolazine, sirolimus, tacrolimus, quinidine, grapefruit juice
- Dihydropyridine (DHP): azole antifungals, barbiturates, carbamazepine, cimetidine, phenytoin, rifampin, anesthetics

Alpha$_2$ Agonists

- Antihypertensives, antipsychotics, tricycle antidepressants

Adrenergic Antagonists

- Antihypertensives, colchicine
- Guanethidine: tricyclic antidepressants, MAOIs

Vasodilators

- Antihypertensives, NSAIDs

Dopamine Agonists

- Antihypertensives

Contraindications, Warnings, and Precautions

Contraindications

- Thiazide diuretics: Persistent anuria/oliguria
- K^+-sparing diuretics: Anuria, pregnancy, hyperkalemia ($K^+ > 5.5$ mEq/L), acute renal insufficiency (SCr > 2 mg/mL)
- Loop diuretics: Sulfa allergy (except for ethacrynic acid), anuria, hepatic coma, severe renal impairment
- ACEIs: Angioedema, pregnancy, bilateral renal artery stenosis
- ARBs: Angioedema, pregnancy, bilateral renal artery stenosis
- Beta blockers: Contraindicated with second- and third-degree heart block, sinus bradycardia, sinus node dysfunction, sick sinus syndrome,

cardiogenic shock, Class IV heart failure, ventricular tachycardia

- Alpha/beta blockers: Contraindicated with second- and third-degree heart block, sinus bradycardia, sinus node dysfunction, sick sinus syndrome, cardiogenic shock, Class IV heart failure, ventricular tachycardia (VT), hypotension (SBP < 90 mm Hg)
- Alpha blockers: Contraindicated with phosphodiesterase inhibitors
- All calcium-channel blockers: Contraindicated with sick sinus syndrome, second- and third-degree heart block, hypotension (SBP < 90 mm Hg)
- Non-DHP calcium-channel blockers: Left ventricular dysfunction, Wolff-Parkinson-White syndrome, VT, acute MI, cardiogenic shock, recent IV beta blocker use
- Alpha$_2$ agonists: Methyldopa is contraindicated with current MAOI therapy, active hepatic disease, abnormal LFTs, hepatitis, hemolytic anemia
- Adrenergic agonists: Active GI disease or depression; current or past electroshock therapy, hypersensitivity to reserpine alkaloids, severe renal failure, ulcerative colitis
- Vasodilators: Contraindicated with dissecting aortic aneurysm; nitroglycerin: anemia, severe early myocardial infarction, increased ICP (sublingual), concurrent use of phosphodiesterase inhibitors such as sildenafil or vardenafil (increased hypotensive effect), constrictive pericarditis, pericardial tamponade, restrictive cardiomyopathy (intravenous)

Warnings and Precautions

- Thiazide diuretics: Caution in patients with sulfa allergy, diabetes, gout, renal failure (CrCl < 30 mL/min), dyslipidemia, photosensitivity, electrolyte imbalances (hypokalemia, hypochloremic alkalosis, hyponatremia, hypomagnesemia, hypercalcemia)
- K^+-sparing diuretics: Caution with potassium intake/supplements, fluid/electrolyte loss, hypotension
- Loop diuretics: Caution with potassium intake/supplements, fluid/electrolyte loss, hypotension, hyperuricemia, ototoxicity with rapid IV administration, photosensitivity, cirrhosis
- ACEIs: Caution with hyperkalemia, orthostatic hypotension, rash, hepatotoxicity, pancreatitis, cholestatic jaundice, renal impairment, development of cough
- ARBs: Caution with hyperkalemia, orthostatic hypotension, renal impairment
- Beta blockers: Caution in patients with diabetes mellitus, hypotension, peripheral vascular disease, reactive airway disease, sinus bradycardia, WPW syndrome, Prinzmetal's angina, emphysema, COPD
- Alpha/beta blockers: Caution in patients with diabetes mellitus, hypotension, peripheral vascular disease, reactive airway disease, sinus bradycardia, WPW syndrome, Prinzmetal's angina, emphysema, COPD
- Alpha blockers: Caution in patients with postural hypotension, syncope with first dose, dizziness, edema, depression
- All calcium-channel blockers: Caution with edema, sinus bradycardia, hypotension
- Alpha$_2$ agonists: Caution with dry mouth, sedation, depression, constipation, rebound hypertension, orthostasis, xerostomia; methyldopa: abnormal LFTs, hepatitis, hemolytic anemia
- Adrenergic antagonists: Caution with asthma, gallstones, renal impairment, Parkinson's disease, gastrointestinal disease
- Vasodilators: Caution with fluid retention, tachycardia, aggravation of angina, fluid/sodium retention; hydralazine: mitral valve rheumatic heart disease, reflex tachycardia, lupus-like syndrome, dizziness, headache; minoxidil: acute MI, hirsuitism, pericardial effusion
- Dopamine agonists: Caution in patients with angina, glaucoma, and increased intracranial pressure

Physiochemical Properties, Solubility, Pharmacodynamics, and Pharmacokinetic Properties

- Hydrochlorothiazide: Ineffective if CrCl < 30 mg/dL
- Amiloride and triamterene: Onset within 2 hours
- Spironolactone: Onset within 24–48 hours
- Oral loop diuretics: Onset in 1–2 hours
- IV loop diuretics: Take action within minutes
- Loop diuretic equivalent oral dosages:
  - Furosemide 40 mg = bumetanide 1 mg = torsemide 10 mg
  - IV dose is generally half the oral dose of loop diuretics
- Beta blockers: Mask the signs of hypoglycemia except for sweating and hunger
- Atenolol: $t_{1/2}$ increased to 28 hours in renal patients
- Propranolol: Food increases absorption by 53%
- Captopril: Take before meals
- Prazosin: Increased incidence of orthostatic hypotension
- Verapamil: Grapefruit juice increases bioavailability by 30%

Table 10-52 Antihypertensive Medications: Biopharmaceutical Principles and Pharmaceutical Characteristics of Dosage Forms

Drug	Dosage Forms	Bioavailability
Thiazide Diuretics		
Chlorothiazide	Oral	65–75%
Chlorthalidone		65%
Hydrochlorothiazide		60-80%
Indapamide		100%
Metolazone		40-65%
K+-Sparing Diuretics:		
Spironolactone	Oral	> 90%
Amiloride		15–25%
Triamterene		30–70%
Eplerenone		69%
Loop Diuretics		
Furosemide	Oral, IV, IM	60–64%
Torsemide	Oral, IV	80%
Ethacrynic acid	Oral, IV	100%
ACEIs		
Benazepril	Oral	37%
Enalapril		60%
Fosinopril		36%
Lisinopril		Decreased with NYHA Class II-IV heart failure
Moexipril		13–22%
Perindopril		75%
Quinapril		50%
Ramipril		28%
Trandolapril		10%
Captopril	Oral	70–75%
Enalaprilat	IV	poorly absorbed
ARBs		
Candesartan	Oral	15%
Eprosartan		13%
Irbesartan		60-80%
Losartan		33%
Telmisartan		42% for 40 mg; 58% for 160 mg
Valsartan		25%
Olmesartan		26%
Beta Blockers		
Acebutolol	Oral	20–60%
Betaxolol		89%
Bisoprolol		80%
Carteolol		85%
Metoprolol succinate		77%
Nadolol		30–50%
Nebivolol		12% of patients are extensive metabolizers; 90% are poor metabolizers
Penbutolol		100%
Pindolol		100%
Timolol		75%
Atenolol	Oral, IV	Oral: 50–60%
Metoprolol tartrate		Oral: 40–50%
Propranolol		30% IR; 9–18% ER
Alpha/Beta Blockers		
Carvedilol	Oral	25–35%
Labetolol	Oral, IV	25%
Alpha Blockers		
Prazosin	Oral	48–68%
Terazosin		90%
Doxazosin		65%
Calcium-Channel Blockers		
Diltiazem	Oral, IV	40%
Verapamil		2–35%
Nicardipine	Oral, IV	35%
Amlodipine	Oral	64–65%
Felodipine		20%
Isradipine		15–24%
Nifedipine		45–75% IR; 84–89% ER
Nisoldipine		5%
Alpha$_2$ Agonists		
Clonidine	Oral, transdermal	75–95%
Guanabenz	Oral	75%
Guanfacine		80% IR; 58% ER
Methyldopa	Oral, IV	50%
Adrenergic Antagonists		
Reserpine	Oral	30-40%
Guanethidine		
Vasodilators		
Hydralazine	Oral, IV	30–50%
Minoxidil	Oral	90%
Sodium nitroprusside	IV	100% (IV)
Nitroglycerin		100% (IV)
Diazoxide		
Dopamine Agonists		
Fenoldopam	IV	–100% (IV)

- Verapamil: Gingival hyperplasia and constipation
- Amlodipine: No reflex tachycardia
- Covera HS (brand of verapamil) and Adalat CC (brand of nifedipine) have "ghost tablets" that can be seen in feces (i.e., the outer shell is visible in feces); however, active drug is absorbed as it passes through the small intestine
- Vasodilators: Typically not used as monotherapy for HTN
- Fenoldopam: Mean plasma levels after a 2-hour infusion (0.5 mcg/kg/min) and after a 100 mg dose are approximately 13 ng/mL and 50 ng/mL, respectively

1.3.0 Monitoring

Pharmacotherapeutic Outcomes

The goal is to reduce elevated blood pressure that could eventually lead to end-organ damage.

Safety and Efficacy Monitoring and Patient Education

- Hypertension has no symptoms. Encourage patients to continue their medications even if they feel well; they will need blood pressure medication for the rest of their life.
- Blood pressure should be checked regularly and physician appointments should not be missed.
- Diet, exercise, weight control, and sodium and alcohol intake play a major role in the treatment of hypertension.

Thiazide Diuretics

- Take as directed, with meals, early in the day to avoid nocturia.

K^+-Sparing Diuretics

- Monitor potassium intake and avoid salt substitutes.
- Take after meals to decrease GI upset.

Loop Diuretics

- Take early in the day to avoid nocturia.
- Monitor potassium intake and avoid salt substitutes.

ACEIs

- Monitor potassium intake and avoid salt substitutes.
- Report any swelling of the lips, mouth, or face. Also report any bothersome, dry cough.
- Take all doses on an empty stomach, 1 hour before or 2 hours after meals. This drug does not eliminate the need for dietary changes or an exercise regimen as recommended by the prescriber.
- Do not take if you become pregnant.

ARBs

- Monitor potassium intake and avoid salt substitutes.
- May be taken with or without food.
- Do not take if you become pregnant.

Beta Blockers and Alpha/Beta Blockers

- Do not suddenly stop taking the medication, as it could worsen the condition.
- These medications mask the signs of hypoglycemia except for sweating and hunger.

Alpha Blockers

- Do not take with phosphodiesterase inhibitors.
- There is an increased incidence of orthostatic hypotension with terazosin. Instruct patients to rise slowly from a sitting position.

Calcium-Channel Blockers

- Take exactly as prescribed; do not skip doses.

$Alpha_2$ Agonists

- If using a clonidine patch, check daily for correct placement; rotate patch sites weekly. Remove the patch while having an MRI scan, as it can cause burns.
- Clonidine: Do not take if you become pregnant.
- Avoid clonidine in patients with altered mental status.
- Do not drink alcohol with methyldopa.

Adrenergic Antagonists

- Do not drink alcohol.
- It may take up to 2 weeks to see the effects of therapy.

Vasodilators

- Hydralazine is the drug of choice for hypertension during pregnancy.
- Do not drink alcohol.
- Sodium nitroprusside to be avoided in patients with renal impairment.

Adverse Drug Reactions

Thiazide Diuretics

- Hypokalemia, hypercalcemia, hyponatremia, hypomagnesemia, hyperuricemia, hypercholesterolemia, hypertriglyceridemia, photosensitivity, skin rash, sexual dysfunction, pancreatitis

K^+-Sparing Diuretics

- Hyperkalemia, hyponatremia, GI disturbances, rash, sexual dysfunction, nephrolithiasis, hyperchloremic metabolic acidosis
- Spironolactone: Gynecomastia, hair loss, menstrual irregularities
- Eplerenone: Hypertriglyceridemia, minimal gynecomastia

Loop Diuretics

- Hypernatremia, hyperuricemia, hyperglycemia, hypokalemia, hypocalcemia, hypomagnesemia, hypochloremia, first-dose orthostatic hypotension (furosemide and torsemide), ototoxicity, blood dyscrasias, metabolic alkalosis, photosensitivity

ACEIs

- Cough, rash, increased SCr, hyperkalemia, first-dose orthostatic hypotension, taste changes, angioedema, fetal abnormalities, hepatotoxicity, pancreatitis, proteinuria

ARBs

- Increased SCr, hyperkalemia, angioedema, hypotension, fetal abnormalities

Beta Blockers

- Fatigue, depression, bradycardia, sexual dysfunction, hypertriglyceridemia, dyslipidemia, orthostatic hypotension, bronchospasm, glucose intolerance, vivid dreams

Alpha/Beta Blockers

- Same as beta blockers, but more orthostatic hypotension

Alpha Blockers

- Postural hypotension, syncope with first dose, dizziness, vertigo, headache, weakness, depression, edema, sexual dysfunction

Calcium-Channel Blockers

- Non-dihydropyridine (non-DHP): CYP 450 3A4 substrates/inhibitors; headache, flushing, hypotension, dizziness, edema, bradycardia, fatigue, nausea, constipation and gingival hyperplasia
- Dihydropyridine (DHP): Peripheral edema, headache, flushing, hypotension, tachycardia, dizziness, rash, gingival hyperplasia

$Alpha_2$ Agonists

- Dry mouth, sedation, orthostasis, bradycardia, constipation, depression, contact dermatitis, sexual dysfunction
- Methyldopa: Can also cause abnormal LFTs, hepatitis, hemolytic anemia, lupus-like syndrome

Adrenergic Antagonists

- Reserpine: Bradycardia, lethargy, nasal congestion, Parkinsonian state, depression
- Guanethidine: Bradycardia, hypotension, weakness, nasal congestion, retrograde ejaculation/impotence

Vasodilators

- Hydralazine: Reflex tachycardia, lupus-like syndrome, fluid retention, dizziness, headache, aggravation of angina
- Minoxidil: Fluid retention, tachycardia, aggravation of angina, pericardial effusion, hirsuitism
- Nitroglycerin: Headache, dizziness, nausea/vomiting, flushing, postural hypotension, reflex tachycardia, coronary steal
- Sodium nitroprusside: Nausea/vomiting, diaphoresis, thiocyanate and cyanide toxicity, tachycardia, sodium retention

Dopamine Agonists

- Tachycardia, headache, facial flushing, angina, and hypokalemia

2.2.0 Select and Dispense Medications in a Manner That Promotes Safe and Effective Use

Table 10-53 Thiazide Diuretics

Drug	Brand Name	Available Strengths
Chlorthiazide	Diuril	250, 500 mg
Chlorthiazide oral suspension	Diuril	250 mg/5 mg
Chlorthiazide IV	Sodium Diuril	500 mg
Chlorthalidone	Thalitone	15, 25, 50, 100 mg
Hydrochlorothiazide	Microzide	12.5 mg
	HydroDiuril	25 mg
	Hydro-Par	50 mg
		100 mg
Indapamide	Lozol	1.25, 2.5 mg
Metolazone	Zaroxolyn	2.5, 5, 10 mg

Table 10-54 K⁺-Sparing Diuretics

Drug	Brand Name	Available Strengths
Spironolactone	Aldactone	25, 50, 100 mg
Amiloride	Midamor	5 mg
Triamterene	Dyrenium	50, 100 mg
Eplerenone	Inspra	25, 50 mg

Table 10-55 Loop Diuretics

Drug	Brand Name	Available Strengths
Furosemide Furosemide oral solution Furosmide IV	Lasix	20, 40, 80 mg 10 mg/mL, 40 mg/5 mL 10 mg/mL
Torsemide	Demadex	5, 10, 20, 10 0mg
Ethacrynic acid tablet Ethacrynic acid IV	Edecrin Edecrin Sodium	25 mg 50 mg

Table 10-56 ACEIs

Drug	Brand Name	Available Strengths
Benazepril	Lotensin	5, 10, 20, 40 mg
Captopril	Capoten	12.5, 25, 50, 100 mg
Enalapril Enalaprilat IV	Vasotec	2.5, 5, 10, 20 mg 1.25 mg/mL
Fosinopril	Monopril	10, 20, 40 mg
Lisinopril	Zestril, Prinivil	2.5, 5, 10, 20, 30, 40 mg
Moexipril	Univasc	7.5, 15 mg
Perindopril	Aceon	2, 4, 8 mg
Quinapril	Accupril	5, 10, 20, 40 mg
Ramipril	Altace	1.25, 2.5, 5, 10 mg
Trandolapril	Mavik	1, 2, 4 mg

Table 10-57 ARBs

Drug	Brand Name	Available Strengths
Candesartan	Atacand	4, 8, 16, 32 mg
Eprosartan	Teveten	600 mg
Irbesartan	Avapro	75, 50, 300 mg
Losartan	Cozaar	25, 50, 100 mg
Olmesartan	Benicar	5, 20, 40 mg
Telmisartan	Micardis	20, 40, 80 mg
Valsartan	Diovan	40, 80, 160, 320 mg

Table 10-58 Beta Blockers

Drug	Brand Name	Available Strengths
Acebutolol	Sectral	200, 400 mg
Atenolol	Tenormin	25, 50, 100 mg
Betaxolol	Kerlone	10, 20 mg
Bisoprolol	Zebeta	5, 10 mg
Carteolol	Cartrol	2.5, 5 mg
Metoprolol tartrate Metoprolol succinate Metoprolol IV	Lopressor Toprol XL Lopressor	25, 50, 100 mg 25, 50, 100, 200 mg 1 mg/mL
Nadolol	Corgard	20, 40, 60, 80, 120, 160 mg
Nebivolol	Bystolic	2.5, 5, 10, 20 mg
Penbutolol	Levatol	20 mg
Pindolol	Visken	5, 10 mg
Propranolol IR Propranolol ER Propranolol ER Propranolol intensol oral solution Propranolol IV	Inderal Inderal LA InnoPran XL Inderal	10, 20, 40, 60, 80, 90 mg 60, 80, 120, 160 mg 80, 120 mg 80 mg/mL 1 mg/mL
Timolol	Blocadren	5, 10, 20 mg

Table 10-59 Alpha/Beta Blockers

Drug	Brand Name	Available Strengths
Carvedilol Carvedilol ER	Coreg Coreg CR	3.125, 6.25, 12.5, 25 mg 10, 20, 40, 80 mg
Labetalol Labetalol IV	Trandate, Normodyne	100, 200, 300 mg 5 mg/mL

Table 10-60 Alpha Blockers

Drug	Brand name	Available Strengths
Prazosin	Minipress	1, 2, 5 mg
Terazosin	Hytrin	1, 2, 5, 10 mg
Doxazosin	Cardura	1, 2, 4, 8 mg
Doxazosin ER	Cardura XL	4, 8 mg

Table 10-61 Calcium-Channel Blockers

Drug	Brand Name	Available Strengths
Diltiazem IR	Cardizem	30, 60, 90, 120 mg
Diltiazem LA	Cardizem LA	120, 180, 240, 300, 360, 420 mg
Diltiazem SR	Cardizem CD	120, 180, 240, 300, 360 mg
	Dilacor XR	120, 180, 240 mg
	Diltia XT	120, 180, 240 mg
	Cartia XT	120, 180, 240, 300 mg
	Tiazac	120, 180, 240, 300, 360, 420 mg
	Taztia XT	120, 180, 240, 300, 360 mg
Diltiazem for injection	Cardizem	5 mg/mL
Diltiazem powder for injection	Cardizem	25 mg
Verapamil	Calan	40, 80, 120 mg
Verapamil SR	Calan SR	120, 180, 240 mg
	Isoptin SR	120, 180, 240 mg
	Verelan	120, 180, 240, 360 mg
	Verelan PM	100, 200, 300 mg
	Covera HS	180, 240 mg
Verapamil for injection		2.5 mg/mL
Amlodipine	Norvasc	2.5, 5, 10 mg
Felodipine	Plendil	2.5, 5, 10 mg
Isradipine	DynaCirc	2.5, 5 mg
Isradipine CR	DynaCirc CR	5, 10 mg
Nicardipine		20, 30 mg
Nicardipine ER	Cardene SR	20, 45, 60 mg
Nicardipine IV	Cardene IV	0.1, 0.2 mg/mL
Nifedipine	Procardia	10, 20 mg
Nifedipine ER	Adalat CC, Procardia XL, Afeditab CR, Nifedical XL	60, 90 mg
Nisoldipine ER	Sular	8.5, 17, 20, 25.5, 30, 34, 40 mg

Table 10-62 Alpha$_2$ Agonists

Drug	Brand Names	Available Strengths
Clonidine	Catapres	0.1, 0.2, 0.3 mg
Clonidine modified release	Jenloga	0.1 mg
Clonidine transdermal	Catapres TTS-1, TTS-2, TTS-3	0.1, 0.2, 0.3 mg
Clonidine for injection	Duraclon	100 mcg/mL, 500 mcg/mL
Guanabenz	Wytensin	4, 8 mg
Guanfacine	Tenex	1, 2 mg
Guanfacine ER	Intuniv	1, 2, 3, 4 mg
Methyldopa	Aldomet	250, 500 mg
Methyldopa for injection		50 mg

Table 10-63 Adrenergic Antagonists

Drug	Brand Name	Available Strengths
Reserpine	Serpasil	0.1, 0.25 mg
Guanethidine	Ismelin	10, 25 mg

Table 10-64 Vasodilators

Drug	Brand Name	Available Strengths
Hydralazine	Apresoline	10, 25, 50, 100 mg
Hydralazine for injection		20 mg/mL
Minoxidil	Loniten	2.5, 10 mg
Sodium nitroprusside IV	Nitropress	50 mg
Nitroglycerin for injection		5 mg/mL
Nitroglycerin in 5% dextrose		100, 200, 400 mcg/mL

Table 10-65 Dopamine Agonists

Drug	Brand Name	Available Strengths
Fenoldopam	Corlopam	10 mg/mL

ANNOTATED BIBLIOGRAPHY

DiPiro JT, Talbert RL, Yee GC, et al. *Pharmacotherapy: A Pathophysiologic Approach*. 6th ed. New York: McGraw-Hill; 2005.

Drug Facts and Comparisons. Wolters Kluwer Health, Inc. Updated periodically.

Micromedex Healthcare Series. Greenwood Village, CO: Thomson Reuters (Healthcare) Inc. Updated periodically.

National Heart, Lung, and Blood Institute, National High Blood Pressure Education Program. *The Seventh*

Report of the Joint National Committee on Prevention, Detection, Evaluation, and Treatment of High Blood Pressure (JNC 7) Express. Bethesda, MD: Author; May 14, 2003. Available at: http://www.nhlbi.nih.gov/guidelines/hypertension/jncintro.htm. Also published in *JAMA*. 2003; 289:2560–2571.

TOPIC: STROKE

Section Coordinator: Teresa K. Hoffmann
Contributor: Teresa K. Hoffmann

Stroke Overview

The proper treatment and management of stroke requires an understanding of the different types of stroke as well as the underlying cause. Pharmacists have a role in ensuring each type of stroke is treated with the most appropriate drugs and that monitoring for side effects as well as drug interactions takes place. Pharmacists can further advise prescribers on the appropriate use of medications to prevent further sequelae and prevent future stroke.

Tips Worth Tweeting

- Stroke is a sudden onset of focal neurologic deficit resulting from interruption of blood flow to the brain.
- It is very important to determine whether a stroke is ischemic (88%) or hemorrhagic (12%), as treatment will vary dramatically depending on the type.
- Consider patient age, past medical history, stroke type, concurrent medications, and duration of symptoms when choosing therapy for acute stroke.
- Consider a transient ischemic attack (TIA) to be a warning sign of eventual stroke.
- Aspirin is effective as secondary prophylaxis but is not as effective as either aspirin + clopidogrel or aspirin + dipyridamole ER in combination.
- Aspirin and dipyridamole separately are not equivalent to the dipyridamole ER + aspirin combination.
- Patients with a history of ischemic stroke should have their blood pressures and cholesterol levels treated regardless of past medical history.

1.1.0 Patient Information

Medication-Induced Causes

- Ischemic stroke: None
- Hemorrhagic stroke: Risk increases with concomitant use of anticoagulants or antiplatelets

Table 10-66 Classification of Stroke

Type	Subtype	Cause
Ischemic	Embolic	Embolism from atrial fibrillation or MI
	Thrombotic	Atherosclerosis
Hemorrhagic	Intracerebral	
	Subarachnoid	
	Subdural	Usually trauma
	Epidural	

Laboratory Testing

- CBC
- Test for a hypercoagulable state only if more common risk factors are not present

Disease States Associated with Stroke

- Hypertension (HTN)
- Heart disease
- Diabetes mellitus (DM)
- TIA
- Previous stroke
- Tobacco abuse
- Hyperlipidemia

Risk Factors

- HTN
- Gender (male > female)
- Ethnicity (higher mortality in blacks)
- Age (incidence doubles with each decade > 55)
- Cardiac disease
- Diabetes
- TIA/prior stroke
- Smoking
- Hyperlipidemia

Signs and Symptoms

See Table 10-67.

Imaging

- CT scan is useful for showing bleeding, which will appear as white areas (hyperintensity). It may

Table 10-67 Symptoms of Stroke (Sudden Onset)

Hemiplegia, hemiparesis
Aphasia
Severe headache
Vision changes
Ataxia
Seizures

take up to 24 hours for an acute ischemic stroke to appear on CT results.
- MRI can show smaller infarcts.
- Carotid ultrasound identifies carotid atherosclerosis.
- Transesophageal echocardiogram is used to identify a structural problem with the heart or an embolus.

Acute Treatment of Ischemic Stroke

- Alteplase (tPA): 0.9 mg/kg (max 90 mg) over 1 hour as continuous infusion
  - Weight ≤ 100 kg: 0.09 mg/kg bolus over 1 minute, followed by 0.81 mg/kg over 1 hour
  - Weight > 100 kg: 9 mg bolus over 1 minute, followed by 81 mg over 1 hour
- Aspirin 160–325 mg daily started within 48 hours of symptom onset

Table 10-68 Criteria for Use of Tissue Plasminogen Activator in Stroke Patients

Inclusion Criteria	Exclusion Criteria
Age greater than 18 years	Minor/rapidly improving stroke symptoms
Symptom onset within 3 hours of presentation (FDA-approved indication)	High clinical suspicion of subarachnoid hemorrhage even if CT scan is normal
Symptom onset within 3–4.5 hours of presentation (unlabeled indication)	Active internal bleeding (GI/GU bleeding within 21 days)
CT of head is negative for hemorrhage	Platelet count < 100,000/mm^3
Clinical diagnosis of acute ischemic stroke with notable neurological deficits	Patient has received heparin within 48 hours and had an elevated APTT
	Recent use of warfarin and INR > 1.7 (PT > 15)
	Intracranial surgery, serious head trauma, or previous stroke in the last 3 months
	Major surgery or trauma in the last 14 days
	Recent arterial puncture at a noncompressible site
	Lumbar puncture within the last 7 days
	History of intracranial hemorrhage, arteriovenous malformation, or aneurysm
	Witnessed seizure at stroke onset
	Recent acute MI
	SBP > 185 mm Hg or DBP > 110 mm Hg

Wellness and Prevention

The following points apply to ischemic strokes:
- Control modifiable risk factors
  - HTN
  - Hyperlipidemia
  - Diabetes mellitus
  - Obesity
  - Tobacco cessation
- Primary prevention
  - Aspirin
    - 75 mg daily if 10-year Framingham Risk ≥ 10%
    - 75–325 mg daily if atrial fibrillation (AF) and $CHADS_2$ score ≤ 1
    - Carotid artery stenosis (symptomatic or asymptomatic)
    - Diabetes mellitus
  - Warfarin with goal INR of 2–3 if AF and $CHADS_2$ score > 2 (optional if score = 1)
- Secondary prevention
  - Noncardioembolic
    - Aspirin 50–325 mg daily + clopidogrel 75 mg daily
    - Aspirin 25 mg + extended-release dipyridamole 200 mg bid
  - Cardioembolic
    - Warfarin with target INR of 2.5 (range 2–3)
  - ACE inhibitor (even if previously normotensive)
  - Statin (even if normal lipids)

1.2.0 Pharmacotherapy

Mechanism of Action of Pharmacologic Agents

- Alteplase: Binds to fibrin in a thrombus and converts plasminogen to plasmin, thereby initiating local fibrinolysis
- Aspirin: Inhibits prostaglandin cyclooxygenase, thereby preventing the production of thromboxane A_2 and inhibiting platelet aggregation
- Clopidogrel
  - Prodrug activated to the active thiol metabolite
  - Metabolite blocks platelet ADP receptors to prevent activation of the GP IIb/IIIa receptor complex and platelet aggregation
- Dipyridamole
  - Inhibits activity of adenosine deaminase and phosphodiesterase, causing an accumulation

of adenosine, adenine nucleotides, and cyclic AMP
    - This accumulation inhibits platelet aggregation
- Warfarin: Inhibits vitamin K epoxide reductase to block the production of vitamin K dependent clotting factors (II, VII, IX, X)
- ACE inhibitors: Block production of angiotensin II (AT II) by the inhibition of angiotensin-converting enzyme, which prevents AT II–mediated vasoconstriction and decreases aldosterone secretion
- Statins: Inhibit 3-hydroxy-3-methylglutaryl coenzyme A (HMG-CoA) reductase, leading to lower LDL and cause upregulation of LDL receptors on the liver

Interaction of Drugs with Foods and Laboratory Tests

Aspirin

- Precautions: NSAIDs, warfarin, corticosteroids, heparin, methotrexate, thrombolytics, uricosuric agents, valproic acid, ACEIs, alcohol
- Lab interactions:
    - False-negative for urinary oxidase glucose tests
    - False-positive for urinary cupric sulfate tests

Table 10-69 Stroke Medications: Drugs, Indications, and Routes of Administration

Drug	Approved Indications	Routes of Administration
Thrombolytics		
Alteplase	Acute ischemic stroke (AIS) within 3 hours of symptom onset	IV
Antiplatelets		
Aspirin	AIS, primary/ secondary prophylaxis	Oral
Clopidogrel	Secondary prophylaxis	Oral
Dipyridamole (ER)	Secondary prophylaxis	Oral
Anticoagulants		
Warfarin	Primary/secondary prophylaxis	Oral, IV
ACEIs		
Ramipril	Prophylaxis	Oral
Statins		
Atorvastatin	Primary/secondary prophylaxis	Oral
Pravastatin	Secondary prophylaxis	Oral
Simvastatin	Primary/secondary prophylaxis	Oral

Clopidogrel

- Precautions: Aspirin, macrolides, proton pump inhibitors, bupropion, warfarin, NSAIDs

Dipyridamole

- Precautions: Cholinesterase inhibitors, adenosine

Contraindications, Warnings, and Precautions

Contraindications

- Aspirin: NSAID-induced asthma, rhinitis, urticaria, inherited or acquired bleeding disorders, children or teenagers with viral illness, GI bleed
- Clopidogrel: Active bleeding, GI bleed, acute intracranial hemorrhage
- Dipyridamole: None

Warnings and Precautions

- Aspirin: Thrombocytopenia, intracranial lesion, chronic alcohol use (more than 3 drinks/day), peptic ulcer disease (PUD), history of GI bleed, GERD, sodium restriction (buffered aspirin only)
- Clopidogrel: Trauma, elective surgery within 5 days, GI ulcer, poor/intermediate CYP2C19 metabolizer, hepatic impairment, ocular disease
- Dipyridamole: PUD, history of GI bleed, bleeding disorder, hypotension

Physiochemical Properties, Solubility, Pharmacodynamics, and Pharmacokinetic Properties

Alteplase

- More than 50% of the drug present in plasma is cleared 5 minutes after infusion is done; more than 80% is cleared within 10 minutes
- Cleared from plasma at a rate of 550–650 mL/min, primarily by the liver

Aspirin

- Hydrolyzed to active salicylate by esterases in GI mucosa, synovial fluid, and blood
- Metabolism by hepatic conjugation

Clopidogrel (75 mg daily)

- Onset: Inhibition of platelet aggregation (IPA) by the second day of treatment
- Peak IPA: 5–7 days
- Half-life: Parent drug: 6 hours; metabolite: 8 hours

Dipyridamole ER

- Metabolism: Hepatic
- Terminal half-life: 10–12 hours

Table 10-70 Stroke Medications: Biopharmaceutical Principles and Pharmaceutical Characteristics of Dosage Forms

Drug	Dosage Form	Bioavailability
Aspirin	Oral	50–75%
Clopidogrel	Oral	50%
Dipyridamole ER/aspirin	Oral	37–66%

1.3.0 Monitoring

Pharmacotherapeutic Outcomes

- Reduce ongoing neurological damage by maintaining or improving perfusion to the ischemic area
- Reduce morbidity and mortality associated with continued infarction
- Prevent future strokes

Safety and Efficacy Monitoring and Patient Education

Aspirin

- Take with food or after meals.
- Take with a full glass of water to reduce the risk of esophageal erosion.
- Do not crush or chew enteric-coated products.
- Do not use if aspirin develops a strong, vinegar odor.
- Call the physician if ringing in the ears or hearing loss occurs.
- Limit alcohol consumption to fewer than 3 drinks/day.

Clopidogrel

- May take longer for bleeding to stop (especially if using with aspirin).
- Notify the dentist of clopidogrel use.

Aspirin/Dipyridamole ER

- Limit alcohol consumption to fewer than 3 drinks/day.
- Do not take with other aspirin-containing products.
- Swallow the capsule whole; do not crush, break, or chew it.

Adverse Drug Reactions

- Aspirin: Dyspepsia, GI ulcer, gastric erosions, duodenal ulcers, bruising, rash, hypernatremia (buffered aspirin), tinnitus
- Clopidogrel: Abdominal pain, vomiting, dyspepsia, gastritis, rash, bleeding, thrombotic thrombocytic purpura (TTP)
- Aspirin/dipyridamole ER: Dyspepsia, GI ulcer, gastric erosions, duodenal ulcers, bruising, rash, hypernatremia (buffered aspirin), tinnitus, headache (39%); tolerance usually develops

Table 10-71 Stroke Medications: Generic Names, Brand Names, and Strengths Available

Generic	Brand Name	Strengths Available
Alteplase powder for reconstitution	Activase	50, 100 mg
Aspirin	Ascriptin, Ecotrin, Halfprin, Bayer Aspirin Regimen, Bufferin, St. Joseph	81, 325 mg
Clopidogrel	Plavix	75, 300 mg
Aspirin/dipyridamole ER	Aggrenox	25/200 mg

ANNOTATED BIBLIOGRAPHY

Drug Facts and Comparisons. Wolters Kluwer Health, Inc. Updated periodically.

Fagan SC, Hess DC. Stroke. In DiPiro JT, Talbert RL, Yee GC, Matzke GR, Wells BG, Posey LM, eds. *Pharmacotherapy: A Pathophysiologic Approach*. 7th ed. Available at: http://www.accesspharmacy.com.polar.onu.edu/content.aspx?aID=3191719.

Goldstein LB, Adams R, Alberts MJ, et al. Primary prevention of ischemic stroke. A guideline from the American Heart Association/American Stroke Association Stroke Council: Cosponsored by the Atherosclerotic Peripheral Vascular Disease Interdisciplinary Working Group; Cardiovascular Nursing Council; Clinical Cardiology Council; Nutrition, Physical Activity, and Metabolism Council; and the Quality of Care and Outcomes Research Interdisciplinary Working Group. *Stroke* 2006;37:1583–1633.

Micromedex Healthcare Series. Greenwood Village, CO: Thomson Reuters (Healthcare) Inc. Updated periodically.

TOPIC: VENOUS THROMBOEMBOLISM

Section Coordinator: Teresa K. Hoffmann
Contributor: Lindsay R. Snyder

Venous Thromboembolism Overview

Pharmacists play an important role in the treatment and prevention of venous thromboembolism (VTE) through anticoagulant selection and monitoring. Vitamin K antagonists such as warfarin require intensive management to maintain therapeutic levels, prevent drug interactions, and ensure patient adherence to the prescribed regimen.

Tips Worth Tweeting

- VTE is a disease characterized by a blood clot in a vein; it includes both deep vein thrombosis (DVT) and pulmonary embolism (PE).
- Risk factors for VTE include increasing age, previous VTE, hypercoagulable states (inherited or acquired), trauma, or major surgery (especially orthopedic surgery).
- Drug therapy can also contribute to VTE risk, especially estrogens, heparin, and erythropoiesis-stimulating agents.
- Prompt diagnosis and initiation of anticoagulation are essential to prevent complications such as post-thrombotic syndrome or death.
- Initiate both vitamin K antagonists (warfarin) and injectable anticoagulants on the first treatment day of acute VTE. Overlap therapy for at least 5 days until INR > 2.
- The goal INR range for warfarin therapy in VTE is 2–3.
- Warfarin therapy requires intensive monitoring for efficacy, safety, and drug–food interactions.
- The most common adverse effect associated with anticoagulation is bleeding.

1.1.0 Patient Information

Medication-Induced Contributors to VTE

- Estrogen-containing oral contraceptives or hormone replacement therapy (HRT)
- Selective estrogen receptor modulators (SERMs)
- Heparin-induced thrombocytopenia (HIT)
- Erythropoiesis-stimulating agents

Laboratory Testing

- d-Dimer: By-product of thrombin generation; usually elevated with VTE
- Erythrocyte sedimentation rate (ESR) and white blood cells (WBC) may also be elevated

Disease States Associated with VTE

Virchow's triad identifies three factors contributing to VTE development:

- Stasis (blood flow alterations)
  - Examples: Bed rest, air travel, paralysis, obesity, prolonged hospitalization, polycythemia vera, varicose veins
- Trauma (vascular endothelial injury)
  - Examples: Major orthopedic surgery, trauma, indwelling venous catheters
- Blood constituent alterations (inherited or acquired hypercoagulable states)
  - Malignancy
  - Antiphospholipid antibodies (found with lupus or inflammatory bowel disease)
  - Nephrotic syndrome
  - Pregnancy/postpartum
  - Hereditary clotting disorders (e.g., protein C or S deficiency, activated protein C resistance/Factor V Leiden)

VTE risk also increases with increasing age and is higher in patients who have previously had a VTE.

Instruments and Techniques Related to Patient Assessment

- Diagnostic tests for DVT
  - Venography: Gold standard; invasive; uses contrast dye
  - Duplex ultrasonography: Most commonly used; noninvasive; can visualize proximal vein clots
- Diagnostic tests for PE
  - Ventilation–perfusion (V/Q) scan: Measures distribution of blood and airflow in the lungs
  - Spiral CT scan: Detects emboli in pulmonary arteries
  - Pulmonary angiography: Gold standard; invasive; uses contrast dye; significant risk of mortality

Signs and Symptoms

Both DVT and PE may be present as part of VTE.

Wellness and Prevention

Prevention of initial or recurrent VTE varies based on the risk factors present. If obesity is a factor, reduction of body weight and regular exercise are recommended. Smoking cessation is encouraged.

Long-distance travel has been associated with increased risk for VTE, although most travelers who develop VTE have additional risk factors.

Table 10-72 Signs and Symptoms of VTE

DVT	PE
Leg pain, swelling, or warmth	Cough (potential hemoptysis)
Dilated superficial veins, or palpable "cord" in leg	Chest pain
Pain in back of knee with foot dorsiflexion	Shortness of breath (SOB)/tachypnea
	Palpitation/tachycardia
	Distention of neck veins
	Cyanosis and hypotension

Recommendations for air travel lasting more than 8 hours include avoiding restrictive clothing, maintaining adequate hydration, and performing frequent calf muscle contraction. For travelers at high risk of VTE, compression stockings may be worn, or a single dose of low-molecular-weight heparin (LMWH) may be administered prior to departure. Aspirin has not been shown to be effective in VTE prevention.

VTE prophylaxis is widely used in the inpatient population for higher-risk groups. Nonpharmacologic strategies include early ambulation following surgery, compression stockings, and intermittent pneumatic compression (IPC) devices. Patients at moderate to high risk of VTE may require pharmacologic thromboprophylaxis with LMWH, unfractionated heparin (UFH), fondaparinux, or warfarin.

1.2.0 Pharmacotherapy

Mechanism of Action by Class

- Unfractionated heparin
  - Binds to antithrombin III, inhibiting activation of clotting factors IX, X, XII, and II; most effect is on thrombin (IIa) and Xa
  - Binds to platelets; may contribute to bleeding independent of anticoagulant effect
- Low-molecular-weight heparins: Anti-Factor Xa activity > anti-Factor II activity
- Fondaparinux: Direct Factor Xa inhibitor
- Warfarin
  - Inhibitor of vitamin K epoxide reductase
  - Decreases available reduced vitamin K, which is required to activate clotting factors II, VII, IX, and X, as well as anticoagulant proteins C and S
- Direct thrombin inhibitors: Interact directly to inhibit thrombin (IIa)

Interaction of Drugs with Foods and Laboratory Tests

All Anticoagulants

Use anticoagulants with caution in conjunction with other medications that could contribute to bleeding risk, such as other anticoagulants, antiplatelet agents (including NSAIDs), or thrombolytics.

Enoxaparin

Risk of bleeding may be increased with SSRIs.

Warfarin

Warfarin has numerous drug and food interactions. Always look for interactions when initiating or discontinuing concomitant therapies, especially those involving CYP 2C9. Some major interactions include the following:

- Enzyme inducers: Rifamycins, carbamazepine, phenytoin, phenobarbital
- Enzyme inhibitors: Azole antifungals, amiodarone, sulfamethoxazole, metronidazole
- Foods that contain vitamin K: Especially leafy, green vegetables; also mayonnaise and oils
- Grapefruit or cranberry juice: May increase INR
- Herbal supplements: Gingko, garlic, vitamin E, fish oil, green tea, ginseng, and St. John's wort, among others
- Smoking: May decrease INR
- Alcohol: Acute ingestion may increase INR

Heparin and LMWHs

These medications are associated with elevated AST/ALT levels.

Table 10-73 VTE Medications: Drugs, Indications, and Routes of Administration

Drug	Approved VTE Indications	Routes of Administration
UFH and LMWHs		
UFH	Prophylaxis treatment	Intravenous (IV), subcutaneous (subQ)
Enoxaparin (Lovenox)	Prophylaxis treatment	subQ
Dalteparin (Fragmin)	Extended treatment of symptomatic VTE (not acute treatment)	subQ
Tinzaparin (Innohep)	Prophylaxis treatment only	subQ
Factor Xa Inhibitors		
Fondaparinux (Arixtra)	Prophylaxis treatment	subQ
Vitamin K Antagonists		
Warfarin (Coumadin)	Prophylaxis (long-term) treatment	Oral, slow IV bolus (rarely used)
Direct Thrombin Inhibitors		
Argatroban (Argatroban)	HIT treatment	IV
Lepirudin (Refludan)	HIT treatment	IV
Bivalirudin (Angiomax)	Heparin alternative for percutaneous coronary intervention (PCI); no VTE indication	IV
Desirudin (Iprivask)	Prophylaxis in hip surgery	subQ

Contraindications, Warnings, and Precautions

Contraindications

- UFH: Severe thrombocytopenia (TCP); any patient for whom suitable blood coagulation tests cannot be performed at appropriate intervals (no need to monitor low-dose heparin)
- LMWHs: TCP and positive test for antiplatelet antibody in presence of LMWH; hypersensitivity to heparin, pork products, or benzyl alcohol (with multidose vials)
  - Dalteparin: Increased bleeding risk in patients undergoing regional anesthesia (for unstable angina or NSTEMI indication), patients with cancer undergoing regional anesthesia (for extended treatment of symptomatic VTE)
  - Fondaparinux: Severe renal impairment (CrCl < 30 mL/min); prophylaxis in patients weighing less than 50 kg who are undergoing hip fracture, hip replacement, knee replacement, or abdominal surgery; bacterial endocarditis; TCP with antiplatelet antibody in presence of fondaparinux
- Warfarin: Pregnancy; recent or upcoming CNS, eye, or traumatic surgery; inadequate laboratory monitoring; noncompliance or unsupervised patients with senility, alcoholism, or psychosis; diagnostic or therapeutic procedures with the potential for uncontrollable bleeding; malignant hypertension
- All: Major bleeding/hemorrhage (except due to DIC); hypersensitivity to the drug

Warnings and Precautions

- Black box warnings:
  - LMWHs and fondaparinux: Spinal and epidural hematoma
  - Warfarin: Bleeding risk
- UFH: Avoid IM administration; hyperlipidemia; benzyl alcohol (certain formulations); heparin resistance; TCP; hyperkalemia; caution in children and the elderly
- LMWH: Neuraxial anesthesia (BBW); PCI/sheath removal; TCP; benzyl alcohol (certain formulations); mechanical heart valves; low-weight patients; renal or hepatic function impairment; avoid IM administration (hematoma)
  - Enoxaparin: Dose adjustment in renal failure
  - Tinzaparin: Priapism, sulfite sensitivity
  - Fondaparinux: Neuraxial anesthesia (BBW); TCP; renal impairment
- Warfarin: Necrosis; atheroemboli/microemboli (purple toes syndrome); HIT (venous limb necrosis/gangrene); concomitant disease states that enhance or decrease anticoagulant effect
- Direct thrombin inhibitors: No antidote
  - Argatroban: Hepatic impairment
  - Lepirudin: Antibodies/reexposure reaction (also desirudin); renal or hepatic impairment (dose adjustment in renal failure)
- All: Potential for hemorrhage, hypersensitivity

Physiochemical Properties, Solubility, Pharmacodynamics, and Pharmacokinetic Properties

- Warfarin: 3–5 days to peak anticoagulant effect
- Enoxaparin: Maximum activity after 3–5 hours
- Dose adjustments in renal failure:
  - Enoxaparin (Lovenox)
  - Dalteparin (Fragmin) (based on anti-Xa level)
  - Lepirudin (Refludan) (based on aPTT)
  - Desirudin (Ipravask) (based on aPTT)

1.3.0 Monitoring

Pharmacotherapeutic Outcomes

- Prevent thrombus extension or embolization
- Prevent VTE recurrence
- Minimize risks of anticoagulation
- Prevent VTE in at-risk patients

Safety and Efficacy Monitoring and Patient Education

- Heparin
  - Monitor activated partial thromboplastin time (aPTT): goal is 1.5–2 times normal
  - Educate on proper subcutaneous injection technique (if necessary)
- LMWHs
  - Monitoring of anti-Factor Xa level is not needed, but may be useful in obesity or renal function impairment
  - Educate on proper subcutaneous injection technique

Table 10-74 VTE Medications: Biopharmaceutical Principles and Pharmaceutical Characteristics of Dosage Forms

Drug	Dosage Form	Bioavailability
Vitamin K Antagonists		
Warfarin	Oral tablet	100%
LMWHs		
Enoxaparin	subQ injection	100%
Dalteparin	subQ injection	87%
Tinzaparin	subQ injection	87%

- Rotate injection sites
- To minimize bruising, do not rub the injection site after injection
- Fondaparinux
  - Do not take NSAIDs or aspirin without consulting a doctor
  - Educate on proper subcutaneous injection technique
- Direct thrombin inhibitors
  - Monitor aPTT; goal is 1.5–2.5 times baseline
- Warfarin
  - INR monitoring is very important to prevent adverse events
  - Strict adherence to prescribed dosage is necessary for safety and efficacy
  - Advise all healthcare providers of warfarin use
    - Carry warfarin identification
    - Notify healthcare providers if starting or discontinuing other medications, including OTCs and supplements
    - Do not take NSAIDs or aspirin without consulting a doctor (increased risk of bleeding without notable increase in INR)
  - Avoid alcohol consumption
  - Avoid activity that could result in injury
  - Vitamin K in food (mostly leafy greens) can affect response to warfarin
  - If warfarin is discontinued, anticoagulant effect persists for about 5 days
- All anticoagulants
  - Notify the healthcare provider immediately and/or go to the emergency department if unusual bleeding or symptoms occur
  - Symptoms that warrant seeking care: Pain, swelling, discomfort, prolonged bleeding from cuts, increased menstrual flow, nosebleeds, bleeding of gums, unusual bruising, red or dark brown urine, red or tarry black stools, headache, dizziness, or weakness

Adverse Drug Reactions

- All anticoagulants: Major or minor bleeding, hypersensitivity reaction
- Heparin: HIT, injection site irritation
- LMWH: HIT, injection site irritation
- Fondaparinux: Thrombocytopenia, injection site irritation
- Warfarin: Purple toe syndrome

Table 10-75 Pharmacotherapeutic Alternatives in VTE

Generic	Brand Name	Strengths Available
Heparin	None	1,000, 2,000, 2,500, 5,000, 7,500, 10,000, 20,000, or 40,000 units/mL
Enoxaparin	Lovenox	Prefilled syringes: 30, 40, 60, 80, 100, 120, 150 mg Multidose vial: 300 mg/3 mL
Dalteparin	Fragmin	Prefilled syringes: 2,500, 5,000, 7,500, 10,000, 12,500, 15,000, 18,000 units/mL Multidose vials: 95,000 units/3.8 mL, 95,000 units/9.5 mL
Tinzaparin	Innohep	Multidose vial: 20,000 units/mL
Fondaparinux	Arixtra	Prefilled syringes: 2.5, 5, 7.5, 10 mg
Argatroban	Argatroban	100 mg/mL in 2.5 mL single-use vials
Lepirudin	Refludan	50 mg vial
Desirudin	Iprivask	15 mg single-use vial
Warfarin	Coumadin, Jantoven (branded generic)	Tablets: 1, 2, 2.5, 3, 4, 5, 6, 7.5, 10 mg Injection: Single-use 5 mg vials

ANNOTATED BIBLIOGRAPHY

Ansell J, Hirsch J, Hylek E, Jacobson A, Crowther M, Palareti G. Pharmacology and management of the vitamin K antagonists. *Chest* 2008;133:160S–198S.

DiPiro JT, Talbert RL, Yee GC, Matzke GR, Wells BG, Posey LM, eds. *Pharmacotherapy: A Pathophysiologic Approach*. 6th ed. New York: McGraw-Hill; 2005.

Drug Facts and Comparisons. Wolters Kluwer Health, Inc. Updated periodically.

Geerts WH, Bergqvist D, Pineo GF, Heit JA, Samama CM, Lassen MR. Prevention of venous thromboembolism. *Chest* 2008;133:381S–453S.

Kearon C, Kahn SR, Agnelli G, Goldhaber S, Raskob GE, Comerota AJ. Antithrombotic therapy for venous thromboembolic disease. *Chest* 2008;133;454S–545S.

Dermatology

CHAPTER

11

TOPIC: PSORIASIS

Contributor: Laura Perry

Tips Worth Tweeting

- Psoriasis is caused by pathogenic T-cell production that leads to increased keratinocyte proliferation and chronic inflammation.
- Psoriasis is characterized by red lesions, or plaques, with silvery-white scales.
- Psoriasis has a strong genetic component, with skin trauma, stress, seasonal changes, and certain drugs acting as triggers for exacerbations or flare-ups.
- Comorbidities associated with psoriasis include anxiety, depression, cardiovascular disease, metabolic disease, and certain types of cancer. Monitoring for and managing these comorbidities is a core component of psoriasis management.
- A variety of topical and systemic therapies are available for the treatment of psoriasis.
- Topical treatment is the usual initial treatment for mild to moderate psoriasis, with systemic therapy and combination therapy with systemic agents, topical agents, and phototherapy typically being reserved for moderate to severe psoriasis.
- Combination, rotational, and sequential therapy are commonly used to increase the effectiveness and decrease the side effects of treatment regimens by allowing for shorter duration of therapy and lower doses of each agent.
- Biological response modifiers are indicated as first-line systemic agents but are typically reserved for patients with a contraindication to or ineffective treatment with other oral systemic agents.
- Responses to treatment may be delayed by 2 to 6 weeks, and complete resolution may not be possible for all patients.
- Nonpharmacological therapy with moisturizers as well as stress reduction and relaxation therapy are important to improve quality of life in psoriatic patients.

Patient Care Scenario: Ambulatory Setting

C. W. is a 45-year-old woman with a history of psoriasis, hypertension, anxiety, and chronic urinary tract infections. She indicates that she was treated for mild psoriasis a while back with over-the-counter coal tar and a prescription steroid cream that resolved all of her lesions. Two weeks ago, C. W. noticed new red plaques covered with whitish silvery scales on each of her elbows (approximately 3 cm in diameter) and a plaque at the base of her hairline on her scalp (approximately 4 cm). Other symptoms she mentions are itching at the plaque sites, aches and pains in her hands, and "dips" in her fingernails.

Date	Physician	Drug	Quantity	Sig	Refills
4/26	Smith	Macrodantin 50 mg	#30	one po HS	3 refills
4/3	Cole	Activella	#28	one po daily	3 refills
4/3	Smith	Diazepam 5 mg	#30	one po daily	0 refills
4/3	Smith	Fosinopril 20 mg	#30	one po daily	5 refills
3/1	Cole	Activella	#28	one po daily	4 refills
3/1	Smith	Diazepam 5 mg	#30	one po daily	1 refill
11/15	Fox	Betamethasone valerate 0.05%	30 g	apply bid	0 refills
11/4	Smith	Diazepam 5mg	#30	one po daily	2 refills

1.1.0 Patient Information

Medication-Induced Causes of Psoriasis

Although there have been no medications associated with the development of psoriasis, several medications do appear to exacerbate existing psoriasis. Some of the medications reported to induce psoriasis flare-ups include lithium, nonsteroidal anti-inflammatory drugs (indomethacin, salicylates), antimalarials (chloroquine, hydroxychloroquine), beta blockers (propranolol, atenolol), quinidine, and withdrawal of corticosteroids.

Laboratory Testing

Diagnosis of psoriasis is based on clinical manifestations during the physical exam rather than on laboratory data. Skin biopsies may be used to confirm the diagnosis.

Disease States Associated with Psoriasis

Psoriatic patients have an increased risk of several psychiatric and medical comorbidities. Psychiatric and psychological comorbidities associated with psoriasis include depression, anxiety, and poor self-esteem. Additionally, the incidence of certain autoimmune disorders, such as inflammatory bowel disorder, Crohn's disease, and ulcerative colitis, is higher in psoriatic patients. Recent data also suggest an increased risk of diabetes, metabolic syndrome, cardiovascular disease, obesity, and lymphoma.

Instruments and Techniques Related to Patient Assessment

First, a physical exam is necessary to classify the type of psoriasis lesion. Next, an accurate patient medical history is important to determine the onset and duration of lesions, family history, presence of exacerbating factors, and treatment history.

Terminology Used in the Classification of Psoriasis

Psoriatic lesions are classified based on characteristics of the lesions as described in Table 11-1. In Auspitz's sign, removal of scales reveals a salmon-pink lesion with pinpoint bleeding. Lesion development at the site of skin trauma (i.e., an insect bite) is known as the Koebner phenomenon.

Table 11-1 Classification of Psoriatic Lesions

Type of Psoriasis	Description
Plaque	Well-defined, sharply demarcated, erythematous plaques varying in size from 1 cm to several centimeters. Typically, they have a dry, thin, silvery-white scale. Plaques tend to be symmetrically distributed across the body.
Inverse	Lesions in the skin folds (axillary, genital, perineal, and intergluteal). Erythematous lesions with minimal scaling occurs due to the moist nature of the areas involved.
Erythrodermic	Generalized erythema covering nearly all of the body surface area. This potentially life-threatening condition involves fever, malaise, thermoregulatory issues, and dehydration.
Pustular	Generalized or localized collections of neutrophils that may be accompanied with toxicity and fever, requiring aggressive systemic therapy.
Guttate	Sudden eruption of small salmon-pink papules and plaques that appear on the trunk and proximal extremities, often preceded by a Group A beta-hemolytic streptococcal infection 2 to 3 weeks prior to the attack.
Nail disease (psoriatic onychodystrophy)	Fingernails are affected in 50% and toenails in 35% of psoriatic patients. Nail disease presents as pitting, subungual hyperkeratosis, and/or yellowing of the nail plate.
Psoriatic arthritis	Inflammatory arthropathy involving mostly the distal interphalangeal joints and adjacent nails. Knees, elbows, wrists, and ankles may also be affected.

Signs and Symptoms of Psoriasis

General characteristics of psoriatic plaques include raised, red to violet lesions with sharp demarcated borders. Plaque lesions are usually covered with silvery-white scales. Plaques appear most commonly on the elbows, knees, scalp, umbilicus, and lumbar areas, but lesions may also extend to the trunk, arms, legs, face, ears, palms, soles, and nails.

Psoriatic lesions may be associated with varying degrees of pruritis and pain. The presence and extent of lesions may wax and wane over time. Patients may experience periods of remission, where no lesions are present, lasting from weeks to years. Approximately 10% to 30% of patients with psoriasis also have psoriatic arthritis.

Wellness and Prevention

Several nonpharmacological treatments may be beneficial as complements to pharmacological treatment to prevent and reduce psoriatic lesions. Oatmeal baths and frequent application of nonmedicated, fragrance-free moisturizers help to soothe the irritation, maintain hydration, and decrease scaling and cracking of lesions. Also, use of lipid-free, fragrance-free cleansers and avoidance of harsh soaps and detergents will help to reduce skin irritation. Balneotherapy is another nonpharmacological therapy that involves bathing in waters that contain certain salts; it is often combined with sun exposure. Other important interventions include reducing psoriasis triggers—for example, emotional stress, skin trauma, and seasonal changes. Although sun exposure may be beneficial to psoriatic lesions, sunscreens with a sun protection factor of 15 to 30 should be worn to prevent sunburn. Skin trauma due to sunburn and scratching may lead to flare-ups. Lastly, emotional support and stress reduction are important interventions to prevent exacerbations of psoriasis.

1.2.0 Pharmacotherapy

Treatments for Psoriasis

Treatment of psoriasis requires modification of the autoimmune response and involves topical therapy, phototherapy, and systemic therapy. The choice of treatment usually depends on the severity of the disease. Initial treatment of mild to moderate psoriasis begins with topical agents, then progresses to add phototherapy and/or systemic agents if necessary.

Treatment of moderate to severe psoriasis involves systemic agents, usually in combination with topical agents or phototherapy. Combination, rotational, and sequential therapy are often used in such treatment to increase its effectiveness and to permit use of lower doses of individual agents. Biological response modifiers are currently recommended as first-line therapies alongside oral systemic agents for moderate to severe psoriasis because they have been shown to induce remission of the disease and improve quality of life. Owing to their relatively high cost, however, biological response modifiers are usually reserved for use when traditional systemic agents are contraindicated or ineffective. In addition to systemic agents, nonsteroidal anti-inflammatory drugs (NSAIDs) and local corticosteroid injections may be employed as adjunctive agents for psoriatic arthritis.

Phototherapy involves the exposure of the skin to ultraviolet A (UVA) or ultraviolet B (UVB) radiation to reduce psoriatic lesions. To increase its efficacy, UVA therapy is usually combined with phostosensitizers called psoralens (i.e., methoxsalen or trioxsalen). This approach, which is known as PUVA, is administered twice monthly. Other topical agents are not usually combined with PUVA treatment, unless treatment proves ineffective. Photochemotherapy is the term used to describe the combination of phototherapy with other topical and systemic psoriasis treatments. Topical agents that may increase the efficacy of PUVA include calcipotriene, tazarotene, coal tar, and corticosteroids. UVB therapy, administered three times weekly, is effective both alone and in combination with topical agents. Additionally, phototherapy with UVA or UVB may be combined with systemic therapies.

Interaction of Drugs with Foods and Laboratory Tests

- Acitretin: methotrexate (increased hepatotoxicity), tetracyclines (increased effects), oral contraceptives (decreased efficacy), ethanol (increased teratogenicity), vitamin A (increased adverse effects)
- Methotrexate: acitretin (increased hepatotoxicity), ciprofloxacin and cyclosporine (increased effects), NSAIDs (may decrease excretion), food (decreased absorption), folate (decrease effectiveness), ethanol (increased risk of liver toxicity)
- Cyclosporine: CYP 3A4 or P-glycoprotein substrates
- Biological response modifiers: live vaccines
- Alefacept: ethanol (may increase liver toxicity)
- Infliximab, adalimumab, etanercept: echinacea (may decrease effects)

Contraindications, Warnings, and Precautions

Contraindications

- Calcipotriene: hypercalcemia or evidence of vitamin D toxicity, use on face, use on acute eruptions

Table 11-2 Drugs to Treat Psoriasis: Indications, Dosing, Dosage Forms, and Routes of Administration

Class	Indication	Generic	Route	Dosage Forms	Dosing Regimen
Corticosteroids: very high potency	Mild to moderate plaque psoriasis (short-term use in thicker plaque areas such as hands and soles)	Augmented betamethasone dipropionate	Topical	Ointment, gel, lotion	Apply to affected area two to four times daily. Do not use for longer than 4 weeks at a time.
		Clobetasol proprionate	Topical	Cream, ointment, gel, foam, lotion, shampoo, scalp application, spray	
		Fluocinonide	Topical	Cream	
		Halobetasol propionate	Topical	Cream, ointment	
Corticosteroids: high potency	Mild to moderate plaque psoriasis (short-term use in thicker plaque areas such as hands and soles)	Augmented betamethasone dipropionate	Topical	Cream	Typical regimens are twice daily, but is dependent on skin type, plaque thickness, and compliance.
		Betamethasone dipropionate	Topical	Ointment, cream	
		Betamethasone valerate	Topical	Ointment	
		Desoximetasone	Topical	Cream, ointment, gel	
		Diflorasone diacetate	Topical	Cream	
		Fluocinonide	Topical	Cream, ointment, gel, solution	
		Halcinonide	Topical	Cream, ointment, solution	
Corticosteroids: medium potency	Mild to moderate plaque psoriasis (most frequently used)	Betamethasone dipropionate	Topical	Lotion	Dosing continues until thick active lesions improve.
		Betamethasone valerate	Topical	Cream, lotion	
		Desoximetasone	Topical	Cream	
		Fluticasone propionate	Topical	Cream, ointment	
		Hydrocortisone butyrate	Topical	Cream, ointment, solution	
		Hydrocortisone valerate	Topical	Cream, ointment	
		Mometasone furoate	Topical	Cream, ointment, lotion	
		Triamcinolone acetonide	Topical	Cream, ointment, lotion	
Corticosteroids: low potency	Mild to moderate plaque psoriasis (used when treatment of the face or flexures is necessary)	Alclometasone dipropionate	Topical	Cream, ointment	Upon clinical improvement application frequency can be decreased.
		Desonide	Topical	Cream, ointment, lotion, foam	
		Fluocinolone acetonide	Topical	Shampoo, solution, cream	
		Hydrocortisone	Topical	Cream, ointment, lotion, topical solution, available OTC	
Vitamin D analogues	Mild to moderate psoriasis	Calcipotriene	Topical	Ointment, cream, solution	Apply to affected skin twice daily; rub in gently and completely.
		Calcitriol	Topical	Ointment	Apply twice daily to affected areas.

Table 11-2 (*continued*)

Class	Indication	Generic	Route	Dosage Forms	Dosing Regimen
Keratolytic agents	Mild to moderate psoriasis, often used as adjunctive agents	Salicylic acid (2–10%)	Topical	Cream, lotion, shampoo, foam, available OTC	Cream/lotion: apply to affected area three to four times daily Ointment: apply to affected area up to four times daily. Shampoo: massage into wet hair or affected area; leave in place for several minutes; rinse thoroughly as directed by healthcare provider. Foam: rub into affected area twice daily.
		Coal tar	Topical	Lotion, cream, shampoo, ointment, gel, solution, available OTC	Shampoo, rub liberally onto wet hair and scalp, leave on for several minutes rinse thoroughly. Repeat and rinse. Bath products, soak 10–20 minutes and then pat dry.
		Anthralin	Topical	Cream, ointment, paste (must be compounded)	Apply once daily for 5–10 minutes. Gradually increase contact time to 20–30 minutes as tolerated. Avoid applying excessive quantities.
		Tazarotene	Topical	Cream, gel	Apply to affected area once daily in the evening.
Oral agents	Moderate to severe psoriasis	Acitretin	Oral	Capsule	25–50 mg once daily. Take with food. Maximum dose: 75 mg daily.
		Methotrexate	Oral, intra-muscular	Tablet, solution	Oral: 2.5–5 mg every 12 hours three times per week or 10–25 mg once week. IM: 10–25 mg once weekly. Lifetime maximum recommended cumulative dose: 2.2 g.
		Cyclosporine	Oral	Capsule	Initial dose: 2.5 mg/kg/day, divided twice daily. Titrate every 2 weeks to if needed (maximum dose: 4 mg/kg/day).
Biologic agents	Moderate to severe chronic plaque psoriasis	Alefacept (CD2-binding monoclonal antibody)	Intra-muscular	Solution reconstituted	15 mg once weekly × 12 weeks
	Moderate to severe chronic plaque psoriasis and psoriatic arthritis	Etanercept (TNF-alpha receptor blocker)	Subcu-taneous	Solution	50 mg twice weekly, 3–4 days apart, × 12 weeks.
	Moderate to severe chronic plaque psoriasis and psoriatic arthritis	Adalimumab (TNF-alpha inhibitor)	Subcu-taneous	Solution	80 mg × 1, then 40 mg every other week starting 1 week after initial dose.
	Moderate to severe chronic plaque psoriasis and psoriatic arthritis	Infliximab (TNF-alpha inhibitor)	Intra-venous	Solution	5 mg/kg at 0, 2, and 6 weeks, then every 8 weeks.
	Moderate to severe chronic plaque psoriasis	Ustekinumab (Interleukin 12–23 inhibitor)	Subcu-taneous	Solution	Weight ≤ 100 kg: 45 mg at 0 and 4 weeks, then every 12 weeks. Weight > 100 kg: 45 mg or 90 mg at 0 and 4 weeks, then every 12 weeks.
Combination products		Calcipotriene and betamethasone	Topical	Cream, ointment	Apply once daily for up to 4 weeks. Do not apply to more than 30% of the total body surface area.
		Coal tar and salicylic acid	Topical	Shampoo	Shampoo: shake well, apply to wet hair for 5 minutes, rinse and repeat.

- Tazarotene: pregnancy, women of childbearing age unable to comply with birth control requirements
- Acitretin: patients who are pregnant or intend on becoming pregnant, ethanol ingestion, severe hepatic or renal dysfunction, chronically elevated blood lipid levels, concomitant use of methotrexate or tetracyclines, hypervitaminosis A
- Methotrexate: pregnancy, breastfeeding, alcoholism, alcoholic liver disease or other chronic liver disease, immunodeficiency syndrome, preexisting blood dyscrasias (i.e., thrombocytopenia)
- Cyclosporine: abnormal renal function, uncontrolled hypertension, malignancies; concomitant treatment with PUVA or UVB therapy, methotrexate, other immunosuppressive agents, coal tar, or radiation therapy
- Alefacept: HIV-positive patients

Warnings/Precautions

- Corticosteroids: HPA-axis suppression
- Calcipotriene, coal tar: application to abraded skin, excessive exposure to natural or artificial sunlight, phototherapy
- Tazarotene: safety and efficacy have not been established in children younger than 12 years of age, photosensitivity
- Biological response modifiers: infections, tuberculosis, malignancy, heart failure (TNF-alpha blockers)
- Methotrexate: renal failure, diarrhea/stomatitis, dermatologic reactions
- Cyclosporine: nephrotoxicity, infections
- Acitretin: blood donation (do not donate blood during therapy or for 3 years following therapy)

Biopharmaceutical Principles and Pharmaceutical Characteristics of Dosage Forms

Ointments are preferred for psoriasis lesions because the occlusive nature of ointments moistens the skin, thereby softening scales for their removal and improving drug penetration. Lotions and creams may be easier to spread onto areas with hair, but may be more drying. Foams have been noted to achieve better drug penetration than creams and lotions and have cosmetic properties that may be more acceptable to patients. Gel formulations are also easy to spread on hairy areas, but are more drying and may cause additional irritation in the presence of dry or abraded skin.

1.3.0 Monitoring

Pharmacotherapeutic Outcomes

The goal of drug therapy is to effect resolution of lesions using regimens of the lowest potency and highest patient acceptability. Avoiding toxicity and choosing regimens that will increase patient compliance are essential.

Safety and Efficacy Monitoring

Reduction in plaque size, redness, scaling, and elevation indicates a positive response to treatment. Treatment may take as long as 2 to 6 weeks to achieve a response, though some patients never achieve a complete response to treatment. In addition to lesion improvement, it is essential to assess improvements in quality of life and other comorbidities. For all treatments, monitor for adverse effects and compliance.

- Acitretin: lipid profile, liver function tests, blood glucose in patients with diabetes
- Methotrexate: CBC with differential and platelets, BUN and serum creatinine, liver function tests (liver biopsy is recommended when the patient reaches a cumulative dose of 1.5 g), baseline chest x-ray, consider PPD for latent TB screening at baseline
- Cyclosporine: blood pressure, serum creatinine, BUN, CBC, serum magnesium, potassium, uric acid, and lipid profile
- Alefacept: CD4+ counts
- TNF-alpha blockers: LFTs, PPD prior to initiating therapy, signs of infection, CBC, vital signs during infusion (infliximab)
- Ustekinumab: PPD prior to initiating therapy, signs/symptoms of infection, CBC
- Phototherapy and photochemotherapy: skin toxicity, nausea, dizziness, headaches, lethargy, basal cell carcinoma, melanoma

Adverse Drug Reactions

- Corticosteroids: skin thinning, telangiectasias, acne, striae, tachyphylaxis, reactivation of psoriasis upon discontinuation (mostly with high-potency agents or long-term use)
- Vitamin D analogs: burning, itching, rash, skin irritation, stinging, tingling, worsening of psoriasis
- Coal tar: burning, stinging, foul-smelling odor, staining of bedding and clothing, photosensitivity
- Anthralin: staining of skin, hair, fingernails, and clothing (wear gloves to apply); skin irritation (apply zinc oxide around lesions to avoid contact with noninfected skin)
- Tazarotene: burning, stinging, desquamation, dry skin, erythema, pruritus, skin pain, worsening of psoriasis
- Acitretin: depression, hepatotoxicity, lipid effects, electrolyte abnormalities, hyperglycemia, decreased hemoglobin and white blood cell counts, photosensitivity, visual disturbances, paresthesia, bone loss (long-term use), hypervitaminosis A (dry lips, mouth, eyes, skin)

Table 11-3 Pharmacotherapeutic Alternatives

Generic	Brand Name	Dosage
Mycophenolate mofetil	Myfortic, CellCept	500 mg orally four times a day, up to a maximum of 4 g/day
Sulfasalazine	Azulfidine, Azulfidine, EN-tabs	3 to 4 g orally daily for 8 weeks
6-Thioguanine	Tabloid	80 mg twice weekly, increased by 20 mg every 2 to 4 weeks; maximum of 160 mg three times per week
Hydroxyurea	Droxia, Hydrea	1 g orally daily, with gradual increase to 2 g/day as needed
Tacrolimus	Prograf, Protopic	0.05 mg/kg orally per day, increased up to 0.15 mg/kg/day as needed

- Methotrexate: nausea, vomiting, diarrhea, mucosal ulceration, leucopenia, thrombocytopenia, dizziness, hepatotoxicity, pulmonary toxicity
- Cyclosporine: hypertension, edema, headache, nausea, tremor, nephrotoxicity, increased potassium, decreased magnesium, elevated lipids, malignancy (use for more than 2 years)
- Alefacept: lymphopenia, malaise, fever, myalgia, pharyngitis, cough, injection site reactions
- Adalimumab, infliximab, etanercept: headache, nausea, diarrhea, upper respiratory tract infections, fatigue, fever, infusion reactions (infliximab—may premedicate with antihistamines, acetaminophen, and/or corticosteroids), hepatotoxicity (infliximab), ocular toxicity (infliximab)
- Ustekinumab: infection, headache, fatigue

Nonadherence, Misuse, or Abuse

Patient counseling should emphasize adherence to medication regimens to ensure they achieve their intended efficacy during the treatment period. Adherence to birth control regimens is essential in women with childbearing potential who are using agents that may be teratogenic.

Pharmacotherapeutic Alternatives

Alternative pharmacotherapeutic options for psoriasis include mycophenolate mofetil, sulfasalazine, 6-thioguanine, hydroxyurea, and tacrolimus. These agents have immunosuppressive effects and are used as add-on or alternative therapy to the preferred treatment regimens.

2.2.0 Dispensing

See Table 11-4.

Table 11-4 Drugs for Psoriasis: Generic Names, Brand Names, and Dosage Form Availability

Generic	Brand Name	Dosage Forms
Augmented betamethasone dipropionate	Diprolene	Ointment, gel, lotion
Clobetasol proprionate	Cormax, Embeline, Embeline E, Temovate, Olux, Clobex, Clobevate	Cream, ointment, gel, foam, lotion, shampoo, scalp application, spray
Fluocinonide	Vanos	Cream
Halobetasol propionate	Ultravate	Cream, ointment
Augmented betamethasone dipropionate	Diprolene AF	Cream
Betamethasone dipropionate	Diprosone	Ointment, cream
Betamethasone valerate		Ointment
Desoximetasone	Topicort	Cream, ointment, gel
Diflorasone diacetate	ApexiCon E, Florone, Psorcon E	Cream
Fluocinonid	Lidex, Lidex-E	Cream, ointment, gel, solution
Halcinonide	Halog	Cream, ointment, solution
Betamethasone dipropionate		Lotion
Betamethasone valerate	Beta-Val	Cream, lotion
Desoximetasone	Topicort LP	Cream
Fluticasone propionate	Cutivate	Cream, ointment
Hydrocortisone butyrate	Locoid, Locoid lipocream	Cream, ointment, solution
Hydrocortisone valerate	Westcort	Cream, ointment

(*continues*)

Table 11-4 (*continued*)

Generic	Brand Name	Dosage Forms
Mometasone furoate	Elocon	Cream, ointment, lotion
Triamcinolone acetonide	Kenalog	Cream, ointment, lotion
Alclometasone diproprionate	Aclovate	Cream, ointment
Desonide	DesOwen, Tridesilon, Verdeso	Cream, ointment, lotion, foam
Fluocinolone acetonide	Synalar, Capex	Shampoo, solution, cream
Hydrocortisone	Ala-Cort, Hydrocortone Phosphate, Solu-Cortef, Hydrocort Acetate, Lanacort, Valerate, Acetate, Probutate, Butyrate	Cream, ointment, lotion, solution
Calcipotriene	Dovonex	Ointment, cream, solution
Calcitriol	Vectical	Ointment
Salicylic acid	Dermarest, Salvax, Akurza, Salitop, Keralyt, Salex	Cream, lotion, shampoo, foam
Coal tar	Ionil, DHS Tar, Denorex, Neutrogena T/Gel	Lotion, cream, shampoo, ointment, gel, solution
Anthralin	Dritho-Scalp	Cream, ointment, paste (must be compounded)
Tazarotene	Tazorac	Cream, gel
Acitretin	Soriatane	Capsule
Methotrexate	Rheumatrex, Trexall	Tablet, solution
Cyclosporine	Gengraf, Neoral	Capsule
Alefacept	Amevive	Solution
Etanercept	Enbrel	Solution
Adalimumab	Humira	Solution
Infliximab	Remicade	Solution
Ustekinumab	Stelara	Solution
Calcipotriene and betamethasone	Taclonex	Cream, ointment
Salicylic acid and coal tar	Tarsum, X-Seb T	Gel, solution

ANNOTATED BIBLIOGRAPHY

Goeser AL. Common skin disorders. In: Chisholm-Burns MA, Wells BG, Schwinghammer TL, et al., eds. *Pharmacotherapy: Principles and Practice*. 2nd ed. New York: McGraw-Hill; 2010:1079–1091.

Lexi-Comp Online. Lexi-Drugs Online., Hudson, OH: Lexi-Comp, Inc.; 2010. Accessed May 22, 2010.

Micromedex Healthcare Series. Greenwood Village, CO: Thomson Reuters (Healthcare) Inc.; updated periodically. Available at http://www.thomsonhc /com/hcs/librarian. Accessed May 22, 2010.

National Psoriasis Foundation. Available at: http://www.psoriasis.org. Accessed May 22, 2010.

West DP, Loyd A, Bauer KA, West LE, Scuderi L, Micali G. Psoriasis. In: DiPiro JT, Tabert RL, Yee GC, et al., eds. *Pharmacotherapy: A Pathophysiologic Approach*. 7th ed. New York: McGraw-Hill; 2008:1603–1617.

TOPIC: ACNE

Contributor: *Laura Perry*

Tips Worth Tweeting

- Acne is a common skin disorder that results from plugging of the pilosebaceous unit of the skin.
- Acne is not a disorder of poor hygiene.
- Acne is most commonly caused by excessive androgen production, leading to increased sebum production, abnormal keratinization, bacterial colonization, and inflammation.
- It is important to tell patients that it is normal to see worsening of acne during the first few weeks of topical acne treatment.

- Treatment should be continued for 6 to 8 weeks for maximal benefit.

Patient Care Scenario: Ambulatory Setting

R. M., a 16-year-old female, complains of worsening acne. It appears she has numerous open comedos and closed comedos on her nose and cheeks. She states she has had acne for a few years, but that it has been worsening over the past 6 months or so, and she is embarrassed at school because of the way her face looks. Although she has acne, R. M. complains that her skin gets very dry in the winter. Aside from her acne, she is otherwise healthy and plays on the varsity girls basketball team at her high school.

Date	Physician	Drug	Quantity	Sig	Refills
3/4	Smith	Triaz 3%	#170.3	apply in A.M.	5 refills
2/28	Cole	Yaz	#28	one po daily	6 refills
11/4	Fox	Augmentin 875 mg	#20	one po bid	0 refills

1.1.0 Patient Information

Medication-Induced Causes of Acne

Acneiform eruptions: adrenocorticotropic hormone, anabolic steroids, azathioprine, danazol, glucocorticoids, halogens (iodides, bromides), isoniazid, lithium, oral contraceptives

Laboratory Testing

There are no laboratory tests available to diagnose acne. Diagnosis is based on clinical signs and symptoms.

Disease States Associated with Acne

- Hormonal influences: androgen excess (puberty)
- Bacteria: Propionibacterium acnes

Instruments and Techniques Related to Patient Assessment

Patient assessment techniques include evaluating the type, number, and distribution of lesions.

- Comedonal or noninflammatory lesions: open comedos ("blackheads"), closed comedos ("whiteheads")
- Inflammatory lesions: papules, pustules, nodules

Terminology Used in the Classification of Acne

The classification of acne is based on lesion type and severity. When determining the severity of acne, the type of lesion should take precedence over the number of lesions. Acne is classified as mild, moderate, or severe.

Signs and Symptoms of Acne

Acne lesions generally appear on the face, but may also be present on the chest, back, and upper arms. Various types of lesions may be present, including both noninflammatory and inflammatory lesions. Inflammatory lesions are typically erythematous and may cause mild discomfort, hyperpigmentation, or scarring.

Wellness and Prevention

Twice-daily facial cleansing with warm water and a gentle, nondrying facial cleanser is preferred. Abrasive cleansers and aggressive washing have not been shown to open or cleanse clogged pores and, in fact, may cause trauma to the skin. Additionally, discourage squeezing or picking at lesions, as this practice may lead to scarring. Use of oil-free moisturizers with or without sunscreen is recommended to improve skin hydration and drug penetration. Avoiding or limiting exposure to dirt, dust, cooking oils, chemical irritants, and oil-based cosmetics or shampoos will also help reduce the occurrence of acne. Warm, humid weather; hats; headbands; and helmets may also precipitate acne.

Table 11-5 Classification of Acne Severity

Severity	Description
Mild (comedonal)	Few to numerous noninflammatory lesions (fewer than 20 lesions) Possible inflammatory lesions (fewer than 15 lesions) No scarring
Moderate (papular and/or pustular)	Few to numerous noninflammatory lesions (20–100 lesions) Numerous inflammatory lesions (30–125 lesions), few nodules Possible scarring
Severe (persistent pustulocystic)	Few to numerous noninflammatory lesions (more than 100 lesions) Extensive inflammatory lesions (more than 50 lesions), including nodules (more than 5 lesions) Extensive scarring

1.2.0 Pharmacotherapy

Treatments for Acne

Treatment of mild to moderate comedonal acne involves single-agent topical therapy with a topical retinoid, benzoyl peroxide, a topical antibiotic, or azelaic acid.

Moderate to severe inflammatory acne requires a combination of topical agents with different mechanisms of action, with or without oral antibiotics. Benzoyl peroxide is both comedolytic and bactericidal, but does not provide an anti-inflammatory effect. Topical retinoids, by comparison, are comedolytic and have anti-inflammatory properties, but are not bactericidal. A common regimen for moderate to severe inflammatory acne involves the application of a topical retinoid in the morning and the application of benzoyl peroxide in the evening. The combination of topical retinoids with benzoyl peroxide provides for a synergistic effect, increasing the efficacy of both agents. Another effective combination used involves a topical antibiotic with benzoyl peroxide; this particular combination also increases the effectiveness of both agents and decreases bacterial resistance. When combination topical treatment is ineffective, an oral antibiotic may be added to the regimen. Topical azelaic acid is used for its anti-inflammatory effects and keratinocyte stabilization.

Severe nodulocystic acne unresponsive to topical agents and oral antibiotics may be treated with oral isotretinoin. Oral isotretinoin works on all four pathologic factors involved in acne—that is, it decreases sebum production, decreases keratinocyte sloughing, decreases bacterial growth, and decreases inflammation.

Interaction of Drugs with Foods and Laboratory Tests

Dairy products and calcium- or magnesium-containing products may decrease absorption of oral tetracyclines (e.g., doxycycline, tetracycline, minocycline). Oral tetracyclines should be administered on an empty stomach and at least 1 to 2 hours prior to, or 4 hours after, antacids. Drug interactions may also potentially occur when administering erythromycin with other agents undergoing hepatic metabolism by CYP 3A4.

Oral isotretinoin may decrease the effects of oral contraceptives. It is recommended that females with childbearing potential use two forms of contraception while on oral isotretinoin. Isotretinoin may also

Table 11-6 Drugs for Acne: Indications, Dosing, Dosage Forms, and Routes of Administration

Class	Indication	Drug	Route	Dosage Forms	Dosing Regimen
Topical agents (miscellaneous)	Mild, noninflammatory acne	Benzoyl peroxide	Topical	Cleanser, cream, foam, gel, liquid, lotion, pad, soap, wash	Apply sparingly once daily. Dose may be increased gradually to two to three times per day until the desired effect is achieved.
	Mild to moderate inflammatory acne	Azelaic acid	Topical	Cream, gel	Gently massage a thin film into the affected areas twice daily (morning and evening).
Retinoids	Mild to moderate non-inflammatory and inflammatory acne	Tretinoin	Topical	Cream, gel	Apply once daily to acne lesions.
		Adapalene	Topical	Cream, gel	Apply once daily before bedtime.
		Tazarotene	Topical	Cream, gel	Apply a thin film once daily (evening).
	Severe nodulocystic acne unresponsive to other topical and oral therapies	Isotretinoin	Oral	Capsule	0.5–1 mg/kg/day in two divided doses.
Antibacterials	Topical: mild to moderate inflammatory acne Oral: moderate to severe acne when topical therapies have failed	Clindamycin	Topical, oral	Gel, lotion, solution, capsule	Topical: apply once daily. Oral: 75–150 mg twice daily.
		Erythromycin	Topical, oral	Gel, ointment, solution, tablet, suspension, capsule	Topical: apply twice daily. Oral: 250–500 mg twice daily.
		Dapsone	Topical	Gel	Apply a thin layer to affected areas twice daily.
		Doxycycline	Oral	Capsule	100 mg twice daily.
		Minocycline	Oral	Capsule	100 mg daily or 50 mg twice daily.
		Tetracycline	Oral	Capsule	500 mg twice daily.

increase the risk of vitamin A toxicity, so it is important to avoid excessive vitamin A intake.

Contraindications, Warnings, and Precautions

Oral tetracyclines are contraindicated in pregnancy and in children younger than 8 years of age. Clindamycin (oral) may be associated with pseudomembranous colitis. Oral tetracyclines and topical retinoids may cause photosensitivity; patients using these medications should avoid sunlamps and excessive sun exposure. Topical retinoids must be used with caution in patients with eczema and in irritated, abraded, or sunburned skin. The safety and efficacy of topical retinoids, azelaic acid, and oral isotretinoin have not been established in children younger than 12 years of age. All individuals receiving oral isotretinoin must register with the iPLEDGE program.

Physiochemical Properties, Pharmacodynamics, and Pharmacokinetics

Minimal systemic absorption occurs with topical drug administration on intact skin. Benzoyl peroxide gel is better absorbed than cream.

Biopharmaceutical Principles and Pharmaceutical Characteristics of Dosage Forms

The choice of topical formulation should be based on skin type:

- Oily to normal skin types: gels, solutions, and lotions
- Normal skin: gels, solutions, lotions, and creams
- Normal to dry skin: lotions and creams
- Ointments are not used (may provoke acne)

Caution should be used with gel formulations, as they are more drying and may cause additional irritation in the presence of dry or abraded skin. Lotions and creams provide moisture, thereby enhancing drug absorption in dry skin.

1.3.0 Monitoring

Pharmacotherapeutic Outcomes

Treatment goals include clearance of acne, prevention of scarring, and coping with psychological stress related to acne and its resultant scarring. Most therapeutic interventions function to prevent the formation of new acne and have minimal impact on existing lesions.

Safety and Efficacy Monitoring

Improvement of symptoms with acne treatment occurs gradually, sometimes taking 6 to 8 weeks to become apparent. Changes in therapy should occur no sooner than every 6 to 8 weeks to allow for an adequate trial. Lesions may worsen in the first 2 to 3 weeks of treatment, especially with topical retinoid therapy. Laboratory monitoring for oral isotretinoin includes a complete blood count with differential and platelet count, baseline sedimentation rate, serum triglycerides, and liver enzymes. All females must also have two negative pregnancy tests prior to beginning oral isotretinoin therapy and then be tested monthly thereafter to rule out pregnancy prior to future prescriptions.

Adverse Drug Reactions

- Topical agents: skin irritation, contact dermatitis, dryness, erythema, peeling, stinging
- Products containing benzoyl peroxide: staining of clothing, bed linens, and hair
- Oral tetracyclines: stomach upset, photosensitivity
- Clindamycin: stomach upset, pseudomembranous colitis
- Erythromycin: stomach upset, diarrhea
- Isotretinoin: teratogenic; dry skin, nose, mouth, and eyes (approximately 90% of patients); peeling skin; itching; photosensitivity; increased triglycerides; increased blood glucose; muscle pain; depression

Nonadherence, Misuse, or Abuse

Patient counseling should emphasize adherence to medication regimens to ensure efficacy during the 6- to 8-week treatment period.

Pharmacotherapeutic Alternatives

Alternative pharmacotherapeutic options for acne include estrogen, progesterone, and aldosterone antagonists. These agents have antiandrogenic activity and are used as add-on therapy to the preferred treatment regimens.

Table 11-7 Pharmacotherapeutic Alternatives

Generic	Brand Name	Dosage
Ethinyl estradiol	Various	20–50 mcg po daily
Norgestimate ethinyl estradiol	Ortho-Cyclen, Ortho Tri-Cyclen, Tri-Sprintec, TriNessa, MonoNessa	0.18–0.35 mg po daily
Norethindrone	Aygestin, Ortho Micronor	0.35 mg po daily
Drosperinone	Yazmin, Yaz	3 mg po daily
Spironolactone	Aldactone	50–200 mg po daily

2.2.0 Dispensing

Table 11-8 Drugs for Acne: Generic Names, Brand Names, and Dosage Form Availability

Generic	Brand Name	Dosage Forms
Benzoyl peroxide	Benzagel, Benzac AC, BenzaShave, BenzEFoam, Benziq, Brevoxyl, PanOxyl, Triaz	Cleanser, cream, foam, gel, liquid, lotion, pad, soap, wash
Azelaic acid	Azelex, Finacea, Finacea Plus	Cream, gel
Tretinoin	Atralin, Avita, Refissa, Renova, Retin-A, Retin-A Micro, Tretin-X	Cream, gel
Adapalene	Differin, Differin XP	Cream, gel
Tazarotene	Avage, Tazorac	Cream, gel
Isotretinoin	Amnesteen, Claravis, Sotret	Capsule
Clindamycin	Cleocin HCl, Cleocyin Phosphate, Cleocin T, ClindaMax, Clindagel	Capsule, gel, lotion, pledget, solution
Erythromycin	Akne-Mycin, E.E.S., Ery-Tab, Erythro-RX, Erythrocin, Romycin	Tablet, suspension, capsule, gel, ointment, solution
Dapsone	Aczone	Gel
Doxycycline	Vibramycin	Capsule
Minocycline	Dynacin, Minocin, Solodyn	Capsule
Tetracycline		Capsule

ANNOTATED BIBLIOGRAPHY

Goeser AL. Common skin disorders. In: Chisholm-Burns MA, Wells BG, Schwinghammer TL, et al., eds. *Pharmacotherapy: Principles and Practice.* New York: McGraw-Hill; 2008:959–973.

Lexi-Comp Online. Lexi-Drugs Online. Hudson, OH: Lexi-Comp, Inc.; 2010. Accessed March 4, 2010.

Micromedex Healthcare Series. Greenwood Village, CO: Thomson Reuters (Healthcare) Inc.; updated periodically. Available at: http://www.thomsonhc.com/hcs/librarian. Accessed March 4, 2010.

West DP, Loyd A, Bauer KA, West LE, Scuderi L, Micali G. Acne vulgaris. In: DiPiro JT, Tabert RL, Yee GC, et al., eds. *Pharmacotherapy: A Pathophysiologic Approach.* 7th ed. New York: McGraw-Hill; 2008: 1591–1602.

Endocrine Disorders

CHAPTER 12

TOPIC: DIABETES

Section Coordinator: Debra Parker
Contributor: Debra Parker

Diabetes Overview

Diabetes is an extremely common metabolic disorder for which pharmacotherapy plays an integral role. Given the existence of nine different medication classes to treat this disease, the necessary patient education and self-monitoring, and the common need for medication adjustments, the pharmacist plays an integral role in the management of this condition.

Tips Worth Tweeting

- Diabetes is a disease affecting metabolism of not only carbohydrates, but also protein and lipids.
- Type 1 diabetes accounts for 5% to 10% of all diabetes cases. It is caused by an absolute insulin deficiency, and its treatment requires insulin; pramlintide may or may not be used as well.
- Type 2 diabetes accounts for more than 90% of all diabetes cases. It is caused by a relative insulin deficiency coupled with insulin resistance. Treatment consists of diet, exercise, and pharmacotherapy, which may or may not include insulin.
- C-peptide levels are indicative of endogenous insulin production.
- The best prevention for type 2 diabetes is diet and exercise, followed by use of metformin.
- Cardinal signs and symptoms of diabetes include polyphagia, polyuria, and polydypsia.
- Nine classes of medications for diabetes exist: (1) sulfonylureas; (2) meglitinides—sulfonylureas and meglitinides are commonly referred to, collectively, as "secretagogues"; (3) biguanides; (4) alpha-glucosidase inhibitors; (5) thiazolidinediones; (6) insulin; (7) incretin mimetics; (8) amylinomimetics; and (9) dipeptidyl peptidase IV inhibitors.
- With the exception of regular (R) insulin and NPH (N) insulin, all classes of diabetes drugs are available by prescription only.
- Acute complications of diabetes may include diabetic ketoacidosis (DKA) in type 1 diabetes and hyperglycemic hyperosmolar syndrome (HHS) in type 2 diabetes.
- Long-term complications of diabetes may be macrovascular (e.g., coronary heart disease, carotid artery disease, peripheral arterial disease) or microvascular (e.g., retinopathy, neuropathy, nephropathy) in nature.

Patient Care Scenario: Ambulatory Setting

57 y/o, 5'3", F, Hispanic, 165 lbs, no known allergies
PMH: DM2 × 10 years, HTN, CAD s/p CABG

Medication Profile

Date	Physician	Drug	Quantity	Sig	Refills
3/2	Lehman	Metformin 1,000 mg	60	1 po bid	11
3/2	Lehman	Actos 30 mg	30	1 po daily	7
3/2	Lehman	Amaryl 4 mg	60	1 po bid	7
4/1	Lehman	Lipitor 40 mg	30	1 po daily	6
4/1	Lehman	Zetia 10 mg	30	1 po daily	6
3/15	Lehman	Metoprolol succinate 50 mg	30	1 po daily	8

Lab Values: A_{1c} 7.8%, BUN 18 mg/dL, SCr 1.6 mg/dL, TC 197 mg/dL, TG 203 mg/dL, HDL 34 mg/dL, LDL 122 mg/dL, AST 21 IU/L, ALT 14 IU/L
Vitals: BP 138/86 mm Hg, HR 72
Over-the-Counter Medications: Occasional acetaminophen.
Social: Denies tobacco use; occasional alcohol.
Notes: 3/2 Discussed signs, symptoms, and appropriate treatment of hypoglycemia.

1.1.0 Patient Information

Definition

Diabetes is a metabolic disorder characterized by hyperglycemia as well as abnormalities in lipid and protein metabolism. Patients may have an absolute lack of insulin (type 1 diabetes) or a combination of a relative insulin deficiency and insulin resistance (type 2 diabetes). Diabetes is characterized by abnormalities in the counter-regulatory hormones glucagon, epinephrine, norepinephrine growth hormone, and cortisol. It currently affects more than 24 million people in the United States, and its incidence on the rise.

Insulin is released from pancreatic beta cells in the islets of Langerhans in response to rising blood glucose. Table 12-1 highlights the role of insulin in normal carbohydrate, fat, and protein metabolism.

Diabetic patients are at a much higher risk for cardiovascular disease. Hyperglycemia itself is rarely a cause of death; instead, diabetes-related mortality is most often due to cardiovascular complications.

Key Terms

- Two main types of **diabetes mellitus**: type 1 (DM1) and type 2 (DM2)
- Other types of diabetes:

Table 12-1 Role of Insulin in Carbohydrate, Fat, and Protein Metabolism

Insulin Promotes	Insulin Inhibits
Fat storage (lipogenesis)	Fat mobilization for energy (lipolysis and ketogenesis)
Liver and muscle storage of glucose as glycogen (glycogenesis)	Glucose release from the liver and muscle (glycogenolysis)
	Glucose formation from amino acids (gluconeogenesis)

  - **Gestational diabetes**: onset of diabetes during pregnancy, which may or may not resolve postpartum; major fetal concern is macrosomia (abnormally large fetal body size); occurs in approximately 7% of all pregnancies
  - **Diabetes insipidus**: not related to diabetes mellitus; is due to a deficiency in antidiuretic hormone (ADH; also known as vasopressin)
- **Diabetic ketoacidosis (DKA)**: severe insulin deficiency in which cells are unable to take up glucose, so proteins and lipids are metabolized as alternative energy sources. Free fatty acids (FFAs) and ketone bodies are formed as by-products of lipolysis; accumulation of ketone bodies leads to metabolic acidosis. Kussmaul respirations (deep and rapid) are a compensatory method to correct the acidosis. Treatment requires insulin, fluid, and electrolyte management.

Table 12-2 Comparison of Type 1 and Type 2 Diabetes

Type 1 Diabetes (DM1)	Type 2 Diabetes (DM2)
Formerly known as juvenile diabetes or insulin-dependent diabetes mellitus (IDDM)	*Formerly* known as adult-onset diabetes or non-insulin-dependent diabetes mellitus (NIDDM)
10% of people with diabetes	90% of people with diabetes
May start at any age (usually before age 30)	Usually starts after age 30
Rapid symptom onset; moderate to severe symptoms	Insidious onset
Usually thin or lean	75% of patients are obese
Inability to produce insulin (caused by destruction of insulin-producing cells)	Caused by insulin resistance or a *relatively* low amount of insulin (may produce insulin, but not enough)
Most likely severe complication of high blood glucose: diabetic ketoacidosis	Most likely severe complication of high blood glucose: hyperglycemic hyperosmolar syndrome

Table 12-3 Diagnosis of Diabetes*

	Fasting Blood Glucose (FBG)	2 Hours after OGTT
Normal	< 100 mg/dL	> 140 mg/dL
IFG	100–125 mg/dL	N/A
IGT	N/A	140–199 mg/dL
Diabetes	≥ 126 mg/dL	≥ 200 mg/dL

*Diabetes may also be diagnosed by an A_{1c} ≥ 6.5% or any blood glucose reading taken without regard to last caloric intake. If the result is greater than 200 mg/dL and the patient has signs and symptoms of DM, this finding is also diagnostic.

- **Hyperglycemic hyperosmolar syndrome (HHS)**: extreme hyperglycemia, osmotic diuresis, dehydration, and electrolyte abnormalities. Ketone bodies are not formed, as some insulin is still present. Treatment requires fluid replacement with or without insulin.

Signs and Symptoms

The cardinal signs and symptoms of diabetes are polyuria, polyphagia, and polydypsia. Others may include fatigue, dry/itchy skin, nonhealing skin infections, blurred vision, and tingling or numbness in hands or feet.

Diagnosis

Diagnosis of diabetes is based on blood tests. Tests may be performed (1) while the patient is fasting (no caloric intake for 8 or more hours), (2) 2 hours after ingestion of 75 g glucose (known as the oral glucose tolerance test [OGTT]), or (3) without regard to last caloric intake using techniques related to patient assessment (known as a "casual" or "random" blood glucose).

Table 12-4 Risk Factors for Type 2 Diabetes

Physical inactivity	Hypertensive (BP > 140/90 mm Hg or on hypertension medications)	History of IGT or IFG on previous testing	Other clinical conditions associated with insulin resistance (e.g., acanthosis nigricans, severe obesity)
High-risk ethnic population*	HDL-C < 35 mg/dL and/or TG > 250 mg/dL	History of GDM or delivery of a baby weighing more than 9 lb	
First-degree relative with diabetes	History of cardiovascular disease	Polycystic ovary syndrome (PCOS)	

* High-risk ethnicities: African American, Latino, Native American, Asian American, Pacific Islander.

Distinguishing Characteristics

Levels of C-peptide (an amino acid chain cleaved during the conversion of pro-insulin to insulin) may be negligible to absent at time of diagnosis of DM1, but may be normal to high at the time of DM2 diagnosis. Routine measurement is not recommended, but such tests may be used to determine whether endogenous insulin is still being produced by a patient with DM2.

Patients with diabetes monitor their own blood glucose with a portable blood glucose machine and accompanying lancets and test strips to which blood is applied.

Risk Factors (Patient, Genetic, and Biosocial)

The cause of DM1 is unknown. Table 12-4 summarizes risk factors for DM2.

Wellness and Prevention

- Type 1 diabetes: Cause of DM1 is unknown. No preventive measures have been identified.
- Type 2 diabetes: Genetic predisposition plays a role in disease development, but diet, exercise, and maintenance of normal body weight have been shown to be *the* most effective way to prevent diabetes. Metformin has also been shown to delay or prevent onset of diabetes in high-risk individuals (e.g., women with a history of gestational diabetes).

Complications

If prevention of disease onset is not possible, prevention of complications is of utmost important. The most common cause of death related to diabetes is cardiovascular complications. Diabetes is also the leading cause of nontraumatic amputations, blindness, and end-stage kidney disease in the United States.

Pneumococcal vaccination and annual influenza vaccination are recommended to decrease mortality associated with these diseases in diabetic patients.

Macrovascular Complications and Recommendations

- Coronary heart disease: Check lipids at least twice a year and check BP at every visit.
  - ACEIs or ARBs: First-line therapies, then diuretics (thiazide diuretics—not loop diuretics—for hypertension control); very common for people to need 3 or more antihypertensives at the same time for adequate BP control
  - Lipids: Statins recommended for all DM2 patients without contraindications, regardless of baseline LDL
  - Smoking cessation

- Carotid artery disease: Check lipids at least twice a year and check BP at every visit.
  - Smoking cessation
- Peripheral arterial disease: Foot exams should take place *at every encounter* with a DM patient. Patients should be advised to examine feet daily.
  - Smoking cessation

Clinical trials suggest decreases in incidence of macrovascular complications can be achieved with glycemic control coupled with control of other cardiovascular risk factors (e.g., hypertension and hyperlipidemia).

Microvascular Complications

- Nephropathy/microalbuminuria: For DM2, urine screening at time of diagnosis is a must; it should be repeated at least annually. ACEIs and ARBs (especially for DM2 patients) have been shown to decrease diabetic nephropathy.
- Neuropathy: May be peripheral (stocking and glove presentation) or central (e.g., gastroparesis, orthostatic hypotension).
- Retinopathy: An annual dilated eye exam is a must. Nothing reverses retinopathy, but laser photocoagulation (laser eye surgery) can "nip damage in the bud" before it progresses. The key is catching it early (hence the annual eye exam).

Every 1% decrease in the A_{1c} level may decrease microvascular complications approximately 20%.

1.2.0 Pharmacotherapy

Pharmacotherapy

Nine medication classes are used to lower blood glucose:

- Sulfonylureas (SURs)
- Meglitinides (sulfonylureas and meglitinides—commonly referred to collectively as secretagogues)
- Biguanides

Table 12-5 American Diabetes Association's Therapeutic Goals

A_{1c}	< 7%	
Blood pressure	≤ 130 mm Hg/≤80 mm Hg	
Urine microalbumin: Cr ratio	< 30 (mg/g)	
Lipids (mg/dL)	LDL	< 100
	HDL	Men, > 40 men; women, > 50
	TG	< 150
	Total cholesterol	< 200

- Alpha-glucosidase inhibitors (AGIs)
- Thiazolidinediones (TZDs)
- Insulin
- Incretin mimetics
- Amylinomimetics
- Dipeptidyl peptidase IV inhibitors

With the exception of regular (R) insulin and NPH (N) insulin, all of these drug classes are available by prescription only.

Hypoglycemia

Patients taking insulin or any other antidiabetic agent that may cause hypoglycemia should know the signs and symptoms of hypoglycemia (tachycardia, shakiness, agitation, and diaphoresis) and the appropriate treatment (15 g of carbohydrates and recheck blood glucose in 15 minutes). A source of carbohydrates should be carried at all times.

Beta blockers may mask the symptoms of hypoglycemia. Patients taking these medications may be less likely to detect hypoglycemic episodes. Beta blockers are *not* contraindicated for patients; in fact, they are frequently utilized, as diabetic patients have a high incidence of cardiovascular disease.

Alcohol impairs gluconeogenesis. For this reason, even though alcoholic beverages contain carbohydrate calories, alcohol may increase the likelihood of hypoglycemia in patients taking antidiabetic medications.

Drug-Induced Hyperglycemia

The drugs listed in Table 12-6 are *not* contraindicated for patients with DM, but monitoring is necessary when they are used. These agents affect blood glucose and demonstrate a pharmacodynamic interaction with glucose-lowering agents. Note that the list in Table 12-6 is not all-inclusive.

General Treatment Approach

Treatment of DM1 absolutely requires insulin, which may or may not combine with pramlintide.

Treatment of DM2 is comprised of a three-pronged approach consisting of diet, exercise, and pharmacotherapy. Pharmacotherapy may or may not include insulin. General guidelines for sequential treatment of DM2 are shown in Table 12-7.

Combination products:

- Metaglip (metformin and glipizide) 2.5/500, 5/500
- Glucovance (glyburide and metformin) 1.25/250, 2.5/500, 5/500
- Duetact (glimepiride and pioglitazone) 30/2, 30/4
- Avandaryl (rosiglitazone and glimepiride) 4/1, 4/2, 4/4, 8/2, 8/4

Combination products: PrandiMet: 1/500, 2/500

Table 12-6 Drugs That May Induce Hyperglycemia

Atypical antipsychotics	Increase insulin resistance by altering receptor-binding characteristics
Beta blockers	Inhibit insulin secretion (especially nonselective agents)
Beta2 agonists	Increase glycogenolysis and lipolysis
Calcium-channel blockers	Inhibit insulin secretion due to inhibition of beta-cell cytosolic calcium
Corticosteroids	Cause peripheral insulin resistance and gluconeogenesis
Fluoroquinolones	Inhibit insulin secretion due to blockade of adenosine triphosphate (ATP)–sensitive potassium channels
Niacin	Increases insulin resistance due to increased free fatty acid mobilization
Phenothiazines	Inhibit insulin secretion
Protease inhibitors	Suppress conversion of proinsulin to insulin via calcium-dependent endopeptidases
Thiazide diuretics	• Inhibit insulin secretion due to hypokalemia • Increase insulin resistance due to free fatty acids

Combination products:

- Actoplus Met (pioglitazone and metformin) 15/500, 15/850
- Avandaryl (rosiglitazone and glimepiride) 4/1, 4/2, 4/4, 8/2, 8/4
- Avandamet (rosiglitazone and metformin) 2/500, 4/500, 2/1,000, 4/1,000

Combination insulins:

- Novolog Mix 70/30 (insulin aspart protamine and insulin aspart)
- Novolin 70/30 (insulin NPH and insulin regular)
- Humalog 75/25 (insulin lispro protamine and insulin lispro)
- Humulin 70/30 (insulin NPH and insulin regular)

Combination products: Janumet (sitagliptin and metformin) 50/500, 50/1,000

1.3.0 Monitoring

The effectiveness of pharmacotherapy is measured via hemoglobin A_{1c} (as often as every 3 months) and measured via patient self-monitoring of blood glucose. Changes in drug therapy should be based on trends and patterns of blood glucose control. Patients with DM2 are often advised to self-monitor blood glucose 2–3 times daily.

Table 12-7 Sequential Treatment for Type 2 Diabetes

Therapy		Drugs	Expected A_{1c} Reduction
1	Therapeutic lifestyle changes (TLC) x 2–3 months	None	
2	TLC and monotherapy with an oral agent or insulin	Met*, SFU, Meg	1–2%
3	TLC, add a second agent (other combinations are also acceptable)	Met + SFU/Meg†	1–3%
		SFU + AGI	0.5–1%
		SFU + TZD	1–1.8%
4	Insulin with an oral agent‡	Any (except AGI or rosiglitazone)	0.2–2.6%
5	Insulin	Insulin alone	2%

Note: The roles of newer agents (e.g., DPP-IV inhibitors and GLP-I analogues) are not yet well defined in the stepwise treatment approach. It is important to reassess the efficacy of any therapeutic lifestyle change or medication in 3 months.

AGI = alpha glucosidase inhibitor; Meg = meglitinide; Met = metformin; SFU = sulfonylurea; TZD = thiazolidinedione.

*Preferred first-line agent unless contraindicated. Has been demonstrated to decrease mortality by approximately 40%.

†Preferred combination when a second oral agent is added.

‡May be considered as second step in therapy if the desired A_{1c} reduction is more than achievable by adding a second oral agent.

2.1.0 Calculations

Creatinine Clearance

The method most often used for calculating creatinine clearance in adults is the Cockcroft-Gault formula:

$$\text{Male: } Cl_{cr} = ([140 - \text{age}] \times \text{weight}) \div (72 \times S_{cr})$$

$$\text{Female: } Cl_{cr}\ ([140 - \text{age}] \times \text{weight})\ (72 \times S_{cr}) \times 0.85$$

- Cl_{cr} = estimated creatinine clearance (mL/min)
- Weight = patient's weight (kg)
- S_{cr} = serum creatinine (mg/dL)

Limitations:

- Only an estimate of renal function
- Not useful if serum creatinine is rapidly changing or the patient is emaciated
- Other factors besides impaired renal function may cause increases in serum creatinine (e.g., dehydration, drug toxicity, exercise)
- May overestimate renal function in the very elderly as well as in obese patients

Table 12-8 Sulfonylureas

- A_{1c} reduction = 1.0–2.0%.
- Mechanism of action: Stimulates pancreatic beta cells to release insulin; binds to SUR1 subunits within the cell to block the ATP-sensitive K^+ channel.
- No difference between agents in terms of long-term efficacy/failure rates.
- First-generation sulfonylureas (chlorpropamide, tolbutamide, acetohexamide, tolazamide) are no longer used; they have longer half-lives (e.g., $t_{1/2}$ for chlorpropamide = 35 hours). A disulfiram-like reaction occurs with chlorpropamide.
- Possible, but *not* absolute cross-reactivity for patients with a "sulfa" allergy.
- Pharmacokinetic/pharmacodynamic considerations: All first-generation SURs are metabolized by the liver and renally excreted. Glipizide is metabolized to inactive metabolites and may be preferred for elderly patients or those with renal impairment.

Agent	Dose (mg) and Dosage Forms	Max/ Day	ADRs/ Warnings/ Precautions	Contraindications	Drug Interactions	Food Considerations
Glipizide	2.5–20 mg qd or bid 5 and 10 mg tabs	40mg	Hypoglycemia Weight gain Hypersensitivity	Known hypersensitivity DM1 Diabetic ketoacidosis (DKA)	Increased risk of hypoglycemia when combined with any other blood glucose–lowering agent	Glyburide and glipizide should be given 30 minutes prior to a meal; others are given without regard to meals NPO patients may need to hold dose to avoid hypoglycemia
Glipizide XL	5–10 mg qd 2.5, 5, and 10 mg tabs	20mg				
Glyburide						
Micronase (Diabeta, Micronase)	1.25–20 mg qd or bid 1.25, 2.5, and 5 mg tabs	20mg				
Micronized (Glynase)	0.75–12 mg qd or bid 1.5, 3, and 6 mg tabs	12mg				
Glimepiride (Amaryl)	1–8 mg qd 1, 2, and 4 mg tabs	8 mg				

Table 12-9 Meglitinides

- A_{1c} reduction = 0.6–1.9% for repaglinide; 0.3–0.5% for nateglinide. Repaglinide is clinically more efficacious than nateglinide.
- Mechanism of action: Similar to SFUs; has faster onset and shorter duration of action, so it affects postprandial hypoglycemia to a greater extent than FBG.
- Extent of insulin release appears to be glucose dependent. More insulin is released when blood glucose is elevated.
- Allows for flexible meal-time dosing.
- Do not use meglinitides in patients who have failed to achieve BG control with SFUs.
- Pharmacokinetic/pharmacodynamic considerations: Hepatic metabolism to inactive metabolites.

Agent	Dose (mg) and Dosage Forms	Max/ Day	ADRs/ Warnings/ Precautions	Contraindications	Drug Interactions	Food Considerations
Repaglinide (Prandin)	0.5–4 mg before meals (ac) 0.5, 1, 2 mg tabs	16 mg	Hypoglycemia Weight gain Hypersensitivity	Hypersensitivity to drug or any of its ingredients Diabetic ketoacidosis (DKA) DM1	Increased risk of hypoglycemia when combined with any other blood glucose–lowering agent Repaglinide: contraindicated with gemfibrozil	Administer 15–30 minutes prior to meals Dose may be omitted if a meal is skipped May need to hold if the patient is NPO or anorexic
Nateglinide (Starlix)	60 –120 mg before meals (ac) 60, 120 mg tabs	360 mg				

Table 12-10 Biguanides

- A_{1c} reduction = 1.0–2.0%.
- Mechanism of action: Decrease hepatic gluconeogenesis and decrease peripheral insulin resistance as the main mechanism of action; may also decrease intestinal glucose absorption.
- Minimal clinical benefit is seen when the dose is increased beyond 2,000 mg/day.
- Immediate release: Only oral agent FDA approved for children 10 years or older.
- Contraindications: SCr > 1.5 mg/dL in males and SCr > 1.4 mg/dL in females; CHF; acute/chronic metabolic acidosis. Hold prior to use of IV contrast and for 48 hours after; reinstitute only after renal function is normal due to the potential of the contrast to induce acute renal failure.
- Pharmacokinetic/pharmacodynamic considerations: 90% unchanged drug is eliminated in urine via active secretion.
- Not recommended in patients with liver disease and alcoholic patients.

Agent	Dose (mg) and Dosage Forms	Max/Day	ADRs/Warnings/ Precautions	Contraindications	Drug Interactions	Food Considerations
Metformin (Glucophage)	Initial: 500 mg bid or 850 mg qd Increase by 500 mg q 2wk 500, 850, 100 mg tabs, 100 mg/mL solution	2550mg (850 TID)	Diarrhea (10–53%) Nausea/vomiting (7–26%) Flatulence Decreases vitamin B_{12} absorption Lactic acidosis (approximately 3 cases per 100,000 patient-years; very rare, but potentially fatal)	SCr > 1.4 mg/dL for men SCr > 1.5 mg/dL for women Hypersensitivity to metformin or any of its ingredients Abnormal creatinine clearance from any cause (e.g., shock, HF, acute MI, septicemia) Metabolic acidosis (any type)	May increase risk of hypoglycemia when used in combination with other blood glucose–lowering agents, but does not cause hypoglycemia when used as monotherapy	Should be taken with food to decrease GI side effects Administer Fortamet with 8 oz water Do not crush, break, or chew XR formulation
Metformin XR (Glucophage XR, Fortamet, Glumetza)	Initial: 500 mg qd Increase by 500 mg q 2wk (give with evening meal) 500, 750, 1,000 mg tabs	2,000 mg				

Table 12-11 Alpha-Glucosidase Inhibitors

- A_{1c} reduction = 0.5–1.0%.
- Mechanism of action: Competitive inhibitor of brush border breakdown of sucrose to glucose and fructose, thereby decreasing postprandial hyperglycemia and serum insulin.
- Allows for flexible meal-time dosing.
- Adjust dose based on 1-hour *postprandial* blood glucose readings. Effect on fasting blood glucose is minimal.

Agent	Dose (mg) and Dosage Forms	Max/d	ADRs/Warnings/ Precautions	Contraindications	Drug Interactions	Food Considerations
Acarbose (Precose)	Initial: 25 tid Increase by 25 q 2 weeks 25, 50, 100 mg tabs	100 mg tid (acarbose: 50 mg tid if ≤ 60 kg)	Flatulence (most common) Diarrhea Increases AST/ALT Not recommended if SCr > 2 mg/dL Use with caution in patients with renal impairment	Hypersensitivity to drug or any ingredients DKA Cirrhosis, IBD, colonic ulceration, partial intestinal obstruction, disorders of absorption/ digestion	Combination with a secretagogue or insulin will increase risk of hypoglycemia, but alpha-glucosidase inhibitors do not cause hypoglycemia when used alone	Should be administered with the first bite of each meal Hypoglycemia must be treated with a monosaccharide (e.g., glucose, lactose, fructose)—not sucrose
Miglitol (Starlix)	Initial: 25 tid Increase by 25 q 2 weeks 25, 50, 100 mg tabs					

Table 12-12 Thiazolidinediones

- A_{1c} reduction = 1.0–1.5%.
- Mechanism of action: Increases insulin sensitivity in muscle, hepatic, and adipose tissue without affecting pancreatic insulin release. (Causes GLUT-4 translocation to cell surface.)
- All agents in this class have comparable efficacy in A_{1c} reduction.
- Effects on cholesterol: Rosiglitazone increases LDL and HDL by 9–19%; pioglitazone increases HDL by 9–19%, but does not increase LDL.
- Pharmacokinetic/pharmacodynamic considerations: Clinical effect on blood glucose may take 3–4 weeks (or longer) to become evident.

Agent	Dose (mg) and Dosage Forms	Max/Day	ADRs/Warnings/Precautions	Contraindications	Drug Interactions	Food Considerations
Rosiglitazone (Avandia)	4–8 mg qd or bid 2, 4, 8 mg tabs	16 mg	Weight gain Edema Lowers Hct/Hgb and may cause megaloblastic anemia Liver toxicity? Decreases bone mineral density Macular edema May induce ovulation Cardiovascular precautions: Black box warning regarding risk of new onset or exacerbation of existing HF Rosiglitazone: believed to increase risk of MI	Liver function tests that are more than 3 times the upper limits of normal (monitor at baseline and q 6–12 months thereafter) NYHA Class III or IV heart failure	Rosiglitazone: Do not use concomitantly with insulin May increase risk of hypoglycemia when used in combination with other blood glucose–lowering agents	May be administered without regard to food
Pioglitazone (Actos)	15–45 mg qd 15, 30, 45 mg tabs	45 mg				

Table 12-13 Insulins

- A_{1c} reduction: Best ability to lower glucose levels, but greatest risk of hypoglycemia.
- Mechanism of action: Exogenous supply of insulin.
- Preparations differ in terms of their onset of action, peak, and duration of action.
- Comparative efficacy: Based on pharmacokinetic differences, some preparations are preferred over others for postprandial blood glucose versus fasting blood glucose control.
- Are the preferred agents for pregnant patients requiring antidiabetic pharmacotherapy.
- Use requires intensive patient education.
- ADRs: Hypoglycemia, weight gain, injection-site reactions.
- Pharmacokinetic/pharmacodynamic considerations: Excreted renally; impaired renal function may result in decreased insulin requirement.
- Protamine is often used to extend the rate of absorption, time to peak, and duration of action.
- Only regular (R) insulin may be given IV. All other formulations are given subcutaneously (SQ). (Note R insulin may also be given SQ.)
- Only rapid-acting insulins (lispro, apidra, aspart) are used for insulin pump therapy.
- Available as U-100 strength, meaning 1 mL of product contains 100 units of insulin.
- R insulin is also available as U-500, meaning 1 mL of product contains 500 units insulin. Extreme caution should be used with this product due to the risk of medication error by overdose.
- Injection sites (in order of preference due to greater and more rapid bioavailability): Abdomen > arm > hip > thigh > buttock
- Sites should be rotated regularly to avoid development of lipohypertrophy.
- Injecting insulin at room temperature decreases likelihood of pain with administration.

Table 12-13 (*continued*)

Insulin	Onset (hr)	Peak (hr)	Duration (hr)	Mix with Other Insulins?	Appearance
Rapid Acting					
Lispro (Humalog)	0.25–0.5	0.5–2.5	3–6.5	Yes	Clear
Aspart (Novolog)	0.17–0.33	1–3	3–5	Yes	Clear
Glulisine (Apidra)	0.25–0.33	1–3	3–5	Yes	Clear
Fast Acting					
Regular	0.5–1	2–5	5–10	Yes	Clear
Intermediate Acting (Should be rolled briskly prior to administration)					
NPH	1–1.5	4–12	16–24	Yes	Cloudy
Long Acting					
Glargine (Lantus)	1	2–20	16–24	No	Clear
Detemir (Levemir)	1	2–20	16–24	No	Clear

Table 12-14 Incretin Mimetics

- A_{1c} reduction = 0.5–0.8%.
- Mechanism of action: Decreases postprandial plasma glucose rise, decreases glucagon secretion following oral caloric intake; slows gastric emptying; increases sense of satiety; inhibits gluconeogenesis.
- Long-acting synthetic version of glucagon-like peptide -1 (GLP-1), which is deficient in DM2, and is normally secreted by intestinal L cells.
- Causes weight gain (1.6 kg [3.5 lb]) over 30 weeks.
- Not approved for use with insulin.

Agent	Dose and Dosage Forms	Max/Day	ADRs/Warnings/ Precautions	Contraindica-tions	Drug Interactions	Food Considerations
Exenatide (Byetta, Bydureon)	5 mcg SQ: bid, 60 min prior to breakfast and evening meal; increase the dose after 1 month OR: with Bydureon 250 mcg/mL; add (1.2 mL [5 mcg/0.02 mL; 60-dose pen]); 2.4 mL [10 mcg/0.04 mL; 60-dose pen]) Vial with 2 mg drug, 0.65 mL diluent	10 mcg SQ bid 2 mg/day once every 7 days	Nausea Vomiting Diarrhea Dyspepsia Pancreatitis has been reported Advise patients to stop use of the drug and contact the prescriber if they develop nausea/vomiting and severe abdominal pain	Hypersensitivity to exenatide or any component of formulation CrCl < 30 mL/ min DM1 GI disease Personal or family history	May enhance hypoglycemic effect of sulfonylureas May enhance effects of warfarin; monitor INR closely	Daily administration: Administer 60 minutes prior to two main meals of the day Extended release: May be administered without regard to food Exenatide slows gastric emptying Can decrease the rate and extent of absorption of other drugs Oral drugs (especially antibiotics and contraceptives) should be taken at least 1 hour before injecting exenatide Medications that should be administered with food should be taken with a meal or snack when exenatide is not administered

(*continues*)

Table 12-14 (*continued*)

Agent	Dose and Dosage Forms	Max/Day	ADRs/Warnings/ Precautions	Contraindications	Drug Interactions	Food Considerations
Liraglutide (Victoza)	0.6 mg daily × 1 week; then 1.2 mg daily Prefilled, multidose pen that delivers doses of 0.6 mg 1.2 mg or 1.8 mg (6 mg/mL, 3 mL)	1.8 mg/day	Nausea Vomiting Diarrhea Dyspepsia Headache Constipation	Hypersensitivity to drug or any of its components Personal or family history of thyroid cancer	Potential to impact the absorption of concomitantly administered oral medications	Potential to impact the absorption of concomitantly administered oral medications

Table 12-15 Amylinomimetic Agents

- A_{1c} reduction = ~ 0.4%.
- Mechanism of action: (1) modulation of gastric emptying; (2) prevention of the postprandial rise in plasma glucagon; (3) satiety leading to decreased caloric intake and potential weight loss; (4) suppression of gluconeogenesis. Synthetic form of endogenous amylin.
- DM1: Indicated as an adjunct to meal-time insulin when optimal insulin therapy is not adequate to achieve the postprandial goal.
- DM2: Indicated as an adjunct to meal-time insulin with or without a sulfonylurea agent and/or metformin when glucose control is not achieved despite optimal insulin therapy.
- Decrease rapid-acting insulins or fixed mixed insulins (e.g., 70/30) by 50% when starting pramlintide.
- Increase dose after 1 week if tolerated (60 to 120 mcg for DM2).
- Dose increases are based on postprandial blood glucose readings.
- Can be used in DM1 and DM2 (DM1: use a lower dose).
- Do *not* mix any insulin product in the same syringe used for the amylinomimetic agent.
- Although an amylinomimetic agent may be administered with an insulin syringe, its dose is measured in *micrograms* (not milliliters or milligrams). Use extreme caution to avoid mistakes in dosage calculation based on units: 15–120 mcg correlates to 0.025–0.2 mL.
- Pharmacokinetic and pharmacodynamic considerations: A significant risk of hypoglycemia arises when amylinomimetic agents are used with insulin. Injection into the arm is discouraged due to a higher variability in absorption versus abdominal or thigh injections.

Agent	Dose and Dosage Forms	Max/Day	ADRs/Warnings/ Precautions	Contraindications	Drug Interactions	Food Considerations
Pramlintide (Symlin)	DM2: 60 mcg before meals DM1: 15 mcg before meals 600 mcg/mL (5 mL); 1,000 mcg/mL (1.5 mL) (60-dose pen-injector); 1,000 mcg/mL (2.7 mL) (120-dose pen-injector)	120 mcg tid	Hypoglycemia (16.8%): Boxed warning regarding risk when used with insulin. If used alone, however, does not cause hypoglycemia, but it is indicated for use *with* insulin. Nausea (28–48%) Vomiting (8–11%) Anorexia (9%)	Gastroparesis Hypoglycemia unawareness History of nonadherence	May enhance the effect of anticholinergic agents, especially as they relate to GI motility	Pramlintide should be administered prior to major meals consisting of ≥ 250 Kcal or ≥ 30 g carbohydrates

Table 12-16 Dipeptidylpeptidase-IV Inhibitors

- A_{1c} reduction = 0.6–0.8%.
- Mechanism of action: Inhibition of dipeptidylpeptidase-IV (the enzyme that degrades endogenous GLP-1). This enhances activity of *endogenous* GLP-I and leads to decreased postprandial glucagon release, improved insulin response, increased feeling of satiety, and slowed gastric emptying.
- Sitagliptin: Not extensively metabolized; transported by p-glycoprotein.
- Saxagliptin: Metabolized by hepatic CYP3A4/5 enzymes to active metabolite with 50% activity of parent drug.

Agent	Dose	Max/Day	ADRs/Warnings/ Precautions	Contraindications	Drug Interactions	Food Considerations
Sitagliptin (Januvia)	100 mg once daily CrCl ≥ 30 and < 50 mL/min: 50 mg daily CrCl < 30: 25 mg daily 25, 50, 100 mg tabs	100 mg	FDA warning regarding possible development of pancreatitis; patients should notify their prescriber immediately if they develop nausea/vomiting, anorexia, or severe abdominal pain Diarrhea (3%) Abdominal pain (2%)	Hypersensitivity to drug or any ingredients DM1 Diabetic ketoacidosis	Serum concentrations may be decreased by p-glycoprotein inducers Serum concentrations may be increased by p-glycoprotein inhibitors.	May be administered with or without food
Saxagliptin (Onglyza)	2.5–5 mg once daily CrCl ≤ 50 mL/min: 2.5 mg daily 2.5, 5 mg tabs	5 mg	Headache (7%) Peripheral edema (4%; risk increases if saxagliptin is used in combination with thiazolidinedione)	Hypersensitivity to drug or any ingredients DM1 Diabetic ketoacidosis	Serum concentration may be increased by strong CYP3A4 inhibitors Serum concentration may be decreased by strong CYP 3A4 inducers	May be administered with or without food
Linagliptin (Tradjenta)	5 mg daily	5 mg	Nasopharyngitis Hypoglycemia (when combined with a sulfonylurea) Pancreatitis (1 in 562 patient-years according to manufacturer's data)	Hypersensitivity to drug or any ingredients DM1 Diabetic ketoacidosis		May be administered with or without food

Table 12-17 Recommended Follow-Up for Diabetes

- Consider aspirin (81 mg daily) therapy for patients with diabetes aged > 40 years or with evidence of CVD risk factors
- Give annual flu vaccine, if indicated
- Give pneumonia vaccine, if indicated

A_{1c} measurements	Every 3 months until stable, annually thereafter
Blood pressure	Every visit
Lipids	Every 3 months until stable, annually thereafter
Micro/macroalbuminuria	Annually
Eye evaluation	Every 1 year
Foot evaluation	Every visit

For obese patients, many clinicians will use an adjusted body weight (IBW + 0.4 [ABW – IBW]) rather than actual body weight.

Adjusting Insulin

500 Rule

The "500 rule" is used to calculate the number of carbohydrate grams covered by 1 unit of insulin of rapid-acting insulin (e.g., lispro, aspart, or apidra):

$$\text{Carbohydrates (g)} = 500 / \text{total daily dose of insulin}$$

Example: A patient who takes 35 units of insulin glargine once daily and 5 units of insulin lispro before each meal takes a total of 50 units of insulin daily.

$$\text{Carbohydrates} = 500 / 50 = 10\text{g}$$

Thus, 1 unit of insulin lispro, aspart, or apidra will be needed to cover 10 grams of carbohydrates.

1,800 Rule

The "1,800 rule" is used to estimate the number of points (in mg/dL) that blood glucose will drop after administration of 1 unit of insulin (e.g., lispro, aspart, or apidra):

Blood glucose drop (mg/dL)
= 1,800 / total daily does of insulin

Example: A patient's total daily insulin dose is 20 units

$$\text{Blood glucose drop} = 1{,}800/20 = 90 \text{ mg/dL}$$

Blood glucose will be estimated to drop approximately 90 mg/dL after administration of 1 unit of insulin lispro, aspart, or apidra.

2.2.0 Dispensing

Insulin: Package, Storage, Handling, and Disposal

Insulin products are available via vial or pen delivery device.

Advise patients to roll any product containing intermediate-acting (N) insulin briskly prior to administration.

Insulin products, incretin mimetics, and amylinomimetics should be kept refrigerated until ready for use. The current pen or vial being used should be kept at room temperature. Products exposed to temperature extremes should be discarded.

Medication Administration and Equipment

- Most antidiabetic agents are orally administered.
- Injectables include insulin products, pramlintide, and exenatide.
- Only insulin regular (R) may be administered intravenously. All other types of insulin (including R) are given subcutaneously via vial and syringe or pen delivery device.

Compounding

With the commercial availability of mixed insulin products (e.g., Humulin 70/30, Novolog 70/30, Humalog 75/25), fewer patients now mix their own insulins. However, those that do should keep in mind the following tips:

- Insulin glargine and insulin detemir may *not* be mixed with other insulins.
- When mixing short-acting insulin and longer-acting insulin, an amount of air equal to the volume that will be withdrawn should be injected into each vial first. Then, the shorter-acting insulin should be withdrawn into the syringe *first*, following by withdrawal of the longer-acting insulin into the syringe. Rule of thumb: Always draw the shorter-acting insulin up first!
- Do not mix any other medication or diluents with insulin intended for SQ injection.

ANNOTATED BIBLIOGRAPHY

American Diabetes Association. Diagnosis and classification of diabetes mellitus. *Diabetes Care* 2010;33:S62–S69. doi: 10.2337/dc10-S062

American Diabetes Association. Standards of medical care in diabetes—2010. *Diabetes Care* 2010;33: S11–S61. doi: 10.2337/dc10-S011

Cook CL, Johnson JT, Wade WE. Diabetes. In: Chisholm-Burns MA, Wells BG, Schwinghammer TL, Malone PM, Kolesar JM, Rotschafer JC, DiPiro JT, eds. *Pharmacotherapy: Principles and Practice*. China: McGraw-Hill, 2008:643–666.

Diabetes data and trends. Department of Health and Human Services, Centers for Disease Control and Prevention. Available at: http://www.cdc.gov/diabetes/statistics/diabetes_slides.htm. Accessed February 20, 2010.

DRUGDEX Information System. Greenwood Village, CO: Thomson Healthcare; 1974–2008. Updated periodically. Available from: https://www.thomsonhc.com. Accessed February 20, 2010.

Lexi-Comp Online. Hudson, OH: Lexi-Comp, 1978–2008. Available at: http://online.lexi.com/crlsql/servlet/crlonline. Accessed February 20, 2010.

Triplitt CL, Reasner CA, Isley WL. Diabetes Mellitus. In DiPiro JT, Talbert RL, Yee GC, Matzke GR, Wells BG, Posey LM, eds. *Pharmacotherapy: A Pathophysiologic Approach*. 7th ed. Available at: http://www.accesspharmacy.com/content.aspx?aID=3207048.

TOPIC: ERECTILE DYSFUNCTION

Section Coordinator: Debra Parker
Contributor: Debra Parker

Erectile Dysfunction Overview

Erectile dysfunction becomes increasing prevalent as the male population ages. Although it is a condition that does not affect morbidity and mortality, it is associated with low self-esteem, depression, and decreased quality of life; it may also cause stress in relationships.

Pharmacotherapy is generally the first-line treatment approach, with PDE-5 inhibitors being the drug class of choice. Pharmacists play an important role in patient counseling and ensuring drug interactions do not result in untoward side effects.

Tips Worth Tweeting

- Erectile dysfunction—the inability to gain and maintain an erection adequate for sexual intercourse—becomes increasingly prevalent as the male population ages.
- Underlying causes may be physiologic, psychological, medications, or comorbid disease states.
- Nonpharmacologic treatments include vacuum erection devices and penile implants.
- Pharmacologic treatments include PDE-5 inhibitors (first-line therapy), alprostadil, phentolamine, and papaverine. Testosterone may be appropriate for documented hypogonadism. Yohimbine is not recommended.
- The goal of therapy is to improve the patient's quality of life and sexual function by using the most cost-effective treatment associated with the fewest side effects.

Patient Care Scenario: Community Pharmacy

66 y/o, 5'7", 239 lbS, M, Caucasian
Allergies: NKA
PMH: Obesity, HTN, "prediabetes," hyperlipidemia, OA
Lab Values: TC 265 mg/dL; HDL 38 mg/dL; LDL 120 mg/dL; TG 270 mg/dL; FBG 185 mg/dL

Medication Profile

Date	Physician	Drug	Quantity	Sig	Refills
5/19	Huber	Viagra 100 mg	30	1 po daily	11
5/19	Huber	HCTZ 25 mg	30	1 po daily	8
5/19	Huber	Atenolol 100 mg	30	1 po daily	8
5/19	–	Multivitamin	30	1 po daily	10
5/19	Huber	Pravastatin 40 mg	30	1 po daily	5
5/19	Huber	Gemfibrozil 600 mg	30	1 po daily	5
5/19	Huber	Ibuprofen 200 mg	100	2 po bid prn	10
5/19	–	Glucosamine chondroitin 500 mg	90	1 po tid	–
4/27	–	St. John's wort 200 mg	30	1 po daily	–

Vitals: 156/88; HR 64
Social Hx: Tobacco: 1 ppd. Alcohol: 3–4 beers each evening. Does not exercise. No specific dietary habits.

1.1.0 Patient Information

Definition

Erectile dysfunction, or the inability to gain and maintain an erection adequate for sexual intercourse, is a condition that becomes increasingly prevalent in men after the age of 40. Although not life threatening, it often contributes to decreased quality of life and depression in affected patients. This condition may be caused by the physiology of aging, medications, lifestyle, or psychological factors, or any combination of these. Treatment may include pharmacotherapy, surgery, psychotherapy, or medical devices, although pharmacotherapy is the most commonly used option.

Key Terms

The following terms are distinct and should not be used interchangeably.

- **Erectile dysfunction (ED):** The inability to gain and maintain an erection.
- **Decreased libido:** Decreased interest in sexual activity.
- **Impotence**: Decreased ability to either gain or maintain an erection and/or inability to ejaculate normally. This term is less specific than erectile dysfunction.

Pathophysiology

Penis Anatomy

There are three discrete components to the anatomy of the penis:

- Two dorsolateral corpora cavernosa, which fill with blood during erection.
- One corpus spongiosum, which surrounds the penile urethra. The corpus spongiosum prevents urethral constriction during erection. At the distal end, it forms the glans penis.

Stimulation of an erection is a function of sympathetic and parasympathetic innervations as well as adequate blood flow to the penis.

- Sympathetic tone: Alpha$_2$-adrenergic receptors maintain arterial resistance and a balance of blood inflow and outflow to maintain the penis's flaccid state. With sexual stimulation, sympathetic tone decreases and parasympathetic tone increases, arterial resistance decreases, and a net increase in arterial blood inflow to the penis occurs.

- Parasympathetic tone: Acetylcholine leads to production of nitric oxide, which increases the production of cyclic guanosine monophosphate (cGMP). Cyclic adenosine monophosphate (cAMP) production is also increased by increased levels of vasoactive peptide and prostaglandins E_1 and E_2. cAMP and cGMP cause penile smooth-muscle relaxation and resultant filling/pooling of blood into the cavities of the corpus cavernosum. With this pooling, venules are compressed, decreasing blood outflow, and the penis increases in length and rigidity.

Following ejaculation, sympathetic discharge leads to detumescence and the return of penile flaccidity.

The ability to gain and maintain an erection is reliant on sexual desire (libido), the response to sexual stimulation (sympathetic and parasympathetic), and normal blood flow. Decreased levels of testosterone not only contribute to decreased libido, but also result in a decreased formation of nitric oxide and, therefore, decreased ability to maintain an adequate erection.

Diagnosis

The diagnosis of erectile dysfunction is often made based only on a detailed patient history.

If more than the usual patient interview is conducted, the International Index of Erectile Dysfunction (IIED) questionnaire is the one most commonly used to assess ED severity. It evaluates libido, erectile function, orgasmic function, and sexual and overall satisfaction. A score of less than 26/30 is considered indicative of ED. The lower the score is, the greater the severity of the ED.

Risk Factors

Cardiovascular disease (CVD) and hyperlipidemia often go hand in hand with ED. In fact, ED may be the first sign of comorbid CVD. Thus risk factors for ED are the same as those for the development of CVD: diabetes, hyperlipidemia, HTN, age greater than 45 years, HDL less than 40, smoking, family history, and known coronary heart disease or peripheral arterial disease.

Low testosterone, increased stress, and use of specific medications may also increase the risk of developing erectile dysfunction.

Medication Classes That Increase Risk of ED

- Antihypertensives: beta blockers (especially nonselective agents), thiazide diuretics, centrally acting agents (e.g., clonidine, methyldopa, and reserpine), spironolactone, alpha blockers
- Antidepressants: TCAs, MAOIs, SSRIs
- Antipsychotics: phenothiazines, risperidone, lithium
- Anticonvulsants: carbamazepine, phenytoin
- Antiandrogens: 5-alpha reductase inhibitors (e.g. finasteride)
- Miscellaneous: cimetidine, gemfibrozil, ethanol, cocaine, marijuana

Other Medical Conditions That May Lead to ED

- Trauma (e.g., spinal cord injury or pelvic fracture)
- Endocrine disorders: hypogonadism, adrenal, pituitary or thyroid disorders
- Neurologic disorders
- Local anatomic conditions (e.g., prostatitis, enlarged prostate, penile disease)

Wellness and Prevention

Given that the risk factors for the development of ED are virtually the same as those of the development of cardiovascular disease, a healthy diet, physical activity, maintenance of a healthy weight, avoidance of excessive alcohol consumption, and avoidance of tobacco use are all expected to decrease the likelihood of ED. In addition, diabetes is associated with decreased microvascular circulation, as well as with autonomic neuropathy as a result of poorly controlled blood glucose. As such, patients with diabetes should be counseled that inadequate control of their disease may lead to ED.

1.2.0 Pharmacotherapy

Treatment

Treatment may be pharmacologic or nonpharmacologic. Nonpharmacologic treatment options include the following:

- Psychotherapy/counseling: Effective only when a physical condition is not the underlying cause of ED
- Lifestyle modifications: Weight loss, smoking cessation, healthy diet, increased exercise, decreased use/avoidance of alcohol, avoidance of illicit drugs

Devices

Vacuum erection devices (VEDs) draw blood into the penis by creating an external vacuum. A constrictive band is then placed at penile base for 30 minutes or less to maintain the erection.

- Advantages: Noninvasive; effective in more than 90% of patients
- Disadvantages: Takes approximately 30 minutes; does not allow for sexual spontaneity; increased risk of priapism in patients with bleeding disorders or on anticoagulants
- Contraindicated for patients with sickle cell disease

Prostheses are an alternative when VED or drug therapy fails. These devices are invasive, so they carry a risk (albeit small) of infection; device failure is also possible. Implants may last up to 10 years in some patients. Two options are available:

- Inflatable rod: The penis remains flaccid until a pump within the scrotum is activated and fluid moves into the rod to create an erection. Detumescence is achieved by pressing a release button on the pump.
- Malleable but firm rod: Inserted into the corpus cavernosa. The penis remains firm at all times; it is bent into position by the patient when desired.

Goals of Therapy

- Assist the patient in the ability to achieve adequate erectile function for sexual intercourse and, as a result, have improved quality of life.
- Use the most effective, most convenient, least costly, and safest method to do so.

Drug Therapy

The most commonly prescribed class of medications for ED is the phophodiesterase-5 (PDE-5) inhibitors. Other drug therapies include alprostadil, papaverine, phentolamine, yohimbine, and testosterone supplementation. Routes of therapy, depending on the drug, may be oral, topical, buccal, intraurethral suppository, or intracavernosal or intramuscular injections.

PDE-5 Inhibitors

- First-line drug therapy due to convenience, ease of administration, and mild side-effect profile.
- Mechanism of action: Inhibition of PDE-5 results in decreased degradation of cGMP. Increased cGMP concentrations enhance smooth-muscle relaxation in the corpus cavernosa and subsequent filling with blood.
- All PDE-5 inhibitors are administered orally.
- Comparative efficacy: 50–80% efficacy, which is presumed to be similar for all agents.
  - Tadalafil: Has a long half-life, allowing for effects to last up to 72 hours; it may be taken as little as 30 minutes prior to intercourse.
- Food and dietary supplement considerations:
  - Grapefruit juice and St. John's wort: Increase PDE-5 concentrations.
  - Sildenafil and vardenafil (but not tadalafil): Bioavailability is decreased by high-fat meals.
- Contraindications: Concurrent use of nitrates in any form—may cause a precipitous drop in blood pressure.
- Other drug interactions: Increased risk of symptomatic hypotension with alpha blockers; use the lowest effective dose of the PDE-5 inhibitor. Dosage reduction is recommended if the patient is also taking strong CYP3A4 inhibitors.
- ADRs/warning/precautions:
  - Most common: Headache, flushing, dyspepsia.
  - Other possible side effects: May cause temporary color vision impairment (dose related), symptomatic hypotension (especially in patients taking alpha blockers, with left ventricular outflow obstruction, or who have consumed significant amounts of alcohol), rare cases of vision loss due to nonarteritic anterior ischemic optic neuropathy (NAION), rare cases of priapism.
- Patient counseling: PDE-5 inhibitors do not directly cause erection, but rather enhance response to sexual stimulation. Seek medical assistance for an erection lasting longer than 4 hours. A single trial of a medication at a specific dose is not adequate to determine efficacy. As many as 6–8 attempts at intercourse are recommended before deciding if a drug and dose are effective.

Other Pharmacotherapy

Alprostadil

- Mechanism of action: Increases cAMP levels and subsequent smooth muscle relaxation
- Two routes of administration:
  - Transurethral suppository: Onset of action 5–10 minutes.
    - ADRs: Aching in penis, legs, perineum, minor urethral spotting, priapism, lightheadedness possible.

Table 12-18 Phophodiesterase-5 Inhibitors

Generic (Brand) Name	Dose and Dosage Forms	Dosing Frequency
Sildenafil (Viagra)	25–100 mg 1 hr before intercourse Tablets: 25, 50, 100 mg	Once daily
Tadalafil (Cialis)	As needed dose: 5–20 mg 30 min before intercourse Once-daily dose: 2.5 mg daily Tablets: 2.5, 5, 10, 20 mg	Once daily (q 72 hr when taken with strong CYP3A4 inhibitors) Once daily
Vardenafil (Levitra)	5–20 mg 1 hr before intercourse Tablets: 2.5, 5, 10, 20 mg	Once daily

- Contraindications: Intercourse with a pregnant patient unless wearing a condom.
  - Intracavernosal injection: Only FDA-approved intracavernosal injection. More effective than transurethral suppository.
    - The medication is injected into the corpus cavernosa, which is massaged to ensure drug distribution.
    - Effective in as many as 90% of patients, but the route of administration, side effects, and lack of spontaneity are deterrents to its use.
    - ADRs: Pain, bleeding or bruising at the injection site, fibrosis, possible priapism. The risk of priapism is increased in patients with sickle cell disease, bleeding disorders, or use of anticoagulants.

Papaverine and Phentolamine

- Non-FDA-approved agents for intracavernosal injection. Used in combination with alprostadil in varying compounded concentrations. Rarely used alone.
- Papaverine mechanism of action: Nonselective phosphodiesterase inhibitor; relaxes smooth muscle and increases blood flow.
- Phentolamine mechanism of action: Competitive alpha-adrenergic antagonist resulting in arterial dilation and net inflow of blood into the penis.

Yohimbine

- Not recommended by FDA for treatment of ED.
- Historically used because it inhibits $alpha_2$ receptors in the brain associated with libido and stimulation of erection.

Testosterone Supplementation

- Recommended and effective only for patients with documented hypogonadism; in these cases, should increase libido and sense of well-being.
- May or may not improve erectile dysfunction.
- Need for additional pharmacotherapy should be assessed after 3 months of therapy.

Table 12-19 Alprostadil

Route	Brand Names	Dose and Dosage Forms	Maximum Dose
Intracavernosal injection	Caverject Edex	1.25–60 mcg 5–20 min prior to intercourse	3 or fewer injections/ week with 24 hr or longer between injections
Transurethral suppository	Muse	125–1,000 mcg	1–2 suppositories/day

- Routes of administration:
  - Intramuscular injection
    - Inexpensive, but injection is needed only every 2–4 months; swings from supratherapeutic to subtherapeutic testosterone levels affect mood and well-being
    - Testosterone cypionate (Depo-Testosterone) and testosterone enanthate (Delatestryl)
  - Topical (gel or patch)
    - More expensive but route is more appealing to patients; applied daily
    - Patients must wash hands thoroughly and avoid baths/showers for 5–6 hours after application
    - Patches: Testoderm, Testoderm TTS, Androderm
    - Gels: AndroGel 1%, Testim
  - Buccal
    - Not recommended; has poor bioavailability due to first-pass metabolism; products formulated to increase bioavailability are associated with increased risk of hepatotoxicity
    - Trade name: Striant

Adverse Effects and Monitoring

- Testosterone ADRs: Gynecomastia, dyslipidemia, acne, polycythemia
- Monitoring: Annual PSA test, digital rectal exam (DRE), LFTs

1.3.0 Monitoring

- Four weeks after therapy was initiated or altered, does the patient report improvement in quality of life and sexual satisfaction? The IIED questionnaire may or may not be used to assess the level of change.
- Laboratory tests and physical exam are not necessary, except if monitoring testosterone blood levels.
- If goals of therapy are not met, reassess the goals to ensure they are realistic, and consider possible comorbid condition contributions. If neither is an issue, titrate the dose of the drug therapy if not maximized, change to another drug class, or add a second class of ED medications if warranted.

2.2.0 Dispensing

- Muse: Keep refrigerated prior to dispensing. It is stable at room temperature up to 14 days.
- Caverject solution: Store frozen prior to dispensing. Once dispensed, it remains stable while frozen for up to 3 months. It is stable while refrigerated

for up to 7 days. The solution may be allowed to warm to room temperature prior to use, but should not be put back in the refrigerator or refrozen.

ANNOTATED BIBLIOGRAPHY

DRUGDEX Information System. Greenwood Village, CO: Thomson Healthcare; 1974–2008. Updated periodically. Available at: https://www.thomsonhc.com. Accessed March 5, 2010.

Lee M. Erectile Dysfunction. DiPiro JT, Talbert RL, Yee GC, Matzke GR, Wells BG, Posey LM, eds. *Pharmacotherapy: A Pathophysiologic Approach*. 7th ed. Available at: http://www.accesspharmacy.com/content.aspx?aID=3207048.

Lexi-Comp Online. Hudson, OH: Lexi-Comp, 1978–2008. Available at: http://online.lexi.com/crlsql/servlet/crlonline. Accessed March 5, 2010.

Liday C, Heyneman C. Erectile Dysfunction. In: Chisholm-Burns MA, Wells BG, Schwinghammer TL, Malone PM, Kolesar JM, Rotschafer JC, DiPiro JT, eds. *Pharmacotherapy: Principles and Practice*. China: McGraw-Hill, 2008:779–789.

TOPIC: HYPERLIPIDEMIA

Section Coordinator: Debra Parker
Contributor: Lori J. Ernsthausen

Hyperlipidemia Overview

Increases in total cholesterol and LDL lead to increased risk of coronary heart disease, cerebrovascular disease, and peripheral vascular disease. In the United States, coronary heart disease is the leading cause of death among men and women. Pharmacists can play a key role in managing hyperlipidemia through patient counseling regarding therapeutic lifestyle changes, medication therapy management, and continued patient risk assessment.

Tips Worth Tweeting

- LDL is considered the primary target for therapy.
- Therapeutic lifestyle changes are an important part of lipid management and should be encouraged in all patients.
- HMG-CoA reductase inhibitors are the most effective agents for lowering LDL and total cholesterol.
- High triglycerides may be managed through lifestyle changes, such as smoking cessation and decreased alcohol intake, as well as agents such as fenofibrate, gemfibrozil and omega-3 fatty acids.

Patient Care Scenario: Outpatient Medication Therapy Management Clinic

61 y/o, 5'2", 134 lb, F, Caucasian
Allergies: NKA
PMH: HTN diagnosed 6 years ago, hypothyroidism, OA
Lab Values: TC 268 mg/dL; HDL 66 mg/dL; LDL 172 mg/dL; TG 150 mg/dL; FBG 88 mg/dL; AST 35 U/L, ALT 28 U/L, BUN 15 mg/dL, SCr 0.9 mg/dL
Vitals: 152/86; HR 68

Medication Profile

Date	Physician	Drug	Quantity	Sig	Refills
10/9	Murphy	HCTZ 12.5 mg	30	1 po q AM	8
10/9	Murphy	Ibuprofen 600 mg	180	1 po three times daily	6
10/9	Murphy	Lisinopril 5 mg	30	1 po daily	8
10/9	–	Multi-vitamin	30	1 po daily	10

Social Hx: Tobacco: nonsmoker. Alcohol: shares a bottle of wine with her husband most evenings. Exercise: swims 5 mornings each week. Diet: no specific dietary habits.

1.1.0 Patient Information

Definition

The three major lipids in the body (cholesterol, triglycerides, and phospholipids) are packaged and transported throughout our bodies via lipoprotein particles. There are three main types of lipoproteins that vary in size and density: low-density lipoprotein (LDL), high-density lipoprotein (HDL), and very low-density lipoprotein (VLDL). An elevation of one or more of the following lipids constitutes hyperlipidemia: cholesterol, cholesterol esters, phospholipids, or triglycerides. Increased total cholesterol, increased LDL, and low HDL have been linked to the development of coronary heart disease (CHD). Coronary atherosclerosis leading to a myocardial infarction (MI) is the most common consequence of hyperlipidemia. An inverse relationship exists with HDL and coronary heart disease; that is, as HDL increases, risk for CHD decreases. Thus, the goal for management of hyperlipidemia may be to decrease one's risk for coronary heart disease (primary prevention) or to decrease the risk for a second coronary heart disease event (secondary prevention).

Laboratory Values

A fasting lipid panel measures total cholesterol, triglycerides, HDL, and LDL.

Diagnosis

The patient's fasting lipid panel is obtained after a 9- to 12-hour fast. Based on the patient interview or history, determine the presence of coronary heart disease (CHD) risk factors, CHD risk equivalents, and other major risk factors; calculate the Framingham risk (if necessary); and determine the patient's goal LDL. Compare the patient's LDL, HDL, and triglyceride levels to goal levels to make a diagnosis and determine treatment.

Risk Factors

- Coronary heart disease or CHD risk equivalents: MI, unstable angina, chronic stable angina, coronary intervention(s), carotid artery disease (stroke, transient ischemic attack), peripheral artery disease, abdominal aortic aneurysm, diabetes mellitus, multiple risk factors with a Framingham 10-year calculated risk > 20%
- Major risk factors: Smoking, hypertension (BP ≥ 140/90 or on antihypertensive medication), low HDL (< 40 mg/dL), age (men ≥ 45 years, women ≥ 55 years), family history of premature CHD event (male first-degree relative < 55 years, female first-degree relative < 65 years)
- Negative risk factor: HDL ≥ 60 mg/dL
- Framingham risk point scale: Used to estimate 10-year CHD risk, when the patient is found to have two or more CHD risk factors; it can be calculated at the following website: http:www.nhlbi.nih.gov/guidelines/cholesterol/index.htm

Secondary Causes of Dyslipidemia

- Disease states: Diabetes mellitus, liver disease, nephritic syndrome, chronic kidney disease, hypothyroidism, smoking, obesity
- Drugs: Estrogen and progestin, antiretroviral agents, thiazide diuretics, beta blockers, glucocorticoids, cyclosporine, retinoids, bile acid sequestrants

1.2.0 Pharmacotherapy

Treatment

Treatment may be pharmacologic or nonpharmacologic. Nonpharmacologic treatment options include therapeutic lifestyle changes (which may decrease LDL by 20–25%):

- Decrease dietary saturated fat, cholesterol, and total calories
- Increase intake of soluble fiber and plant stanols/sterols
- Decrease/avoid alcohol
- Increase physical activity
- Stop smoking
- Lose weight

Goals of Therapy

Treatment goals and therapy for the management of hyperlipidemia are determined by assessing the fasting lipoprotein levels, calculating coronary heart disease and coronary heart disease risk equivalents, and identifying other major risk factors. All patients with hyperlipidemia should initiate therapeutic lifestyle changes (TLC). The patient's risk category will determine whether pharmacotherapy should be initiated as well.

Patients with elevated LDL are typically treated with therapeutic lifestyle changes and an agent from the HMG-CoA reductase inhibitor class as first-line therapy; however, bile acid sequestrants, ezetimibe, and nicotinic acid may also be used as monotherapy for LDL reduction. HMG-CoA reductase inhibitors may also be combined with ezetimibe and/or a bile acid sequestrant for additional LDL lowering, while bile acid sequestrants may be combined with ezetimibe in patients who cannot tolerate HMG-CoA reductase inhibitors.

When triglycerides reduction is needed, agents such as nicotinic acid, fibrates, or omega-3 fatty acids are considered. High triglycerides are managed through lifestyle changes, such as smoking cessation and decreased alcohol intake, as well as agents such as fenofibrate, gemfibrozil, and omega-3 fatty acids. Niacin does have a favorable effect on TG, but it is typically prescribed in combination dyslipidemias rather than isolated hypertriglyceridemia.

While drugs such as niacin or fibrates (niacin > fibrates) may raise a patient's HDL, the most effective treatment option for low HDL levels remains lifestyle changes. Increased physical activity, weight loss, and smoking cessation are all recommended to increase HDL.

Treatment of LDL

In general, drug therapy should be considered when LDL is more than 30 mg/dL above the goal.

Treatment of Elevated Triglycerides

When triglycerides are less than 150 mg/dL, the following measures are considered:

1. Primary goal: Achieve LDL goal
2. Weight management and increase physical activity

Table 12-20 LDL Goals and Recommendations for Beginning Therapeutic Lifestyle Changes and Drug Therapy

Risk Category	LDL Goal	Begin Therapeutic Lifestyle Changes	Consider Drug Therapy
Optional category: Very high risk	Optional goal: < 70 mg/dL	≥ 70 mg/dL	≥ 70 mg/dL
High risk: CHD or CHD risk equivalent (10-year risk > 20%)	< 100 mg/dL	≥ 100 mg/dL	≥ 100 mg/dL
Moderately high risk: 2+ risk factors (10-year risk 10–20%)	< 130 mg/dL Optional goal: < 100 mg/dL	≥ 130 mg/dL Optional: ≥ 100 mg/dL	≥ 130 mg/dL
Moderate risk: 2+ risk factors (10-year risk < 10%)	< 130 mg/dL	≥ 130 mg/dL	≥ 160 mg/dL
Lower risk: 0–1 risk factors	< 160 mg/dL	≥ 160 mg/dL	≥ 190 mg/dL

Modified from: U.S. Department of Health and Human Services, Public Health Service, National Institutes of Health, National Heart, Lung, and Blood Institute, NIH Publication No. 01-3305, May 2011. Update from: Grundy SM, Cleeman JI, Merz NB, et al. Implications of recent clinical trials for the National Cholesterol Education Program Adult Treatment Panel III guidelines. *Circulation*. 2004;110:227–239.

3. If TG ≥ 200 mg/dL after LDL goal is reached
    a. Secondary goal: non-HDL cholesterol (total-HDL) 30 mg/dL higher than LDL
4. If TG is 200–499 mg/dL after LDL goal is reached
    a. Intensify LDL-lowering agent or add nicotinic acid or fibrate
5. If TG ≥ 500 mg/dL
    a. Primary goal: lower TG
    b. Very low-fat diet
    c. Weight management and physical activity
    d. Use fibrate or nicotinic acid
    e. When TG < 500 mg/dL, return to LDL lowering as primary goal

Treatment of Low HDL

When HDL is less than 40 mg/dL, the following measures should be considered:

1. Primary goal: Achieve LDL goal
2. Weight management and increase physical activity
3. If TG is 200–400 mg/dL, achieve non-HDL goal
4. If TG < 200 mg/dL (isolated low HDL) in a patient with CHD or a CHD equivalent, consider nicotinic acid or fibrate

Drug Therapy

HMG-CoA Reductase Inhibitors

- The HMG-CoA reductase inhibitors, commonly referred to as "statins," are the most effective agents for lowering LDL and total cholesterol.
- Depending on the agent and dose chosen, statins will lower LDL by approximately 20–60%. With each additional increase in dose, only about a 6% further decrease may be seen.
- Rhabdomyolysis is a severe, life-threatening adverse effect of statin therapy that is a result of skeletal muscle breakdown (although not all rhabdomyolysis is due to statin therapy). Myopathy is not the same as rhabdomyolysis. Myopathy refers to muscle weakness, pain/soreness, cramping, or stiffness that is not accompanied by muscle breakdown and is not life threatening.
- Mechanism of action: Inhibition of the rate-limiting enzyme in cholesterol synthesis, 3-hydroxy-3-methylglutaryl coenzyme A (HMG-CoA) reductase. Inhibition of HMG-CoA reductase also results in increased LDL catabolism.

Drug and food interactions:

- Lovastatin, simvastatin, and atorvastatin are metabolized by CYP 3A4. Drugs and juices that inhibit CYP3A4 (e.g., amiodarone, erythromycin, clarithromycin, ketoconazole, verapamil, diltiazem, and grapefruit juice) may increase the levels of the statin.
- Fluvastatin is metabolized by CYP 2C9.
- All statins are substrates of p-glycoprotein and may have their blood concentrations increased by drugs that inhibit p-glycoprotein (e.g., diltiazem, cyclosporine, digoxin) or by fruit juices such as grapefruit juice.
- Pravastatin, rosuvastatin, and pitavastatin are not significantly metabolized by CYP450 enzymes and, therefore, are less likely to be involved in drug interactions.

ADRs, contraindications, warnings, and precautions:

- Potential ADRs include increased serum aminotransferase levels (primarily ALT), elevated creatinine kinase, myopathy, rhabdomyolysis. Limit grapefruit juice intake.
- Do not exceed simvastatin 20 daily mg with verapamil or amiodarone.
- Do not exceed simvastatin 40 mg with diltiazem or Niaspan.

Pharmacodynamic and pharmacokinetic properties:

- HMG-CoA reductase inhibitors reach their maximal effectiveness in 2–4 weeks. See the list of drug and food interactions for more information regarding differences in metabolism among agents in the class.
- HMG-CoA reductase inhibitors have different potencies and require different doses to achieve the LDL goal. Estimated equivalent doses of currently available statins: rosuvastatin 5 mg, pitavastatin 2 mg, atorvastatin 10 mg, simvastatin 20 mg, pravastatin 40 mg, lovastatin 40 mg, fluvastatin 80 mg.

Patient counseling:

- Take the dose in the evening or at bedtime.
- May take the dose with or without food.
- Avoid excessive alcohol.
- Report any unusual muscle pain, stiffness, or cramping to the physician.
- Avoid consuming large amounts of grapefruit juice (i.e., more than 1 quart/day).

Cholesterol Absorption Inhibitors

- Ezetimibe is generally used in combination with a statin for patients who need additional LDL lowering beyond what may be provided by the HMG-CoA reductase inhibitor.
- Clinical outcome data are currently lacking for ezetimibe. For this reason, it should not be recommended as monotherapy unless the patient is intolerant or has a contraindication to a statin.
- Mechanism of action: Blocks the absorption of both biliary and dietary cholesterol across the brush border of the small intestine.

Drug and food interactions:

- The risk of cholelithiasis is increased with concomitant use of fibric acid derivatives.

ADRs, contraindications, warnings, and precautions:

- Potential ADRs include arthralgia, fatigue, diarrhea, and upper respiratory tract infection.
- Do not use in patients with moderate to severe hepatic impairment.

Pharmacodynamic and pharmacokinetic properties:

- Ezetimibe undergoes glucuronidation in the intestinal wall, forming an active metabolite that is enterohepatically circulated. This enterohepatic circulation limits systemic exposure to the drug and is thought to contribute to the low incidence of ADRs with ezetimibe.

Patient counseling:

- Take at the same time each day.
- May be taken at the same time as the statin.

Bile Acid Sequestrants

- Bile acid sequestrants are useful when combined with statins if additional LDL lowering is needed or as monotherapy if the patient does not tolerate or has a contraindication to statin therapy.
- The use of these agents is often limited due to their gastrointestinal side effects.
- Cholestyramine is available only as a powder that must be suspended by the patient.
- Mechanism of action: Bind to bile acids, forming an insoluble complex that prevents reabsorption and increases fecal elimination of bile acid–bound LDL.

Table 12-21 HMG-CoA Reductase Inhibitors

Drug	Dosage Forms	Dosing Frequency	LDL Reduction
Atorvastatin (Lipitor)	Tablets: 10 mg, 20 mg, 40 mg, 80 mg	Once daily	35–60%
Fluvastatin (Lescol, Lescol XL)	Capsules (Lescol): 20 mg, 40 mg Tablets (Lescol XL): 80 mg	Once daily (may administer 40 mg capsule twice daily)	22–35%
Lovastatin (Altoprev, Mevacor)	Tablets, extended release (Altoprev): 20 mg, 40 mg, 60 mg Tablets (Mevacor): 10 mg, 20 mg, 40 mg	Once daily	21–42%
Pitavastatin (Livalo)	Tablets: 1 mg, 2 mg, 4 mg	Once daily	38–45%
Pravastatin (Pravachol)	Tablets: 10 mg, 20 mg, 40 mg, 80 mg	Once daily	22–37%
Rosuvastatin (Crestor)	Tablets: 5 mg, 10 mg, 20 mg, 40 mg	Once daily	45–63%
Simvastatin (Zocor)	Tablets: 5 mg, 10 mg, 20 mg, 40 mg, 80 mg	Once daily	26–47%

Table 12-22 Cholesterol Absorption Inhibitors

Drug	Dosage Forms	Dosing Frequency	LDL Reduction
Ezetimibe (Zetia)	Tablet: 10 mg	Once daily	18%

Drug and food interactions:

- All bile acid sequestrants may interfere with the absorption of other drugs such as digoxin, thyroxine, thiazide diuretics, fat-soluble vitamins, beta blockers, folic acid, and acetaminophen.

ADRs, contraindications, warnings, and precautions:

- Potential ADRs include constipation (in more than 10% of patients), abdominal pain and distention, belching, and flatulence.
- Avoid in patients with high triglycerides, as bile acid sequestrants may further increase the level.

Pharmacodynamic and pharmacokinetic properties:

- No systemic absorption
- Fecal excretion

Patient counseling:

- Administer other medications 1 hour before or 1 hour after administration of bile acid sequestrants.
- Use the manufacturer's measuring scoop, if provided by the pharmacy, for bulk powder.
- Mix the powder with 6–8 oz of a noncarbonated beverage such as juice (e.g., orange juice) or water. Alternatively, cholestyramine may be mixed with applesauce, pudding, or gelatin (e.g., Jello).
- Patients experiencing constipation may increase fluid and fiber intake or use a stool softener.

Nicotinic Acid

- Niacin (nicotinic acid, vitamin B_3) is an extremely useful agent in that it can be used to treat high LDL, high triglycerides, and low HDL. While niacin does have a favorable effect on TG, it is typically prescribed for the treatment of combination dyslipidemias rather than isolated hypertriglyceridemia.
- Niacin should always be titrated upward from the lowest dose.
- Slo-Niacin is a SR formulation that can be purchased as an OTC product. IR niacin (Niacor) and ER niacin (Niaspan) are prescription products.
- Mechanism of action: Decreases hepatic synthesis of VLDL.

Drug and food interactions:

- The combination of nicotinic acid and HMG-CoA reductase inhibitors increases the risk for myopathy.
- Concurrent use with bile acid sequestrants may decrease the absorption of niacin.
- Prothrombin time may be increased in patients taking anticoagulants.

ADRs, contraindications, warnings, and precautions:

- Potential ADRs include flushing, hyperglycemia, hyperuricemia, GI complaints, and hepatotoxicity.
- Flushing is most common with the immediate-release formulations and less common with the extended- or sustained-release formulations. Flushing may cause some temporary discomfort, but it does not cause permanent harm or damage.

Pharmacodynamic and pharmacokinetic properties:

- Niacin undergoes extensive first-pass metabolism.
- Peak serum concentrations are reached within 30–60 minutes for the immediate-release formulation and 4–5 hours for the extended-release formulation.

Patient counseling:

- Flushing can be minimized by titrating the dose with gradual increases; administering aspirin 325 mg, ibuprofen 200 mg, or another NSAID 30–60 minutes before niacin; administering ER niacin at bedtime with a small, low-fat snack; or administering IR niacin in the middle of the meal. Flushing usually diminishes over weeks to months with consistent dosing. Flushing can be exacerbated by hot baths or showers, hot or spicy foods, and alcohol.
- Do not crush sustained-release tablets.
- Over-the-counter "flush-free" niacin contains inositol hexanicotinate and has not been shown to improve lipid levels.

Table 12-23 Bile Acid Sequestrants

Drug	Dosage Forms	Dosing Frequency	LDL Reduction
Cholestyramine (Prevalite, Questran)	Powder for suspension: 4 g/packet or 4 g/dose	Powder: once or twice daily	15–30%
Colesevelam (Welchol)	Granules for suspension: 3.75 g/packet Tablet: 625 mg	Granules: one packet once daily Tablet: 3 tablets (1.875 g) twice daily	8–15%
Colestipol (Colestid)	Granules for suspension: 5 g/scoop, 5 g/packet Tablet: 1 g	Granules: once daily or divided 2–4 times daily Tablets: once or twice daily	15–30%

Table 12-24 Nicotinic Acid

Drug	Dosage Forms	Dosing Frequency	Expected Decrease in LDL	Expected Increase in HDL	Expected Decrease in Triglycerides
Niacin	Tablet, extended release (Niaspan): 500 mg, 750 mg, 1,000 mg Tablet, controlled release (Slo-Niacin): 250 mg, 500 mg, 750 mg Tablet, immediate release (Niacor): 500 mg	Once daily (at bedtime or with evening meal)	5–25%	15–35%	20–50%

Fibric Acid Derivatives

- The most effective role for fibric acid derivatives is in the management of a patient with increased triglycerides and low HDL.
- The use of fenofibrate in combination with a statin is preferred over gemfibrozil in combination with a statin. Most statins have recommendations on the maximum dose appropriate when used in combination with gemfibrozil.
- Mechanism of action: PPAR-α agonist that decreases apolipoproteins B, C-III, and E while increasing apolipoproteins A-I and A-II. Overall, these changes result in a reduction of VLDL and an increase in HDL.

Drug and food interactions:

- The risks of myopathy and rhabdomyolysis are increased with concomitant use of fibrates and statins and/or the presence of renal insufficiency due to inhibition of glucuronidation and delayed renal excretion of statins. This combination may be used with caution, and the patient should be counseled regarding signs and symptoms of myopathy. Fenofibrate inhibits the glucuronidation to a lesser extent than gemfibrozil and is preferred in combination with HMG-CoA reductase inhibitors.
- Fibric acid derivatives carry an increased risk for bleeding in patients using warfarin.

ADRs, contraindications, warnings, and precautions:

- Potential ADRs: Dyspepsia, abdominal pain, diarrhea, flatulence, rash, fatigue, cholelithiasis, increased liver function tests, myopathy, rhabdomyolysis.
- Contraindicated in patients with gallbladder disease, biliary cirrhosis, and hepatic or renal dysfunction.

Pharmacodynamic and pharmacokinetic properties:

- Gemfibrozil: Inhibits 2C8, 2C9, 2C19, and 1A2; metabolized by hepatic oxidation and undergoes enterohepatic recycling.
- Fenofibrate: Metabolized in the tissue and plasma to the active form; inactivated by hepatic or renal glucuronidation.
- Absorption of gemfibrozil and fenofibrate is increased when these drugs are taken with meals.

Patient counseling:

- Gemfibrozil: Administer 30 minutes prior to meals.
- Fenofibrate: If you are diabetic, monitor your blood glucose closely when starting this medication.
- Fenoglide, Lofibra, and Lipofen: Take with meals.
- Antara, TriCor, and Triglide: May administer with or without food.

Omega-3 Fatty Acids

- Omega-3 fatty acids are considered to be essential fatty acids and are recommended for the treatment of high triglycerides (greater than 500 mg/dL).
- Essential fatty acids cannot be made by mammalian cells and must be obtained through dietary sources such as coldwater fish.

Table 12-25 Fibric Acid Derivatives

Drug	Dosage Forms	Dosing Frequency	Triglyceride Reduction
Fenofibrate	Capsule (Lipofen): 50 mg, 150 mg Capsule (Antara): 43 mg, 130 mg Capsule (Lofibra): 67 mg, 134 mg, 200 mg Tablet (Lofibra): 54 mg, 160 mg Tablet (TriCor): 48 mg, 145 mg Tablet (Triglide): 50 mg, 160 mg	Once daily	23–54%
Gemfibrozil	Tablet (Lopid): 600 mg	Twice daily (before meals)	20–60%

- The efficacy of fish oil depends on the amount of omega-3 fatty acids—specifically, eicosapentaenoic acid (EPA) and doxosahexaenoic acid (DHA).
- Dietary supplements with omega-3 fatty acids in them are often called fish oil supplements.
- Mechanism of action: The mechanism by which triglyceride levels are reduced is not completely understood.

Drug and food interactions:

- May enhance the effects of antiplatelet agents and the anticoagulant effect of warfarin.

ADRs, contraindications, warnings, and precautions:

- Potential ADRs: Diarrhea, prolonged bleeding time.
- Use with caution in patients with fish allergy.
- May increase LDL.

Patient counseling:

- Patients concomitantly taking antiplatelet or anticoagulant therapy should be monitored closely for bleeding.
- Some patient guidelines may suggest refrigerating or freezing prescription or nonprescription omega-3 fatty acids to improve the palatability and decrease any fish taste or smell. Prescription Lovaza capsules should *not* be frozen.

Pharmacotherapeutic alternatives:

- Many fish oil dietary supplements are available without a prescription, but those formulations often require the administration of multiple capsules due to smaller amounts of active ingredients.

1.3.0 Monitoring

Pharmacotherapeutic Outcomes

- Check fasting lipoprotein levels at baseline, and then 4–6 weeks (minimum) after initiation of therapy.
- If goals are not attained, consider titrating therapy or adding a second agent.

Table 12-26 Omega-3 Fatty Acids

Drug	Dosage Forms	Dosing Frequency	Triglyceride Reduction
Omega-3 fatty acid ethyl esters	Capsule (Lovaza): 1 g (contains approximately 375 mg DHA and 465 EPA per capsule)	Once daily (or in two divided doses)	20–50%

- If initiating therapeutic lifestyle changes without drug therapy, assess fasting lipoprotein levels 12–18 weeks after the trial of TLC.

Safety and efficacy monitoring

- Obtain liver function tests at baseline and then at 6–12 weeks for all statins, fibrates, and niacin.
- Obtain baseline CPK for patients taking statins, fibrates, and/or niacin. Recheck this test if the patient experiences symptoms of myopathy.
- Monitor fasting blood glucose in diabetic patients taking niacin.
- Monitor INR closely in patients taking omega-3 fatty acids and anticoagulants.

2.2.0 Dispensing

Bioequivalence

- Niacin formulations are not interchangeable.
- Not all fenofibrate formulations are considered therapeutically equivalent.

ANNOTATED BIBLIOGRAPHY

Ito MK. Hyperlipidemia. In: Chisholm-Burns MA, Wells BG, Schwinghammer TL, Malone PM, Kolesar JM, Rotschafer JC, DiPiro JT, eds. *Pharmacotherapy: Principles and Practice.* China: McGraw-Hill, 2008:175–193.

Lexi-Comp Online. Hudson, OH: Lexi-Comp, 1978–2008. Available at: http://online.lexi.com/crlsql/servlet/crlonline. Accessed December 23, 2010.

Pharmacists Letter Online. Stockton, CA: Therapeutic Research Center, 1995–2010. Available at: http://pharmacistsletter.therapeuticresearch.com/home.aspx?cs=&s=PL. Accessed December 27, 2010.

Talbert RL. Hyperlipidemia. DiPiro JT, Talbert TL, Yee GC, Matzke GR, Wells BG, Posey LM. *Pharmacotherapy: A Pathophysiologic Approach*, 7th ed. Available at: http://www.accesspharmacy.com/content.aspx?aid=3199458.

TOPIC: OBESITY

Section Coordinator: Debra Parker
Contributor: Lori J. Ernsthausen

Obesity Overview

The proportion of the U.S. population (children, teenagers, and adults) considered either overweight or obese is a significant health concern. In 2007–2008, the overall prevalence of overweight and obese persons among U.S. adults was 68%. Childhood and teenage obesity has more than doubled in the past 30 years. Obesity contributes to an increased risk of death in the presence of hypertension, hyperlipidemia, diabetes mellitus, coronary artery disease, stroke, and sleep apnea. Patients with these comorbidities require aggressive management of their risk factors as well as weight loss.

Tips Worth Tweeting

- Obesity is a chronic disease.
- Management of obesity includes a combination of diet modification, increased physical activity, and behavior modification.
- Pharmacologic therapy, in addition to lifestyle modifications, is reserved for patients who are considered obese or who are overweight with other risk factors or comorbidities.

Patient Care Scenario: Outpatient Medication Therapy Management Clinic

57 y/o, 5'3", 302 lbs, F, Caucasian

P. H. is a 57-year-old female who has been obese for as long as she can remember. Other than her obesity and "mild" arthritis, she states that she was always healthy until she felt a lump in her breast 2 years ago. After presenting to her PCP for this problem, she was diagnosed with and treated for breast cancer. P. H. says that this scare has motivated her tremendously and she is now ready to get her weight under control. She has been through diabetes education, where she learned healthy eating habits. Prior to this program, she ate whatever she wanted, often going out several times per week, and had never tried any specific diet. She now goes out to eat about once per week, preferring to cook healthy meals at home for herself and her husband, who is also obese. P. H. recently purchased a treadmill, but does not like to use it because her knees get so sore.

Medication Profile

Date	Physician	Drug	Quantity	Sig	Refills
1/6	Green	Lantus SoloStar Pen	15 mL	48 units SC daily	4
1/6	Green	Metformin ER 850 mg	90	1 po three times daily	4
12/22	Freeman	Enalapril 10 mg	60	1 po twice daily	8
12/22	Freeman	HCTZ 25 mg	30	1 po daily	10
12/22	Cooper	Tamoxifen 20 mg	30	1 po daily	3
11/14	–	Tylenol Arthritis		1 po q 6 h prn knee pain	

Allergies: NKA

PMH: DM type 2, hypertension, breast cancer (s/p mastectomy, chemotherapy, and radiation), osteoarthritis of bilateral knees

Lab Values: FBG 132 mg/dL; HgbA_{1c} 7.9%, BUN 16 mg/dL, SCr 1.0 mg/dL, Na 139 mEq/L, K 3.9 mEq/L, Cl 99 mEq/L, CO2 25 mEq/L

Vitals: 142/70; HR 82, RR 15, waist circumference 46 in.

Social Hx: Tobacco: quit 8 years ago. Alcohol: denies use.

1.1.0 Patient Information

Diagnosis and Assessment

Evaluation of body mass index (BMI), waist circumference, risk factors, and comorbidities is part of overweight and obese patient assessment. Body mass index (BMI) is a measure of body fat based on height and weight. It may overestimate excess body fat in certain conditions such as edema, muscular build, or very short or very tall individuals.

$$\text{BMI (kg/m}^2\text{)} = \text{weight (kg)} / [\text{height (m)}]^2$$

$$\text{BMI (kg/m}^2\text{)} = \text{weight (lb)} \times 703 / [\text{height (in)}]^2$$

- BMI < 25 kg/m^2: Maintain weight; prevent weight gain.
- BMI 25–29.9 kg/m^2 or elevated waist circumference with 2 or more comorbidities: Weight loss is indicated.
- BMI ≥ 30 kg/m^2: Weight loss is indicated.

Waist circumference reflects distribution of body fat and is used to evaluate central obesity. Central obesity increases the likelihood of development of hypertension, diabetes, dyslipidemia, and cardiovascular disease. Persons with high-risk waist circumference meet the following criteria:

- Men: waist circumference greater than 40 in (102 cm)
- Women: waist circumference greater than 35 in (89 cm)

Table 12-27 BMI Classification

Underweight	Less than 18.5 kg/m^2
Normal weight	18.5–24.9 kg/m^2
Overweight	25–29.9 kg/m^2
Obesity (class 1)	30–34.9 kg/m^2
Obesity (class 2)	35–39.9 kg/m^2
Extreme obesity (class 3)	Greater than or equal to 40 kg/m^2

Comorbidities

- Coronary heart disease
- Atherosclerosis
- Type 2 diabetes
- Sleep apnea

Risk Factors

- Smoking
- Hypertension
- Elevated LDL
- Low HDL
- Impaired fasting glucose
- Family history of premature CHD

Weight loss is recommended for the following individuals:

- Patients with BMI ≥ 30 kg/m^2
- Patients with BMI between 25–29.9 kg/m^2
- Patients with high-risk waist circumference and two or more risk factors

Treatment Goals

- Prevent any additional weight gain
- Reduce and maintain lower body weight
- Control risk factors

Initial weight loss goals:

- Loss of 10% body weight over 6 months
- 1- to 2-lb weight loss each week until goal is reached

Dietary Therapy and Physical Activity

Dietary modifications for weight loss and weight maintenance should include a diet balanced in carbohydrates, protein, and fat, such as the low-calorie Step 1 Diet. A reduction in total daily caloric intake of 500 to 1,000 kcal will help achieve a weight loss of 1 to 2 pounds per week. Consumption of complex carbohydrates from vegetables, fruits, and whole grains contributes to a balanced diet and increases intake of soluble fiber. The primary sources of protein should be from plants and lean sources of animal protein. It is important to maintain adequate intake of vitamins and minerals, especially calcium.

Pharmacists can help their patients adjust to a low-calorie diet by providing dietary education and counseling. Patients may need instruction on reading and interpreting nutrition labels and recognizing food composition (e.g., fats, carbohydrates, protein). Additional considerations for dietary modification include decreasing alcohol consumption and increasing water intake. Patients may also be counseled in determining correct portion size and healthy methods of food preparation. Decreasing caloric intake may be more easily managed by avoiding eating out and packing meals for work or school that contain healthy foods. Pharmacists may guide patients to online educational resources and support groups, as well as recipes and cookbooks for healthy living.

A low-calorie diet combined with physical activity results in a greater weight loss than diet alone. Patients who have not been engaging in physical activity should slowly increase the amount and intensity of physical activity over several weeks. Patients should consider starting with 10–30 minutes of moderate physical activity 3 days per week, with a target goal of 60 minutes on most or all days of the week. Moderate physical activity, such as gardening for 30–45 minutes, walking 2 miles in 30 minutes, washing windows and floors for 45–60 minutes, or swimming laps for 20 minutes burns approximately 150 calories per day or 1,000 calories per week.

1.2.0 Pharmacotherapy

Treatment

Pharmacotherapy, in addition to lifestyle modifications, is reserved for patients with a BMI ≥ 30 kg/m^2 or BMI ≥ 27 kg/m^2 with other risk factors. Nondrug therapy should be tried for at least 6 months before starting drug therapy. Weight is likely to be regained if lifestyle changes do not continue indefinitely. Surgical intervention may be considered for patients with extreme obesity (BMI ≥ 40 or BMI ≥ 35 with comorbidities).

Drug Therapy

Orlistat

- Orlistat (Xenical, Alli) is available in both a prescription and a nonprescription formulation.
- Mechanism of action: Inhibits pancreatic and gastric lipases as well as triglyceride hydrolysis, resulting in a caloric deficit and weight loss.
- Efficacy: After 1 year of treatment, approximately 60% of patients have lost at least 5% of baseline weight when taking a 120 mg, three times daily, dose.
- Drug interactions and food and dietary supplement considerations: Separate doses of orlistat and levothyroxine by at least 4 hours and cyclosporine by at least 2 hours. Daily fat intake should be approximately 30% of total caloric intake and separated over three meals. Gastrointestinal side effects may increase with a high-fat diet or with any meal containing a very large amount of fat.
- ADRs: Minimal systemic effects have been reported with orlistat due to the local action of the drug in the GI tract. Potential adverse drug effects include oily spotting, flatus with discharge, fecal urgency, fatty/oily stools, increased defecation,

Table 12-28 Orlistat

Drug	Dose and Dosage Form	Dosing Frequency
Orlistat (Xenical, Alli)	Xenical: 120 mg capsule; Alli: 60 mg capsule	Three times daily with each meal containing fat

fecal incontinence, cholelithiasis, hepatitis, and pancreatitis. Orlistat also decreases the absorption of fat-soluble vitamins such as A, D, E, K, and beta-carotene.
- Patient counseling: Orlistat may be taken up to 1 hour after a meal. If a meal is missed or contains little fat, no dose needs to be given. Supplement the diet with a multivitamin. Administer the multivitamin 2 hours prior to or 2 hours after an orlistat dose. Patients taking warfarin should have their INR monitored closely when initiating orlistat.

Phentermine

- Phentermine is a controlled substance (C-IV) with abuse potential due its structural similarity to amphetamines.
- Phentermine is indicated only for short-term use and should be discontinued within the first 4 weeks of treatment if satisfactory weight loss has not occurred.
- Mechanism of action: Sympathomimetic amine that increases norepinephrine and dopamine release in the CNS, leading to reduced appetite.
- Efficacy: Average weight loss over 2- to 24-week studies was 3.6 kg.
- Drug interactions and food and dietary supplement considerations: Avoid phentermine in patients taking MAO inhibitors, as concomitant use may lead to hypertensive crisis.
- ADRs: Heart palpitations, tachycardia, increased blood pressure, restlessness, insomnia, tremor, dysphoria, headache, and constipation. More serious, but rare, potential adverse effects include pulmonary hypertension and valvular heart disease.
- Patient counseling: Administer in the morning before breakfast or 1–2 hours after breakfast. Avoid late-evening administration. Phentermine is approved only for short-term use, and patients who do not experience weight loss within the first month of treatment should discontinue phentermine. Weight loss medications, such as phentermine, are meant to be prescribed along with dietary modifications. Those patients with a history of cardiovascular disease should avoid phentermine.

Table 12-29 Phentermine

Drug	Dose and Dosage Form	Dosing Frequency
Phentermine (Adipex-P)	15 mg, 30 mg, 37.5 mg capsule 37.5 mg tablet	Once or twice daily

Diethylpropion

- Diethylproprion is also a controlled substance (C-IV) with abuse potential due its structural similarity to amphetamines.
- Mechanism of action: Sympathomimetic amine that increases norepinephrine and dopamine release in the CNS, leading to reduced appetite.
- Efficacy: Average weight loss during 6- to 12-month administration is 3 kg.
- ADRs: Heart palpitations, tachycardia, increased blood pressure, restlessness, insomnia, tremor, dysphoria, headache, constipation, and bone marrow suppression. More serious, but rare, potential adverse effects include pulmonary hypertension and valvular heart disease.
- Patient counseling: Administer the dose at midmorning. Do not crush controlled-release tablets. Do not take the dose at bedtime. Diethylpropion is approved only for short-term use, and patients who do not experience weight loss within the first month of treatment should discontinue diethylpropion. Weight loss medications, such as diethylpropion, are meant to be prescribed along with dietary modifications. Patients may need to undergo baseline cardiac evaluation, and those with a history of cardiovascular disease should avoid diethylpropion.

Other Pharmacologic Agents

Other agents that have been used or studied off-label for weight loss include bupropion, caffeine, ephedrine, exenatide, fluoxetine, pramlintide, topiramate, thyroid hormone, and zonisamide. Natural products such as 5-hydroxytryptophan (5-HTP), barley, chromium, chitosan, conjugated linoleic acid, bitter orange, glucomannan, hoodia, and pyruvate are commonly used for weight loss, although many of these products lack evidence showing a clinically significant effect on body weight and composition or long-term safety data.

Table 12-30 Diethylpropion

Drug	Dose and Dosage Form	Dosing Frequency
Diethylpropion, controlled release	75 mg tablet	Once daily

1.3.0 Monitoring

Safety and Efficacy Monitoring

- Weight and waist circumference: Measure every 1–2 weeks. Waist circumference may decrease even if weight does not decrease due to changes in lean body mass.
- Blood pressure: Adjust medications as needed.
- Patients with diabetes may require close blood glucose monitoring and adjustment of medications.
- Monitor for adverse effects of drug therapy.
- Assess weight loss at 4 weeks for patients taking phentermine or diethylpropion. Discontinue these medications if weight loss is less than 1.8 kg or if tolerance develops.

2.2.0 Dispensing

Be familiar with your state law as it relates to prescribing and dispensing Schedule III or IV controlled substances for weight loss.

Physicians may prescribe an FDA-approved Schedule III or IV controlled substance for weight loss only after obtaining a thorough medical and weight loss or gain history, performing a complete physical examination, and determining that the patient is obese. Physicians must review their own records of prior treatment or another physician's records of prior treatment and must document that the patient has made a good-faith effort to lose weight with caloric restriction, nutritional counseling, behavior modification, and exercise without the utilization of controlled substances, and that the treatment has been ineffective.

Limitations may exist for quantity dispensed and course of treatment. Pharmacists should perform a prospective drug review prior to dispensing to ensure patient safety and compliance with state law. In some states, the State Board of Pharmacy may require the pharmacist to document the patient's BMI or weight loss since the last prescription. Pharmacists should also be familiar with the prescribing authority of mid-level practitioners in their state, as prescribing authority varies from state to state.

ANNOTATED BIBLIOGRAPHY

Graham MR, Lindsey CC. Overweight and obesity. In: Chisholm-Burns MA, Wells BG, Schwinghammer TL, Malone PM, Kolesar JM, Rotschafer JC, DiPiro JT, eds. *Pharmacotherapy: Principles and Practice.* China: McGraw-Hill, 2008:1529–1539.

Lexi-Comp Online. Hudson, OH: Lexi-Comp, 1978–2008. Available at: http://online.lexi.com/crlsql/servlet/crlonline. Accessed January 7, 2011.

National High Blood Pressure Education Program. *The Fourth Report on the Diagnosis, Evaluation, and Treatment of High Blood Pressure in Children and Adolescents.* Rev. ed. NIH Publication No. 05-5267. Bethesda, MD: National Heart, Lung, and Blood Institute, 2005.

Pharmacists Letter Online. Stockton, CA: Therapeutic Research Center, 1995–2010. Available at: http://pharmacistsletter.therapeuticresearch.com/home.aspx?cs=&s=PL. Accessed January 5, 2011.

TOPIC: THYROID DISORDERS

Section Coordinator: *Debra Parker*
Contributor: *Debra Parker*

Thyroid Disorders Overview

Thyroid hormones are necessary for normal fetal development and adult metabolism. Thyroid hormones (T_3 and T_4) affect almost every organ system. More than 8 million Americans have a thyroid disorder, with hypothyroidism being the most common and requiring lifelong pharmacotherapy. Levothyroxine, the agent of choice, is subject to food, mineral, and multiple drug interactions. The pharmacist plays an important role in promoting lifelong adherence to the therapeutic regimen and educating patients regarding food, mineral, and drug interactions.

Tips Worth Tweeting

- Thyroid disorders affect more than 8 million Americans.
- Hypothyroidism and hyperthyroidism are the two main thyroid disorders, with hypothyroidism being far more prevalent.
- TSH level (which is elevated in hypothyroidism and decreased in hyperthyroidism) is the most sensitive blood test to diagnose hypothyroidism.
- Treatment of hypothyroidism generally requires lifelong pharmacotherapy.
- Levothyroxine (T_4) is the agent of choice in the treatment of hypothyroidism.
- Treatment of hyperthyroidism may or may not involve initial pharmacotherapy, but the course of the disease and its treatment eventually result in hypothyroidism.
- If drug therapy is used to treat hyperthyroidism, methimazole is preferred over propylthiouracil (PTU).
- Liver toxicity and agranulocytosis are the two most serious side effects of antithyroid drugs (methimazole and PTU).

Patient Care Scenario: Community Pharmacy

67 y/o, 5'2",176 lbs F, Caucasian
Allergies: shellfish—anaphylaxis
PMH: HTN, osteoporosis, atrial fibrillation
Lab Values

Na: 145 mEq/L	Hgb: 13.6 g/dL
K: 4.0 mEq/L	Hct: 44%
Cl: 101 mEq/L	MCV: 80 μm^3
CO_2: 26 mEq/L	TSH: 16.2 mU/L
BUN: 10 mg/dL	FT_4: 0.32 ng/dL
SCr: 0.8 mg/dL	Tot Chol: 225 mg/dL
Glu: 96 mg/dL	TG: 212 mg/dL
HDL: 35 mg/dL	ALT: 15 IU/L
LDL: 148 mg/dL	AST: 21 IU/L

Vitals: BP 142/82; P 64; RR 18; T 97.5°F

Medication Profile:

Date	Physician	Drug	Quantity	Sig	Refills
4/3	Frey	Docusate 100 mg	30	1 bid prn	9
4/5	Frey	Lisinopril 20 mg	30	1 po daily	7
4/5	Frey	Toprol XL 50 mg	30	1 po daily	7
4/16	Spencer	Fosamax 70 mg	4	1 tablet q Monday	6
5/5	Frey	Levothyroxine 100 mcg	30	1 po daily	11
5/5	—	Aspirin 81 mg	30	1 po daily	
5/5	—	Calcium 500 mg	60	1 po bid	
5/5	—	Claritin OTC	30	1 po daily prn	

Social Hx: divorced. Waitress. Denies tobacco use, alcohol, and illicit drug use.
Notes: 5/5: Patient c/o feeling "really run down" recently, and is seeking a recommendation for something to give her more energy. She comments she feels worse than when she went through menopause (6 yrs ago) and hopes her new prescription will help.

1.1.0 Patient Information

Definition

Thyroid disorders are common in the United States. The two most common types are hypothyroidism and hyperthyroidism. If left untreated, these conditions can result in long-term effects, including increased mortality. Treatment of either condition generally results in the lifelong need for pharmacotherapy.

Thyroid Hormones (T_3 and T_4)

- Infants: Responsible for fetal growth and development, especially CNS development. Deficiency leads to irreversible mental retardation (cretinism).
- Adults: Maintain metabolic homeostasis. Affects almost all organ systems.

Stimulation of Thyroid Hormone Release

- Hypothalamus: Releases thyrotropin-releasing hormone (TRH).
- Pituitary: Stimulated by TRH to release thyroid-stimulating hormone (TSH).
- Thyroid gland: Stimulated by TSH to release T_4 (inactive form, which is converted peripherally to T_3) and T_3. T_4 and T_3 are released in a 4:1 ratio.
- T_4 inhibits the release of TSH, forming a negative feedback loop.

Production of Thyroid Hormones

Iodine:

- Ingested in diet
- Reduced to iodide in the intestine
- Transported to the thyroid gland and converted to iodine
- Incorporated into T_3 (triiodothyronine) and T_4 (thyroxine)

T_3 and T_4 are released in a 4:1 ratio from the thyroid gland. T_4 is converted to the active form (T_3) peripherally at the site of action.

Key Terms

- **Primary hypothyroidism/hyperthyroidism:** Problem stems from the thyroid gland; most common types of thyroid disorders.
- **Secondary hypothyroidism/hyperthyroidism:** Problem stems from the pituitary gland
- **Tertiary hypothyroidism/hyperthyroidism:** Problem stems from the hypothalamus; least common types of thyroid disorders.

Diagnosis

The diagnosis of either hypothyroidism or hyperthyroidism is made based on plasma TSH, T_4, and T_3 concentrations.

Thyroid Function Tests

- TSH level: Most sensitive index of hypothyroidism. Can be abnormal before an alteration of FT_4 or T_3 is detected. TSH is carried in blood bound to thyroid-binding globulin (TBG). Alterations in TBG may affect the ability to interpret TSH concentrations.

Table 12-31 Hypothyroidism Versus Hyperthyroidism

Hypothyroidism	Hyperthyroidism
Underproduction of thyroid hormones	Overproduction of thyroid hormones
Prevalence: approximately 8 million Americans Females: 5–7x > males	Less common than hypothyroidism (0.02–0.4% in the United States) Female > males
Most common type: Primary hypothyroidism Hashimoto's disease (more than 90%): Autoimmune attack of the thyroid gland	Most common type: Primary hyperthyroidism Graves' disease: IgG antibodies act like TSH and stimulate the thyroid gland; frequent spontaneous remission
Risk factors: • Female gender • Family history of any thyroid illness • Autoimmune diseases (e.g., rheumatoid arthritis or diabetes) • Advanced age (greater than 60 years)	Risk factors: None identified
Iatrogenic causes: Thyroidectomy or other treatment of hyperthyroidism, amiodarone, iodine deficiency (fish, dairy products), enzymatic effects, iodine, lithium and interferon-alpha, nitroprusside	Iatrogenic causes: Amiodarone, iodine
Clinical presentation: • CNS: Difficulty concentrating; loss of interest/pleasure in sex, pleasurable activities; feeling "worthless"; altered mental status, depression, fatigue • CV: Hypertension • Dermatologic: brittle or thin hair and nails, and skin changes (edema, dryness, yellowish tint) can occur with severe/prolonged hypothyroidism • GI: Unexplained weight gain, constipation • GU: Heavy menses • Miscellaneous: Cold intolerance, hoarseness, muscle aches • Elderly: May be asymptomatic	Clinical presentation: • CNS: Anxiety, nervousness, irritability, insomnia, weakness, fatigue, tremors • CV: Palpitations, bruits, thrills, wide pulse pressure, atrial fibrillation, heart failure • Dermatologic: Heat intolerance, diaphoresis, pretibial myxedema, pedal edema, flushed moist skin, thinning of hair, plumber's nails, diffusely enlarged goiter • GI: Weight loss with increased appetite, diarrhea • GU: Amenorrhea or light menses • Ophthalmologic: Proptosis, lid lag, lid retractions, stare, periorbital edema, loss of extraocular movements, diplopia, photophobia, eye irritation, change in visual acuity • Miscellaneous: Heat intolerance, osteoporosis (if long-standing)
Goiter: May or may not be present	Goiter: May or may not be present
Medical emergency: • Myxedema coma: Mortality rate of approximately 80% if untreated; represents terminal stage of hypothyroidism • Hallmark symptoms: Hypothermia, lethargy, respiratory acidosis, CV shock, coma	Medical emergency: • Thyroid storm: Exaggerated symptoms of hyperthyroidism; coma, death in 20% of thyroid storm cases; usually precipitated by illness or injury • Presentation: Fever, tachycardia (out of proportion to fever), tachypnea, N/V/D, delirium, coma; no specific labs to distinguish from uncomplicated hyperthyroidism • Treatment: Supportive measures and administering antithyroid medications immediately

- Thyroid antibodies (to detect autoimmune disease):
  - Not diagnostic/specific
  - May be used to monitor response to therapy or onset/end of disease remission
- Long-acting thyroid stimulator (LATS): Used to monitor therapy for Graves' disease.
- TSAb: Diagnostic of Graves' disease, but not useful in following progression of disease.
- Alterations in thyroid function tests may be caused by alterations in TBG levels:
  - TBG is increased by prostaglandins, acute and chronic hepatitis, estrogens, clofibrate, and methadone

Table 12-32 Thyroid Levels Associated with Thyroid Disorders

Diagnosis	T_4	FT_4	TSH
Normal	Normal	Normal	Normal
Hyperthyroid	Increased	Increased	Decreased
Hypothyroid	Decreased	Decreased	Increased
TBG	Increased	Normal	Normal
TBG	Decreased	Normal	Normal

- TBG is decreased by severe illness (protein synthesis shunted to fight illness), nephrotic syndrome, Cushing syndrome, hepatic failure (cirrhosis), as well as androgens, anabolic steroids, and glucocorticoids

Risk Factors (Patient, Genetic, and Biosocial)

See Table 12-34.

Wellness and Prevention

- No recommendations are made for prevention.
- Treatment of either hypothyroidism or hyperthyroidism is geared toward achieving and maintaining a euthyroid state to avoid long-term complications, including increased mortality.

1.2.0 Pharmacotherapy of Hypothyroidism

Treatment

- Lifelong pharmacotherapy is required in most patients.
- Pharmacotherapy is *not* indicated for weight loss/obesity, menstrual irregularities, PMS, or "euthyroid sick syndrome" (abnormal thyroid function tests may result from many nonthyroid illnesses).

Goals of Therapy

- Normal TSH (most accurate indicator of adequate replacement)
- Normal or slightly elevated FT_4 level
- Reversal of hypothyroid symptoms

Pharmacotherapy

ADRs/Precautions/Warnings for All Thyroid Hormone Replacements

Generally, these medications are well tolerated when a euthryoid state is achieved. If excess supplement is taken, symptoms similar to hyperthyroidism may appear:

- CNS: Anxiety, nervousness, irritability, insomnia, weakness, fatigue, tremors

Table 12-33 Diagnosis of Thyroid Disorders

Hypothyroidism	Hyperthyroidism
Standard tests: Measure TSH and FT_4* TSH: Most reliable laboratory test to confirm hypothyroidism Diagnosis: Elevated TSH and low FT_4; TSH may be elevated before the development of hypothyroid symptoms	Increased T_4 index and decreased TSH *May* measure T_3 for "T_3 thyrotoxicosis"
Other laboratory findings: ↑TSH ↓Na ↑CPK ↓Hgb/Hct ↑cholesterol[†] ↑LFTs ↑ESR	Other laboratory findings: ↓TSH ↑all other thyroid indices ↑calcium + TSI (Graves') ↓cholesterol ↑LFTs

*FT_4 = free T_4.

[†]Increased cholesterol levels occur because of decreased conversion of cholesterol to bile acids. In addition, thyroid hormones increase the binding of LDL cholesterol to liver cells.

- CV: Palpitations, bruits, thrills, wide pulse pressure
- Dermatologic: Heat intolerance, diaphoresis, pretibial myxedema, pedal edema, flushed moist skin, thinning of hair, plumber's nails, diffusely enlarged goiter
- GI: Weight loss with increased appetite, diarrhea
- GU: Amenorrhea or light menses
- Ophthalmologic: Proptosis, lid lag, lid retraction, stare, periorbital edema, loss of extraocular movements, diplopia, photophobia, eye irritation, change in visual acuity,

Table 12-34 Risk Factors for Thyroid Disorders

Hypothyroidism	Hyperthyroidism
Annual screening should be considered for the following groups: • Patients older than age 65 • Women older than age 40 with a suspicious complaint • Patients with positive thyroid antibodies • After any treatment for hyperthyroidism, or thyroid or neck surgery or irradiation • Patients with evidence of autoimmune disease (e.g., RA, DM1)	Toxic multinodular goiter Toxic adenoma Excess exogenous thyroid hormone ingestion

- Miscellaneous: Heat intolerance, osteoporosis (if long-standing)

Contraindications for All Thyroid Hormone Replacements

None. Lower doses may be necessary for elderly patients or individuals with preexisting arrhythmias or coronary artery disease.

Drug Interactions for All Thyroid Hormone Replacements

- Bind to thyroxine and decrease absorption: Aluminum, sucralfate, cholestyramine, colestipol, ferrous sulfate, kayexelate
- Induce metabolism of thyroxine: Darbamazepine, phenobarbital, phenytoin, rifabutin, rifampin
- Block T_4 to T_3 conversion: Amiodarone, beta blockers
- Increase TBG: Prostaglandins, acute and chronic hepatitis, estrogens, clofibrate, methadone
- Decrease TBG: Androgens, anabolic steroids, glucocorticoids
- Known to cause hypothyroidism: Lithium, interferon-alpha, nitroprusside

Food Interactions for All Thyroid Hormone Replacement

- Food may decrease absorption. Take supplements 30 minutes before or 2 hours after eating.
- Absorption is decreased by antacids, calcium, and iron. Avoid their use within 4 hours of thyroid supplement.

1.3.0 Monitoring for Hypothyroidism

Clinical Response

Improvement in well-being, energy level, and puffiness should be noticed within 2–3 weeks. Skin, hair, and voice improvements may take months to become apparent.

Laboratory Monitoring

- Monitor the patient for 2–3 months after therapy initiation and every 6–12 months thereafter.
- Must measure trough levels of FT_4.

1.2.0 Pharmacotherapy of Hyperthyroidism

Goals of Therapy

- Lower thyroid hormones to reestablish a euthyroid and eumetabolic state
- Duration of therapy: 6 months to more than 2 years
- Primary control: Latent period to improvement; euthyroid in 4–8 weeks
- Perioperative: Achieve euthyroid state prior to surgery
- Adjunct to radiation: Hasten recovery

Treatment

Treatment for hyperthyroidism may include thioamides (antithyroid medications, also known as goitrogens), radioactive iodide (RAI), or surgery (thyroidectomy).

Radiation

The underlying principle is to destroy part, but not all, of the thyroid gland.

Radioactive Iodine

Radioactive iodine becomes concentrated in the thyroid gland just like a stable isotope.

- ^{131}I: Most commonly used form of therapy in the United States
- SE: Early or late development of hypothyroidism
- Contraindicated during pregnancy or while breastfeeding
- Monitoring: At 4- to 6-week intervals for the first 3 months of therapy; at least annual checkups thereafter; hypothyroidism usually develops after therapy within 6–12 months

Pharmacotherapy

See Table 12-37.

Other Pharmacotherapy

Beta blockers:

- May be used with iodide or other thioamides. Block catecholamine action on the heart sensitized by hormones, thereby decreasing the cardiac effects of hyperthyroidism.
- Have no effect on disease. Other beta blockers are used, but propranolol is the most common choice because it also blocks the conversion of T_4 to T_3.

1.3.0 Monitoring for Hyperthyroidism

- Patients treated with antithyroid drugs should be seen initially at 4- to 12-week intervals until euthyroidism is achieved.
- Once euthyroidism is achieved, the ATD dose may be reduced. Patients are then monitored every 3–4 months.
- Monitor: TSH, FT_4, BP, weight, HR, thyroid and eye exam.
- TSH levels may remain low for several months, even after T_4 and T_3 levels become normalized.
- Once antithyroid drugs are discontinued, monitor the patient every 4–6 weeks for 3–4 months, then at increasing intervals for 1 year.
- If the patient remains euthyroid, monitor yearly for the next 3–4 years, and at increasing intervals thereafter.

Table 12-35 Thyroid Hormone Replacement Agents

Levothyroxine Sodium	
• Replacement hormone of choice. • Typical dose is 100–125 mcg po daily. • Lower starting doses (e.g., 25–50 mcg daily) are recommended for the elderly and for individuals with preexisting cardiac disease. • Although weight-based dosing may be used, it is not typically done in clinical practice. • Pharmacokinetic/pharmacodynamic considerations: The FDA states that all levothyroxine products should be considered *inequivalent* unless AB rated as bioequivalent in the FDA "Orange Book." • Levo-T, Levoxyl, Levothroid, Synthroid, Unithroid, and some generics have been AB rated as bioequivalent. • Half-life: 7 days; allows for once-daily dosing. • IV dose is 50% of oral dose.	
Brand Names	**Dosage Forms**
Synthroid Levothroid Levoxyl Unithroid	Tablets: 0.025, 0.05, 0.075, 0.088, 0.1, 0.112, 0.125, 0.137, 0.15, 0.175, 0.2, 0.3 mg Injection: 0.2, 0.5 mg
Levothyroxine Sodium (Triiodothyronine; T_3)	
• Typical dose: 25 mcg po daily. • More costly than T_4. • Half-life: 1.5 hours; requires multiple daily doses. • Greater potential for cardiac symptoms. • More difficult to monitor therapeutic and toxic responses.	
Brand Names	**Dosage Forms**
Cytomel	Tablets: 5, 25, 50 mcg
Triostat	Injection: 10 mcg/mL
Desiccated Thyroid (USP)	
• Typical dose: 60–120 mg po daily. • Derived from porcine or bovine thyroid. • Standardized by iodine content, so there is unacceptable variability in potency and ratios of T_4 to T_3. • Inexpensive, but variability is a major disadvantage. • Contraindication: Hypersensitivity to beef or pork.	
Brand Names	**Dosage Forms**
Armour Thyroid Nature-Throid Westhroid	Tablets: 15, 16.25, 30, 32.5, 60, 65, 90, 120, 130, 180, 195, 240, 300 mg
Liotrix	
• Typical dose: 60–120 mg po daily. • Mixture of T_4 and T_3 in a 4:1 ratio. • Thought to be the "agent of choice" before it was realized that a significant amount of T_4 is converted peripherally to T_3. • No real advantage/need to use this medication due to its cost and the problems inherent to T_3-containing preparations.	
Brand Names	**Dosage Forms**
Thyrolar	Tablets: 15, 30, 60, 120, 180 mg

Table 12-36 Therapy for Hyperthyroidism

	Thioamides	RAI*	Surgery
Therapy of choice	• Children • Young adults • Graves' disease • PTU *only* if pregnant/lactating	• Adults • Elderly/cardiac • Poor surgical risk • Failed treatment with thiamides • Status post thyroid surgery	• Second trimester of pregnancy • Recurrent thyrotoxicosis • Malignancies • Large goiters • Refuses alternative treatment options • Alternative for children
Advantages	• Onset: 2–4 weeks • No radiation exposure • No surgical risks • Safer in pregnancy • PTU preferred for thyroid storm	• Onset: 2–4 weeks • No surgical risks • Option when surgery is not possible • Permanent solution	• Immediate onset • No radiation • Removes malignancy • Permanent solution
Disadvantages (possible)	• Agranulocytosis • SLE-like syndrome • Must avoid concurrent iodides (salt, topical, x-ray) • Hypersensitivity	• Long-term monitoring • Cannot be used if the patient is pregnant • Thyroid cancer/genetic damage?	• Surgical risks • Hypoparathyroidism • Hypothyroidism • Scarring

May postpone use until it is determined that the patient's condition is not self-limiting.

Table 12-37 Antithyroid Agents

Also known as thioamides, thionamides, or goitrogens.

- Mechanism of action: Inhibit thyroid peroxidase and hence the iodination and coupling reactions in thyroid synthesis; block synthesis of T_3 and T_4. Propylthiouracil (PTU) also inhibits the conversion of T_4 to T_3.
- ADRs/warnings/precautions: Fever, headache, paresthesias, skin rash, agranulocytosis, hepatitis, GI symptoms (liver toxicity, jaundice).
- Safety alert: In June 2009, FDA issued a statement indicating increased risk of serious liver injury (including failure and death) with PTU use; approximately six times greater incidence is reported with PTU compared to methimazole. Avoid PTU use unless the patient has Graves' disease and is in the first trimester of pregnancy, or in the case of any patient with Graves' disease who is allergic to or intolerant of methimazole.
- Drug interactions: Hyperthyroidism itself increases the metabolism of clotting factors; consequently, patients taking warfarin may require lower doses. Treatment of hyperthyroidism slows metabolism of clotting factors, and may result in higher doses for patients taking warfarin.
- Pharmacokinetic/pharmacodynamic considerations: Methimazole is approximately 10 times as potent as PTU. PTU has a much shorter half-life, requiring multiple daily dosing.

Agent	Dosage Forms	Usual Dose	Precautions
Methimazole (Tapazole, Northyx)	Tablets: 5, 10, 20 mg	Initial therapy: 15–60 mg/day in divided doses based on the severity of the patient's condition Maintenance dose: 5–15 mg/day as a single dose or in divided doses	Avoid during the first trimester of pregnancy; secreted in breastmilk
Propylthiouracil (PTU) (Propacil)	Tablets: 50 mg	300–400 mg q 6–8 hr	See the FDA safety alert mentioned above

Table 12-38 Iodides

- Lugol's solution: 5% iodine and 10% potassium iodide.
- SSKI (saturated solution of potassium iodide): 1 g/mL; contains 38 mg iodine per drop.
- Mechanism of action: Paradoxically decrease hormone synthesis and release. Iodides act as a negative feedback, overwhelming the thyroid and decreasing hormone synthesis. May be used prior to surgery to decrease the vascularity and size of the thyroid gland or in cases of thyroid storm where rapid reversal of symptoms is required.
- May be used with beta blockers to decrease the cardiac effects of hyperthyroidism. (Other beta blockers are used, but propranolol is the most common choice; may also be used with a calcium-channel blocker such as diltiazem.)
- ADRs/warnings/precautions:
  - Lugol's solution: Prolonged use can lead to hypothyroidism. Can cause acne flare-ups and dermatitis.
  - SSKI: Irregular heartbeat, confusion, tiredness, fever, rash, salivary gland swelling/tenderness, swelling of neck/throat, myxedema, lymph node swelling, abdominal discomfort, nausea, vomiting, diarrhea, hyperthyroidism/hypothyroidism, metallic taste.
- Contraindications: Avoid if the patient has hypersensitivity to iodine or any component of the formulation; hyperkalemia; pulmonary edema; impaired renal function; hyperthyroidism; or iodine-induced goiter.
- Food considerations: May dilute these medications in water, fruit juice, or milk. Take with food to decrease gastric irritation.

Agent	Dosage Form	Usual Dose
Lugol's solution (strong iodine solution)	Solution, oral: Potassium iodide 100 mg/mL and iodine 50 mg/mL (480 mL)	Perioperative dose: 0.1–0.3 mL (35 drops) tid × 10 days prior to surgery
SSKI (saturated solution of potassium iodide)	1 g/mL	50–250 mg (1–5 drops) tid × 10 days prior to surgery

2.1.0 Calculations

Dosage Conversion

Equivalent doses: Levothyroxine sodium (T_4) 100 mcg is usually considered equivalent to desiccated thyroid 60 mg, thyroglobulin 60 mg, or liothyronine sodium (T_3) 25 mcg. This is a general guideline only, however; each patient must be carefully evaluated when switching thyroid hormone replacement products as well as when switching from one brand-name agent to another. Close monitoring of TSH and FT_4 levels is required.

Table 12-39 Effects of Thyroid Status on Actions of Other Drugs

Drug	Thyroid Status	Mechanism	Effect
Sympathomimetic	Hyper	↑ Sensitivity to catecholamines	↑ Thyrotoxic symptoms
Digitalis	Hyper	↑ VD of digitalis	Requires more digitalis
	Hypo	↓ VD of digitalis	Requires less digitalis
Insulin	Hyper	↑ Metabolism of insulin	Requires more insulin
	Hypo	↓ Metabolism of insulin	Requires less insulin
Warfarin	Hyper	↑ Metabolism of clotting factors (CF)	Requires less warfarin
	Hypo	↓ Metabolism of CF	Requires more warfarin

2.2.0 Dispensing

- Lugol's solution and SSKI: Store at controlled room temperature. Protect from light and keep the container tightly closed.
- SSKI: If exposed to cold, crystallization may occur. Warm and shake the solution to redissolve any crystals. If the solution becomes brown/yellow, it should be discarded.

Compounding

SSKI reconstitution:

- May be mixed with water, fruit juice, infant formula, flat soda, or milk.
- Formulas for making a 16.25 mg/5 mL solution as well as an 8.125 mg/5 mL oral solution suggest the resulting product is stable for up to 7 days under refrigeration.

ANNOTATED BIBLIOGRAPHY

DRUGDEX Information System. Greenwood Village, CO: Thomson Healthcare, 1974–2008. Updated periodically. Available at: https://www.thomsonhc.com. Accessed February 20, 2010.

Katz MD. Thyroid disorders. In: Chisholm-Burns MA, Wells BG, Schwinghammer TL, Malone PM, Kolesar JM, Rotschafer JC, DiPiro JT, eds. *Pharmacotherapy: Principles and Practice.* China: McGraw-Hill, 2008:667–683.

Lexi-Comp Online. Hudson, OH: Lexi-Comp, 1978–2008. Available at: http://online.lexi.com/crlsql/servlet/crlonline. Accessed February 20, 2010.

Gastrointestinal

CHAPTER

13

TOPIC: CONSTIPATION

Section Coordinator: Tracy K. Pettinger
Contributor: Gina Davis

Tips Worth Tweeting

- Prescription and over-the-counter (OTC) medications can cause constipation. Therefore, it is always important to rule out medication-induced constipation and provide alternative recommendations to the patient's primary care provider (PCP).
- Treatment for constipation accompanied by certain alarm symptoms should be referred to a PCP for evaluation before recommending an OTC laxative.
- Most cases of constipation can be treated with gradual increases of fiber in the diet, fluid intake, and physical activity.
- Fiber laxatives are recommended as first-line therapy to prevent and treat constipation when dietary fiber is not increased.
- Watch and educate patients on laxative overuse or abuse.

Patient Care Scenario: Community Setting

B. M.: 60 y/o, 5'6", F, 154 lbs
History:

- Hypothyroidism
- Insomnia
- GERD
- CVA 5 years ago

Labs: normal TSH

Date	Physician	Drug	Quantity	Sig	Refills
5/23	Watson	diphenhydramine 50 mg	30	one tablet hs	0
5/23	Watson	levothyroxine 75 mcg	30	one tablet q A.M.	3
5/23	Watson	omeprazole 20 mg	30	one tablet q day	4
5/23	Watson	amoxicillin 500 mg	30	one tablet tid	0

1.1.0 Patient Information

Causes of Constipation

To optimize treatment, secondary etiologies must be considered. Constipation can result from numerous causes, such as medications (see Table 13-1), medical conditions (see Table 13-2), diet, fluid intake, and exercise characteristics. When secondary causes are ruled out, idiopathic or functional (primary) constipation can be considered and evaluated.

Laboratory and Diagnostic Testing

A detailed medical history, a physical exam, blood and electrolyte testing, and colonoscopy

Table 13-1 Common Medications That May Cause Constipation[1,2,7]

Opioids	Anticholinergics
Tricyclic antidepressants	Calcium-channel blockers
Chemotherapy agents	Antiparkinsonian agents
Sympathomimetics	Antipsychotics
Diuretics	Sedating antihistamines
Aluminum- or calcium-containing antacids	
Calcium supplements	Clonidine
Iron supplements	Antidiarrheal agents
Benzodiazepines	Beta blockers
Cholestyramine	Nonsteroidal anti-inflammatory drugs

Table 13-2 Medical Conditions That May Cause Constipation[1,2,7]

Disorders of the Gastrointestinal Tract
Irritable bowel syndrome (IBS)
Diverticulitis
Anal fissures or strictures
Tumors
Hemorrhoids
Hernia
Helminthic infections
Metabolic Disorders
Diabetes mellitus neuropathy
Uremia
Hypokalemia
Hypomagnesemia
Endocrine Disorders
Hypothyroidism
Hypercalemia
Panhypopituitarism
Pheochromocytoma
Neurogenic Causes
CNS diseases
Spinal cord injury
Cerebral vascular accidents (CVA)
CNS tumor
Dementia
Pregnancy
Psychogenic Causes
Psychiatric diseases (e.g., anxiety, depression)

should be done by the physician when constipation is accompanied by alarming symptoms, such as blood in the stools, weight loss, or anorexia (see Table 19-4).

Lab/diagnostic tests that can be used for constipation include the following:

- Electrolyte: potassium and calcium level
- Dehydration: BUN to CR ratio, sodium and chloride, ins and outs (I&Os)
- Blood in stool
- Anemias: CBC
- Proctoscopy
- Sigmoidoscopy and colonoscopy
- Radiography and barium enema
- Marker studies: colonic transit time
- Defecography
- Balloon insertion
- Anorectal manometry
- Rule out medical conditions (i.e., check thyroid function, serum glucose) or medications causing constipation
- Physical exam: abdomen, rectal

Signs and Symptoms

Constipation is a common medical complaint from patients. However, the manifestations or the meaning of constipation differs from one patient to another. A patient with constipation may complain of one or more of the following:

- Decrease in frequency of bowel movements
- Hard, dry stools or small stools
- Straining or pain while having a bowel movement
- Bloating
- Feelings of an incomplete bowel movement

A physical exam by a physician is needed if constipation is a chronic problem or accompanied by other pertinent alarm signs or symptoms, such as weight loss or blood in the stools (see Table 13-4).

Wellness and Prevention

Patient education on lifestyle modifications is one of the first steps that can be taken to improve and prevent constipation. Lifestyle modifications include increasing fiber in the diet, increasing fluid intake, and engaging in regular physical activity.

Increase fiber intake gradually over a period of 7 to 10 days to help with tolerance to GI side effects. The total daily fiber amounts recommended by the Institute of Medicine are as follows:

- Men younger than age 50: 38 grams
- Women younger than age 50: 25 grams
- Men older than age 50: 30 grams
- Women older than age 50: 21 grams

Dietary fiber can be increased in the diet by eating wheat grains, oats, fruits, and vegetables. Be cautious

Table 13-3 Questions to Ask the Patient[1,2]

- Medical history?
- Current medications?
- Bowel movements: How often? Consistency of stools? Accompanying symptoms (e.g., nausea, abdominal pain)? How long have you been experiencing these symptoms?
- Any history of constipation? Which medications were used to treat it? Length of use of previous medications?
- Family history of medical conditions that could cause constipation?
- Allergies?
- Age of patient?
- Lifestyle characteristics (diet, exercise, fluid intake)?

when recommending fiber to the diets of patients with hypocalemia and low iron levels because some fibers can inhibit absorption of these supplements.

Generally, drinking 6 to 8 glasses of water per day (about 2 liters) can help with constipation. Watch for fluid overload in patients who have fluid restrictions (i.e., kidney disease, congestive heart failure).

Encourage patients to immediately respond to the feeling of needing to have a bowel movement and educate them to make time for a regular bathroom visit. Tell patients to try having a bowel movement soon after waking in the morning or 30 minutes after meals. A stool diary can help to record the details (e.g., frequency, consistency) of the bowel movement.

1.2.0 Pharmacotherapy

Self-care options can be recommended in some cases, but the pharmacist should recognize when the patient should be referred to the PCP (Table 13-4).

When secondary causes are ruled out, empiric treatment can be tried. First, lifestyle modifications can be made to improve and prevent constipation. Lifestyle modifications include increasing fiber in the diet, increasing fluid intake, and engaging in regular physical activity. After increasing dietary fiber, patients should notice an effect on bowel function 3 to 5 days after initiation of this intervention; however, it should be continued for at least 1 month before determining the effect on relief of constipation. Encourage patients to immediately respond to the feeling of needing to have a bowel movement and educate them to make time for a regular bathroom visit.

Table 13-4 When to Refer Patients to a Physician[1,2]

- No relief after 1 week of using OTC laxatives
- Constipation accompanied by nausea, vomiting, weight loss, rectal pain, fever, cramping, abdominal pain, blood in the stool, marked flatulence, or anorexia
- Recurring constipation (over 3-month period)
- Fecal impact or obstruction
- Constipation caused by a medical condition or a medication
- Constipation and a family history of inflammatory bowel disease or colon cancer
- Sudden changes in stool

For patients who are not able to get enough fiber in their diet, concentrated fiber sources, also known as bulk-forming agents (e.g., psyllium, calcium polycarbophil, methylcellulose), are available. In most cases of constipation, bulk-forming agents are usually recommended as first-line therapies because they most closely mimic the natural physiologic process of bowel evacuation. Synthetic colloidal cellulous products (calcium polycarbophil and methylcellulose) tend to cause less flatulence than natural fiber. Other agents are used when the bulk-forming laxative is not effective, when it is contraindicated, or when a more rapid effect is needed. Consider that making lifestyle modifications or using bulk-forming agents can take 3 or more days to help with constipation. If constipation is not relieved after 1 week of self-care, an evaluation by a PCP should be recommended.

The next options may include a saline laxative (i.e., milk of magnesia) or polyethylene glycol. If constipation is still present, consider a stimulant laxative or lactulose. Be aware that lactulose can cause gas, and stimulant laxatives can cause gas and abdominal cramping.

Stimulants should not be used daily and should be used only intermittently. It is important to monitor how long the laxative is used for each episode of constipation and how often it is repeated. Overuse of laxatives can lead to alteration of the normal functioning of the gut, which in turn can cause dependence on the laxative to produce a bowel movement.

Acute Constipation

Because the bulk-forming agents have a delayed onset of affect, a tap-water enema or glycerin suppositories can be used if immediate results are needed. If these options do not provide relief, oral sorbitol, bisacodyl, senna, or saline laxatives (milk of magnesia) can be tried.

Chronic Constipation

First, lifestyle medications should be optimized. If pharmacotherapy is needed, consider a bulk-forming agent—specifically, psyllium—first. Alternative agents that can be used include polyethylene glycol or lactulose. Polyethylene glycol may be slightly more effective than lactulose. Lubiprostone (Amitiza) is indicated for chronic idiopathic constipation and can be considered for patients who do not respond to other agents.

Constipation Secondary to Opiate Use

Use a stimulant laxative in combination with a stool softener. Prevention of constipation is necessary when starting an opiate, especially in an elderly patient. Bulk-forming laxatives are not helpful to manage constipation induced by opiates.

In a hospitalized patient, for immediate resolution of constipation related to the use of opiates, a tap-water enema, glycerin suppository, or oral milk of magnesia can be used.

Prevention of Constipation When Straining Can Be Dangerous

Stool softeners are used to prevent constipation when straining is not allowed, such as following abdominal surgery. Stool softeners may also be helpful in patients who have anal fissures to decrease pain when having a bowel movement.

Drug Indications, Dosing Regimens, and Routes of Administration

It is important to look at the active ingredients in the products because some brand names may be used for multiple products.

Table 13-5 Drug Categories, Dosing Regimens, and Dosage Forms

	Examples of Brand Names	Dosing Regimens	Dosage Forms
Fiber/Bulk-Forming Laxatives (OTC)			
Psyllium	Metamucil and others	See individual products Follow each dose with 8 oz of water	Capsule Powder Wafer
Methylcellulose	Citrucel	Caplet: 2–4 caplets 1–3 times /day; follow each dose with 8 oz of water Powder: 1 heaping tablespoon (19 g) in 8 oz of water, 1–3 times/day	Caplet Powder
Calcium polycarbophil	Fibercon and others	1,250 mg 1–4 times/day; follow each dose with 8 oz of water	Caplet, captab Tablet Chewable tablet
Emollients/Stool Softeners (OTC)			
Docusate sodium	Colace and others	Oral: 50–200 mg in 1–4 divided doses	Capsule Liquid Syrup Rectal enema
Docusate calcium	Surfak and others	Oral: 240 mg once daily	Capsule Liquid
Lubricant Laxatives (OTC)			
Mineral oil	Fleet and others	See individual products	Oral microemulsion Rectal oil enema Oral oil
Hyperosmolar Agents			
Sorbitol	N/A (OTC)	Oral: 30–45 mL daily (as 70% solution)	Oral solution
Lactulose	Constulose and others	Oral: 15–30 mL daily to twice a day	Crystals for oral solution Oral solution Rectal solution
Polyethylene glycol (PEG)	Miralax and others	17 g of powder (1 heaping tablespoon) daily dissolved in 4–8 oz of water, juice, coffee, soda, or tea	Powder for oral solution
PEG and electrolytes	CoLyte, GoLYTELY, and others	See individual products: for bowel cleansing prior to GI exam	Powder for oral solution

Table 13-5 (*continued*)

	Examples of Brand Names	Dosing Regimens	Dosage Forms
Stimulants (OTC)			
Bisacodyl	Dulcolax Correctol	Oral: 5–15 mg once daily Rectal suppository: 10 mg once daily	Rectal solution enema Rectal suppository Tablet (EC, DR)
Senna (sennosides A and B)	Senokot Ex-Lax and others	See individual products	Oral liquid Orally disintegrating strip Oral syrup Tablet Chewable tablet
Saline Laxatives (OTC)			
Magnesium citrate	Generic	Oral: 150–300 mL (give daily or in 2 divided doses); used as a cathartic agent	Oral solution
Magnesium hydroxide	Milk of Magnesia	See individual products	Oral suspension Chewable tablet
Sodium biphosphate	Fleet Phospho-Soda	Oral: 15 mL single dose (maximum dose: 45 mL/day) on an empty stomach; dilute dose with 4 oz of water and then follow dose with 8 oz water	Oral solution Rectal solution enema Tablet
Chloride-Channel Activators			
Lubiprostone	Amitiza	24 mcg twice a day with food (swallow whole; do not break or chew)	Capsule

Table 13-6 Drug and Food Interactions

	Drug Interactions	Food Interactions
Fiber/bulk-forming laxatives	Separate administration of bulk-forming medications with other medications by 2 hours due to binding and decreasing absorption.	N/A
Emollients/stool softeners	Do not take with mineral oil because docusate can emulsify the mineral oil and, therefore, increase the mineral oil absorption. This can lead to accumulation in the hepatic lymphoid tissue.	N/A
Lubricant laxatives	Use with caution in patients taking anticoagulants due to possibility of decreasing vitamin K absorption and, therefore, increasing the risk of bleeding. Avoid use with docusate.	Decreases absorption of fat-soluble vitamins; separate from meals by 2 hours.
Hyperosmolar agents	Avoid the use of sorbitol with calcium or sodium polystyrene sulfonate.	N/A
Stimulants	Bisacodyl: separate with antacids and H3 blockers and PPI by 1 hour.	Bisacodyl: separate with milk/dairy products by 1 hour.
Saline laxatives	Avoid the use of laxatives containing magnesium with calcium or sodium polystyrene sulfonate (may increase the risk for metabolic alkalosis). Separate with medications where magnesium could decrease their absorption.	Take on an empty stomach.
Chloride-channel activators	N/A	N/A

Table 13-7 Contraindications, Warnings, and Precautions

	Contraindications, Warnings, and Precautions
Fiber/bulk-forming laxatives	Must take with fluid (at least 8 oz). Adequate water intake is important when used in conjunction with fiber to help alleviate constipation and prevent obstruction. Esophageal obstruction can occur in patients who have swallowing difficulties or in patients who have esophageal strictures or ulcers and ingest a bulk laxative in the dry form. Do not use if the patient has narrowing of the esophagus. Do not use in patients with fecal impaction or GI obstruction. Watch for hypercalcemia when calcium polycarbophil is used. Avoid use in patients on severe fluid restriction, such as renal dysfunction and heart failure. Watch the sugar content of certain bulk-forming agents if the patient is diabetic; conversely, do not use the sugar-free formulation that contains aspartame in patients with phenylketonuria.
Emollients/ stool softeners	Avoid use in patients with intestinal obstruction. Ensure that hydration is adequate.
Lubricant laxatives	Do not use in patients with appendicitis, undiagnosed rectal bleeding, dysphagia, colonoscopy, ileostomy, ulcerative colitis, or diverticulitis. Oral ingestion may cause aspiration and lead to lipid pneumonia; therefore do not administer these laxatives before lying down; to the young, elderly, or bedridden; or to patients who have conditions that result in trouble swallowing. Also, do not administer with food. Do not use in pregnant women or elderly population.
Hyperosmolar agents	Use caution in patients with renal impairment or cardiopulmonary disease. Intake of large volumes may cause fluid overload and/or electrolyte imbalances. Lactulose solution contains sugar; use with caution in diabetic patients. Avoid in patients with bowel obstruction.
Stimulants	Avoid in patients with abdominal obstruction. Senna: avoid use in patients with acute intestinal inflammation, colitis ulcerosa, appendicitis, or pregnancy.
Saline laxatives	Magnesium citrate, magnesium hydroxide: avoid use in patients with renal dysfunction (watch for hypermagnesemia). Long-term use can cause electrolyte disturbances. Sodium phosphate: avoid use in patients with renal dysfunction (watch for hyperphosphotemia). Watch use in sodium-restricted patients. Saline laxatives are contraindicated or require caution in patients with ulcerative colitis, diverticulitis, intestinal obstruction, appendicitis, ileostomy, colostomy, dehydration, renal impairment, cardiovascular disease (i.e., congestive heart failure), or diabetes.
Chloride-channel activators	Use caution in patients with hepatic or renal impairment because safety in these individuals has not been established. Avoid use in patients with gastrointestinal obstruction or with severe diarrhea.

Interaction of Drugs with Foods and Laboratory Tests

See Table 13-6.

Contraindications, Warnings, and Precautions

Do not give laxatives to children younger than the age of 6, unless prescribed by a physician. See Table 13-7.

1.3.0 Monitoring

Pharmacotherapeutic Outcomes

Desired outcomes of pharmacotherapy include relief of the constipating symptoms (i.e., decreased straining, increased frequency of bowel movement, decreased abdominal bloating or distention), prevention of any further constipation, no drug side effects, and avoidance of laxative abuse or misuse.

Safety and Efficacy Monitoring

Educate the patient to watch for drug-related side effects (see Table 13-9). For ambulatory patients who start by increasing dietary fiber or use a bulk-forming laxative, follow-up should occur in 1 week. Educate patients to seek medical attention if alarming symptoms arise. If patients do not obtain relief, refer them to the PCP. Monitor for electrolyte imbalances due to diarrhea, dehydration, or toxicity of laxatives that contain electrolytes.

Table 13-8 Mechanism of Action and Onset of Action

	Mechanism of Action	Onset of Action
Fiber/bulk-forming laxatives	Absorb water and increase bulk of stool; increase gastrointestinal motility; decrease colonic transit time	12–24 hours but can take up to 3 days (calcium polycarbophil: 24–48 hours)
Emollients/stool softeners	Decrease surface tension, which allows the stool to absorb more water and soften	24–72 hours
Lubricant laxatives	Coat the stool to allow the stool to pass through the GI tract more easily	1–3 days (oral)
Hyperosmolar agents	Draw water into the rectum, which increases intestinal motility	24–72 hours (glycerin suppositories: 30 minutes)
Stimulants	Stimulate the mucosal nerve plexus of the colon to increase motility	6 hours for oral bisacodyl; 6–12 hours for senna
Saline laxatives	Draw fluid into the GI tract through an osmotic gradient, increasing intraluminal pressure and motility; decrease colon transit time; cholecystokinin production may be stimulated, which causes accumulation of fluid and electrolytes within the intestinal lumen	0.5–3 hours for magnesium citrate and sodium phosphate; 0.5–6 hours for magnesium hydroxide; 2–5 minutes rectally
Chloride-channel activators	Activate chloride channels locally to increase chloride-rich intestinal fluid secretion	Within 24 hours

Table 13-9 Side Effects

	Side Effects
Fiber/bulk-forming laxatives	Flatulence and bloating Few to no systemic side effects because the laxatives are not absorbed
Emollients/stool softeners	Diarrhea and mild abdominal cramping Prolonged and frequent use may cause dependence or electrolyte imbalance
Lubricant laxatives	Other agents used to soften the stool, such as docusate, may be safer Diarrhea, nausea and vomiting, abdominal cramps Minimal systemic absorption; with prolonged use, oil droplets may be found on organs, such as the liver or spleen, and trigger an antibody response Watch for oil that may leak through the anus, causing anal pruritus
Hyperosmolar agents	Bloating, abdominal discomfort, cramping, and gas May cause electrolyte imbalances with routine use
Stimulants	Gas and abdominal cramping Neurologic damage with chronic use of senna, but unproven Bisacodyl: incontinence, hypokalemia, abdominal cramping
Saline laxatives	Abdominal cramps, diarrhea, gas Watch for electrolyte imbalances
Chloride-channel activators	Headache, diarrhea, and nausea (take with food)

Adverse Drug Reactions

See Table 13-9.

Nonadherence, Misuse, or Abuse

Laxatives may be abused by patients. These products should always be used at the smallest effective dose for the shortest period of time that they are needed. Some patients may not realize the long-term effects of laxative use. Notably, patients may overuse laxatives when they think that they need to "stay regular" by having a daily bowel movement. These patients may think that absence of daily bowel movements can lead to buildup of toxic substances in the bowel.

Laxatives may also be abused by patients to produce weight loss. These patients may also suffer from anorexia or bulimia nervosa. Overuse can lead to loss of smooth and striated muscle tonicity. The diarrhea

Table 13-10 Techniques for Drug Preparation, Compounding, and Quality Assurance

Medication	Tips That Can Improve Palatability
Sodium biphosphate	Chilled and take with citrus-flavored carbonated beverage
Magnesium citrate	Chilled and take with a glass of water, fruit juice, or citrus-flavored carbonated beverage
Liquid senna	Take with fruit juice or milk
Docusate syrup	Take with milk or juice
Mineral oil	Chill
Lactulose	Take with milk, juice, water, or citrus-flavored beverage
PEG	Stir powder in water, juice, soda, coffee, or tea
Senna	Take with fruit juice or milk

may be watery, and the patient may have accompanying symptoms of abdominal pain, weight loss, nausea, and vomiting. Other features may include electrolyte imbalance (i.e., hypokalemia), steatorrhea, liver disease, protein loss, and osteomalacia.

When stopping a laxative after it has been used chronically or abused, the patient should be weaned off the medication and lifestyle modifications (increased fiber and fluid in the diet, plus exercise) should be implemented.

Bioequivalence

Bulk-forming agents may contain phenylalanine, potassium, and sodium, and may contain varying amounts of calories. Consequently, individual packaging should be checked.

Docusate calcium and docusate sodium can be interchangeable because the amount of sodium, calcium, or potassium salts per dosage form is clinically insignificant.

Polyethylene glycol (PEG) comes in a formulation that does not contain electrolytes (PEG 3350 or Miralax), and a formulation that does contain electrolytes (CoLyte or GoLYTELY).

Package, Storage, Handling, and Disposal

Drugs should be stored at room temperature and away from light and humidity. Some medications can be refrigerated after being mixed. Always refer to the product labeling for the expiration time after reconstitution. For example, CoLyte and GoLYTELY are stored at room temperature before reconstitution and can be refrigerated after being reconstituted. The reconstituted solution should be used within 48 hours of preparation.

ANNOTATED BIBLIOGRAPHY

1. Spruill W, Wade W. Diarrhea, constipation, and irritable bowel syndrome. In: Dipiro JT, et al., eds. *Pharmacotherapy: A Pathophysiological Approach*. 7th ed. New York, NY: McGraw-Hill; 2008: 617–632.
2. Curry C Jr, Butler D. Constipation. In: *Handbook of Nonprescription Drugs: An Interactive Approach to Self-Care*. 16th ed. Washington, DC: American Pharmacist Association; 2009:263–288.
3. Medications for constipation. *Pharmacist's Letter/Prescriber's Letter* 2007;23(5):230503.
4. Lexi-Comp Online. Available at: http://online.lexi.com/crlsql/servlet/crlonline. Accessed February 27, 2010.
5. Micromedex Healthcare Series. Available at: http://www.thomsonhc.com/hcs/librarian. Accessed March 10, 2010.
6. American Gastroenterological Association. AGA Institute medical positional statement on constipation. *Gastroenterology* 2000;119:1761–1778.
7. Hsieh C. Treatment of constipation in older adults. *Am Fam Physician* 20051;72(11):2277–2284.
8. Arce D, Ermocilla C, Costa H. Evaluation of constipation. *Am Fam Physician* 2002;65(11):2283–2290.

TOPIC: DIARRHEA

Section Coordinator: *Tracy K. Pettinger*
Contributors: *Tanner W. Higginbothom and Kevin W. Cleveland*

Tips Worth Tweeting

- Diarrhea can be classified as acute or chronic, infectious or noninfectious, and mild, moderate, or severe.
- Stool cultures are recommended in patients with moderate to severe diarrhea who have had recent antibiotic use, hospitalization, or daycare attendance, or who have concurrent fever, bloody stools, or signs of systemic illness.
- Diarrhea can be due to altered intestinal transit and can be secretory, osmotic, and/or exudative in nature.
- Noninfectious diarrhea is symptomatically treated with agents that decrease secretion, decrease gut motility, and/or adsorb intestinal contents.
- Infectious diarrhea is usually self-limiting but may require antibiotic use based on the specific pathogen.

- All moderate to severe diarrhea treatment should be accompanied by fluid and electrolyte replacement therapy.

Patient Care Scenario: Hospital

Chief Complaint

K. C. is a 5-year-old boy brought to the ER with complaints of abdominal pain, nausea, and diarrhea over the past 2 days. He admits feeling "weak" and "tired."

History of Present Illness

K. C. has had stomach pains, loss of appetite, and numerous watery stools for the past 48 hours. The diarrhea has progressed from nonbloody to bloody over the past day. Approximately 5 days before the diarrhea started, K. C.'s daycare center celebrated another child's birthday, during which the children ate hamburgers cooked by the daycare staff. K. C.'s father is concerned that perhaps the hamburgers were not cooked thoroughly.

Medication Record

None; NKDA

Physical Examination

- Gen: pale, ill-appearing white male
- VS: BP 104/69, P 90, RR 22, T 37°C, Ht 3'3", Wt 44 lbs
- Skin: loose skin turgor
- HEENT: PERRLA; dry and pale mucous membranes
- Chest: RRR, clear to A & P
- Abd: hyperactive bowel sounds; diffuse tenderness; no guarding or rebound; no organomegaly
- Genit/rect: heme (+) stool

Laboratory and Diagnostic Tests

Na	137 mEq/L	BUN	29 mEq/L	Hct	32%	AST	30 IU/L
K	2.8 mEq/L	SCr	1.1 mg/dL	Plt	400 × 10^3/mm^3	ALT	20 IU/L
Cl	95 mEq/L	Glu	92 mg/dL	WBC	16.5 × 10^3/mm^3	Stool negative (–) for fecal leukocytes	
CO_2	23 mEq/L	Hgb	11 mg/dL	60% PMNs			
				48% Lymphs			
				2% Monos			

Diagnosis

- Infectious diarrhea; *E. coli* O157:H7 likely pathogen
- Dehydration

1.1.0 Patient Information

Disease States Associated with Diarrhea

- Intestinal infection
- Crohn's disease
- Ulcerative colitis
- Irritable bowel syndrome
- Hyperthyroidism
- Diabetes mellitus
- Lactose intolerance
- Secretory hormonal tumor

Instruments and Techniques Related to Patient Assessment

- Dietary history, weight assessment, and dehydration assessment: colonoscopy if diarrhea is chronic or the patient has blood in the stool
- Endoscopy and biopsy may be helpful in conditions such as colitis or cancer
- Radiography may be helpful in inflammatory conditions

Laboratory Testing

- Stool analysis can examine blood, mucus, fat, mineral, and electrolyte content as well as osmolality, pH, and daily stool volume.
- Specific pathogen screens should be requested depending on the patient's history and presentation; they are recommended in patients with moderate to severe diarrhea who have had recent antibiotic use, hospitalization, or daycare attendance, or concurrent fever, bloody stools, or signs of systemic illness.
- Pseudomembranous colitis (*Clostridium difficile*) should be suspected in cases of diarrhea following antibiotic use within the previous 2 weeks or within 72 hours of hospital discharge.

Table 13-11 Medication-Induced Causes of Diarrhea

Alpha-glucosidase inhibitors	Antineoplastics	Quinidine	Reserpine	Bethanechol
Magnesium compounds	5-Aminosalicylates	Digitalis	Hydralazine	Neostigmine
Laxatives	NSAIDs	Digoxin	ACE inhibitors	Metoclopramide
Antibiotics	Proton pump inhibitors	Methyldopa	Misoprostol	Metformin
	H2-receptor blockers	Guanabenz	Colchicine	Theophylline

- Immunocompromised patients should be tested for a variety of bacterial, viral, and parasitic pathogens.

Signs and Symptoms of Diarrhea

- Frequent loose, watery stools
- Abdominal cramps
- Abdominal pain
- Nausea, vomiting
- Malaise
- Chills, fever
- Bloating
- Possibly bloody/painful stool
- Audible bowel sounds
- Hyperperistalsis
- Localized or general tenderness

Terminology Used in Classification of Diarrhea

- Acute diarrhea: lasting less than 14 days
- Persistent diarrhea: lasting more than 14 days but less than 30 days
- Chronic diarrhea: lasting more than 30 days
- Mild diarrhea: does not hinder normal activities
- Moderate diarrhea: limits normal activities
- Severe diarrhea: completely prevents normal activities
- Infectious diarrhea: diarrhea caused by viruses, bacteria, or protozoa
- Noninfectious diarrhea: diarrhea in which no infectious organism can be identified as the cause
- Traveler's diarrhea: syndrome with an onset during or after travel, most commonly caused by consumption of food or water contaminated with bacterial pathogens and, less commonly, with viruses or parasites
- Gastroenteritis: inflammation of the stomach and intestines; often called the "stomach flu," as it is commonly accompanied by vomiting and diarrhea
- Dysentery: form of infectious diarrhea accompanied by symptoms such as fever, bloody/mucoid stool, and tenesmus; it is most often caused by infection with *Shigella* spp.

Noninfectious Diarrhea

There are four subgroups of clinical diarrhea:

- *Secretory.* Substances cause an increase in secretion of extra water and electrolytes, often via inhibition of Na+/K+ ATPase or stimulation of intracellular cAMP, or substances inhibit absorption of water and electrolytes. Unlike osmotic diarrhea, secretory diarrhea continues even when the individual is in a fasting state, and the stool maintains its normal ionic contents.
- *Osmotic.* Exogenous substances that are poorly absorbed from the lumen cause increased secretion of water and electrolytes so as to match the osmolality of the lumen contents with that of the plasma. Malabsorption of carbohydrates, lactose intolerance, chronic pancreatitis, cystic fibrosis, and consumption of magnesium compounds can all result in osmotic diarrhea. Osmotic diarrhea ceases with fasting and has an abnormally high electrolyte concentration.
- *Exudative.* Inflammatory diseases (e.g., ulcerative colitis, Crohn's disease, diverticulitis) lead to large amounts of mucus, blood, and serum proteins in the gut. Absorption, secretion, and motility can also be affected by inflammatory diseases.
- *Altered intestinal transit.* This condition may be caused by bypass surgery, intestinal resection, and drugs.

Infectious Diarrhea

See Table 13-12.

Wellness and Prevention

Viral infectious diarrhea can be prevented by avoiding person-to-person contact, as this is the main method for transmission.

Bacterial and protozoal infectious diarrhea is usually due to poor environmental hygiene practices, such as food and water contamination and poor sanitation techniques. Drinking water can be treated, and uncooked foods of any kind (including fresh vegetables and fruits) should be avoided while traveling.

Vaccines are available for typhoid fever and rotavirus.

Antibiotic or bismuth subsalicylate prophylaxis can be used to help prevent traveler's diarrhea.

1.2.0 Pharmacotherapy

Drug Indications

- If diarrhea remains acute without fever or systemic symptoms, symptomatic treatment is indicated,

Table 13-12 Common Pathogens in Infectious Diarrhea

Viruses	Bacteria	Protozoa
Norovirus	*Salmonella*	*Giardia*
Sapovirus	*Shigella*	*Cryptosporidium*
Rotavirus	*Campylobacter*	*Cyclospora*
	Staphylococcus	*Isospora belli*
	Escherichia coli	
	Clostridium difficile	

along with fluid and electrolyte replacement therapy.

- If fever or systemic symptoms accompany diarrhea, and the stool is negative for infection, continue symptomatic treatment.
- If diarrhea becomes chronic, a history and physical examination are necessary to determine its possible causes.
- If infection is suspected or determined, different antimicrobial agents may be used, depending on the causative organism.
- Antimicrobial agents can treat certain infectious diarrheas.
  - Use is not necessary in most cases of mild diarrhea.
  - Reduces risk of morbidity and mortality in certain infections.
- *Escherichia coli*
  - Enterotoxigenic: empirical use of antibiotics may shorten the disease duration.
  - Enterohemorrhagic: no specific drug therapy; supportive care is recommended without antibiotic use.
- Pseudomembranous colitis (*Clostridium difficile*)
  - Antimotility agents should be avoided.
  - Antibiotics are indicated.
- Shigellosis (*Shigella* spp.)
  - Usually self-limiting (4–7 days).
  - Antibiotic use is reserved for the elderly, children, and healthcare workers.
- Salmonellosis (*Salmonella*)
  - Infection can lead to enterocolitis, bacteremia, enteric fever, or localized infections at any site.
  - Antimotility agents increase the risk of complications in enterocolitis and should be avoided.
  - Antibiotics are not useful in treating salmonellosis-associated enterocolitis in otherwise healthy adults.
- Campylobacteriosis (*Campylobacter jejuni*)
  - Antimotility agents should be avoided.
  - Antibiotics shorten the duration of toxin excretion from bacteria but do not lessen the severity or duration of diarrhea.
  - Antibiotics may be used only if started within the first 4 days of illness or in patients with fevers, bloody diarrhea, pregnancy, or immunodeficiency.
- Rotavirus infection
  - Bismuth subsalicylate, antimotility agents, and antibiotics are not recommended.
  - RotaTeq is a live, oral vaccine that may help prevent infection.
- Other viral infections
  - Oral rehydration therapy is the cornerstone of therapy.
- Traveler's diarrhea
  - Treatment should include antibiotics with a spectrum of activity against the invading pathogen.
  - Symptom relief can be achieved with loperamide or bismuth subsalicylate in nonbloody diarrhea.
  - Prophylactic antibiotic use depends on the area of travel and the likely pathogens in the location.

Other Treatments

Food Considerations

Generally, feeding should be continued as tolerated. Fasting has not been widely studied as a treatment for any form of diarrhea buy may alleviate osmotic diarrhea.

Table 13-13 Pharmacotherapy for Symptomatic Treatment of Diarrhea

Drug	Mechanism of Action	Dose	Adverse Effects	Interactions (Drug, Food, Lab, Disease)	Pearls
Bismuth subsalicylate	Directly inhibits microbial activity and binds to bacterial enterotoxins Antiprostaglandin effects of the salicylate component inhibit secretion and hypermotility	Oral: 525 mg every 30 min to 1 hr up to a maximum of 8 doses daily	Constipation, darkened tongue and stools; tinnitus, nausea, and vomiting with toxic levels of salicylate	May increase risk of bleeding in patients taking anticoagulants Toxic levels of salicylate may accumulate in patients with renal dysfunction or those taking aspirin	Useful in prevention and treatment of both infectious and noninfectious diarrhea

(*continues*)

Table 13-13 (*continued*)

Drug	Mechanism of Action	Dose	Adverse Effects	Interactions (Drug, Food, Lab, Disease)	Pearls
Octreotide	Inhibits release of vasoactive substances (e.g., serotonin, gastrin, vasoactive intestinal peptide) from intestinal or pancreatic tumor	IV or subQ: 200–300 mcg/day in 2–4 divided doses for 2 weeks; adjust up to 600 mcg/day in 2–4 divided doses to achieve a therapeutic response Depot IM: 20 mg intragluteally at 4-week intervals for 2 months, after which the dose may be titrated, depending on symptom control; continue subcutaneous injections for at least 2 weeks during the switch to IM injection	Nausea, diarrhea, abdominal pain, local injection pain; cholelithiasis is possible with prolonged use; steatorrhea is possible with high doses	May augment QTc-prolonging effect of QTc-prolonging medications	Treats diarrhea associated with peptide-secreting tumors
Loperamide	Decreases secretions by inhibiting calmodulin, a calcium-binding protein that controls chloride secretion Decreases peristalsis through inhibition of local neuronal mechanisms	Oral: 4 mg, followed by 2 mg after each loose stool, up to a maximum of 16 mg/day	Dizziness, constipation, or fatigue	Avoid in diarrhea accompanied by fever or dysentery Use in children is discouraged	Opioid agonist that does not cross the blood–brain barrier
Diphenoxylate/atropine	Decreases motility via stimulation of opioid receptors in the intestines	Oral: 5 mg 4 times daily until diarrhea is controlled; adjust dose to response; maximum dose is 20 mg/day	Blurred vision, drowsiness, dizziness, urinary retention, dry mouth, constipation	Avoid in diarrhea accompanied by a fever or dysentery Use in children is discouraged Avoid in bacterial enteritis caused by *E. coli*, *Shigella*, or *Salmonella*	Atropine is added to help prevent abuse of diphenoxylate
Difenoxin	Same as diphenoxylate	Oral: 2 mg initially, 1 mg after each loose stool thereafter; maximum dose is 8 mg/day	Same as diphenoxylate	Same as diphenoxylate	Atropine is added to help prevent abuse of difenoxin
Kaolin/pectin	Kaolin component adsorbs bacteria and toxins and reduces water loss	Oral: 60–120 mL at the first sign of diarrhea and after each bowel movement as needed	Constipation	Avoid use in pseudomembranous enterocolitis or toxigenic bacteria	

Table 13-13 (*continued*)

Drug	Mechanism of Action	Dose	Adverse Effects	Interactions (Drug, Food, Lab, Disease)	Pearls
Polycarbophil	Adsorbs bacteria and toxins and reduces water loss	Oral: 1 g 4 times daily or after each loose stool; maximum dose is 12 tablets/day	Constipation		Useful for diarrhea and constipation Should be taken with adequate fluid to avoid swelling and blockage of the throat or esophagus
Probiotics	Replaces normal depleted intestinal flora; restores intestinal function and suppresses colonization of pathogenic organisms	Varies widely with different products; should be administered with water, milk, juice, or other light snack	Stomach and intestinal upset, including gas and bloating	Patients with hypersensitivity to lactose or milk should avoid lactobacillus	Product selection is important, as some probiotics are more effective than others in certain conditions
Lactase enzyme	Necessary for the breakdown of carbohydrates found in dairy products	Oral: 9,000 FCC lactase units with the first bite of dairy food; may be adjusted for individual response			Useful for prevention and treatment of lactose-intolerant diarrhea

Table 13-14 Antibiotic Pharmacotherapy for Treatment of Diarrhea

Antibiotic	Mechanism of Action	Dose	Adverse Effects	Interactions (Drug, Food, Lab, Disease)	Pearls
Doxycycline	Bacteriostatic: inhibits protein synthesis by binding to bacterial ribosomes	Cholera: 300 mg tablet once or 100 mg tablet twice daily for 3 days	Photosensitivity, GI upset (nausea, diarrhea)	Avoid dairy, antacids, and iron preparations within 2 hours of drug administration Anticonvulsants can decrease serum concentrations May increase chance of bleeding when taken with warfarin Oral contraception effectiveness may be decreased with co-administration Contraindicated in pregnancy, breastfeeding, and children younger than 8 years because of possible tooth discoloration and bone growth interference	Taking with food can minimize GI upset

(*continues*)

Table 13-14 (*continued*)

Antibiotic	Mechanism of Action	Dose	Adverse Effects	Interactions (Drug, Food, Lab, Disease)	Pearls
Trimethoprim-sulfamethoxazole DS	Bacteriostatic: sulfamethoxazole inhibits bacterial folic acid synthesis; trimethoprim blocks synthesis of essential nucleic acids and proteins	Cholera: 800/160 mg tablet twice daily for 3 days *E. coli,* salmonellosis: 800/160 mg tablet twice daily for 5 days Shigellosis: 800/160 mg tablet twice daily for 3–5 days Traveler's diarrhea: 800/160 mg daily	Possible rash, urticaria, or Stevens-Johnson syndrome, nausea, vomiting	Contraindicated with sulfa allergy	
Ciprofloxacin	Bactericidal: inhibits bacterial DNA topoisomerase; displays post-antibiotic effect	Cholera: 500 mg tablet twice daily for 3 days or 1 g tablet once *E. coli,* shigellosis: 500 mg tablet twice daily for 3 days Salmonellosis, campylobacteriosis: 500 mg tablet twice daily for 5 days (3–14 days for enteric fever) Traveler's diarrhea: 500 mg daily	Nausea, insomnia, dizziness, QT prolongation, tendonitis, photosensitivity, rash, urticaria	Avoid dairy, antacids, and iron preparations within 2 hours of drug administration May increase risk of bleeding in patients receiving oral anticoagulants Avoid in patients with preexisting QT prolongation Dosage adjustment is required when CrCl is less than 40 mL/min Should be avoided in children and pregnant women	Associated with an increased risk of tendon rupture and tendinitis; however, use of fluoroquinolones in pediatric patients is increasing for multidrug-resistant infections
Metronidazole	Increases intracellular concentration of bacterial cells; free-radical production destroys cellular components	Pseudomembranous colitis: 250 mg tablet 4 times daily for 10 days or 500 mg tablet 3 times daily for 10 days	GI discomfort, nausea, vomiting, *Candida* infection of genital area, dizziness, headache	May increase risk of bleeding in patients receiving oral anticoagulants	Disulfiram-like reaction may occur with concurrent alcohol ingestion
Vancomycin	Inhibits peptidoglycan synthesis by binding to the cell wall	Pseudomembranous colitis: 125 mg tablet 4 times daily for 10 days	Ototoxicity, thrombophlebitis, nephrotoxicity	Use cautiously in patients with renal dysfunction and patients with previous hearing loss	"Red man syndrome" is not an allergic reaction and can be minimized with slow infusion
Ceftriaxone	Bactericidal: inhibits cell wall synthesis by inhibition of mucopeptide synthesis	Salmonellosis: 2 g IV daily for 5 days	Hypersensitivity reactions including fever, rash, pruritus, urticaria, anaphylaxis, nausea, vomiting, diarrhea, *C. difficile* colitis, blood dyscrasias (rare)	Probenecid may increase serum levels	Requires dosage adjustment in renally impaired patients if doses exceed 2 g/day or if the patient has concurrent hepatic dysfunction Cross-sensitivity with penicillins is possible

Table 13-14 (*continued*)

Antibiotic	Mechanism of Action	Dose	Adverse Effects	Interactions (Drug, Food, Lab, Disease)	Pearls
Azithromycin	Bacteriostatic: inhibits RNA synthesis by binding to the 50S RNA subunit	Salmonellosis: 1 g for 1 day, followed by 500 mg daily for 5 days	Nausea, vomiting, diarrhea, cramping, abdominal pain, QT prolongation and torsades de pointes (rare)	Aluminum- or magnesium-containing antacids decrease absorption	
Erythromycin	Bacteriostatic: inhibits RNA synthesis by binding to the 50S RNA subunit	Campylobacteriosis: 500 mg tablet twice daily for 5 days	Nausea, vomiting, diarrhea, cramping, abdominal pain, QT prolongation and torsades de pointes (rare)	Aluminum- or magnesium-containing antacids decrease absorption	Avoid grapefruit juice Take on an empty stomach

If diarrhea is accompanied by vomiting and/or nausea, eating mild foods that reduce the frequency of stools (e.g., low fiber foods) and intestinal transit time may be helpful.

Water Considerations

Correction of fluid and electrolyte disturbances is the cornerstone therapy for infectious and noninfectious diarrhea. In the absence of vomiting and severe dehydration, oral rehydration with water or other oral rehydration preparations is preferred.

- Mild dehydration in children (a loss of 3–5% of baseline body weight) should be treated with 50 mL/kg over 2 to 4 hours, after which 10 mL/kg should be administered after each loose stool.
- Moderate dehydration in children (a loss of 6–9% of baseline body weight) should be treated with 100 mL/kg over 2 to 4 hours, after which 10 mL/kg should be administered after each loose stool.
- Parenteral Ringer's lactate or normal saline can be used in cases of severe dehydration, uncontrolled vomiting, shock, or loss of consciousness.

1.3.0 Monitoring

Pharmacotherapeutic Outcomes

Most medications used for diarrhea are palliative, not curative. They include agents that decrease secretion, decrease gut motility, and adsorb intestinal contents. Most acute diarrhea is self-limiting within 3 to 7 days.

Safety Monitoring

- Adequate hydration
- Proper diet
- Electrolyte and acid–base balances
- Adverse drug reactions

Efficacy Monitoring

- Symptomatic relief
- Elimination of curable infections

ANNOTATED BIBLIOGRAPHY

Abraham B, Sellin JH. Drug-induced diarrhea. *Curr Gastroenterol Rep* 2007;9:365–372.

Adams PF, Benson V. *Current Estimates from the National Health Interview Survey, 1989*. Washington, DC: U.S. Government Printing Office; 1990:1–221.

Ansdell VE, Ericsson CD. Prevention and empiric treatment of traveler's diarrhea. *Med Clin North Am* 1999;83:945–973, vi.

Binder HJ. Causes of chronic diarrhea. *N Engl J Med* 2006;355:236–239.

DuPont HL. Guidelines on acute infectious diarrhea in adults: The Practice Parameters Committee of the American College of Gastroenterology. *Am J Gastroenterol* 1997;92:1962–1975.

Everhart JE. Overview. In: Everhart JE, ed. *Digestive Diseases in the United States: Epidemiology and Impact*. U.S. Department of Health and Human

Services, Public Health Service, National Institutes of Health, National Institute of Diabetes and Digestive and Kidney Diseases. Washington, DC: U.S. Government Printing Office; 1994:1–53.

Farthing M, Lindberg G, Dite P, et al. *World Gastroenterology Organisation Practice Guideline: Acute Diarrhea*. March 2008.

Fine KD, Schiller LR. AGA technical review on the evaluation and management of chronic diarrhea. *Gastroenterology* 1999;116:1464–1486.

Guerrant RL, Van Gilder T, Steiner TS, et al.; Infectious Diseases Society of America. Practice guidelines for the management of infectious diarrhea. *Clin Infect Dis* 2001;32:331–351.

Martin S, Jung R. Gastrointestinal infections and enterotoxigenic poisonings. In: DiPiro JT, Talbert RL, Yee GC, et al., eds. *Pharmacotherapy: A Pathophysiologic Approach*. 7th ed. New York, NY: McGraw-Hill; 2008:1857-1873.

Sandler RS, Stewart WF, Liberman JN, et al. Abdominal pain, bloating, and diarrhea in the United States: prevalence and impact. *Dig Dis Sci* 2000;45:1166–1171.

Spruill WJ, Wade WE. Diarrhea, constipation, and irritable bowel syndrome. In: DiPiro JT, Talbert RL, Yee GC, et al., eds. *Pharmacotherapy: A Pathophysiologic Approach*. 7th ed. New York, NY: McGraw-Hill; 2008:617–32.

TOPIC: GASTROESOPHAGEAL REFLUX DISEASE (GERD)

Section Coordinator: Tracy K. Pettinger
Contributor: Brooke Pugmire

Tips Worth Tweeting

- Gastroesophageal reflux disease (GERD) is a common condition affecting approximately 20% of the population.
- Typical GERD symptoms include heartburn, regurgitation, and belching.
- Several drugs are known to induce or exacerbate GERD and should be avoided, if possible, in patients with symptoms of this disease.
- Lifestyle modifications should be implemented along with drug therapies in all patients with GERD symptoms.
- Antacids and H2 receptor antagonists are indicated in patients with mild GERD symptoms. PPIs are more effective for moderate to severe GERD symptoms.
- GERD treatment should be administered for 8 weeks; long-term maintenance therapy may be needed.
- Antacids, H2-receptor antagonists, and PPIs are generally well tolerated; GI adverse effects are the most common complaints.
- Many antacids, H2-receptor antagonists, and PPIs are available generically and OTC in convenient dosage forms at a low cost.

Patient Care Scenario: Ambulatory Setting

A 66 y/o white man with NKDA c/o heartburn and belching after the evening meal and over last 1–2 months has had some difficulty sleeping due to these symptoms when lying down at night. Hypertension, atrial fibrillation, seasonal allergic rhinitis, and depression. Clinic VS today: BP 126/66, P 60, wt 198 lbs, ht 5'10". Today BUN 20 mg/dL, Cr 1.1 mg/dL, Glu 98 mg/dL, Na 138 mEq/L, K 4.4 mEq/L, Cl 102 mmol/L, CO2 25 mmol/L.

Date	Physician	Drug	Quantity	Sig	Refills
1/15	Price	Diltizazem ER 120 mg	90	One po qd	1
1/15	Price	Warfarin 5 mg	90	One po qd or ud	1
1/15	Price	Digoxin 0.125 mg	90	One po qd	1
10/11	Price	Loratadine 10 mg	90	One po qd	1
12/20	Cliff	Sertraline 50 mg	90	One po qd	1

1.1.0 Pharmacotherapy

Medications, Laboratory Testing, and Disease State

GERD occurs as a result of an imbalance between aggressive (acid, pepsin, bile acids) and defensive (luminal clearance, lower esophageal sphincter [LES] tone, tissue resistance) factors leading to abnormal reflux of gastric contents into the esophagus and subsequent mucosal damage. Drugs known to induce or aggravate GERD by decreasing LES tone include calcium-channel blockers, nitrates, beta agonists, theophylline, benzodiazepines, and anticholinergics (which include urinary incontinence drugs, tricyclic antidepressants, and antihistamines). Bisphosphonates, NSAIDs, corticosteroids, potassium chloride, tetracyclines, and iron may directly irritate esophageal mucosa. The risk of GERD likely increases with the number of GERD-inducing medications taken. Alcohol consumption and nicotine dependence also contribute to LES relaxation.

Instruments and Techniques Related to Patient Assessment

GERD is usually diagnosed based on patient symptoms. Resolution of symptoms after a 1- to 2-week proton pump inhibitor (PPI) trial is a sensitive, cost-effective diagnostic test. Upper GI endoscopy to assess mucosal injury is indicated in patients with alarm symptoms, those with refractory GERD, and those suspected to have complications. In contrast, 24-hour ambulatory pH monitoring is reserved for patients with endoscopic-negative, refractory GERD to determine the frequency and duration of episodes and for patients with atypical symptoms to rule out other disease states. A barium esophagram can be used to detect ulcers, strictures, or obstructions in patients suspected to have these complications.

Terminology, Signs, and Symptoms

GERD is classified into three types: nonerosive reflux disease (NERD), erosive esophagitis (EE), and Barrett's esophagus (BE). Typical, atypical, and alarm symptoms associated with GERD are shown in Table 13-15. Typical (classic) symptoms usually occur after meals or when reclining/lying. Alarm symptoms indicate more severe disease and a need for physician evaluation. Symptom severity does not correlate well with the severity of mucosal damage, however. Esophageal ulceration and stricture are potential complications of GERD. Patients with Barrett's esophagus are at increased risk of developing adenocarcinoma.

Wellness, Prevention, and Treatment

Approximately 20% of the population experiences GERD symptoms weekly—a pattern that can significantly affect quality of life. As many as 50% of pregnant women have esophageal reflux, with half of them experiencing heartburn daily. Avoiding drugs known to cause GERD whenever possible and promoting healthy lifestyle habits are key in preventing GERD. Lifestyle changes to eliminate factors that exacerbate GERD include the following:

- Smoking cessation
- Eating small meals
- Avoiding reclining or lying within 3 hours after food consumption
- Avoiding foods that reduce LES pressure (e.g., alcohol, chocolate, fatty foods, peppermint), irritate the gastric mucosa (e.g., spicy, citrus, or tomato foods, coffee), or increase acid production (e.g., cola, beer)
- Elevating the head of the bed 6 inches

Table 13-15 Symptoms Associated with GERD

Typical Symptoms	Atypical Symptoms	Alarm Symptoms
Heartburn	Hoarseness	Dysphagia
Regurgitation	Asthma	Odynophagia
Belching	Chronic cough	Choking
	Chest pain that resembles angina	Bleeding or anemia
		Weight loss

Early treatment with OTC or prescription products will help in the prevention of complications associated with GERD.

1.2.0 Pharmacotherapy

Drug Indications

Medications used in the treatment of GERD are shown in Table 13-6 later in this section. Acid suppression is the mainstay of GERD treatment using PPIs or histamine$_2$ (H2)-receptor antagonists (H2RAs). PPIs provide more rapid relief of symptoms and esophageal healing than H2RAs. Patients with mild symptoms should be treated with lifestyle modifications and antacids or H2RAs initially, with progression to PPI therapy if symptoms persist. Standard doses of PPIs are appropriate initially in conjunction with lifestyle modifications in patients with moderate to severe symptoms or documented esophagitis. High-dose PPIs are recommended for individuals with ulcers, strictures, or Barrett's esophagus. PPIs at equivalent doses produce similar symptom relief and healing of esophagitis. H2RAs are also equally effective at equivalent doses. Acid suppressant therapy should continue for 8 weeks to allow for maximal healing and may be required on a long-term basis as maintenance therapy in patients with more severe symptoms. Maintenance therapy is also preferred in individuals with complications of GERD.

Mechanism of Action

Antacids neutralize gastric acid by inhibiting the conversion of pepsinogen to pepsin, resulting in increased LES tone and the pH of gastric contents. PPIs suppress gastric acid secretion by inhibiting the binding of the H+-K+-ATPase enzyme on gastric parietal cells. H2RAs suppress gastric acid secretion by blocking H2 receptors on gastric parietal cells.

Interaction of Drugs with Foods and Laboratory Tests

Antacids reduce the absorption of ferrous sulfate, tetracyclines, fluoroquinolones, azoles, quinidine, digoxin, and phenytoin. Cimetidine is a potent inhibitor of cytochrome P450 enzymes and decreases the metabolism of numerous drugs, including phenytoin, theophylline, and warfarin. PPIs may reduce levels of clopidogrel's active metabolite through CYP2C19 inhibition, resulting in decreased clinical efficacy of clopidogrel and increased risk of thrombosis. PPIs and H2RAs decrease the absorption of itraconazole, and may also cause false-negative results on *Helicobacter pylori* breath tests.

Contraindications, Warnings, and Precautions

Patients with renal failure who take antacids on a chronic basis may develop magnesium or aluminum toxicity. H2RAs should be used with caution in the elderly and in patients with renal insufficiency due to their increased risk of experiencing CNS adverse effects. Most H2RAs and PPIs are pregnancy Category B drugs and likely safe during pregnancy.

Physiochemical Properties, Pharmacodynamics, and Pharmacokinetic Properties

PPIs should be administered daily 30 to 60 minutes prior to the first meal of the day to allow for maximum acid suppression. When given with food, the absorption of PPIs may be reduced or delayed. For patients with difficulty swallowing, the contents of esomeprazole, lansoprazole, and omeprazole capsules may be mixed with applesauce or juice and immediately swallowed.

Pharmacokinetic Dosage Calculations

PPIs are typically dosed once daily. By comparison, twice-daily dosing of H2RAs is usually required. The oral dose of ranitidine and nizatidine should be reduced to 150 mg once daily in patients with a creatinine clearance less than 50 mL/min. The recommended dose of famotidine in renal impairment is 20 mg once daily.

Biopharmaceutical and Pharmaceutical Characteristics of Dosage Forms

The bioavailability of many calcium carbonate products has been questioned and should be home-tested by placing one tablet in 6 ounces of vinegar stirred every 2 to 3 minutes. Disintegration should occur within 30 minutes.

1.3.0 Monitoring

Pharmacotherapeutic Outcomes

The goals of therapy are to provide cost-effective treatment for relief of symptoms; to decrease symptom frequency, duration, and severity; to promote healing; and to prevent complications.

Safety and Efficacy Monitoring

The patient should be assessed for relief of postprandial and nocturnal heartburn and regurgitation and improvement in quality of life after 4 to 8 weeks of treatment. Symptom frequency and duration should be determined in those patients who do not achieve complete relief. Use of antacids for symptom relief should also be identified. Assessing adherence to drug and nondrug treatments as well as the presence of GERD-inducing drugs is important. Laboratory and other tests are usually not needed to evaluate efficacy.

Adverse Drug Reactions

Patients should be monitored for adverse effects of therapy when such treatment is initiated, and then periodically throughout treatment. PPIs and H2RAs are generally well tolerated but can cause headache, dizziness, nausea, abdominal pain, and diarrhea. Long-term use of PPIs may cause respiratory tract infections, vitamin B_{12} deficiency due to malabsorption of cobalamin, and increased risk of fractures due to malabsorption of calcium. Vitamin B_{12} levels and fracture risk should be assessed periodically during long-term treatment. Aluminum-containing antacids may cause constipation, whereas magnesium-containing antacids may cause diarrhea. Aluminum also binds phosphate, which can lead to bone demineralization. Antacids can cause acid–base disturbances as well.

Pharmacotherapeutic Alternatives

Many PPIs and H2RAs are available generically at a reduced cost relative to brand-name products with equal efficacy. Cimetidine is not a preferred H2RA because of its numerous drug interactions.

2.2.0 Dispensing

Generic and Brand Names

Generic and brand names of medications used in the treatment of GERD are shown in Table 13-16.

Dosage Forms Availability

Dosage strength and form for GERD medications are shown in Table 13-16. Agents available without a prescription are included.

Physical Attributes of Commercial Products

Esomeprazole capsules are purple in color with three pale stripes at one end and often called the "purple pill." Generic availability may result in different capsule color.

Packaging, Storage, Handling, and Disposal

PPI capsules and tablets should be swallowed whole without chewing, crushing, or splitting. PPIs and H3RAs should be stored at room temperature in an air-tight container away from light and moisture.

Table 13-16 Selected Medications Used in Gastroesophageal Reflux Disease

Drug—Generic (Brand Name)	Class	Dosage and Frequency	Dosage Forms	Rx or OTC
Esomeprazole (Nexium)	PPI	20–40 mg qd	C, IV	Rx
Lansoprazole (Prevacid)	PPI	15 mg qd–30 mg bid	C, L, IV	OTC
Omeprazole (Prilosec)	PPI	20–40 mg qd	C, T	OTC
Pantoprazole (Protonix)	PPI	40–80 mg qd	T, IV	Rx
Rabeprazole (Aciphex)	PPI	10–20 mg qd	T	Rx
Cimetidine (Tagamet)	H2RA	300 mg qid–800 mg qhs	T, L, IV	OTC
Famotidine (Pepcid)	H2RA	20 mg bid–40 mg qhs	T, L, IV	OTC
Nizatidine (Axid)	H2RA	150 mg bid–300 mg qhs	C, L	OTC
Ranitidine (Zantac)	H2RA	150 mg bid–300 mg qhs	T, L, IV, C	OTC
Aluminum hydroxide (Amphogel)	Antacid	5–10 mL prn	T, L	OTC
Aluminum hydroxide + magnesium carbonate (Gaviscon)	Antacid	15–30 mL prn	T, L	OTC
Aluminum hydroxide + magnesium hydroxide (Maalox)	Antacid	10–20 mL prn	T, L	OTC
Aluminum hydroxide + magnesium hydroxide + simethicone (Mylanta)	Antacid	10–45 mL prn	T, L	OTC
Calcium carbonate (Tums, Titralac)	Antacid	2–4 tabs prn	T, L	OTC
Calcium carbonate + magnesium hydroxide (Rolaids)	Antacid	2–4 tabs prn	T, L	OTC
Magnesium hydroxide (Milk of Magnesia)	Antacid	15–30 mL prn	T, L	OTC

T = tablet; C = capsule; L = liquid; IV = intravenous.

ANNOTATED BIBLIOGRAPHY

Ali T, Roberts DN, Tierney WM. Long-term safety concerns with proton pump inhibitors. *Am J Med* 2009;122:896–903.

DeVault KR, Castell DO, et al. Updated guidelines for the diagnosis and treatment of gastroesophageal reflux disease. *Am J Gastroenterol* 2005;100:190–200.

Facts & Comparisons. Available at: http://online.factsandcomparisons.com/index.aspx. Accessed February 26, 2010.

Kahrilas PJ, Shaheen NJ, et al. American Gastroenterological Association medical position statement on the management of gastroesophageal reflux disease. *Gastroenterology* 2008;135:1383–1391.

Micromedex Healthcare Series. Available at: http://www.thomsonhc.com/hcs/librarian. Accessed February 26, 2010.

Williams DB, Schade RR. Gastroesophageal reflux disease. In: Dipiro JT, Talbert RL, Yee GC, et al., eds. *Pharmacotherapy: A Pathophysiologic Approach.* 7th ed. New York: McGraw-Hill; 2008:555–568.

TOPIC: HEPATITIS

Section Coordinator: Tracy K. Pettinger
Contributor: Adam D. Porath

Tips Worth Tweeting

- Viral hepatitis can be caused by several viruses, including hepatitis A, B, C, D, and E.
- Hepatitis B (HBV) and hepatitis C (HCV) are responsible for the majority of morbidity and mortality associated with infectious hepatitis.
- Hepatitis B, C, and D are transmitted through exposure to infected body fluids.
- Chronic infection with HBV and HCV can lead to chronic liver disease, hepatocellular carcinoma, and subsequent death in a minority of patients.
- Response to HBV therapy is variable, based on viral resistance.
- HBV infection can be prevented by immunization with an interferon-based regimen.
- Response to hepatitis D (HDV) is unique, in that transmission of the virus requires coinfection with hepatitis B.
- HDV is the rarest but also the most pathogenic form of viral hepatitis, leading to cirrhosis in roughly 80% of infected patients.
- Hepatitis A and E are typically contracted through fecal–oral transmission via contaminated food or water.
- There is no specific treatment for hepatitis A and E, but infection with hepatitis A (HAV) can be prevented by immunization.

- Drug-induced liver disease can be caused by numerous drugs, with the most common culprit being alcohol.
- Infection with viral hepatitis is preventable through immunization, with the exception of HCV.
- Chronic hepatitis B and C can be treated with pharmacotherapy, but response rates vary.

Patient Care Scenario: Ambulatory Setting

- 60 y/o, 5'10", M, 176 lbs. Quit drinking 2 years ago. Previously a heavy drinker.
- History of hepatitis C and depression.
- Labs: ALT 80 units/L, Serum Cr 1.3, Hg 9.0 g/dL, HCV RNA undetectable.

Date	Physician	Drug	Quantity	Sig	Refills
6/18	Smith	Ribavirin 200 mg	180	3 tabs twice daily	3
6/18	Smith	Peginterferon alfa-2a 180 mcg	4	1 subQ once weekly	3
7/20	Smith	Sertraline 50 mg	30	1 tab once daily	2

1.1.0 Patient Information

Medication-induced liver injury is associated with numerous drugs via a variety of mechanisms. The incidence of drug-induced liver disease is estimated to be between 1 in 10,000 and 1 in 100,000 patients. Alcohol is the drug most commonly associated with drug-induced liver disease, accounting for more than 90% of patients hospitalized for elevated transaminases.

Table 13-17 Medications Associated with Liver Injury

Drug	Proposed Mechanisms of Liver Injury
Acetaminophen	Centrolobular necrosis
ACE inhibitors	Cholestatic injury
Alcohol	Steatohepatitis
Amiodarone	Phospholipidosis
Amoxicillin/clavulanic acid	Cholestatic injury
Androgens	Liver vascular disorders
Aspirin	Centrolobular necrosis
Azathioprine	Liver vascular disorders
Azole antifungals	Hepatocellular necrosis
Carbamazepine	Cholestatic injury
Comfrey	Liver vascular disorders
Cytotoxic chemotherapeutic agents	Liver vascular disorders
Danazol	Liver vascular disorders
Erythromycin	Cholestatic injury
Estrogens	Liver vascular disorders
HMG-CoA reductase inhibitors	Cholestatic injury
Isoniazid	Hepatocelluar necrosis
Methotrexate	Toxic cirrhosis
Parenteral nutrition (TPN)	Cholestatic injury
Phenothiazines	Cholestatic injury
Protease inhibitors	Mitochondrial toxicity
Sulfonamides	Cholestatic injury
Sulfonylureas	Cholestatic injury
Tamoxifen	Liver vascular disorders
Tetracycline	Steatohepatitis
Valproic acid	Centrolobular necrosis, steatohepatitis

Laboratory Testing

Liver function tests (LFTs) are often the first sign of chronic hepatitis. Alanine aminotransferase (ALT) is usually elevated to a greater extent than aspartate aminotransferase (AST) in viral hepatitis. The opposite (AST > ALT) is most often the case in drug-induced hepatitis, including, most commonly, alcoholic hepatitis.

Patients presenting with unexplained elevations in LFTs should be screened for viral hepatitis, especially if they are at high risk for infection based on history. A thorough medication history should also be obtained to rule out drug-induced liver injury.

Patients suspected of possible viral hepatitis infection should receive serologic screening for viral hepatitis. Screening for viral hepatitis should include: hepatitis A antibody (anti-HAV), hepatitis B surface antigen (HBsAg), antibody to hepatitis B core antigen (anti-HBc), antibody to hepatitis B surface antigen (anti-HBs), and hepatitis C antibody (anti-HCV). Serologic screening for suspected acute viral infection should include specific testing for IgM antibodies to HAV (IgM anti-HAV) and hepatitis B core antigen (IgM anti-HBc). Positive results for anti-HCV should be followed by hepatitis C recombinant immunoblot assay (RIBA).

Hepatitis B "e" antigen (HBeAg) is a marker of active viral replication in HBV infection. An inactive carrier of chronic HBV will eventually lose HBeAg positivity with the production of anti-HBe. Loss of HBeAg, either through the natural disease course or as a result of antiviral pharmacotherapy, is a positive prognostic marker. HBV and HCV viral loads are also routinely

Table 13-18 Persons Who Should Be Screened for Viral Hepatitis

- Any history of illicit injection drug use, even those who have used such drugs only once
- Children born to mothers with known viral hepatitis infection
- Healthcare workers exposed to blood or body fluids of a patient with viral hepatitis
- HIV-positive patients
- Household or current sexual partners of a patient with known viral hepatitis
- Inmates of correctional facilities
- Men who have sex with men
- Patients who received a blood product prior to 1992
- Patients who have ever been on hemodialysis
- Patients who have received an organ transplant
- Patients who were born, or whose parents were born, in areas of high viral hepatitis endemicity
- Patients needing immunosuppressive therapy

Table 13-19 Interpretation of Viral Hepatitis Serology

Hepatitis A	
Anti-HAV (+), IgM anti-HAV (–)	Resolved HAV or prior vaccination, immune to HAV infection
Anti-HAV (+), IgM anti-HAV (+)	Acute HAV infection
Hepatitis B	
HBsAg (–), anti-HBc (–), anti-HBs (–)	Susceptible to HBV infection
HBsAg (–), anti-HBc (–), anti-HBs (+)	Immune to HBV due to vaccination
HBsAg (–), anti-HBc (+), anti-HBs (+)	Immune due to natural infection
HBsAg (+), IgM anti-HBc (+), anti-HBs (+)	Acute HBV infection
HBsAg (+), anti-HBc (+), anti-HBs (–)	Chronic HBV infection
HBsAg (–), anti-HBc (+), anti-HBs (–)	Variable interpretation
Hepatitis C	
Anti-HCV (+), RIBA (+)	HCV Infection
Anti-HCV (+), RIBA (–)	HCV exposure; results should be followed up in 6 months to rule out chronic infection

measured via PCR to determine treatment decisions and response to therapy.

Disease states associated with hepatitis include alcoholism, intravenous illicit drug use, and HIV infection. Patients with disease states or injuries that required blood transfusion prior to 1992 are also at increased risk for exposure to viral hepatitis. It is estimated that 25% of HIV-positive patients are coinfected with HCV. Coinfection with HIV and concomitant alcohol abuse increase the risk of the development of cirrhosis.

Instruments and Techniques Related to Patient Assessment

Liver biopsy is considered the gold standard for assessing the extent of liver disease secondary to viral hepatitis. Liver biopsy should be considered by patients and their physicians in the setting of chronic HCV for the purpose of prognosis and to help guide treatment decisions. Although several noninvasive alternative diagnostic tests are available, their ability to differentiate between the various stages of fibrosis is inferior to traditional biopsy.

Key Terms

Anti-HAV: hepatitis A antibody
Anti-HBc: antibody to hepatitis B core antigen
Anti-HBs: antibody to hepatitis B surface antigen
Anti-HCV: hepatitis C antibody
HBeAg: hepatitis B "e" antigen
HBIG: hepatitis B immune globulin
HBsAg: hepatitis B surface antigen
IgM anti-HAV: IgM antibodies to HAV
IgM anti-HBc: IgM antibodies to hepatitis B core antigen
PCR: polymerase chain reaction
RIBA: recombinant immunoblot assay

Signs and Symptoms

Acute hepatitis can present with a variety of nonspecific symptoms, including anorexia, nausea, vomiting, fever, fatigue, and abdominal pain. Other signs and symptoms that may be present include dark urine, light-colored stools, joint pain, and jaundice.

Chronic hepatitis is often asymptomatic. Patients rarely present with signs and symptoms similar to those seen in acute hepatitis; rather, chronic hepatitis is often detected by laboratory abnormalities (i.e., elevated ALT).

Wellness and Prevention

With the exception of hepatitis C, transmission of viral hepatitis can be prevented through immunization. The Centers for Disease Control and Prevention (CDC) Advisory Committee on Immunization Practices (ACIP) regularly releases updated recommended immunization schedules for both adult and pediatric patients.

Infection with hepatitis C can be minimized by avoiding high-risk behaviors—particularly illicit injection drug use, which is the primary mode of transmission in the United States.

Avoidance of excessive alcohol consumption can minimize the long-term risk of alcohol-related liver disease.

1.2.0 Pharmacotherapy

Drugs for Hepatitis: Indications and Mechanisms of Action

Hepatitis A

Most cases of acute HAV infection are self-limiting. Treatment consists of supportive care for associated symptoms. The pharmacotherapeutic approach to prevention of HAV is similar for both pre- and post-exposure prophylaxis, consisting of a series of two vaccinations.

Hepatitis B

Similar to HAV, HBV is a vaccine-preventable disease. Routine vaccination is now advocated for all infants born in the United States. Unvaccinated patients (including infants of HBsAg-positive mothers) who are exposed to HBV should receive a dose of hepatitis B immune globulin (HBIG) in addition to the three-dose vaccine series.

Pharmacotherapy is typically not indicated in acute HBV infection given that more than 95% of immunocompetent patients will recover without intervention. Antiviral therapy should be initiated in select chronically HBV-infected patients based on their HBeAg status, HBV viral load, and extent of ALT elevation. Selection of antiviral regimen should be undertaken by clinicians experienced in the treatment of HBV.

Hepatitis C

The decision to treat chronic HCV should be based on a variety of factors, including patient adherence, degree of liver fibrosis, and concomitant disease states (i.e., uncontrolled depression). The treatment of choice for chronic HCV is peginterferon-alfa plus ribavirin.

Dosing Regimens/Routes of Administration

See Table 13-20 and 13-21.

Interaction of Drugs with Foods and Laboratory Tests

Entecavir should be taken on an empty stomach. All other oral nucleoside analogues may be taken without regard for food.

Contraindications, Warnings, and Precautions

In general, there are no contraindications to viral hepatitis-related vaccine and immune globulin products other than known hypersensitivity to vaccine components. Patients whose serology indicates previous immunity through either natural infection or vaccination should not be reimmunized.

There are no specific contraindications to the oral nucleoside analogues used in the treatment of chronic HBV infections. Patients should be screened for HIV

Table 13-20 Vaccine Preparations

	Brand Name	Adult Dosing	Pediatric Dosing
Hepatitis A	Havrix	1440 ELISA units (1 mL) IM, with a booster dose of 1 mL 6–12 months after primary immunization	12 months to 18 years old: 720 ELISA units (0.5 mL) IM, with a booster dose of 0.5 mL 6–12 months after primary immunization
	Vaqta	50 units (1 mL) IM, with a booster dose of 1 mL 6–18 months after primary immunization	12 months to 18 years old: 25 units (0.5 mL) IM, with a booster dose of 0.5 mL 6–18 months after primary immunization
Hepatitis A/ hepatitis B	Twinrix	Three doses (1 mL) IM given at 0, 1, and 6 months *Accelerated regimen:* four doses (1 mL) IM given at day 0, 7, and 21–30, and a booster at 12 months	1–18 years old: three doses (0.5 mL) IM given at 0, 1, and 6 months *Alternative regimen:* 1–15 years old: two doses (1 mL) IM given at 0 and 6–12 months
Hepatitis B	Engerix-B, Recombivax-B	Three doses (1 mL) IM given at 0, 1, and 6 months*	Three doses (0.5 mL) IM given at 0, 1, and 6 months
Diphtheria, tetanus, pertussis, hepatitis B, and polio	Pediarix		6 weeks to younger than 7 years old: 0.5 mL IM q 6–8 weeks × 3 doses
Hepatitis B immune globulin	HepaGam B, HyperHep B, Nabi-HB	Younger than 12 months: 0.5 mL IM Older than 12 months: refer to adult dosing	0.06 mL/kg IM within 14 days of exposure

*Dosage adjustments required for patients on hemodialysis.

Table 13-21 Antiviral Medications for the Treatment of Chronic HBV

Generic Name (Brand Name)	Dosing	Common Adverse Effects
Adefovir (Hepsera)	10 mg po once daily*	Headache, abdominal pain, diarrhea, hepatitis exacerbation upon discontinuation, weakness, hematurina
Entecavir (Baraclude)	0.5 mg po once daily*	Minimal
Lamivudine (Epivir-HBV)	100 mg po once daily*	Headache, fatigue, insomnia, nausea, diarrhea, pancreatitis, neutropenia, mylagias, neuropathy, infections
Peginterferon alfa-2a (Pegasys)	180 mcg sq once weekly	Depression, anxiety, flu-like symptoms, bone marrow suppression
Telbivudine (Tyzeka)	600 mg po once daily*	Headache, fatigue, CPK increases
Tenofovir (Viread)	300 mg po once daily*	Neuralgias, diarrhea, nausea, weakness

*Dosage adjustments required for CrCl less than 50 mL/min.

Table 13-22 Contraindications to Peginterferon and Ribavirin Therapy

- Uncontrolled depression
- History of solid-organ transplant
- Untreated thyroid disorder
- Pregnancy or nonadherence to two forms of contraception
- Severe concurrent medical conditions, including CHF, uncontrolled HTN, COPD, and uncontrolled diabetes

coinfection prior to initiating antiviral therapy due to the risk of development of viral resistance in persons with unrecognized HIV.

Numerous relative contraindications to peginterferon/ribavirin therapy have been identified through clinical trial experience. Individual treatment decisions must be made on a case-by-case basis after weighing the risks and benefits of treatment.

Pharmacokinetic Dosage Calculations

All of the oral nucleoside analogues used in the treatment of chronic HBV require renal dosage adjustment. Ribavirin is not recommended in patients with a CrCl less than 50 mL/min.

1.3.0 Monitoring

Pharmacotherapeutic Outcomes

Hepatitis B

Response to therapy for chronic HBV infection is measured through a variety of laboratory tests. In general, the goals of therapy are seroconversion (HBeAg-negative), an undetectable HBsAg level, and an undetectable HBV viral load.

Hepatitis C

The general treatment goal for treatment of chronic HCV is an undetectable HCV viral load. Timing of the patient's response (undetectable HCV viral load) will dictate the duration of therapy. Depending on the viral genotype, nonresponse at 12 to 24 weeks indicates treatment failure and discontinuation of therapy is indicated.

Safety and Efficacy Monitoring and Patient Education

Patients receiving oral nucleoside analogues should have baseline and periodic monitoring of renal function. Additionally, patients taking telbivudine should be monitored for myalgias and CPK elevations.

Patients receiving peginterferon products should be monitored closely for depressive symptoms and suicidal ideation, and treatment should be discontinued for severe or persistent psychiatric symptoms. Patients on peginterferon should also be monitored for bone marrow suppression. Treatment should be discontinued for an ANC less than 500 or a platelet count less than 25,000/mm^3.

Patients on ribavirin should be monitored for hemolytic anemia, especially within the first few weeks of the initiation of treatment. Ribavirin is a known teratogen, so female patients should be screened for pregnancy prior to initiating treatment with this agent. Two forms of birth control should be used while patients are on ribavirin and for 6 months after discontinuation of treatment.

Patients with any form of viral hepatitis should be counseled about measures to prevent viral transmission, including abstinence from blood donation and illicit injection drug use. Patients should also be advised about the risk of sexual transmission of HBV and HCV. Household and sexual contacts of HAV- and HBV-positive patients should be offered vaccination if not previously vaccinated.

Adverse Drug Reactions

Viral hepatitis vaccine and immune globulin products are generally well tolerated. Common adverse reactions to these products include injection-site tenderness, headache, and fatigue. Rarely, anaphylaxis can occur with these products. Epinephrine should be available at the time of administration.

The oral nucleoside analogues are also generally well tolerated. Rare cases of lactic acidosis, severe hepatomegaly, and steatosis have been reported. Severe, acute exacerbations of HBV infection have been reported with discontinuation of these products.

Peginterferon and ribavirin combination therapy commonly results in adverse reactions. Specifically, adverse neuropsychiatric effects and bone marrow suppression are often noted. Subsequent discontinuation of chronic HCV therapy secondary to adverse effects of peginterferon/ribavirin prior to planned duration of therapy is also common.

Nonadherence, Misuse, or Abuse

Nonadherence to peginterferon therapy is common due to the high incidence of adverse effects associated with this treatment.

2.2.0 Dispensing

Calculations

Dosing of HBIG and ribavirin is weight based.

Bioequivalence

Two FDA-approved peginterferon products are available for the treatment of chronic HCV; peginterferon-alfa 2a (Pegasys) and peginterferon-alfa 2b (PegIntron). These products are dosed differently and are not bioequivalent.

Packaging, Storage, Handling, and Disposal

All of the oral nucleoside analogues used in the treatment of chronic HBV should be stored at room temperature. Viral hepatitis-related vaccine and immune globulin products should be refrigerated until immediately prior to use. Similarly, peginterferon products should be refrigerated until immediately prior to use. Syringes used in the administration of peginterferon products should be disposed of in an appropriate sharps container.

ANNOTATED BIBLIOGRAPHY

Farci P, Chessa L, Balestrieri C, Serra G, Lai ME. Treatment of chronic hepatitis D. *J Viral Hepatitis* 2007;14(suppl 1):58–63.

Ghany MG, Strader DB, Thomas DL, Seeff LB; American Association for the Study of Liver Diseases. Diagnosis, management, and treatment of hepatitis C: an update. *Hepatology* 2009;49(4):1335–1374.

Gilbert DN, Moellering RC, Eliopoulos GM, Chambers HF, Saag MS, eds. *The Sanford Guide to Antimicrobial Therapy*. 39th ed. Sperryville, VA: Antimicrobial Therapy, Inc.; 2009.

Hooper J, Martin A. Overview of hepatitis B and C management. *US Pharmacist* December 2009; 32–41.

Kirchain WR, Allen RE. Drug-induced liver disease. In: Dipiro JT, Talbert RL, Yee GC, Matzke GR, Wells BG, Posey LM, eds. *Pharmacotherapy: A Pathophysiologic Approach*. 7th ed. New York, NY: McGraw-Hill Medical; 2008.

Lok ASF, McMahon BJ; American Association for the Study of Liver Diseases. Chronic hepatitis B: update 2009. *Hepatology* 2009;50(3):1–36.

TOPIC: INFLAMMATORY BOWEL DISEASE

Section Coordinator: Tracy K. Pettinger
Contributor: Christopher T. Owens

Tips Worth Tweeting

- Inflammatory bowel disease (IBD) is a generic term used to describe two major types of idiopathic, chronic, inflammatory conditions of the GI tract characterized by sporadic exacerbations and remission: Crohn's disease (CD) and ulcerative colitis (UC).
- IBD and irritable bowel syndrome (IBS) are sometimes confused, but they are distinct clinical entities.
- Smoking is associated with a twofold increased risk for CD, but a 50% decreased risk for UC.
- CD and UC may be differentiated based on clinical and endoscopic findings, such as anatomic site and depth of bowel wall involvement.
- Histologically, the presence of granulomas is important for a diagnosis of CD, whereas crypt abscesses are found in UC.
- Although idiopathic, IBD onset and severity may be related to a number of factors, including infectious, genetic, immunologic, psychological, and lifestyle issues.
- Mesalamine-containing drugs (5-ASA) are the cornerstone of treatment of IBD. The site and severity of disease influences the selection of pharmacotherapy.
- Aminosalicylates (5-ASA) drugs all share the same base structure, but differences in their side chains or pharmaceutical formulation affect their site of activity in the bowel.

- Corticosteroids are effective at inducing remission of IBD, but should not be used to maintain remission.
- Immunosuppressants and TNF-alpha inhibitors are often reserved for more severe or refractory disease.

Patient Care Scenario: Ambulatory Setting

27 y/o, 6'2", M, 159 lbs, college student. No current medical history or regular medications. Reports occasional use of loperamide OTC for diarrhea in past 2 weeks. Recently gave up smoking (about 6 months ago).

B. G. presents to the student health center clinic complaining of episodic diarrhea, abdominal pain, and cramping with unformed stools, increasing over past 2 weeks. He reports that the frequency of unformed stools has increased from 2/day to 6–8/day, with mucus and blood in stool and hemorrhoids. PE findings include pain, erythema, swelling of both knees, and no abdominal masses. Temp = 101.2° F, pulse = 112, ESR = 70 mm/hr; LFTs are within normal limits; stool cultures are negative; colonoscopy shows evidence of granular, edematous mucosa with continuous ulcerations extending from the anus to the terminal ileum.

1.1.0 Patient Information

Laboratory Testing

Elevated ESR, increased temperature, and increased pulse rate strengthen the suspicion of IBD. The evaluation of suspected IBD should include a stool culture to rule out bacterial or parasitic causes, blood work to evaluate markers of systemic inflammation (erythrocyte sedimentation rate, C-reactive protein), a complete blood count (CBC) and electrolytes, and colonoscopy to visualize the inflamed mucosa.

Table 13-23 Disease States Associated with Extra-intestinal Symptoms of IBD

Ophthalmic
Iritis or uveitis
Episcleritis
Musculoskeletal
Arthritis
Ankylosing spondylitis
Dermatologic
Erythema nodosum
Pyoderma gangrenosum
Hepatic
Cholangitis
Hematologic
Anemia
Deep vein thrombosis

Table 13-24 Terminology Used in Classification of Ulcerative Colitis Based on Symptoms

Mild
• Fewer than 4 stools per day, with or without blood
• No systemic disturbances
• Normal ESR
• Minimal abdominal tenderness
Moderate
• More than 4 stools per day, with or without blood
• Minimal systemic disturbances
• Elevation in ESR possible
• Abdominal tenderness possible
Severe
• More than 6 stools per day, with blood frequently present
• Systemic disturbances (fever, tachycardia, anemia)
• ESR > 30
• Abdominal tenderness likely
Fulminant
• More than 10 stools per day, bloody
• Systemic disturbances (fever, tachycardia, anemia)
• ESR > 30
• Colon dilated
• Abdominal tenderness and distention

Instruments and Techniques Related to Patient Assessment

Colonoscopy is the diagnostic tool of choice for confirming IBD and for differentiating CD from UC.

Signs and Symptoms

Increased bowel movements and blood/mucus in the stool indicate possible IBD.

Although CD and UC are both types of IBD, these conditions must be differentiated from each other to optimize treatment and therapeutic outcomes. The clinical presentation of CD more often includes fever, malaise, abdominal pain, and evidence of malnutrition, although these findings may also be present in patients with UC. Complications such as strictures (narrowing of the intestinal lumen) and fistulas (abnormal connections between epithelial surfaces) are more common with CD, as it involves a transmural inflammatory process that affects all layers of the intestine wall.

Table 13-25 Comparison of Crohn's Disease and Ulcerative Colitis

Feature	Crohn's Disease	Ulcerative Colitis
Malaise, fever	Common	Uncommon
Abdominal pain	Very common	Common
Rectal involvement	About 20%	Almost 100%
Continuous disease	Rare	Common
Strictures	Common	Rare
Fistulae	Common	Rare
Granulomas	Common	Rare
Crypt abscesses	Rare	Common
Extra-intestinal symptoms	Possible	Possible
Malabsorption/ malnutrition	Common	Uncommon

Wellness and Prevention

Smokers have a lower incidence of ulcerative colitis, and nicotine has been studied as a treatment. Patients who are ex-smokers have a higher incidence of UC than do nonsmokers. Interestingly, the incidence of CD is higher in smokers than in nonsmokers.

The risk of colonic cancer is increased particularly in UC patients, such that increased cancer surveillance is recommended starting within 10 years of diagnosis.

The clinical course of IBD varies considerably. Most patients will experience intermittent bouts of symptoms or flares of disease, interspersed among times of remission. Others may have a single flare that, once treated appropriately, ends with complete remission. A few patients will have continuous, unremitting symptoms that necessitate surgical intervention (i.e., colectomy for UC or bowel resection for CD).

Although drug therapy is the mainstay of treatment for IBD, several nonpharmacologic interventions may be effective, including patient education and participation in support groups through organizations such as the Crohn's and Colitis Foundation of America (CCFA), proper diet to maintain nutrition and avoidance of foods that exacerbate symptoms, and surgical management, if necessary, for uncontrollable disease. A number of alternative treatments may be beneficial as well, but more research is needed to determine the appropriate dosage and their place in therapy.

Table 13-26 Complementary and Alternative Approaches for IBD

Acupuncture
Bromelain
Nicotine
Omega-3 fatty acids (fish and flaxseed oils)
Probiotics

1.2.0 Pharmacotherapy

Drugs for IBD: Indications and Mechanisms of Action

Several classes of drugs are used in the treatment of IBD, including corticosteroids, 5-ASA (mesalamine) drugs, immunomodulators, tumor necrosis factor inhibitors, and antibiotics. The exact choice of drug depends on a number of factors, including the severity, extent, and location of bowel involvement; past response; patient dosage form preference (oral versus rectal); financial status; patient tolerance and adverse-effect profile; compliance (number of tablets/capsules needed to be taken and schedule); and the presence of complications.

The cornerstone of IBD treatment for maintaining disease remission is the mesalamine-containing drugs (also known as 5-ASA or aminosalicylates). These drugs act as topical anti-inflammatory agents in the bowel and exert their effects on cyclooxygenase and lipoxygenase much as other anti-inflammatory drugs do. They may also be employed to induce remission in patients whose disease is not severe. Aminosalicylates are available in a variety of oral and rectal formulations.

Biopharmaceutical Principles and Pharmaceutical Characteristics of Dosage Forms

The location of anti-inflammatory activity for different mesalamine products is related to their formulation. Some have pH-dependent release (Asacol, Pentasa, Lialda), whereas others are linked to active or inert carrier molecules via an azo bond that is cleaved by colonic bacterial activity (sulfasalazine, olsalazine, and balsalazide). Mesalamine products that are pH coated or have other delayed-release formulations should not be chewed or crushed to ensure the maximum benefit is realized.

Mesalamine Products

Any of the agents except olsalazine is acceptable as first-line therapy. Historically, sulfasalazine has been the treatment of choice for mild-to-moderate IBD due to its relatively high efficacy and lower cost. It consists of a sulfpyridine molecule bonded to 5-ASA, with the sulfa part acting as a carrier. Unfortunately, most of the adverse effects and hypersensitivity associated with this drug result from the presence of sulfpyridine. Olsalazine is composed of two 5-ASA molecules bonded

Table 13-27 Aminosalicylate Comparison

Product	Brand Name	Formulation	Bowel Location
Sulfasalazine	Azulfadine	Enteric-coated tablet	Terminal ileum and large intestine
Mesalamine	Asacol	Delayed-release tablet	Terminal ileum and large intestine
	Pentasa	Microgranule capsule	Jejunum, ileum, and large intestine
	Lialda	Multi-matrix system	Terminal ileum and large intestine
	Rowasa	Enema or suppository	Rectum
Olsalazine	Dipentum	Capsule	Terminal ileum and large intestine
Balsalazide	Colazal	Capsule	Terminal ileum and large intestine

together, but has a high incidence of GI adverse effects and is not considered a first-line drug. Oral mesalamine or balsalazide have become the aminosalicylates of choice due to their better safety profiles and increased patient tolerability.

Corticosteroids

Corticosteroids have powerful anti-inflammatory and immune system effects and are most commonly used for inducing a remission in patients with moderate-to-severe disease at presentation. Oral, rectal, and parenteral corticosteroids are effective for inducing, but not retaining, IBD remission. The choice of product depends on the location and severity of the disease, with intravenous steroids being reserved for more severe or fulminant presentations. The rectal route offers the advantage of more rapid response time and lower risk of systemic adverse effects, but may be unacceptable to many patients. Although IV steroids are used in patients with severe disease, these individuals are often switched to oral steroids within 3 to 7 days. Oral prednisone is the treatment of choice for inducing remission in patients with moderate-to-severe disease and is often initiated at a dose of 40 to 60 mg/day and tapered over 2 to 3 months, with 5-ASA drugs being started mid-taper.

Adverse Effects

The adverse effects of corticosteroids are of the greatest concern, especially with long-term use. They include sleep disturbances, mood alteration, increased appetite, glucose intolerance, osteoporosis, infections, and edema.

Budesonide

Oral budesonide (Entocort EC) is a newer option approved for active CD, especially in steroid-dependent patients. Because of its significant first-pass metabolism, this drug has low systemic bioavailability, is associated with fewer adverse effects, and may be repeated for recurrences.

Immunosuppressants

Immunosuppressant medications are an option for patients who are steroid dependent and who experience disease flares when steroids are discontinued. Agents used for IBD include oral azathioprine and 6-mercaptopurine. IV cyclosporine and tacrolimus are reserved for refractory cases in whom corticosteroids prove ineffective; they may be given a trial prior to surgical options being pursued. Oral immunosuppressant agents may take as long as 6 months to produce their full response and are effective at maintaining remission.

Tumor necrosis factor-alpha inhibitors such as infliximab and adalimumab are indicated for the treatment of moderately to severely active CD in patients who have shown an inadequate response to other agents. These drugs are also particularly useful in the management of fistulizing CD, but must not be used in individuals with active or latent tuberculosis.

Adverse Effects

Adverse effects of immunosuppressants may be severe, and include nausea and vomiting, malaise, bone marrow suppression, and hepatotoxicity.

Antimicrobials

Antimicrobial agents are used predominantly in the management of CD, particularly in fistulizing disease. The agents used most frequently include ciprofloxacin and metronidazole. They are thought to reduce bacterial activity in the small intestine in areas of stricture, fistulae, or recent surgery. They may also have an effect on the immune response in the gut.

1.3.0 Monitoring

Pharmacotherapeutic Outcomes

The goals of IBD pharmacotherapy are to induce and maintain disease remission, heal eroded mucosa, restore and maintain nutrition, control extra-intestinal symptoms, prevent complications, maintain quality of life, minimize drug-related adverse effects, and provide cost-effective care.

Resolution of symptoms, nutrition status, adverse effects of drug therapy, and endoscopic findings indicating healing mucosa and disease control should be routinely monitored in patients with IBD.

Safety and Efficacy Monitoring

Patients should experience a resolution of active disease as indicated by a return to normal or near-normal bowel habits (i.e., two to three formed to semi-formed stools per day), no blood or mucus in the stool, and no abdominal pain; these conditions should be assessed at all clinical visits. Normal daily functioning should accompany improvement in bowel and extra-intestinal symptoms. Extra-intestinal symptoms often correlate with extent and severity of bowel disease, but not always. Assessment of these manifestations should be made at every visit. Regular ocular exams are recommended as well. Quality of life assessments should also be conducted.

Adverse Drug Reactions

Laboratory monitoring—to include CBC and LFTs—should be performed periodically, at least yearly. If immunosuppressant drug therapy is initiated, a CBC should be performed weekly for the first month of treatment, then every 2 weeks for 2 more months, and then monthly thereafter.

Potential adverse effects of 5-ASA drug therapy may be similar to disease symptoms such as diarrhea and abdominal pain. Because drug regimens may necessitate up to three times daily dosing and include nine or more tablets/capsules per day, compliance should be assessed as well.

Adverse effects of corticosteroids require monitoring of signs and symptoms experienced by the patient, including weight gain and mood disorders as well as laboratory findings (hyperglycemia, increased WBC).

Interaction of Drugs with Foods and Laboratory Tests

Patients should be counseled on lifestyle and dietary changes that may help them manage their condition and prevent exacerbations. Careful consideration should be given to potential trigger foods, and an association should be confirmed prior to eliminating specific dietary components.

Corticosteroids should be taken with food to minimize stomach upset. These medications are associated with insomnia, increased appetite, skin thinning, changes in mood, edema, glucose intolerance, and osteoporosis.

Fluoroquinolones must not be taken within 4 to 6 hours of liquid antacids, multivitamins, iron, or zinc-containing products to avoid decreased absorption and decreased efficacy. Metronidazole should be taken with food to avoid stomach upset, and patients must avoid alcohol consumption to prevent the severe nausea and vomiting that accompanies the disulfiram reaction. Live vaccines should not be administered to patients receiving infliximab therapy.

Contraindications, Warnings, and Precautions

Certain medications should be used with great caution in IBD, including loperamide, diphenoxylate, antispasmodics, and anticholinergics. These agents may precipitate a life-threatening complication known as toxic megacolon.

Patient Education

Rectal formulations should be used as directed. Suspension enemas should be shaken prior to use. Suppositories must be unwrapped prior to insertion and not handled excessively.

Parasthesias have been reported with long-term use of IBD medications, and patients must be counseled to report numbness or tingling in the extremities immediately.

Tumor necrosis factor inhibitors such as infliximab may increase the risk of infections; the patient should be instructed to report this complication promptly if it occurs. Infusions reactions are also possible and may include itching, flushing, and changes in blood pressure.

ANNOTATED BIBLIOGRAPHY

DiPiro JT, Schade RR. Inflammatory bowel disease. In: DiPiro JT, Talbert RL, Yee GC, et al., eds. *Pharmacotherapy: A Pathophysiologic Approach*. 6th ed. Stamford, CT: Appleton & Lange, 2005:649–664.

Farrell RJ, Peppercorn MA. Ulcerative colitis. *Lancet* 2002;359:331–340.

Garnett WR, Yunker NS. The treatment of inflammatory bowel disease. In: Mueller BA, Bertch KE, Dunsworth TS, et al., eds. *Pharmacotherapy Self-Assessment Program: Book 8. Gastroenterology*. 4th ed. Kansas City: American College of Clinical Pharmacy, 2002:29–64.

Knutson D, Greenberg G, et al. Management of Crohn's disease: a practical approach. *Am Fam Physician* 2003;68:707–714, 717–718.

Langan RC, Gotsch PB, Krafczyk MA, et al. Ulcerative colitis: diagnosis and treatment. *Am Fam Physician* 2007;76:1323–1330.

Ragunath K, Williams JG. Balsalazide therapy in ulcerative colitis. *Aliment Pharmacol Ther* 2001;15: 1549–1554.

Wall GC. Lower gastrointestinal disorders. In: Koda-Kimble MA, Young LY, Kradjan WA, Guglielmo BJ, eds. *Applied Therapeutics: The Clinical Use of Drugs*. 8th ed. Baltimore: Lippincott Williams & Wilkins, 2004:28.1–28.24.

TOPIC: PANCREATITIS

Section Coordinator: *Tracy K. Pettinger*
Contributors: *Tracy K. Pettinger and Nicole Murdock*

Tips Worth Tweeting

- Pancreatitis—the inflammation of the pancreas—can occur on an acute or chronic level.
- Both conditions are associated with severe abdominal pain.
- Acute pancreatitis (AP) is most often self-limiting, but is treated with bowel rest, fluid resuscitation, and pain relief measures (most often in the form of narcotics).
- Chronic pancreatitis (CP) is defined as permanent damage to the pancreatic cells due to chronic inflammation.
- CP is characterized by pain, malabsorption, and steatorrhea.
- Pain is treated with both non-narcotic and narcotic therapies.
- Pancreatic enzymes are used to treat the pain and steatorrhea associated with pancreatitis.
- The most common causes of AP and CP are alcohol abuse and mechanical blockages (especially gallstones).
- Many medications have been reported to cause AP.
- Lipase is more specific than amylase in the diagnosis of AP.
- Recurrent cases of AP may lead to CP.

Patient Care Scenario: Ambulatory Setting

- 36 y/o, 6'4", M, 220 lbs, 1 beer per day
- History of hyperlipidemia, asthma
- History of present illness: woke up to sudden and intense pain radiating to the back + nausea and vomiting

Date	Physician	Drug	Quantity	Sig	Refills
5/31	Watson	Albuterol inhaler	1	2 puffs q 6 hr prn for SOB	2
5/23	Watson	Simvastatin 40 mg	90	one daily	1
4/21	Watson	Advair 250/50	1	inhale 1 puff twice daily	2

Table 13-28 Drugs Associated with Acute Pancreatitis

Cannabis
Codeine
Dexamethasone*
Enalapril*
Estrogens
Exenatide*
Furosemide
Losartan
Metronidazole
Omeprazole
Pravastatin*
Saw palmetto
Sulfamethoxazole
Tetracycline
Thiazides
Trimethoprim-sulfamethoxazole
Valproic acid

*Other drugs in this class have also been implicated.

1.1.0 Patient Information

Medication-Induced Causes of Acute Pancreatitis

Drug-induced pancreatitis accounts for approximately 2% of AP cases. Individuals at higher risk include persons with HIV, cancer, inflammatory bowel disease, and polypharmacy. Female and pediatric patients are also at higher risk. Several medications and herbal supplements have been associated with pancreatitis.

Laboratory Testing

Acute Pancreatitis

Two enzymes are released from the pancreas when damage has occurred and can confirm the diagnosis of AP—namely, amylase and lipase. Amylase levels increase within 24 hours of the onset of symptoms, but may be normal in those persons with alcoholism. Amylase levels greater than three times the upper limit of normal are consistent with AP; however, other conditions may cause such elevation. Lipase is more sensitive and specific compared to amylase for diagnosing AP; it also remains elevated in the serum for a longer period of time.

Other laboratory tests can be performed to determine the severity and etiology of AP, including a complete metabolic panel, lipid panel, complete blood count, and arterial blood gases. Levels of C-reactive protein (CRP) may be elevated 48 hours after the onset of pain and may help distinguish between mild and severe cases.

Chronic Pancreatitis

Amylase and lipase are often normal in CP unless an acute attack is occurring. Increased levels of these enzymes are generally neither diagnostic nor prognostic. A 72-hour fecal fat test is the gold standard for the diagnosis of steatorrhea, with the excretion of more than 7 grams of fat per day indicating malabsorption. Fecal elastase measurements may provide another means of determining pancreatic exocrine dysfunction. A complete blood count, electrolytes, and liver function should also be evaluated.

Disease States Associated with Pancreatitis

See Table 13-29 and 13-30.

Instruments and Techniques Related to Patient Assessment

Acute Pancreatitis

Imaging can be used to determine the cause and severity of AP. An abdominal ultrasound is performed to assess for gallstones. An abdominal CT with contrast is the best test to determine severity, identify complications, and exclude potential causes of the abdominal pain.

Vital signs should be assessed frequently (every 4 hours), as the patient with AP may become hypoxic and dehydrated. A pain scale should be used to determine the effectiveness of pain treatment.

Table 13-29 Conditions Associated with Acute Pancreatitis

Mechanical blockage: gallstones
Infection: bacterial, viral, parasitic, fungal
Metabolic: hypercalcemia, hypertriglyceridemia (level > 1,000 mg/dL)
Autoimmune: systemic lupus erythematosus, Sjögren's syndrome
Procedure complication: ERCP
Genetic
Anatomic or functional disorders
Other: pregnancy, tumor, vasculitis

Table 13-30 Conditions Associated with Chronic Pancreatitis

Ductal obstruction: stones, trauma, pseudocysts
Metabolic: hyperparathyroidism, hypertriglyceridemia
Autoimmune: inflammatory bowel disease, systemic lupus erythematosus, cystic fibrosis
Genetic
Autoimmune pancreatitis
Tropical pancreatitis

To predict adverse outcomes and the severity of AP, validated scoring systems may be used. They include Ranson's criteria, the Imrie scoring system, the APACHE II scale, and the CT Severity Index.

Chronic Pancreatitis

A variety of imaging studies are used in CP. Plain films can be used to identify calcification within the pancreatic duct. A transabdominal ultrasound, computed tomography (CT) scan, or magnetic resonance imaging (MRI) may also be used to show calcifications, obstructions, and other abnormalities of the pancreas as well as to differentiate CP from cancer. An ERCP can be used, but is invasive and may cause pancreatitis. MRCP is another option. A pain scale should be used to determine the effectiveness of pain treatment. The degree of malabsorption should be monitored.

Key Terms

APACHE II: Acute Physiology and Chronic Health Evaluation

ERCP: endoscopic retrograde cholangiopancreatography

MRCP: magnetic resonance cholangiopancreatography

Endocrine function of the pancreas: hormone production and release—most notably, insulin, glucagon, and somatostatin

Exocrine function of the pancreas: aids in digestion and includes production and release of amylase, lipase, and other enzymes

Signs and Symptoms

The classic presentation symptom of AP is acute, severe, upper abdominal pain that can radiate to the back. It may be accompanied by nausea, vomiting, and tenderness. Common signs of AP include a low-grade fever, hypotension, tachypnea, shallow respirations, jaundice, abdominal distention, and guarding. AP is usually exacerbated by eating and by alcohol consumption.

Wellness and Prevention

Acute Pancreatitis

Alcohol abuse accounts for approximately 35% of AP cases, making it and gallstones the most common causes of AP. Ten percent of chronic alcohol abusers (who consume more than 80 g of alcohol daily) develop AP.

Chronic Pancreatitis

Alcohol abuse is responsible for 70% to 80% of CP cases. The risk of developing CP is related to the duration of abuse and the amount of alcohol consumed. Patients who abuse alcohol should seek counseling.

Table 13-31 Signs and Symptoms of Chronic Pancreatitis

Sign or Symptom	Comment
Abdominal pain	• Described as dull, epigastric, and radiating to the back • Usually worse at night and 15–30 minutes after eating • Can be discrete at first, then progressively worse
Fat and protein malabsorption	• Steatorrhea ○ Associated with diarrhea and bloating ○ Loose, greasy, foul-smelling stools ○ Occurs early • Azotorrhea • Vitamin B_{12} and fat-soluble vitamin malabsorption • Malnutrition • Weight loss
Pancreatic diabetes	• Can also lead to weight loss • Usually occurs with pancreatic calcification • Usually a complication late in the disease • Begins more with glucose intolerance
Nausea and vomiting	• Dehydration • Potential electrolyte disturbances

1.2.0 Pharmacotherapy

Drugs for Pancreatitis: Indications and Mechanisms of Action

Acute Pancreatitis

Most cases of AP are mild, with minimal organ dysfunction, and are self-limiting. Therapy focuses on bowel rest, volume repletion, oxygen administration, pain management, and antiemetics. The cause of the AP should be determined and corrected, if possible—for example, through discontinuation of the offending medication or removal of gallstones. In more severe cases of AP, therapy may include antibiotics, enteral nutrition, and surgical interventions.

In mild AP, the patient should receive nothing orally so as to decrease the pancreatic secretions and complications. However, intravenous fluids should be administered to maintain hydration and blood pressure. Enteral (preferred) or parenteral nutrition should be considered if the patient is not likely to receive any nutrition orally for more than 7 days.

Pain management primarily relies on narcotics. Merperidine historically has been preferred because it does not cause spasm of the sphincter of Oddi. The clinical relevance of this effect is unknown. Due to its potential toxicities, merperidine is not recommended as first-line therapy, however. Instead, morphine and fentanyl are commonly used for this indication.

There is no preferred antiemetic for use in AP. Patient-specific factors such as comorbid disease states and allergies as well as the potential adverse effects of each medication class should be taken into consideration prior to initiation.

Chronic Pancreatitis

Therapy focuses on pain management and treatment of malabsorption and steatorrhea. With regard to pain, scheduled, non-narcotic medications, such as acetaminophen, NSAIDs, or tramadol, should be considered first. Most patients, however, will require narcotic medications for pain control.

Pancreatic enzyme replacement is used for the treatment of both pain and malabsorption. As their mechanism of action in relieving pain, the enzymes provide negative feedback inhibition to the pancreas. Efficacy trials regarding pain control have yielded mixed results. Pancreatic enzyme replacement also supplies lipase, protease, and amylase to facilitate absorption. Generally, 25,000 to 40,000 IU of pancreatic lipase should be consumed with each meal. The dose should be titrated to reduce steatorrhea to less than 15 g/day. Patients should be encouraged to discontinue alcohol consumption and to eat meals that contain around 20 g of fat.

Dosing Regimens and Routes of Administration

Acute Pancreatitis

Avoid oral administration of medication until the pancreatitis is stable.

Chronic Pancreatitis

See Table 13-32.

Interaction of Drugs with Foods and Laboratory Tests

As a treatment for CP, pancreatic enzymes should be taken before or with each meal with a full glass of water. The enzymes should not be taken with calcium- or magnesium-containing antacids or dairy products. The absorption of iron salts and l-methylfolate may be decreased when such therapy is administered; the effectiveness of acarbose and miglitol may be decreased as well. Conversely, immediate-release pancreatic enzyme formulations may be inactivated by an acidic pH and may require acid suppression therapy (i.e., H3 blocker or proton pump inhibitor).

Table 13-32 Chronic Pancreatitis Enzyme Preparations

Product	Lipase Content (USP units)	Protease Content (USP units)	Amylase Content (USP units)	Comments
Immediate Release				
Pancrelipase tablets Panokase tablets Viokase 8 tablets	8,000	30,000	30,000	Various manufacturers; all porcine derived Not interchangeable
Pancrelipase tablets Viokase 16 tablets	16,000	60,000	60,000	Various manufacturers; all porcine derived Not interchangeable
Viokase powder	16,800	70,000	70,000	Porcine derived Amount in ¼ teaspoon (0.7 g)
Enteric-Coated Microspheres				
Pancrecarb MS-4 DR capsules	4,000	25,000	25,000	Has bicarbonate buffer Porcine derived
Pancrelipase capsules Panocaps DR capsules Ultrase capsules	4,500	25,000	20,000	Various manufacturers Not interchangeable
Creon DR capsules	6,000	19,000	30,000	Porcine derived
Pancrecarb MS-8 DR capsules	8,000	45,000	40,000	Has bicarbonate buffer Porcine derived
Palcaps 10 DR capsules	10,000	37,500	33,200	Porcine derived
Creon DR capsules	12,000	38,000	60,000	Porcine derived
Lipram-UL 12 DR capsules	12,000	39,000	39,000	Porcine derived
Pancrelipase capsules Panocaps MT 16 DR capsules	16,000	48,000	48,000	Porcine derived Not interchangeable
Pancrecarb MS-16 DR capsules	16,000	52,000	52,000	Has bicarbonate buffer Porcine derived
Lipram-UL 18 DR capsules	18,000	58,500	58,500	Porcine derived
Panocaps MT 20 DR capsules	20,000	44,000	56,000	Porcine derived
Lipram-UL 20 DR capsules	20,000	65,000	65,000	Porcine derived
Palcaps 20 DR capsules	20,000	75,000	66,400	Porcine derived
Creon DR capsules	24,000	76,000	120,000	Porcine derived
Enteric-Coated Microtablets				
Pancrease MT capsules	4,000	12,000	12,000	Porcine derived
Pancrease MT 10 capsules	10,000	30,000	30,000	Porcine derived
Ultrase MT 12 capsules	12,000	39,000	39,000	Porcine derived
Pancrease MT 16 capsules	16,000	48,000	48,000	Porcine derived
Ultrase MT 18 capsules	18,000	58,500	58,500	Porcine derived
Pancrease MT 20 capsules	20,000	44,000	56,000	Porcine derived
Ultrase MT 20 capsules	20,000	65,000	65,000	Porcine derived
Enteric-Coated Beads				
Zenpep DR capsules	5,000	17,000	27,000	Porcine derived
Zenpep DR capsules	10,000	34,000	55,000	Porcine derived
Zenpep DR capsules	15,000	51,000	82,000	Porcine derived
Zenpep DR capsules	20,000	68,000	109,000	Porcine derived

MS = microspheres; MT = microtablets; DR = delayed release.

Contraindications, Warnings, and Precautions

Contraindications to pancreatic enzyme replacement in CP patients include hypersensitivity to porcine proteins or enzymes, acute pancreatitis, and exacerbation of chronic pancreatitis. Caution is warranted in those patients with oral mucosa irritation, who will not be able to swallow the dose. Individuals with a history of gout, hyperuricemia, or renal impairment may experience increased blood levels of uric acid.

Physiochemical Properties, Solubility, Pharmacodynamics, and Pharmacokinetics

All products for CP are oral medications available in various dosage forms.

Pharmacokinetic Dosage Calculations

The doses of enzyme preparations for CP do not need to be adjusted in patients with renal or hepatic dysfunction.

Biopharmaceutical Principles and Pharmaceutical Characteristics of Dosage Forms

- Clinically significant variability may arise even between batches of the same formulation.
- Capsules should not be crushed, chewed, or mixed with foods with a pH greater than 4, as this practice will lead to premature release of the enzyme.
- Creon capsules, Pancrease MT DR capsules, and Zenpep capsules can be opened and mixed with an acidic food that does not require chewing, such as applesauce.
- Avoid inhalation of Viokase powder, as this may cause nasal and respiratory tract irritation.

1.3.0 Monitoring

Pharmacotherapeutic Outcomes

Acute Pancreatitis

Outcomes to be assessed include pain control, fluid and nutritional status, electrolytes, adverse effects of therapy, and signs and symptoms of worsening clinical status. Alcohol use should be monitored.

Chronic Pancreatitis

Outcomes to be assessed include reduction in pain, steatorrhea, symptoms of malabsorption (a 72-hour stool test for fecal fat may need to be used), and constipation. Consider a serum uric acid, complete blood count, vitamin B_{12} measurement, and folic acid level yearly. Alcohol use should be monitored.

Safety and Efficacy Monitoring and Patient Education

Enzyme supplements should be taken with meals and should be taken as directed by the provider. The dosage may need to be adjusted frequently until the best dose is found. If a dose is missed, the patient should take the medication as soon as possible unless it is almost time for the next dose; in that case, the patient should skip the missed dose.

The enzymes are made from the pancreas of pigs.

Adverse Drug Reactions

Overall, enzyme replacement for CP at therapeutic doses is well tolerated. Hypersensitivity reactions can occur due to the use of porcine proteins, however. Hyperuricouria and hyperuricemia, leading to kidney stones and gout, have been reported at high doses. Gastrointestinal effects vary with the dose and the dosage form, but can include diarrhea, constipation, flatulence, nausea, abdominal pain, oral irritation, and abnormal feces. On rare occasions, stricture of the colon and distal intestinal obstruction syndrome may occur. Skin reactions such as rash, pruritus, and urticaria have been noted as well. Fibrosing colonopathy can occur with high doses and prolonged use of enzyme replacement therapy.

Nonadherence, Misuse, or Abuse

Overdose of pancreatic enzymes may cause diarrhea and stomach upset.

2.2.0 Dispensing

Calculations

Dosage recommendations are in international units (IU) but the enzyme preparations are expressed in USP units. One IU is equivalent to 2 to 3 USP units.

Physical Attributes of Commercial Products

A variety of dosage forms are available, with varying amounts of enzymes in each.

Bioequivalence

The products are not bioequivalent and cannot be interchanged without discussion with the healthcare provider.

Package, Storage, Handling, and Disposal

Drugs should be stored at room temperature, away from light and humidity.

ANNOTATED BIBLIOGRAPHY

American Gastroenterological Association. AGA Institute medical positional statement on acute pancreatitis. *Gastroenterology* 2007;132:2019–2021.

Badalov N, Baradaria R, Iswara K, Li J, et al. Drug-induced acute pancreatitis: an evidence-based review. *Clin Gastroenterol Hepatol* 2007;5:648–661.

Banks PA, Freeman ML. Practice parameters committee of the American College of Gastroenterology. *Am J Gastroenterol* 2006;101:2379–2400.

Carroll JK, Herrick B, Gipson T, Lee SP. Acute pancreatitis: diagnosis, prognosis, and treatment. *Am Fam Physician* 2007;75:1513–1520.

Facts & Comparisons. Available at: http://online.factsandcomparisons.com/index.aspx. Accessed February 15, 2010.

Ferrone M, Raimondo M, Scolapio JS. *Pharmacotherapy* 2007;27:910–920.

Frossard J, Steer ML, Pastor CM. Acute pancreatitis. *Lancet* 2008;371:143–152.

Lexi-Comp Online. Available at: http://online.lexi.com/crlsql/servlet/crlonline. Accessed February 15, 2010.

Micromedex Healthcare Series. Available at: http://www.thomsonhc.com/hcs/librarian. Accessed February 15, 2010.

Tattersall SJN, Apte MV, Wilson JS. A fire inside: current concepts in chronic pancreatitis. *Intern Med J* 2008;38:592–598.

TOPIC: PEPTIC ULCER DISEASE (PUD)

Section Coordinator: Tracy K. Pettinger
Contributor: Thomas G. Wadsworth

Tips Worth Tweeting

- *H. pylori* and NSAIDs are the most common causes of duodenal and gastric ulcers, respectively.
- PPI-based triple therapy that includes clarithromycin and amoxicillin has the highest eradication rate when directed against peptic ulcer disease (PUD).
- All NSAIDs can cause PUD, although more COX-2 preferential agents may carry a lower risk of disease development.
- PPIs are the drugs of choice for treatment and prevention of NSAID-induced ulcers.
- PUD is an erosive condition of the gastric or duodenal geography, typically extending deep into the muscularis mucosa.
- PUD can result in life-threatening upper GI bleeding, perforation, or obstruction. It is characterized by episodic periods of exacerbation and remission.
- PUD can be categorized into three causative subtypes with identified risk factors: *H. pylori*–associated ulcers, NSAID-induced ulcers, and stress ulcers.
- Treatment is aimed at relieving symptoms, healing ulcers, preventing ulcer complications, and preventing recurrent ulceration.
- *H. pylori*–positive patients are treated with PPI-based triple, quadruple, or sequential drug therapies that include select antimicrobials.
- *H. pylori*–negative NSAID ulcers are treated with PPIs, which are preferred in this indication over H2-receptor antagonists or sucralfate.
- Prophylactic NSAID cotherapy with PPIs, prostaglandins, or H2RAs can prevent recurrence of ulceration. Prevention also includes risk factor modification, including dietary and lifestyle changes.

Patient Care Scenario: Community

M. W. is a 52-year-old carpenter who presents to his PCP complaining of sharp epigastric pain/burning, along with fatigue for the last several weeks. His stomach pain is relieved when he eats, but it returns a few hours later and often awakens him during the night. M. W. is taking OTC antacids and OTC ranitidine, which produce some relief, but wonders if he is taking too much.

Past medical history: hypertension, hyperlipidemia, CAD (MI 2 years ago), chronic low back pain, constipation
SH: smokes ½ ppd, drinks 1–2 beers/day
Allergies: penicillin
Vitals: BP 110/82, HR 68, Wt 185 lbs, Ht 6'1"
Labs: SCr 1.1 mg/dL, BUN 10 mg/dL, Hct 28%, Hgb 10.2 g/dL, urea breath test—negative, *H. pylori* antibody—positive

Date	Physician	Drug	Sig	Quantity	Refills
2/3	Thompson	Pravastatin 40 mg	1 po hs	90	1
2/3	Thompson	Clopidogrel 75 mg	1 po qd	90	3
1/03	Thompson	Atenolol 50 mg	1 po qd	90	3
12/14	Jackson	Norco 5/325 mg	1–2 po q4–6 hr prn	100	0
12/5	Thompson	Lodine XL 500 mg	1 po bid prn	60	9

1.1.0 Patient Information

Medication-Induced Causes of PUD

NSAIDs are the most common cause of medication-induced upper GI bleeding. Some agents are less toxic to the GI tract than others, such as COX-2 preferential

Table 13-33 Drugs Associated with Upper GI Ulceration/Bleeding

Selective serotonin reuptake inhibitors (SSRIs)
Oral potassium chloride
Bisphosphonates
Ethanol
Anticoagulants
Platelet inhibitors
NSAIDS

NSAIDs (e.g., etodolac, nabumetone, meloxicam). Piroxicam and ketoralac are the NSAIDs considered to carry the highest risk of PUD development.

Laboratory Testing

H. pylori status can be determined by a number of tests that differ in terms of their invasiveness, sensitivity, and specificity. Hematocrit and hemoglobin levels should be measured to detect significant blood loss, or a stool hemoccult (guaiac card) performed to detect smaller occult (hidden) bleeding.

Disease States Associated with PUD

- Zollinger-Ellison syndrome: gastric acid hypersecretion and recurrent peptic ulcers resulting from gastrin-producing tumors
- Radiation/chemotherapy
- Vascular insufficiency
- Other chronic diseases expressing a strong association with PUD: mastocytosis, multiple endocrine neoplasia type 1, chronic pulmonary diseases, chronic renal failure, kidney stones, hepatic cirrhosis, and alpha$_1$-antitrypsin deficiency

Instruments and Techniques Related to Patient Assessment

- Upper GI radiography: Single barium contrast or double contrast is often the initial procedure when uncomplicated PUD is suspected. It is less costly and less invasive.
- Endoscopy: Fiberoptic upper endoscopy permits direct visualization of ulceration. It is more sensitive and is often used to confirm radiographic findings.

Key Terms

***Helicobacter pylori (H. pylori)*:** spiral shaped, pH-sensitive, gram-negative, microaerophilic bacterium that resides between the mucosal layer and epithelial cells of the stomach or duodenum.

Classification of PUD

H. pylori is the most common cause of non-NSAID ulcers; thus eradication of *H. pylori* significantly decreases ulcer recurrence. However, only 20% of patients will experience symptomatic PUD. The prevalence of *H. pylori* infection in the United States ranges from 30% to 40% in adults, but is higher in ethnic

Table 13-34 *H. pylori* Diagnostic Tests

Test	Description	Specificity	Sensitivity	Comments
Invasive (Endoscopic)				
Histology	Microbiologic staining	98–99%	90–95%	Gold standard; costly and time consuming.
Culture	Cultured biopsy	100%	100%	Takes time; allows for abx sensitivity/resistance testing; use only after treatment failure.
Rapid urease (biopsy)	Detects presence of NH4 generated by *H. pylori* urease	95–100%	80–95%	Rapid results; false negatives may occur due to partial treatments, or use of H3RAs, PPIs, or bismuth. Patient should be off these agents 1 week prior to testing.
Noninvasive				
Serological antibody detection	Detects IgG to *H. pylori* in serum or whole blood (ELISA)	79%	85%	Can be done in lab or office; cannot distinguish between active or previous infection. Do not use to test from eradication following treatment.
Urea breath test	Detects radioactive CO_2 exhalation after ingestions of urea radiolabeled with ^{13}C or ^{14}C	95%	97%	Can be used to test for diagnosis and eradication; recent use of antibiotics, H3RAs, bismuth, and PPIs can result in false negatives. Patients must be off 2 weeks before and 4 weeks after treatment prior to testing.
Stool antigen	Detects *H. pylori* in stool using polyclonal or monoclonal antibody test	87%	88–92%	Can be used for diagnosis and to confirm eradication. PPIs, bismuth, H3RAs, and antibiotics can cause false negatives but to a lesser extent than in other tests.

groups (African Americans and Latin Americans) and in developing countries. Transmission primarily occurs via the fecal–oral route but can involve the oral–oral route (unlikely) and gastro–oral route (endoscopes). Risk factors for infection include consumption of raw vegetables, contaminated water, crowded living conditions, and large numbers of children.

NSAID-Induced PUD

Approximately 15% to 30% of regular NSAID users will develop gastroduodenal ulcers, with gastric ulcers being the most common form. Such disease can occur as soon as a week after NSAID use or with continued treatment. All NSAIDs are implicated (including low-dose ASA), but incidence may be lower with use of COX-2 preferential NSAIDs (e.g., salsalate, etodolac, nabumetone, meloxicam, celecoxib, diclofenac). NSAIDs cause gastric mucosal damage both by direct topical irritation and—more importantly—through the inhibition of cyptoprotective mucosal prostaglandin synthesis. Loss of the protective mucosal layer exposes gastric tissue to endogenous erosive acids and enzymes (pepsin). Although ulceration can occur at any time during therapy, its risk increases with dose and duration of use.

Other risk factors for NSAID-induced PUD are listed in Table 13-36. Combinations of risk factors are additive.

Stress Ulcers

Stress ulcers involve ulcerations due to the physiologic stress of severe illness. They occur primarily in the fundus of the stomach and are the most common cause of GI bleeds in the ICU. Two major independent risk factors for stress ulcers are mechanical ventilation for more than 48 hours (OR 15.6) and existing coagulopathy (platelets < 50,000, INR > 1.5, apt > 2× control). Stress ulcers are often asymptomatic but could include one or more of the symptoms listed in Table 13-37.

Table 13-36 Risk Factors for NSAID-Induced Ulcer

Age > 60 years
Previous peptic ulcer
Existing coagulopathy
High NSAID dose
Chronic use of NSAIDs
Concomitant corticosteroid use
Concomitant SSRI use
Concomitant anticoagulant use
Concomitant antiplatelet use
Chronic illness
H. pylori infection
Alcohol consumption
Cigarette smoking

Table 13-37 Symptoms of Ulcers

Abdominal/epigastric pain, fullness, cramping
Nocturnal pain that awakens the patient from sleep
Heartburn, belching, bloating
Nausea, vomiting, anorexia (gastric > duodenal) Symptoms worsened by food (gastric)
Symptoms relieved by food (duodenal)
Chronic fatigue or malaise (suggest active bleed)
Hematemesis (vomiting blood)
Melena (black-colored stools)

Signs and Symptoms of PUD

Approximately 20% of patients with chronic PUD will develop upper GI bleed, perforation, or obstruction.

Table 13-35 Classification of PUD

	Duodenal Ulcer	Gastric Ulcer
Common causes	*H. pylori* (95%), NSAIDs	NSAIDs, *H. pylori*
Uncommon causes	Zollinger-Ellison syndrome Hypercalcemia Granulomatous diseases Neoplasia Infections (CMV, HSV, TB) Ectopic pancreatic tissue	Crohn's disease Infections (CMV, HSV)
Differentiating symptoms	Epigastric pain worse at night Pain 1–3 hours following meal Pain relieved by eating	Epigastric pain worse with eating

Signs

Signs of PUD that are possible but not always present include weight loss, microcytic anemia (low hematocrit and hemoglobin), guiac positive (occult blood), and *H. pylori*–positive status.

Symptoms

Although most patients are asymptomatic, the emergence of symptoms depends on the severity of ulceration and the loss of blood. Ulcer pain and symptoms vary and may occur in clusters for weeks, with this time then followed by an asymptomatic period lasting weeks to years. Epigastric pain is often associated with *H. pylori* infection. NSAID-induced ulcers can be associated with dyspepsia but most often asymptomatic. Ulceration should be suspected when NSAID-related dyspepsia is not relieved by antiulcer medications. If bleeding is occurring, patients can develop acute/chronic anemia with associated lethargy/fatigue.

Wellness and Prevention

Although the role of diet and stress is unclear in PUD, patients with PUD or at risk for PUD should make efforts to eliminate/reduce their psychological stress, use of cigarettes, over-consumption of alcohol, consumption of spicy foods, and consumption of caffeinated beverages. NSAIDs should be eliminated or used at the lowest effective doses for the shortest period of time. If NSAID therapy is necessary, then the following guidelines are suggested: (1) COX-2 preferential agents are preferred, and (2) cotherapy with PPIs or misoprostol is effective for primary/secondary prevention.

1.2.0 Pharmacotherapy

Drug Indications, Dosing Regimens, and Routes of Administration

NSAID-Induced PUD

The causative agent should be discontinued, with daily use of a PPI being undertaken for 6 to 8 weeks, or 8 to 12 weeks if use of the NSAID is continued. Eradicate *H. pylori* if present. If continued NSAID use is needed, prophylactic cotherapy with PPI or misoprostol is indicated. Misoprostol is a synthetic prostaglandin E_1 analog that replaces prostaglandins inhibited by NSAIDs.

H. pylori–Induced PUD

Eradication of *H. pylori* is the foundation of treatment because it promotes ulcer healing and prevents recurrence. The primary treatment goal is eradication of the organism using PPI-based triple medication therapy as the first-line regimen; this combination includes a PPI plus two selected antibiotics for 7 to 14 days. If a second course of treatment is required, a PPI-based triple medication regimen should be used again, but with different antibiotics; alternatively, a four-drug regimen, consisting of a PPI plus bismuth subsalicylate, metronidazole, and tetracycline, should be used. (See Table 13-38 for a list of regimens.) Any PPI is acceptable and can be dosed once daily, although twice-daily dosing may be more effective. The PPI should be continued at least 2 weeks after eradication to ensure complete ulcer healing. H2RAs should not be used in place of PPIs in this indication because they are associated with reduced eradication rates. If an H2RA is used, the duration of treatment should be lengthened to 14 days with continuation of the H2RA for 3 weeks after antibiotics are completed. Sequential therapy should not be used as the first-line option, but has shown eradication rates superior to PPI-based triple therapy.

Interaction of Drugs with Foods and Laboratory Tests

- PPIs may reduce the effectiveness of clopidogrel by inhibiting the hepatic isoenzyme CYP 2C9, which prevents clopidogrel's conversion to its active metabolite.
- Proton pump inhibitor absorption may be delayed by food.
- Sucralafate may bind to other medications and should be separated from them in terms of administration.
- Use of H2RAs, PPIs, bismuth, or antibiotics 2 weeks before or 4 weeks after a urea breath test, stool antigen, or rapid urease test can lead to false-negative results.

Contraindications, Warnings, and Precautions

- Misoprostol is contraindicated in pregnancy (Category X).
- Bismuth subsalicylate is contraindicated in patients with salicylate allergies.

Physiochemical Properties, Solubility, Pharmacodynamics, and Pharmacokinetics

PPI formulations are enteric coated because they are degraded rapidly by gastric acid. They include pH-sensitive granules (omeprazole, esomeprazole, lansoprazole) and delayed-release tablets (rabeprazole, pantoprazole, OTC omeprazole).

1.3.0 Monitoring

Pharmacotherapeutic Outcomes

Desirable outcomes include resolution of symptoms, ulcer healing, *H. pylori* eradication, and prevention of ulcer complications and reoccurrence.

Table 13-38 *H. pylori* Treatment Regimens

Regimen	Antibiotic #1	Antibiotic #2	Comments
Triple-Drug Therapy			
PPI (7–14 days)	Clarithromycin* 500 mg bid	Amoxicillin† 1 g bid **or** Metronidazole 500 mg bid	First-line therapy. The amoxicillin/metronidazole combination may be less effective. The clarithromycin/metronidazole combination is preferred in patients with penicillin allergies.
Quadruple-Drug Therapy			
PPI **or** H3-antagonist **and** bismuth subsalicylate 525 mg qid (7–14 days)	Metronidazole 250–500 mg qid	Tetracycline‡ 500 mg qid **or** Amoxicillin 500 mg qid **or** Clarithromycin 250–500 mg qid	For people who have recently used a macrolide. Used as salvage therapy. Can be used as first-line therapy, but is generally reserved for second-line use because of poor compliance and tolerability.
Sequential Therapy			
PPI (10 days)	Amoxicillin† 1 g bid (First 5 days)	Clarithromycin* 500 mg bid **and** Metronidazole 500 mg bid (For additional 5 days)	Second-line therapy. Achieved superior eradication rates compared to PPI-based triple therapy.

* *Do not* substitute with azithromycin or erythromycin.

† *Do not* substitute with ampicillin.

‡ *Do not* substitute with doxycyclin or minocycline.

Table 13-39 Proton Pump Inhibitors: Generic and Brand Names and Dosage Form Availability

Generic Name (Brand Name)	Dosage Forms	*H. pylori* Eradication	PUD Healing	PUD Maintenance	CYP
Rabeprazole (Aciphex)	20 mg tablets	20 mg qd	20 mg qd	20 mg qd	2C19, 3A4
Omeprazole (Prilosec, Prilosec OTC)	10, 20, and 40 mg capsules 2.5 and 10 mg suspensions	20–40 mg bid	20–40 mg qd	20–40 mg qd	2C19, 2C9, 3A4
Omeprazole/sodium bicarbonate (Zegrid, Zegrid OTC)	20 and 40 mg capsules (1,100 mg $NaHCO_3$) 20 and 40 mg powdered suspensions (1,680 mg $NaHCO_3$)	20–40 mg bid	20–40 mg qd	20–40 mg qd	2C19, 2C9, 3A4
Esomeprazole (Nexium)	20 and 40 mg capsules 10, 20, and 40 mg suspensions 20 and 40 mg injections	40 mg qd	20–40 mg qd	20 mg qd	2C19, 3A4
Lansoprazole (Prevacid)	15 and 30 mg capsules 15 and 30 mg suspensions 15 and 30 mg orally disintegrating tablet 30 mg injection	30 mg bid	15–30 mg qd	15–30 mg qd	2C9, 3A4
Dexlansoprazole (Kapidex)	30 and 60 mg capsules	60 mg qd (not approved)	30–60 mg qd (not approved)		2C19, 2C9, 3A4
Pantoprazole (Protonix)	20 and 40 mg tablets 40 mg suspension 40 mg injection	40 mg bid	40 mg qd	40 mg qd	2C19, 3A4

Table 13-40 H2 Antagonists: Generic and Brand Names and Dosage Form Availability

Generic Name (Brand Name)	Dosage Forms	*H. pylori* Eradication (Requires Combo Therapy)	PUD Healing	PUD Maintenance	CYP
Cimetidine (Tagamet)	200, 300, 400, and 800 mg tablets 300 mg/5 mL solution	400 mg bid	300 mg qid 400 mg bid 800 mg qhs	400–800 mg qhs	1A2
Famotidine (Pepcid, Pepcid AC, others)	10, 20, and 40 mg tablets 40 mg/5 mL solution	40 mg qd	20 mg bid 40 mg qhs	20–40 mg qhs	–
Nizatidine (Axid)	75, 150, and 300 mg capsules 15 mg/mL solution	150 mg bid	150 mg bid 300 mg qhs	150–300 mg qhs	–
Ranitidine (Zantac)	75, 150, and 300 mg tablets 150 and 300 mg capsules 15 mg/mL syrup 25 mg/mL injection 25 mg effervescent	150 mg bid	150 mg bid 300 mg qhs	150–300 mg qhs	–

Table 13-41 Other Drugs for PUD: Generic and Brand Names and Dosage Form Availability

Generic Name (Brand Name)	Dosage Forms	*H. pylori* Eradication (Requires Combination Therapy)	PUD Healing	PUD Maintenance	CYP	Comments
Misoprostol (Cytotec, Athrotec)	100 and 200 mcg tablets	Not indicated	Not indicated	200 mcg qid	–	
Sucralfate (Carafate)	1 g tablets 1 g/10 mL suspension	Not indicated	1 g qid 2 g bid	1–2 g bid 1 g qid	–	1 hr before meals and bedtime
Bismuth subsalicylate (Pepto-Bismol, Kaopectate)	262 mg tablets 262 mg/5 mL suspension 525 mg/15 mL suspension	525 mg qid	Not indicated	Not indicated		

Safety and Efficacy Monitoring and Patient Education

- PPIs should be taken ½ to 1 hour prior to meals.
- Misoprostol should be taken with food to minimize the risk of GI upset and diarrhea.
- Sucralfate should be taken on an empty stomach.

Adverse Drug Reactions

Misoprostol is known to cause significant GI distress, diarrhea, and abdominal cramping.

2.2.0 Dispensing

Compounding

- Extemporaneous oral preparations: pellets from PPI capsules can be mixed in various vehicles for suspensions
- Water: esomeprazole
- Apple sauce: omeprazole, lansoprazole
- Juice: omeprazole, esomeprazole, lansoprazole
- Sodium bicarbonate 8.4%: omeprazole, lansoprazole, pantoprazol

Table 13-42 Combination Packs for PUD: Brand Names and Dosage Form Availability

Combination Pack	Type	Components	Dose	Days per Pack	Cost	Comments
Prevpac (triple regimen)	Combination package *Blister cards*	Each blister card contains: *30 mg lansoprazole—2 capsules* *500 mg clarithromycin—2 tablets* *500 mg amoxicillin—4 capsules*	1 card/day (bid)	14 days	$356	
Helidac (quadruple regimen)	Combination package *Blister cards*	Each blister card contains: *250 mg metronidazole—4 tablets* *500 mg tetracycline—4 capsules* *262.4 mg bismuth subsalicylate—8 tablets*	1 card/day (qid)	14 days	$350	Separate PPI Rx needed
Pylera (quadruple regimen)	3-in-1 capsule	1 capsule contains: *125 mg metronidazole* *125 mg tetracycline* *140 mg bismuth subcitrate potassium*	3 capsules (qid)	10 days	$350	Separate PPI Rx needed Can be used in patients with ASA allergies (no salicylates)

ANNOTATED BIBLIOGRAPHY

Berardi RR, Welage LS. Peptic ulcer disease. In: Dipiro JT, ed. *Pharmacotherapy: A Pathophysiologic Approach*. 7th ed. New York, NY: McGraw-Hill Medical; 2008:569–587.

Bhatt DL, Scheiman J, Abraham NS, Antman EM, Chan FKL, et al. ACCF/ACG/AHA 2008 expert consensus document on reducing the gastrointestinal risks of antiplatelet therapy and NSAID use: a report of the American College of Cardiology Foundation Task Force on Clinical Expert Consensus Documents. *Circulation* 2008;118. Available at: http://circ.ahajournals.org. Accessed January 13, 2010.

Chey WD, Wong BCY, et al. American College of Gastroenterology guideline on the management of *Helicobacter pylori* infection. *Am J Gastroenterology* 2007;102:1808–1825.

Hematology

CHAPTER 14

TOPIC: ANEMIA

Section Coordinator: Barb Mason
Contributor: Barb Mason

Tips Worth Tweeting

- Anemia is a decrease in hemoglobin or number of red blood cells, which results in decreased oxygen-carrying capacity of the blood, with nonspecific symptoms.
- Anemia is not a disease itself, but rather a sign of a disease whose severity and cause guide treatment.
- Consider cell size (normo, micro, macro), color (Hgb content, hypo, normo) when classifying anemia prior to treatment.
- More than one anemia can be present concurrently.
- Rule out vitamin B_{12} deficiency before treating folic acid deficiency.
- Iron salts are absorbed similarly but differ in their elemental iron percentage content.
- Treatment for anemia needs to continue until stores are replaced—that is, not just until symptoms disappear.
- Anemia of chronic disease (ACD) is not treated with iron; iron overload can result if this distinction is not recognized.

Patient Care Scenario: Ambulatory Setting

69 y/o, 5'7", F, white, 154 lbs, allergies to sulfas, two beers daily

Vitamin B_{12} deficiency, coronary artery disease, arthritis, Parkinson's disease, hypertension

Bun 15 mg/dL, Cr 1.0 mg/dL, TSH 5.30 IU/mL, vitamin B_{12} 78 pg/mL, hemoglobin 12 g/dL, hematocrit 36%, MCV 120 fL, RBC folate 300 ng/mL

Date	Physician	Drug	Quantity	Sig	Refills
1/8	Mann	Felodipine	5 mg #30	one po daily	4
1/8	Mann	Metoprolol	50 mg #30	one po daily	4
1/31	Mann	Carbidopa/levodopa	50/100 #120	one three times daily	2
10/26	Mod	Cyanocobalamin	1,000 mcg/mL 10 mL	one mL injection sq monthly	prn
10/31	Mod	Isosorbide	10 mg #90	take one tablet tid	2
10/1	Mod	Needle	26 G ½ in #4	dispensed	2
10/2	Mod	Ferrous sulfate	325 mg #30	take one tablet daily	3

8/28 discussed disposal of needles and provided sharps container

Wife administers B_{12}, patient unable to do so

1.1.0 Pharmacotherapy

Medication-Induced Causes of Anemia

Macrocytic anemias: hydroxyurea, zidovudine, colchicine, paraminosalicylic acid, alcohol, 5-FU, metformin, phenytoin, methotrexate, trimethoprim, triamterene, phenobarbital

Microcytic anemias: iron deficiency, nonsteroidal anti-inflammatory drugs

Laboratory Testing

Complete blood count (CBC) measures hemoglobin (Hgb), hematocrit (Hct), and red blood cells (RBs) and, therefore, transport of oxygen to tissue.

Mean cell hemoglobin (MCH; MCHC) detects the amount of hemoglobin in cells

- Decreased: microcytosis
- Increased: macrocytosis

Reticulocytes: young immature erythrocytes indicate new RBC production; a normal value may indicate inability of the bone marrow to respond

Serum ferritin: indicates iron storage

Serum iron level: measures amount of iron bound to transferrin

Total iron binding capacity (TIBC): measures the capacity of transferrin to bind iron

RBC Indices

Mean cell volume (MCV): detects changes in cell size

- Decreased: microcytosis (iron)
- Increased: macrocytosis (vitamin B_{12}, folic acid)

Disease States Associated with Anemia

Disease states associated with anemia include chronic infections, chronic inflammation, malignancies, congestive heart failure, and kidney disease. Pernicious anemia is caused by the absence of intrinsic factor and may occur post gastric resection. Vitamin B_{12} deficiency may be caused by inadequate intake, malabsorption, and inadequate utilization; it takes several years to develop. Folic acid deficiency may be caused by inadequate intake, decreased absorption, or hyperutilization or inadequate utilization. Folic acid deficiency can occur within 4 to 5 months of cessation of folic acid intake.

Table 14-1 Lab Interpretation of Anemia

	Vitamin B_{12}	Folic Acid	Iron Deficiency	ACD
Iron	Normal	Normal	Low	Low
Ferritin	Normal	Normal	Low	Normal or high
TIBC	Normal	Normal	High	Normal or low
MCV, MCH	High	High	Low	Normal or low

Table 14-2 Classification of Anemia

Morphology	Etiology	Pathophysiology
Macrocytic: pernicious, B_{12}, folate, megaloblastic	Deficiency	Excess blood loss
Microcytic hypochromic: iron deficiency	Central	Excess RBC destruction
Normocytic: recent blood loss, hemolysis, anemia of chronic disease	Peripheral	Inadequate RBC production

Instruments and Techniques Related to Patient Assessment

Dietary histories are needed to determine whether patients are meeting the recommended dietary allowances. Stool guaiac cards may be used to detect occult blood loss leading to iron deficiency.

Key Terms

Folic acid (folic acid–deficiency anemia)
Iron (iron–deficiency anemia)
Vitamin B_{12} (vitamin B_{12}–deficiency anemia, pernicious anemia)

Wellness and Prevention

Many persons have anemia but are unaware of that condition. Screening guidelines differ based on patient

Table 14-3 Signs and Symptoms of Anemia

Mild to Moderate Anemia	Severe Anemia	Most Severe
Asymptomatic	Tachycardia	Koilonychias
Fatigue	Palpitations	Angular stomatitis
Pallor	Angina	Glossitis
Weakness	High-output cardiac failure	Pica
Irritability	Dizziness	
Sensitivity to cold	Cheilosis	
Headache	Shortness of breath	
Loss of appetite, abnormal taste and smell		
Smooth, sore tongue		
Diarrhea or constipation		
Paresthesias, tremor		
Loss of coordination		

Table 14-4 Drugs for Anemia: Indications, Dosing, and Routes

Drug	Indications	Dosing Regimens	Routes of Administration
Iron dextran (InFed)	Iron-deficiency anemia	Cumulative 1,000 mg	IV, IM DexFerrum IV only
Iron sucrose (Venofer)	Anemia associated with chronic kidney disease	100–300 mg; cumulative dose of 1,000 mg	IV
Sodium ferric gluconate (Ferrlecit)	Anemia associated with chronic kidney disease	125 mg elemental over 1 hour; cumulative dose of 1,000 mg	IV
Ferumoxytol (Feraheme)	Iron-deficiency anemia Chronic kidney disease	510 mg IV injection, then second dose 5–8 days later	IV single-use vial 510 mg/17 ml elemental iron 30 mg/ml
Vitamin B_{12}	Nutritional vitamin B_{12} deficiency	100 mcg daily for 1 week, then 100 mcg on alternate days for 7 doses, then every 3 days for 2–3 weeks, then 100 mcg monthly for life, or 1,000 mcg/day for 1 week, then 1,000 mcg/week for 1 month	IM or deep SC or PO
	Pernicious anemia	1000 mcg daily for 1 month, 1,000 mcg/month	
Folic acid	Nutritional folate deficiency	0.4 mg day deficiency, 1 mg day, 0.8 mg/day pregnancy	PO

age. Groups at higher risk for iron deficiency include children younger than age 2 years, adolescent girls, pregnant females, and individuals older than 65 years. Folic acid intake is essential in women of childbearing age to decrease the risk of neural tube defects in their offspring. Anemia among elderly persons, though quite prevalent, is not an inevitable consequence of aging and is associated with increased risk of hospitalization, mortality, reduced quality of life, and decreased physical function. Iron-deficiency anemia is a leading cause of infant morbidity and mortality. Primary prevention is the key.

1.2.0 Pharmacotherapy

Drug Indications, Dosing Regimens, and Routes of Administration

Parenteral iron indications include malabsorption syndromes, duodenal or upper small intestine resection, inflammatory bowel disease, patients with continued blood loss in which the amount of iron lost exceeds oral replacement, inadequate response to oral iron therapy, inability to tolerate oral iron supplements, patient noncompliance with oral iron therapy (the most common cause of oral iron supplementation failure), and patients with high intake of antacids. The iron dose depends on the patient's tolerance, with the goal being 200 mg of elemental iron daily, usually in two to three divided doses.

Parenteral vitamin B_{12} indications include noncompliance with oral therapy or neurological symptoms.

Interaction of Drugs with Foods and Laboratory Tests

Food decreases iron absorption by as much as 40% to 50%. Drugs that decrease iron absorption include calcium antacids, H_2 antagonists, proton pump inhibitors, tetracycline, captopril, cefdinir, fluoroquinolones, levothyroxine, and levodopa. Eggs, milk, coffee, and tea decrease iron absorption; their consumption should be separated from iron intake by 2 hours. Iron may cause falsely elevated bilirubin levels and decreased serum calcium. Doses of dextran greater than 5 mL may give a brown color to skin.

Drugs that decrease vitamin B_{12} absorption include colchicine, para-aminosalicyclic acid, and alcohol. Hot foods can decrease intranasal vitamin B_{12} absorption, so separate dosing and hot food ingestion by 1 hour. Use of methotrexate and antibiotics can invalidate the results of a vitamin B_{12} assay.

Contraindications, Warnings, and Precautions

Folic acid and vitamin B_{12} are not substitutes for each other, but their use may improve symptoms and hematological response. Avoid folic acid and folinic acid confusion.

Unnecessary therapy with parenteral iron can cause hemosiderosis and iron overload. Iron dextran should be used cautiously in patients with asthma or history of allergies. Parenteral use of complexes of iron and carbohydrates has resulted in anaphylactic reactions, and even deaths. Iron dextran should be given only when resuscitation techniques and treatment of anaphylaxis and shock are readily available, with the infusion rate being monitored. "Black box" warnings have been applied to iron dextran and oral iron-containing products. For the oral agents, this warning is prompted by the risk of accidental overdose in children.

Physiochemical Properties, Solubility, Pharmacodynamics, and Pharmacokinetics

IM iron is absorbed into the capillaries and lymph. Circulating dextran is removed by the RES, which splits the complex into iron and dextran. Iron is bound to protein to form hemosiderin, ferritin, or transferrin. IM absorption occurs within 72 hours, with IV half-life being 5 to 20 hours. Iron absorption is highest (25–35 mg/day) during the first month, but decreases gradually (4 mg/day after 3–4 months). Iron is absorbed from the duodenum and upper jejunum by active transport. Ferrous salt is absorbed three times more readily than the ferric form.

Folic acid is completely absorbed following its administration, even in malabsorption syndromes due to the glutamate form of the drug used in therapy. Increasing the dosage does not enhance the hematologic effect, as the excess is excreted unchanged in the urine.

An intrinsic factor from parietal cells regulates vitamin B_{12} absorption in the terminal ileus. Oral supplements have 25% bioavailability. Vitamin B_{12} is stored in the liver and enters the enterohepatic circulation. In blood, it is bound to transcobalamin II. Nasally administered vitamin B_{12} is absorbed through blood vessels in the nasal passage. Nascobal needs to be protected from light.

Pharmacokinetic Dosage Calculations

Tables and formulas exist for calculating iron replacement doses. Ferrous fumarate consists of 33% iron; ferrous gluconate, 11.6%; and ferrous sulfate, 30%. Knowledge of the percentage of elemental iron present in the therapy will allow for dosage calculations.

Biopharmaceutical Principles and Pharmaceutical Characteristics of Dosage Forms

- Oral bioavailability iron absorption: 10% to 35%
- Intravenous iron absorption: 80% to 95%

If the patient has nasal congestion, defer intranasal vitamin B_{12} administration due to the erratic absorption. IV iron preps differ in their molecular size, degradation kinetics, and bioavailability.

1.3.0 Monitoring

Pharmacotherapeutic Outcomes

The goals of therapy are to correct the cause of the anemia, prevent recurrence, and replace depleted stores.

Safety and Efficacy Monitoring and Patient Education

Oral iron therapy produces reticulocytosis in 5–7 days. The reticulocyte levels return to normal in 15 days, with Hgb initially increasing at a rate of 1–2 g/dL every week, but then slowing until levels are normalized.

If the patient has an inadequate response to the therapy, reconsider the diagnosis. Also, assess the patient for noncompliance, continual blood loss, and poor absorption.

Continue iron therapy for 2–3 months after the correction of anemia to replenish stores. Monitoring iron therapy needs to continue until serum ferritin returns to normal, which may take 3–6 months.

Response to parenteral therapy does not occur any more rapidly than the response to oral iron therapy.

The rate of Hgb generation is essentially equivalent whether iron is given orally, IM, or IV.

In cases involving folic acid deficiency, with therapy Hct rises within weeks and reaches normal levels in 1–2 months; MCV will initially increase due to the increase in reticulocytes but will gradually decrease to normal. Monitor the patient's serum folate levels. Reticulocytosis should occur in 2–3 days, and RBC morphology should normalize in 24–48 hours.

It is vital to rule out vitamin B_{12} deficiency when folic acid deficiency is suspected. Vitamin B_{12} deficiency responds quickly to replacement. Reticulocytosis is evident in 2–5 days and peaks around day 7. Hgb begins to rise after the first week, and returns to normal within 2 months. CBC and vitamin B_{12} level should be assessed after 1–2 months of therapy and at 6 months. Neuropsychiatric signs and symptoms may be reversed if treated early. Neurological function can improve in 24–48 hours. If neurological dysfunction is long-standing, however, it can be irreversible. Poor response to therapy may indicate infection, uremia, and bone marrow suppression. Slow therapy response or failure to observe normalization of lab results may suggest concurrent iron deficiency or misdiagnosis. It may be necessary to continue vitamin B_{12} therapy for the rest of the patient's lifetime.

Adverse Drug Reactions

Oral iron GI tolerance improves with small doses and gradual increases. The side-effect profile, which may include nausea, abdominal cramps, diarrhea, and constipation, is related to the amount of elemental iron rather than the iron salt form. Iron can cause black stools; oral tablets may lead to drug-induced esophagitis; and liquid products can stain teeth and dentures. Parenteral iron is used if adverse reactions limit oral use.

Keep iron out of the reach of children, Accidental overdose of iron-containing products is a leading cause

Table 14-5 Drugs for Anemia: Generic Names, Brand Names, and Dosage Forms

Generic	Brand Name	Dosage Form Availability
Vitamin B_{12}	Cobolin-M, Cyomin, Depo-Cobolin	PO: 100 mcg, 500 mcg, 1,000 mcg, sublingual 1,000 mcg, 5,000 mcg Lozenge: 50 mcg, 100 mcg, 100 mcg, 250 mcg, 500 mcg Injection: 100 mcg/mL, 1,000 mcg/mL
Folic acid	Folvite, Folacin-800, FA-8	Intranasal spray: 25 mcg/ 0.1 mL, 500 mcg/0.1 mL 0.4 mg, 0.8 mg Tablets: 1 mg Injection: 5 mg/mL

of fatal poisoning in children younger than age 6. A "black box" warning applies to parenteral iron dextran.

Adverse effects from folic acid use are minimal because this compound is water soluble. Rare hypersensitivity reactions, GI effects, confusion, irritability, and sleep disturbance may occur.

Vitamin B_{12} supplementation may cause hyperuricemia, hypokalemia, rebound thrombocytosis leading to thrombotic events, and sodium retention—especially in those patients with compromised cardiovascular function due to expansion of intravascular volume secondary to an increase in RBC production.

Nonadherence, Misuse, or Abuse

Hematinics are often misused by patients for "energy" replacement. Nonadherence may occur when patients' anemia symptoms go away, but counseling needs to emphasize the importance of continued therapy to replace stores. Nonadherence to oral replacement for iron and vitamin B_{12} deficiency may justify the need for parenteral treatment.

Pharmacotherapeutic Alternatives

Ferrous sulfate, fumarate, and gluconate are all absorbed similarly.

2.2.0 Dispensing

Calculations

Rationale for oral iron dose in the treatment of iron-deficiency anemia:

$$\frac{0.25 \text{ g Hgb}}{100 \text{ mL blood}} \times 5000 \text{ ml of blood} / 70 \text{ kg} \times \frac{3.4 \text{ mg Fe}}{\text{g Hgb}} = 40 \text{ mg Fe (elemental)}$$

Because only a maximum of 20% of elemental iron is absorbed, it is necessary to give 5 times the 40 mg dose of iron to have 40 mg absorbed—that is, 200 mg elemental iron. Because ferrous sulfate is only 20% elemental iron, it is necessary to give 5 times the amount of ferrous sulfate: 1,000 mg/day or 325 mg tid.

For the dose calculation for parenteral iron, see the appendix.

Physical Attributes of Commercial Products

The IM formulation of vitamin B_{12} is red in color.

Bioequivalence

There is a potential for erratic absorption with nasal vitamin B_{12}, so it is important to monitor serum vitamin B_{12} levels when this formulation is employed. Use nasal therapy only for maintenance therapy after the patient is stabilized.

Package, Storage, Handling, and Disposal

Protect vitamin B_{12} injection products from light. Avoid freezing them.

Table 14-6 Iron Replacement Therapy: Generic Names, Brand Names, and Dosage Form Availability

Generic Name (Brand name)	Dosage Form Availability
Ferrous sulfate (Feosol)	225 mg (465 mg iron)
Ferrous sulfate, anhydrous	300 mg (60 mg iron) 240 mg (65 mg iron)
Ferrous sulfate elixir	220 mg/5 mL
Polysaccharide iron complex	150 mg iron/capsule
Ferrous gluconate (Fergon)	300 mg (37 mg iron)
Slow Fe (slow release)	Tablets, slow release 160 mg (50 mg iron) 142 mg (45 mg iron)
Fer-In-Sol drops	15 mg/mL
Fer-Gen-Sol concentrated drops	75 mg per 0.6 mL
Ferrous sulfate syrup liquid	300 mg/5 mL
Ferrous carbonyl suspension (Icar)	15 mg carbonyl per 1.25 mL
Ferrous aspartate	112 mg (18 mg elemental iron)
Ferrous fumarate	90 mg (29.5 mg elemental), 324 mg (106 mg elemental)
Ferro-Sequels	Time-release tablets 150 mg (50 mg iron)

Medication Administration Equipment

Nasal vitamin B_{12} requires pump priming. Nascobal has a safety clip, which should be discarded after the eighth dose. Discard CaloMist after 30 days. With sublingual formulations, the patient should keep the medication under the tongue for 30 seconds before swallowing it.

ANNOTATED BIBLIOGRAPHY

Hutson P. Hematology: Red and white blood cell tests. In: Lee M, ed. *Basic Skills in Interpreting Laboratory Data*. Bethesda, MD: ASHP, 2004:441–469.

Ineck B, Mason B, Lytons W. Anemia. In: Dipiro JT, Talbert TL, Yee GC, Matzke GR, Wells BG, Posey LM, eds. *Pharmacotherapy: A Pathophysiologic Approach*. 7th ed. New York, NY: McGraw Hill 2008:1639–1664.

TOPIC: ANEMIA OF CHRONIC KIDNEY DISEASE

Section Coordinator: Barb Mason
Contributor: Michelle L. Steed

Tips Worth Tweeting

- Anemia of chronic kidney disease (CKD) presents with low hemoglobin (Hgb) and hematocrit (Hct); MCV is generally low to normal.
- First-line treatment for anemia of CKD is erthyropoiesis-stimulating agents (ESAs).
- Goal Hgb levels should be maintained between 10 and 12 g/dL.
- Secondary iron deficiency (ferritin levels less than 100 ng/mL) should be replaced in combination with ESA therapy.
- Treatment of anemia reduces the cardiovascular complications of anemia and may slow progression of CKD.
- The National Kidney Foundation (NKF) provides guidelines for management of CKD.
- Anemia is the most common complication of chronic kidney disease.
- Anemia of CKD is caused by a decline in erythropoietin production by the kidneys.

Patient Care Ambulatory Setting Scenario

A. P. is a 68-year-old male diagnosed with type 2 diabetes, hypertension, hyperlipidemia, depression, hypothyroidism, diabetic nephropathy, and diabetic neuropathy.

Vitals: BP 122/70, P 58, height 5'7", weight 197.8 lbs, SpO_2 95%, R 22

Laboratory tests:

WBC 6.1×10^{-3}/mcL
RBC 4.3×10^{-6}/mcL
Hgb 7.7 g/dL
Hct 32%
Plt 198×10^{-3}/mcL
MCV 92 fL
Ferritin 20 ng/mL
SCr 2.3 mg/dL
BUN 22 mg/dL
Na 129 mEq/L
K 4.5 mEq/L
Cl 102mmol/L
CO_2 24 mmol/L
GFR < 60 mL/min

Date	Physician	Drug	Quantity	Sig	Refills
2/3	Kyle	Novolin 70/30	1	40 units bid	5
12/1	Kyle	Furosemide 20 mg	30	one 20mg q A.M.,	5
11/1	Kyle	Clonidine 0.1 mg	60	one 0.1 mg bid,	4
10/1	Kyle	Simvastatin 20 mg	30	20, mg one qhs	3
12/14	Black	Fluoxetine 40 mg qd	30	40 mg one daily	1
12/1	Kyle	Levothyroxine 125 mcg	30	one q A.M.,	2
2/3	Kyle	Gabapentin 300 mg	90	one 300 mg Tid	2
6/1	Kyle	Aspirin 81 mg	30	one daily in A.M.	5
12/1	Kyle	Potassium chloride 10 mEq	10	one 10 mEq q A.M.	5

Allergies: Atenolol (rash), penicillin (anaphylactic)

1.1.0 Patient Information

Laboratory Testing Used in Classification of Anemia of CKD

The current NKF guidelines define anemia as a hemoglobin level less than 11 g/dL. Vitamin B_{12} deficiency, folic acid deficiency, hemolysis, bleeding, and bone marrow suppression also need to be considered in the differential diagnosis. Lab test findings in anemia of CKD include decreased RBC, Hgb and Hct, serum iron, TIBC, ferritin, and erythropoietin levels.

Disease States Associated with Anemia

Uremia due to declining renal function decreases the life span of RBCs. Hemodialysis and blood loss from laboratory testing can contribute to the anemia of CKD.

Treat the patient for iron deficiency, hyperparathyroidism, infection, inflammatory disease, and hypertension as appropriate.

Signs and Symptoms

Patients with anemia of CKD may experience fatigue, decreased quality of life, cold intolerance, shortness of breath, decreased exercise capacity, left ventricular hypertrophy, congestive heart failure, and impaired mental status.

Wellness and Prevention

Evaluate CKD patients for anemia when the GFR falls below 60 mL/min or serum creatinine rises above 2 mg/dL. Dietary intake should be maintained but still may not be adequate to maintain iron stores.

1.2.0 Pharmacotherapy

Drug Indications, Dosing Regimens, and Routes of Administration

Starting doses of ESAs depends on the starting Hgb level and the target Hgb level.

- Epoetin alfa: 50–100 IU/kg three times a week
- Darbepoetin alfa: 0.45 mcg/kg every week or 0.75 mcg/kg every 2 weeks

Dose adjustments for both ESA agents (for increases and decreases) should be done every 2–4 weeks by 25% increments.

To switch between ESAs, add up the total weekly units or dose in micrograms, and use the following conversion factor: 222 IU epoetin alfa = 1 mcg darbepoetin alfa.

Contraindications, Warnings, and Precautions

Increased blood pressure occurs with use of ESAs. ESAs can lead to iron deficiency if iron stores are not adequately maintained. Iron dextran has been associated with anaphylactic reactions.

Physiochemical Properties, Pharmacodynamics, and Pharmacokinetics

Subcutaneous ESA administration produces a more predictable and sustained response than intravenous administration. Oral iron is less expensive but poor absorption usually necessitates IV iron administration.

1.3.0 Monitoring

Monitor Hgb every 1–2 weeks when ESA therapy is initiated, and then every 2–4 weeks after the goal is attained. Iron stores should be evaluated monthly if the patient is not receiving iron supplementation, and every 3 months if the patient is taking iron.

Table 14-7 Erthyropoiesis-Stimulating Agents

Agent	Class	Route of Administration*	Dosage Forms
Epoetin alfa† (Epogen, Procrit)	First generation, short acting	SQ IV	Single-dose vials (2,000, 3,000, 4,000, 10,000, or 40,000 U/mL) Multidose vials (10,000 or 20,000 U/mL)
Darbepoetin alfa† (Aranesp)	Second generation, long acting	SQ IV	Single-dose vials (25, 40, 60, 100, 150, 200, 300, or 500 mcg vials) Single-dose prefilled syringes (SingleJect) (SureClick Autoinjector) (25, 40, 60, 100, 150, 200, 300, or 500 mcg syringes)

*NKF-K/DOQI guidelines recommend the SQ method of administration, but IV administration is sometimes used for patients on dialysis as they have easy administration through the dialysis port.

†"Black box" warning: Increased mortality, serious cardiovascular events, thromboembolic events, stroke, and increased risk of tumor progression or recurrence.

Table 14-8 Oral Iron Replacement Agents

Agents	Percent Elemental Iron	Tablet Strengths Available
Ferrous sulfate—exsiccated (dried) (multiple brand names)	20	50–325 mg
Ferrous gluconate (multiple brand names)	12	50–325 mg
Ferrous fumrate (multiple brand names)	33	50–325 mg
Carbonyl iron (Feosol)	100	225 mg
Polysaccharide iron complex + ferrous bis-glycinate chelate (Niferex)	100	150 mg

1. The total daily dose for iron replacement should be 200 mg of elemental iron per day.

2. Oral replacement is generally sufficient for patients not on dialysis; for patients on dialysis, intravenous administration of iron is recommended.

3. Oral iron supplementation absorption can be enhanced by dosing ascorbic acid (250–500 mg) with each dose.

Table 14-9 Injectable Iron Replacement Agents

Agent	Strength	Administration and Dosing	Allergy Potential
Iron dextran (DexFerrum)	50 mg/mL	IV: 50 mg/min IV push; dilute in 250 mL of 0.9% normal saline	Higher allergy potential—requires a test dose for both brand names (0.5 mL test dose over 30 seconds IV push or 0.5 mL IM)
(InFed)	50 mg/mL	IV: 50 mg/min IV push or IM; dilute in 250 mL of 0.9% normal saline Dose (mL) = 0.0442 (desired Hgb − observed Hgb) × LBW + (0.26 × LBW)	
Sodium ferric gluconate (Ferrlecit)	12.5 mg /mL	IV: 12.5 mg/min IV; dilute in 100 mL of 0.9% normal saline Dose: cumulative to target dose of 1,000 mg (8 × 125 mg IV doses)	Lower allergy potential; no test dose required
Iron sucrose (Venofer)	20 mg/mL	IV: 20–50 mg/min IV; diluted in 100 mL of 0.9% normal saline Dose: cumulative repletion to target dose of 1,000 mg (various doses and frequency based on severity of CKD and type of dialysis, if any)	Lower allergy potential; no test dose is required
Ferumoxytol (Feraheme)	30 mg/mL	IV: undiluted, 30 mg /sec IV push Dose: 510 mg × 2 doses	Higher allergy potential

2.2.0 Dispensing

Iron replacement is recommended for serum ferritin levels less than 100 ng/mL in combination with ESAs.

ANNOTATED BIBLIOGRAPHY

Abboud H, Henrich WL. Clinical practice: Stage IV chronic kidney disease. *N Eng J Med* 2010;362–356.

Abu-Alfa AK. CKD series: evaluation and treatment of chronic kidney disease. *Hosp Physician* July 2003:31–38, 46.

National Kidney Foundation. KDOQI clinical practice guidelines for anemia of chronic kidney disease: update 2000. *Am J Kidney Dis* 2001;37 (suppl 1):S182–S238.

O'Mara NB. Anemia in patients with chronic kidney disease. *Diab Spectrum* 2008;21(1):13–19.

Snively CS, Gutierrez C. Chronic kidney disease: prevention and treatment of common complications. *Am Fam Physician* 2004;70:1921–1930.

Infectious Disease

CHAPTER

15

TOPIC: ANTIBIOTIC RESISTANCE

Section Coordinator: Michael Klepser
Contributor: Connie Valente

Tips Worth Tweeting

- Factors leading to antibiotic resistance include inappropriate use of antibiotics, inadequate patient education, and antimicrobial use in food-producing animals.
- Types of antibiotic resistance include intrinsic and acquired.
- Mechanisms of antibiotic resistance include enzymatic inactivation of the antibiotic, target alteration, altered permeability to the drug, development of an altered metabolic pathway, and development of an altered enzyme.
- Examples of pathogens associated with antibiotic resistance include methicillin-resistant *Staphylococcus aureus* (MRSA), vancomycin-resistant enterococcus (VRE), and penicillin-resistant *Streptococcus pneumoniae*.
- Prevention of antibiotic resistance can occur through vaccination, appropriate infection diagnosis and treatment, transmission prevention, patient education, and antibiotic guideline development.

Key Terms

Antibiotic resistance: The ability of bacteria to grow in the presence of an antibiotic that would normally cause inhibition of cell growth or cell death.

Factors Leading to Antibiotic Resistance

- Inappropriate use of antibiotics
  - Treatment of nonbacterial or undiagnosed infections
  - Inappropriate use of broad-spectrum antibiotics for unknown infections
  - Inappropriate use of antimicrobial prophylaxis
- Hospitals
  - Overuse of antibiotics among inpatients, which spreads highly resistant bacteria
- Inadequate patient education
  - Self-medication
  - Lack of patient compliance—do not complete regimen or forget doses, which leads to selection of more resistant bacteria that were not initially inhibited by the antibiotic
- Antimicrobial use in food-producing animals for disease control and growth promotion

Types of Antibiotic Resistance

Intrinsic Resistance

- Natural
- The organism is inherently resistant to the antibiotic
- Does not require previous antibiotic exposure

- Example: the use of vancomycin, a cell-wall synthesis inhibitor, for treatment of *E. coli* infection; *E. coli* is a gram-negative bacterium
  - Gram-negative bacteria have a membrane covering their cell walls, creating a barrier to antibiotic permeability

Acquired Resistance

- Requires previous antibiotic exposure
- A microorganism that was once susceptible to a drug changes and becomes less susceptible or resistant
- Occurs through genetic mechanisms
  - Mutation
  - Gene transfer
    - Transformation: Bacterial uptake of genetic material from the external environment
    - Transduction: Extrachromosomal DNA is enclosed in a plasmid and transferred between bacteria by a bacteriophage
    - Conjugation: Genetic material located in a plasmid is transferred between cells by direct contact

Mechanisms of Antibiotic Resistance

Enzymatic Inactivation That Destroys the Antibiotic

- Beta-lactamases
  - Cleave the amide bond of the beta-lactam ring
  - Constitutively produced: *Bacteroides, Acinetobacter*
  - Inducible: *Enterobacter, Citrobacter, Pseudomonas*
    - Extended-spectrum beta-lactamases
      - Can destroy all beta-lactams except cephamycins
      - Most common in *Klebsiella pneumoniae* and *Escherichi coli*
      - Beta-lactamase inhibitors will halt the spread of these bacteria
      - Genes are found on plasmids
    - AmpC beta-lactamases
      - Resistant to beta-lactamase inhibitors
      - Found in *K. pneumonia, C. freundii, M. morganii, S. marcescens,* and *P. aeruginosa*
      - Genes are found on chromosomes—inducible
  - Treatment strategies
    - Larger doses of beta-lactams
    - Carbapenems
    - Beta-lactamase inhibitors: Tazobactam, clavulanate, sulbactam
- Aminoglycoside-modifying enzymes
  - Modification blocks the entry of the drug into the cell
  - Acetylation, phosphorylation, and adenylation
  - Enterococci with high-level resistance
- Chloramphenicol acetyl transferase
- Erythromycin esterase

Target Alteration

- Altered penicillin-binding proteins (PBP): Penicillin resistance in *Streptococcus pneumoniae* and enterococci
- Altered ribosomal binding sites: Erythromycin-resistant organisms with altered 50S ribosomal protein
- Altered cell-wall precursors: Enterococcal resistance to vancomycin due to decreased affinity
- Alterations in DNA gyrase: *Pseudomonas aeruginosa* resistance to ciprofloxacin
- Altered amount of drug receptor: Some bacteria can increase or decrease synthesis of dihydrofolate reductase so to overcome and become resistant to trimethoprim

Altered Permeability to the Drug Through Bacterial Cell Membranes

- Efflux pumps: Active efflux systems
  - Primary mechanism for resistance to tetracyclines
  - Example: *E. coli* resistance to tetracyclines and fluoroquinolones
- Change in quantity or size of porin channels: Decreased transport of the drug into the cell
- Changes in transport proteins

Development of an Altered Metabolic Pathway

- Allows bacteria to bypass the reaction that the antibiotic inhibits
- Example: Sulfonamide-resistant bacteria use preformed folic acid instead of PABA

Development of an Altered Enzyme That Can Still Function and Is Less Affected by the Antibiotic

- Example: Trimethoprim-resistant bacteria develop a dihydrofolic acid reductase enzyme that is less affected by trimethoprim

Examples of Pathogens Associated with Antibiotic Resistance:

- Methicillin-resistant *Staphylococcus aureus* (MRSA)
  - Hospital-acquired MRSA (HA-MRSA): Most common

- Community-acquired MRSA (CA-MRSA): Occurring with increasing frequency, especially in IV drug users
- The mechanism of resistance is the production of an altered PBP
- Drug of choice: IV vancomycin
- Trimethoprim-sulfamethoxazole (TMP/SMX) or minocycline can be used in sensitive strains
- Other treatment options: Linezolid, daptomycin
- Vancomycin-intermediate-susceptibility (VISA) and -resistant (VRSA) organisms have been isolated
    - TMP/SMX is a treatment option

- Vancomycin-resistant enterococcus (VRE)
    - Has become common in Europe and North America
    - Enterococcus has intrinsic resistance to penicillin, ampicillin, and low-level aminoglycoside resistance
    - Enterococcus also has acquired resistance to beta-lactams through altered PBPs; fluoroquinolones; macrolides; tetracyclines; and high-level aminoglycoside resistance through aminoglycoside-modifying enzymes
    - Shows two types of resistance to vancomycin
        - Acquired: *E. faecalis* and *E. faecium*
        - Intrinsic: Seen in more uncommon strains
    - Mechanism of resistance: Alterations in the D-ala-D-ala linkages in the cell-wall precursors
    - Treatment options:
        - Linezolid, daptomycin, streptogramins
- Penicillin-resistant *Streptococcus pneumoniae*
    - *S. pneumoniae* was consistently susceptible to penicillin until 1963
    - Approximately 5–10% of pneumococci are resistant to penicillin in the United States
    - Resistant strains are commonly found in children younger than age 6 years
    - A result of overuse, resulting in selection for resistant organisms
    - Mechanism of resistance: Altered PBPs
    - Pneumococci have been frequently found resistant to (TMP-SMX) and have developed resistance to tetracyclines and macrolides
    - Treatment options:
        - High-dose IV penicillin, extended-spectrum cephalosporins, carbapenems
        - Prevention of infection with vaccination

Prevention of the Spread of Antibiotic Resistance

- Vaccination: Pneumococcal vaccine, annual influenza vaccine
- Diagnose and treat infection appropriately, by targeting the pathogen
    - Culture and sensitivity
    - Use the narrowest-spectrum antibiotic based on susceptibility results
- Proper use of antimicrobials
    - Prescriber education
    - Knowledge of local susceptibility data
    - Stop treatment:
        - When the infection is cured
        - When cultures are negative
        - When infection is not diagnosed
- Prevent transmission
    - Isolation of the pathogen
    - Infection control precautions
    - Hand washing
- Patient education
    - Compliance with medication
    - Finish antibiotic therapy
- Develop guidelines for the appropriate use of antibiotics

ANNOTATED BIBLIOGRAPHY

12 steps to prevent antimicrobial resistance among hospitalized adults. Available at: http://www.cdc.gov/drugresistance/healthcare/ha/12steps_HA.htm. Accessed February 21, 2010.

Antimicrobial (drug) resistance. Available at: http://www3.niaid.nih.gov/topics/antimicrobialResistance/. Accessed February 21, 2010.

Bacterial resistance to antibiotics. Available at: http://www.textbookofbacteriology.net/resantimicrobial_2.html. Accessed February 21, 2010.

Brooks GF, Butel JS, Morse SA. Antimicrobial chemotherapy. In Brooks GF, Butel JS, Morse SA, eds. *Jawetz, Melnick, and Adelberg's Medical Microbiology,* 24th ed. Available at: http://0-www.accesspharmacy.com.libcat.ferris.edu/content.aspx?aID=2756055.

Chambers HF, Deck DH. Beta-lactam and other cell wall- and membrane-active antibiotics. In Katzung BG, Masters SB, Trevor AJ, eds. *Basic and Clinical Pharmacology,* 11th ed. Available at: http://0-www.accesspharmacy.com.libcat.ferris.edu/content.aspx?aID=4510232.

Gold HS, Moellering RC. Antimicrobial-drug resistance. *New Engl J Med.* 1996;335(19):1445–1453.

Scholar EM, Pratt WB. *The Antimicrobial Drugs,* 2nd ed. New York: Oxford University Press; 2000.

World Health Organization. Antimicrobial resistance. Available at: http://www.who.int/mediacentre/factsheets/fs194/en/. Accessed February 21, 2010.

TOPIC: ANTIVIRALS

Section Coordinator: Michael Klepser
Contributors: Greg Hall and Amber Norris

Tips Worth Tweeting

- There are five types of hepatitis: A, B, C, D, and E.
- Antiviral therapy is typically used in the treatment of hepatitis B and C.
- Hepatitis C is the most common cause of chronic infections. Hepatitis B is less prone to causing chronic infections, and hepatitis D can cause chronic infections only in the presence of hepatitis B.
- Ganciclovir is a potentially carcinogenic and mutagenic agent; it should be handled using proper procedures for chemotherapy handling and disposal.
- Pegylated interferon-alfa has a longer half-life because polyethylene glycol (PEG) slows metabolism.
- Monitoring for interferon-alpha 2b includes depression and suicidal ideation.
- The adamantines are not active against influenza B.
- Oseltamivir capsules can be opened and mixed with liquids.
- Acyclovir topical should be dosed at 0.5 inch for every 4 square inches of surface area per application.
- Cytomegalovirus (CMV) can cause birth defects and illness in healthy and immunocompromised individuals; first-line treatment for this infection includes ganciclovir and valganciclovir.
- Influenza comes in two types, A and B. Vaccination is key to prevention of this infection.
- Influenza treatment includes adamantines and neuraminidase inhibitors.
- The herpes family of viruses includes herpes simplex virus 1 (HSV-1; cold sores), herpes simplex virus 2 (HSV-2; genital herpes), varicella zoster (shingles and chickenpox), CMV, and the Epstein-Barr virus (EBV; mononucleosis).
- Treatment and suppressive therapy do not eradicate the virus but rather suppress and reduce the severity of viral infection.
- Antiviral agents include acyclovir, valacyclovir, famcicyclovir, penciclovir, and docosanol.

Patient Care Scenario: Ambulatory Setting

A 34 y/o M, 5'10" patient presents to the pharmacy with complaints of extreme fatigue, weakness, dark urine and abdominal pain. You also notice he is slightly jaundiced. Upon further investigation, you find the patient has a history of IV drug abuse. You refer him to the hospital right away because you suspect he is suffering from a viral infection.

Hepatitis

Key Terms

There are five types of hepatitis: A, B, C, D, and E. Types A and E are transmitted through fecal–oral contamination and tend not to cause chronic infections. In contrast, types B, C, and D are spread through contaminated blood and can cause chronic infections. Hepatitis C is the most common cause of chronic infections, while hepatitis B is less prone to causing chronic infections and hepatitis D can cause chronic infections only in the presence of hepatitis B. Antiviral therapy is typically used in the treatment of hepatitis B and C.

Hepatitis B

1.1.0 Patient Information

Hepatitis B is caused by the hepatitis B virus (HBV) and causes inflammation of the liver.

Signs and Symptoms

In acute infections, HBV causes liver inflammation, jaundice, vomiting, and possibly death. Chronic infections may develop from HBV that can result in cirrhosis and liver cancer.

Disease States Associated with Hepatitis B

An individual can become infected with HBV by exposure to infected blood or body fluids.

Prevention and Wellness

A hepatitis B vaccine is available to prevent infection with HBV.

1.2.0 Pharmacotherapy

Treatment is not needed in most acutely infected patients. Pharmaceutical treatment is needed in chronic disease and in immunocompromised individuals. The immune modulators interferon-alpha 2b and pegylated interferon-alpha 2a and the antivirals adefovir, entecavir, lamivudine, tenofovir, and telbivudine can be used to treat chronic infections caused by HBV.

Hepatitis C

1.1.0 Patient Information

Hepatitis C virus (HCV) is the most common bloodborne pathogen. It causes approximately 10,000 deaths per year.

Signs and Symptoms

Acute infection may present with fatigue, jaundice, dark urine, weakness, anorexia, and abdominal pain in approximately one-third of infected adults. Persistent fatigue is the most common symptom of a chronic infection. Nearly 85% of patients will go on to develop chronic HCV infections. As many as 5–20% of chronically infected patients may progress to cirrhosis.

Disease States Associated with Hepatitis C

The biggest risk factor for acquiring HCV is IV drug use, while sexual transmission is possible but not a major risk factor.

1.2.0 Pharmacotherapy

Treatment usually involves a combination of Peginterferon-alfa 2a or 2b or interferon-alpha 2b and ribavirin.

Table 15-1 Adefovir Dipivoxil

Brand name: Hepsera
Generic: No
Supplied: 10 mg tabs
Indication: Chronic hepatitis B
Mechanism of action: HBV DNA polymerase inhibitor
Drug/lab/food interactions: Tenofovir; renally eliminated drugs may increase concentration
Contraindications: Hypersensitivity to adefovir or any component of product
Pharmacokinetics:
• Half-life: 7.5 hours
• Bioavailability: 59%
• Metabolism: Rapidly metabolized to active metabolite
• Excretion: 45% found in urine; glomerular filtration and active tubular secretion
• Protein binding: 4% or less
Adverse effects:
• Common: Asthenia, elevated serum creatinine
• Serious: Hypophosphatemia, lactic acidosis, pancreatitis, elevated ALT, hepatomegaly with steatosis, renal failure
Safety/monitoring:
• Symptomatic improvement
• ALT
• Hepatic function during therapy and repeatedly for several months after therapy
• HBV DNA
• HBeAg, HBsAg
• Renal function
• Symptoms of lactic acidosis or severe hepatomegaly with steatosis
Administration: Take with or without food

Contraindications, Precautions, and Warnings

Contraindications to this combination therapy include autoimmune hepatitis, pregnant female or male with a pregnant partner, CrCl less than 50 mL/min, hemoglobinopathies, hemodialysis, and ischemic heart disease or cerebrovascular disease.

Cytomegalovirus

1.1.0 Patient Information

Part of the herpes family, CMV can be latent or lytic and causes disease characterized by the production of enlarged cells.

Table 15-2 Entecavir

Brand name: Baraclude
Generic: No
Supplied: 0.05 mg/mL oral solution, 0.5 mg and 1 mg tabs
Indication: Chronic hepatitis B
Mechanism: HBV DNA polymerase inhibitor
Drug/lab/food interactions: Renally eliminated drugs may increase concentrations; food delays absorption and decreases concentration
Contraindications: None known
Pharmacokinetics:
• Half-life: 128–149 hours
• Bioavailability: 100%
• Metabolism: Not a substrate or inhibitor of CYP450 system
• Excretion: 62–73% unchanged
• Protein binding: 13%
Adverse effects:
• Common: Nausea, dizziness, headache, fatigue
• Serious: Lactic acidosis, severe hepatomegaly with steatosis, anaphylaxis
Safety/monitoring:
• ALT/hepatic function during therapy and repeatedly for several months after therapy
• HBV DNA
• HBeAg, HBsAg
• Renal function
• Symptoms of lactic acidosis or severe hepatomegaly with steatosis
Administration:
• Take at least 2 hours after a meal and 2 hours before the next meal.
• Do not dilute the solution.
• Use the calibrated dosing spoon supplied with the medication, and rinse the spoon with water after each dose.

Table 15-3 Lamivudine

Brand name: Epivir
Generic: No
Supplied: 5 mg/mL or 10 mg/mL oral solution; 100 mg, 150 mg, and 300 mg tabs
Indications: HIV, chronic hepatitis B
Mechanism of action: Nucleoside reverse transcriptase inhibitor (NRTI)
Drug/lab/food interactions: Interferon-alpha, ribavirin, zalcitabine
Contraindications: Hypersensitivity to lamivudine or any component of lamivudine product
Pharmacokinetics: • Half-life: Children: 2 hours; adults: 5–7 hours • Bioavailability: Children: 66%; adults: 88% • Metabolism: Approximately 5% • Excretion: Primarily urine • Protein binding: 36% or less
Adverse effects: • Common: Lipodystrophy, decreased appetite, nausea, headache, fatigue • Serious: Lactic acidosis, pancreatitis, hepatomegaly
Safety/monitoring: • ALT • Liver function in patients coinfected with HIV • Several months after discontinuation • HBV DNA • HBeAg, HBsAg • Symptoms of lactic acidosis • Pancreatic panel (in patients with history of pancreatitis)
Administration: Take with or without food

Signs and Symptoms

Cytomegalovirus is an important human pathogen that can cause birth defects in newborns and a wide variety of illnesses in both healthy and immunocompromised older children and adults. CMV causes systemic infections that can result in mononucleosis-like illness, retinitis, colitis, and esophagitis. Infants, immunosuppressed individuals, and organ transplant patients are at higher risk for contracting the virus. Transmission of the virus requires close human-to-human contact; the virus can be shed in urine, semen, saliva, breastmilk, and cervical secretions and is carried in circulating white blood cells.

1.2.0 Pharmacotherapy

Treatment of CMV infection involves antiviral agents, including ganciclovir and valganciclovir as first-line choices, and foscarnet and cidofovir as second-line therapies.

Table 15-4 Tenofovir Disoproxil Fumarate

Brand name: Viread
Generic: No
Supplied: 300 mg tabs
Indications: HIV, chronic hepatitis B
Mechanism of action: Reverse transcriptase inhibitor
Drug/lab/food interactions: Adefovir, didanosine, atazanavir (increase concentrations)
Contraindications: None known
Pharmacokinetics: • Half-life: 17 hours • Bioavailability: 25% (fasting); increases by 40% with food • Metabolism: Not a CYP substrate; converted by hydrolysis to tenofovir, then phosphorylated to active tenofovir diphosphate • Excretion: 70–80% unchanged via glomerular filtration and active tubular secretion • Protein binding: 7%
Adverse effects: • Common: Rash, diarrhea, flatulence, nausea, vomiting, asthenia • Serious: Lactic acidosis, hepatomegaly with steatosis, hypersensitivity, osteopenia, acute renal failure, renal impairment
Safety/monitoring: • ALT • HBV DNA • HBeAg, HBsAg • During treatment and for at least several months after discontinuing therapy • Symptomatic improvement and quality of life • Hepatic function for at least several months after therapy is discontinued; renal function at baseline and at appropriate intervals during therapy • Bone mineral density in patients with a history of pathologic bone fracture or risk for osteopenia
Administration: Take orally with or without food

Influenza

1.1.0 Patient Information

The influenza virus causes thousands of deaths each year in the United States, and approximately 500,000 deaths worldwide each year. The young and the elderly are the most susceptible to mortality from these infections. Two types of influenza affect humans: Type A and Type B. Type A is usually responsible for the seasonal influenza and pandemics, whereas Type B is responsible for more random outbreaks. Type A is categorized by two surface antigens: hemagglutinin and neuraminidase. Hemagglutinin allows entry of the virus into host cells, and neuraminidase allows the virus to break out of the host cell.

Signs and Symptoms

Signs and symptoms of influenza include fever, myalgias, malaise, headache, runny nose, and sore throat, as well as nausea and vomiting.

Prevention and Wellness

Vaccination is used to prevent the infection.

1.2.0 Pharmacotherapy

Two classes of antiviral agents are used to prevent against and treat influenza: adamantines, which include amantadine and rimantadine, and neuraminidase inhibitors, which include oseltamavir and zanamavir.

Table 15-5 Telbivudine

Brand name: Tyzeka
Generic: No
Supplied: 600 mg oral tabs
Indication: Chronic hepatitis B
Mechanism of action: Inhibits HBV DNA polymerase
Drug/lab/food interactions: None
Contraindications: Previous hypersensitivity to telbivudine
Pharmacokinetics: • Half-life: 40–49 hours • Bioavailability: 52% • Metabolism: None • Excretion: 42% unchanged • Protein binding: 3.3%
Adverse effects: • Common: Headache, cough, fatigue • Serious: Lactic acidosis, hepatomegaly with steatosis, rhabdomyolysis
Safety/monitoring: • Clinical response to therapy (ALT, HBeAg, HBV DNA, HBsAg) • Creatinine kinase • Symptoms of myopathy • Symptoms of lactic acidosis; evaluate regularly during treatment • Exacerbation of hepatitis at least several months after discontinuing treatment • Liver function • Renal function • Peripheral neuropathy symptoms • Routine complete physical exam (weight, temperature, energy levels, appetite)
Administration: May be taken with or without food

Table 15-6 Peginterferon-Alfa 2b

Brand name: PEG-Intron
Generic: No
Supplied: 50 mcg, 80 mcg, 120 mcg, and 150 mcg kit
Indications: Chronic hepatitis C; can be used in combination with ribavirin
Mechanism of action: Pegylated interferon-alfa has a longer half-life than regular interferon-alpha; immunomodulator; enhances phagocyte and lymphocyte activity
Drug/lab/food interactions: Theophylline (increase in theophylline conc.), myelosuppressive agents
Contraindications: Must not be used in combination with ribavirin in pregnant women; men with pregnant partners; and patients with autoimmune hepatitis, hemoglobinopathies, CrCl less than 50 mL/min, hemodialysis, or ischemic heart disease or cerebrovascular disease
Pharmacokinetics: • Half-life: 40 hours • Metabolism: PEG conjugation slows metabolism • Excretion: Urine—30%
Adverse effects: • Common: Alopecia, dry skin, injection-site reaction, hyperuricemia, abdominal pain, decreased appetite, diarrhea, nausea, vomiting, weight loss, arthralgia, myalgia, dizziness, headache, insomnia, reduced concentration pharyngitis, fatigue, fever, rigor • Serious: Colitis, pancreatitis, autoimmune thrombocytopenia, blindness, thrombosis of retinal vein, aggressive behavior, depression, homicidal/suicidal thoughts
Safety/monitoring: • Evidence of depression and other psychiatric symptoms • CBC, including platelets; baseline and at week 2 and week 4 of therapy or more frequently if clinically indicated • ECG, prior to concomitant treatment with ribavirin, in patients with preexisting cardiac disease • Blood chemistry, including ALT, AST, bilirubin, and uric acid; baseline and during therapy • Hepatic function and signs of liver toxicity • Renal function and signs of toxicity, in patients with renal impairment • Triglyceride levels • Blood glucose, serum amylase, and thyroid function • Ophthalmologic exams; baseline for all patients, and then during therapy for patients with preexisting ophthalmologic disorders • Pregnancy tests, during therapy and 6 months after therapy • Pulmonary function tests • Signs and symptoms of colitis and pancreatitis

(*continues*)

Table 15-6 (*continued*)

Administration: • Pen: To reconstitute, hold the pen upright and press the two halves together until they click. Gently invert the pen to mix the agents, but do not shake it, and use immediately. Keeping the pen upright, attach the supplied needle. To select the dose, pull back on the dosing button until the dark bands are visible and turn the button until the dark band is aligned with the correct dose. The pen is for single use only and cannot be stored for more than 24 hours at 2–8°C; discard any unused portion. • Vials: Reconstitute with 0.7 mL of supplied diluent only and swirl gently, then use immediately. Do not add other medications or diluents to the solution. The vials are intended for single use only and cannot be stored for more than 24 hours at –8°C; discard any unused diluent and solution.

The adamantines are not active against influenza B, and high levels of resistance have been shown to these drugs. Thus the neuraminidase inhibitors are the drugs of choice for influenza.

Herpes Viruses

1.1.0 Patient Information

The herpes family of viruses includes many members that infect humans, including herpes simplex virus types 1 (HSV-1; cold sores) and 2 (HSV-2; genital herpes). Varicella zoster (shingles and chickenpox), CMV, and the Epstein-Barr virus (mononucleosis) are also included in the herpes family. These viruses can be lytic or latent and often cause recurrent infections.

Table 15-7 Interferon-Alpha 2b

Brand name: Intron-A
Generic: No
Supplied: 3, 5, 10, 18, 25, and 50 million unit powder for injection solution
Indications: Chronic hepatitis B and hepatitis C
Mechanism of action: Immunomodulator; enhances lymphocyte and phagocyte activity
Drug/food/lab interactions: Aldesleukin (increased risk of renal and myocardial toxicity), ribavirin, theophylline derivatives, zidovudine (decreased metabolism)
Contraindications: Hypersensitivity to interferon-alfa or any component of the formulation; decompensated liver disease; autoimmune hepatitis
Pharmacokinetics: • Half-life: 2–3 hours (IV, IM, SubQ) • Bioavailability: IM: 83%; SubQ: 90% • Metabolism: Primarily renal
Adverse effects: • Common: Infusion-related effects (fever, chills myalgia), alopecia, rash, nausea and vomiting, fatigue, headache, neutropenia, dizziness, depression, dry mouth • Serious: Cardiomyopathy, vasculitis, erythema multiforme, injection-site necrosis, Stevens-Johnson syndrome, toxic epidermal necrolysis, hypertriglyceridemia, thrombocytopenia, hepatotoxicity, myositis, rhabdomyolysis, cerebrovascular accident, optic disc edema, optic neuritis, retinal hemorrhage, retinopathy, thrombosis of retinal artery, thrombosis of retinal vein, hearing loss, suicidal ideation (less than 5%), pneumonia, pneumonitis, pulmonary infiltrate
Safety/monitoring: • Evidence of depression and other psychiatric symptoms • CBC, including platelets; baseline and at week 2 and week 4 of therapy or more frequently if clinically indicated • ECG, prior to concomitant treatment with ribavirin, in patients with preexisting cardiac disease • Blood chemistry, including ALT, AST, bilirubin, and uric acid; baseline and during therapy • Hepatic function and signs of liver toxicity • Renal function and signs of toxicity in patients with renal impairment • Triglyceride levels • Blood glucose, serum amylase, and thyroid function • Ophthalmologic exams; baseline for all patients, and during therapy for patients with preexisting ophthalmologic disorders • Pregnancy tests, during therapy and 6 months after therapy • Pulmonary function tests • Signs and symptoms of colitis and pancreatitis

Table 15-7 (*continued*)

Administration: Dosage forms and strengths are indication specific and are not interchangeable. Administer injections in the evening if possible to enhance tolerability. Acetaminophen may be administered at the time of injection to reduce the incidence of certain adverse reactions.
• Powder for injection: Reconstitute with sterile water for injection and use immediately; discard any unused portion; for IM, SubQ, IV, or intralesional use
• Solution for injection: Do not dilute; not recommended for IV use
• Multidose pen solution: For SubQ use only

Table 15-8 Peginterferon-Alfa 2a

Brand name: Pegasys
Generic: No
Supplied: 180 mcg/mL and 180 mcg/0.5 mL kits
Indications: Chronic hepatitis B and hepatitis C
Mechanism of action: Pegylated interferon-alfa has a longer half-life; immunomodulator; enhances phagocyte and lymphocyte activity
Drug/lab/food interactions: Transient increase in ALT; decreased WBC, ANC, and platelets; abnormal thyroid lab values; increased theophylline levels
Contraindications: Autoimmune hepatitis, decompensated liver disease, use in neonates and infants (contains benzyl alcohol)
Pharmacokinetics:
• Half-life: 80 hours
• Metabolism: PEG slows metabolism compared to interferon-alfa; inhibits CYP1A2
Adverse effects:
• Common: Alopecia, dermatitis, dry skin, injection-site inflammation/reaction, weight loss, abdominal pain, diarrhea, appetite loss, nausea and vomiting, thrombocytopenia, arthralgia, myalgia, dizziness, headache, insomnia, decreased concentration, anxiety, irritability, cough, dyspnea, fatigue, fever, influenza-like symptoms
• Serious: Angina, dysrhythmias, Stevens-Johnson syndrome, diabetes mellitus, colitis, gastrointestinal hemorrhage, pancreatitis, peptic ulcer disease, anemia, severe cytopenia, cholangitis, liver failure/steatosis, severe hypersensitivity reaction, cerebral hemorrhage/ischemia, peripheral neuropathy, corneal ulcer, aggressive behavior, depression, psychotic disorder
Safety/monitoring:
• Symptomatic improvement
• CBC with differential
• Blood pressure
• ECG
• Hepatic function
• Pulmonary function
• Renal function
• Thyroid-stimulating hormone (TSH), every 12 weeks
• Blood glucose
• Uric acid
• Serum amylase
• Serum triglyceride
• Hematological tests (at 2 weeks and 4 weeks) and biochemical tests (at 4 weeks)
• Evidence of neuropsychiatric reactions, such as depression or suicidal ideation
• Ophthalmologic exams; baseline for all patients and during therapy for patients with preexisting ophthalmologic disorders
• Pregnancy test; monthly during combination therapy with ribavirin and for 6 weeks after therapy
Administration:
• When used in combination with ribavirin, administer ribavirin orally with food.
• Administer as a subcutaneous injection in the thigh or abdomen, on the same day of the week at about the same time.

Table 15-9 Ribavirin

Brand names: Rebetol, Ribasphere, Virazole, Copegus, RibaPak, RibaTab
Generic: Yes
Supplied: 200 mg capsules; 200 mg, 400 mg, and 600 mg tabs; 40 mg/mL oral solution; 6 g inhalation powder for solution
Indications: Chronic hepatitis C infections (in combination with peginterferon-alfa 2b)
Mechanism of action: Unknown; may act as a competitive inhibitor for viral enzymes
Drug/food/lab interactions: Didanosine (increases toxicity), decreases effects of stavudine and zidovudine
Contraindications (when used in combination with peginterferon-alfa 2b): Autoimmune hepatitis, pregnant female or male with a pregnant partner, CrCl less than 50 mL/min, hemoglobinopathies, hemodialysis, patients with ischemic heart disease or cerebrovascular disease
Pharmacokinetics:
• Half-life: Oral: 298 hours; inhalation: 9.5 hours
• Bioavailability: 64%; increases with consumption of a high-fat meal
• Metabolism: Hepatic
• Excretion: Urine
• Protein binding: None
Adverse effects:
• Common: Pruritus, rash, indigestion, loss of appetite, nausea, headache, fatigue
• Serious: Bradyarrhythmia, cardiac arrest, hypotension, pancreatitis, hemolytic anemia, hepatotoxicity, hyperammonemia, hyperbilirubinemia, suicidal ideation, respiratory complications
Safety/monitoring:
• Virologic response (hepatitis C RNA levels) after 12 and 24 weeks of therapy
• Improvement in hepatic function tests and signs and symptoms
• CBC with differential (Hgb or Hct at weeks 2 and 4, or more frequently if clinically warranted) prior to initiating therapy, then periodically
• Biochemical test before initiation, at week 4, and periodically
• Pregnancy test before initiating therapy, on a monthly basis during therapy, and for 6 months after discontinuation
• Liver function tests before initiating therapy and periodically thereafter
• TSH test before initiating therapy and periodically thereafter
• ECG in patients with preexisting heart disease, prior to initiating therapy and periodically thereafter
• Eye exam at baseline in all patients, and periodically during therapy in patients with preexisting ophthalmologic disorders
• Respiratory function during inhalation therapy
• Fluid status during inhalation therapy
Administration:
• Minimize exposure to pregnant women.
• To reconstitute the powder for inhalation, mix with a minimum of 75 mL sterile water for injection or inhalation (preservative-free) in the original vial and shake well; transfer to a 500-mL SPAG-2 reservoir and further dilute to a final volume of 300 mL with sterile water for injection or inhalation (preservative-free) to a concentration of 20 mg/mL. Administer with a SPAG-2 small particle aerosol generator only. Do not mix with other medications.
• Inspect the solution for particles and discoloration before administration. Discard the solution in the SPAG-2 unit at least every 24 hours.
• Take the oral formulation with food. Capsules should not be opened, crushed, or broken.

1.2.0 Pharmacotherapy

Treatment and suppressive therapy of herpes viral infections are achieved with several antiviral agents, including acyclovir and valacyclovir, famciclovir, penciclovir, and docosanol. These treatments do not kill or eradicate the virus, but rather suppress the virus and reduce the severity and number of breakouts.

Table 15-10 Valganciclovir

Brand name: Valcyte
Generic: No
Supplied: 50 mg/mL powder for solution, 450 mg oral tabs
Indications: CMV retinitis treatment; CMV prophylaxis in kidney, heart, or pancreas transplant patients
Mechanism of action: Inhibits viral DNA polymerase
Drug/food/lab interactions: Didanosine (increases didanosine concentration and toxicity); food increases absorption
Contraindications: Hypersensitivity to valganciclovir, ganciclovir, or any component of product
Pharmacokinetics:
• Half-life: 4–7 hours; increases with renal impairment
• Bioavailability: 60% with food
• Metabolism: Converted to ganciclovir by intestinal mucosal cells and hepatocytes
• Excretion: Urine (as ganciclovir)
• Protein binding: 1–2%
Adverse effects:
• Common: Diarrhea, nausea, vomiting, anemia, neutropenia, thrombocytopenia, tremor, cough, upper respiratory infection, fever
Safety/monitoring:
• Improvement in signs and symptoms
• Ophthalmic follow-up exams at least every 4–6 weeks during treatment
• CBC with differential and platelet counts frequently, especially in patients with a history of leukopenia or neutrophil counts less than 1,000 cells/mcL at treatment initiation; more frequently if oral ganciclovir is switched to valganciclovir
• Renal function in elderly patients and patients with impaired renal function
Administration:
• Do not substitute for ganciclovir capsules on a one-to-one basis because oral doses of valganciclovir produce a much higher bioavailability of the active ganciclovir than the ganciclovir capsules do.
• This drug is potentially carcinogenic and mutagenic; it should be handled using proper procedures for chemotherapy handling and disposal. Avoid direct contact of broken or crushed tablets with the skin or mucous membranes.
• Take this medication with food.
• Do not break or crush tablets.
• The solution is not recommended for use in adult patients.

Table 15-11 Ganciclovir

Brand names: Cytovene, Vitrasert, Zirgan
Generic: Yes
Supplied: 250 mg and 500 mg capsules, 4.5 mg intraocular implant
Indications: CMV retinitis treatment, CMV prophylaxis in transplant patients
Mechanism of action: Inhibits viral DNA polymerase
Drug/food/lab interactions: Imipenem, lamivudine, didanosine
Contraindications: Hypersensitivity to ganciclovir or acyclovir
Pharmacokinetics:
• Half-life: 2–6 hours
• Bioavailability: 5%; increases with food; increases to 30% with consumption of a high-fat meal
• Metabolism: Minimal
• Excretion: 80–99% unchanged in feces and urine
• Protein binding: 1–2%

(*continues*)

Table 15-11 (*continued*)

Adverse effects:
• Common: Pruritus, sweating, diarrhea, loss of appetite, vomiting, anemia, neutropenia, thrombocytopenia, neuropathy, blurred vision, eye irritation, elevated serum creatinine, fever, shivering
• Serious: Cardiac arrest, torsades de pointes, Stevens-Johnson syndrome, gastrointestinal perforation, pancreatitis, liver failure, anaphylaxis, rhabdomyolysis, cerebrovascular accident, renal failure
Safety/monitoring:
• CBC with differential; twice a week during induction and once a week after that, especially in patients with a history of leukopenia and in those with neutrophil counts less than 1,000 cells/mcL at the beginning of treatment
• Renal function; twice a week during induction of therapy and once a week after that especially in patients with impaired renal function
• Serum electrolytes; twice a week during induction and once a week after that
• Herpes simplex keratitis: Efficacy is apparent by the resolution of ulcers
• CMV retinitis: Ophthalmic exams immediately before initiation of therapy, at the end of induction (or reinduction) therapy, and monthly after that; more frequent follow-up may be required, but should be at least every 4–6 weeks
Administration:
• Proper procedures need to be used for handling and disposal of chemotherapy, because this drug is potentially carcinogenic and mutagenic.
• Aseptic technique must be used at all times when handling the intravitreal implant. Handle only by the suture tab to avoid damage to the polymer coating, which can result in an increased rate of drug release from the implant.
• With the oral formulation, try to avoid direct contact between the powder in the capsules and the skin or mucous membranes. The medication should be taken with food, and the capsules should not be opened or crushed.

Table 15-12 Cidofovir

Brand name: Vistide
Generic: No
Supplied: 75 mg/mL IV solution
Indications: CMV retinitis (administer with probenecid)
Mechanism of action: Inhibits viral DNA polymerase
Drug/food/lab interactions: Nephrotoxic agents
Contraindications: Sulfa allergy, renal impairment (CrCl < 55 mL/min; SCr > 1.5, or 2+ proteinuria), administration with other nephrotoxic drugs
Pharmacokinetics:
• Half-life: 2.5 hours
• Metabolism: Minimal; phosphorylation occurs intracellularly
• Excretion: Urine
• Protein binding: Less than 6%
Adverse effects:
• Common: Rash, nausea, vomiting, headache
• Serious: Metabolic acidosis, neutropenia, decreased intraocular pressure, iritis, severe nephrotoxicity
Safety/monitoring:
• Symptomatic improvement
• Ophthalmic exam
• WBC with differential prior to each dose
• Renal function and urine protein within 48 hours prior to each dose
• Intraocular pressure and ocular symptoms of uveitis/iritis
• Signs of metabolic acidosis
Administration: This agent should be given only as an intravenous infusion, not as an intraocular injection. Dilute the appropriate dose in 100 mL normal saline (NS) and administer at a constant rate over 1 hour, using a standard infusion pump.

Table 15-13 Foscarnet Sodium

Brand name: Foscavir
Generic: Yes
Supplied: 24 mg/mL IV solution
Indications: CMV retinitis; in patients with acyclovir-resistant herpes simplex virus
Mechanism of action: Inhibits viral DNA polymerase and reverse transcriptase
Contraindications: Hypersensitivity to foscarnet
Pharmacokinetics:
• Half-life: 3 hours
• Metabolism: None
• Excretion: Renal
• Protein binding: 14–17%
Adverse effects:
• Common: Diarrhea, nausea, vomiting, anemia, headache, fever
• Serious: Electrolyte imbalances, seizures, nephrotoxicity
Safety/monitoring:
• Symptomatic improvement
• Ophthalmologic exam
• CBC
• Renal function, especially creatinine clearance; baseline, 2–3 times per week during initiation, and every 1–2 weeks during maintenance
• Electrolyte panel; baseline, 2–3 times per week during initiation, and every 1–2 weeks during maintenance
• Signs and symptoms of electrolyte abnormalities
Administration: Should be given intravenously using a standard infusion pump. The recommended infusion rate should not be exceeded, and a central venous line or peripheral vein catheter should be used. For a peripheral line infusion, dilute the solution with D_5W or NS to a concentration of 12 mg/mL. No dilution is needed for a central line infusion. Administer hydration therapy of 750–1,000 mL of NS or D_5W before giving the first dose. For the remaining doses, give 750–1,000 mL of hydration fluid concurrently with a 90–120 mg/kg dose and 500 mL of hydration fluid concurrently with a 40–60 mg/kg dose.

Table 15-14 Amantadine

Brand name: Symmetrel
Generic: Yes
Supplied: 100 mg tabs, 100 mg capsules, 100 mg liquid capsules, 50 mg/mL oral solution, 50 mg/mL oral syrup
Indications: Influenza A treatment and prophylaxis
Mechanism of action: Inhibits release of viral DNA into host by interfering with the viral M2 protein
Drug/food/lab interactions: Drugs that cause QT prolongation, anticholinergics, potassium chloride, influenza vaccine (reduces vaccine effectiveness)
Contraindications: Breastfeeding, hypersensitivity to amantadine or rimantadine, narrow-angle glaucoma
Pharmacokinetics:
• Half-life: 24 hours
• Bioavailability: 86–90%
• Metabolism: Minimal
• Excretion: 80–90% unchanged in urine
• Protein binding: 67%
Adverse effects:
• Common: Orthostatic hypotension, peripheral edema, constipation, diarrhea, appetite loss, nausea, xerostomia, ataxia, confusion, dizziness, headache, insomnia, somnolence, agitation, anxiety, depression, irritability, fatigue

(*continues*)

Table 15-14 (*continued*)

- Serious: Cardiac arrest, cardiac dysrhythmia, congestive heart failure, hypotension, tachycardia, malignant melanoma, agranulocytosis, leukopenia, neutropenia, hypersensitivity reaction, neuroleptic malignant syndrome, suicidal ideation, acute respiratory failure, pulmonary edema

Safety/monitoring:

- Signs and symptoms of infection
- Changes in mental state, which may occur with or without a prior history of psychiatric illness, and during short courses of treatment; watch for disorientation, confusion, depression, personality changes, agitation, aggressive behavior, hallucinations, paranoia, somnolence, or insomnia
- Central nervous system (CNS) adverse events, especially in patients also receiving CNS stimulants
- Congestive heart failure history or preexisting peripheral edema; may exacerbate condition
- Neuroleptic malignant syndrome during dose reduction or discontinuation; watch for fever, muscle rigidity, involuntary movements, altered consciousness, mental status changes, autonomic dysfunction, tachycardia, tachypnea, and hypertension or hypotension
- Patients with preexisting epilepsy or history of seizures may be at increased risk for seizures
- Compulsive urges (gambling, sexual); may require a dose reduction or discontinuation
- May exacerbate preexisting psychiatric disorders or substance abuse
- Frequently and regularly examine skin for signs of melanoma

Table 15-15 Rimantadine

Brand name: Flumandine

Generic: Yes

Supplied: 100 mg tabs

Indications: Influenza A treatment and prophylaxis

Mechanism of action: Inhibits viral replication of influenza A via interference with the M2 viral protein

Drug/food/lab interactions: Live influenza vaccine (reduces the vaccine's effectiveness); acetaminophen and aspirin (both decrease absorption of rimantidine)

Contraindications: Hypersensitivity to rimantadine or amantadine

Pharmacokinetics:

- Half-life: 25 hours
- Bioavailability: Approximately 90–100%
- Metabolism: Extensive hepatic
- Excretion: Less than 25% unchanged in urine
- Protein binding: Approximately 40%

Adverse effects:

- Common: Appetite loss, nausea, vomiting, dry mouth, dizziness, insomnia, anxiety
- Serious: Seizure

Safety/monitoring: Fever, symptomatic improvement

Administration: Start within 48 hours of symptoms for treatment of influenza

Table 15-16 Oseltamivir Phosphate

Brand name: Tamiflu

Generic: No

Supplied: 30, 45, and 75 mg oral tabs; 12 mg/mL oral powder for suspension

Indications: Treatment and prophylaxis of influenza A and B in adults and children older than age 1 year

Mechanism of action: Neuraminidase inhibitor

Drug/food/lab interactions: Live influenza vaccine (diminishes the effectiveness of the vaccine)

Table 15-16 (*continued*)

Contraindications: Hypersensitivity to oseltamivir
Pharmacokinetics:
• Half-life: 6–10 hours
• Bioavailability: Oseltamivir carboxylate (active drug): 75%
• Metabolism: Extensively metabolized to oseltamivir carboxylate (active drug) by liver esterases; not a CYP450 substrate or inhibitor
• Excretion: Urine
• Protein binding: Oseltamivir carboxylate: 3%
Adverse effects:
• Common: Abdominal pain, nausea, vomiting
• Serious: Cardiac dysrhythmias, Stevens-Johnson syndrome, toxic epidermal necrolysis, GI hemorrhage, hemorrhagic colitis, hepatitis, anaphylaxis, seizure, delirium
Safety/monitoring: Fever, symptomatic improvement
Administration:
• This medication can be taken with or without food. The capsules may be opened and mixed with sweetened liquids, such as regular or sugar-free chocolate syrup. Shake the suspension well before measuring each dose, and dispense it with an appropriate measuring device.
• Compounded suspension during Tamiflu suspension shortage: Transfer contents of the required oseltamivir 75 mg capsules into a clean mortar and triturate to a fine powder; add one-third of the volume of the vehicle (cherry syrup or Ora-Sweet sugar-free; 29 mL for six capsules—total volume, 30 mL; 38.5 mL for eight capsules—total volume, 40 mL; 48 mL for 10 capsules—total volume, 50 mL; 57 mL for 12 capsules—total volume, 60 mL) and triturate to form a uniform suspension. Transfer the suspension to an amber glass bottle. Rinse the mortar and pestle with one-third of the vehicle two more times, transferring the vehicle to the bottle each time. Shake well to dissolve the active drug. The suspension is stable for 35 days when refrigerated (at 2–8°C) or for 5 days at room temperature. The compounded suspension concentration is 15 mg/mL.

Table 15-17 Zanamavir

Brand name: Relenza
Generic: No
Supplied: 5 mg/actuation inhalation disk
Indications: Treatment for influenza A and B in adults and children older than age 7 years; prophylaxis for influenza A and B in adults and children older than age 5 years
Mechanism of action: Neuraminidase inhibitor
Drug/food/lab interactions: Live influenza vaccine (diminishes the effectiveness of the vaccine)
Contraindications: Underlying airway disease (asthma, COPD); hypersensitivity to zanamivir or any component of the product, including lactose
Pharmacokinetics:
• Half-life: 2.5–5 hours
• Bioavailability: 4–17% (inhalation)
• Metabolism: None
• Excretion: Urine (as unchanged drug)
• Protein binding: Less than 10%
Adverse effects:
• Common: Arthralgia, dizziness, cough, pain in throat, sinusitis, fever with chills
• Serious: Cardiac dysrhythmias, facial edema, rash, anaphylaxis, seizure, delirium
Safety/monitoring: Fever, symptomatic improvement, respiratory function in patients with underlying airway disease
Administration: Administer only with the provided Diskhaler device. Do not reconstitute the inhalation powder in any liquid formulation. This medication is not recommended for use in a nebulizer or mechanical ventilator. If administered concurrently, use the inhaled bronchodilator first.

Table 15-18 Acyclovir

Brand name: Zovirax

Generic: Yes

Supplied: 200 mg capsules; 400 mg and 800 mg tablets; 200 mg/5 mL oral suspension

Indications: HSV (genital herpes, cold sores) treatment and suppressive therapy; shingles and chickenpox (varicella zoster)

Mechanism of action: Inhibits viral DNA polymerase

Drug/food/lab interactions: Varicella virus vaccine (decreased vaccine effectiveness), tizanidine (increased concentrations of tizanidine), probenecid (increased acyclovir levels), and hydantoins (decreased levels with acyclovir administration)

Contraindications: Hypersensitivity to acyclovir

Pharmacokinetics:

- Half-life: Neonates: 4 hours; children: 1–12 hours; adults: 3 hours
- Bioavailability: 15–30%
- Metabolism: Small amount of hepatic metabolism
- Excretion: Urine (30–90% unchanged)
- Protein binding: 9–33%

Adverse effects:

- Common: Injection-site phlebitis, sensation of burning skin, diarrhea, nausea, vomiting, agitation, confusion, dizziness, hallucinations, somnolence, elevated BUN and SCr, malaise
- Serious: Thrombocytopenic purpura, confusion, tremor agitation, renal impairment

Safety/monitoring: Symptomatic improvement, renal function

Administration:

- Do not administer as a subcutaneous or intramuscular injection.
- The injectable formulation should be administered intravenously, only as an infusion and not as a rapid bolus injection.
- The IV solution should be reconstituted with sterile water for injection and used within 12 hours of reconstitution. Be sure not to use bacteriostatic water for injection that contains benzyl alcohol or parabens. After reconstitution, dilute the appropriate dose in D_5W or NS (biologic or colloidal fluids are not recommended for dilution) to a concentration of 7 mg/mL or less, and infuse over 1 hour.
- The oral formulations can be taken with or without food. Be sure to shake the suspension well before measuring each dose.
- Apply a sufficient quantity of the topical formulation with a finger cot or rubber glove to adequately cover any lesions. The dose size per application should be approximately 0.5 inch for every 4 square inches of surface area.

Table 15-19 Valacyclovir

Brand name: Valtrex

Generic: Yes

Supplied: 500 mg, 1 g tabs

Indications: Herpes labialis (cold sores), genital herpes, herpes zoster (shingles)

Mechanism of action: Converted to acyclovir; inhibits viral DNA polymerase

Drug/food/lab interactions: Probenecid (increased valacyclovir levels), mycophenolate, and mycophenolic acid (increased risk of neutropenia)

Contraindications: Hypersensitivity to valacyclovir or acyclovir or any component of the product

Pharmacokinetics:

- Half-life: 2.5–3.3 hours
- Bioavailability: 55% when converted to acyclovir
- Metabolism: Extensively metabolized to acyclovir
- Excretion: Urine and feces
- Protein binding: 13–18%

Adverse effects:

- Common: Rash, abdominal pain, nausea, vomiting, headache, fatigue
- Serious: Thrombocytopenia, hemolytic uremia syndrome

Table 15-19 (*continued*)

Safety/monitoring:

- Symptomatic improvement
- Ophthalmologic exam
- CBC
- Renal function (CrCl) baseline
- BIW to TIW during initiation, then once every 2–3 weeks during maintenance
- Electrolyte panel

Administration: Take orally with or without food

Table 15-20 Famciclovir

Brand name: Famvir

Generic: Yes

Supplied: 125, 250, and 500 mg tabs

Indications: Treatment of HSV infections, treatment of herpes zoster

Mechanism of action: Transformed to penciclovir; penciclovir inhibits HSV DNA polymerase

Drug/food/lab interactions: Drugs eliminated by active tubular secretion may increase concentrations of famciclovir; food decreases absorption

Contraindications: Hypersensitivity to famciclovir, penciclovir, or any component of the product

Pharmacokinetics:

- Half-life: 1.6–3 hours; longer in patients with renal failure
- Bioavailability: 77%
- Metabolism: Deacetylated and oxidized to form penciclovir, not via CYP450
- Excretion: 73% urine, 27% feces
- Protein binding: Less than 20%

Adverse effects:

- Common: Diarrhea, flatulence, nausea, vomiting, headache, dysmenorrheal
- Serious: Erythema multiforme

Safety/monitoring: Symptomatic improvement

Administration: Take orally with or without food

Table 15-21 Penciclovir

Brand name: Denavir

Generic: No

Supplied: 1% topical cream

Indications: Herpes labialis (cold sores)

Mechanism of action: Inhibits HSV DNA polymerase

Drug/food/lab interactions: None known

Contraindications: Hypersensitivity to penciclovir or any component of the product

Pharmacokinetics: Not absorbed

Adverse effects:

- Common: Erythema
- Safety/monitoring: Symptomatic improvement

Administration: Apply only to lips and face

Table 15-22 Docosanol

Brand name: Abreva

Generic: No

Supplied: 10% topical cream OTC

Indications: Herpes labialis (cold sores)

Mechanism of action: Inhibits fusion of the viral envelope with the host cell's membrane, thereby inhibiting viral entry

Drug/food/lab interactions: none known

Contraindications: Hypersensitivity to docosanol or any component of product

Pharmacokinetics: Not absorbed

Adverse effects: Application-site reactions, headache

Safety/monitoring: Improvement in lesions

Administration: Gently rub in to completely cover the affected area

Table 15-23 Patient Education

Medications	Patient Education
Hepatitis Agents	
Adefovir dipivoxil	• Safe sex practices to reduce disease transmission; the drug does not prevent transmission. • Do not abruptly discontinue. • May experience abdominal pain, diarrhea, dyspepsia, flatulence, nausea, asthenia, and headaches. • Report signs and symptoms of nephrotoxicity, nausea, vomiting, abdominal pain, tachypnea, or hepatic impairment.
Entecavir	• Do not engage in activities requiring mental alertness or coordination until the drug effects are realized. • Safe sex practices; the medication does not prevent disease transmission. • May experience nausea, dizziness, headache, or fatigue. • Report nausea, vomiting, abdominal pain, tachypnea, signs and symptoms of decreased renal or liver function. • After discontinuing this medication, watch for and report signs of hepatitis. Discontinuation can cause severe hepatitis exacerbations. • Do not abruptly discontinue this medication. • Take at least 2 hours before and 2 hours after a meal.
Peginterferon-alfa 2a	• Avoid activities that require mental alertness or coordination until the drug effects are known, as this agent may cause dizziness. • May experience alopecia, myalgia, headache, insomnia, anxiety, irritability, fatigue, fever, flu-like symptoms, and rigor. • Report any visual disturbances, unusual bleeding/bruising, signs or symptoms of pulmonary disorder, depression, suicidal ideation, or unusual changes in behavior. • Proper technique and placement of injections are important. Patients should rotate injection sites. • If a dose is missed or given up to 2 days late, the patient should take the dose as soon as possible. However, if the missed dose is more than 2 days late, the patient should contact the physician.
Lamivudine	• Safe sex practices; the medication does not prevent disease transmission. • May experience lipodystrophy, decreased appetite, nausea, vomiting, headache, or fatigue. • Report nausea, vomiting, abdominal pain, tachypnea, hepatic dysfunction, fever, light-headedness, infections, or disease exacerbation.
Tenofovir disoproxil fumarate	• Safe sex practices; the medication does not prevent disease transmission. • May experience lipodystrophy, diarrhea, flatulence, and asthenia. • Report nausea, vomiting, abdominal pain, tachypnea, jaundice, dark urine, or pale stools.
Peginterferon-alfa 2b	• May experience an influenza-like illness. • Report any visual disturbances, depression, suicidal ideation, unusual changes in behavior, dark urine, abdominal pain, bloody diarrhea, fever, or signs and symptoms of pancreatitis. • Proper technique and placement of injections are important; rotate injection sites.
Ribavirin	• Pregnant women should avoid exposure to inhalation therapy. • Need reliable contraception, because this medication can harm the fetus. Contraception must be used during treatment and up to 6 months after therapy in male and female patients. • May experience rash, pruritus, dyspepsia, anorexia, nausea, headache, conjunctivitis, rigors, insomnia, depression, fatigue, and dry mouth. • Report severe depression, suicidal ideation, respiratory deterioration, pancreatitis, hemolytic anemia, or cardiac deterioration. • Do not open, crush, or break the capsules. • Take the oral formulation consistently with regard to food. • Teach the proper inhalation technique. Do not mix with other medications.

Table 15-23 (*continued*)

Medications	Patient Education
Hepatitis Agents (*continued*)	
Telbivudine	• Safe sex practices; the drug does not prevent disease transmission. • May experience abdominal pain, headache, nasopharyngitis, upper respiratory infection, malaise, or fatigue. • Report nausea, vomiting, abdominal pain, tachypnea, decreased renal function, or decreased liver function. • Report hepatitis exacerbations after discontinuation of therapy.
Influenza Agents	
Amantadine hydrochloride	• Avoid activities that require mental alertness or coordination until the drug effects are known. • May experience anticholinergic symptoms, orthostatic hypotension, peripheral edema, diarrhea, loss of appetite, nausea, confusion, headache, insomnia, agitation, anxiety, depression, hallucinations, irritability, fatigue, blurred vision, increased compulsive behaviors, or mental disorder exacerbation. • Report sweating, fever, stupor, unstable blood pressure, muscle rigidity, or autonomic dysfunction, especially with a sudden dose decrease or discontinuation. • Advise the patient to watch for and report signs of melanoma. • Avoid alcohol with this medication.
Oseltamivir phosphate	• Not a substitute for an annual flu vaccine. • May experience nausea, vomiting, insomnia, and bronchitis. • Counsel patients that if they miss a dose, to take it as soon as possible, unless the next dose is within 2 hours; in that case, skip the missed dose.
Peramivir	• This medication does not seem to minimize the risk of influenza transmission, and this is not an FDA-approved indication for the drug. The patient can accept or refuse this therapy. • May experience diarrhea, nausea, vomiting, bacterial infection, anaphylaxis, serious skin reactions, and neutropenia. • Watch for signs of unusual behavior.
Rimantadine Hydrochloride	• Avoid activities requiring mental alertness and coordination until the drug effects are known, because it may cause dizziness. • May experience anorexia, nausea, vomiting, xerostomia, insomnia, and nervousness. • Report seizures. • Start taking this drug within 48 hours of the first sign of the flu. • Patients can take this medication with food to minimize gastric irritation.
Zanamivir	• Not to be used in a nebulizer; should be used only with the provided Diskhaler. Instruct patients on proper inhalation technique. • May experience diarrhea, nausea, headache, cough, and nasal symptoms. • Report signs and symptoms of bronchospasm and respiratory depression.
Herpes Agents	
Acycolvir	• Maintain adequate hydration with oral therapy to minimize the risk of renal toxicity. • This medication does not prevent reinfection or disease transmission with genital herpes. Patients should abstain from sex during acute outbreaks and always use condoms. • Warn patients who are taking the oral formulation that they may experience diarrhea, nausea, vomiting, or renal impairment. Elderly patients may experience more neurological adverse effects. • Patients using the topical form of the drug may experience local application reactions such as burning, dryness, pruritus, or stinging. • When used intermittently, initiate treatment at the first sign of a breakout. • Make sure the patient is aware that topical formulations are not to be used in the eye, mouth, or nose. • Topical application should be done with a finger cot or rubber glove to reduce the risk of viral transmission.

(*continues*)

Table 15-23 (*continued*)

Medications	Patient Education
Herpes Agents (*continued*)	
Famciclovir	• Safe sex practices; the medication does not prevent disease transmission. • May experience diarrhea, nausea, headache, dysmenorrhea, flu-like symptoms, or a spreading red rash that may progress to blistering. • Report signs and symptoms of renal impairment.
Valacyclovir hydrochloride	• Counsel patients to avoid sex during outbreaks, and inform them that the medication does not prevent disease transmission. • Do not suddenly discontinue the medication without consulting the prescriber. • Maintain adequate hydration to prevent precipitation of acyclovir in the renal tubules.
Foscarnet sodium	• Avoid activities that require mental alertness or coordination until the drug effects are known. • Maintain adequate hydration to avoid kidney damage during therapy. • May experience diarrhea, nausea, vomiting, or headaches. • Report signs and symptoms of renal impairment or electrolyte abnormalities.
Docosanol	• For herpetic lesions on the lips and face only; not to be used on genital herpes. • Avoid contact with the eyes. • May experience an application-site reaction or headache.
Penciclovir	• May experience erythema. • Apply the drug to the lips and face only; avoid drug contact with mucous membranes and the eyes. • Use at the first sign of a cold sore.
Cytomegalovirus Agents	
Cidofovir	• Warn patients that this medication may cause infertility in men. Both male and female patients need to use reliable contraception, because the medication has the potential to cause fetal harm. Contraception should be used during treatment and up to 3 months after therapy for men and for 1 month after therapy for women. • May experience nausea, vomiting, headache, neutropenia, or iritis. • Report signs and symptoms of metabolic acidosis, nephrotoxicity, or infections. • A full course of probenecid should be taken as prescribed with each dose of cidofovir.
Ganciclovir	• Both male and female patients need to use reliable contraception, because this medication has the potential to cause fetal harm. Contraception should be used during treatment and up to 3 months after therapy. Patients should also be warned that this drug may cause infertility in both men and women. • May experience appetite loss or fever. • Report signs and symptoms of pancytopenia. • Patients with the implant should expect a decrease in visual acuity, especially within 2–4 weeks after implantation. However, they should report a problem if their vision does not improve after this time. • Inform patients that this medication is not a cure, but should help reduce symptoms. • Instruct patients to take the capsules with food. • Teach patients the proper procedures for handling and disposing of chemotherapy. • Warn patients that this drug is an irritant, so they should avoid direct contact of skin or mucous membranes with the powder or solution.
Valganciclovir hydrochloride	• Counsel patients on the need for reliable contraception to prevent fetal harm. Contraception should be used during therapy and for at least 1 month after treatment in women, and at least 3 months following therapy in men. • Patients need to be instructed on proper handling to avoid direct contact of skin and mucous membranes with broken or crushed tablets. • May experience abdominal pain, diarrhea, nausea, vomiting, headache, insomnia, cough, constipation, and fever. • Patients should maintain adequate hydration to avoid renal toxicity. • Advise patients to take this medication with food.

TOPIC: BIOTERRORISM AND CHEMOTERRORISM

Section Coordinator: Michael Klepser
Contributor: Mindy Jock

Tips Worth Tweeting

- Biologic agents associated with bioterrorism are classified into three categories—A, B, and C—based on their ease of dissemination, public health impact, and requirement of preparedness.
- Classes of chemical agents likely to be used in a terrorist attack include biotoxins, vesicants, blood agents, or nerve agents.
- Atropine is used in patients exposed to nerve gases (sarin, tabun, soman, and VX).
- Amyl nitrate is part of a cyanide antidote kit. It increases formation of methemoglobin, which binds cyanide to form nontoxic cyanomethemoglobin.
- Prolidoxime is used in individuals with symptoms of exposure to nerve gases because it reactivates cholinesterase.

Patient Care Scenario

An intern for a U.S. senator opened a letter that was covered with a white powder. The intern came down with a low-grade fever, sweats, and myalgias NKA. The powder was identified as *Bacillus anthracis.*

Bioterrorism

Bioterrorism is the release of a biologic substance (bacterial, viral, or toxin) to intentionally cause harm to a population. The biologic agents used for this purpose are generally found in the natural environment, but often have been manipulated to be more harmful.

Biologic agents are classified into three categories based on their ease of dissemination, public health impact, and requirement of preparedness.

Key Terms

Category A: High-priority agents that present the highest risk to public security.

- Easily spread from person to person
- High morbidity and mortality
- May cause public panic
- Special action and public health preparedness needed
- Agents in this category: *Bacillus anthracis* (anthrax), *Clostridium botulinum* toxin (botulism), *Yersinia pestis* (plague), Variola virus (smallpox), *Francisella tularensis* (tularemia), filioviruses and arenaviruses (viral hemorrhagic fever)

Category B: Second-highest-priority agents

- Moderately easy to disseminate
- Moderate mortality and low morbidity
- Require enhancement of the Centers for Disease Control and Prevention laboratory capacity
- Agents in this category: alphaviruses (encephalomyelitis), *Brucella* species (brucellosis), *Burkholdera* species (glanders and melioidosis), *Coxiella burnetii* (Q fever), *Chlamydia psittaci* (psittacosis), staphylococcal enterotoxin B and ricin (toxic syndromes), *Rickettsia prowazekii* (typhus fever)
- Food safety threats: *Salmonella* species, *Escherichia coli*
- Water safety threats: *Vibrio cholerae, Cryptosporidium parvum*

Category C: Emerging agents that could be engineered for mass destruction

- Easily available
- Easily produced and disseminated
- Have potential for high morbidity and mortality
- Agents in this category: emerging threats, hantaviruses, multidrug-resistant tuberculosis, Nipah virus (encephalitis), tick-borne hemorrhagic fever viruses, yellow fever

1.1.0 Patient Information

See Table 15-24.

1.2.0 Pharmacotherapy

In treating pregnant patients and children, the benefits of treatment outweigh the risks (see Table 15-25).

Chemoterrorism

Chemical agents may be used in attacks to kill, seriously injure, or physiologically incapacitate people through various mechanisms. Classes of chemical agents that might be used in such an attack include biotoxins, vesicants, blood agents, and nerve agents. Additional classes of chemical agents that have been used during warfare include choking agents, incapacitating agents, and tear gases. These agents are unlikely to be used during terrorist attacks, but definitions are included here for completeness.

Table 15-24 Biologic Agents and Diseases

Disease	Systems Affected	Transmission	Incubation Period	Signs and Symptoms
Anthrax (*Bacillus anthracis*)	Cutaneous	Direct contact with spores	Up to 1 day	• Localized itching • Papular lesions that turn vesicular • Black eschar at days 7–10
	Respiratory	Inhalation of aerosolized spores	Less than 1 week up to 2 months	• Initial phase: nonspecific symptoms: malaise, fatigue, myalgias, chest discomfort, low-grade fever, sweats • Possible symptomatic improvement for 1–3 days • Subsequent phase: high fever, severe respiratory distress, shock and death
	Gastrointestinal	Consumption of undercooked meats or dairy of infected animals	1–7 days	• Initial phase: nausea, vomiting, fever, severe abdominal pain, hematemesis, (bloody) diarrhea • Subsequent phase: at 2–4 days, abdominal pain decreases, ascites develops, shock and death occur after 2–5 days
	Oropharyngeal		1–7 days	• Fever, neck swelling, regional lymphadenopathy, throat pain, ulcers on the tongue may progress to necrosis
Botulism (*Clostridium botulinum* toxin)	Muscular	Foodborne Wound Intestinal colonization Inhalation	6 hours to 10 days	• Symmetrical cranial neuropathies • Descending weakness • Descending paralysis
Plague (*Yersinia pestis*)	Pneumonic plague	Aerosol attack, respiratory droplets	1–6 days	• Fever, weakness, rapidly developing pneumonia, possible bloody sputum, possible respiratory failure, shock and death
	Bubonic plague	Bite from infected flea	2–6 days	• Swollen, tender lymph glands (buboes) • Fever, headache, chills, and weakness • Bacteria can spread through the bloodstream to the lungs
	Septicemic plague	Bacteremia		• Fever, chills, abdominal pain, shock • Bleeding • May occur with pneumonic or bubonic plague
Smallpox (Variola virus)	Cutaneous	Aerosol, direct contact with infected individual	7–17 days	• Initial phase: high fever, malaise, head and body aches, vomiting • Early rash: initially in tongue and mouth, which break open as a rash appears on the body • Pustular rash • Pustules and scabs • Resolving scabs
Tularemia (*Francisella tularensis*)		Handling infected animal, eating/drinking contaminated food, aerosol	3–14 days	• Sudden fever, chills, headaches, diarrhea, muscle aches, joint pain, dry cough, progressive weakness, pneumonia possibly with bloody sputum
Viral hemorrhagic fevers (filoviruses and arenaviruses)		Aerosol, rodents, mosquitoes, and ticks	2–21 days	• Initial phase: sudden fever, myalgia, malaise, headache, vomiting, abdominal pain, maculopapular rash • Late phase: hepatic failure, renal failure, neurologic deficits, hemorrhagic diathesis, shock, and multi-organ dysfunction

Table 15-25 Treatment and Prophylaxis for Illness due to Biologic Agents

Disease	Type	Treatment	Duration	Prophylaxis
Anthrax (*Bacillus anthracis*)	Cutaneous	• Ciprofloxacin 500 mg po bid *or* • Doxycycline 100 mg po bid	60 days	• Immunization • Ciprofloxacin 500 mg po bid *or* • Doxycycline 100 mg po bid
	Respiratory	• Ciprofloxacin 400 mg IV q 12 hr *or* • Doxycycline 100 mg IV q 12 hr • Switch to po when clinically appropriate	60 days	
	Gastrointestinal	Use respiratory protocol	60 days	
	Oropharyngeal	Use respiratory protocol	60 days	
Botulism (*Clostridium botulinum* toxin)		• Antitoxin • Supportive care		• Neutralizing antibody • Antitoxin • Immunization
Plague *(Yersinia pestis*)		• Streptomycin 30 mg/kg/day divided IM bid *or* • Gentamicin 5 mg/kg IM or IV daily *or* • Doxycycline 200 mg IV, then 100 mg IV bid until clinically improved, then 100 mg po bid *or* • Ciprofloxacin 400 mg IV bid until clinically improved, then 750 mg po bid	10–14 days	• Doxycycline 100 mg bid × 7 days *or* • Ciprofloxacin 500 mg bid × 7 days
Smallpox (Variola virus)		• Supportive care		• Immunization
Tularemia *(Francisella tularensis*)	Contained	**Preferred:** • Streptomycin 1 g IM bid *or* • Gentamicin 5 mg/kg IM or IV daily **Alternative:** • Doxycycline 100 mg IV bid *or* • Chloramphenicol 15 mg/kg *or* • Ciprofloxacin 400 mg IV bid	• Gentamicin × 10 days • Doxycycline or Chloramphenicol × 14 days	• Vaccine under review by FDA • Postexposure prophylaxis is the same as for a mass-casualty event
	Mass casualty	• Doxycycline 100 mg po bid *or* • Ciprofloxacin 500 mg po bid	• Ciprofloxacin × 10 days • Doxycycline × 14–21 days	
Viral hemorrhagic fevers (filoviruses and arenaviruses)		• Ribavirin 30 mg/kg once; 16 mg/kg q 6 hr × 4 days, then 8 mg/kg q 8 hr × 6 days	10 days	• None available

Table 15-26 Chemical Agents

	Substance	Form	Symptom Onset	Signs and Symptoms	Treatment
Biotoxins	Abrin	Inhalation	Within 8 hours	• Respiratory distress • Fever • Cough • Nausea • Heavy sweating • Pulmonary edema	Supportive care
		Ingestion	6 hours to 3 days	• Bloody vomit and diarrhea • Severe dehydration • Hypotension • Hallucinations • Seizures	Supportive care
	Ricin	Inhalation	4–8 hours	• Irritation of throat and nose • Respiratory distress • Pulmonary edema • Flu-like symptoms*	Supportive care
		Ingestion	1–6 hours	• Gastrointestinal symptoms • Persistent vomiting • Voluminous diarrhea • Dehydration • Hypovolemic shock	• Activated charcoal • Gastric lavage • Supportive care, if needed
Blister agents/ vesicants	Nitrogen mustard (HN-1, HN-2, HN-3)	Inhalation	Up to several hours	• Sinus pain • Sore throat • Cough • Shortness of breath • Tremors • Incoordination • Seizures	• Externally flush with water and 0.5% sodium hypochlorite solution • Ocular lubricants • Bronchodilators • Atropine sulfate 0.4–0.6 mg IM or IV for nausea and vomiting • Do *not* induce vomiting • Supportive care
		Skin/eye contact	Up to several hours	• Ophthalmic irritation, pain, swelling, and tearing • Blindness • Redness • Blistering • CNS symptoms may occur with large exposure	
		Ingestion		• Abdominal pain • Nausea/vomiting • Diarrhea	
	Sulfur mustard (H)	Inhalation	2–24 hours	• Sinus pain • Laryngitis • Cough • Wheezing • Necrosis of respiratory epithelium, leading to pseudomembrane • Hypotension • Atrioventricular block • Tremors	• Externally flush with water and 0.5% sodium hypochlorite solution • Ocular lubricants • Bronchodilators • Atropine sulfate 0.4–0.6 mg IM or IV for nausea and vomiting • Milk may be helpful for ingestion

Table 15-26 (*continued*)

	Substance	Form	Symptom Onset	Signs and Symptoms	Treatment
Blister agents/ vesicants (*continued*)				• Convulsions • Ataxia	• Do *not* induce vomiting • Supportive care
		Skin/eye contact	Skin: 4–8 hours Eye: 1 hour or more	• Erythema • Blistering • Second- to third-degree burns • Pain • Swelling • Lacrimation • Photophobia	
		Ingestion	2–24 hours	• Abdominal pain • Nausea/vomiting • Hematemesis • Diarrhea	
	Phosgene oxime	Inhalation		• Rhinorrhea • Hoarseness • Sinus pain • Pulmonary edema • Necrotizing bronchiolitis • Pulmonary thrombosis	Supportive care
		Skin/eye contact	Immediate	• Pain • Conjunctivitis • Necrosis	
Blood agents	Arsine Stibine	Inhalation	2–24 hours	• Weakness • Fatigue • Headache • Drowsiness • Confusion • Dyspnea • Tachypnea • Hypotension • Gastrointestinal symptoms • Kidney failure • Hemoglobinuria • Jaundice	• Supportive care • Blood transfusions • Hemodialysis
	Cyanide	• Inhalation • Skin/eye contact • Ingestion	Immediate	• Tachypnea • Restlessness • Dizziness • Weakness • Headache • Nausea/vomiting • Tachycardia/bradycardia • Convulsions • Hypotension • Respiratory failure	Cyanide antidote kit[†]: amyl nitrite perles, parenteral sodium nitrite, parenteral sodium thiosulfate

(*continues*)

Table 15-26 (*continued*)

	Substance	Form	Symptom Onset	Signs and Symptoms	Treatment
Nerve agents	Sarin Tabun Soman VX	• Inhalation • Skin/eye contact • Ingestion	Immediate	• Rhinorrhea • Blurred vision • Miosis • Irritability • Nervousness • Fatigue • Insomnia • Memory loss • Bronchial secretions • Chest tightness • Respiratory failure • Bradycardia • Bradyarrhythmia • Hypertension • Muscle twitching • Paralysis	• Atropine 2–6 mg IM; repeat every 5–10 minutes with 2 mg until ventilation improves • Pralidoxime chloride 600–1,800 mg IM • Diazepam 5–10 mg as needed for seizures • Supportive care

*Flu-like symptoms: fever, nausea, weakness, myalgia, arthralgia.

†See the text for further information about the cyanide antidote kit.

Key Terms

Biotoxins: Toxins that come from a biologic source (plants or animals).

Vesicants: Chemicals that severely blister the skin, eyes, and respiratory tract.

Blood agents: Chemicals that are absorbed into the blood.

Nerve agents: Chemicals that prevent the nervous system from working.

Choking agents: Chemicals that irritate or cause swelling of the respiratory tract.

Incapacitating agents: Chemicals that cause people to have an altered state of consciousness,

Tear gases: Highly irritating agents often used for crowd control.

1.1.0 Patient Information

See Table 15-26.

1.2.0 Pharmacotherapy

Treatment Agents

Atropine

Atropine is a competitive antagonist for the muscarinic receptors. To improve ventilation in patients exposed to nerve gases (sarin, tabun, soman, and VX), give atropine 2–6 mg IM, repeating the treatment every 5–10 minutes with 2 mg atropine until the desired response is achieved. Atropine may also be used to treat nausea and vomiting in patients who experience nitrogen mustard and sulfur mustard exposure at a dosage of 0.4–0.6 mg IM or IV.

Cyanide Antidote Kits

Cyanide antidote kits contain amyl nitrite perles, parenteral sodium nitrite, and parenteral sodium thiosulfate. Oxygen should be supplied initially.

With an unconscious patient and a strong suspicion of cyanide poisoning, the amyl nitrate perles maybe be broken onto a gauze pad, held under the nose or over the mouth by a mask, and left there for 30 seconds of every minute. Every 3 minutes, a new perle should be used until sodium nitrite infusions are initiated. Amyl nitrite increases the formation of methemoglobin, which binds cyanide to form nontoxic cyanmethemoglobin.

Sodium nitrite should be initiated intravenously as soon as possible to unresponsive patients at an adult dose of 300 mg (10 mL of a 3% solution) infused over at least 5 minutes. Patients should be monitored for hypotension. Sodium nitrite works by the same mechanism as amyl nitrite.

Sodium thiosulfate is administered last at an adult dose of 12.5 g (50 mL of a 25% solution) to be given over 10–20 minutes. Allow the patient 30 minutes to respond to this medication. If the clinical response is inadequate, repeat the treatment with a dose of 6.25 g of sodium thiosulfate. The sulfur provided by sodium thiosulfate increases the reaction rate of rhonanese, an enzyme that detoxifies cyanide by converting it to thiocyanate.

Pralidoxime Chloride

Individuals with symptoms of exposure to nerve gases (sarin, tabun, soman, and VX) should be treated with pralidoxime chloride 600 mg IM every 15 minutes up to 3 doses. Pralidoxime reactivates cholinesterase.

Supportive Care

In many cases of exposure to chemical agents, there are no available antidotes. In these situations, patients are treated with supportive care based on their symptoms. The patient's airway, breathing, and circulation (ABCs) are the initial factors that must be stabilized. Some chemicals may lead to hepatic or renal failure, so medications must be adjusted as necessary. Seizures may be treated with diazepam 5–10 mg as needed.

ANNOTATED BIBLIOGRAPHY

Agency for Toxic Substance and Disease Registry. Centers for Disease Control and Prevention. Available at: http://atsdr.cdc.gov. Accessed February 2010.

Emergency Preparedness and Response. Centers for Disease Control and Prevention. Available at: http://emergency.cdc.gov. Accessed February 2010.

Evison D, Hinsley D, Rice P. Chemical weapons. *BMJ* 2002;324:332–335.

Kales SN, Christiani DC. Acute chemical emergencies. *N Engl J Med* 2004;350:800–808.

Karwa M, Currie B, Kvetan V. Bioterrorism: preparing for the impossible or the improbable. *Crit Care Med* 2005;33:S75–S95.

Micromedex Heath Care Series. Available at: http://www.thomsonhc.com. Accessed February 2010.

O'Brien KK, Higdon ML, Halverson JJ. Recognition and management of bioterrorism infections. *Am Fam Physician* 2003;67:1927–1934.

TOPIC: BONE AND JOINT INFECTIONS

Section Coordinator: *Michael Klepser*
Contributors: *Curtis D. Collins and Jerod L. Nagel*

Tips Worth Tweeting

- Osteomyelitis and septic arthritis are difficult-to-treat infections requiring long courses of antimicrobials.
- Empiric therapy should cover likely pathogens based on patient risk factors, with subsequent therapy being guided by culture and susceptibility results.
- Osteomyelitis is commonly caused by *Staphylococcus aureus*, and to a lesser extent by coagulase-negative staphylococci, streptococci, and aerobic gram-negative bacilli (mainly *Klebsiella, Escherichia coli, Pseudomonas aeruginosa,* and *Proteus*).
- Bone concentrations of antibiotics are significantly less than corresponding serum concentrations, which is the main reason why intravenous therapy is preferred in bone and joint infections.

Patient Care Scenario: Hospital Setting

A 57 y/o M (HR 78, BP 138/84, Temp 99.0, RR 14), with type 2 diabetes is admitted for evaluation of a foot ulcer with possible osteomyelitis. The patient states that he cut his foot approximately 3 weeks ago, and shortly afterward developed a red, swollen, painful, and purulent ulcer, which has increased in size to 4 × 2 cm.

Date	Physician	Drug	Quantity	Sig	Refills
5/4	Jane	Lantus Insulin	1	18 units q am	4
5/4	Jane	Regular Insulin	1	5 units before each meal	3
3/2	Jane	Metformin 500 mg	60	1 bid	3
4/2	Jane	Lisinopril 20 mg	30	1 daily	4
4/3	Jane	Warfarin 5 mg	30	1 daily	3

Labs:

- Glucose: 189
- Creatinine: 1.1
- WBC: 16.2
- ESR: 85

Osteomyelitis

Key Terms

Osteomyelitis is an infection of the bone caused by one of three mechanisms: hematogenous seeding from bacteremia, spread of bacteria from adjacent infected tissue, or direct inoculation following trauma or surgery.

1.1.0 Patient Information

Disease States Associated with Osteomyelitis

Intravenous drug use, sickle cell disease, and bacteremia are risk factors for osteomyelitis from hematogenous seeding. The common sites of infection in adults are the vertebrae, stenoclavicular bone, and sacroiliac bone.

Osteomyelitis can occur in patients following trauma, and it develops in approximately 25% of open fractures. The blunted immune response, plus altered blood flow and soft-tissue inflammation resulting from severe trauma, make it difficult for the body to fight any bacteria that might have been introduced.

The last and most common cause of osteomyelitis is spread of bacteria from adjacent tissue to the bone, which is primarily seen in diabetic foot infections and, to a lesser extent, in decubitis ulcers. Patients with uncontrolled or advanced diabetes can develop peripheral neuropathy and peripheral vascular disease, which can contribute to slow identification of wound infections and poor wound healing.

Hematogenous seeding is the primary cause of pediatric osteomyelitis in patients younger than age 17 years, and commonly affects the long bones (femur, tibia, and humerus). In contrast, hematogenous seeding accounts for approximately 20% of all osteomyelitis in adult patients.

Causative Organisms

Osteomyelitis is commonly caused by *Staphylococcus aureus*, and to a lesser extent by coagulase-negative staphylococci, streptococci, and aerobic gram-negative bacilli (mainly *Klebsiella, Escherichia coli, Pseudomonas aeruginosa,* and *Proteus*). However, infection is possible with numerous other organisms, including enterococci, anaerobes, other gram-negative bacilli, *Candida*, molds, and mycobacteria. Patients with chronic diabetic foot ulcers and multiple courses of broad-spectrum antibiotic exposure are at higher risk of acquiring a resistant or uncommon pathogen.

Osteomyelitis secondary to open fracture is commonly caused by skin flora, such as staphylococci and streptococci, but may also include bacteria from soil or bacteria on other innate objects. Additionally, patients with open fractures generally require surgery and have significant hospital stays, which could result in infection with nosocomial pathogens, including methicillin-resistant *Staphylococcus aureus, Pseudomonas, Enterobacter, Klebsiella, Serratia* and *Citrobacter*. Osteomyelitis following surgery involving bones or in close proximity to bones (such as spinal surgery) could be caused by nosocomial pathogens or skin flora listed previously. *Staphylococcus aureus, Pseudomonas,* and *Serratia* are pathogens often associated with infections linked to intravenous drug use. Generally, hematogenous seeding in pediatric and adult patients is commonly monomicrobial, whereas osteomyelitis from direct inoculation and contiguous spread can be polymicrobial.

Signs and Symptoms

Common symptoms associated with osteomyelitis include bone pain, local erythema, redness, warmth, fever, malaise, and nausea. These symptoms may be blunted in patients with advanced diabetes.

Instruments and Techniques Related to Patient Assessment

Diagnosis is commonly made by evaluating symptoms and imaging studies, such as computed tomography (CT), magnetic resonance imaging (MRI), or radiography (x-ray). In certain situations, these imaging studies may not be conclusive, such as in very acute infection, bone tumor, or acute trauma to the bone.

Bone biopsy, elevated sedimentation rate, elevated C-reactive protein, and cultures from blood or bone will help aid in diagnosis in such cases. Patients with diabetic foot ulcers are at higher risk of developing osteomyelitis, and physical examination, including probing for bone, can be helpful in making their diagnosis. Additionally, osteomyelitis is likely if the patient has an ulcer greater than 2 × 2 cm in size, a wound infection for longer than 2 weeks, and a sedimentation rate greater than 70 mm/hr. If the bone can be seen or palpated on examination, then osteomyelitis is highly probable.

A bone biopsy with culture, using sterile technique, is strongly encouraged if the patient has symptoms and imaging study results consistent with osteomyelitis. A positive bone biopsy culture is the definitive result for diagnosis, and will both help identify the causative organism and provide guidance for appropriate antibiotic therapy. A bone biopsy is preferred over a superficial swab, as the later method may yield colonizing bacteria of the wound that are not actually responsible for the osteomyelitis.

1.2.0 Pharmacotherapy

Treatment involves a prolonged course of intravenous antibiotics (4–6 weeks), and usually requires surgical debridement of necrotic bone tissue. If osteomyelitis arises adjacent to surgically implanted hardware or prosthetic material, then removal of these materials is strongly encouraged. If the materials cannot be removed, the patient will complete 4–6 weeks of intravenous therapy, and then require lifelong suppression of infection with an oral antibiotic.

Drug Indications, Dosing Regimens, and Routes of Administration

Empiric intravenous therapy for osteomyelitis should be active against Staphylococcus aureus and streptococci. Additional broad-spectrum empiric coverage should be considered for patients with osteomyelitis from chronic diabetic foot ulcers, or when a nosocomial pathogen is suspected. Ideally, empiric therapy should be started after cultures are obtained from the bone biopsy. However, if the patient is bacteremic or unstable, then therapy should be started immediately. Nafcillin, cefazolin, and vancomycin are reasonable empiric options for osteomyelitis, depending on patient-specific conditions and risk factors. Ampicillin/sulbactam and piperacillin/tazobactam are empiric options for osteomyelitis secondary to diabetic foot infections. Piperacillin/tazobactam or other anti-pseudomonal agents should be prescribed for nosocomial osteomyelitis. Therapy should be tailored once culture and sensitivity results are obtained.

Physiochemical Properties, Solubility, Pharmacodynamics, and Pharmacokinetic Properties

Antibiotic bone concentrations are significantly less than corresponding serum concentrations, which is the main reason why intravenous therapy is preferred for osteomyelitis. Advanced diabetes can alter the microvascular and macrovascular blood circulation, which affects antibiotic bone concentrations and, ultimately, the probability of successful outcomes. Nafcillin, cefazolin, ampicillin/sulbactam, and piperacillin/tazobactam reach a bone concentration that is approximately 10–35% of their serum concentration, which is adequate to treat most common osteomyelitis organisms. Vancomycin's bone concentration is slightly lower, at 5–15% of its serum concentrations. The goal vancomycin serum concentration of 15–20 mcg/mL is recommended by current vancomycin dosing guidelines supported by the Infectious Diseases Society of America, Society of Infectious Diseases Pharmacists, and American Society of Health-System Pharmacists.

1.3.0 Pharmacotherapy Monitoring

Weekly monitoring for resolution of infection and potential adverse effects from antibiotic therapy should be performed during therapy. Inflammatory makers, such as C-reactive protein and sedimentation rate, should decrease and become normalized by the end of therapy (assuming the patient does not have other disease states that would increase these inflammatory markers). Imaging studies are generally not helpful to monitor resolution of infection.

Patients should be educated about potential adverse effects of antibiotic therapy, and weekly lab tests should be obtained. At minimum, the patient should have a weekly complete blood count (CBC) and chemistry-7 panel (which includes serum creatinine, BUN, and electrolytes). Additional monitoring may be needed depending on the specific antibiotic used for therapy, and any patient-specific disease–drug or drug–drug interactions. Generally, there are no food–drug interactions, as patients are usually on intravenous therapy. Fluoroquinolones, linezolid, metronidazole, and rifampin could be administered orally instead of intravenously, however. Table 15-27 lists adverse effects and drug–drug interactions associated with common osteomyelitis therapy.

Septic Arthritis

Key Terms

Septic arthritis, also known as infectious arthritis, is an infection of the fluid and tissues of a joint usually caused by bacteria, but sometimes caused by viruses or fungi. Like osteomyelitis, septic arthritis can be caused from multiple mechanisms, including direct inoculation following trauma or surgery, spread via adjacent infected tissue, or hematogenous seeding. Hematogenous seeding is the most common mechanism of infection.

1.1.0 Patient Information

Disease States Associated with Septic Arthritis

The following individuals are at increased risk for developing septic arthritis: patients older than 80 years of age, or those with a history of arthritis, IV drug abuse, diabetes mellitus, prosthetic joints, recent joint surgery, immunosuppressive therapy, or previous intra-articular injection. In addition, this infection also occurs in 2 to 5 of every 100,000 patients without risk factors annually. The presence of risk factors, however, increases the incidence of septic arthritis significantly. For example, individuals with rheumatoid arthritis experience 28 to 38 infections per 100,000 patients annually. Patients with multiple risk factors are at even greater risk.

Causative Organisms

Septic arthritis is usually caused by a singular organism; polymicrobial infections are rare. The most common causes of septic arthritis are gram-positive organisms

Table 15-27 Pharmacotherapy of Commonly Prescribed Antibiotics for Bone and Joint Infections

	Nafcillin	Cefazolin	Vancomycin	Ceftriaxone	Piperacillin/ Tazobactam	Ampicillin/ Sulbactam
Brand name	Nafcil Unipen Nallpen	Kefzol Ancef	Vancocin	Rocephin	Zosyn	Unasyn
Adult dosage regimen	2 g every 4 hr	2 g every 8 hr	10–15 mg/kg every 8–12 hr	1–2 g daily	4.5 g every 6–8 hr	3 g every 6 hr
Renal dose adjustment needed	No	Yes	Yes	No	Yes	Yes
Common adverse effects	Rash Phlebitis	Rash Pruritus	Red man's syndrome Phlebitis	Rash	Rash GI disturbance	Rash
Serious or life-threatening adverse effects	Anaphylaxis Hypokalemia Interstitial nephritis Hepatotoxicity Neutropenia	Anaphylaxis Neutropenia Thrombocyt-openia Seizures Drug fever	Neutropenia Eosinophilia Thrombocyto-penia Ototoxicity Allergic reactions	Anaphylaxis Hepatotoxicity Neutropenia Eosinophilia Thrombocytopenia Biliary lithiasis	Anaphylaxis Neutropenia Eosinophilia Thrombocytopenia Hepatotoxicity Seizure Interstitial nephritis	Anaphylaxis Hepatotoxicity Neutropenia Eosinophilia Thrombocyto-penia Seizure GI disturbance
Monitoring	Complete blood count Liver function tests Electrolytes Serum creatinine	Complete blood count Serum creatinine	Vancomycin levels Complete blood count Electrolytes Serum creatinine	Complete blood count Liver function tests	Complete blood count Liver function tests Electrolytes Serum creatinine	Complete blood count Liver function tests Electrolytes Serum creatinine
Contraindi-cations	Allergy to penicillin Allergy to corn	Allergy to cephalosp-orins	Allergy to vancomycin	Concurrent administration of calcium-containing IV solutions, including continuous calcium-containing infusions such as parenteral nutrition, in neonates (aged 28 days or less) Allergy to cephalosporins	Allergy to penicillin	Allergy to penicillin
Precautions	Hepatoxicity Acute renal failure Allergy to cephalosporins History of *C. difficile* colitis Warfarin therapy	Allergy to penicillin History of *C. difficile* colitis Warfarin therapy History of seizure	Concomitant nephrotoxic, ototoxic, and anesthetic drugs	Allergy to penicillin History of *C. difficile* colitis Warfarin therapy History of seizure Malnutrition Biliary stasis	Allergy to cephalosporins History of *C. difficile* colitis Warfarin therapy History of seizure	Allergy to cephalosporins History of *C. difficile* colitis Warfarin therapy History of seizure

Table 15-27 (*continued*)

	Nafcillin	Cefazolin	Vancomycin	Ceftriaxone	Piperacillin/ Tazobactam	Ampicillin/ Sulbactam
Major drug–drug interactions	Cyclosporine	None	None	Calcium-containing products and Ringer's solution in neonates	Methotrexate Vecuronium	None
Moderate drug–drug interactions	Warfarin Nifedipine	Warfarin Probenecid	Gentamicn Streptomycin Succinylcholine Warfarin	Cyclosporine Typhoid vaccine	Oral contraceptives Probenecid Warfarin	Oral contraceptives Probenecid Warfarin

such as *Staphylococcus aureus* and *Streptococcus. S. aureus* is especially common in patients with rheumatoid arthritis and intravenous drug users. Much as with osteomyelitis, however, a wide variety of pathogens can cause infection. Gram-negative infections are also common in intravenous drug abusers with septic arthritis, and *Neisseria gonorrhoeae* is a common cause in younger patients.

Signs and Symptoms

Patients will often present with symptoms including fever, along with joint pain and swelling that may limit joint motion. Infections of any joint is possible, although manifestations in the knee, hip, and wrist are most common. Lyme disease, arthritis, and gout are disease states where patients can present with similar symptoms and should be considered in the differential diagnosis.

Instruments and Techniques Related to Patient Assessment

Synovial fluid joint aspirations prior to antimicrobial therapy are a key component in diagnosing and guiding treatment of septic arthritis. Aspirated infected fluid often appears purulent with an elevated leukocyte count. Joint drainage is a necessary adjunct to antimicrobial therapy. Closed-needle aspiration is used in most cases, although septic arthritis cases involving the hip require open surgical drainage.

Laboratory Testing

Monitoring for clinical response involves demonstration of sterile fluid and a declining leukocyte count. The Gram stain is both a diagnostic tool and a therapy guide.

1.2.0 Pharmacotherapy

Initial empiric antimicrobial treatment should cover the most likely possible pathogens.

Drug Indications, Dosing, and Routes of Administration

Vancomycin is an appropriate first choice for therapy in patients with gram-positive cocci on a Gram stain of the aspirated synovial fluid. Vancomycin is also a good choice in patients without organisms present on Gram stain but with concomitant risk factors such as rheumatoid arthritis or systemic lupus erythematosus. Cefazolin and nafcillin are appropriate options for de-escalation from vancomycin if susceptibilities return in the form of methicillin-susceptible *S. aureus*.

Ceftriaxone and other third- or fourth-generation cephalosporins are common treatments if the Gram stain is positive for gram-negative organisms. Fluoroquinolones with gram-negative activity (i.e., ciprofloxacin or levofloxacin) are treatment options in patients with severe cephalosporin allergies. Combinations of vancomycin and ceftriaxone are often used in patients with negative Gram stains and a remaining high suspicion for septic arthritis. Table 15-27 provides information on medications commonly used to treat bone and joint infections, including septic arthritis and osteomyelitis.

1.3.0 Pharmacotherapy Monitoring

Patients should be educated on the potential adverse effects of their treatments, and specific counseling on the parameters of outpatient parenteral therapy may be needed if therapy will be delivered in the home setting. Additional monitoring (including therapeutic concentration monitoring) may be needed depending on the specific antibiotic and on any patient-specific disease–drug or drug–drug interactions. Food–drug interactions may become an issue if the patient is prescribed fluoroquinolone oral therapy.

As with many infectious disease states, clinical trial data on the specific duration of therapy for septic arthritis are lacking. Patients with septic arthritis caused by *S. aureus* and *Pseudomonas aeruginosa* are often treated for 4 weeks. If the infectious agent is susceptible to them, antimicrobial agents with high oral bioavailability are therapeutic options for oral therapy following a 2-week course of intravenous therapy.

The prognosis for septic arthritis is highly patient specific. Patients with preexisting joint disease, those with an infected joint containing synthetic material, elderly patients, and patients with infections caused by *S. aureus* tend to have a worse prognosis for complete recovery. Mortality rates are accentuated by immunosuppression, coexisting disease states, and age (in older patients). Mortality from this cause has been reported to range from 10 to 19%.

ANNOTATED BIBLIOGRAPHY

Berbari EF, Steckelberg JM, Osmon DR. Osteomyelitis. In Mandell GL, Bennett JE, Dolin R, ed. *Mandell, Douglas and Bennett's Principles and Practice of Infectious Disease,*. 6th ed. New York: Churchill and Livingstone; 2005;1322–1337., Eds

Gerding DN, Huges CE, Bamberger CM, et al. Extravascular antimicrobial distribution and the respective blood concentrations in humans. In: Larian V, ed. *Antibiotics in Laboratory Medicine,* 4th ed. Baltimore: Williams & Wilkins; 1996:835–899.

Kaandorp CJE, Kriknen P, Moens HJB, et al. The outcome of bacterial arthritis: a prospective community-based study. *Arthritis Rheum* 1997;40:884.

Kaandorp CJE, van Schaardenburg D, Krijnen P, et al. Risk factors for septic arthritis in patients with joint disease. *Arthritis Rheum* 1995;38:1819–1825.

Lipinsky BA, Berendt AR, Derry HG, et al. Diagnosis and treatment of diabetic foot infections. *Clin Infect Dis* 2004;39:885–910.

Ross JJ, Saltzman CL, Carling P, Shapiro DS. Pneumococcal septic arthritis: review of 190 cases. *Clin Infect Dis* 2003;36:319.

Ross JJ. Septic arthritis. *Infect Dis Clin N Am* 2005;19: 799–817.

TOPIC: FUNGAL INFECTIONS

Section Coordinator: Michael Klepser
Contributors: Scott J. Bergman, Michaela M. Doss, and Halley Connor-Hustedde

---

Tips Worth Tweeting

- Pathogenic fungi can be divided into general categories of molds, yeasts, and dermatophytes
- Some fungi can change their morphology depending on their environment.
- Recognition of fungal infections can be challenging because only some will appear on the Gram stain of routine cultures performed in clinical microbiology laboratories.
- The cell walls of fungi consist of a chitin and/or cellulose; these elements are identified with special tests and different types of stains.
- Typically, blood cultures must be incubated for at least 24 hours before fungal growth is detected. Usually only yeasts are identified with this technique.
- Identification of a specific organism may occur while the sample is grown on agar, but only after at least 48 to 72 hours.
- Speciation and susceptibility testing of fungus is not always performed by clinical laboratories unless there is a special request for such information, because it can be technically difficult to obtain.
- Amphotericin B can be used to treat almost every fungal infection. Nevertheless, because of its side effects, this agent is usually reserved for the most serious or refractory cases.
- Voriconazole is a drug of choice for *Aspergillus* infection.
- Itraconazole is effective for infections involving endemic dimorphic fungi.
- Fluconazole has predictable pharmacokinetics and is active against most *Candida* species.
- Posaconazole has a broad spectrum of activity, but at this time is approved only for prevention of fungal infections. Echinocandins such as caspofungin are well tolerated and used for both *Candida* and *Aspergillus* infections.
- Dermatophyte infections can be treated with topical azoles or terbinafine depending on their severity. Cryptococcal meningitis should be treated with amphotericin B plus flucytosine, followed by fluconazole for a total of at least 10 weeks.
- Molds such as *Aspergillus*, Zygomycetes, *Fusarium,* and *Scedosporium* species grow in branch-like patterns and have filamentous extensions called hyphae.
- Yeasts are round in shape and tend to gather together in colonies. *Candida* and *Cryptococcus* are examples of pathogenic yeasts.
- Dermatophytes are fungi that live on skin and can cause superficial infections.
- Fungal treatment should be based on the most likely infectious organism; its susceptibility pattern; drug properties, including distribution to the site of infection and interaction potential; and patient-specific factors such as renal or hepatic disease.

Patient Care Scenario: Community Setting

K. T. is a 26-year-old female who presents to the community pharmacy where you work with a 3-day history of vaginal itching and painful urination. She tells you that this is the second time she has experienced this problem, and that her doctor told her she had a vaginal yeast infection when she experienced similar symptoms.

Molds

Aspergillus is a ubiquitous hyaline mold capable of causing a variety of both invasive and noninvasive infections as well as allergic bronchopulmonary aspergillosis (ABPA). Clinically significant infections are most commonly caused by *A. fumigatus, A. flavus, A. niger,* and *A. terreus. Aspergillus* typically enters the human body through inhalation and proceeds to invade the lung or paranasal sinuses, thereby causing respiratory disease. *Aspergillus* can disseminate to various organs or the CNS via hematogenous spread.

1.1.0 Patient Information

Disease States Associated with Aspergillus *Infections*

Although *Aspergillus* infections occasionally occur in otherwise healthy individuals, patients who are immunocompromised are at highest risk because of their impaired phagocyte and macrophage function.

Signs and Symptoms

Patients with *Aspergillus* infection commonly present with chest pain, fever, hemoptysis, and dyspnea.

Laboratory Testing

A definitive diagnosis by biopsy or positive culture from a sterile site is required for *Aspergillus* infections. Other diagnostic measures, such as the galactomannan antigen blood test, CT scans, and bronchial alveolar lavage (BAL), may assist in identifying the infection as well. Surgical removal of fungal balls, called aspergillomas, in the lungs is required for the optimal outcome. Species identification and drug susceptibilities should be requested when possible, as antifungal therapy has the potential to be toxic and ineffective. Because *Aspergillus* is a slow-growing and difficult-to-treat fungus, therapy needs to be continued for 6–12 weeks or even longer if immunosuppression continues.

1.2.0 Pharmacotherapy

Voriconazole is recommended as first-line therapy for invasive *Aspergillus* infections.

Mechanism of Action

Voriconazole is a broad-spectrum triazole antifungal that, like all agents in the class, increases ergosterol synthesis and inhibits fungal cells' membrane development.

Drug Indications, Dosing Regimens, and Routes of Administration

The typical dose for invasive fungal infections is 6 mg/kg intravenously (IV) every 12 hours × 2 doses, followed by 4 mg/kg IV every 12 hours. The oral dose is 200 mg orally every 12 hours in a tablet or suspension.

Physiochemical Properties, Solubility, Pharmacodynamics, and Pharmacokinetic Properties

The route of administration may be switched to an oral formulation as tolerated, as voriconazole has very high bioavailability. It is best to take the oral medication at least 1 hour before or after meals, as this practice will increase absorption. Unlike other azole antifungals, voriconazole does not require an acidic environment in the stomach for optimal absorption. This agent possesses 96% oral bioavailability, has 58% protein binding with a Vd = 4.6 L/kg, and undergoes extensive liver metabolism via CYP 2C19, 2C9 and 3A4. The half-life is dose dependent due to the nonlinear pharmacokinetics of the drug. Wide interpatient variability in serum concentrations occurs, so therapeutic drug monitoring may be necessary in some situations. The proposed therapeutic range in severely ill patients is approximately 2–6 mcg/mL.

1.3.0 Monitoring

Contraindications, Warnings, and Precautions

After the loading dose is complete, administration of the IV formulation of voriconazole should be avoided in patients with moderate to severe renal insufficiency (CrCl < 50 mL/min). This is due to the accumulation of a cyclodextrin carrier vehicle that could potentially result in toxicity. Additionally, this medication should not be used in patients with severe hepatic insufficiency.

Adverse Drug Reactions

Visual disturbances and hallucinations are common adverse drug reactions (ADRs) experienced with voriconazole use, especially when it is given at high concentrations. Other serious ADRs include prolonged QT syndrome, torsades de pointes, Stevens-Johnson syndrome, toxic epidermal necrolysis, pancreatitis, and anaphylactoid reactions.

Interactions with Drugs, Foods, and Laboratory Tests

Any medication metabolized by CYP 2C19, 2C9, or 3A4 may be altered by voriconazole (e.g., cyclosporin, tacrolimus, sirolimus, efavirenz, phenytoin). Contraindications include use of carbamazepine, CYP3A4 substrates (terfenadine, astemizole, cisapride, pimozide, quinidine), ergot alkaloids, long-acting barbiturates, rifabutin, rifampin, high-dose ritonovir, sirolimus, and St. John's wort. Precautions for use include proarrhythmic conditions (monitor with electrocardiograms), concomitant use of efavirenz or ritonovir, hypersensitivity to other azole antifungals, hepatic insufficiency, and renal dysfunction.

1.2.0 Pharmacotherapy

Drug Indications, Dosing Regimens, and Routes of Administration

Fluconazole and ketoconazole are considered clinically ineffective for aspergillosis, but other triazole antifungals—namely, itraconazole and posaconazole—have been used to treat *Aspergillus* infections. Unfortunately, they have little value in cases resistant to voriconazole. Posaconazole was approved by the Food and Drug Administration (FDA) for prophylaxis of patients at high risk of fungal infections in 2006. It is available in oral suspension only, and the dosing is 200 mg three times per day for this indication. For treatment of *Aspergillus* infections, 200 mg four times daily has been recommended, followed by 400 mg twice daily when the patient is stable.

Physiochemical Properties, Solubility, Pharmacodynamics, and Pharmacokinetic Properties

Posaconazole has dose-dependent oral bioavailability, which limits its absorption at high doses and prevents a high load from being given. An IV formulation does not yet exist because of the agent's water insolubility. Both areas under the curve and maximum concentration averages are increased when posaconazole is administered with a high-fat meal as compared with the fasted state. Before being excreted in feces, posaconazole is not metabolized but still strongly inhibits CYP3A4 because its mechanism of action interferes with CYP450-dependent fungal growth.

1.3.0 Monitoring

Contraindications, Warnings, and Precautions

Posaconazole is contraindicated with concomitant use of sirolimus, ergot alkaloids, and the CYP3A4 substrates terfenadine, astemizole, cisapride, pimozide, halofantrine, and quinidine. Hepatic reactions have been reported, so monitoring of liver function tests is recommended with use of posaconazole. In addition, QTc may be prolonged, so monitoring with frequent electrocardiograms and serum electrolyte levels is recommended.

1.2.0 Pharmacotherapy

Amphotericin B (AmB) is a well-studied alternative to voriconazole for treatment of *Aspergillus* infections.

Mechanism of Action

Amphotericin B acts by binding to sterols in the fungal cell membrane. This binding produces a change in membrane permeability, thereby allowing leakage of intracellular components and cell death.

Drug Indications, Dosing Regimens, and Routes of Administration

Amphotericin is available in both conventional and lipid-based formulations. The original deoxycholate formulation is usually dosed at 0.7 mg/kg/day IV, but 1–1.5 mg/kg/day can be used for *Aspergillus* infection. Doses exceeding 1.5 mg/kg place the patient at risk for potentially fatal cardiac or cardiorespiratory arrest.

Interaction with Drugs, Foods, and Laboratory Tests

All formulations of amphotericin B should be compounded in dextrose 5% solution. Sodium chloride–containing solutions should not be used, as precipitation may occur. Formulations of amphotericin B are *not* interchangeable with one another, and verification of the formulation to be administered is essential to prevent harmful medication errors.

1.3.0 Monitoring

Adverse Drug Reactions

Common ADRs with amphotericin B are nephrotoxicity, hypokalemia, hypomagnesemia, hypocalcemia, hypotension, and rash, plus acute infusion reactions including anaphylaxis, headache, dizziness, seizure, and asthenia. For patients who experience other infusion-related reactions such as fever, chills, hypotension, or nausea with amphotericin B, a premedication regimen consisting of acetaminophen plus diphenhydramine or hydrocortisone may be administered. Meperidine has also been used in patients experiencing rigors during the infusion. It is important for patients to be adequately hydrated prior to amphotericin B infusion to reduce the agent's nephrotoxicity. A bolus of normal saline (250 mL over 2 hours) immediately preceding the dose is recommended. Generally, amphotericin B lipid formulations dosed at 3–5 mg/kg/day IV are preferred because they are considered less nephrotoxic and better tolerated compared to the conventional amphotericin B formulation.

Contraindications, Warnings, and Precautions

Use of amphotericin B with other nephrotoxic medications should be avoided if possible, and close monitoring of serum electrolytes is necessary. Although the medication is not widely eliminated via the kidneys, dose adjustments are crucial for patients with renal impairment because of the high risk of nephrotoxicity.

Physiochemical Properties, Solubility, Pharmacodynamics, and Pharmacokinetic Properties

Amphotericin B engages in significant drug interactions with digoxin and cyclosporine, and toxicity from these medications can result due to their concentrations being increased.

1.2.0 Pharmacotherapy

The echinocandins are an antifungal class that can be used for salvage therapy in *Aspergillus* infections if other medications are not tolerated or simply cannot be used. Although only caspofungin is FDA approved for treatment of invasive *Aspergillosis* infections, micafungin and anidulafungin may also be useful.

Mechanism of Action

These agents act by inhibiting β (1,3)-d-glucan synthase, an essential component of fungal cell walls. Because of their large molecular size, these agents come only in IV formulations.

Drug Indications, Dosing Regimens, and Routes of Administration

Caspofungin is dosed 70 mg on day 1, followed by 50 mg daily for all indications. No adjustment is needed for any of the echinocandins in renal impairment, although caspofungin doses should be adjusted in patients with moderate hepatic impairment (i.e., a Child-Pugh score of 7–9). The recommended dose in this population is 70 mg on day 1, then 35 mg daily. Patients with severe liver failure have not been studied sufficiently as candidates for caspofungin or micafungin treatment, but anidulafungin can be used safely in this group.

Physiochemical Properties, Solubility, Pharmacodynamics, and Pharmacokinetic Properties

Caspofungin is highly protein bound (97% to albumin) and achieves extensive tissue distribution.

1.3.0 Monitoring

Adverse Effects

Adverse effects with echinocandins are uncommon and generally mild, including hypotension, rash, diarrhea, increased levels of hepatic liver transaminases, fever, and shivering. Other serious ADRs, such as pancreatitis, liver failure, septic shock, and respiratory complications, have been reported as well.

Monitoring of liver transaminases is recommended during therapy, although changes in this biomarker are usually minimal compared to the triazole antifungals.

Interaction with Drugs, Foods, and Laboratory Tests

Concomitant use of caspofungin with cyclosporine generally is not recommended due to the combination's potential to result in a large increase in liver function tests and drug interactions. Tacrolimus levels have been found to be decreased when administered with caspofungin, so monitoring serum levels of tacrolimus is necessary to ensure appropriate therapeutic effects. Caspofungin should be diluted only with normal saline—not with dextrose-containing solutions. Because of the high mortality rate associated with aspergillosis even with current treatments, combination therapy with voriconazole plus an echinocandin or liposomal amphotericin B is being studied, but insufficient data exist to fully recommend this combination.

Dimorphic Fungi

Histoplasma capsulatum, Blastomyces dermatitides, and *Coccidioides immitis* are referred to as endemic dimorphic fungi because they are molds found in the environment of different regions of the world; when these organisms are aerosolized (into conidia) and enter the human body, however, they germinate and convert to yeasts. The yeast form tends to reside in the pulmonary cavity where it entered the body through inhalation.

1.1.0 Patient Information

Signs and Symptoms

A patient who is exposed to dimorphic fungi could develop an infectious process in the lungs or remain asymptomatic for years. Some patients might present with pulmonary or systemic symptoms, but many others might not even know they are colonized depending on their immune status. Hematogenous dissemination of yeasts may also allow these fungi to reach numerous other organs in the body, where development of granulomatous lesions can take place.

Diseases States and Conditions Associated with Dimorphic Fungi

Dimorphic fungal infection occurs more often in immunocompromised patients and can be seen on radiographic images. *H. capsulatum* is endemic to the Ohio and Mississippi River valleys in the United States, whereas *Blastomyces* tends to be endemic in the southeastern United States and Great Lakes region. In contrast, *Coccidioides* is typically found in the southwestern United States. Disruption of soil is responsible for many outbreaks involving endemic, dimorphic fungi, especially *Cocciciodes*. Bat and bird droppings accelerate sporulation of *Histoplasma* and facilitate the spread of this organism into new habitats.

1.2.0 Pharmacotherapy

Drug Indications, Dosing Regimens, and Routes of Administration

Treatment for histoplasmosis should be initiated for patients who experience hypoxemia or who have illness lasting greater than 1 month. For moderate to severe cases, therapy with amphotericin B (preferably the liposomal formulation) should be initiated for 1–2 weeks. Treatment with itraconazole 200 mg po daily should then follow for a total of 12 weeks. For chronic pulmonary disease, itraconazole 200 mg po once or twice daily for at least 12 months is recommended. Itraconazole is now available only in an oral formulation, as the IV version has been discontinued. A loading dose of 200 mg every 8 hours for three doses can be attempted to reach a steady state faster. This consideration is especially important if the patient is being treated for aspergillosis or other serious infections.

Physiochemical Properties, Solubility, Pharmacodynamics, and Pharmacokinetic Properties

Itraconazole capsules require an acidic environment for absorption, and it is recommended that they be taken with food. The oral suspension, in contrast, should be taken in a fasting state, as it has a cyclodextrin carrier. Because itraconazole absorption varies, therapeutic drug monitoring can be performed. Serum trough concentrations of greater than 0.5 mcg/mL after 7 days of therapy have been associated with success. Itraconazole undergoes extensive liver metabolism by CYP3A4 and has many significant drug interactions.

1.3.0 Monitoring

Contraindications, Warnings, and Precautions

Contraindications for itraconazole include use of medications that are metabolized by CYP3A4 (e.g., cisapride, dofetilide, ergot alkaloids, HMG CoA-reductase inhibitors, oral midazolam, nisoldipine, pimozide, quinidine, and triazolam). Proceed with caution in patients with congestive heart failure because of the negative inotropic effect associated with itraconazole. Hepatic insufficiency is a relative contraindication as well. Common ADRs include rash, hypokalemia, and GI upset.

1.2.0 Pharmacotherapy

Drug Indications, Dosing Regimens, and Routes of Administration

Although posaconazole is not yet FDA indicated for infections caused by *Histoplasma,* in vivo tests have demonstrated that this agent has good activity against this organism. As a consequence, posaconazole has been used as salvage therapy in dimorphic fungal infections. Fluconazole and ketoconazole have been used to treat *Histoplasma* but are less effective than itraconazole.

The suggested ketoconazole dosing is 200 mg po once daily, but for serious infections it may be increased to 400 mg po daily.

Interaction with Drugs, Foods, and Laboratory Tests

Such an acidic environment is required for proper absorption that ketoconazole should be administered with a cola beverage. Concomitant use of antacids, histamine-2 receptor blockers, or proton pump inhibitors should be delayed until 2 hours after ketoconazole administration—or preferably not given at all. Many significant drug interactions also occur with ketoconazole, as this agent inhibits CYP 1A2, 2A6, 2C9, 2C19, 2D6, and 3A4. Medications that are metabolized through these pathways or are substrates should be evaluated for interaction potential. Concomitant use of terfenadine, astemizole, and cisapride is contraindicated with ketoconazole because of the risk of increased QT prolongation, torsades de pointes, ventricular tachycardia, ventricular fibrillation, and other serious cardiovascular events. Use with triazolam is also contraindicated.

1.3.0 Monitoring

Contraindications, Warnings, and Precautions

Along with its poor oral absorption, another reason why ketoconazole is not readily used for dimorphic fungal infections is that it has been associated with hepatic toxicities. Given this relationship, liver transaminases must be closely monitored during treatment.

Adverse Effects

Adverse effects associated with ketoconazole use include nausea, vomiting, diarrhea, pruritus, hypersensitivity reactions, and hepatotoxicity. No dose adjustment is needed for renal impairment, although dose reductions should be considered in those patients with severe liver disease, as ketoconazole undergoes significant liver metabolism.

1.2.0 Pharmacotherapy

Drug Indications, Dosing Regimens, and Routes of Administration

Similar regimens of amphotericin B and itraconazole are followed for the treatment of *Blastomyces* and *Coccidioides* infections. Fluconazole is active against endemic dimorphic fungi but has a limited role in the treatment of dimorphic fungal infections because studies have reported greater relapse rates when this agent is used than with itraconazole treatment. Clinically, fluconazole is used for *Coccidiodes* because of its more predictable pharmacokinetics and its usefulness in CNS infections due to its enhanced penetration of the blood–brain barrier as compared to the other azoles. Likewise, voriconazole is able to achieve adequate CNS concentrations and, therefore, is also an alternative agent, but it has less activity for dimorphic fungi. Some patients may require lifelong suppression with an azole following infection with dimorphic fungi if immunosuppression cannot be reversed.

1.3.0 Monitoring

Azoles should never be used in pregnant women, as they are teratogenic.

Dermatophytes

Infection of the skin or nail can be caused by the dermatophytic fungi known as *Trichophyton, Epidermophyton,* and *Microsporum*. These organisms cause several common superficial infections that affect various regions of the body.

1.1.0 Patient Information

Infections caused by dermatophytes include tinea pedis (athlete's foot), tinea cruris (jock itch), tinea mannum (hands), tinea corporis (trunk and extremities), tinea capitis (scalp hair follicles), and tinea barbae (facial hair follicles). No matter which variant of tinea occurs, all of these infections are treated similarly.

1.2.0 Pharmacotherapy

Mechanism of Action

Terbinafine (Lamisil) is an allylamine that inhibits the biosynthesis of ergosterol in the fungal cell membrane.

Drug Indications, Dosing Regimens, and Routes of Administration

For fingernail infections, the required dose of terbinafine is 250 mg po × 6 weeks.

For toenail infections, the duration of therapy is extended to 12 weeks. Topical imidazoles (such as ketoconazole, clotrimazole, econazole, and miconazole), tolnaftate, or allylamines (terbinafine and butenafine) are all recommended first-line treatments for dermatophyte infections. In general, topical therapy should continue for 2–4 weeks. One week of an allylamine administered twice daily, however, is equivalent to 2 weeks of a once-daily imidazole or 2 weeks of a twice-daily imidazole. If systemic therapy is needed because of refractory infection, fluconazole 150 mg once per week × 1–4 weeks, itraconazole 200–400 mg/day × 1 week, ketoconazole 200 mg daily × 4 weeks, and terbinafine 250 mg/day × 2 weeks are all therapeutic options. In some cases of tinea capitis, an antifungal shampoo such as ketoconazole is indicated in addition to oral therapy. Mild topical steroids such as hydrocortisone may be used for severe cases of inflammation, but care should be taken not to use such a medication for more than a few days, as infection can spread due to the steroid's immunosuppressive properties.

Onchomycosis, or tinea unguium, is an infection of the nails that may affect either fingers or toes. Infections involving the toenails typically require longer treatment as compared to infections of the fingernails. The treatment of choice for onchomycosis is systemic therapy with terbinafine; itraconazole is an alternative.

Terbinafine is supplied in a variety of formulations, including tablets, oral granules, and a topical solution or cream. As an alternative, itraconazole is recommended to be dosed in twice daily for 1 week per month (a "pulse") or once daily continuously for 2–4 months. In addition to terbinafine and itraconazole, ciclopirax (Penlac) nail lacquer is a treatment option for onchyomycosis, albeit a less effective one. This topical antifungal is applied evenly over the nail and surrounding skin at bedtime (must allow 8 hours before washing). Applications may be made over the previous coat for 7 days, but after that the lacquer should be removed with alcohol and the cycle should be restarted.

1.3.0 Monitoring

Contraindications, Warnings, and Precautions

Terbinafine is not recommended in patients with renal impairment (CrCl < 50 mL/min) or in patients with chronic or active liver disease. Due to this agent's rapid and extensive liver metabolism, monitoring of liver transaminases throughout the course of therapy is important.

Adverse Effects

Adverse effects noted with this medication may include headache, fever, rash, diarrhea, vomiting, nausea, increased liver enzymes, nasopharyngitis, and nasal congestion. Reports of acute pancreatitis, severe dermatological reactions (Stevens-Johnson syndrome and toxic epidermal necrolysis), pancytopenia, neutropenia, hepatic failure, exacerbation of lupus erythematosus, and ocular changes have been noted.

Patients with onchyomycosis may experience a burning sensation, irritation, redness, and shape or color change of nail when they use ciclopirax. This medication is most often used in patients with hepatic dysfunction or adverse reactions to both terbinafine and itraconazole.

Interaction with Drugs, Foods, and Laboratory Tests

Terbinafine is a strong CYP2D6 inhibitor as well as a weak CYP3A4 inducer; therefore, it has the potential for significant drug interactions. Some CYP2D6 interactions have been noted with atomoxetine, codeine, nebivolol, tamoxifen, thioridazine, tramadol, and tricyclic antidepressants. When administered with terbinafine, rifampin has a 100% increased clearance rate.

Yeasts

Candida Infections

Most people are familiar with *Candida albicans* and its associated conditions, as this organism is part of normal skin, gastrointestinal tract, and females' vaginal flora. *Candida* yeasts are unicellular, thin-walled organisms that reproduce by budding. Many species of *Candida* exist, all of which have morphological similarities, though they can have differing susceptibility patterns. The most common species that cause disease in humans are *C. albicans, C. glabrata, C. parapsilosis,* and *C. tropicalis*. Many other species also exist, such as *C. krusei, C. dubliniensis, C. guillermondii,* and *C. lusitaniae*; these variants cause only 1–2% of invasive infections, however.

Candida infections can range in severity from a very mild vaginal candidiasis to a life-threatening candidemia (infection of the blood). Typically, *Candida* come from an endogenous source and infections are precipitated by disruption of normal flora.

When patients develop *Candida* infections, the symptoms vary immensely depending on the organs involved. For example, a patient with vaginal candidiasis might have itching and burning in the affected area, while a patient with candidemia is likely to develop sepsis-like symptoms such as fever, tachycardia, tachypnea, and hypotension. If the *Candida* infection is isolated to only one site, such as a catheter, the patient may be asymptomatic.

Patients at risk for *Candida* bloodstream infections include not only those who are immunosuppressed and have taken broad-spectrum antibiotics, but also patients with indwelling catheters. *Candida* has a propensity to stick to medical devices and form biofilms that are difficult to eradicate. Patients with diabetes, those receiving total parenteral nutrition, and patients on long-term corticosteroid therapy are at increased risk of candidemia due to elevated glucose levels circulating in their blood and neutrophil dysfunction. Patients without intact integumentary systems are also at high risk for such infections because their first line of containment defense is damaged and they often receive broad-spectrum antibiotics that select out yeast.

When treating patients for invasive *Candida* infections, it is important to remember that if venous and urinary catheters are not removed, it is unlikely the patient will improve with antifungal therapy.

1.1.0 Patient Information

Disease States and Conditions Associated with Candida *Infections*

Antibiotic use is a major contributing factor to vaginal candidiasis, because such therapy means that beneficial bacteria that are part of the normal flora are killed and balance is disrupted, thereby allowing *C. albicans* overgrowth. Vaginal candidiasis is more common in specific disease states such as diabetes, pregnancy, obesity, and HIV/AIDS, all of which are favorable conditions for the yeast to grow.

Signs and Symptoms

The typical symptoms of *Candida* infection upon presentation include itching, white clumpy discharge, vulvovaginal tenderness or redness, pain with intercourse, and pain with urination. In most cases, patients can safely treat vaginal candidiasis with topical over-the-counter (OTC) products, given that prescription treatments are no more effective than the OTC therapies. However, there are certain circumstances that warrant seeking a physician's opinion. Referral to a physician is advisable if it is the patient's first yeast infection, if the patient is pregnant, or if sexually transmitted diseases are suspected. Recurrent vaginal yeast infections are concerning because contributing factors may go unresolved if the patient self-treats each infection.

It is important to remember several points when counseling patients on the use of OTC yeast infection products. First, ask patients if they have had a yeast infection previously. If it is their first occurrence, they should seek medical attention to rule out other causes. If the patient has diabetes or is immunocompromised, then the scenario is considered a complicated yeast infection. It is still reasonable to use an OTC product in such patients, but the infection should be treated for no less than 7 days. In these cases, 10–14 days of therapy is ideal. Also, let the patient know that uncontrolled blood glucose is a risk factor for yeast infection, so they should notify their physician about improving their underlying disease.

Topical products work better if applied at bedtime so that they have more time to act at the site of infection. An important point to stress to patients is avoidance of vaginal penetration throughout the course of treatment—including both sexual intercourse and tampon use. Avoidance of tight clothing and nylon or silk underwear can help prevent new infections.

1.2.0 Pharmacotherapy

Vaginal candidiasis can be treated with nonprescription topical azole antifungals such as butoconazole, clotrimazole, miconazole, and ticonazole for 1–7 days, depending on the potency. Prescription creams such as nystatin and terconazole also exist, but their efficacy is no better than that of the cheaper OTC alternatives. A one-time dose of oral fluconazole 150 mg can also be used if it is more convenient for the patient. For refractory cases, fluconazole may need to be given weekly.

1.3.0 Pharmacotherapy Monitoring

The only side effects of topical products for vaginal candidiasis are occasional burning, stinging, or irritation.

Oropharyngeal Candidiasis

Oropharyngeal candidiasis—commonly referred to as oral thrush—is also caused by *C. albicans*. The risk factors for oral candidiasis are very similar to the risk factors for vaginal candidiasis. Those persons with previous antibiotic exposure or in an immunocompromised state are at the highest risk for developing this type of infection. An additional risk factor to consider with oral candidiasis is inhaled corticosteroids.

Table 15-28 Products Available for Treatment of Vaginal Candidiasis

Generic Product Name	Common Brand Names
Butoconazole nitrate (available as cream)	Mycelex-3
Clotrimazole (available as cream, tablet)	Gyne-Lotrimin 7, Mycelex-7, Gyne-Lotrimin 3
Miconazole (available as cream, suppository)	Monistat 1, Monistat 3, Monistat 7, Femizole-M, M-zole 3, M-zole 7
Ticonazole (available as ointment)	Vagistat-1
Prescription-Only Products	
Terconazole (available as cream, suppository)	Terazol 7, Terazol 3, Zazole
Fluconazole (available as tablet, suspension, IV solution)	Diflucan 150 mg × 1

1.1.0 Patient Information

With oropharyngeal candidiasis, the yeast may appear in spots or patches upon the throat, tongue, cheeks, or borders of the mouth. It is usually yellowish to white in appearance, and has a fluffy or chunky texture. Much like the case with vaginal candidiasis, the mucosa may appear irritated and inflamed, and the patient may experience tenderness.

Oral candidiasis should not be treated with OTC medications or remedies. Patients with recent chemotherapy exposure, HIV/AIDS, or other immunocompromising factors should seek prompt medical attention, because the yeast could spread to the bloodstream.

1.2.0 Pharmacotherapy

Oral thrush often responds to clotrimazole troches or nystatin suspensions, both of which can target the infection locally. Nevertheless, systemic treatment with fluconazole 200 mg daily is recommended for immunosuppressed patients. This group has a high relapse rate, and difficulty swallowing can occur. In this scenario, an alternative IV therapy, such as one of the echinocandins or amphotericin B, may be needed in severe cases.

Candida species differ in their susceptibilities to antifungal agents, so identification of the precise organism is clinically important for appropriate treatment. Nearly 100% of *Candida albicans, C. parapsilosis*, and *C. tropicalis* remain susceptible to fluconazole and the rest of the azole antifungals. Roughly 50% of all invasive *Candida* infections are due to *C. albicans*, 20% to *C. parapsilosis*, and 10% to *C. tropicalis*, although not all institutions have similar rates. In contrast, *C. krusei* is known to have resistance inherently to fluconazole, and some *C. glabrata* (20%) have developed such resistance over time. Amphotericin B (preferably a lipid formulation) is an alternative to fluconazole with these species are involved in infections, but some resistance exists in some of the same species, as well as in *C. lusitaniae*. The echinocandins can be used to treat these fluconazole-resistant *Candida* species instead. Current guidelines recommend these medications for initial treatment of critically ill or neutropenic patients suspected of having invasive candidiasis. *Candida parapsilosis*, however, has shown decreased susceptibility to the otherwise broad-spectrum echinocandin class, so caution should be used when treating infections involving this species.

Drug Indications, Dosing Regimens, and Routes of Administration

The dose of caspofungin for invasive candidiasis is the same as for aspergillosis: 70 mg × 1, then 50 mg daily. Micafungin 100 mg daily has been shown to be equivalent to caspofungin and liposomal amphotericin B, while anidulafungin 200 mg × 1, then 100 mg, compares favorably to fluconazole.

Fluconazole is an effective therapy that is recommended in patients with less serious disease. Because echinocandins are only available via the IV route, fluconazole is a logical oral step-down therapy for clinically stable patients with susceptible species. For candidemia, a one-time loading dose of fluconazole 800 mg (or 12 mg/kg), followed by 400 mg (or 6 mg/kg) daily, is recommended. Fluconazole has more predictable pharmacokinetics than other azole antifungals, and its absorption is not affected by stomach acidity. This agent also has fewer significant drug interactions because CYP3A4 is disrupted only when it is given at high doses. Fluconazole primarily inhibits CYP2C9 and CYP2C19, instead of CYP3A4. It is generally well tolerated, but hepatic transamines can become elevated while patients are receiving therapy.

Cryptococcal Infections

Cryptococcus neoformans is an encapsulated yeast responsible for causing the systemic disease known as cryptococcosis. This organism is found in pigeon droppings and soil everywhere, from which it is then transmitted through inhalation. Dissemination from the lungs into the CNS is the most common route of *C. neoformans* infection. Other regions of dissemination include skin and bone marrow.

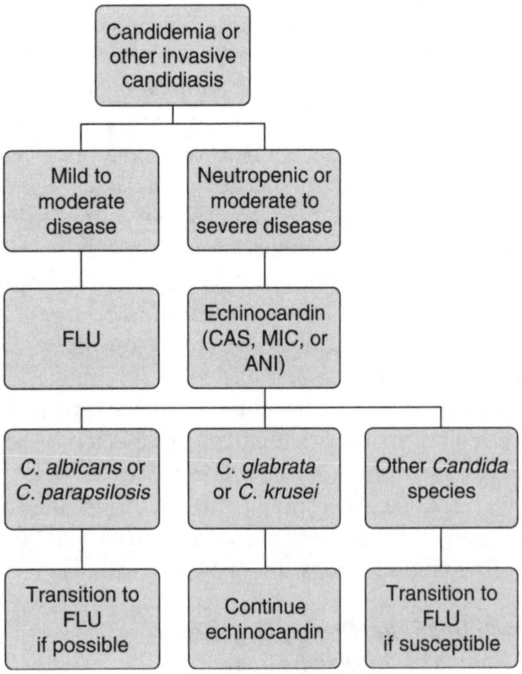

Figure 15-1 Treatment of Candidemia and Invasive Candidiasis
FLU = fluconazole; CAS = caspofungin; MIC = micafungin; ANI = anidulafungin. Refer to text for dosing.
Note: Amphotericin B (lipid formulation) is a valid alternative to echinocandins. All patients with recent azole exposure should be started on an echinocandin or amphotericin B.

1.1.0 Patient Information

Signs and Symptoms

Patients are rarely symptomatic when first infected with *C. neoformans* because this yeast does not release harmful toxins, and minimal inflammatory responses occur. However, the organism is not easily killed by phagocytosis due to its resistant polysaccharide capsule. Rates of clinically significant infections have risen in recent years due an increased number of immunocompromised hosts.

1.2.0 Pharmacotherapy

Drug Indications, Dosing Regimens, and Routes of Administration

Treatment of pulmonary infection may not be necessary if patients are asymptomatic, but for mild to moderate disease, oral fluconazole 200–400 mg can be used. In more severe cases or whenever there is dissemination to the CNS, amphotericin B 0.7 mg/kg/day is recommended. For more rapid eradication of the infection from the CNS, flucytosine (5-FC) should be added if possible. Flucystosine is an oral thymidine analog that inhibits DNA synthesis after being taken into cells by a fungal specific enzyme. For patients with normal renal function, flucytosine 100 mg/kg/day should be divided in four equal doses.

In patients who are intolerant of amphotericin B, combinations of fluconazole plus flucytosine have been studied but are not preferred. After patients are treated for cryptococcal with 2 weeks of induction therapy, a consolidation period can take place with fluconazole 400–800 mg/day for a minimum of 8 weeks. Refractory disease may need intrathecal or intraventricular doses of amphotericin B (usually 0.5 mg) instilled into the brain before resolution occurs. Suppressive therapy after infection with fluconazole 200–400 mg is standard as long as patients are immunocompromised. This secondary prophylaxis is especially important in HIV-positive patients because relapse rates are very high in this group.

1.3.0 Pharmacotherapy Monitoring

Adverse Effects

Flucystosine is related to the cancer chemotherapy agent 5-fluorouracil (5-FU) and, therefore, can cause bone marrow suppression at higher doses. Otherwise, it is well tolerated, but resistance develops quickly in fungi if it is used alone.

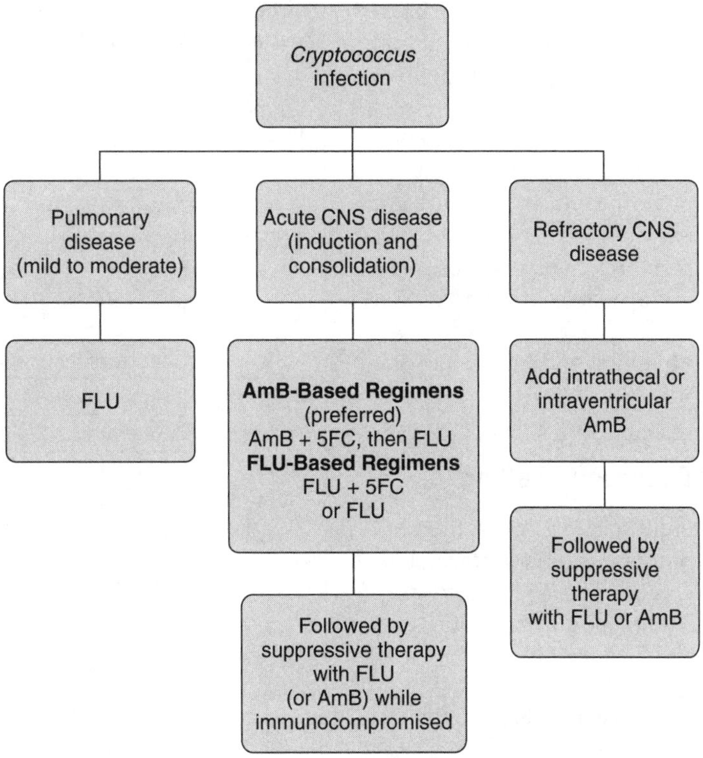

Figure 15-2 Treatment of Cryptococcal Infections
CNS = central nervous system; FLU = fluconazole; 5FC = flucytosine; AmB = amphotericin B. Refer to text for dosing.

ANNOTATED BIBLIOGRAPHY

Berardi RR, Kroon LA, McDermott JH, et al. Vaginal and vulvovaginal disorders. In *Handbook of Nonprescription Drugs*. Minneapolis: APhA Publications; 2006.

Brown T, Chin T. Superficial fungal infections. In DiPiro JT, Talbert RL, Yee GC, eds. *Pharmacotherapy: A Pathophysiologic Approach*. New York: McGraw-Hill Medical; 2008. 1957–1972

Carver P. Invasive fungal infections. In DiPiro JT, Talbert RL, Yee GC, eds. *Pharmacotherapy: A Pathophysiologic Approach*. New York: McGraw-Hill Medical; 2008. 1973–2002

Chapman SW, Dismukes WE, Proia LA, et al. Clinical practice guidelines for the management of blastomycosis: 2008 update by the Infectious Disease Society of America. *Clin Infect Dis* 2008;46:1801–1812.

Galgiani JN, Ampel NM, Blair JE, et al. Coccidioidomycosis. *Clin Infect Dis* 2005;41:1217–1223.

Pappas PG, et al. Infectious Diseases Society of America. Clinical practice guidelines for the management of candidiasis: 2009 update by the Infectious Diseases Society of America. *Clin Infect Dis* 2009;48:503–535.

Perfect JR, et al. Clinical practice guidelines for the management of cryptococcal disease: 2010 update by the Infectious Diseases Society of America. *Clin Infect Dis* 2010;50(3):291–322.

Walsh TJ, Anaissie EJ, Denning DW, et al. Treatment of aspergillosis: clinical practice guidelines of the Infectious Diseases Society of America. *Clin Infect Dis* 2008;46:327–360.

Wheat JL, Freifeld AG, Kleiman MB, et al. Clinical practice guidelines for the management of patients with histoplasmosis: 2007 update by the Infectious Disease Society of America. *Clin Infect Dis* 2007;45:807–825.

TOPIC: HIV/AIDS

Section Coordinator: *Michael Klepser*
Contributors: *Nathan Everson, Jean C. Lee, and H. Stephen Lee*

Tips Worth Tweeting

- Drug therapy for treatment-naïve patients differs from therapy of those patients who have previously received highly active antiretroviral therapy (HAART).
- Medication adherence is critical to the success of antiretroviral regimens.
- HIV possesses several unique enzymes, and many of those enzymes have been identified as targets of therapy.
- HIV reverse transcriptase transcribes viral RNA into DNA.

- Nucleoside reverse transcriptase inhibitors (NRTIs) mimic natural nucleotides and inhibit the action of reverse transcriptase through competitive inhibition.
- Lactic acidosis and hepatic steatosis are considered side effects of the NRTI drug class.
- Didanosine and tavudine have significant overlapping toxicities.
- Many non-nucleoside reverse transcriptase inhibitors (NNRTIs) are available as combination medications.
- Some NNRTIs can both inhibit and induce hepatic metabolism.

Patient Care Scenario: Community Setting

B. T., a 42 y/o M, 5'7", recently started HAART therapy. His regimen contains the protease inhibitor atazanavir. You review this patient's medications list and find a major drug interaction that should be addressed promptly.

Date	Physician	Drug	Quantity	Sig	Refills
2/4	Top	ASA	100	1 daily	4
2/4	Top	Omeprazole 20 mg	60	1 bid	3
2/4	Top	Acetaminophen 325 mg	100	1 qid prn	3
2/4	Top	Citalopram 20 mg	30	1 daily	4
2/4	Top	Cetirizine 10 mg	30	1 daily	3

Highly Active Antiretroviral Therapy

The current standard of care for HIV therapy utilizes a multidrug approach and is traditionally referred to as highly active antiretroviral therapy (HAART). The accepted class abbreviations and currently available drugs are listed in the Key Terms and in Table 15-29.

Key Terms

NRTI: Nucleoside reverse transcriptase inhibitor
NNRTI: Non-nucleoside reverse transcriptase inhibitor
PI: Protease inhibitor
INSTI: Integrase strand transfer inhibitor

As recommended by treatment guidelines (issued in March 2012), drug therapy for treatment-naïve patients, or those who have not received HAART previously, includes a combination of three different drugs over a least two classes. These drug regimens are listed in Table 15-30.

Table 15-29 Currently Marketed Antiretroviral Drugs (as of June 2012)

Class	Generic	Brand	Abbreviation
NRTI	Abacavir	Ziagen	ABC
	Didanosine	Videx EC	ddI
	Emtricitabine	Emtriva	FTC
	Lamivudine	Epivir	3TC
	Stavudine	Zerit	d4T
	Tenofovir	Viread	TDF
	Zidovudine	Retrovir	AZT, ZDV
NNRTI	Delavirdine	Rescriptor	DLV
	Efavirenz	Sustiva	EFV
	Etravirine	Intelence	ETR
	Nevirapine	Viramune	NVP
	Rilpivirine	Edurant	RPV
PI	Atazanavir	Reyataz	ATV
	Darunavir	Prezista	DRV
	Fosamprenavir	Lexiva	FPV
	Indinavir	Crixivan	IDV
	Lopinavir (w/ ritonavir)	Kaletra	LPV/r
	Nelfinavir	Viracept	NFV
	Ritonavir	Norvir	RTV
	Saquinavir	Invirase	SQV
	Tipranavir	Aptivus	TPV
INSTI	Raltegravir	Isentress	RAL
Fusion inhibitor	Enfurvitide	Fuzeon	T-20, ENF
Entry CCR5 inhibitor	Maraviroc	Selzentry	MVC

1.1.0 Patient Information

Adherence/Resistance

Proper adherence is critical to the success of an antiretroviral regimen. Not only does poor adherence result in a lack of efficacy, but it also allows for the development of resistance. In the event of nonadherence, different medication classes will have different rates of resistance. Consequently, some regimens can be quite unforgiving to nonadherent patients, whereas others may allow slightly more room for error. Regardless, proper counseling and assessment are essential to determine whether patients are ready to begin therapy and which barriers to adherence need to be addressed.

Antiretroviral treatment is recommended in HIV-positive patients who present with an acquired immunodeficiency syndrome (AIDS)–defining illness or a CD4 count of fewer than 350 cells/mm^3.

Table 15-30 Currently Marketed Combination Antiretroviral Drugs (as of June 2012)

Brand	Generic	Abbreviation
Atripla	Efavirenz + emtricitabine + tenofovir	ATR
Combivir	Zidovudine + lamivudine	CBV
Complera	Rilpivirine + emtricitabine + tenofovir	
Epzicom	Abacavir + lamivudine	EPZ
Trizivir	Abacavir + zidovudine + lamivudine	TZV
Truvada	Tenofovir + emtricitabine	TRV

Table 15-31 Initial Drug Regimens in Treatment-Naïve Patients

2 NRTIs + 1 NNRTI
2 NRTIs + 1 PI (often boosted with ritonavir)
1 NRTIs + 1 INSTI

Antiretroviral treatment is recommended in all HIV-positive patients. The current guidelines differ on the strength of this recommendation based on CD4 count. Treating patients with fewer than 350 cells/mm^3 is an AI strong recommendation, treating those with 350–500 cells/mm^3 is an AII strong recommendation, and treating patients with more than 500 cells/mm^3 is a BIII moderate recommendation. Treatment for HIV is strongly recommended irrespective of CD4 count in the presence of pregnancy, an AIDS-defining illness, HIV-associated nephropathy, or hepatitis B/C coinfection.

Antiretroviral Medications for the Treatment of HIV Infection

1.2.0 Pharmacotherapy

Mechanism of Action

HIV possesses several unique enzymes, many of which have been identified as targets for therapy. HIV reverse transcriptase is one example; it transcribes viral RNA into DNA. The new viral DNA is then incorporated into the host genome and propagates the life cycle of the virus. The NRTIs, which mimic natural nucleotides, inhibit the action of reverse transcriptase through competitive inhibition. The drug inserts itself in the place of a nucleoside, preventing the creation of a viral DNA strand.

1.3.0 Monitoring

Adverse Drug Events

The side-effect profile of the NRTIs has improved with newer agents. Lactic acidosis and hepatic steatosis are considered side effects of the entire NRTI class, although they are less common with newer agents. Other side effects are drug specific and outlined in Table 15-32.

Drug Interactions

While the NRTIs do not induce or inhibit metabolism like other antiretroviral classes, they are still associated with significant drug and toxicity interactions.

2.2.0 Dispensing

Many of the NRTIs are available as combination medications. These are used quite often in practice, and they provide a lower pill burden, which facilitates adherence

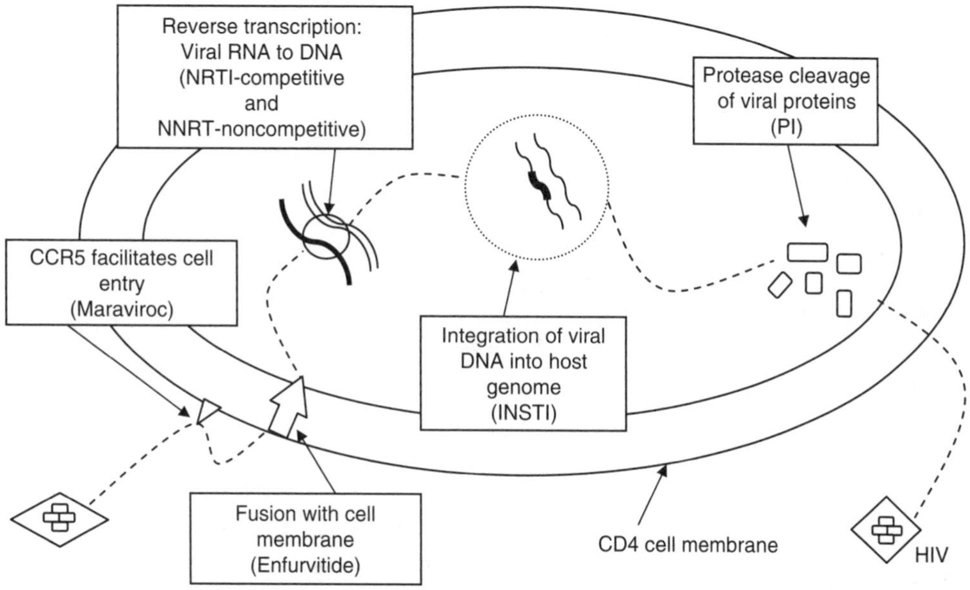

Figure 15-3 Antiretroviral Targets in the HIV Life Cycle: Nucleoside Reverse Transcriptase Inhibitors

Table 15-32 NRTI Monitoring

NRTI	Adverse Events	Warnings/Contraindications
Abacavir	Hypersensitivity reaction	Presence of HLA-B 5701 allele is associated with hypersensitivity. Potential increase in MI risk.
Didanosine	Pancreatitis, peripheral neuropathy, higher risk of lactic acidosis	Contraindication with ribavirin and allopurinol. Avoid with stavudine (significant overlapping toxicities).
Emtricitabine	Usually well tolerated	Potential for exacerbation of hepatitis upon discontinuation of FTC in hepatitis B–coinfected patients.
Lamivudine	Usually well tolerated	Potential for exacerbation of hepatitis upon discontinuation of 3TC in hepatitis B–coinfected patients.
Stavudine	Pancreatitis, peripheral neuropathy, higher risk of lactic acidosis lipodystrophy (lipoatrophy)	Avoid with didanosine (significant overlapping toxicities).
Tenofovir	Renal insufficiency, GI (NVD,* gas, bloating)	Possible transient decrease in bone mineral density. Potential for exacerbation of hepatitis upon discontinuation of TDF in hepatitis B–coinfected patients.
Zidovudine	Macrocytic anemia, neutropenia, GI discomfort, nail discoloration, higher risk of lactic acidosis	None noted

*NVD = nausea, vomiting, diarrhea.

Table 15-33 NRTI Dispensing Information

NRTI	Recommended Dosage	Elimination	Food Requirements
Abacavir	300 mg q 12 hr or 600 mg daily	Hepatic (non-CYP) Adjust the dose in patients with hepatic insufficiency	With or without food
Didanosine	400 mg daily or with TDF 250 mg daily	Renal Adjust the dose in patients with renal insufficiency	Take without food 30 minutes before or 2 hours after meal Disregard food restriction with TDF
Emtricitabine	200 mg daily	Renal Adjust the dose in patients with renal insufficiency	With or without food
Lamivudine	150 mg q 12 hr or 300 mg daily	Renal Adjust the dose in patients with renal insufficiency	With or without food
Stavudine	Weight based: ≥ 60 kg: 40 mg q 12 hr < 60 kg: 30 mg q 12 hr	Renal Adjust the dose in patients with renal insufficiency	With or without food
Tenofovir (nucleotide analog)	300 mg daily	Renal Adjust the dose in patients with renal insufficiency	With or without food
Zidovudine	300 mg q 12 hr or 200 mg q 8 hr Available IV	Renal Adjust the dose in patients with renal insufficiency	With or without food
Combinations			
Combivir	1 tablet q 12 hr	Renal: see individual agents	With or without food
Epzicom	1 tablet daily	Renal and hepatic: see individual agents	With or without food
Trizivir	1 tablet q 12 hr	Renal and hepatic: see individual agents	With or without food
Truvada	1 tablet daily	Renal: see individual agents	With or without food

to the regimen. Table 15-30 summarizes the currently marketed combination medications. Most antiretrovirals are available only in oral form. Dosages are all given for the oral route of administration unless otherwise specified.

Non-nucleoside Reverse Transcriptase Inhibitors

1.1.0 Pharmacotherapy

Mechanism of Action

NNRTIs, unlike NRTIs, do not act as nucleosides. They bind to reverse transcriptase noncompetitively at a hydrophobic pocket away from the active site, leading to a conformational change that reduces reverse transcriptase activity and produces termination of DNA chain elongation.

1.2.0 Pharmacotherapy Monitoring

Adverse Drug Events

Rash is considered a class side effect of the NNRTIs. Stevens-Johnson syndrome has been reported rarely with all NNRTIs, although more often with nevirapine.

Drug Interactions

Some NNRTIs may have complex drug interactions. The fact that several can both inhibit and induce hepatic metabolism may be problematic when trying to treat other conditions.

Table 15-34 NNRTI Monitoring

NNRTI	Adverse Events	Warnings/ Contraindications	CYP Effects/ Drug Interactions
Delavirdine	Rash, HA, increase in transaminases	Not used commonly	Inhibitor: 3A4 Substrate: 3A4
Efavirenz	Rash, CNS effects (range from mild to severe; most resolve or lessen in 2–4 weeks), increase in transaminases	Possible teratogenicity (avoid in pregnancy) Can cause false-positive results with some drug screens	Inhibitor: 3A4 Inducer: 3A4 Substrates: 3A4, 2B6
Etravirine	Rash, hypersensitivity reactions	None noted	Inhibitors: 2C9, 2C19 Inducer: 3A4 Substrates: 3A4, 2C9, 2C19
Nevirapine	Rash, hepatitis	None noted	Inducer: 3A4
Rilpivirine	Rash, depression, headache, insomnia	Not recommended to start in patients with a viral load greater than 100,000	Substrate: 3A4 Acid-lowering drugs significantly lower RVP absorption; refer to guidelines for dosing

2.2.0 Dispensing

See Table 15-35.

Protease Inhibitors

1.2.0 Pharmacotherapy

Mechanism of Action

Protease is a viral enzyme that works in the late stages of viral replication. The precursor *gag-pol* polyprotein molecules are cleaved, allowing the virus to mature. PIs work in the active site of the protease enzyme, preventing cleavage of the protein. The consequent virus particles are immature and noninfective.

Boosting

The PI ritonavir is rarely given to patients at full treatment doses, but is instead given in low doses with other protease inhibitors. Ritonavir is a potent CYP 3A4 and 2D6 inhibitor. It effectively inhibits most other protease inhibitors, increasing their plasma levels and half-lives, and thereby allowing for a reduced pill burden and less frequent dosing. Ritonavir also demonstrates increased efficacy and reduces the development of drug resistance.

1.3.0 Monitoring

Adverse Drug Events

PIs have several class side effects. Effect frequencies are not universal, however, and the newer agents are generally more tolerable for patients. GI effects, especially diarrhea, are associated with this class. PIs are also associated with metabolic complications such as negative effects on the lipid profile, increases in LDL and triglycerides, fat maldistribution, and hyperglycemia and insulin resistance.

Drug Interactions

PIs have very complex drug interactions. All of these drugs are CYP inhibitors and substrates, with some being inducers as well. The interaction list is extensive, and patients on PIs should be screened carefully for drug interactions.

Table 15-35 NNRTI Dispensing Information

NNRTI	Recommended Dosage	Elimination	Food Requirements
Delavirdine	400 mg q 8 hr	Hepatic	With or without food
Efavirenz	600 mg daily Taking the drug at bedtime may help patients with CNS side effects	Hepatic	Avoid with fatty meals; foods with high fat content can increase absorption, leading to greater side effects
Etravirine	200 mg q 12 hr	Hepatic	Take after a meal
Nevirapine	200 mg daily × 14 days, then 200 mg q 12 hr 400 mg XR daily; CD4 requirements for initiation: Men: CD4 < 400 Women: CD4 < 250	Hepatic	With or without food
Rilpivirine	25 mg daily	Hepatic	Take with meal; minimum 500 calories of solid food
Combination			
Atripla	1 tablet daily Taking the drug at bedtime may help patients with CNS side effects	Renal and hepatic: see individual agents	Avoid with fatty meals; foods with high fat content can increase absorption, leading to greater side effects
Complera	1 tablet daily	Renal and hepatic: see individual agents	Take with meal; minimum of 500 calories of solid food

Table 15-36 PI Monitoring

PI	Adverse Events	Warnings/Contraindications	CYP Effects/Drug Interactions
Atazanavir	Hyperbilirubemia, hyperglycemia, fat maldistribution, nephrolithiasis	Prolonged PR interval: use with caution with other PR-lengthening drugs	Inhibitors: 3A4, UGT1A1 Substrate: 3A4 Acid-lowering drugs significantly lower ATV absorption; refer to guidelines for dosing options
Darunavir	GI (ND), hyperlipidemia, hyperglycemia, fat maldistribution, hepatotoxicity, skin rash	Sulfonamide moiety; use caution in patients with allergy	Inhibitor: 3A4 Substrate: 3A4
Fos-amprenavir	GI (NVD), hyperlipidemia, hyperglycemia, fat maldistribution, increase in transaminases, skin rash, nephrolithiasis	Sulfonamide moiety; use caution in patients with allergy	Inhibitor: 3A4 Inducer: 3A4 Substrate: 3A4
Indinavir	Nephrolithiasis, GI (N), hyperbilirubemia, hyperlipidemia, hyperglycemia, fat maldistribution,	Need adequate hydration (suggested 48 oz of water daily)	Inhibitor: 3A4 Substrate: 3A4
Lopinavir (with ritonavir)	GI (NVD), asthenia, hyperglycemia, hyperlipidemia (especially triglyceridemia), fat maldistribution	Prolonged PR and QT intervals; use other interval-lengthening drugs with caution	Inhibitor: 3A4 Substrate: 3A4
Nelfinavir	GI (D), hyperlipidemia, hyperglycemia, fat maldistribution, increase in transaminases	None noted	Inhibitor: 3A4 Substrates: 3A4, 2C19 (converted to active metabolite)
Ritonavir	GI (NVD), hepatitis, hyperglycemia, fat maldistribution, hyperlipidemia (especially triglyceridemia), asthenia, paresthesias	Many adverse effects not seen at low PI- boosting doses	Inhibitors: 3A4 (potent), 2D6 Substrates: 3A4, 2D6 (lesser)
Saquinavir	GI (ND), hyperlipidemia, hyperglycemia, fat maldistribution, increase in transaminases	None noted	Inhibitor: 3A4 Substrate: 3A4
Tipranavir	Hepatotoxicity, skin rash, hyperlipidemia (especially triglyceridemia), hyperglycemia, fat maldistribution	Cases of intracranial hemorrhage (rare)	Inhibitor: 3A4 (2D6 with ritonavir) Substrate: 3A4

Table 15-37 PI Dispensing Information

PI	Recommended Dosage	Elimination	Food Requirements
Atazanavir	Drug naïve: • 400 mg daily • 300 mg with RTV 100 mg daily Drug experienced: • 300 mg with RTV 100 mg daily	Hepatic Adjust dose in patients with hepatic insufficiency	With food Acid needed for absorption
Darunavir	Drug naïve: • 800 mg with RTV 100 mg daily Drug experienced: • 600 mg with RTV 100 mg q 12 hr	Hepatic	With food
Fosamprenavir	Drug naïve: • 1,400 mg daily • 1,400 mg with RTV 100–200 mg daily Drug experienced: • 1,400 mg with RTV 100 mg q 12 hr	Hepatic Adjust dose in patients with hepatic insufficiency	With or without food
Indinavir	800 mg q 12 hr or 800 mg with RTV 100 mg q 12 hr	Hepatic Adjust dose in patients with hepatic insufficiency	1 hour prior or 2 hours post food With RTV: With or without food
Lopinavir (with ritonavir)	400 mg/100 mg q 12 hr or 800 mg/200 mg daily (naïve only)	Hepatic	Tablet: With or without food Solution: With food
Nelfinavir	1,250 mg q 12 hr or 750 mg q 8 hr	Hepatic	With food
Ritonavir	Boosted dose: Refer to other PIs	Hepatic	With food (improves drug tolerability)
Saquinavir	1,000 mg with RTV 100 mg q 12 hr	Hepatic	Within 2 hours following a meal
Tipranavir	500 mg with RTV 200 mg q 12 hr	Hepatic	With or without food

2.2.0 Dispensing

See Table 15-37.

Integrase Strand Transfer Inhibitors

1.2.0 Pharmacotherapy

Mechanism of Action

Integrase is a viral enzyme that incorporates the viral DNA (converted from RNA via reverse transcriptase) into the host DNA. The INSTIs work primarily on the third step of integration—that is, strand transfer. Blocking this transfer stops the viral DNA from being merged with the host DNA and halts creation of viral components.

1.3.0 Monitoring

Adverse Drug Events

Raltegravir is generally well tolerated. Caution should be used in patients already on drugs that may be affecting CPK, such as HMG CoA inhibitors.

Table 15-38 INSTI Monitoring

INSTI	Adverse Events	Warnings/ Contraindications
Raltegravir	GI (ND), HA	May cause CPK elevation

2.2.0 Dispensing

Table 15-39 INSTI Dispensing Information

INSTI	Recommended Dosage	Elimination	Food Requirements
Raltegravir	400 mg q 12 hr Recommended change to 800 mg q 12 hr when coadministered with rifampin	Glucuronidation (UGT1A1 substrate)	With or without food

Table 15-40 Fusion Inhibitor Monitoring

Fusion Inhibitor	Adverse Events	Warnings/ Contraindications
Enfurvitide	Local injection-site reactions (*very* common)	Risk of hypersensitivity reaction

Fusion Inhibitors

1.1.0 Pharmacotherapy

Method of Action

To enter the CD4 cell, the virus must first bind and then fuse with the cell membrane. Enfurvitide is a synthetic peptide designed to attach to glycoproteins on the HIV viral envelope. This attachment prevents a conformational change in the membrane necessary for viral fusion.

1.2.0 Monitoring

The most common side effects from enfurvitide are local injection-site reactions, pain, swelling, and even permanent cysts and nodules. Enfurvitide is reserved for treatment-experienced patients who have failed previous treatments or have contraindications to other therapies.

2.2.0 Dispensing

Enfurvitide is a peptide, making the subcutaneous route the preferable route of administration. Unfortunately, this route may cause significant problems in relation to adherence. Enfurvitide requires twice-daily injections and in most patients leaves nodules in the skin after each dose.

Entry Inhibitors

1.2.0 Pharmacotherapy

Mechanisms of Action

Glycoproteins on the virus must bind to a CD4 receptor as well as a chemokine receptor to begin entry into the cell. Two chemokine receptors are possible sites for HIV binding: CXCR4 and CCR5. The virus can use CCR5, CXCR4, or both receptors (called dual tropism).

Table 15-41 Fusion Inhibitor Dispensing Information

Fusion Inhibitor	Recommended Dosage	Elimination
Enfurvitide	90 mg SC q 12 hr	Break down into amino acids

Table 15-42 Entry Inhibitor Monitoring

Entry Inhibitor	Adverse Events	Warnings/ Contraindications	CYP Effects/ Drug Interactions
Maraviroc	Hepatotoxicity, rash, cough, abdominal pain, muscle pain, dizziness, postural hypotension	Tropism	Substrate: 3A4 Dosage is based on the presence of strong CYP 3A inducers/ inhibitors; see the recommended dosage

Table 15-43 Entry Inhibitor Dispensing Information

Entry Inhibitor	Recommended Dosage	Elimination	Food Requirements
Maraviroc	300 mg q 12 hr 150 mg q 12 hr (with inhibitors) 600 mg q 12 hr (with inducers)	Hepatic	With or without food

period to enter the cell. Maraviroc is a CCR5 antagonist that prevents CCR5 tropic viruses from binding to the cell and entering it.

1.3.0 Monitoring

Tropism

Testing the virus's tropism is crucial to determine whether maraviroc can be used. Tropism tests should be obtained before initiation of maraviroc therapy. If the patient has a CXCR4 or dual tropism, virus therapy with maraviroc is not recommended. Maraviroc is currently indicated only for CCR5 tropism.

2.2.0 Dispensing

Maraviroc is approved for both treatment-experienced and treatment-naïve patients.

ANNOTATED BIBLIOGRAPHY

Anderson PL, Kakuda TN, Fletcher CV. Human immunodeficiency virus infection. In DiPiro JT, Talbert RL, Yee GC, et al., eds. *Pharmacotherapy: A Pathophysiologic Approach,* 7th ed. Available at: http://0-www.accesspharmacy.com.libcat.ferris.edu/content.aspx?aID=3217664.

Brooks GF, Butel JS, Morse SA. Pathogenesis and control of viral diseases. In Brooks GF, Butel JS, Morse SA, eds. *Jawetz, Melnick, and Adelberg's Medical Microbiology,* 24th ed. Available at: http://0-www.accesspharmacy.com.libcat.ferris.edu/content.aspx?aID=2760305.

Jamjian MC, McNicholl IR. Enfuvirtide: first fusion inhibitor for treatment of HIV infection. *Am J Health Syst Pharm* 2004;61(12):1242–1247.

Lieberman-Blum SS, Fung HB, Bandres JC. Maraviroc: a CCR5-receptor antagonist for the treatment of HIV-1 infection. *Clin Ther* 2008;30(7):1228–1250.

Panel on Antiretroviral Guidelines for Adults and Adolescents. Guidelines for the use of antiretroviral agents in HIV-1-infected adults and adolescents. Department of Health and Human Services. November 3, 2008; 1–139. Available at http://www.aidsinfo.nih.gov/ContentFiles/AdultandAdolescentGL.pdf. Accessed December 1, 2009.

Safrin S. Antiviral agents. In Katzung BG, Masters SB, Trevor AJ, eds. *Basic and Clinical Pharmacology,* 11th ed. Available at: http://0-www.accesspharmacy.com.libcat.ferris.edu/content.aspx?aID=4521594.

TOPIC: MENINGITIS

Section Coordinator: Michael Klepser
Contributors: Katie Hinkle and Heather L. VandenBussche

Tips Worth Tweeting

- Acute bacterial meningitis is the most common infection of the central nervous system and may be caused by spread from a primary infection, trauma, or congenital defects.
- Meningitis leads to inflammation within the meninges, subarachnoid space, and brain parenchyma and can result in decreased levels of consciousness, seizures, increased intracranial pressure, and stroke.
- Mortality and morbidity for meningitis are high; nearly 20% of patients die and 30–50% of survivors develop neurologic disabilities, including seizures and hearing loss.
- Meningitis is caused by a number of different organisms that vary based on age and comorbid conditions.
- Signs and symptoms of bacterial meningitis vary with age and are often nonspecific.
- The introduction of Hib vaccine has significantly decreased the incidence of *Haemophilus influenzae* meningitis.
- Antibiotic therapy is most often empiric, based on the patient's age, predisposing factors, and common pathogens.
- There may be a role for use of adjunctive dexamethasone in some types of meningitis and specific age groups.
- Appropriate bactericidal antibiotic selection is based on the drug's spectrum of activity and extent of penetration into the cerebrospinal fluid.

Patient Care Scenario: Hospital Setting

B. H. is a 4-month-old male who was born at full term. His mother brings him to the emergency department with a fever and unusual stiffness. The doctor suspects bacterial meningitis.

Organisms

The pathogens that mostly commonly cause bacterial meningitis include *Streptococcus pneumoniae* (approximately 50% of cases), *Neisseria meningitidis* (25%), group B streptococci (15%), and *Listeria monocytogenes* (10%). *Haemophilus influenzae* was previously the number one cause of bacterial meningitis, but increased utilization of the *H. influenzae* type b (Hib) vaccine has reduced the incidence to less than 10%. *L. monocytogenes* and group B streptococcal infections are more common in neonates, and *N. meningitidis* accounts for as many as 60% of these infections in children and young adults.

1.1.0 Patient Information

Signs and Symptoms

Signs and symptoms of bacterial meningitis vary with age and are often nonspecific. Patients usually present with fever, nuchal rigidity, altered mental status, chills, vomiting, photophobia, and severe headache. Kernig and Brudzinski signs are more common in adults than in children, whereas seizures are more frequent in children than in adults. Irritability, delirium, drowsiness, lethargy, and coma may also be present. Young children may present with bulging fontanelles, apnea, purpuric rash, and convulsions.

Neurologic complications associated with bacterial meningitis are not the direct result of infection, but rather result from the inflammatory response that the pathogens provoke. The cascade of events that ensues may lead to cerebral edema, elevated intracranial pressure, decreased cerebral blood flow, cerebral ischemia, and death.

Laboratory Testing

If a patient presents with symptoms suggestive of bacterial meningitis, blood and cerebrospinal fluid (CSF)

Table 15-44 Empiric Antibiotic Therapy for Bacterial Meningitis

Age or Predisposing Factor	Common Pathogens	Empiric Antimicrobial Therapy
Age < 1 month	Group B streptococci, *E. coli, L. monocytogenes, Klebsiella* spp.	Ampicillin **plus** (cefotaxime **or** aminoglycoside)
Age: 1–23 months	*S. pneumoniae, N. meningitidis,* group B streptococci, *H. influenzae, E. coli*	Vancomycin **plus** (ceftriaxone **or** cefotaxime)
Age: 2–50 years	*N. meningitidis, S. pneumoniae*	Vancomycin **plus** (ceftriaxone **or** cefotaxime)
Age > 50 years	*S. pneumoniae, N. meningitidis, L. monocytogenes,* aerobic gram-negative bacilli	Vancomycin **plus** ampicillin **plus** (ceftriaxone **or** cefotaxime)
Basilar skull fracture	*S. pneumoniae, H. influenzae,* group A β-hemolytic streptococci	Vancomycin **plus** (ceftriaxone **or** cefotaxime)
Penetrating head trauma	*S. aureus,* coagulase-negative staphylococci, aerobic gram-negative bacilli (including *P. aeruginosa*)	Vancomycin **plus** (cefepime **or** ceftazidime **or** meropenem)
Post-neurosurgery	Aerobic gram-negative bacilli (including *P. aeruginosa*), *S. aureus,* coagulase-negative staphylococci	Vancomycin **plus** (cefepime **or** ceftazidime **or** meropenem)
CSF shunt	Coagulase-negative staphylococci, *S. aureus,* aerobic gram-negative bacilli (including *P. aeruginosa*), *Propionibacterium acnes*	Vancomycin **plus** (cefepime **or** ceftazidime **or** meropenem)

cultures must be obtained and empiric antibiotic therapy started immediately. Diagnosis is made by lumbar puncture (LP) and CSF analysis, looking for elevated white blood cell (WBC) and protein content and decreased glucose levels. Computed tomography (CT) or magnetic resonance imaging (MRI) may or may not be necessary.

Wellness and Prevention

As mentioned earlier, introduction of the Hib vaccine has significantly decreased the incidence of *H. influenzae* meningitis. In addition, the increased use of conjugate vaccines has reduced the rates of pneumococcal and meningococcal meningitis across all age groups in developed countries.

1.2.0 Pharmacotherapy

Treatment of bacterial meningitis includes early initiation of appropriate antibiotics, along with supportive care with fluids, electrolytes, antipyretics, and analgesics. Antibiotic therapy is most often empiric based on the patient's age, predisposing factors, and common pathogens.

Once the causative organism has been identified by CSF Gram stain and culture, antibiotic therapy should be adjusted to target the specific organism, keeping susceptibility testing (if available) or local susceptibilities in mind at all times.

Adjunctive Therapy

Current guidelines recommend the use of adjunctive dexamethasone in adults with pneumococcal meningitis, as well as infants and children with *H. influenzae* type b meningitis. Additionally, the American Academy of Pediatrics recommends considering dexamethasone treatment for infants and children with pneumococcal meningitis. Dexamethasone inhibits the production of IL-1 and TNF, thereby decreasing the inflammatory reaction secondary to the release of bacterial cell-wall components after exposure to bactericidal antibiotics. This inflammatory response is believed to be a major cause of the neurologic damage and mortality associated with meningitis, so its inhibition should significantly decrease these negative outcomes.

Drug Indications, Dosing Regimens, Routes of Administration

Dexamethasone (0.15 mg/kg) should be administered 10–20 minutes before the first antibiotic dose and continued every 6 hours for 2–4 days. If not given before the first dose of antibiotics, dexamethasone is not indicated due to the unlikelihood of improved outcomes.

There is insufficient evidence to recommend the use of adjunctive dexamethasone in neonates and in children and adults with meningitis due to other bacterial organisms. Nevertheless, some experts recommend initiating dexamethasone in all patients who

Table 15-45 Targeted Therapy for Bacterial Meningitis Based on the Isolated Pathogen

Microorganism	First-Line Therapy	Alternatives	Recommended Duration
S. pneumoniae			
Penicillin-sensitive	Penicillin (PCN) G or ampicillin	Ceftriaxone, cefotaxime, chloramphenicol	10–14 days
Penicillin-intermediate	Ceftriaxone or cefotaxime	Cefepime, meropenem	
Penicillin-resistant	Vancomycin **plus** ceftriaxone or cefotaxime	Moxifloxacin	
N. meningitides			
Penicillin-sensitive	PCN G or ampicillin	Ceftriaxone, cefotaxime, chloramphenicol	7 days
Penicillin-resistant	Ceftriaxone or cefotaxime	Chloramphenicol, moxifloxacin, meropenem	
Group B streptococci	Ampicillin or PCN G ± aminoglycoside	Ceftriaxone, cefotaxime	14–21 days
L. monocytogenes	Ampicillin or PCN G ± aminoglycoside	Trimethoprim-sulfamethoxazole (TMP-SMZ), meropenem	≥ 21 days
H. influenzae			
β-lactamase negative	Ampicillin	Ceftriaxone, cefotaxime, cefepime, chloramphenicol, moxifloxacin	7–10 days
β-lactamase positive	Ceftriaxone or cefotaxime	Cefepime, chloramphenicol, moxifloxacin	
E. coli **and** *Klebsiella*	Ceftriaxone or cefotaxime	Aztreonam, moxifloxacin, meropenem, TMP-SMZ, ampicillin	21 days
P. aeruginosa	Cefepime or ceftazidime ± aminoglycoside	Aztreonam, ciprofloxacin, meropenem	21 days
S. aureus			
Methicillin-sensitive	Nafcillin or oxacillin	Vancomycin, meropenem	14–21 days
Methicillin-resistant	Vancomycin ± rifampin	TMP-SMZ, linezolid	
S. epidermidis	Vancomycin ± rifampin	Linezolid	14–21 days
***Enterococcus* spp.**			
Ampicillin-susceptible	Ampicillin **plus** gentamicin	—	Not established
Ampicillin-resistant	Vancomycin **plus** gentamicin	—	
Vancomycin-resistant	Linezolid	—	

present with meningitis, provided the potential benefits outweigh the associated risks.

Prophylaxis for Close Contacts

Chemoprophylaxis is recommended for close contacts of patients with *N. meningitidis* and *H. influenzae* meningitis. Close contacts include all individuals who have been exposed to respiratory or oral secretions through coughing, sneezing, kissing, or sharing toys, beverages, or cigarettes.

Drug Indications, Dosing Regimens, Routes of Administration

Prophylaxis against *N. meningitidis* is usually a 2-day course of rifampin. Dosing is 600 mg every 12 hours in adults, 10 mg/kg every 12 hours in children and infants older than 1 month, and 5 mg/kg every 12 hours in infants younger than 1 month. Alternatives for adults include single-dose ciprofloxacin (500–750 mg PO), single-dose azithromycin (500 mg PO), or single-dose ceftriaxone (250 mg IM). Children younger than 12 years old may receive a single 125-mg dose of intramuscular ceftriaxone as an alternative to rifampin.

Close contacts of patients with *H. influenzae* meningitis should receive a 4-day course of rifampin: 600 mg/day in adults and 20 mg/kg/day in children. In addition, unvaccinated children aged 12–48 months should receive one dose of the Hib vaccine, and unvaccinated children aged 2–11 months should receive three doses. Fully vaccinated children and adults do not require chemoprophylaxis.

Special Dosing Considerations

Many factors need to be considered when designing a treatment regimen for a patient with bacterial meningitis. As with initiation of any medication, patient-specific characteristics (e.g., age, allergies, comorbid conditions) must be considered. Appropriate antibiotic selection is then based on the medication's spectrum of activity (for both empiric and targeted therapy) as well as its extent of penetration into the cerebrospinal fluid.

Physiochemical Properties, Solubility, Pharmacodynamics, and Pharmacokinetic Properties

Bactericidal antibiotics are preferred over bacteriostatic agents because host defenses cannot effectively eradicate the pathogens from the meninges as quickly as is typically necessary to resolve this infection. CSF penetration depends on the physicochemical and pharmacokinetic properties of the drug, as well as the degree of inflammation of the patient's meninges. For example, antibiotics with low molecular weight, high lipid solubility, and limited protein binding will be more capable of crossing into the CNS. Inflammation of the meninges loosens junctions between capillary endothelial cells and inhibits efflux pumps, allowing for increased access of some antibiotics to the CNS. In general, maximum antibiotic doses are required in bacterial meningitis to obtain adequate access to the site of infection, and intravenous antimicrobial therapy is recommended to maintain sufficient concentrations of drug in the CSF throughout treatment. Some antibiotics (i.e., aminoglycosides) may be administered intrathecally or intraventricularly to increase penetration; however, a thorough evaluation of potential risks and benefits must be carried out prior to administering antibiotics via these routes.

1.3.0 Pharmacotherapy Monitoring

Therapeutic outcomes are evaluated largely based on clinical improvement. Vital signs are monitored diligently, and patients are assessed for signs and symptoms including headache, fever, nuchal rigidity, mental status, and Brudzinski and Kernig signs on a regular basis, especially during the first 72 hours of treatment. Emphasis is placed on progressive improvement, rather than individual assessments.

Table 15-46 Antibiotics for Meningitis: Spectrum, Penetration, and Dose

Drug	Spectrum	CSF Penetration*	Intravenous Adult Dose
Ampicillin	Gram (+), Gram (–)	1	2 g q 4 hr
Aztreonam	Gram (–)	1	2 g q 6–8 hr
Cefepime	Gram (+), Gram (–)	1	2 g q 8 hr
Cefotaxime	Gram (–) > Gram (+) with good *S. pneumoniae*	1	2 g q 4–6 hr
Ceftazidime	Gram (–) > Gram (+), *P. aeruginosa*	1	2 g q 8 hr
Ceftriaxone	Gram (–) > Gram (+) with good *S. pneumoniae*	1	2 g q 12–24 hr
Chloramphenicol	Gram (+), Gram (–)	2	1–1.5 g q 6 hr
Ciprofloxacin	Gram (–) including *P. aeruginosa*	1	400 mg q 8–12 hr
Gentamicin	Gram (–), Gram (+) including group B streptococci and *Listeria*; synergistic with β-lactams	0†	2.5 mg/kg q 8–12 hr†
Linezolid	Gram (+) including MRSA	1	600 mg q 12 hr
Meropenem	Gram (+), Gram (–), anaerobes	1	2 g q 8 hr
Moxifloxacin	Gram (+), Gram (–)	1	400 mg q 24 hr
Nafcillin/oxacillin	Gram (+)	1	2 g q 4 hr
Penicillin G	Gram (+), *N. meningitidis*	1	4 million units q 4 hr
Rifampin	Gram (+), Gram (–)	2	600 mg q 24 hr
TMP-SMZ	Gram (+), Gram (–)	2	5 mg/kg TMP q 6–12 hr
Vancomycin	Gram (+) including MRSA	1	15 mg/kg q 8–12 hr

*Degree of CSF penetration identified:

0: subtherapeutic levels in CSF regardless of inflammation.

1: therapeutic levels in presence of inflammation.

2: therapeutic levels regardless of inflammation.

†Aminoglycosides have increased penetration into the CNS in neonates and are typically reserved for empiric therapy in these patients. Gentamicin is given as a loading dose of 4–5 mg/kg, followed by 2.5 mg/kg every 8 to 36 hours depending on the patient's gestational and postnatal age.

Initial blood and CSF Gram stains, cultures, and susceptibility testing are used to direct and streamline antibiotic therapy. Repeat cultures should be performed in certain patients to help identify when sterilization has occurred and determine the appropriate duration of antibiotic therapy.

ANNOTATED BIBLIOGRAPHY

Assiri AM, AlAsmari FA, Zimmerman VA, et al. Corticosteroid administration and outcome of adolescents and adults with acute bacterial meningitis: a meta-analysis. *Mayo Clin Proc* 2009 May;84(5):403–409.

Mitropoulos IF, Hermsen ED, Schafer JA, Rotschafer JC. Central nervous system infections. In Dipiro JT, Talbert RL, Yee GC, et al., eds. *Pharmacotherapy: A Pathophysiologic Approach,* 7th ed. New York, McGraw-Hill; 1743–1760

Roos KL, Tyler KL. Meningitis, encephalitis, brain abscess, and empyema. In Fauci AS, Braunwald E, Kasper DL, et al., eds. *Harrison's Principles of Internal Medicine.* 17th ed. New York: McGraw-Hill; 2621–2641

Tunkel AR, Hartman BJ, Kaplan SL, et al. Practice guidelines for the management of bacterial meningitis. *Clin Infect Dis* 2004;39:1267–1284.

TOPIC: PARASITES

Section Coordinator: Michael Klepser
Contributor: Amy C. Bower

Tips Worth Tweeting

- A parasite is an organism dependent upon a host organism for survival.
- The parasite feeds, grows, and multiplies inside its host while generally causing harm.
- A vector is an organism that carries disease from one host to another. Examples include mosquitoes and ticks.

Patient Care Scenario: Community Setting

A. L. is a 32 y.o., 5'6", M, 154 lbs, who presents to the pharmacy counter requesting something to help alleviate his "horrible diarrhea" and abdominal cramping. Upon questioning A. L., you learn that he recently took a 5-day camping trip with his friends. A.L. attests to eating only prepackaged foods from home, but occasionally drank from streams that appeared very clean. He reaches for a box of Imodium and asks if it will help.

Key Terms

Three main categories of parasites cause disease in humans:

- **Protozoa:** Microscopic, single-celled organisms that replicate inside the infected host.
- **Helminthes:** Large, multicellular organisms. There are three main groups:
  - Platyhelminthes (flatworms)
  - Nematodes (roundworms)
  - Acanthocephalans (thorny-headed worms)
- **Ectoparasites:** Organisms that attach or burrow into the skin of the host to gain nourishment and cause disease on their own or by acting as a vector. Examples include ticks, mites, and lice.

Ivermectin (Stromectol)

1.2.0 Pharmacotherapy

Indication

Ivermectin is used for treatment of the following infections:

- Strongyloidiasis of the intestinal tract due to the nematode *Strongyloides stercoralis*
- Onchocerciasis due to the nematode *Onchocerca volvulus*
- Unlabeled uses: Scabies and pediculosis pubis

Mechanism of Action

Ivermectin interferes with the nervous system and muscle function of the parasite. It binds to chloride ion channels in invertebrate nerve and muscle cells, leading to increased permeability of the membranes to chloride ions. This causes hyperpolarization of the cells and subsequent death of the parasite.

1.3.0 Monitoring

Adverse Drug Reactions

The most common potential adverse drug reactions with ivermectin are minor and include pruritus, urticarial rash, and lymph node tenderness/enlargement. Ivermectin may also cause tachycardia, dizziness, diarrhea, and nausea. Ophthalmological reactions can occur in patients with onchocerciasis, a parasitic infection that can lead to blindness.

Monitoring Parameters

Periodic ophthalmic exams (onchocerciasis) and follow-up stool examinations should be performed.

Patient Instructions

Ivermectin should be administered on an empty stomach with water.

Albendazole (Albenza)

1.2.0 Pharmacotherapy

Indication

Albendazole is used for treatment of the following infections:

- Parenchymal neurocysticercosis caused by *Taenia solium* and cystic hydatid disease caused by *Echinococcus granulosus*
- Unlabeled uses: Treatment of giardiasis, hookworms, pinworms, and roundworm infections

Mechanism of Action

Albendazole decreases ATP production of intestinal helminthes and larvae by causing degeneration of cytoplasmic microtubules in intestinal and tegmental cells. As a result, glycogen is depleted and glucose uptake is reduced, which eventually leads to immobilization and death of the pathogen.

1.3.0 Monitoring

Adverse Drug Reactions

The most common potential reactions with albendazole involve the central nervous system and include headache and dizziness. Albendazole can also cause increased LFT's, abdominal pain, nausea, vomiting, and alopecia.

Monitoring Parameters

Monitor fecal specimens for parasites for 3 weeks post treatment. CBC and LFTs should be obtained prior to initiating treatment and every 2 weeks during therapy.

Patient Instructions

Albendazole should be administered with a high-fat meal to increase absorption.

Mebendazole (Vermox)

1.2.0 Pharmacotherapy

Indication

Mebendazole is used for treatment of pinworms, whipworms, roundworms, and hookworms.

Mechanism of Action

Mebendazole selectively blocks uptake of glucose and other essential nutrients in susceptible helminths.

1.3.0 Monitoring

Adverse Drug Reactions

The most serious potential adverse effect of mebendazole therapy is bone marrow suppression. Neutropenia and agranulocytosis have been reported with high doses and prolonged use. Mebendazole may also cause diarrhea, nausea, headache, dizziness, and rash.

Monitoring Parameters

Fecal samples should be assessed for ova within several weeks after initiation of therapy.

Patient Instructions

Mebendazole may be taken without regard to food. This drug is available only as chewable tablets and may be swallowed whole, crushed, or mixed with food.

Nitazoxanide (Alinia)

1.2.0 Pharmacotherapy

Indications

Nitazoxanide is indicated for the treatment of diarrhea caused by *Giardia lamblia* and *Cryptosporidium parvum*.

Mechanism of Action

Nitazoxanide interferes with enzyme-dependent reactions that are essential to anaerobic metabolism.

1.3.0 Monitoring

Adverse Drug Reactions

Rates of drug reactions with nitazoxanide were similar to those associated with placebo. The most common drug reactions include headache, abdominal pain, diarrhea, nausea, and vomiting.

Monitoring Parameters

Symptomatic improvement should be monitored closely.

Patient Instructions

- Nitazoxanide should be taken with food. It is available as a suspension and tablet.
- The suspension should be shaken before administration, stored at room temperature, and discarded after 7 days.

Tinidazole (Tindamax)

1.2.0 Pharmacotherapy

Indications

Tinidazole is indicated for the treatment of trichomoniasis caused by *T. vaginalis*, giardiasis, bacterial vaginosis, and intestinal amebiasis.

Table 15-47 Treatment of Parasitic Infections

Pathogen	Transmission	Symptoms	Diagnosis	Treatment (Adult)	Comments
Protozoa					
Giardia lamblia (giardiasis)	• Fecal–oral • Ingestion of contaminated food/water	• Diarrhea, flatulence, abdominal cramping, nausea • Onset: 1–2 weeks after initial infection	• Ova and parasite exam of multiple stool samples or • Presence of **Giardia** antigen in stool sample	• Tinidazole 2 g po × 1 or • Nitazoxanide 500 mg po bid × 3 days	• Campers/hikers at highest risk
Cryptosporidium parvum (cryptosporidiosis)	• Fecal–oral • Ingestion of contaminated food/water	• Acute, self-limiting watery diarrhea, abdominal cramping, low-grade fever • Onset: 1 week after initial infection	• Acid-fast stain or fluorescence test of stool samples	• No widely accepted treatment • Extended-spectrum macrolides may be used • Nitazoxanide 500 mg po × 3 days	• Infection most severe in patients with AIDS • Nitazoxanide not indicated for immunocompromised patients
Toxoplasma gondii (toxoplasmosis)	• Ingestion of cysts through contaminated cat feces or undercooked meat	• Asymptomatic cervical lymphadenitis, mononucleosis syndrome • Congenital: high risk of vertical transmission • May result in neurological sequelae and chorioretinitis of newborn • Pulmonary, ocular, and CNS involvement in patients with AIDS	• Serological tests and biopsy	• Acute infection: sulfadiazine 1–1.5 g po q 6 hr + pyrimethamine 50–100 mg daily + leucovorin or • Sulfamethoxazole/trimethoprim 10 mg/kg/day q 12 hr	• Pregnant women should avoid changing cat litter, and meats should be heated to more than 60°C
Trichomonas vaginalis (trichomoniasis)	• Sexually transmitted	• Thin, frothy, yellowish-gray vaginal discharge • Vulvar pruritus, dyspareunia, dysuria	• Wet mount and microscopic evaluation of vaginal/cervical swab	• Metronidazole 2 g po × 1 or • Metronidazole 500 mg po bid × 7 days or • Tinidazole 2 g po × 1	• Treat male sexual partners (metronidazole/tinidazole 2 g po × 1)
Helminthes					
Hookworm (*Necator americanus, Ancylostoma duodenale*)		• Iron deficiency caused by hookworm parasitizing blood in the intestine • Localized erythema in area of initial hookworm penetration	• Examination of stool for presence of eggs	• Albendazole 400 mg po × 1 or • Mebendazole 100 mg po bid × 3 days or 500 mg × 1	• Albendazole must be taken with food to increase bioavailability
Pinworm (*Enterobius vermicularis*)	• Direct person-to-person spread	• Perianal pruritus due to the eggs laid at night on perianal folds	• "Scotch-tape test": tape is placed on perianal area in the morning before bathing • Eggs easily adhere to tape and are visible to naked eye and under microscope	• Albendazole 400 mg po × 1 • Mebendazole 100 mg po ×1, then repeat in 1 week	• Nearly 100% cure rate • Most common in school-aged children

(*continues*)

Table 15-47 (*continued*)

Pathogen	Transmission	Symptoms	Diagnosis	Treatment (Adult)	Comments
Helminthes (*continued*)					
Intestinal tapeworm (*Diphyloo-borthrium latum*)	• Ingestion of poorly cooked meats • Licking of mucous membranes of human by infected animals	• Abdominal cramping, "hunger pains," abnormal-appearing stools, change in mental status	• Ova and parasite examination of stool • CT or MRI of infected organ	• Praziquantel 5–10 mg/kg po × 1 dose (adult and children) • Albendazole: dose/duration depend on the specific pathogen and site of infection	• Most infections are asymptomatic; infection may last decades
Ectoparasites					
Lice (head/body) (*Pediculus humanus*) Pubic lice (crabs) (*Phthirus pubis*)	• Humans are reservoir for lice • Lice reside on soiled clothing and attach to skin for blood meal • Transmission occurs via combs/brushes	• Severe pruritus of infected area (scalp, body) • Erythematous papules found on the body	• Diagnosis is confirmed when nits are identified on a hair shaft or lice are found on the body	• Permethrin 1% cream rinse: apply to clean dry hair for 10 min; repeat in 1 week • Malathion: apply to dry hair for 8–12 hr • Launder bed sheets and clothing in hot water and hot dry cycle • Combs/brushes should be discarded • Permethrin: apply to pubic hair • Occlusive ophthalmic ointment is applied to infected eyelashes/brows to smother the parasite	• Lindane is no longer recommended as first-line therapy due to the risk of neurotoxicity and aplastic anemia
Scabies (*Scarcoptes scabiei*)	• Person-to-person by direct contact	• Intense pruritus occurring along the beltline, genital region, wrists, knees, elbows, or feet	• Identification of pruritic papules and compatible clinical history	• Permethrin 5%: apply to skin for 8–14 hr; repeat in 1 week • Alternative: ivermectin 200 mcg/kg × 1, repeat in 2 weeks	• Safe for children older than age 2 months

Mechanism of Action

Tinidazole causes cytotoxicity by damaging DNA and preventing its synthesis.

1.3.0 Monitoring

Adverse Drug Reactions

Tinidazole should be reserved for only its FDA-approved indications due to concerns regarding carcinogenicity (black box warning). Reported adverse effects are numerous and include fatigue, headache, metallic taste, and mild gastrointestinal disturbance. Seizures and peripheral neuropathy have also been reported.

Monitoring Parameters

Symptomatic improvement should be monitored closely.

Patient Instructions

Avoid alcohol and preparations containing alcohol while taking tinidazole and for 3 days following completion of therapy due to a possible disulfiram-like reaction. The patient should avoid intercourse if being treated for trichomoniasis. Tinidazole should be taken with food to minimize epigastric disturbance.

Praziquantel (Biltricide)

1.2.0 Pharmacotherapy

Indications

Praziquantel is indicated for treatment of schistosomiasis. Unlabeled indications include treatment of tapeworm infections.

Mechanism of Action

Praziquantel increases cell permeability to calcium, causing paralysis of worm musculature and eventually leading to the worm's detachment from blood vessels and, therefore, its dislodgement.

1.3.0 Monitoring

Adverse Drug Reactions

The majority of adverse reactions develop due to the death of the parasites and the consequent immune reaction of the host. Adverse effects include abdominal cramping, dizziness, headache, malaise, and diarrhea.

Monitoring Parameters

Symptomatic improvement should be monitored closely.

Patient Instructions

All close family members should be treated for worm infestations. Praziquantel may be taken without regard to food.

ANNOTATED BIBLIOGRAPHY

Centers for Disease Control and Prevention. Parasitic diseases. 2008. Available at: http://www.cdc.gov/ncidod/dpd/aboutparasites.htm. Accessed February 2, 2012.

Liu LX, Weller PF. Antiparasitic drugs. *N Engl J Med* 1996;334(18):1178–1184.

Tindamax [Package insert]. San Antonio, TX: Mission Pharmaceuticals; 2010.

TOPIC: SEPSIS

Section Coordinator: Michael Klepser
Contributors: Payal K. Gurnani and Christopher W. Crank

Tips Worth Tweeting

- The increasing incidence of sepsis demonstrates the need to immediately recognize sepsis and initiate therapy as soon as possible.
- Recognition of sepsis should trigger the initiation of sepsis protocols directing early goal-directed fluid resuscitation, administration of antimicrobial therapy, hemodynamic stabilization, and, where applicable, source control.
- Systemic inflammatory response syndrome, severe sepsis, and septic shock all are terms that fall under sepsis and have precise definitions.
- Potential reasons for a rise in the incidence of sepsis include increased use of cytotoxic and immunosuppressive drugs and procedures such as chemotherapy and transplantation; increased frequency of use of invasive devices; increased longevity of patients prone to sepsis; emergence of the human immunodeficiency virus (HIV) infection; and increasing microbial resistance.

Patient Care Scenario: Hospital Setting

A 65 y/o M, 180 lbs, presents to the medical intensive care unit with septic shock and a baseline APACHE II score of 26.

Key Terms

In 1992, the American College of Chest Physicians/Society of Critical Care Medicine conference convened with the goal of providing a conceptual and practical framework to define sepsis. Systemic inflammatory response syndrome, severe sepsis, and septic shock—all terms that fall under the "sepsis" heading—were defined as well.

Systemic inflammatory response syndrome (SIRS), or the systemic activation of the immune response, can result from a variety of infectious and noninfectious causes, including trauma, pancreatitis, ischemia, tissue injury, and immune-mediated organ injury. SIRS involves two or more of the following clinical manifestations:

- Body temperature greater than 38°C or less than 36°C
- Heart rate greater than 90 beats per minute
- Tachypnea, evidenced by a respiratory rate greater than 20/min or $PaCO_2$ lower than 32 mm Hg
- White blood cell count greater than 12,000 cells/µL, lower than 4,000 cells/µL, or greater than 10% immature cells

Sepsis is the inflammatory response to infection. The inflammatory response includes two or more clinical manifestations of SIRS, resulting from an infectious process.

Infection is a pathological process caused by invasion of a normally sterile tissue, fluid, or body cavity by pathogenic or potentially pathogenic microorganisms. It is often strongly suspected even without an evident source of infection.

Severe sepsis includes sepsis and associated organ dysfunction or hypoperfusion abnormalities such as lactic acidosis, oliguria, and acute alterations in mental status.

Septic shock is defined as sepsis-induced hypotension, persisting despite fluid resuscitation to maintain a central venous pressure between 8 and 12 mm Hg,

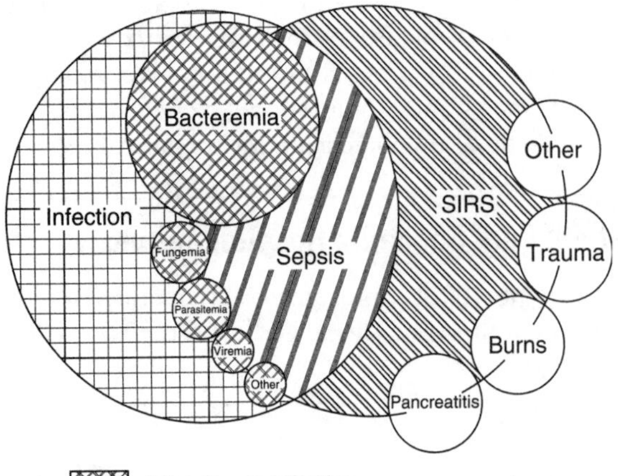

Figure 15-4 Sepsis

with the presence of organ dysfunction and hypoperfusion abnormalities. **Sepsis-induced hypotension** is defined as a systolic blood pressure (SBP) less than 90 mm Hg or a decrease of 40 mm Hg or more from baseline in the absence of other causes for hypotension.

Definitions of sepsis have led to greater recognition of the disease. Due to the broad nature of these definitions, however, bedside evaluation of the patient has remained vital in the diagnosis of the disease.

Pathogenesis of Sepsis

Sepsis is a result of the activation of the immune response following the introduction of microorganisms into the local or systemic environment of the host. The pathophysiology of sepsis also involves the activation and dysregulation of the inflammatory and coagulation systems. Dysregulation of these systems ultimately affects organ function and subsequently, the overall outcome of the patient. This outcome can, however, be strongly influenced by additional factors such as burden of infection as well as virulence and resistance patterns of infecting organisms.

Role of the Immune System

The immune response to infection consists of both innate and adaptive immunity. The innate immune system includes macrophages and natural killer cells, which may act directly on pathogens or trigger adaptive immune responses by activating T and B cells. In addition, the innate immune system identifies pathogens by means of pattern-recognition receptors, called toll-like receptors (TLRs); these proteins bind to macromolecules of microbial pathogens. Stimulation of TLRs induces a signaling pathway that involves the production of inflammatory mediators such as TNF-α, interleukin-1β, and nuclear factor-κB (NF-kb), as well as anti-inflammatory cytokines such as IL-10. In addition to the upregulation of cytokines, activation of TLRs results in the upregulation of microbial killing mechanisms, including the production of reactive nitrogen species.

The release of cytokines and expression of costimulatory molecules as a result of the activation of TLRs are essential for activation of cells of the adaptive immune system. Cells of the adaptive immune system differ from those of the innate immune system in that they possess specificity for recognition and remembrance of antigens by humoral and cell-mediated responses.

Role of the Inflammatory Cascade

Previous theories of sepsis have identified this disease as an uncontrolled inflammatory response. More recent evidence suggests that initially sepsis may be characterized by increases in inflammatory mediators; as it persists, however, there is a shift toward the production of anti-inflammatory mediators.

Macrophages and dendritic cells are activated by the ingestion of bacteria and by cytokines secreted by CD4 T cells. CD4 cells secrete cytokines with inflammatory properties (type 1 helper T cells), including TNF-α, interferon-γ, and IL-2, as well as cytokines with anti-inflammatory properties (type 2 helper T cells), including IL-4 and IL-10. Whether cytokines with inflammatory or anti-inflammatory properties are secreted is influenced by the type of pathogen, bacterial burden, and site of infection.

Role of the Coagulation Cascade

The pathophysiology of sepsis also involves an alteration in the balance of the coagulation systems. The increase in cytokines released during sepsis promotes the expression of tissue factor on endothelial cells, monocytes, and neutrophils. Tissue factor signals the extrinsic coagulation pathway by activation of Factor VII and, ultimately, the formation of thrombin. In addition to the activation of the extrinsic pathway, the intrinsic pathway is signaled by the activation of Factor XI, which leads to further production of thrombin. Under normal circumstances, procoagulant factors are balanced by anticoagulant factors; however, during sepsis, a decrease in anticoagulant factors such as antithrombin III, protein C, protein S, and tissue factor pathway inhibitor promotes a procoagulant state. In addition, this pro-inflammatory and procoagulant state is augmented during periods of ischemia and hypoxia as a result of the release of tissue factor and plasminogen-activator inhibitor 1.

1.1.0 Patient Information

Signs and Symptoms

Patients presenting with sepsis and septic shock are hypotensive, and typically tachycardic, owing to major fluid deficits. As a result of this hypovolemia, cardiac output decreases and contributes to poor systemic oxygen delivery, or a low central venous oxygen saturation (SvO_2), as well as failure of the circulatory system to adequately perfuse vital organs. Hypoperfusion manifests as mental status changes, oliguria, and increased serum lactate levels due to the presence of anaerobic metabolism. In addition to hypovolemia, dysfunction on a cellular level from the release of inflammatory mediators contributes to multi-organ failure.

Table 15-48 Receptor Binding

Drug	Dose Range	α_1 β_1 β_2 DA Dopamine	Adverse Effects
Catecholamines			
Dopamine	2–20 mcg/kg/min	Low dose: ++ Intermediate dose: ++++ ++ High dose: +++	• Tachyarrhythmias • Tissue ischemia • Marked hypotension (with rapid discontinuation)
Dobutamine	2.5–20 mcg/kg/min	+ +++++ +++ N/A	• Hypotension • Tachycardia • Ventricular arrhythmias • Cardiac ischemia
Norepinephrine	2–20 mcg/min	+++++ +++ ++ N/A	• Reflex bradycardia • Arrhythmias • Peripheral ischemia
Epinephrine	1–10 mcg/min	+++++ ++++ +++ N/A	• Ventricular arrhythmias • Cardiac ischemia
Phenylephrine	25–200 mcg/min	+++++ 0 0 N/A	• Reflex bradycardia
Vasoactive Agents			
Vasopressin	0.04 unit/min	V_1 receptors	• Hyponatremia • Hypertension • Cardiac ischemia • Severe peripheral vasoconstriction • Splanchnic vasoconstriction

1.2.0 Pharmacotherapy

The Surviving Sepsis Campaign Guidelines for the management of severe sepsis and septic shock were published to provide evidence-based recommendations in an effort to improve outcomes for critically ill patients. These guidelines include recommendations on early goal-directed resuscitation, early administration of broad-spectrum antimicrobial therapy, and an emphasis on source control, among others.

Fluid Therapy

The Surviving Sepsis Campaign Guidelines recommend early fluid resuscitation of a patient with sepsis-induced hypoperfusion, as studies have demonstrated improved survival for these patients. During the first 6 hours, the goals of resuscitation include central venous pressure (CVP) between 8 and 12 mm Hg, mean arterial pressure (MAP) greater than or equal to 65 mm Hg, urine output greater than or equal to 0.5 mL/kg/hr, and a central venous or mixed venous oxygen saturation of greater than or equal to 70% or 65%, respectively (grade 1C). Fluid resuscitation with either crystalloids (i.e., normal saline or lactated Ringer's solution) or colloids (i.e., albumin) should be administered. Hypovolemic patients should receive a fluid challenge of 1 L of crystalloid or 300–500 mL of colloids over 30 minutes.

Antibiotic Therapy

As the epidemiology of sepsis continues to change, trends in antibiotic therapy have changed as well. Increasing microbial resistance and varying microbiologic etiologies have led to the use of a wide variety of antimicrobial agents. The choice of antimicrobial agent has also been influenced by a shift in the predominance of gram-positive organisms over gram-negative organisms as the primary pathogens responsible for sepsis as well as the recent emergence of fungal pathogens.

Laboratory Testing

At least two blood cultures should be obtained—one peripheral and one drawn through each vascular device in place for greater than 48 hours—prior to initiation of antimicrobial therapy. In addition, at least one culture from all suspected sites of infection as well as sterile sites should be obtained, if such cultures do not result in significant delay in antibiotic administration (grade 1C). Prompt attainment of cultures is critical to increase the likelihood of identifying potential pathogens—information that will aid in optimizing antimicrobial therapy. It is essential to obtain cultures prior to the administration of antibiotics, as antibiotics may result in rapid sterilization of cultures within a few hours after the first antibiotic dose.

Drug Indications, Dosing Regimens, and Routes of Administration

Intravenous antibiotic therapy should be initiated within the first hour of recognition of severe sepsis and septic shock (grade 1B). Initially, empiric therapy should include broad-spectrum antimicrobials targeting the pathogens most likely responsible for the patient's infection. Antimicrobials should also be selected on an individual basis by taking into account the patient's history, drug allergies, underlying comorbidities, previous infections, antimicrobial history, resistance patterns within the community and institution, and potential for adverse reactions.

Vasopressors and Inotropes

Vasopressors should be initiated to maintain a MAP greater than or equal to 65 mm Hg (grade 1C). Vasopressor therapy is essential to ensure adequate perfusion of tissues and organs in the face of persistent hypotension. Norepinephrine or dopamine is recommended as the first choice of vasopressor in septic shock (grade 1C). Epinephrine should be reserved as the first alternative in septic shock unresponsive to norepinephrine or dopamine (grade 2B).

Drug Indications, Dosing Regimens, and Routes of Administration

- *Dopamine.* Dopamine, a precursor to norepinephrine and epinephrine and an endogenous central neurotransmitter, possesses dose-dependent pharmacologic effects. At doses less than 5 mcg/kg/min, dopamine stimulates dopaminergic DA_1 and DA_2 receptors, resulting in vasodilation in the renal, mesenteric, and coronary beds. At doses of 5–10 mcg/kg/min, dopamine stimulates β_1-adrenergic receptors, increasing cardiac contractility and heart rate. At doses greater than 10 mcg/kg/min, α_1-adrenergic effects predominate, resulting in arterial vasoconstriction and, subsequently, an increase in blood pressure.
- *Norepinephrine.* Norepinephrine, an endogenous mediator of the sympathetic nervous system, increases blood pressure through potent α_1-mediated vasoconstriction. With minimal inotropic and chronotropic effects, this vasoactive agent has been shown to be useful in situations where increases in heart rate are undesirable.
- *Epinephrine.* Epinephrine is an endogenous catecholamine with β_1, β_2, and α_1-adrenergic effects. Beta-adrenergic effects predominate at lower doses and α_1-adrenergic effects at higher doses. In addition, epinephrine increases oxygen delivery in septic shock by increasing cardiac index without affecting system vascular resistance (SVR).

Table 15-49 Other Supportive Pharmacologic Therapies (Adapted from the Surviving Sepsis Campaign Guidelines)

Recommendation	Drug Therapy	Rationale	Considerations
Stress ulcer prophylaxis	H2 blocker (grade 1A) or PPI (grade 1B)	• Trials confirming the benefit of stress ulcer prophylaxis include patients with sepsis. • Conditions shown to benefit from stress ulcer prophylaxis (coagulopathy, mechanical ventilation, and hypotension) are present in patients with severe sepsis and septic shock.	• Patients should be routinely assessed for continued need for prophylaxis.
Venous thromboembolism prophylaxis	Low-molecular-weight heparin (LMWH) or unfractionated heparin (UFH) (grade 1A)	• ICU patients are at high risk for thromboembolic events.	• UFH is preferred over LMWH in patients with moderate to severe renal dysfunction. • Mechanical methods (intermittent compression devices and graduated compression stockings) are recommended when anticoagulation is contraindicated or as an adjunct to anticoagulation in high-risk populations.
Analgesia/sedation/neuromuscular blockade		• To facilitate mechanical ventilation of critically ill patients	• The use of sedation protocols with a sedation goal should be used. Studies have demonstrated utilization of these protocols can reduce the duration of mechanical ventilation and ICU and hospital length of stay (grade 1B). • Intermittent bolus sedation or continuous infusion sedation to predetermined endpoints with daily interruption is recommended (grade 1B). • The use of neuromuscular blockers should be avoided if possible due to the risk of prolonged neuromuscular blockade following discontinuation (grade 1B).
Glycemic control	Intravenous insulin (grade 1B)	• Based on randomized controlled trials in medical and surgical patients, glucose control demonstrated improved outcomes in these subsets of patients.	• Insulin should be titrated to a goal blood glucose less than 150 mg/dL (grade 2C). • All patients receiving intravenous insulin should have their blood glucose initially monitored every 1–2 hours (grade 1C).

- *Phenylephrine.* Phenylephrine possesses potent α-adrenergic activity, resulting in its ability to increase blood pressure through vasoconstrictive effects. This agent should not be administered as an initial vasopressor, but instead should be used as adjunct therapy to dopamine or norepinephrine. In addition, phenylephrine, due to its negligible activity on β-receptors, is useful in cases where cardiac stimulation is not warranted.
- *Dobutamine.* Dobutamine, a synthetic catecholamine, possesses a strong affinity for both β_1 and β_2 receptors in a 3:1 ratio, respectively. The β_1 effects of dobutamine result in its potent inotropic activity and weak chronotropic activity. At low doses (less than or equal to 5 mcg/kg/min), the combined α_1-adrenergic agonism and antagonism and β_2 stimulation result in mild vasodilatory effects. At doses greater than 15 mcg/kg/min, dobutamine stimulates both α_1 and β_2; however, the vasoconstrictive effects predominate at these higher doses. Dobutamine is utilized in instances where cardiac output and systemic oxygen delivery remain low.
- *Vasopressin.* Vasopressin, known as antidiuretic hormone, is stored in the posterior pituitary gland. Vasopressin stimulates V_1, V_2, and V_3 receptors; however, its vasoconstrictive effects are mediated through its effects on the V_1 receptor. At doses of 0.03 unit/min, vasopressin has shown to be effective in reversing catecholamine-resistant hypotension in septic shock patients; thus it is used as an adjunct agent to other vasopressors.

Controversial Therapies

Recombinant Human Activated Protein C (rhAPC)

Increases in cytokines such as TNF-α during sepsis decrease the synthesis of thrombomodulin, which is essential for the activation of protein C. The impaired activity of protein C results in an increase in the synthesis in plasminogen-activator inhibitor 1, thereby impairing fibrinolysis. The guidelines recommend that rhAPC be used in patients with sepsis-induced organ dysfunction, and an APACHE II score greater than or equal to 25, in the absence of contraindications (grade 2B).

Corticosteroids

Intravenous hydrocortisone should be administered as 50 mg every 6 hours to patients with septic shock unresponsive to fluid resuscitation and vasopressor therapy (grade 2C). The role of corticosteroids in shock has not been fully elucidated. Steroids should, therefore, be utilized on an individualized basis.

Sepsis Protocols

A recent approach to improve adherence to guidelines and help improve outcomes in sepsis patients has been the implementation of institutional-driven protocols for the management of sepsis and septic shock. The purpose of these protocols is to provide timely and appropriate care to patients presenting with sepsis and to create a continuum of management during the course of care. Protocols are initiated as soon as sepsis-induced hypoperfusion is identified and target hemodynamic stabilization of the patient is determined. These protocols include goals for fluid resuscitation, recommendations for antibiotic selection, and collection of laboratory data, cultures, and source control information.

1.3.0 Pharmacotherapy Monitoring

The adverse effects of vasopressor agents largely depend on their physiologic actions. For instance, the potent vasoconstrictive effects of norepinephrine, epinephrine, dopamine, phenylephrine, and vasopressin increase the likelihood of peripheral and gut ischemia. In addition, norepinephrine, epinephrine, dobutamine, and dopamine have the potential to lead to development of arrhythmias due to their cardiac effects. Extravasation of the drug can potentially occur in all cases where vasopressor therapy is used. Antimicrobial therapy should be reassessed daily and de-escalated upon clinical improvement of the patient or susceptibility patterns of the given drugs to the infecting pathogen(s). The duration of therapy should take into consideration the source of infection and the clinical improvement of the patient.

Emergent source control is imperative and should occur within an appropriate time frame. Identification of the site of infection and recognition of adequate source control measures, including the drainage of an abscess, debridement of necrotic tissue, and removal of an infected device, should be performed (grade 1C).

ANNOTATED BIBLIOGRAPHY

Dellinger RP, et al. Surviving Sepsis Campaign: international guidelines for management of severe sepsis and septic shock 2008. *Crit Care Med* 2008;36(1):296–327.

Guyatt G, et al. Applying the grades of recommendation for antithrombotic and thrombolytic therapy: the seventh ACCP conference and antithrombotic and thrombolytic therapy. *Chest* 2004;126(3):179S–189S. Available at: http://www.gradeworkinggroup.org/.

Hollenberg SM. Vasopressor support in septic shock. *Chest* 2007;132:1678–1687.

Hollenberg SM, et al. Practice parameters for hemodynamic support of sepsis in adult patients: 2004 update. *Crit Care Med* 2004;32(9):1928–1948.

Hotchkiss RS, Karl IE. The pathophysiology and treatment of sepsis. *N Engl J Med* 2003;348(2):138–150.

Leone M, Martin C. Vasopressor use in septic shock: an update. *Curr Opin Anesthesiol* 2008;21:141–147.

Levy MM, et al. 2001 SCCM/ESICM/ACCP/ATS/SIS International Sepsis Definitions Conference. *Intens Care Med* 2003;29:530–538.

Overgaard CB, Dzavik V. Inotropes and vasopressors: review of physiology and clinical use in cardiovascular disease. *Circulation* 2008;118:1047–1056.

Remick DG. Biological perspectives: pathophysiology of sepsis. *Am J Pathol* 2007;170:1435–1444.

Rivers E, et al. Early goal-directed therapy in the treatment of severe sepsis and septic shock. *N Engl J Med* 2001;345(19):1368–1377.

Russell JA. Management of sepsis. *N Engl J Med* 2006; 355:1699–1713.

TOPIC: SEXUALLY TRANSMITTED INFECTIONS

Section Coordinator: *Michael Klepser*
Contributors: *Jill A. Covyeou and Jennifer K. Hagerman*

Tips Worth Tweeting

- Special populations with sexually transmitted infections, such as pregnant women or immunocompromised patients, may require modification in recommended therapy, or additional follow-up or screening.

- Syphilis infection is characterized by four distinct stages.
- The pharmacist should be cautious when choosing the preparation of penicillin G for syphilis treatment, as combinations of benzathine and procaine penicillin or oral penicillin are not appropriate for some types of syphilis.
- Causative organisms of bacterial vaginosis include bacteria such as *Gardneralla vaginalis, Mobiluncus* spp., *Mycoplasma hominis*, and *Prevotella* spp.
- Human papillomavirus (HPV) strains that cause genital warts are not associated with cervical cancer.
- Patients receiving episodic treatment for herpes simplex virus (HSV) should begin within 1 day of symptom onset (or during the prodrome period) for greatest efficacy.
- Although fluoroquinolones (FQs) have frequently been used for the management of gonococcal infections, this class of medications is no longer recommended for treatment due to an increase in bacterial resistance.

The term "sexually transmitted infection" (STI) encompasses a wide array of bacterial and viral infections. STIs are most common in young adults (ages 15–24) and minority populations (specifically African Americans). If left untreated, STIs can cause serious long-term health consequences such as infertility, pelvic inflammatory disease (PID), and cancer.

Wellness and Prevention

The most reliable way to prevent the transmission of STIs is to abstain from sex (including oral, vaginal, and anal sex). Other methods include being in a mutually monogamous long-term relationship with an uninfected partner or using a barrier method such as the male condom with each sexual encounter. While the male condom can help prevent the transmission of some STIs, it might not provide complete protection against genital herpes or genital warts if the infected area is not protected by the condom. Patients should be counseled to use a latex product instead of "natural" or "lambskin" products, as the pore size of latex is much smaller, allowing fewer particles to penetrate the membrane. Other forms of contraception (diaphragms, spermacide, emergency contraception, and surgical sterilization) can protect against unplanned pregnancy but do not reliably protect against STIs.

Syphilis

Syphilis is an infection caused by the bacterium *Treponema pallidum.*

1.1.0 Patient Information

Signs and Symptoms

Syphilis infection is characterized by four distinct stages. In the primary stage, the patient develops a small, painless sore (chancre) on the genital area 10 days to 3 months after exposure; this chancre resolves without treatment in 3–6 weeks. Secondary syphilis is characterized by a generalized nonpruritic skin rash days to weeks after the chancre has resolved and may be accompanied by flu-like symptoms. The early latent stage is the first year after exposure, and the late latent stage is greater than 1 year after exposure; patients are usually asymptomatic in these stages. Twenty-five to 30% of patients with latent syphilis will go on to develop tertiary syphilis, which results in cardiac or central nervous system symptoms or gummatous lesions in organs and tissues.

1.2.0 Pharmacotherapy

Patients with primary or secondary syphilis should be counseled that treatment may induce the Jarisch-Herxheimer reaction, which is characterized by flu-like symptoms, for the first 12–24 hours. The pharmacist should be cautious when choosing the preparation of penicillin G, as combinations of benzathine and procaine penicillin or oral penicillin are not appropriate. Alternative treatments should be reserved for patients with a penicillin allergy.

1.3.0 Monitoring

The goal of treatment is to completely eradicate *T. pallidum*. Transmission of *T. pallidum* occurs only during symptomatic periods of the disease; however, partners of patients in any stage of syphilis should be evaluated clinically and serologically and treated appropriately. Patients should be reevaluated at 6 and 12 months after treatment (for primary and secondary syphilis) or at 6, 12, and 24 months (for latent syphilis) to ensure successful treatment.

Genital HSV

Genital HSV (herpes) is an infection caused by the herpes simplex viruses type 1 (HSV-1) or type 2 (HSV-2). Most genital infections are caused by HSV-2.

1.1.0 Patient Information

Signs and Symptoms

Genital HSV is characterized by painful blisters that form on or around the genitals, which break open, leaving ulcers that heal in 2–4 weeks. The primary episode may be accompanied by flu-like symptoms. The patient may continue to have recurrences throughout their life, although those episodes may be further apart and less intense.

1.2.0 Pharmacotherapy

Therapy with IV medications should be reserved for immunocompromised patients or patients with severe symptoms requiring hospitalization. Patients receiving episodic treatment should begin therapy within 1 day of symptom onset (or during the prodrome period) for greatest efficacy.

1.3.0 Pharmacotherapy Monitoring

Treatment goals are to relieve symptoms, shorten duration of flare-ups, and decrease viral shedding (transmission); these goals can be achieved through episodic or suppressive therapy. Patients should be counseled that they can still shed the virus even when they are asymptomatic; thus many patients chose to take suppressive therapy to decrease viral shedding and risk of transmitting the infection.

Genital HPV

Genital human papillomavirus (HPV) is the most common STI.

1.1.0 Patient Information

Signs and Symptoms

Most strains of HPV are asymptomatic; however, several are associated with genital warts or linked to cervical cancer. Strains that cause genital warts are not associated with cervical cancer; therefore, patients should be counseled that genital warts do not cause cervical cancer.

Warts can appear as small bumps or groups of bumps and can be raised, flat, or cauliflower shaped. In most cases, the patient's immune system will clear the virus within 1 year, and treatment is not recommended in asymptomatic patients. Symptomatic patients can treat the warts; however, if left untreated, genital warts can resolve, remain unchanged, or increase.

1.2.0 Pharmacotherapy

Patients should monitor for wart recurrences and follow-up with their provider. Only approximately 10% of women with a high-risk HPV strain (nonwart causing) will go on to develop a chronic infection that can put them at risk for cervical cancer.

1.3.0 Pharmacotherapy Monitoring

The goal of treatment is to remove the warts; however, this does not eradicate the virus and the warts may return.

Wellness and Prevention

Two vaccines are currently on the market for the prevention of cervical, vulvar, and vaginal cancers:

- Gardasil protects against HPV strains 6, 11, 16, and 18.
- Cervarix protects against HPV strains 16 and 18.

Both vaccines require a series of 3 immunizations.

Women should continue to get regular Pap screening regardless of their HPV status.

Chlamydia

1.1.0 Patient Information

In 2008, the CDC received more than 1.2 million reports of sexually transmitted chlamydial infections. This number likely underestimates the true prevalence of disease because patients with such infections are often asymptomatic. If left untreated, infections caused by the organism *Chlamydia trachomatis* can spread from the lower genital tract and lead to complications such as PID and infertility.

Laboratory Testing

Tests such as the nucleic acid amplification test (NAAT) can be used for screening and diagnosis.

Signs and Symptoms

Symptoms, if present, typically occur within 1–3 weeks of contact with an infected person and may include vaginal or penile discharge and dysuria.

1.2.0 Pharmacotherapy

A single dose of azithromycin or 7 days of doxycycline are the recommended first-line treatment options for uncomplicated urogenital *Chlamydia* infections in adults. Management of sex partners is crucial to prevent further transmission of the disease. The most recent sex partner (regardless of time frame) and all sex partners within the 60 days prior to diagnosis or onset of symptoms should be evaluated and receive treatment.

Wellness and Prevention

Chlamydia screening is indicated for all sexually active women 25 years of age or younger and for all pregnant women. Women older than the age of 25 years at high risk for *Chlamydia* infections should also be screened.

Gonorrhea

Gonorrhea is caused by the gram-negative bacterium *Neisseria gonorrhoeae*.

1.1.0 Patient Information

Signs and Symptoms

Women with gonorrhea are frequently asymptomatic and may be unaware that they are infected. Similar to *Chlamydia* infections, untreated gonococcal infections may result in complications such as PID; therefore, women at high risk should be screened for infection. Symptoms (when present) typically emerge 2–5 days after contact with an infected individual; however, onset may be delayed up to a month. Symptoms in women may include vaginal discharge or dysuria. Infected men may present with dysuria and penile discharge.

Laboratory Testing

Tests such as the NAAT can be used to diagnose gonococcal urogenital infections in both men and women. A Gram stain of a urethral specimen positive for polymorphonuclear leukocytes and intracellular gram-negative diplocci is also diagnostic for gonococcal infection. In addition to urogenital infections, disseminated infections, conjunctivitis, and pharyngeal infections can be caused by *N. gonorrhoeae*.

1.2.0 Pharmacotherapy

Although fluoroquinolones (FQs) have frequently been used for the management of gonococcal infections, this class of medications is no longer recommended for treatment due to an increase in bacterial resistance. For uncomplicated infections, first-line therapy is a single intramuscular dose of ceftriaxone pluz azithromycin or doxycycline. Dosing and alternative treatments are outlined in Table 15-50.

Gonococcal infections commonly occur simultaneously with *Chlamydia* infections and, unless ruled out, both infections should be treated. This, as well as increasing N. *gonorrhoeae* reistance is why azithromycin or doxycycline dual therapy is the recommended regimen for treatment of gonococcal infections. As with *Chlamydia* infections, management of sex partners is important to curb further transmission of gonorrhea. The most recent sex partner (regardless of time frame) and all sex partners within the 60 days prior to diagnosis or onset of symptoms should be evaluated and receive treatment.

1.3.0 Patient Monitoring

Patients with *Chlamydia* infection and/or gonorrhea should be counseled to avoid sex until both they and their sex partners have completed treatment and are asymptomatic to help prevent the spread of infection.

Bacterial Vaginosis

Bacterial vaginosis (BV) is a polymicrobial infection that occurs in women. Causative organisms include bacteria such as *Gardneralla vaginalis, Mobiluncus* spp., *Mycoplasma hominis*, and *Prevotella* spp. Women who are sexually active are more likely to acquire BV; however, other activities such as douching may also increase the risk of contracting BV.

1.1.0 Patient Information

Laboratory Testing

Bacterial vaginosis can be diagnosed by Gram stain or by meeting three out of four clinical criteria:

- Homogenous, white, adherent vaginal discharge
- Clue cells (vaginal epithelial cells coated with bacteria) seen by microscopy
- Vaginal fluid pH > 4.5
- Vaginal discharge with a fishy odor with or without adding potassium hydroxide to the sample (positive "whiff" test)

1.2.0 Pharmacotherapy

Recommended treatment of bacterial vaginosis is outlined in Table 15-50. Empiric treatment of sex partners is not warranted.

Trichomoniasis

Trichomoniasis is a protozoan infection caused by *Trichomonas vaginalis.*

1.1.0 Patient Information

Signs and Symptoms

Women with BV commonly present with foul-smelling discolored (e.g., yellow-green) vaginal discharge and irritation within a month of contact with an infected person. Some women may be asymptomatic. Men may also be asymptomatic or may present with urethritis.

Laboratory Testing

In women, available methods of diagnosis of vaginal trichomoniasis include microscopic evaluation of wet mount or culture of vaginal secretions. In men, culture of urethral swab, urine, and semen is recommended for diagnosis.

1.2.0 Pharmacotherapy

Options for treatment include metronidazole or tinidazole. Doses and duration of treatment are outlined in Table 15-50. Treatment of the infected patient's sex partners is recommended.

Table 15-50 Management of Common STIs

Disease	First-Line Therapy*	Alternative Treatment*
Syphilis	*Primary, Secondary, and Early Latent:* Benzathine penicillin G 2.4 million units IM (single dose) *Late Latent or Latent of Unknown Duration:* Benzathine penicillin G 2.4 million units IM every week × 3 weeks *Tertiary:* Benzathine penicillin G 2.4 million units IM every week × 3 weeks *Neurosyphilis:* Aqueous crystalline penicillin G 3-4 million unit IV every 4 hr × 10–14 days	*Primary, Secondary, and Early Latent:* Doxycycline 100 mg po bid × 14 days Tetracycline 500 mg po qid ×14 days *Late Latent or Latent of Unknown Duration:* Doxycycline 100 mg po bid × 28 days Tetracycline 500 mg po qid × 28 days *Tertiary:* Procaine penicillin 2.4 million units IM daily **plus** probenecid 500 mg po qid × 10–14 days *Neurosyphilis:* Ceftriaxone 2 g daily IM or IV × 10–14 days
Genital HSV	*Episodic:* Acyclovir 400 mg po tid × 5 days Acyclovir 800 mg po bid × 5 days Acyclovir 800 mg po tid × 2 days Famciclovir 125 mg po bid × 5 days Famciclovir 1 g po bid × 1 day Valacyclovir 500 mg po bid × 3 days Valacyclovir 1 g po daily × 5 days *Suppressive:* Acyclovir 400 mg po bid Famciclovir 250 mg po bid Valacyclovir 500 mg po daily Valacyclovir 1g po daily	Acyclovir 5–10 mg/kg IV every 8 hr × 2–7 days until clinical improvement occurs, then oral therapy to complete 10 days of total therapy
Genital HPV	*Patient Administered:* Podofilox 0.5% solution or gel applied to visible warts bid × 3 days, followed by 4 days of rest (cycle may be repeated to up to 4 cycles) Imiquimod 5% cream applied daily at bedtime 3 times per week (up to 16 weeks), then washed with soap and water 6–10 hr later Sinecatchins 15% ointment applied tid (0.5 cm strand to each wart) up to 16 weeks	*Provider Administered:* Cryotherapy with liquid nitrogen Podophyllin resin 10%–25% Trichloroacetic acid or bichloroacetic acid 80%–90% Surgical removal Intralesional interferon Laser surgery
Chlamydia	Azithromycin 1 g po in a single dose Doxycycline 100 mg po bid for 7 days	Erythromycin base 500 mg po qid for 7 days Erythromycin ethylsuccinate 800 mg po qid for 7 days Ofloxacin 300 mg po bid for 7 days Levofloxacin 500 mg po daily for 7 days
Gonorrhea	Ceftriaxone 125 mg IM in a single dose PLUS Azithromycin 1 g po in a single dose OR Doxycycline 100mg po bid × 7 days	† If ceftriaxone is not available: Cefixime 400mg po in a single dose PLUS Azithromycin 1 g po in a single dose OR Doxycycline 100mg po bid × 7 days PLUS Test of cure in 1 week

Table 15-50 (*continued*)

Disease	First-Line Therapy*	Alternative Treatment*
Gonorrhea (*continued*)		For severe penicillin allergy: Azithromycin 2 g po in a single dose PLUS Test of cure in 1 week
Bacterial vaginosis	Clindamycin cream 2%, 5g intravaginally at bedtime for 7 days Metronidazole 500 mg orally bid for 7 days Metronidazole gel 0.75%, 5 g intravaginally, daily for 5 days	Clindamycin 300 mg po bid for 7 days Clindamycin ovules 100 mg intravaginally HS for 3 days Tinidazole 2 g po daily × 2 days Tinidazole 1 g po daily × 5 days
Trichomoniasis	Metronidazole 2 g po in a single dose Tinidazole 2 g po in a single dose	Metronidazole 500 mg po bid for 7 days

Notes: bid: twice daily; HS: at bedtime; IM: intramuscularly; IV: intravenously; po: orally; tid: three times daily; qid: four times daily.

*For nonpregnant, non-HIV-positive patients.

†Azithromycin preferred over doxycycline as second agent

Table 15-51 Characteristics of Medications Commonly Utilized in the Management of STIs

Drug	Mechanism of Action	Adverse Effects	Comments
Penicillins • Benzathine penicillin G • Aqueous crystalline penicillin G • Procaine penicillin	Beta-lactam: interferes with bacterial cell-wall synthesis	Rash, anemia, injection-site pain, confusion, drowsiness, seizure	• Use caution in patients with impaired renal function
Tetracyclines • Doxycycline • Tetracycline	Inhibits bacterial protein synthesis	Photosensitivity, rash, nausea/vomiting, diarrhea, tooth discoloration (children), anemia	• Contraindicated in children younger than 8 years • Take with food to decrease GI effects • Take with full glass of water • Multivalent cations can decrease serum levels (most relevant with tetracycline)
Probenicid	Competitively inhibits the renal tubular secretion of beta-lactams (increasing plasma levels)	Flushing, dizziness, fever, headache, rash, nausea/vomiting, anemia, hepatic necrosis, gouty arthritis (acute)	• Contraindicated in patients with a history of uric acid kidney stones • Salicylates can decrease serum levels
Cephalosporins • Ceftriaxone • Cefixime	Inhibits bacterial cell-wall synthesis	Injection-site pain and induration (ceftriaxone), rash, nausea/vomiting/diarrhea, anemias	• Use caution in patients with penicillin allergy • Do not reconstitute ceftriaxone with a calcium-containing solution
Antivirals • Acyclovir • Famciclovir • Valacyclovir	Inhibits viral DNA synthesis and viral replication	Malaise, headache, nausea/vomiting/diarrhea, rash, increased liver function tests, acute renal failure	• Use caution in patients with renal disease • Maintain adequate hydration (acyclovir)
Imiquimod	Unknown	Application-site reactions, edema, flaking, itching, crusting, dryness, vesicles, weeping, burning, fever, malaise, myalgia	• Avoid using live vaccines

(*continues*)

Table 15-51 (*continued*)

Drug	Mechanism of Action	Adverse Effects	Comments
Podofilox	Antimitotic	Localized pain, irritation, and inflammation	• Solution should be applied with a cotton swab • Gel should be applied with finger
Macrolides • Azithromycin • Erythromycin	Inhibits bacterial protein synthesis by binding to the 50S ribosomal subunit	Diarrhea, nausea/vomiting, abdominal pain, QT prolongation, elevated liver transaminases	
Fluoroquinolones • Ofloxacin • Levofloxacin	Inhibits bacterial DNA gyrase and topoisomerase IV	Nausea/vomiting, diarrhea, photosensitivity, tendinitis, QT prolongation	• Multivalent cations can decrease serum levels • Adjust dosing frequency in patients with renal impairment • Increased incidence of FQ-resistant *N. gonorrhoeae* strains
Clindamycin	Inhibits bacterial protein synthesis by binding to the 50S ribosomal subunit	Oral: diarrhea, *Clostridium difficile*–associated diarrhea, nausea/vomiting, abdominal pain Cream/intravaginal ovules: vulvovaginitis, vulvovaginal candidiasis, vaginal discharge	• Clindamycin cream might weaken latex condoms and diaphragms
Metronidazole	Exact mechanism unknown; disrupts DNA and inhibits nucleic acid synthesis	Oral: Reddish-brown color to urine, metallic taste, "furry" tongue, nausea/vomiting/diarrhea Intravaginal gel: vulvovaginal candidiasis, headache, vaginal pruritus, nausea	• Disulfiram-like reaction may occur if taken with alcohol (flushing, headache, abdominal cramps, nausea/vomiting); alcohol should be avoided (including alcohol-containing mouthwash/cold medicine) during therapy and for at least 1 day after • Pregnancy category B; however, should be avoided in first trimester
Tinidazole	Exhibits antiprotozoal and antibacterial activities; exact mechanism unknown	Metallic/bitter taste, nausea/vomiting, anorexia	• Disulfiram-like reaction may occur if taken with alcohol; alcohol should be avoided during therapy and for 3 days after • Patients should take with food to minimize gastrointestinal effects
Sinecatechins	Unknown	Erythema, pruritis, burning, pain, ulceration, edema, enduration, vesicular rash	• Use finger to ensure coverage with a thin layer of ointment • Do not wash off after use, may weaken condoms and diaphragm

ANNOTATED BIBLIOGRAPHY

Centers for Disease Control and Prevention. Notice to readers: discontinuation of spectinomycin. *Morb Mortal Wkly Rep* 2006;55(13):370.

Centers for Disease Control and Prevention. Sexually transmitted diseases treatment guidelines, 2010 *MMWR Recomm Rep* 2010;59RR-12:1–114.

Centers for Disease Control and Prevention. Sexually transmitted diseases trends in the United States: 2010 national data for gonorrhea, chalmydia and syphylis. Available at: http://www.cdc.gov/std/stats2010/trends2010.pdf. Accessed June 21, 2012.

Centers for Disease Control and Prevention. Update to CDC's sexually transmitted diseases treatment guidelines, 2010: Oral cephalosporins no long a recommended treatment for gonococcal infections. *Morb Mortal Wkly Rep* 2012;61:590-594.

Centers for Disease Control and Prevention. Update to CDC's sexually transmitted diseases treatment guidelines, 2006: fluoroquinolones no longer recommended for treatment of gonococcal infections. *Morb Mortal Wkly Rep* 2007;56:332–336.

DiPiro JT, Talbert RL, Yee GC, et al, eds. *Pharmacotherapy: A Pathophysiologic Approach*. 7th ed. New York: McGraw Hill, 2008.

Egan ME, Lipsky MS. Diagnosis of vaginitis. *Am Fam Physician* 2000;62:1095-1104.

Fatahzadeh M, Schwartz R. Human herpes simplex virus infections: epidemiology, pathogenesis, symptomatology, diagnosis, and management. *J Am Acad Dermatol* 2007;57(5):737–763.

Kent M, Romanelli F. Reexamining syphilis: an update on epidemiology, clinical manifestations, and management. *Ann Pharmacother* 2008;42:226–236.

Miller KE. Diagnosis and treatment of *Chlamydia trachomatis* infection. *Am Fam Physician* 2006;73:1411–1416.

Ogunmodede F, Yale S, Krawisz B, et al. Human papillomavirus infections in primary care. *CM&R* 2007;5(4):210–217.

Owen MK, Clenney TL. Management of vaginitis. *Am Fam Physician* 2004;70:2125–2132.

TOPIC: SKIN AND SOFT-TISSUE INFECTIONS

Section Coordinator: Michael Klepser
Contributor: Matt Beachnau

Tips Worth Tweeting

- Skin and soft-tissue infections can range from mild and self-limiting (cellulitis) to severe and complex (necrotizing fasciitis).
- Three forms of impetigo are possible, each of which has a unique presentation. Streptococci and/or *Staphylococcus aureus* (MSSA/MRSA) typically cause these infections.
- Cellulitis is a common skin infection typically caused by *Streptococcus* and *S. aureus* (MSSA/MRSA). Cellulitis can be a simple self-limiting infection, or it can lead to complications including systemic infection.
- Community-acquired MRSA is an emerging pathogen that must be considered with skin and soft-tissue infections, especially in areas of higher prevalence and at-risk patient populations.
- Necrotizing fasciitis is a rare but life-threatening subcutaneous infection. Emergent surgical intervention is the primary treatment. This infection may be monomicrobial or polymicrobial in nature.
- Consider normal mouth flora for causative organisms of bite wounds. Empirically treat bites with antibiotics regardless of the wound appearance.

Key Terms

Skin and soft tissue infections (SSTIs) refer to any infections that involve the epidermis, dermis, subcutaneous fat, fascia, or muscle. Gram-positive organisms typically cause simple infections.

Impetigo

Impetigo is a contagious skin infection that typically affects infants and children.

Table 15-52 Treatment Regimens for Impetigo

Antibiotics	Spectrum of Activity	Class	Dose*	Comments
Dicloxacillin (generic only)	*Staphylococcus aureus* (MSSA), *Streptococcus*	Penicillin (penicillinase-resistant)	250 mg po 4 times daily	
Cephalexin (Keflex)	*S. aureus, S. pyogenes, S. pneumoniae*, gram (–)	First-generation cephalosporin	250 mg po 4 times daily	
Erythromycin (Ery-Tab)	Gram (+), especially *Streptococcus*; gram (–), atypicals (e.g., *Mycoplasma, Legionella*)	Macrolide	250 mg po 4 times daily	Some *Staphylococcus* and *Streptococcus* resistance
Clindamycin (Cleocin)	Gram (+), anaerobes		300–400 mg po 3 times daily	
Amoxicillin/clavulanate (Augmentin)	*S. aureus* (MSSA), gram (–): *E. coli*, anaerobes	Aminopenicillin	250–500 mg po twice daily	
Mupirocin ointment (Bactroban)	*S. aureus* (MSSA/MRSA), *Streptococcus*, gram (–)		Apply topically to lesions 3 times daily	

Note: Treatment duration is typically 7–10 days for oral antibiotic therapy and 5 days for topical antibiotic therapy.

*Adult dose; pediatric dose not included.

Data from: Stevens DL, Bisno AL, Chambers HF, Everett ED, Dellinger P, Goldstein EJ, Gorbach SL, Hirschmann JV, Kaplan EL, Montoya JG, Wade JC. Practice guidelines for the diagnosis and management of skin and soft-tissue infections. *Clin Infect Dis* 2005 Nov 15;41(10):1373–406.

1.1.0 Patient Information

Signs and Symptoms

There are three forms of impetigo:

- *Impetigo Contagiosa:* The most common form of impetigo, this variant presents as itching red sores near the nose and mouth that may rupture and ooze.
- *Bullous Impetigo:* This form of impetigo affects children younger than 2 years old. It can present as itchy blisters on the trunk, arms, and legs. These blisters may break and crust over and may last longer than other forms of impetigo.
- *Ecthyma:* This more serious form of impetigo typically penetrates deep into the dermis. It presents with painful sores/blisters, usually on the legs and feet.

Causes

Impetigo is caused by skin bacteria that enter through cuts, scrapes, or insect bites.

Organisms

Streptococci and/or *S. aureus* (some infections involve MRSA)

1.2.0 Pharmacotherapy

See Table 15-52.

Cellulitis

Cellulitis is an acute infection that affects the epidermis and dermis.[1,2]

1.1.0 Patient Information

Signs and Symptoms

Cellulitis is characterized by redness, swelling, tenderness, pain, and warmth.

Causes

Cellulitis typically occurs when bacteria enter through a break in the skin. Cracking between the toes is a common cause of lower extremity cellulitis.

Organisms

The most common organisms that cause cellulitis are *S. aureus* (including methillicin-sensitive *S. aureus* [MSSA] and methicillin-resistant *S. aureus* [MRSA]) and *Streptococcus* species. Group A beta-hemolytic *Streptococcus* (*S. pyogenes*) is most often the cause of cellulitis. Other infectious organisms include *Pastuella multocida* (dog/cat bites). In addition, some gram-negative organisms such as *Pseudomonas* can cause infection in immunocompromised patients.

1.2.0 Pharmacotherapy

- Cleaning a wound with soap and water is all that is necessary for patients with mild cellulitis. This type of infection is typically self-resolving.

Table 15-53 Treatment Regimens for MSSA

Antibiotics	Spectrum of Activity	Class	Dose*	Comments
Nafcillin or oxacillin (generic only)	*Staphylococcus aureus* (MSSA), *Streptococcus*	Penicillin (penicillinase-resistant)	1–2 g IV every 4 hr	IV drug of choice
Dicloxacillin (generic only)	*S. aureus* (MSSA), *Streptococcus*	Penicillin (penicillinase-resistant)	500 mg po 4 times daily	Oral agent of choice for MSSA
Cefazolin (Ancef)	*S. aureus, S. pyogenes, S. pneumoniae, gram* (–)	First-generation cephalosporin	1 g IV every 8 hr	
Cephalexin (Keflex)	*S. aureus, S. pyogenes, S. pneumoniae*, gram (–)	First-generation cephalosporin	500 mg po 4 times daily	
Clindamycin (Cleocin)	Gram (+), anaerobes		600 mg/kg IV every 8 hr; or 300–600 mg po 3 times daily	Potential for emergence of resistance; inducible resistance in MRSA
Doxycycline (Vibramycin)	Gram (+), gram (–), atypicals	Tetracycline	100 mg po twice daily	
TMP-SMZ (Bactrim)	Gram (+) MSSA/MRSA, gram (–)	Sulfonamide	1–2 double-strength tablets po twice daily	

Note: Treatment duration is typically 7 days depending on clinical response.

*Adult dose, pediatrics dose not included.

Data from: Stevens DL, Bisno AL, Chambers HF, Everett ED, Dellinger P, Goldstein EJ, Gorbach SL, Hirschmann JV, Kaplan EL, Montoya JG, Wade JC. Practice guidelines for the diagnosis and management of skin and soft-tissue infections. *Clin Infect Dis* 2005 Nov 15;41(10):1373–406

Table 15-54 Treatment Regimens for MRSA

Antibiotics	Spectrum of Activity	Class	Dose*	Comments
Vancomycin (Vancocin)†	Gram (+) MSSA/MRSA		30 mg/kg IV in 2 divided doses	IV drug of choice for MRSA
Linezolid (Zyvox)	Gram (+), MSSA/MRSA, *E. faecalis* (VRE)	Oxazolidinone	600 mg IV or po every 12 hr	Very expensive
Clindamycin (Cleocin)	Gram (+), anaerobes		600 mg/kg IV every 8 hr, or 300–450 mg po 3 times daily	Emergence of resistance, inducible resistance in MRSA
Daptomycin (Cubicin)	Gram (+) MSSA/MRSA, *E. faecalis* (VRE)	Cyclic lipopeptides	4 mg/kg IV every 12 hr	
Doxycycline (Vibramycin)	Gram (+), gram (–), atypicals	Tetracycline	100 mg po twice daily	Not recommended for children
TMP-SMZ (Bactrim)	Gram (+), MSSA/MRSA, gram (–)	Sulfonamide	1 or 2 double-strength tablets twice daily	

Note: Treatment duration is typically 7 days depending on clinical response.

*Adult dosing; pediatrics dosing not included.

†Dose based on the patient's renal function. Dosing may depend on institution policy. Target serum trough concentration is 10–15 mcg/dL.

Data from: Stevens DL, Bisno AL, Chambers HF, Everett ED, Dellinger P, Goldstein EJ, Gorbach SL, Hirschmann JV, Kaplan EL, Montoya JG, Wade JC. Practice guidelines for the diagnosis and management of skin and soft-tissue infections. *Clin Infect Dis* 2005 Nov 15;41(10):1373–406.

- Patients with evidence of systemic infections (e.g., fever, increasing pain, tachycardia, hypotension) should be treated empirically based on the site of infection and triggering event (e.g., scrape, cut, bite) to target organisms that we suspect are causing the infection.

Community-Acquired MRSA

S. aureus commonly colonizes the skin, axillae, and nares. Since the introduction of antibiotics, this bacterium has developed resistance to some commonly used antibiotics, including beta-lactams and macrolides. MRSA has typically been linked to hospitalized patients or patients in nursing homes. Recently, community-acquired MRSA (CA-MRSA) has emerged in patients with no association to healthcare exposure. This organism commonly causes SSTIs and presents as abscesses and cellulitis, although it does have the potential to cause serious bacteremias and pneumonia. CA-MRSA may be found in less than 1% of the population; however, the incidence varies among certain populations.

1.1.0 Patient Information

Disease States and Conditions Associated with CA-MRSA

Populations at high risk for CA-MRSA include children younger than 2 years (especially in child care), Native Americans, and Alaskan Natives. Transmission occurs mainly by person-to-person exposure. In the past, CA-MRSA has caused outbreaks among sports teams, prisoners, military personnel, men who have sex with men, tattoo recipients, and IV drug users. Certain geographical locations may have a higher prevalence of MRSA infections.

1.2.0 Pharmacotherapy

1. Incision and drainage (I&D) of abscess or other lesions. Be sure to culture the aspirate.
2. If infection does not resolve:
   2a. Mild infections: Local care with topical antibiotics (Mupirocin) or oral antibiotics. Adjust the treatment based on the sensitivity results from cultures.
   2b. Moderate infection (patient may have a fever but appears stable): If MRSA is suspected, then administer empiric antibiotics and adjust based on the sensitivity results from cultures.
   2c. Severe or critically ill (patient appears unstable; sepsis; necrotizing fasciitis): Admit the patient to a hospital for treatment with broad-spectrum antibiotics, including treatment of MRSA. Adjust the treatment based on the sensitivity results from cultures.

Cultures

Drain the wound or biopsy area of inflammation. If the culture results in identification of *S. aureus,* then request a D-test to determine resistance to clindamycin. A D-test is conducted by placing erythromycin

Table 15-55 Signs, Symptoms, and Risk Factors for CA-MRSA

Signs and Symptoms	Risk Factors
• Looks like spider bite • Pustular lesions • Boils • Abscess • Impetigo • Infected wound	• IV drug use • Incarceration • Participation in contact sports • Contact with someone colonized by MRSA • High prevalence of MRSA in the community

and clindamycin disks on an agar plate that includes the isolates in questions. Flattening of the clindamycin zone (D shaped) indicates inducible resistance.

Necrotizing Fasciitis

Necrotizing fasciitis is a rare but potentially fatal subcutaneous infection that runs along superficial tissue between the skin and underlying muscle. It is sometimes referred to as flesh-eating bacteria.

1.1.0 Patient Information

Signs and Symptoms

Approximately 80% of patients with necrotizing fasciitis present with skin lesions that might include minor abrasions, insect bites, surgical sites, or boils. These lesions often appear insignificant or as minor cellulitis. The remaining 20% of patients may have no visible presentation. As the infection progresses, patients may present with fevers, lethargy, edema, pain, and skin discoloration. A unique clinical feature is a wooden-hard feel to the subcutaneous tissue.

Causes

Necrotizing fasciitis occurs when bacteria enter through a break in the skin.

Organisms

The infectious organisms may be monomicrobial or polymicrobial: *Streptococcus* (group A; *S. pyogenes*), *S. aureus* (MSSA and MRSA), *Vibrio vulnificus*, *Clostridium perfringes*, and *Bacteroides fragilis*.

1.2.0 Pharmacotherapy

Emergent surgical intervention is the primary treatment in cases of necrotizing fasciitis. Because this infection often presents as cellulitis, early empiric treatment with antibiotics is recommended. Always adjust therapy based on cultures and sensitivity results.

Bites

Human Bite

Human bites may be a result of teeth biting skin, or a closed-fist injury where a fist strikes teeth.

1.1.0 Patient Information

Organisms

Infectious organisms in case of human bites may include the normal oral flora: *Streptococcus* species (especially *viridans*), *Staphylococcus*, *Haemophilus* species, *Eikenella corrodens*, and anaerobes (*Fusobacterium* species, peptostreptococci, *Prevotella* species, and *Porphyromonas* species). Human bites also have the potential to spread viral infections including: herpes, hepatitis B and C, and HIV.

1.2.0 Pharmacotherapy

Topical wound care and irrigation are recommended. Empiric antibiotics should be given to all patients with bite wounds regardless of the wound appearance.

Animal Bites

Dog and cat bites account for a majority of animal bites; however, we will consider other animals as a cause of infection.

1.1.0 Patient Information

- Dog bites typically cause a crushing injury. This can cause deep structure damage to bones, tendons, muscles, and nerves.
- Cat bites are typically puncture wounds that may allow bacteria to enter through the skin directly. These infections usually develop faster than dog bites.

Organisms

- Dog bites: *Staphylococcus, Streptococcus, Eikenella, Pasteurella, Proteus, Klebsiella, Haemophilus, Enterobacter, Bacteroides, Moraxella, Neisseria, Prevotella, Porphyromonas*
- Cat bites: *Pasteurella, Actinomyces, Bacteroides, Clostridium, Peptostreptococcus, Staphylococcus, Streptococcus*
- Others (swine, rodent, primates, reptiles): *Pasteurella, Bacteroides, Proteus, Streptococcus, Mycoplasma, Streptobacillus, Spirillum, Enterococcus, Enterobacteriaceae, Pseudomonas, Clostridium*

Table 15-56 Dosing Regimens for Necrotizing Fasciitis

Disease State	Antibiotics	Spectrum of Activity	Class	Dose*	Comments
Mixed infections	Ampicillin-sulbactam (Unasyn) **or** Piperacillin-tazobactam (Zosyn) **plus** Ciprofloxacin (Cipro) **plus** Clindamycin (Cleocin)	*Staphylococcus aureus* (MSSA), gram (–), anaerobes *S. aureus* (MSSA), gram (–), anaerobes, *Pseudomonas* Gram (+), gram (–), atypicals Gram (+), anaerobes	Aminopenicillin Antipseudomonal penicillin Fluoroquinolone	1.5–3 g IV every 6 hr 3.375–4.5 g IV every 6–8 hr 400 mg IV every 12 hr 600–900 mg/kg IV every 8 hr	For patients with penicillin allergy: clindamycin **or** metronidazole with an aminoglycoside **or** fluoroquinolone
	Imipenem/cilastatin (Invanz)	Gram (+), gram (–), anaerobes	Carbapenem	500 mg IV every 6 hr	
	Meropenem (Merrem)	Gram (+), gram (–), anaerobes	Carbapenem	1 g IV every 8 hr	
	Ertapenem	Gram (+), gram (–), anaerobes	Carbapenem	1 g IV daily	
	Cefotaxime (Claforan) **plus** Metronidazole (Flagyl) **or** Clindamycin (Cleocin)	Gram (–) > gram (+) Anaerobes Gram (+), anaerobes	Third-generation cephalosporin	2 g IV every 6 hr 500 mg IV every 6 hr 600–900 mg/kg IV every 8 hr	
Streptococcus infections	Penicillin **plus** Clindamycin (Cleocin)	*Streptococcus* species Gram (+), anaerobes	Penicillin	4 MU IV every 4–6 hr 600–900 mg/kg IV every 8 hr	For penicillin-allergic patients; vancomycin, daptomycin, or linezolid
S. aureus infections	Nafcillin or oxacillin (generics only)	*S. aureus*, *Streptococcus* species	Penicillin (penicillinase-resistant)	2 g IV every 4 hr	For penicillin-allergic patients; vancomycin, daptomycin, or linezolid
	Cefazolin (Ancef)	*S. aureus, S. pyogenes,* Gram (–)	First-generation cephalosporin	2 g IV every 8 hr	
	Vancomycin†	Gram (+) MSSA/MRSA		30 mg/kg IV in 2 divided doses	
	Clindamycin (Cleocin)	Gram (+), anaerobes		600–900 mg/kg IV every 8 hr	
Clostridium infections	Clindamycin (Cleocin)	Gram (+), anaerobes		600–900 mg/kg IV every 8 hr	
	Penicillin	*Streptococcus* species	Penicillin	4 MU IV every 4–6 hr	

Note: Continue antibiotics until repeat operative procedures are no longer necessary, the patient has shown clinical improvement, and the patient has been afebrile for 48–72 hours.

*Adult dosing; pediatrics dosing not included.

†Dose based on the patient's renal function. Dosing may depend on the institution's policy. Target serum trough concentration is 10–15 mcg/dL.

Data from: Stevens DL, Bisno AL, Chambers HF, Everett ED, Dellinger P, Goldstein EJ, Gorbach SL, Hirschmann JV, Kaplan EL, Montoya JG, Wade JC. Practice guidelines for the diagnosis and management of skin and soft-tissue infections. *Clin Infect Dis* 2005 Nov 15;41(10):1373–406.

Table 15-57 Dosing Regimen for Bites

Disease State	Antibiotics	Spectrum of Activity	Class	Dose*	Comments
Animal Bites					
	Amoxicillin-clavulana (Augmentin)	Gram (+), gram (–), anaerobes	Aminopenicillin	500/875 mg po twice daily	
	Ampicillin-sulbactam (Unasyn)	Gram (+), gram (–), anaerobes	Aminopenicillin	1.5–3 g IV every 6–8 hr	
	Piperacillin-tazpbactam (Zosyn)	*Staphylococcus aureus* (MSSA), gram (–), anaerobes	Antipseudomonal penicillin	3.375 g IV every 4–6 hr	Good activity against *Pasteurella multocida*
	Imipnem/cilastatin	Gram (+), gram (–), anaerobes	Carbapenem	500 mg IV every 6 hr	
	Meropenem (Merem)	Gram (+), gram (–), anaerobes	Carbapenem	1 g IV every 8 hr	
	Ertapenem (Invanz)	Gram (+), gram (–), anaerobes	Carbapenem	1 g IV daily	
	Doxycycline (Vibramycin)	Gram (+), gram (–), atypicals, anaerobes	Tetracycline	100 mg po twice daily	
	Penicillin **plus** Dicloxacillin	*Streptococcus* *Streptococcus, Staphylococcus* (MSSA)	Penicillin	500 mg po twice daily 500 mg po 4 times daily	
	TMP-SMZ (Bactrim)	Gram (+) MSSA/MRSA, gram (–)	Sulfonamide	160–180 mg po twice daily	No anaerobes
	Metronidazole (Flagyl)	Anaerobes		250–500 mg po 3 times daily	No aerobes
	Clindamycin (Cleocin)	Gram (+), anaerobes		300 mg po 3 times daily	No activity against *Pasteurella multocida*
	Cephalexin (Keflex): Oral	*S. aureus, S. pyogenes,* gram (–)	First-generation cephalosporin	500 mg po 3 times daily	No activity against *Pasteurella multocida*
	Cefazolin (Ancef): IV			1 g IV every 8 hr	
	Ceftriaxone (Rocephin)	Gram (–) > Gram (+)	Third-generation cephalosporin	1 g IV every 24 hr	
	Ciprofloxacin (Cipro)	Gram (+), gram (–), atypicals	Fluoroquinolones	500 mg po twice daily, or 400 mg IV every 12 hr	Good activity against *Pasteurella multocida*
Human Bites					
	Amoxicillin-clavulanate (Augmentin)	Gram (+), gram (–), anaerobes	Aminopenicillin	500/875 mg po every 8 hr	
	Ampicillin-sulbactam (Unasyn)	Gram (+), gram (–), anaerobes	Aminopenicillin	1.5–3 g IV every 6 hr	
	Imipnem/cilastatin	Gram (+), gram (–), anaerobes	Carbapenem	500 mg IV every 6 hr	
	Meropenem (Merrem)	Gram (+), gram (–), anaerobes	Carbapenem	1 g IV daily	
	Ertapenem (Invanz)	Gram (+), gram (–), anaerobes	Carbapenem	1 g IV daily	
	Doxycycline (Vibramycin)	Gram (+), gram (–), atypicals, anaerobes	Tetracycline	100 mg po twice daily	Good activity against *Eikenella*

Table 15-57 (*continued*)

Disease State	Antibiotics	Spectrum of Activity	Class	Dose*	Comments
Human Bites (*continued*)					
	TMP-SMZ (Bactrim)	Gram (+) MSSA/MRSA, gram (–)	Sulfonamide	2 DS tabs po twice daily	No anaerobes
	Metronidazole (Flagyl)	Anaerobes		500 mg po 3 times daily	No aerobes
	Clindamycin (Cleocin)	Gram (+), anaerobes		300 mg po 3 times daily	No activity against *Eikenella*
	Cephalexin (Keflex): Oral	*S. aureus, S. pyogenes,* gram (–)	First-generation cephalosporin	500 mg po 3 times daily	No activity against *E. corrodens*
	Cefazolin (Ancef): IV			1 g IV every 8 hr	

Note: Duration of antibiotic treatment is typically 7–10 days. Therapy may be extended to 4–6 weeks in cases of septic arthritis and osteomyelitis.

*Adult doses only; pediatric doses not included.

Data from: Stevens DL, Bisno AL, Chambers HF, Everett ED, Dellinger P, Goldstein EJ, Gorbach SL, Hirschmann JV, Kaplan EL, Montoya JG, Wade JC. Practice guidelines for the diagnosis and management of skin and soft-tissue infections. Clin Infect Dis 2005 Nov 15;41(10):1373–406.

ANNOTATED BIBLIOGRAPHY

1. McCormack, J. Traumatic skin and soft tissue infections. In Koda-Kimble MA, Young LY, Kradjen WA, Gluglielmo BJ, eds. *Applied Therapeutics: The Clinical Use of Drugs*. Philadelphia: Lippincott Williams, & Wilkins; 2005;65:1–66.
2. Stevens DL, Bisno AL, Chambers HF, et al. Practice guidelines for the diagnosis and management of skin and soft-tissue infections. *Clin Infect Dis* 2005;41(10):1373–1406.
3. Kowalski TJ, Berbari EF, Osmon DR. Epidemiology, treatment, and prevention of community-acquired methicillin-resistant *Staphylococcus aureus* infections. *Mayo Clin Proc* 2005;80(9):1201–1208.
4. *Community Associated Methicillin Resistant* Staphylococcus aureus *(CA-MRSA): Guidelines for Management and Control of Transmission.* PPH 42160. Wisconsin DFHS; October 2005.
5. King MD, Humphrey BJ, Wang YF, et al. Emergence of community-acquired methicillin-resistant *Staphylococcus aureus* USA 300 clone as the predominant cause of skin and soft-tissue infections. *Ann Intern Med* 2006;144(5):309–318.

Musculoskeletal

CHAPTER

16

TOPIC: GOUT

Section Coordinator: Katherine Kelly Orr
Contributor: Barb Mason and Kendall M. Crane

Tips Worth Tweeting

- Patients with gout can be classified as being either overproducers of uric acid or underexcretors—a distinction that may help guide therapy decisions.
- Gout results from altered purine metabolism or uric acid excretion.
- Use of drugs such as low-dose aspirin, alcohol, cytotoxic drugs, niacin, and hydrochlorothiazide can precipitate gout symptoms.
- A positive response to colchicine in an acute attack of gout supports the diagnosis of gout.
- Although indomethacin is most commonly used for acute gout treatment, any of the nonsteroidal anti-inflammatory agents will work in this indication.
- Colchicine causes diarrhea; it is administered orally, but rarely intravenously due to its potential for bone marrow depression and local extravasation.
- Uricosuric therapy should not be started during an acute attack.
- Two xanthine oxidase inhibitors—allopurinol and febuxostat—are on the market as gout therapies.
- Gout, which can be acute or chronic, is characterized by urate crystal–induced arthritis attacks.
- Gout risk increases with elevated serum uric acid levels; some patients may be asymptomatic with hyperuricemia.
- Elitek (rasburicase) can result in methemoglobinemia.
- Treatment is directed toward prevention and acute treatment of an attack.
- Drugs that lower the level of uric acid should not be used during an acute attack.
- Nonsteroidal anti-inflammatory drugs, colchicine, and steroids are used to treat acute attacks.
- Drugs that inhibit the synthesis of urate (allopurinol, febuxostat) and uricosurics that increase excretion of urate (probenecid, sulfinpyrazone) are used to prevent recurrent gout attacks.
- Fluid intake and dosage adjustment for renal impairment are important components of care to remember for gout.

Patient Care Scenario: Ambulatory Setting

47 y/o, 5'11", M, 176 lbs, two glasses of wine daily

Hypertension, history of gout, hyperlipidemia

Bun 25 mg/dL, Cr. 1.6 mg/dL, serum uric acid 10 mg/dL

Date	Physician	Drug	Quantity	Sig	Refills
12/1	Lowe	Allopurinol 300 mg	30	one daily	5
3/27	Lowe	Losartan 100 mg	30	one daily	5
2/1	Lowe	Hydrochlorothiazide 50 mg	30	one daily	5

1.1.0 Patient Information

Medication-Induced Causes of Hyperuricemia/Gout

Hydrochlorothiazide increases uric acid levels. Cyclosporine and levodopa decrease renal urate clearance. Niacin and ethambutol compete with urate for tubular secretion. Cytototoxic drugs increase nucleic acid turnover. Nucleotide reverse transcriptase inhibitors, like ritonavir may increase urate concentrations.

Laboratory Testing

Hyperuricemia is the biochemical diagnosis based on lab tests, and gout is the clinical diagnosis. An elevated serum uric acid lab value does not always equate to gout.

Hyperuricemia is just one of 12 criteria for gout diagnosis; six of these criteria must be met to confirm the presence of gout. Other lab tests needed to assess a patient with presumed gout include BUN and serum creatinine, plus a WBC count to rule out an infection that may mimic gout. Synovial fluid aspirate can be performed to identify the monosodium crystals and distinguish gout from pseudogout (calcium pyrophosphate).

Disease States

Secondary hyperuricemia and gout are myeloproliferative disorders.

Instruments/Techniques Related to Patient Assessment

A 24-hour urine collection can be performed to distinguish overproducers of uric acid from underexcreters.

Key Terms

- The **American College of Rheumatology** (ACR) has developed criteria for gout diagnosis.
- The **European League Against Rheumatism** (EULAR) has developed evidence-based guidelines for treatment.

Signs and Symptoms

Gout is characterized by abrupt, severe, acute pain of a single joint with inflammation. The pain frequently occurs at night.

Wellness, Prevention, and Treatment

Risk factors for gout include hypertension, hyperlipidemia, impaired fasting glucose, and obesity. Uric acid excretion is decreased in patients with renal impairment and in patients with alcohol abuse. Obese patients have a higher elevated uric acid, and weight reduction can decrease gout attacks. Purine-rich diets can elevate serum urate; likewise, the type of protein that is consumed can affect urate levels.

1.2.0 Pharmacotherapy

Mechanism of Action

- Colchicine: impairs leukocyte migration
- Allopurinol and febuxostat: xanthine oxidase inhibitors
- Probenecid and sulfinpyrazone: block uric acid reabsorption at the proximal convoluted tubule

Table 16-1 Drugs for Gout: Indications and Dosing Regimens

Drug	Indication	Dosing Regimen
Allopurinol	Urate reduction	CrCl > 90mL/min: 300 mg day 60–90 mL/min: 200 mg day 30–60 mL/min: 100 mg day <30 mL/min: 50 mg day
Probenecid	Block uric acid reabsorption	250 mg bid for 1 week, then 500 mg bid; titrate based on serum uric acid level
Sulfinpyrazone	Block uric acid reabsorption	50 mg bid, increase by 100 mg weekly
Febuxostat	Urate reduction	40 mg once daily up, to 80 mg once daily
Rasburicase	Recombinant urate oxidase enzyme	Available as 1.5 mg and 7.5 mg injections
NSAIDs	Acute treatment of gout	Indomethacin: 50 mg tid Naproxen: 1,000 mg daily for 3 days, then 500 mg daily for 7 days Sulindac: 200 mg bid
Colchicine	Acute treatment of gout	1.2 mg initially, then 0.6 mg every 2 hr until pain relief, diarrhea, or maximum of 8 mg
Corticosteroids	Acute treatment of gout	Intra-articular injection: triamcinolone hexacetonide 20–40 mg Prednisone: 30–50 mg daily po

Interaction of Drugs with Foods and Laboratory Tests

Febuxostat can be taken with or without food; probenecid may be taken with food, milk, or antacids. Colchicine may cause false-positive results in testing for bleeding or bruising,

- Febuxostat interactions: azathioprine, mercaptopurine, theophylline.
- Allopurinol interactions: azathioprine, captopril, cyclophosphamide, enalapril, mercaptopurine,
- Probenecid interactions: doripenem, methotrexate, zalcitabine, citalopram, ciprofloxacin, aspirin, ketorolac.
- Colchicine interactions: cyclosporin, itraconazole, nefazodone, ranolozine, clarithromycin, diltiazem, verapamil. Colchicine is inhibited by acidifying agents and potentiated by alkalinizing agents. Grapefruit juice can increase colchicine's effects.

Contraindications, Warnings, and Precautions

Colchicine should not be used concomitantly with *p*-glycoprotein or strong CYP 3A4 inhibitors or in patients with hepatic or renal impairment. In patients with hepatic or renal disease, the dose or frequency of colchicine should be decreased. Probenecid should be used with caution in patients with peptic ulcer disease and renal impairment (less than 50 mL/min).

Physiochemical Properties, Pharmacodynamics, and Pharmacokinetic Properties

- Febuxostat: 49% bioavailability; T_{max} = 1–1.5 hr; PB 99%; hepatic UGT enzymes, CYP 450 enzymes, and non-CYP 450 enzymes; active metabolite hydroxyfebuxostat; half-life = 5–8 hr.
- Allopurinol: Metabolite is oxypurinol, which inhibits hepatic microsomal enzyme activity. Dose-dependent elimination occurs due to self-inhibition of allopurinol. Bioavailability 80–90%; hepatic metabolite 15 hr; renal excretion 12%.
- Probenecid: Complete absorption; hepatic metabolism; 5–10% urinary unchanged; half-life = 3–8 hr, increasing to 6–12 hr with larger doses.
- Colchicine: 45% bioavailability; half-life = 26–31 hr; 40–65% renal excretion; T_{max} = 1.3 hr.

In pharmacokinetic dosage calculations, adjust the dose of allopurinol based on the patient's renal function.

1.3.0 Monitoring

- Probenecid: Monitor CBC with differential, platelets, renal function, and hepatic enzymes periodically.
- Colchicine: Monitor blood count periodically, as well as renal function and hepatic function.
- Rasburicase: Monitor for methemoglobinemia and hemolytic reactions. Educate the patient to report swelling of the lips or tongue, chest pain, shortness of breath, and bluish skin or lips.

Pharmacotherapeutic Outcomes

Treatment goals are to relieve pain and inflammation. Acute attacks of gout may increase when allopurinol is started due to mobilization of tissue stores of uric acid.

Safety and Efficacy Monitoring

Patients on colchicine should report skin rash, sore throat, fever, bleeding, bruising, tiredness, weakness, numbness, or tingling; they should also have blood counts performed periodically. Myopathy and neuropathy may occur with colchicine use in patients with impaired renal function. Patients on febuxostat should have liver function tests monitored at 2 and 4 months after initiating therapy, then periodically thereafter. Probenecid should not be used in patients with creatinine clearance less than 50 mL/min. Allopurinol is dosed based on renal function; thus periodic renal function testing should be done to assess the need for dosage adjustment.

Adverse Drug Reactions

- Colchicine: diarrhea, nausea, vomiting, and (possible) impaired fertility
- Febuxostat: patients should report signs and symptoms of myocardial infarction or stroke
- Probenecid: rash, GI effects, headache, and hematologic side effects
- Allopurinol: rash, immune hypersensitivity, myelosuppression, agranulocytosis
- Rasburicase: diarrhea, abdominal pain

Pharmacotherapeutic Alternatives

Febuxostat is more potent than allopurinol and works by the same mechanism of action; thus these medications can be used as alternatives for each other.

Table 16-2 Drugs for Gout: Generic Names, Brand Names, and Dosage Forms Availability

Generic	Brand Name	Dosage Forms
Colchicine	Colcrys	0.6 mg tabs
Probenecid	Benemid, Probalan	500 mg tabs
Allopurinol	Zyloprim	100 and 300 mg tabs
Febuxostat	Uloric	40 and 80 mg
Sulfinpyrazone	Anturane	300 mg

Rasburicase Elitek Single-use vial of lyophilized powder: 1.5 and 7.5 mg (used off-label for gout)

Nonsteroidal medications for symptomatic therapy with FDA-approved indications for gout were listed previously, but any NSAID may be effective.

Packaging, Storage, Handling, and Disposal

Do not refrigerate reconstituted or diluted solutions of allopurinol.

ANNOTATED BIBLIOGRAPHY

American College of Rheumatology. Gout. 2008. Available at: http://www.rheumatology.org/public/factsheets/diseases_and_conditions/gout.asp.

Rott KT, Agudelo CA. Gout. *New Engl J Med* 2003; 349:1647–1655.

Schlesinger N. Management of acute and chronic gouty arthritis. *Drugs* 2004;64:2399–2416.

Terkeltaub RA, Edwards NL, Pratt PW, et al. Gout. In: Klippel JH, Weyand CM, Wortmann RL, eds. *Primer on the Rheumatic Diseases.* 11th ed. Atlanta: Arthritis Foundation; 1998:230–243.

TOPIC: OSTEOARTHRITIS

Section Coordinator: Katherine Kelly Orr
Contributor: Katherine Kelly Orr

Tips Worth Tweeting

- Osteoarthritis is the most prevalent form of arthritis in the United States.
- Osteoarthritis is the result of synovial joint destruction.
- Localized pain to the affected joint may be accompanied by tenderness, bony enlargement, or crepitus.
- Genetic predisposition, trauma, excess body weight, and age are risk factors for osteoarthritis.
- Drug management focuses on use of analgesics for pain relief, starting with nonprescription medications such as acetaminophen or NSAIDs.
- Patients with an increased risk for stomach bleeds or cardiovascular events should avoid NSAID use.
- Tramadol and opioid analgesics should be reserved for patients with moderate to severe osteoarthritis.
- Topical analgesics applied to the affected joints may be used as monotherapy or as an adjunct to oral therapies.
- Intra-articular injections of corticosteroids or hyaluronic acid are an additional treatment option for osteoarthritis of the knee and hip.
- Treatment outcomes include pain relief, improvement of mobility, and maintaining activities of daily living.

Patient Care Scenario: Ambulatory Setting

78 y/o, 5'6" F, 176 lbs, occasional EtOH, NKDA
PMH high cholesterol, atrial fibrillation, hypertension, and osteoarthritis
Increasing pain in her right knee upon walking, which improves with rest
INR 2.2; BP 134/80 mm Hg; HR 80

Date	Physician	Drug	Quantity	Sig	Refills
3/1	Sun	Warfarin 2 mg	30	once daily	5
3/1	Sun	Metoprolol succinate 50 mg	30	once daily	11
3/1	Sun	Lisinopril 10 mg	30	once daily	11
3/1	Sun	Atorvastatin 10 mg	30	once daily	11
3/11	OTC	Acetaminophen	120	650 mg every 4–6 hr	prn

1.1.0 Patient Information

Diagnosis is made upon patient clinical assessment of symptoms and/or laboratory or radiological findings.

Laboratory Testing

Joint fluid analysis (clear, viscous, or white blood cell count less than 2,000/mm^3) and other blood tests (ESR < 20–40 mm/hr or RF < 1:40) will help rule out infection, gout, or rheumatoid arthritis.

Instruments

X-ray or MRI can show narrowing of joint spaces, signifying cartilage breakdown and growth of new bony formations.

Key Terms

- The **American College of Rheumatology** (ACR) has developed criteria for hand, hip, and knee osteoarthritis diagnosis and practice guidelines for the management of knee and hip.
- The **American Academy of Orthopaedic Surgeons** (AAOS) has developed evidence-based guidelines.
- **Crepitus:** a crackling, popping, or grating noise and/or sensation produced by joints.
- **Patellar taping procedures:** correct knee position, reducing pain and improving range of motion.

Signs and Symptoms

Osteoarthritis is more common in patients of advancing age and females. Localized pain to the affected joint may be accompanied by tenderness, bony enlargement, or crepitus. The condition is present in one or multiple joints of the hands, hips, knees, neck, or lower back. Symptoms worsen upon activity, whereas relief is felt upon resting. Joint stiffness is common in the morning or after periods of inactivity, but quickly dissipates. Patients may have bone deformity and limited functionality of joints, resulting in loss of ability to perform activities of daily living.

Wellness, Prevention, and Treatment

Risk factors for osteoarthritis include increasing age, genetic predisposition, trauma, excess body mass, female gender, repetitive motions of the joints, and specific occupations. Incorporation of nonpharmacologic measures into treatment is as important as drug therapy. Options include patient education, self-management programs, social support, exercise (e.g., low-impact aerobic, range of motion, strength training), weight loss for those patients who are overweight, assistive devices for walking (e.g., canes, walkers) or other activities, good footwear, joint protection (braces or splints), patellar taping, and physical and occupational therapy.

1.2.0 Pharmacotherapy

Mechanism of Action

- Acetaminophen: analgesic; central nervous system inhibition of prostaglandin synthesis and inhibition of pain impulses peripherally

Table 16-3 Drugs for Osteoarthritis: Indications and Dosing Regimens

Drug	Indication	Dosing Regimen
Acetaminophen	Mild to moderate pain, considered first-line therapy due to its safety profile	650–1,000 mg every 4–6 hr, not to exceed 4 g/day
NSAIDs[1,2]	Mild to moderate pain	Ibuprofen: 400–800 mg every 4–6 hr, not to exceed 3,200 mg/day Naproxen: 250–500 mg twice per day, not to exceed 1,500 mg/day Nambutone: 1,000 mg once per day, then up to 1,000 twice per day Diclofenac EC tablets: 50–75 mg 2–3 times per day Diclofenac extended release tablets: 100 mg once per day, 200 mg maximum Diclofenac gel: apply 2 g to upper extremities or 4 g to lower extremities 4 times per day, not to exceed 8 or 16 g per joint
COX-2 inhibitor	Mild to moderate pain	Celecoxib: 100 mg twice per day or 200 mg once per day
Tramadol	Moderate to severe pain	Tramadol: start at 25 mg per day and increase 25 mg every 3 days up to 25 mg four times per day; may increase by 50 mg every 3 days up to 50 mg 4 times per day; maintenance: 50–100 mg every 4–6 hr, not to exceed 400 mg/day Tramadol ER: 100 mg once daily, may titrate up 100 mg every 5 days, not to exceed 300 mg/day
Glucocorticoids[3]	Monotherapy or adjunct for short-term acute pain relief of joint	Triamcinolone hexacetonide: up to 40 mg intra-articular injection Beclomethasone: 3–12 mg intra-articular injection
Hyaluronic acid	Pain relief in knee for those patients who do not respond to nonpharmacologic measures or acetaminophen	16–30 mg per 2 mL once weekly for a total of 3–5 intra-articular knee injections; inject subcutaneous local anesthetic (lidocaine) prior to administration
Opioid analgesics	Cannot tolerate tramadol or continue with severe pain	Acetaminophen with codeine: 300–1,000 mg acetaminophen/15–60 mg codeine every 4 hr as needed, not to exceed 4 g or 360 mg per day Acetaminophen/hydrocodone: 1 or 2 tablets every 4–6 hr as needed, not to exceed 4 g acetaminophen
Topical analgesics	Monotherapy or adjunct to oral therapy	Capsaicin: apply to affected joint 3–4 times/day Methyl salicylate: apply to affected joint 2–4 times/day

1. ACR recommends that NSAIDs be paired with misoprostil or a proton pump inhibitor in patients at risk of upper GI bleeding.

2. OTC NSAIDs should not be used for more than 10 days without provider oversight.

3. Glucorticoids may be mixed with 1–2% lidocaine not containing parabens or phenols.

- NSAIDs: analgesic; anti-inflammatory by inhibiting both cyclooxgenase-1 and cyclooxgenase-2, thereby reducing prostaglandin synthesis
- COX-2 inhibitors: analgesic; anti-inflammatory by inhibiting cyclooxgenase-2, thereby reducing prostaglandin synthesis
- Tramadol: centrally acting oral analgesic; a synthetic opioid agonist that inhibits reuptake of norepinephrine and serotonin
- Glucocorticoids: analgesic; anti-inflammatory
- Hyaluronic acid: protective buffer; assists in absorbing mechanical stress in the knee
- Opioids: analgesic; centrally acting on opioid receptors, resulting in pain relief
- Capsaicin: analgesic; depletes substance P, a primary mediator of pain, thereby blocking pain impulses
- Methyl salicylate: analgesic; counterirritant/rubifacient, producing sensations of mild inflammation; some NSAID properties

Interaction of Drugs with Foods and Laboratory Tests

- Acetaminophen interactions: may prolong half-life of warfarin, therefore increasing bleeding risk. Coadministration with carbamazepine, diflusinal, isoniazid, phenytoin, fosphenytoin, and sulfapyrizone results in increased hepatic toxicity. May increase levels of chloramphenicol, busulfan, and fenoldopam.
- NSAIDs, COX-2 inhibitor interactions: may increase bleeding when given with warfarin, heparin, low-molecular-weight heparins, clopidogrel, pentoxifylline, selective serotonin reuptake inhibitors (SSRIs), serotonin–norepinephrine reuptake inhibitors (SNRIs), gingko biloba, and other platelet-inhibiting medications or natural products. NSAIDs can decrease secretion of methotrexate, cyclosporine, lithium, and pemetrexed, resulting in toxicity. Coadministration with tacrolimus has resulted in renal failure. Can interfere with the effectiveness of antihypertensive medications such as diuretics, ACE inhibitors, ARBs, calcium-channel blockers, and beta blockers. Hypoglycemia may occur when used with sulfonylureas. Can cause false-positive results for fecal occult blood tests with upper GI bleeding.
- Tramadol: SSRIs, SNRIs, tricyclic antidepressants, monoamine inhibitors, triptans, and opioids lower the seizure threshold. CNS depressants such as benzodiazepines, opioids, sedatives, phenothiazines, tranquilizers, or alcohol will further decrease respiratory depression. Previously mentioned serotonergic medications or inhibitors of CYP 2D6 and CYP 3A4 increase the risk of serotonin syndrome.
- Opioid analgesics: anticholinergic medications will worsen constipation. Coadministration with additional opioids, benzodiazepines, tranquilizers, kava, valerian, other sedative medications or natural products, and alcohol may exacerbate central nervous system depression or respiratory depression. Opioid antagonists will precipitate withdrawal and negate the effects of narcotic analgesics.

Contraindications, Warnings, and Precautions

Acetaminophen use could result in hepatotoxicity at higher doses (exceeding 4 g/day) and is contraindicated in patients with liver failure. It should be used with caution in patients who have hepatic insufficiency or who consume three or more alcoholic drinks per day. Watch for hidden sources of acetaminophen in combination products.

NSAIDs (oral and topical) and COX-2 inhibitors include warnings regarding stomach bleeds. The risk is increased in individuals with the following characteristics: age greater than 60 years; with a previous history of stomach ulcers or bleeding; taking concomitant anticoagulants, corticosteroids, or other NSAIDs; consuming three or more alcoholic drinks per day while using NSAIDs; or exceeding the recommended daily dose of NSAIDs or using them for longer than directed. The risk of heart attack and stroke also increase if the patient exceeds the recommended dose or uses it for longer than recommended. Renal toxicity may occur; risk factors for reversible renal failure include age of 65 years or older, hypertension, and/or congestive heart failure with administration of diuretics or angiotensin-converting enzyme inhibitors. Avoid use of ketoralac due to the increased risk of renal and gastrointestinal complications in elderly patients; ketoralac is also not appropriate for chronic use. Avoid use if the patient has an allergy to aspirin or other NSAIDs.

Tramadol may lower the seizure threshold and cause respiratory depression. Precautions are necessary with its use in patients with epilepsy, history of seizures, or other medications or conditions that increase risk for seizures. Tramadol is contraindicated in cases of respiratory depression, conditions, and medications that increase risk of CNS depression. Serotonergic medications and inhibitors of CYP 2D6 and CYP 3A4 increase the risk of serotonin syndrome. Anaphylaxis has occurred after the first dose of tramadol; avoid use of this medication in patients with allergies to opioids.

Hyularonic acid should not be used in patients with joint infection or skin conditions present at the injection site. Allergic reactions have been reported with Hyalgan; exercise caution if the patient has an allergy to eggs, feathers, or birds.

Intra-articular glucocorticoids should be avoided in patients with joint infection.

Maximum dosages of acetaminophen or NSAIDs should not be exceeded when using fixed-combination products of opioid analgesics. Take precautions in patients with pulmonary disease, Addison's disease, head injuries, dependence on alcohol, or severe hepatic or renal disease. Patients with hypersensitivity to metabisulfites should avoid use of these products.

Patients should apply capsaicin in a well-ventilated area, avoid contact with eyes and mucous membranes, and wash areas subjected to unintended contact immediately after exposure. Latex gloves will not offer protection—only nitrile gloves. Application of topical analgesics should be limited to the affected joint. Do not apply these products to broken or abraided skin, and do not wrap the area or apply a heating pad.

Physiochemical Properties, Pharmacodynamics, and Pharmacokinetic Properties

- Acetaminophen: 60–98% bioavailability, half-life = 4 hr, T_{max} = 1–2 hr, 10–30 % PB, 90–95% metabolized hepatically by glucouronidation and sulfate to conjugate metabolites.
- Celecoxib: half-life = 11 hr, T_{max} = 3 hr, PB 97%, extensively hepatically metabolizes CYP 450 2C9 to inactive metabolites.
- Ibuprofen: half-life = 2 hr, T_{max} = 1–2 hr, 99% PB, renally metabolized, two major metabolites: (+)-2-(*p*-[2-hydroxymethyl-propyl] phenyl) propionic acid and (+)-2-(*p*-2-(p-[2-carboxy-propyl] phenyl) propionic acid.
- Diclofenec (oral): 55% bioavailability, half-life = 2 hr, T_{max} = 1–6 hr (delayed by food for up to another 4 hr), 99% PB, hepatically metabolized by first-pass metabolism, conjugation, and hydroxylation.
- Diclofenec (gel): 6% bioavailability compared to oral formulation, T_{max} = 10–14 hr, half-life = 1–2 hr.
- Naproxen: 99% bioavailability, half-life = 12-24 hr, T_{max} = 2–4 hr (4–6 hr with delayed release), 99% PB, renally metabolized, major metabolite 6-0-desmethyl naproxen.
- Nambutone: prodrug hepatically metabolized to active 6-methoxy-2-naphthylacetic acid (6MNA); half-life = 24 hr, T_{max} 3–6 hr, 99% PB; food increases rate of absorption.
- Tramadol: 75% bioavailability, half-life = 6.5 hr, T_{max} = 1–2.3 hr (IR), 4–12 hr (ER), PB 20%, 60% renal metabolite, hepatically metabolized CYP 450 2D6 and 3A4, conjugation, demethylation, glucuronidation, sulfation; active metabolite *O*-desmethyltramadol has half-life = 7 hr.
- Capsaicin: T_{max} = 60 min (topical patch).
- Codeine: half-life = 3 hr, extensively metabolized by liver, demethylation 10% to morphine.
- Hydrocodone: half-life = 4 hr, T_{max} = 1 hr, extensively metabolized by liver, demethylation, and other metabolites.

Pharmacokinetic Dosage Calculations

- Tramadol: Do not use the ER formulation in patients with hepatic or renal impairment; use dose reduction IR in patients with cirrhosis or CrCl < 30 cc/min; start elderly patients in a lower dosage range.
- Celecoxib: Reduce the dose to 50% of the normal dose in patients with hepatic insufficiency.
- Codeine: Dosages should be reduced to 75% of the normal dose in patients with moderate renal failure and to half of the normal dose in patients with severe renal failure. Consider reducing the dose in patients with hepatic insufficiency.

1.3.0 Monitoring

Pharmacotherapeutic Outcomes

Treatment goals are reduction in pain, improvement of mobility, and maintaining activities of daily living.

Safety and Efficacy Monitoring

Adverse Drug Reactions

Patients on NSAIDs should be aware of the signs or symptoms of a stomach bleed, including faintness, hematemesis, and dark or bloody stools. Patients should report signs or symptoms of cardiovascular events. Monitor blood pressure in at-risk patients.

Hyularonic acid can lead to injection site pain; increases in swelling and joint pain may also occur. Monitor for signs and symptoms of infection, septic arthritis, or pseudogout.

Tramadol can result in nausea, vomiting, dry mouth, constipation, drowsiness, dizziness, headache, flushing, and pruritus. Monitor for respiratory depression or seizure.

Intra-articular glucocorticoids are controversial because their use may result in further destruction of the joint. Monitor for signs and symptoms of infection or septic arthritis.

Opioid analgesics can cause rash, pruritus, constipation, nausea, vomiting, sedation, and respiratory depression.

Capsaicin results in a burning or stinging to the area of application that may last for months, but will lessen over time. Local treatment pain can be relieved with an ice pack.

On some products, methyl salicylate is labeled as an NSAID with the warnings previously discussed.

Nonadherence, Misuse, or Abuse

Tramadol should be tapered, as its abrupt discontinuation can result in withdrawal symptoms. It is not a scheduled medication, but dependence and abuse may occur. Codeine and hydrocodone in combination with acetaminophen or ibuprofen are Schedule III or IV drugs. Their use may lead to tolerance and abuse.

Pharmacotherapeutic Alternatives

Any NSAID besides those listed may be used, except ketoralac. Other opioids or opioid–analgesic combinations may be used instead depending on the severity of the patient's condition.

Glucosamine sulfate, with or without chondroitin, has been used as an alternative to or in conjunction with the medications previously discussed. Its purposed mechanism of action is stimulation of cartilage and synovial fluid production. General dosing is 1,500 mg daily orally, once or in divided dosages; an effect may not be seen until 6–8 weeks of treatment. Common side effects are gastrointestinal symptoms. Glucosamine sulfate should be avoided in patients with a history of shellfish allergy. Patients with diabetes should monitor their blood glucose when initiating therapy. Chondroitin can increase risk of bleeding and should be used in caution in conjunction with antiplatelet or anticoagulant agents.

Table 16-4 Drugs for Osteoarthritis: Generic Names, Brand Names, and Dosage Forms Availability

Generic	Brand Name	Dosage Forms
Acetaminophen	Tylenol	325 mg, 500 mg, and 650 mg tablets or capsules Liquid
Ibuprofen	Motrin, Advil, Nuprin	200 mg, 400 mg, 600 mg, and 800 mg tablets; 100 mg chewable tablet 100 mg/5 mL suspension
Naproxen	Aleve, Naprosyn, EC Naprosyn	250 mg, 375 mg, and 500 mg tablets 375 mg and 500 mg EC tablets 25 mg/mL suspension
Diclofenec	Voltaren, Voltaren XR, Voltaren Gel	25 mg, 50 mg, and 75 mg EC tablets; 75 mg and 100 mg XR tablets 1% gel
Diclofenec/misoprostil	Arthrotec	50 mg and 75 mg tablets with 200 mcg misoprostil
Nabumetone	Relafen	500 mg and 750 mg tablets
Celexicob	Celebrex	50 mg, 100 mg, 200 mg, and 400 mg capsules
Tramadol hydrochloride	Ultram	50 mg tablets
Tramadol hydrochloride ER	Ultram ER, Ryzolt	100 mg, 200 mg, and 300 mg tablets
Tramadol hydrochloride/ acetaminophen	Ultracet	37.5 mg/325 mg tablets
Triamcinolone hexacetonide	Aristospan	5 mg/mL and 20 mg/mL injection suspension
Betamethasone	Celestone Soluspan	6 mg/mL injection suspension
Hyaluronic acid	Synvisc, Hyalgan, Supartz, Orthovisc	16, 20, 25, and 30 mg per 2 mL prefilled syringes; 10 mg/mL injection solution
Capsaicin	Zostrix, Capsagesic-HP Arthritis Relief	Cream, lotion, patch, powder 0.025–0.25%
Methyl salicylate	BenGay, Icy Hot, Salonpas, Salonpas Arthritis Pain	Cream, patch up to 10%
Acetaminophen/codeine	Tylenol with Codeine, Tylenol with Codeine #3, Tylenol with Codeine #4, Cocet	300 mg/15 mg, 300 mg/30 mg, 300 mg/60 mg, and 650 mg/30 mg tablets 120 mg/12 mg per 5 mL solution or elixir
Acetaminophen/ hydrocodone	Norco, Vicodin, Vicodin ES, Vicodin HP, Lortab, Lortab 5/500, Lortab 7.5/500, Lortab 10/500	325 mg/5 mg, 325 mg/7.5 mg, 325 mg/10 mg, 500 mg/5 mg, 500 mg/7.5 mg, 500 mg/10 mg, 750 mg/7.5 mg, and 660 mg/10 mg tablets 500 mg/7.5 mg per 15 mL elixir

2.1.0 Dispensing

See Table 16-4.

ANNOTATED BIBLIOGRAPHY

ACR Subcommittee on Osteoarthritis Guidelines. Recommendations for medical management of osteoarthritis of the hip and knee. *Arthritis Rheum* 2000;43(9):1905–1915.

AGS Panel on Pharmacologic Management of Persistent Pain in Older Persons. Pharmacological management of persistent pain in older persons. *JAGS* 2009;57:1331–1346.

American Academy of Orthopaedic Surgeons. *Clinical Practice Guideline on the Treatment of Osteoarthritis of the Knee (Non-Arthropathy)*. Rosemont, IL: Author; 2008.

Antman EM, Bennett JS, Daugherty A, Furberg C, Roberts H, Taubert KA; American Heart Association. Use of nonsteroidal antiinflammatory drugs: an update for clinicians: a scientific statement from the American Heart Association. *Circulation* 2007;115(12):1634–1642.

McQueen CM, Orr KK. Natural products. In: *Handbook of Nonprescription Drugs: An Interactive Approach to Self-Care*. 16th ed. 2009.

Micromedex® Healthcare Series. Greenwood Village, CO: Thomson Reuters. Available at: http://csi.micromedex.com. Accessed February 17, 2010.

TOPIC: ARTHRITIS

Section Coordinator: Katherine Kelly Orr
Contributors: Jennifer D. Smith and Jeffrey M. Tingen

Tips Worth Tweeting

- Rheumatoid arthritis (RA) presents with symmetrically affected joints and morning stiffness lasting longer than 1 hour.
- A rheumatoid factor test is typically negative during the early stages of RA. Thus a diagnosis of RA should not be excluded based on this laboratory value alone.
- Methotrexate (MTX) dosing for RA is once weekly, not daily. Folic acid (not folinic acid) is added to MTX to prevent adverse effects.
- Biologic DMARDs (Disease-Modifying AntiRheumatic Drugs) should not be used in combination due to the increased risk of adverse effects.
- Hydroxychloroquine can cause retinal toxicity. Patients should have an ophthalmic examination every 6–12 months while using this agent.
- Prodromal symptoms of RA include anorexia and fatigue.
- Conditions associated with RA include anemia, cardiovascular disease, osteoporosis, and pulmonary infections.
- Treatment for RA is more aggressive now because it is recognized that early treatment can retard joint erosion. Treatments target inflammatory mediators—prostaglandins, cytokines, and/or tumor necrosis factor.
- Methotrexate is the most commonly used DMARD and can be used as monotherapy or in combination with other nonbiologic or biologic DMARDs.

Patient Care Scenario: Ambulatory Setting

C. P. is a 32-year-old, 119 lb female who presents to her primary care provider complaining of constant fatigue and painful swollen joints in her wrists and fingers. She states that she feels weaker in the mornings and it seems to take a long time to get going during the morning hours. She has noticed a recent continued weight loss, though her diet has not changed. She has been smoking for the past 10 years.

Allergic to sulfonamides.
Laboratory values: A_{1C}: 5.2; TSH: 1.09; C-reactive protein: 10.2; rheumatoid factor: (–); WBC: 15; PLT: 500; Hgb: 11.3; Hct: 33.8; Scr: 1.05; AST/ALT: 27/15; TC: 211; TG: 107; HDL: 80; LDL: 110
Physical exam: (+) warm, swollen tender joints bilaterally in finger and wrist joints; (+) rheumatoid nodules

C. P.'s physician initiates therapy for RA with MTX and leflunomide. When C. P. does not show any improvement after 3 months, she is switched to therapy with MTX and adalimumab. Over the course of the next 6 months of therapy with MTX and adalimumab, C. P. presents with continuously elevated systolic blood pressure readings and recurring urinary tract infections. C. P. had previously never experienced urinary tract infections.

Date	Physician	Drug	Quantity	Sig	Refills
4/2	Green	Oral contraceptive	30 mcg ethinyl estradiol	30 one daily	5
5/1	Rapp	Methotrexate	2.5 mg po #12	three tablets weekly on Wed	3
5/1	Rapp	Adalimumab kit	40 mg/0.8mL	40 mg subQ every other week	2

1.1.0 Patient Information

Laboratory Testing

- Complete blood cell count with differential: increased platelets and white blood cells and decreased hemoglobin/hematocrit
- Rheumatoid factor: negative early in disease
- Erythrocyte sedimentation rate: increased
- C-reactive protein: increased
- Urinalysis: microscopic hematuria or proteinuria
- Immunoglobulins: increased α-1 and α-2 globulins
- Hepatic and renal function evaluated to guide medication decisions

Disease States Associated with Rheumatoid Arthritis

RA is associated with anemia, osteoporosis, cardiovascular disease, lymphoma, and pulmonary infections.

Instruments and Techniques Related to Patient Assessment

Recommendations for treatment are based on three factors:

- Disease duration: early (less than 6 months), intermediate (6–24 months), or longer (more than 24 months)
- Disease activity assessment: low, moderate, or high
- Poor prognostic factors: functional limitations, extra-articular disease, positive anti-CCP antibodies, bony erosions by radiography

Terminology Associated with Rheumatoid Arthritis

- Rheumatoid nodules
- Proximal interphalangeal joints
- Metacarpophalangeal joints
- Metatarsophalangeal joints
- Biologic DMARDs (agents derived from human genes, designed to target specific immune system components that cause inflammation)
- Nonbiologic DMARDs (traditional antirheumatic drugs that modify the disease progression)

Signs and Symptoms

- Prodromal symptoms (anorexia, weakness, fatigue)
- Morning stiffness of affected joints for at least 1 hour
- Symmetric arthritis of one or more joint areas: wrist, proximal interphalangeal (PIP), metacarpophalangeal (MCP), elbow, knee, ankle, metatarsophalangeal (MTP) joints
- Rheumatoid nodules
- Serum rheumatoid factor positive
- Radiographic changes of affected joints

Wellness and Prevention of Rheumatoid Arthritis

- Risk factors: female, family history, increased age, exposure to silica dust, cigarette smoking
- Preventive measures: high vitamin D intake, oral contraceptive use

Treatment of Rheumatoid Arthritis

- Analgesics: pain control only with no effect on inflammation or disease modification.
- Anti-inflammatory agents (NSAIDs and COX-2 inhibitors): reduce inflammation, but can contribute to CV and GI complications; limited use or reduced doses in patients of advanced age; no effect on disease modification.
- Glucocorticoids (intra-articular and oral): low-dose oral therapy effective for moderate to severe RA; intra-articular glucocorticoids effective if inflammation is limited to one to two affected joints. Extended use or high doses of glucocorticoids may contribute to osteoporosis, hypertension, diabetes, and dyslipidemia.
- Nonbiologic disease–modifying antirheumatic drugs (DMARDs):
  - Antimalarials: hydroxychloroquine—most commonly used and tolerated. Administer the lowest possible dose due to its potential for retinal toxicity.
  - Leflunomide: slows progression of structural damage; alternative to MTX or sulfasalazine for patients with high disease activity or poor prognosis; boxed warning for severe liver injury; use with caution in patients with preexisting liver disease, elevated liver enzymes, or receiving hepatotoxic agents.
  - Methotrexate (MTX): most commonly used; long-term efficacy for disease modification; avoid use in patients with hepatic disease and use cautiously in patients with renal disease.
  - Sulfasalazine: limited long-term data for use in RA and should not be used as monotherapy. An immediate response is not seen with this agent.
- Biologic DMARDs:
  - TNF-α-blocking agents (infliximab, adalimumab, etanercept, golimumab, certolizumab pegol): recommended for patients with high disease activity and poor prognosis or failure on MTX; use as monotherapy or in addition to MTX.
  - Recombinant fusion protein (abatacept): recommended for inadequate response to MTX + DMARD or sequential use of other nonbiologic DMARDs.
  - Chimeric human–murine anti-human antigen CD20 monoclonal antibody (rituximab):

recommended for inadequate response to MTX + DMARD or sequential use of other nonbiologic DMARDs.
    - Recombinant human interleukin-1 (IL-1) receptor antagonist (anakinra): recommended for patients with moderate to severe disease activity or inadequate response with one or more DMARDs; used alone or with DMARDs, except TNF blockers.
    - Interleukin-6 receptor antagonist (tocilizumab): recommended for patients with moderate to severe disease activity with inadequate response to one or more TNF blockers.

Treatment Indications

- Single-agent use: Recently, a reverse pyramid approach has been used to treat symptoms of RA early and aggressively to prevent disease progression. Single-agent therapy may be effective if used early in the disease and/or a disease-modifying agent is used. MTX remains the backbone of therapy, either as monotherapy or combination therapy.
- Dual nonbiologic DMARD combination recommendations:
    - MTX + hydroxychloroquine: moderate to high disease activity
    - MTX + leflunomide: intermediate or long duration of disease
    - MTX + sulfasalazine: high disease activity and poor prognosis
- Triple-nonbiologic DMARD combination: MTX + hydroxychloroquine + sulfasalazine: moderate to high levels of disease activity and poor prognosis
- Biologic DMARD combination: The combination of biologic DMARDs may lead to serious adverse events and is not recommended at this time.

1.2.0 Pharmacotherapy

See Table 16-5.

Physiochemical Properties, Pharmacodynamics, and Pharmacokinetics

- Hydroxychloroquine: mechanism of action (MOA) is unclear and little pharmacokinetic information is available.
- Leflunomide: prodrug, converted to A77 1726, an active metabolite. The MOA in RA treatment is unclear. The elimination half-life of A77 1726 is 14–18 days, but it can take up to 2 years for metabolite concentrations to become undetectable in urine. Activated charcoal or cholestyramine can be used to hasten metabolite clearance.
- MTX: exact MOA in RA unknown. Oral bioavailability is 50% or less, and elimination follows a biphasic excretion pattern.
- Sulfasalazine: prodrug, metabolized to sulfapyridine and mesalamine in vivo. Sulfasalazine is well absorbed and distributed extensively. The half-life is 5–6 hours, but is extended in geriatric patients. The MOA in RA is unclear.
- Anti-TNFα agents: bind to and neutralize TNF, thereby inhibiting TNF-mediated inflammation. Infliximab is given by IV infusion, whereas adalimumab, etanercept, golimumab, and certolizumab pegol are SQ injections.
- Recombinant fusion protein (abatacept): prevents activation of T cells and inhibits the production of TNF, IF-γ, and IL-2. Half-life elimination is 8–25 days.
- Rituximab: monoclonal antibody that targets the CD20 antigen on B lymphocytes, thereby delaying progression of structural damage. IV absorption is immediate, and mean elimination half-life is 19 days.
- Anakinra: blocks IL-1, which is responsible for inflammatory and immunologic responses, as well as bone resorption and cartilage degradation. SQ bioavailability is 95%; half-life elimination is 4–6 hours.
- Tocilizumab: blocks IL-6, which appears to be responsible for acute and chronic inflammation. Elimination is concentration dependent.

1.3.0 Monitoring

Pharmacotherapeutic Outcomes

The desired outcomes are improved quality of life, decreased swelling and joint pain, improved physical functioning, decreased morning stiffness, improved range of motion, and improved grip strength.

Safety and Efficacy Monitoring and Patient Education

- With hydroxychloroquine and sulfasalazine, it may take 4–12 weeks to see a response.
- With MTX, initiate folic acid 5–10 mg po once weekly (except on the day of MTX dosing) to reduce side effects.
- With TNF-α blocking agents, monitor CBC; look for signs and symptoms of TB or other infections; perform HBV screening; and measure LFTs. Infliximab can produce acute and delayed infusion reactions; pretreatment with APAP, antihistamine, or prednisone is recommended to prevent acute infusion reactions.
- Monitor neutrophils and platelets every 4–8 weeks for patients taking tocilizumab. Discontinue

Table 16-5 Drugs for Rheumatoid Arthritis

Drug	Dosing	Administration Route	Drug/Food Interactions	Contraindications or Reasons for Caution
Nonbiologic DMARDs				
Hydroxychloroquine	Initial: 400–600 mg daily Maintenance: 200–400 mg daily	Oral	Vaccines (live and inactivated); echinacea; leflunomide; mefloquine; natalizumab; lumefantrine; BCG	Retinal/visual field changes; hepatic disease; alcoholism; G-6-PD deficiency; psoriasis; porphyria
Leflunomide	100 mg once daily for 3 days, then 20 mg once daily thereafter	Oral	Hepatotoxic agents; anticoagulants; cholestyramine; MTX; NSAIDs; rifampin; live vaccines	Renal impairment; hepatic impairment
Methotrexate	7.5–20 mg once weekly	Oral	Protein-bound drugs; weak organic acids; NSAIDs; penicillins live vaccines; hepatotoxic agents; theophylline	Infection; PUD; ulcerative colitis; malignant disease; renal dysfunction; blood dyscrasias; immunodeficiency; alcoholism or liver disease attributed to alcoholism
Sulfasalazine	2–3 g daily in equally divided doses	Oral, delayed release	Digoxin, folic acid, iron: ↓ absorption; MTX: ↑ GI effects	Renal or hepatic dysfunction; blood dyscrasias; salicylate or sulfonamide allergy
Biologic DMARDs				
Infliximab	3 mg/kg given at 0, 2, and 6 weeks, then once every 8 weeks	IV infusion over 2 hr	Other biologic DMARDs; echinacea; live vaccines	Heart failure; lymphoma or malignancies; seizure disorders; hematologic abnormalities; Crohn's disease; active infection; tuberculosis; live vaccines
Adalimumab	40 mg once weekly without MTX; 40 mg every other week with MTX	SQ injection		
Etanercept	50 mg once weekly	SQ injection		
Golimumab	50 mg once monthly in combination with MTX	SQ injection		
Certolizumab pegol	400 mg (2 injections of 200 mg) at 0, 2, and 4 weeks; 200 mg every other week thereafter	SQ injection		
Abatacept	IV: <60 kg: 500 mg; 60–100 kg: 750 mg; >100 kg: 1 g Given at 0, 2, and 4 weeks, then every 4 weeks SQ: 125 mg with 24 hr of infusion, then once weekly	IV infusion SQ injection	Other biologic DMARDs; live vaccines	Active infection; tuberculosis; hepatitis B; live vaccines; COPD; lymphoma or malignancies
Rituximab	1,000 mg days 1 and 15 (2 total doses) (Flat dose for RA)	IV infusion	Cisplatin; live vaccines	Hepatitis B; CV disease; pulmonary disease
Anakinra	100 mg daily	SQ injection	Biologic DMARDs; live vaccines	Active infection, asthma; renal impairment
Tocilizumab	4 mg/kg every 4 weeks; may increase to 8 mg/kg; maximum dose: 800 mg per infusion	IV	Echinacea; live vaccines; leflunomide; biologic DMARDs	Thrombocytopenia; active infection; neutropenia; active hepatic disease or hepatic impairment; gastric perforation

therapy for ANC < 500/mm³ or platelets < 50,000/mm³.

- With biologic DMARDs (except rituximab), monitor for signs and symptoms of infection.

Adverse Drug Reactions

- Hydroxychloroquine: retinopathy; gastrointestinal disorders; CNS; dermatologic disorders
- Leflunomide: hepatotoxicity; reversible alopecia; gastrointestinal disorders; allergic reaction; headache; hypertension; respiratory and urinary tract infections
- MTX: hematologic (leucopenia; thrombocytopenia; anemia); gastrointestinal disorders; acute and chronic hepatotoxicity; pulmonary toxicity; sensitivity reactions

- Sulfasalazine: gastrointestinal disorders; rash; LFT abnormalities; orange-yellow skin and urine
- TNF-α: pancytopenia; heart failure; malignancies and lymphoproliferative disorders; reactivation of hepatitis B infection; new-onset psoriasis; lupus-like syndrome (infliximab); hypertension (adalimumab, etanercept, certolizumab); renal dysfunction (infliximab)
- Abatacept: HA; URTI; nausea

Table 16-6 Dispensing Information for Rheumatoid Arthritis Drugs

Generic	Brand Name	Availability	Package, Storage, Handling, and Disposal	Physical Attributes of Commercial Products	Administration Equipment
Hydroxychloroquine	Plaquenil	Tablets	Protect from light and store at room temperature		
Leflunomide	Arava	Tablets	Protect from light		
Methotrexate	Rheumatrex Dose Pack Trexall	Tablets; solution for injection	Protect from light and store at room temperature		
Sulfasalazine: enteric-coated	Azulfidine EN-tabs	Tablets	Store at room temperature		
Infliximab	Remicade	Powder for reconstitution	Initiate IV infusion within 3 hours of preparation	Colorless to light yellow solution; translucent particles may be present because infliximab is a protein	Intravenous infusion equipment
Adalimumab	Humira	Prefilled syringes; injection pen	Store injection at 2–8°C and protect from light; prefilled syringes and injection pens are for single use; discard unused portions		
Etanercept	Enbrel	Prefilled syringes; prefilled auto-injectors; powder for reconstitution	Prefilled syringes and auto-injectors should be protected from light and refrigerated; powder for injection should be refrigerated and is stable for 24 months following manufacturing; if not refrigerated, powder is stable for only 45 days from manufacturing; once reconstituted, powder formulation should be used within 14 days	Colorless to light yellow solution	
Golimumab	Simponi	Prefilled auto-injector syringes	Refrigerate and protect from light; syringe should be at room temperature for 30 min prior to injection		
Certolizumab pegol	Cimzia	Powder for reconstitution or prefilled syringes	Refrigerate; bring to room temperature prior to use with syringes or reconstitution of vials; reconstituted vials should be used within 24 hours if refrigerated or within 2 hours if left at room temperature		Provided 20-gauge needle for reconstitution; provided 23-gauge needle for administration
Abatacept	Orencia	Powder for reconstitution or prefilled syringes	Use the silicone-free disposable syringe provided by the manufacturer when reconstituting the powder and gently swirl to minimize foaming; NS should be used for reconstitution SQ: Refrigerate; protect from light	Colorless to pale yellow reconstituted solution; translucent particles may develop if a silicone-free disposable syringe is not used for reconstitution, in which case the solution should be discarded.	Intravenous infusion equipment; low-protein-binding filter with pore diameter of 0.2–1.2 micron; silicone-free disposable syringe
Rituximab	Rituxan	Injection solution	Refrigerate vials; protect from sunlight and shaking; infusion solution is stable for 24 hours when refrigerated and for 48 hours at room temperature		Intravenous infusion equipment
Anakinra	Kineret	Single-use prefilled syringe	Store in refrigerator and protect from sunlight; do not shake		
Tocilizumab	Actemra	Injection solution	Store in refrigerator and protect from sunlight; after dilution, use within 24 hours whether refrigerated or at room temperature		Intravenous infusion equipment

- Rituximab: neurologic manifestations (consider progressive multifocal leukoencephalopathy)
- Anakinra: sensitivity reactions; infection; abdominal pain
- Tocilizumab: hypertension; increased LFTs; URTI; infusion-related reactions; neutropenia; thrombocytopenia; gastrointestinal perforation

Biologic DMARDs should not be used together due to the increased risk of adverse effects.

Pharmacotherapeutic Alternatives

Alternatives to pharmacotherapy include Mediterranean diet; exercise therapy; sufficient rest; herbal medicines (γ-linolenic acid [GLA], evening primrose oil, feverfew, flaxseed oil, and *Tripterygium wilfodii* Hook F.), though the evidence is inconclusive regarding their safety and efficacy.

2.1.0 Calculations

ANC calculation for tocilizumab: (segmented neutrophils [+] band neutrophils) × (white blood cell count)

2.2.0 Dispensing

See Table 16-6.

ANNOTATED BIBLIOGRAPHY

AHFS On-line. Available at: http://online.statref.com.libproxy.lib.unc.edu/document.aspx?fxid=18&docid=105. Accessed January 19, 2010 and February 10, 2010.

Cash JM. Antirheumatic drugs. In: Stein JH, et al., eds. *Internal Medicine*. 5th ed. Mosby; 1998. Available at: http://online.statref.com.lib.unc.edu/document.aspx?fxid=9&docid=1585. Accessed January 19, 2010.

Dayer JM, Choy E. Therapeutic targets in rheumatoid arthritis: the interleukin-6 receptor. *Rheumatology* 2010;49:15–24.

Klareskog L, Catrina AI, Paget S. Rheumatoid arthritis. *Lancet* 2009;373:659–672.

Lexi-Drugs On-line. Available at: http://www.crlonline.com.proxy.campbell.edu/crlsql/servlet/crlonline. Accessed January 19, 2010 and February 10, 2010.

National Collaborating Centre for Chronic Conditions. *Rheumatoid Arthritis: National Clinical Guideline for Management and Treatment in Adults*. London: Royal College of Physicians; February 2009.

Rindfleisch JA, Muller D. Diagnosis and management of rheumatoid arthritis. *Am Fam Physician* 2005;72(6):1037–1047.

Saag KG, Teng GG, Patkar NM, et al. American College of Rheumatology 2008 recommendations for the use of nonbiologic and biologic disease-modifying antirheumatic drugs in rheumatoid arthritis. *Arthritis Rheum* 2008;59(6):762–784.

Soeken KL, Miller SA, Ernst E. Herbal medicines for the treatment of rheumatoid arthritis: a systematic review. *Rheumatology* 2003;42:652–659.

Whittle SL, Hughes RA. Folate supplementation and methotrexate treatment in rheumatoid arthritis: a review. *Rheumatology* 2004;43:267–271.

TOPIC: SYSTEMIC LUPUS ERYTHEMATOSUS

Section Coordinator: Katherine Kelly Orr
Contributors: Jeffrey M.Tingen and Jennifer D.Smith

Tips Worth Tweeting

- Systemic Lupus Erythematosus (SLE) may present with manifestations in the musculoskeletal, mucocutaneous, nervous, pulmonary, cardiovascular, renal, gastrointestinal, and lymph systems.
- Common manifestations include arthralgia, arthritis, butterfly rash, photosensitivity, discoid lesions, psychosis, hypertension, and anemia.
- SLE is caused by immunologic abnormalities, including antibodies of an antinuclear, anticytoplasmic, and antiphospholipid nature.
- Treatment of SLE may include nonsteroidal anti-inflammatory drugs (NSAIDs), corticosteroids, antimalarials, immunosuppressants, and cytotoxic agents.
- With hydroxychloroquine therapy, it may take 3–6 months for SLE manifestations to respond to treatment.

Patient Care Scenario: Ambulatory Setting

R. J. is a 27-year-old woman who presents to the health center with a primary complaint of a rash. The rash has spread across the bridge of her nose and cheeks; the patient reports no itching associated with the rash. R. J. also

Date	Physician	Drug	Quantity	Sig	Refills
3/4	Wilson	Multivitamin	30	one tablet daily	6
2/21	Wilson	Calcium carbonate 500 mg	100	one tablet TID	6
1/2	Pend	Paroxetine 20 mg	30	one tablet daily	2

complains of tiredness and decreased appetite that have progressively worsened. She reports no allergies.

> Laboratory assays: anti-dsDNA antibodies: (+); antiphospholipid antibodies: (+); hematocrit: 37%; hemoglobin: 13 g/dL; white blood cell count: 3,700/mm^3; platelet count: 300,000/mm^3; serum creatinine: 1.0 mg/dL; liver function tests: within normal limits
> Physical exam: (+) malar rash

R. J.'s physician initiates therapy for her new systemic lupus erythematosus (SLE) diagnosis. R. J. is started on hydroxychloroquine 200 mg bid and prednisone 5 mg qd. R. J. comes in one week later for a follow-up appointment. She reports nausea and fatigue, but states that the rash has improved.

1.1.0 Patient Information

Medication-Induced Causes

Medications that are more associated with SLE include chlorpromazine, hydralazine, isoniazid, methyldopa, procainamide, and quinidine. If a patient presents with symptoms of SLE, all medications should be reviewed to determine if the symptoms are medication induced.

Laboratory Testing

Complete blood cell count with differential—normal platelet count with decreased white blood cell count and normal hemoglobin/hematocrit; anti-dsDNA antibodies present and antiphospholipid antibodies present; hepatic and renal function evaluated to guide medication decisions.

Disease States Associated with Systemic Lupus Erythematosus

Pleuritis, nephropathy, anemia, antiphospholipid syndrome, neuropathy, and depression have all been found in conjunction with SLE.

Instruments and Techniques Related to Patient Assessment

An extensive patient history is key to assessment of the patient. No single symptom or finding is able to determine a diagnosis of SLE. Laboratory assays are important for aiding in the diagnosis of the disease, including a complete blood count, platelet count, erythrocyte sedimentation rate, antinuclear antibodies, and urinalysis. Diagnosis is based on the patient's clinical symptoms and laboratory findings. If a patient is diagnosed by a primary care physician or other healthcare provider, the patient should also be evaluated by a rheumatologist for confirmation.

Key Terms

- **Malar rash:** fixed erythema, flat or raised, spreading across the bridge of the nose and cheeks.
- **Discoid rash:** erythematous–raised patches with scaling.

Signs and Symptoms

- Constitutional: fatigue, fever, weight loss
- Musculoskeletal: arthritis, arthralgia, myositis
- Skin: malar rash, photosensitivity, alopecia, Raynaud's phenomenon, purpura, urticaria, vasculitis
- Renal: hematuria, proteinuria, nephritic syndrome
- Gastrointestinal: nausea, vomiting, abdominal pain
- Pulmonary: pleurisy, pulmonary hypertension
- Cardiac: pericarditis, endocarditis, myocarditis
- Reticuloendothelial: lymphadenopathy, splenomegaly, hepatomegaly
- Hematologic: anemia, thrombocytopenia, leukopenia
- Neuropsychiatric: psychosis, seizures, cranial neuropathy, peripheral neuropathy

Wellness and Prevention

- Risk factors: family history (especially first-degree relatives with SLE), gender (women are more greatly affected than men with an estimated 10:1 ratio), ethnicity (African Americans are more likely to develop SLE than Caucasians and also develop more severe complications), pharmacological therapy (some medications may induce SLE)
- Preventive measures: none are known but avoidance of tobacco products may help prevent SLE

Treatment

- NSAIDs: given for initial treatment in patients who experience fever and arthritis. There is no preferred NSAID for the treatment of SLE, but the NSAID should be dosed appropriately to provide anti-inflammatory effects. NSAIDs should be used with caution in patients with SLE nephritis because NSAIDs can decrease renal blood flow and the glomerular filtration rate.
- Corticosteroids: given for treatment of more severe manifestations of SLE that are not controlled by other treatments such as NSAIDs or antimalarial agents. Corticosteroids are generally used in the management of CNS disease, pneumonitis, vasculitis, thrombocytopenia, dermatitis, and other more severe complications. The lowest dose able to suppress the disease and maintain suppression is recommended for SLE. Topical corticosteroids may be used with dermatitis manifestations. Patients may need to be on maintenance therapy

with corticosteroids and/or may require steroid pulse therapy during SLE flares.

- Antimalarial agents: used for various SLE manifestations such as rash, arthralgia, pleuritis, fatigue, mild pericardial inflammation, and leucopenia. Hydroxychloroquine is often the antimalarial agent of choice and is best used for long-term management of SLE manifestations; antimalarial agents do not provide immediate relief and take around 3–6 months to provide their maximum effect.
- Immunosuppressants: Azathioprine and mycophenolate mofetil are the two most commonly used immunosuppressants for SLE; these agents are generally used for more severe manifestations that have not adequately responded to glucocorticoid treatment. Azathioprine and mycophenolate mofetil have been studied more extensively as a treatment option for SLE nephritis.
- Cytotoxic agents: reserved for very severe cases of SLE. Cyclophosphamide is the most studied cytotoxic agent used in this indication and is generally used for severe nephritis and CNS manifestations. It is administered intravenously, and mesna is commonly administered before therapy to prevent hemorrhagic cystitis associated with cyclophosphamide's bladder-related toxic effects.

1.2.0 Pharmacotherapy

Drug Indications

- NSAIDs: mild disease including fever, arthritis, skin rash, and serositis (tissue lining of the organs)
- Corticosteroids: initial control of severe disease; control of mild disease or maintenance after administration of higher doses to suppress disease; and life-threatening disease (intravenous corticosteroids)

Table 16-7 Drugs for Systemic Lupus Erythematosus

Drug	Dosing	Administration Route	Drug/Food Interactions	Contraindications or Reasons for Caution
NSAIDs (various agents)	Anti-inflammatory dosing for the individual agent	Oral	ACE inhibitors (renal impairment), antiplatelets/anticoagulants (bleeding risk), ethanol (GI irritation)	Aspirin-sensitive asthma, bleeding or risk of bleeding
Hydroxychloroquine	200–400 mg daily	Oral	Phenothiazines, BCG, echinacea, leflunomide, mefloquine, natalizumab, trastuzumab, vaccines, ethanol (GI irritation)	Visual/retinal changes, long-term use in children
Prednisone	Initial control of severe symptoms: 1–2 mg/kg/day Control of mild disease: < 1 mg/kg/day	Oral	Antidiabetic agents, antacids, echinacea, leflunomide, macrolides (except azithromycin), natalizumab, quinolones, vaccines, warfarin, ethanol (GI irritation)	Systemic fungal infections, psychiatric disorders, immunosuppression
Methylprednisolone	500–1,000 mg daily for 3–6 days	Intravenous	Antidiabetic agents, antacids, echinacea, leflunomide, macrolides (except azithromycin), natalizumab, quinolones, vaccines, warfarin	Systemic fungal infections, psychiatric disorders, immunosuppression
Azathioprine	1–3 mg/kg/day	Oral	Allopurinol, BCG, febuxostat, leflunomide, mercaptopurine, sulfamethoxazole-trimethoprim, vaccines, warfarin, echinacea	Pregnancy, hepatic impairment, renal impairment,
Mycophenolate mofetil	1–3 g daily	Oral	Acyclovir, valacyclovir, antacids, BCG, cholestyramine, cyclosporine, echinacea, leflunomide, magnesium salts, metronidazole, natalizumab, oral contraceptives (estrogens and progestins), penicillins, probenecid, proton pump inhibitors, quinolones, rifamycin derivatives, sevelamer, vaccines	Pregnancy, renal impairment
Cyclophosphamide	0.5–1 g/m^2 IV monthly for 6 months, then every 3 months × 2 years or for 1 year after remission 1–3 mg/kg po daily	Intravenous, oral	Allopurinol, BCG, digoxin, CYP2 inducers/inhibitors, echinacea, etanercept, leflunomide, natalizumab, succinylcholine, vaccines, warfarin	Hepatic impairment, renal impairment, pregnancy

- Antimalarial agents: mild disease including arthritis, skin rash, and serositis
- Immunosuppressants: more severe disease including nephritis or other severe manifestations
- Cytotoxic agents: more severe disease including nephritis or other severe manifestations

The agents used for SLE may be used in combination to control manifestations of the disease.

Pharmacotherapy

See Table 16-7.

Physicochemical Properties, Pharmacodynamics, and Pharmacokinetics

- NSAIDs (various): decreases cyclooxygenase-1 and -2, which decreases prostaglandin precursors and decreases inflammation; pharmacokinetics: specific to each individual agent
- Hydroxychloroquine: unclear MOA; pharmacokinetics: hepatically eliminated
- Prednisone: decreases inflammation by suppressing immune system activity; pharmacokinetics: hepatic metabolism and renal excretion
- Azathioprine: interferes with cellular metabolic processes; pharmacokinetics: hepatic metabolism and renal excretion
- Mycophenolate mofetil: suppresses T and B lymphocytes involved in causing SLE manifestations; pharmacokinetics: bioavailability—94%, hepatic metabolism
- Cyclophosphamide: alkylating agent that cross-links DNA strands to decrease DNA synthesis; pharmacokinetics: prodrug that is activated by hepatic metabolism

1.3.0 Monitoring

Pharmacotherapeutic Outcomes

The goals of therapy are to improve quality of life, effectively manage symptoms, and induce SLE remission during flares, while maintaining remission periods for as long as possible between flares.

Safety and Monitoring and Patient Education

- NSAIDs: risk of GI bleeding, renal impairment, and hypertension; monitor CBC, serum creatinine, urinalysis, AST, and ALT
- Hydroxychloroquine: vision change/damage; monitor vision and ocular changes every 6–12 months
- Corticosteroids: hyperglycemia, hypertension, osteoporosis, weight gain, and fluid retention; monitor glucose and bone mineral density
- Azathioprine: myelosuppression, hepatotoxicity, and lympoproliferative disorders; monitor CBC, platelet count, serum creatinine, AST, and ALT
- Mycophenolate mofetil: myelosuppression, hepatotoxicity, and lymphoproliferative disorders; monitor CBC, hepatic function tests, BUN, and serum creatinine
- Cyclophosphamide: myelosuppression, myeloproliferative disorders, and hemorrhagic cystitis; monitor CBC with differential, platelet count, and urinalysis

Adverse Drug Reactions

- NSAIDs: bleeding, edema, hypertension
- Hydroxychloroquine: CNS effects, rash, pigmentary changes of skin and hair, GI upset, ocular toxicity
- Corticosteroids: infection, GI upset, blood pressure elevation, blood glucose disturbance, seizures, loss of bone mineral density
- Azathioprine: GI upset, leukopenia, thrombocytopenia, infection
- Mycophenolate mofetil: abdominal pain, anemia, GI upset, hypertension, infection, rash
- Cyclophosphamide: alopecia, infertility, GI upset, acute hemorrhagic cystitis or urinary fibrosis, anemia, thrombocytopenia

Table 16-8 Drugs for Systemic Lupus Erythematosus: Generic Names, Brand Names, and Dosage Forms Availability

Generic	Brand Name	Dosage Forms/Strengths
NSAIDs	Various	Oral solids, injectables
Hydroxychloroquine	Plaquenil	200 mg tablet
Prednisone		2.5, 5, 10, 20, and 50 mg tablets
Methylprednisolone	Medrol, Solu-Medrol, Depo-Medrol	4 mg tablet Powder for reconstitution (sodium succinate): 40 mg, 125 mg, 500 mg, 1 g, and 2 g Injection (acetate): 20 mg/mL, 40 mg/mL, 80 mg/mL
Azathioprine	Azasan, Imuran	50, 75, and 100 mg tablets
Mycophenolate mofetil	Cellcept	250 mg capsule 500 mg tablet Powder for suspension: 200 mg/mL
Cyclophosphamide	Cytoxan	25 and 50 mg tablets Powder for reconstitution: 500 mg, 1 g, and 2 g

Pharmacotherapeutic Alternatives

Limitation of sun exposure is recommended. Dehydroepiandosterone (DHEA) has been used experimentally as a steroid-sparing regimen in patients with mild disease.

2.1.0 Dispensing

See Table 16-8.

Calculations

Body surface area for cyclophosphamide:

$$\text{BSA (m}^2\text{)} = \sqrt{[(\text{height in cm}) \times \text{weight in kg})/3{,}600]}$$

ANNOTATED BIBLIOGRAPHY

American College of Rheumatology, Ad Hoc Committee on Systemic Lupus Erythematosus Guidelines. Guidelines for referral and management of systemic lupus erythematosus. *Arthritis Rheum* 1999; 42:1785–1796.

Ansel HC, Stoklosa MJ. *Pharmaceutical Calculations*. 11th ed. Baltimore, MD: Lippincott Williams & Wilkins; 2001:79.

Clinical Pharmacology. Available at: http://www.clinicalpharmacology-ip.com.proxy.campbell.edu. Accessed February 20, 2010.

Delafuente JC, Cappuzzo KA. Systemic lupus erythematosus and other collagen-vascular diseases. In: DiPiro JT, Talbert RL, Yee GC, Matzke GR, Wells BG, Posey LM, eds. *Pharmacotherapy: A Pathophysiologic Approach*. 6th ed. New York: McGraw-Hill; 2005:1581–1597.

LexiComp. Available at: http://www.crlonline.com.proxy.campbell.edu. Accessed February 20, 2010.

Parham P. *The Immune System*. 2nd ed. New York: Garland Science Publishing; 2005:351–352.

Neurologic

CHAPTER

17

TOPIC: ALZHEIMER'S DEMENTIA

Section Coordinator: Rex S. Lott
Contributor: Seth Thomas

Tips Worth Tweeting

- Medications with significant anticholinergic properties can worsen the cognitive disturbances seen in Alzheimer's dementia.
- Delirium can occur in patients from a variety of causes and may be confused with dementia.
- Age is one of the most significant risk factors for development of Alzheimer's dementia.
- Early initiation of treatment with acetylcholinesterase inhibitors and memantine will not prevent progression of Alzheimer's dementia, but this treatment may delay the onset of serious disability.
- When patients with Alzheimer's dementia develop significant behavioral or psychotic symptoms, treatment with antipsychotic medications may be necessary, although these medications may increase risk of morbidity and mortality.
- Failure to respond to or tolerate one acetylcholinesterase inhibitor should not rule out a therapeutic trial of another agent in this class.

Patient Care Scenario: Ambulatory Setting

J. L., 67 y.o. female Vietnam vet, 68 inches, 143 lbs, NKDA

PMH: Depression, anxiety, PTSD, h/o alcoholism, mild transaminitis, h/o "Robo tripping" (dextromethorphan abuse), peptic ulcer disease, hypertension, osteoporosis, hysterectomy 25 years ago

Lab values: AST = 65 IU/L, ALT = 47 IU/L, SrCr = 1.2 mg/mL, MCV = 81 μm^3, RBC = 4.2 × 10^6/mm^3, TSH = 2.5 mIU/L, Na = 137 mEq/L, K = 3.8 mEq/L, C-reactive protein = 15 mg/dL

Medication list: Alprazolam 0.25 mg po tid prn anxiety, omeprazole 20 mg po qd, lisinopril 10 mg po qd, alendronate 70 mg po once weekly, paroxetine 40 mg po qhs (increased 2 months ago from 20 mg)

J. L.'s daughter is with her today and reports her mother has been more confused the last few weeks, forgetting meetings with her daughter, misplacing her keys frequently, and having problems concentrating. Evaluating J. L.'s medication refill history, you notice she has become increasingly more noncompliant the last few months with her maintenance medications.

1.10 Patient Information

Patient History

Medication-Induced Delirium

Avoid or limit anticholinergic medications or agents with strong anticholinergic properties in the elderly. These agents can cause delirium, which mimics the dementia found in Alzheimer's disease (AD). Examples include benztropine, tolterodine, oxybutynin, solifenacin, dicyclomine, hyoscyamine, scopolamine patches, paroxetine, certain antipsychotics (chlorpromazine, thioridazine, loxapine, olanzapine, clozapine, and quetiapine), and antihistamines such as diphenhydramine and doxylamine. Blood pressure medications, muscle relaxants, opioid agonists, antineoplastics, and sedative hypnotics can also worsen dementia acutely.

Laboratory Testing

Initial workup should include thyroid panel, liver function tests, and a CBC with differential.

Disease States That Can Mimic AD

- Alcoholism
- Parkinson's
- Hypothyroidism
- Hepatic encephalopathy
- Infection
- Hypoglycemia
- Vascular disease
- Acute renal failure

Patient Assessment and Diagnosis

Instruments/Techniques

Comprehensive evaluations and family history are 90% accurate in diagnosing "probable AD." DSM-IV criteria for probable AD include identification of gradual onset of decreased mental abilities resulting in social/occupational functioning problems, impairment of recent memory (inability to learn new things), and presence of at least one of the following:

- Aphasia
- Apraxia
- Agnosia
- Anomia
- Executive functioning deficiencies and cognitive deficits not due to any other disease state, medication, or lab abnormality

The only definitive diagnosis for AD is upon autopsy with visualization of β-amyloid plaques or neurofibrillary tangles in brain neurons.

Key Terms

- **Delirium versus dementia:** Delirium involves an *acute* change in consciousness or cognitive abilities (hours to days) and is almost always attributable to disease states or medications. Delirium is reversible. Mild cognitive impairment is normal as we age; dementia is a chronic, progressive dysfunction (months to years) in cognitive abilities and is not a normal part of aging (e.g., AD, Lewy body dementia, vascular multi-infarct dementia, Pick's disease, and HIV/AIDS-induced dementia)
- **Early-onset versus late onset AD:** Early-onset AD occurs between the ages of 40 and 64 and is uncommon. Late-onset AD covers the vast majority of cases and occurs after the age of 65.

Signs and Symptoms

- **Cognitive symptoms:** Short-term memory loss, difficulty performing familiar tasks, language problems, disorientation to time and place, poor or decreased judgment, problems with abstract thinking, misplacing things frequently, change in mood or personality, loss of initiative.
- **Noncognitive symptoms:** Psychosis (paranoia, visual/auditory hallucinations, aggression), depression, behavioral disturbances, insomnia or sundowning. These symptoms are the most common reasons for nursing home placement.
- **Functional symptoms:** Inability to function independently (i.e., no longer able to get dressed, take a shower, clean the house or feed oneself).

Maintenance of Wellness and Prevention/ Treatment of AD

Age is the biggest risk factor for development of AD. This risk doubles every 5 years after age 65 (from 2% up to 30% by age 85). AD affects women twice as often as men. The presence of the apolipoprotein E4 genotype (Apo-E4) confers higher risk for AD. Environmental factors that may increase risk for AD include previous stroke, alcohol abuse, small head circumference or decreased education, repeated head trauma, Down syndrome, and heavy metal toxicity.

There is no cure for AD, but agents such as acetylcholinesterase inhibitors (donepezil, rivastigmine, galantamine) and memantine may slow the progression of the disease if initiated early. The best preventative strategy is "use it or lose it." Higher education and exercises that stimulate cortical function appear to offset the cognitive decline seen in AD. Statins (pravastatin and lovastatin, but *not* simvastatin) may be protective by decreasing cholesterol levels. Estrogen, vitamin E, and selegiline are *not* useful treatments due to their high risk-to-benefit profiles.

1.2.0 Pharmacotherapy

Uses and Indications for Drug Products

Donepezil (Aricept/Aricept ODT), rivastigmine (Exelon, Exelon patch), and galantamine (Razadyne/Razadyne ER)

Table 17-1 Medications to Treat Alzheimer's Disease

Drug Name	Drug Type and Indications	Mechanism	Common Side Effects	Manufacturer's Recommended Dosage	Notes
Memantine (Namenda) Tablets, extended-release tablets, oral solution	*N*-Methyl D-aspartate (NMDA) inhibitor Moderate to severe Alzheimer's	Blocks toxic effects associated with excess glutamate and regulates glutamate activation	Dizziness, headache, constipation, confusion	• Tablets/solution: Initial dose of 5 mg once a day • May increase dose to 10 mg/day (5 mg twice a day), 15 mg/day (5 mg and 10 mg as separate doses), and 20 mg/day (10 mg twice a day at minimum 1-week intervals if well tolerated • Extended-release tablet: Initial dose of 7 mg once a day; may increase dose to 14 mg/day, 21 mg/day, and 28 mg/day at minimum 1-week intervals if well tolerated	• Renal excretion • Maximum 5 mg twice daily if creatinine clearance less than 30 mL/min • Renal tubular acidosis/UTI—can increase urine pH and serum concentrations
Galantamine (Razadyne)	Cholinesterase inhibitor Mild to moderate Alzheimer's	Prevents the breakdown of acetylcholine in the brain	Nausea, vomiting, diarrhea, weight loss, loss of appetite	• Tablets/solution: Initial dose of 8 mg/day (4 mg twice daily) • May increase dose to 16 mg/day (8 mg twice daily) and 24 mg/day (12 mg twice daily) at minimum 4-week intervals if well tolerated • Extended-release capsule: Same dosage as above but taken once daily	• Generic preparations available • Food delays absorption by 1.5 hours and decreases C_{max} by 25% • Do not use if CrCl < 9 mL/min or Child-Pugh score of 10–15 • Maximum of 16 mg/day in patients with mild renal/liver impairment
Rivastigmine (Exelon)	Cholinesterase inhibitor Mild to moderate Alzheimer's	Prevents the breakdown of acetylcholine and butyrylcholine (a neurotrans-mitter similar to acetylcholine) in the brain	Nausea, vomiting, diarrhea, weight loss, loss of appetite, muscle weakness	• Capsules/oral solution: Initial dose of 3 mg/day (1.5 mg twice daily) • May increase dose to 6 mg/day (3 mg twice daily), 9 mg/day (4.5 mg twice daily) and 12 mg/day (6 mg twice daily) at minimum 2- week intervals if well tolerated • Patch: Initial dose of 4.6 mg once daily; may increase to 9.5 mg once daily after minimum of 4 weeks if well tolerated	• Capsules available as generic preparation • Food delays oral absorption by 1.5 hours, but improves tolerability • Patch: ↓body weight predicts increased side effects • Oral doses < 6 mg/day = 4.6 mg patch • Oral doses 6–12 mg = 9.5 mg patch
Donepezil (Aricept)	Cholinesterase inhibitor Mild to moderate and moderate to severe Alzheimer's	Prevents the breakdown of acetylcholine in the brain	Nausea, vomiting, diarrhea	• Tablets/orally disintegrating tablets: Initial dose of 5 mg once daily • May increase dose to 10 mg/day after 4–6 weeks if well tolerated, then to 23 mg/day after at least 3 months • 23-mg dose available as brand-name tablet only	

(*continues*)

Table 17-1 (*continued*)

Drug Name	Drug Type and Indications	Mechanism	Common Side Effects	Manufacturer's Recommended Dosage	Notes
Gingko biloba	Nutritional supplement Not FDA approved for Alzheimer's	May decrease β-amyloid plaque formation, which may in turn slow neuronal degeneration	Minimal	• 120–240 mg/day in 2–3 divided doses • Need extract with 24% ginkgoflavon-glycosides and 6% terpenes (high variation in herbal products)	• Avoid with concurrent antiplatelet/ anticoagulant therapy (may increase bleeding risk)

Modified from: *Alzheimer's Disease Medications Fact Sheet.* NIH Publication No. 08-3431, Alzheimer's Disease Education and Referral (ADEAR) Center, National Institute on Aging, National Institutes of Health, U.S. Department of Health and Human Services; November 2008 (updated December 2010). Available at: http://www.nia.nih.gov/alzheimers/publication/alzheimers-disease-medications-fact-sheet. Accessed August 8, 2012.

are all FDA-approved medications for mild to moderate AD. Tacrine (Cognex) is no longer in widespread use due to its significant risk for elevated liver enzymes. Memantine (Namenda) is approved for moderate to severe AD as monotherapy or as add-on therapy with an acetylcholinesterase (AchE) inhibitor. Gingko biloba may be as effective as AchE inhibitors in mild to moderate AD.

None of the available agents is curative. Realistically, they are intended to prolong long-term care placement for 6–24 months.

Antipsychotics, anxiolytics, hypnotics and antidepressants are used to treat various noncognitive behaviors.

Mechanisms of Action

The AchE inhibitors prevent the breakdown of acetylcholine (Ach), increasing the amount of Ach available for synaptic transmission. They do *not* reverse or halt neuronal degeneration, but can improve cognitive signaling for several months in mild to moderate cases.

Namenda is a NMDA receptor antagonist. It lowers neuronal excitation and slows cell death by inhibiting excitatory glutamate and aspartate pathways in the central nervous system (CNS).

Gingko biloba may decrease β-amyloid plaque formation, which may in turn slow neuronal degeneration. Agents to treat noncognitive problems are primarily used for symptom control and do not affect disease development or progression.

Drug, Food, and Lab Test Interactions

Rivastigmine has the highest incidence of nausea and vomiting and should be taken with food. Donepezil and galantamine may be given with food if stomach upset occurs. There are few drug–drug interactions (DDI) with this pharmacologic class, but anticholinergic agents make AchE inhibitors less effective and can adversely affect cognitive symptoms.

Memantine should be used with caution in conjunction with dextromethorphan, which is also a NMDA antagonist. Theoretically, nicotine in tobacco smoke may compete with memantine for renal elimination via tubular secretion. This potential interaction has not been documented. Carbonic anhydrase inhibitors (acetazolamide) and sodium bicarbonate alter urine pH and may cause retention of memantine.

Gingko biloba can increase the risk of bleeding. Monitor patients closely for signs and symptoms of bleeding and bruising with concurrent use of antiplatelet and anticoagulation agents.

Many antipsychotics are metabolized through the CYP 1A2 and 2D6 pathways; thus there is a potential for DDI. Many antipsychotics also possess varying degrees of anticholinergic activity. Examine the patient profile closely when initiating therapy.

Contraindications, Warnings, and Precautions

AchE inhibitors may have vagotonic effects leading to bradycardia or heart block. Monitor patients for syncopal episodes or supraventricular cardiac conduction abnormalities. Do not use donepezil in patients with a history of allergy to piperidine derivatives. Rivastigmine should be avoided in patients with allergy to carbamate derivatives. Dose-related nausea, vomiting, and diarrhea is common. Use rivastigmine with caution in patients with asthma, COPD, and peptic ulcer disease/NSAID use, and in patients with seizure disorders. Monitor patients for weight loss with rivastigmine. Do not use galantamine in patients with severe liver or renal dysfunction. Avoid memantine or adjust its dose in patients with severe renal impairment.

Antipsychotics may increase the risk of cardiac death in the elderly, and some of these medications negatively affect the patient's metabolic profile. The FDA has issued a warning regarding use of antipsychotics for behavioral symptoms in elderly patients with dementia.

Physiochemical Properties, Solubility, Pharmacodynamics, and Pharmacokinetic Properties

Donepezil is the only AchE inhibitor that is highly protein bound. Memantine excretion is entirely renal and is reduced by alkaline urine pH. All agents should be slowly increased every 2 weeks (rivastigmine) to 4 weeks (donepezil, galantamine). Memantine dosage can be increased weekly.

1.3.0 Monitoring

Pharmacotherapeutic Outcomes and Endpoints

The goal of therapy is to maintain cognitive function and independent living as long as possible, to improve quality of life, and ultimately to delay placement in a long-term healthcare facility.

Patient Evaluation and Monitoring to Determine the Safety and Efficacy of Pharmacotherapy

Improvement should be assessed through cognitive evaluation tools (2–4 points for MMSE and ADAS-Cog in 6 months—if no change, switch therapeutic agents) and ADL scores (subjective measure usually assessed by family members or social workers).

Mechanism of Adverse Reactions, Allergies, Side Effects, and Iatrogenic Illness and Remedies

The main adverse reactions to the AchE inhibitors include hypertension, insomnia, GI side effects (rivastigmine > galantamine > donepezil), chest pain, abnormal dreaming, fatigue, headache, and urinary incontinence.

Memantine can cause hypertension, syncope, dizziness, headache, and confusion. Watch for sudden weight loss, jaundice, or development of stroke or TIA. Monitor patients for signs and symptoms of bleeding and bruising with gingko biloba.

Antipsychotics often have anticholinergic side effects that can worsen cognitive functioning and lead to constipation, urinary retention, and dry mouth. Watch for movement disorders with these agents (e.g., tremor, myoclonic jerks, rigidity). Patients need to be monitored for oversedation while on benzodiazepines (avoid long-acting agents such as diazepam and librium in the elderly). SSRIs should be started at low doses for depression and increased slowly to minimize side effects such as sleep disturbance, nausea, and tremor.

Prevention of Medication Nonadherence, Misuse, and Abuse

Because memory loss is usually present with AD, it is important to maintain patients on a familiar schedule and in a comfortable environment. Utilize weekly medication boxes to decrease medication errors and ensure compliance. Frequent visits from the same family members and healthcare workers also aid in this endeavor. Overall, keep demands on the patient simple, try to remain calm and supportive, and provide constant reminders, explanations, and orientation cues to minimize confusion.

Pharmacotherapeutic Alternatives

Failure with any one agent does not preclude using other agents in the same pharmacological class. If no improvement occurs within 6 months or if intolerance develops, consider another agent or combination therapy with memantine. For aggressive behavior, several agents can be used. Although risperidone, olanzapine, quetiapine, and aripiprazole have been studied most often in clinical trials (e.g., the CATIE-AD study), other antipsychotics can be considered if these agents fail to provide benefit.

Dispensing

See Table 17-2.

Dosage Form Availability

Bioequivalence

When converting patients from oral rivastigmine to the transdermal patch:

- For oral doses less than 6 mg/day: switch to the 4.6 mg/24 hr patch
- For doses between 6–12 mg/day, use a 9.5 mg/24 hr patch

Table 17-2 Medications for Alzheimer's Dementia: Generic Names, Brand Names, and Dosage Forms

Generic	Brand Name	Dosage Forms
Donepezil	Aricept and Aricept ODT	Oral tablets: 5 mg, 10 mg Orally disintegrating tablets: 5 mg, 10 mg
Rivastigmine	Exelon	Oral capsules: 1.5 mg, 3 mg, 4.5 mg, 6 mg Oral solution: 2 mg/mL Transdermal patch: 4.6 mg/24 hr, 9.5 mg/24 hr
Galantamine	Razadyne and Razadyne ER	Oral capsule, extended release: 8 mg, 16 mg, 24 mg Oral tablets: 4 mg, 8 mg, 12 mg Oral solution: 4 mg/mL
Memantine	Namenda	Oral tablets: 5 mg, 10 mg Oral solution: 2 mg/mL
Gingko biloba		Variable (lack of standardization can be problematic)

Packaging, Storage, Handling, and Disposal

Dispose of used rivastigmine patches by folding them together along the adhesive side, inserting them back in their original container, and throwing them in the garbage. All oral Alzheimer's dementia medications are best stored at room temperature, away from excessive moisture; store orally disintegrating tablets (ODTs) in their original packaging until just prior to administration to avoid deterioration of the product.

Medication Administration Equipment

Apply rivastigmine transdermal patches to hairless areas (the back is preferable to prevent removal by the patient, but the upper arms or chest is also acceptable). Patients can bathe with the patch on, but excessive heat increases release of medication. Rotate the application site daily.

For the donepezil ODT formulation, instruct the patient to allow the tablet to dissolve fully on the tongue, followed by drinking a glass of water.

Access, Evaluate, and Apply Information to Promote Optimal Health Care

The Alzheimer's Association (www.alz.org) is an authoritative source for up-to-date information for patients suffering from Alzheimer's disease, their family members, and healthcare workers. The American Psychiatric Association offers detailed information for practitioners, including information on administering cognitive evaluation tools. Family members of someone with AD can also seek out local support groups.

Educate the Public and Healthcare Professionals Regarding Medical Conditions, Wellness, Dietary Supplements, and Medical Devices

No environmental factors have been definitively proved to cause AD, but evidence indicates that higher education and constant memory and cognition exercises can strengthen synaptic connections in the brain and potentially delay development of AD in susceptible individuals. While onset of disability from AD can be delayed for several years, there is currently no cure and cognitive deterioration is inevitable. Most people with AD will die of an unrelated complication, rather than the disease itself, such as pneumonia, infection, malnutrition or dehydration.

ANNOTATED BIBLIOGRAPHY

Alzheimer's Association. Diagnosing Alzheimer's. Available at: http://www.alz.org/alzheimers_disease_diagnosis.asp. Accessed January 10, 2010.

American Psychiatric Association. Practice guideline for the treatment of patients with Alzheimer's disease and other dementias. Available at: http://www.psychiatryonline.com/pracGuide/loadGuidelinePdf.aspx?file=AlzPG101007. Accessed January 10, 2010.

Cummings JL. Alzheimer's disease. *N Engl J Med* 2004;351:56–67.

Faulkner JK, Bartlett J, Hicks P. Alzheimer's disease. In: DiPiro JT, Talbert RL, Yee GC, et al., eds. *Pharmacotherapy: A Pathophysiological Approach*. Stamford: Appleton & Lange; 1999: 1157–1173.

Mace NL, Rabins PV. *The 36-Hour Day: A Family Guide to Caring for Persons with Alzheimer's Disease, Related Dementing Illnesses, and Memory Loss in Later Life*. 4th ed. New York: John Hopkins University Press; 2008.

Vitamin Research Products. Ginkgo: Study explores its cognitive-enhancing mechanism of action. Available at: http://www.vrp.com/articles.aspx?page=LIST&ProdID=1590&zType=2. Accessed December 13, 2009.

TOPIC: HEADACHES

Section Coordinator: Rex S. Lott
Contributor: Jolie Jantz

Tips Worth Tweeting

Migraine Headache

- Acute treatment with any of the triptans is appropriate if NSAIDs are ineffective.
- Non-oral routes of triptans or DHE should be used for patients experiencing nausea and vomiting.
- In patients who cannot use triptans or DHE because of contraindications, antiemetics or intranasal opioids should be considered.
- If debilitating migraines occur more than once per month, prophylaxis is indicated with propranolol, amitriptyline, valproic acid, or topiramate.

Tension-Type Headache

- Most commonly experienced headache.
- Acute treatment with acetaminophen, aspirin, and NSAIDs.
- Prophylaxis with amitriptyline or mirtazapine.

Cluster Headache

- Rare, excruciating headache, experienced mostly by men.
- Acute treatment includes oxygen plus SC or IN sumatriptan.
- Preventive treatment should be started along with acute treatment, and includes verapamil, lithium, oral steroid taper, or DHE.

Headache Drug Information

- Triptans possess various contraindications and drug interactions that pharmacists should be aware of.
- For all headaches, acute medication therapy should be minimized to avoid medication overuse headache (MOH).

Patient Care Scenario: Ambulatory Setting

A 25-year-old female presents to a pharmacy with a transferred prescription for hydromorphone 4–8 mg po q 4 hr prn migraine pain. When the pharmacist counsels the patient about her prescription, the patient tells him she has an allergy to sumatriptan, but the hydromorphone works well for her migraines. Upon further counseling, her allergy is described as a 5-minute experience of chest pain/tightness after an injection in the emergency room of sumatriptan 6 mg SC × 1. In the past, treatment with ibuprofen has helped only minimally. The patient admits that she needs hydromorphone 2–3 times per week, which is more than previously needed to control her migraines. The patient has no comorbidities and takes no other medications.

1.1.0 Migraine

- Chronic neurovascular disorder with severe headache (HA) and autonomic nervous system dysfunction
- Strong genetic component
- More common and more severe in women than in men
- Onset usually in adolescence or early adulthood
- Migraine headache diagnosis requires:
  - Exclusion of secondary causes and other primary HA disorders
  - Five attacks of HA lasting 4–72 hours with at least two of the following:
    - Unilateral location and pulsating quality
    - Intensity that inhibits daily activities
    - Aggravation by physical activity
    - Nausea and/or vomiting
    - Photophobia and phonophobia
- Migraine with aura
  - Experienced by approximately 30% of patients with migraine
  - Auras are focal neurological symptoms that precede or accompany migraine and include fully reversible visual, sensory, or speech symptoms:
    - Seeing flickering lights, spots, or lines or loss of vision
    - Feeling "pins and needles" or numbness
    - Experiencing dysphasic speech disturbances
- Goals of treatment
  - Rapid and consistent treatment to avoid recurrence
  - Restore the patient's ability to function
  - Minimize the need for backup or rescue medications
  - Guard against medication overuse headache

1.2.0 Pharmacologic Acute Therapy

NSAIDs

- First-line therapy—usually effective for mild to moderate pain.
- Ibuprofen, naproxen sodium, aspirin.
- Aspirin + acetaminophen + caffeine (Excedrin Migraine).
- Caffeine works as an adjunctive agent via analgesic and possibly anti-inflammatory properties. It also may increase the absorption of other coadministered medications.

"Triptans": Selective Serotonin$_{1B/1D}$ Agonists

- The mechanism of action is thought to be cranial vasoconstriction, interruption of vasoactive peptide release from perivascular trigeminal neurons, blockage of neurotransmission from the dorsal horn to the thalamus, and facilitation of descending pain inhibitory systems.
- Indications include severe migraine and migraine in patients who fail NSAID therapy.
- Select a non-oral route for patients with nausea and vomiting.
- All agents in this class should be avoided by patients with cardiovascular disease, uncontrolled HTN, or hemiplegic or basilar migraines.
- All agents except rizatriptan should be avoided in patients with cerebrovascular and peripheral vascular disease.
- Triptans cannot be used concomitantly with other triptans or ergotamine.

Table 17-3 Selected Acute Migraine Therapies

Drug	Route	Dosing	Adverse Effects	Contraindications	Comments
Ergot Alkaloids: nonselective 5-HT$_1$ agonists, α-adrenergic antagonists					
Dihydroergotamine (DHE)	IM, SQ	0.5–1 mg in 1 hr	N/V, peripheral ischemia, paresthesias, diarrhea	Coronary, cerebral or peripheral vascular disease, sepsis, pregnancy, hepatic or renal impairment, serotonin agonist within 24 hr	Maximum 3 mg/day (2 mg/day IV).
	Nasal	0.5 mg (1 spray) each nostril			May repeat dose in 15 min; maximum 3 mg/day
Serotonin Agonists (Triptans): *selective 5-HT$_{1B}$/5-HT$_{1D}$ agonists*					
Sumatriptan (Imitrex)	Oral	25–100 mg, may repeat in 2 hr; maximum 200 mg/day	Paresthesias, chest pain, warm/hot sensation	All triptans: ischemic heart disease, uncontrolled HTN, other triptans or ergot derivatives, MAOIs (unless noted); cerebrovascular and peripheral vascular disease (except Maxalt)	Needle-free SQ device available, SQ preferred for rapid onset and presence of N/V
	Nasal	5-20 mg, max 40 mg/d	Bad taste, N/V, nasal discomfort, flushing		
	SQ	4–6 mg; maximum 12 mg/day	Injection-site pain, tingling, dizziness, chest discomfort		
Naratriptan (Amerge)	Oral	2.5 mg, may repeat in 4 hr; maximum 5 mg/day	Nausea, dizziness, flushing		Not contraindicated with MAOIs
Almotriptan (Axert)	Oral	6.25 mg or 12.5 mg; maximum 25 mg/day	Nausea, dizziness		Not contraindicated with MAOIs; contains sulfonyl group
Eletriptan (Relpax)	Oral	20 mg or 40 mg, may repeat in 2 hr; maximum 80 mg/day	Paresthesias, N/V, chest tightness, dizziness	Watch CYP3A4 interactions	Not contraindicated with MAOIs; long half-life
Frovatriptan (Frova)	Oral	2.5 mg, may repeat in 2 hr; maximum of 7.5 mg/day	Dizziness, paresthesias, flushing, chest pain		Longest half-life; slow onset; low HA recurrence
Rizatriptan (Maxalt)	Oral, ODT	5–10 mg, may repeat in 2 hr; maximum 30 mg/day (15 mg/day if taking propranolol)	Dizziness, pressure sensations, N/V, abdominal pain, dry mouth		Best efficacy of oral medications, but high recurrence rate
Zolmitriptan (Zomig)	Oral, ODT	2.5–5 mg, may repeat in 2 hr; maximum 10 mg	Increased BP, coronary spasm, chest pain		
	Nasal	5 mg, may repeat in 2 hr; maximum 10 mg			

- Most triptans cannot be used concomitantly with MAOIs; exceptions include eletriptan, naratriptan, and frovatriptan.
- Side effects such as chest and neck pain/tightness, paresthesias, and flushing occur commonly and are known as "triptan sensations." Switching to a different agent is encouraged if they occur.
- Because of the risk of serious—albeit rare—cardiovascular events, consider CV workup in patients experiencing triptan sensations.

Ergotamine: Nonselective Serotonin Agonist, α-Adrenergic Antagonist

- Dihydroergotamine (DHE)
  - Dosage forms: SC, IM, IV, intranasal (with or without an antiemetic).
  - Contraindicated in renal or hepatic failure; coronary, cerebral, or peripheral vascular disease; uncontrolled HTN; pregnancy.
  - Do not use in the presence of CYP3A4 inhibitors, triptans, or MAOIs.

Antiemetics

- Metoclopramide, prochlorperazine, IV.
- Some evidence to support monotherapy.
- Useful as adjunct therapy when nausea and vomiting are present.

Opioids

- Butorphanol intranasal: Good evidence to support its use
- Oral opioids: Weak evidence for effectiveness and increased risk of dependence

Table 17-4 Selected Preventive Drug Therapies

Drug*	Dosing	Adverse Effects	Contraindications	Comments
Propranolol	20 mg bid-tid (maximum 320 mg/day)	Fatigue, bradycardia, depression, hypotension, hyperglycemia, bronchospasm	Asthma, diabetes, Raynaud's syndrome, depression	Drugs of choice for migraine prophylaxis. Do not discontinue abruptly.
Timolol	10 mg tid (maximum 30 mg/day)			
Divalproex sodium	250 mg q HS titrated to effective dose	N/V, tremor, weight gain, alopecia, thrombocytopenia, hepatotoxicity	Hepatotoxicity	Watch for drug interactions. Useful for comorbid bipolar disorder
Topiramate	25 mg/day titrated to 50 mg bid	Paresthesias, weight loss, N/V, diarrhea, confusion, fatigue	Hypersensitivity	May be useful for comorbid bipolar disorder
Amitriptyline	25–150 mg/day	Anticholinergic effects	Glaucoma, dementia, BPH	Drug of choice for tension-type HA
Verapamil	80 mg tid (maximum 480 mg/day)	Constipation, bradycardia, hypotension	Second- or third-degree AV block, aortic stenosis, CHF	Drug of choice for cluster HA. Watch for drug interactions.

* FDA-approved agents for migraine prophylaxis appear in bold.

Other Therapies

- Isometheptene + dichloralphenazone + acetaminophen (Midrin): vasodilator + sedative + analgesic

Pharmacologic Preventive Therapy

Initiate preventive therapy in patients who satisfy the following criteria:

- Two or more debilitating attacks per month
- Contraindication to, or failure of, acute treatments
- Use of acute treatments more than 2 times per week
- Presence of uncommon migraine
- Hemiplegic migraine, prolonged aura, or migrainous infarction

Streamline the drug therapy by choosing an agent based on the patient's comorbid conditions—HTN, psychiatric disorder, seizure disorder, peripheral neuropathy.

Consider a prophylactic drug holiday after 6 months if no comorbid indication is present or after 12 months if a comorbid indication is present.

Alternative/Adjunctive Therapies

- Minimize triggers (see Table 17-5)
- Maintain headache diary
- Sleep hygiene
- Stress management
- Regular exercise
- Natural medicines: Therapies with at least one positive randomized placebo-controlled trial to support their use as preventive agents
    - Riboflavin (vitamin B_2)
    - Coenzyme Q10
    - Butterbur (*Petasites hybridus*)
    - Feverfew (*Tanacetum parthenium*)
- Botulinum Toxin A: Its manufacturer is seeking an FDA indication for treatment of chronic migraine based on several positive studies
- Calcitonin gene-related peptide (CGRP) antagonists: Non-serotonergic, non-vasoconstricting, migraine-specific medication in Phase III trials

Table 17-5 Common Triggers of Migraine

Food Triggers
Alcohol
Caffeine
Chocolate
Monosodium glutamate
Tyramine-containing foods
Nitrate-containing foods
Behavior/Physiologic Triggers
Too much or too little sleep
Skipped meals
Stress or post stress
Menstruation
Fatigue
Physical activity
Environmental Triggers
Loud noises
Weather changes
Perfumes or fumes
High altitude
Exposure to glare or flickering lights

Tension-Type Headache

- Most common headache disorder
- Lifetime prevalence of 30–78%
- Characteristics:
  - Bilateral, dull ache
  - Nonpulsating quality
  - Hatband distribution of pain around head
  - Contraction of neck/scalp muscles
  - Not aggravated by physical activity
- Diagnosis requirements:
  - Bilateral HA with pressing, tightening, nonpulsating pain lasting from minutes to days
  - Pericranial tenderness with palpation
  - No nausea or vomiting
  - Photophobia or phonophobia, but not both, may occur

Pharmacologic Acute Therapy

- Acetaminophen
- Aspirin
- NSAIDs
- Triptans: For severe cases or patients with primary migraine disorder

Pharmacologic Preventive Therapy

- First line: Amitriptyline 50–100 mg/day (and other TCAs)
- Second line: Mirtazapine
- Other possibly effective strategies:
  - SSRIs: Sertraline, fluoxetine
  - Botulinum Toxin A: Local injections in frontal, temporal, occipital, or trapezius area every 3–4 months
  - Propranolol
  - Benzodiazepines

Cluster Headache

- Prevalence 0.1–0.4%
- Mostly occurs in men (male-to-female ratio = 6:1)
- Characteristics:
  - Unilateral pain around eye or temple
  - Severe, excruciating pain
  - Sudden onset and short duration
- Diagnosis requirements:
  - Five severe unilateral HA with orbital, supraorbital, or temporal pain lasting 15–180 minutes
  - Accompanying restlessness and ipsilateral facial swelling, lacrimation, sweating, sinus congestion, or rhinorrhea
  - Frequency ranges from 1 episode every other day to 8 episodes per day
- Initial treatment should include both acute therapy and preventive therapy to achieve and maintain remission.

Pharmacologic Acute Therapy

- Oxygen therapy via nonrebreathing mask
- Sumatriptan 6 mg SQ or 20 mg IN
- Dihydroergotamine IV: Also used for preventive therapy
- Steroids (oral or suboccipital injection): Also used for preventive therapy

Pharmacologic Preventive Therapy

- Verapamil
- Lithium
- Topiramate

Medication Overuse Headache

- Also known as analgesic-rebound headache or rebound headache
- Prevalence is 0.7–1.7%
- Diagnosis requirements: HA present on 15 or more days per month in the presence of the following:
  - HA medication overuse for 3 or more months
  - Worsening HA during medication overuse
  - Resolving HA within 2 months after discontinuation of medication overuse
- Often associated with nonrestorative sleep, neck pain, and vasomotor instability (sinus headache symptoms)
- Common comorbidities include depression and anxiety
- Any drugs used for treatment of HA can cause MOH
  - Ergotamine derivatives
  - Barbiturates
  - Triptans—possibly the most common culprit
  - Simple and combined analgesics
  - Opioids
  - Benzodiazepines
  - Caffeine (possibly)

Treatment

- Goals of therapy
  - Patient detoxification: Wean off of overused HA medications
  - Halting of chronic HA
  - Improvement of patient responsiveness to medications
- "Cold turkey" technique: Abrupt withdrawal therapy
  - May need transitional medications to bridge therapy: Corticosteroids, NSAIDs, DHE, triptans
  - Avoid abrupt withdrawal therapy if excessive usage of opioids or benzodiazepines may precipitate severe withdrawal symptoms
  - Quickly titrate preventive drug therapy to goal

Table 17-6 Comparison of Headache Characteristics

Symptom	Migraine	Tension Type	Cluster
Pain location	Unilateral or bilateral	Bilateral, hatband distribution	Always unilateral near eye or temple
Character-istics	Gradual, crescendo, pulsating, moderate or severe intensity	Pressure, tightness, nonpulsating, dull ache, neck/scalp muscle tightness	Quick crescendo to excruciating, explosive, throbbing pain
Patient epidemiol-ogy	18% women 6% men	88% women 69% men	Less than 2% of population, mostly men (6:1)
Duration	5 hours to 3 days	30 minutes to 7 days	30 minutes to 3 hours
Associated symptoms	Nausea, vomiting, photopho-bia, aura	None	Ispsilateral lacrimation, eye redness, rhinorrhea, nasal congestion

- "Slow weaning" technique: Gradual withdrawal therapy
  - Medication tapering over several weeks
  - Consider adding preventive drug therapy before weaning
- Withdrawal HA usually occurs, with clinical features depending on which medication is overused
- Advise the patient to avoid treating nonsevere headaches if possible
- Consider an inpatient program for monitoring if the patient is at risk for severe drug withdrawal symptoms with severe comorbid medical and/or psychiatric illnesses

ANNOTATED BIBLIOGRAPHY

Ailani J. Chronic Tension-type headache. *Curr Pain Headache Rep* 2009;13:479–483.

Comparison of available triptans. *Pharmacist's Letter /Prescriber's Letter* 2009;25(5):250509.

Evers S, Marziniak M. Clinical features, pathophysiology, and treatment of medication-overuse headache. *Lancet Neurol* 2010;9:391–401.

Evers S, Marziniak M. Clinical features, pathophysiology, and treatment of medication-overuse headache. *Lancet Neurol* 2010;9:391–401.

Francis GJ, Becker WJ, Pringsheim TM. Acute and preventive pharmacologic treatment of cluster headache. *Neurology* 2010;75:463–473.

Goadsby PJ, Sprenger T. Current practice and future directions in the prevention and acute management of migraine. *Lancet Neurol* 2010;9: 285–298.

Headache Classification Committee of the International Headache Society. *The International Classification of Headache Disorders*: 2nd ed. *Cephalgia* 2004;24(suppl 1):1–60.

Headache Classification Subcommittee of the International Headache Society. *The International Classification of Headache Disorders*: 2nd ed. *Cephalgia* 2004;24(suppl 1):9–160.

Katsarava Z, Fritsche G, Muessig M, et al. Clinical features of withdrawal headache following overuse of triptans and other headache drugs. *Neurology* 2001;57(9):1694–1698.

Limmroth V, Katsarava Z, Fritsche G, et al. Features of medication overuse headache following overuse of different acute headache drugs. *Neurology* 2002;59(7):1011–1014.

Loder E. Triptan therapy in migraine. *N Engl J Med* 2010;363:63–70.

Loder E. Triptan therapy in migraine. *N Engl J Med* 2010;363:63–70.

Matchar DB, Young WB, Rosenberg JH, et al. Evidence-based guidelines for migraine headache in the primary care setting: pharmacologic management of acute attacks. 2000. Available at: http://www.aan.com/professionals/practice/guidelines.cfm. Accessed January 13, 2011.

May A, Leone M, Afra J, et al. EFNS guidelines on the treatment of cluster headache and other trigeminal-autonomic cephalgias. *Eur J Neurol* 2006;13:1066–1077.

Noel JM. Neurologic disorders. In: *BCPP Examination Review and Recertification Course*. College of Psychiatric and Neurologic Pharmacists; 2010.

Rapoport AM. New acute treatments for headache. *Neurol Sci* 2010;31(suppl 1):S129–S132.

Silberstein SD. Migraine: preventive treatment. *Curr Med Res Opin* 2001;17(suppl 1):s87–s93.

Silberstein SD. Practice parameter: evidence-based guidelines for migraine headache (an evidence-based review): report of the Quality Standards Subcommittee of the American Academy of Neurology. *Neurology* 2000;55;754.

Stewart WF, Wood C, Reed ML, et al. Cumulative lifetime migraine incidence in women and men. *Cephalgia* 2008;28:1170–1178.

Tepper SJ, Bigal, M, Rapoport A, Sheftell F. Alternative therapies: evidence based evaluation in migraine. *Headache Care* 2006;3:57–64.

Tepper SJ, Tepper DE. Breaking the cycle of medication overuse headache. *Cleveland Clin J Med* 2010;77(4):236–242.

Vincenza S, Weiss K, Wall EM, Mottur-Pilson C. Pharmacologic management of acute attacks of migraine and prevention of migraine headache. *Ann Intern Med* 2002;137:840–849.

TOPIC: PAIN

Section Coordinator: Rex S. Lott
Contributor: Anna Ratka

Tips Worth Tweeting

- Pain is subjective in nature, and there are many categories of pain.
- Consequences of untreated pain are detrimental.
- Pain management should include frequent assessment and individualized therapy.
- Opioid analgesics are used for severe acute pain and for moderate to severe chronic pain.
- Tolerance and dependence to opioids should be expected and differentiated from addiction.
- Increase in opioid dose should be no less than 25% of the patient's present 24-hour opioid dose.
- Rotate opioids if inadequate pain relief is obtained despite dose increases or if intolerable adverse effects develop.
- Opioid analgesics differ in their analgesic potency, adverse-effect profile, and dosage forms.

Patient Care Scenario: Ambulatory Setting

At 10 PM, Mr. Black, a 32-year old male, came to the emergency department very upset, with elevated blood pressure and pulse, and profound grimaces on his face. He said that he had aching pain all over his abdomen; the pain had started in the afternoon. When asked to assess the intensity of his pain, Mr. Black said that his pain was at level 6 (on scale of 0–10). The attending physician gave Mr. Black a prescription for hydrocodone with APAP, 5/325 mg), #10, to take every 4–6 hours as needed for pain, and sent him home.

1.1.0 Patient Information

Pain is inherently subjective in nature. It is an unpleasant sensation disturbing the patient's comfort, thoughts, sleep, or normal activities of daily living. Pain is a multipart syndrome including three components: sensory-discriminative, motivational-affective, and cognitive-evaluative. There are many different types of pain.

Laboratory Testing

There are no diagnostic laboratory tests for pain.

Disease States Associated with Pain

Pain is associated with a variety of diseases. Recent studies suggest that chronic pain can become a disease of its own.

Key Terms

- **Analgesia:** The relief of pain without loss of consciousness.
- **Hyperalgesia:** Exaggerated response to noxious stimuli.
- **Allodynia:** Innocuous stimulus perceived as painful.
- **Opiates:** Compounds derived from the exudates of the poppy plant.
- **Opioids:** Both naturally occurring and synthetic drugs with similar actions.

Classification of Pain

- *Somatic (nociceptive)*: Arises from activation of nociceptors; localized, constant, aching or throbbing.
- *Visceral*: Originates in smooth musculature or sympathetically innervated organs; difficult to localize, dull, aching, referred.
- *Neuropathic (deafferentiation pain, paresthesia)*: Caused by peripheral nerve injury/damage; burning, shooting, tingling, limited response to opioid analgesics; requires an adjuvant.
- *Acute*: Duration of hours to days; rapid nerve conduction, predictable associated problems.
- *Chronic*: Duration of months to years; slow nerve conduction; associated with problems such as anxiety and depression.
- *Breakthrough pain*: A transitory elevation of pain intensity in patients with chronic pain; more severe than the background pain; idiopathic or precipitated by an incident.

Signs and Symptoms

Pain is associated with obvious distress or noticeable suffering. Symptoms depend on the type of pain (as discussed earlier) and may change over time. Signs of pain may include hypertension, tachycardia, mydriasis, and diaphoresis, or there may be no obvious signs.

Consequences of Untreated Pain

- Physiological: Increased catabolic demand, impaired respiratory effort, water retention, inhibited GI motility, hypertension, tachycardia, tachypnea, elevated adrenal corticosteroid secretion, altered brain neurochemistry and neuroprocessing, impaired immune system

- Psychological: negative emotions (anxiety, depression), sleep disturbance, difficulty making decisions, distress

Instruments and Techniques Applied to Pain Assessment

Pain is considered the fifth vital sign and must be assessed routinely. There are many techniques available to assess pain intensity and pain distress. The standard method is the Numeric Pain Intensity Scale: 0 = no pain, 1–4 = mild pain, 5–6 = moderate pain, 7–9 = severe pain, 10 = worst possible pain. A pain assessment inventory should include the following elements: pain level (intensity), pain tolerance (acceptable pain level), location of pain, variation in pattern of pain, pain's effect on activities of daily living, personal belief about pain, and goal for satisfactory pain relief.

Approaches to Relieving Pain

Adequate and thorough pain assessment based on the patient's reports is the first step to effective relief of pain. Approaches to relieve pain include the following:

- Eliminate the cause(s) of pain (e.g., treat inflammation, treat ulcer)
- Prevent pain transmission (e.g., with local anesthetics)
- Affect the way pain is perceived (e.g., with general anesthetics, opioids)
- Affect the patient's reaction to pain (e.g., tranquilizers, opioids)

Pharmacologic Therapies of Pain

- Opioid analgesics (agonists, antagonists, agonists-antagonists, opioid analgesic combinations)
- Adjuvants (e.g., antirheumatic agents, muscle relaxants, non-opioid analgesics, NSAIDs, anticonvulsants)

Opioid analgesics are recommended for severe acute pain and moderate to severe chronic pain. Pain therapy with opioid analgesics should be individualized, especially in the elderly, children, patients with chronic pain, opioid-naïve patients, and patients with hepatic/renal insufficiency. Increase of the opioid dose should be always made as a percentage of the present 24-hour dose. Opioid rotation based on equianalgesic conversion ratios is recommended to improve analgesia and/or minimize adverse effects.

Nonpharmacologic Therapies of Pain (Examples)

- Psychological techniques
- Cognitive-behavioral therapy
- Acupuncture
- Nerve stimulation or blockade
- Orthopedic procedures

Pain management needs to take precedence over other therapies. It should include periodic assessment, reassessment, monitoring, and adjustments of therapy until adequate relief of pain is achieved.

1.2.0 Pharmacotherapy

Opioid analgesics are used for severe acute pain and for moderate to severe chronic pain.

Drug, Food, and Lab Test Interactions

Opioids can interact with sedative-hypnotics (increased CNS depression and respiratory depression), antipsychotic tranquilizers (increased sedation, respiratory depression, and cardiovascular effects), and MAO inhibitors (hypertension, hyperpyretic coma). The analgesic effects of codeine, oxycodone, and tramadol may be decreased by CYP2D6 inhibitors (sertraline, bupropion, diphenhydramine, paroxetine, fluoxetine), by CYP3A4 inhibitors (macrolides), and in CYP2D6 deficiency. Concurrent use of tramadol with TCAs increases the risk of seizures; when this agent is combined with serotonergic agents, it may result in serotonin syndrome.

Food has a relatively profound effect on absorption of oral opioids. Proper timing of doses in relation to meals may improve bioavailability of oral analgesics.

Contraindications, Warnings, and Precautions

Examples of clinical conditions in which opioids should be avoided include pulmonary dysfunction (opioids increase the risk of respiratory compromise), hypovolemia (opioids result in orthostatic hypotension), asthma (opioids cause bronchospasm), and head trauma (opioids cause respiratory depression and increase intracranial pressure). Caution should be exercised if opioids are given to opioid-naïve patients with no pain (adverse effects are more prominent). Avoid withdrawal in patients on chronic opioids; do not stop opioids abruptly, and avoid simultaneous administration of antagonist or mixed agonist-antagonists. Expect tolerance and physical dependence; differentiate these conditions from addiction.

Pharmacodynamics and Pharmacokinetics

The chief action of opioids is to impair the normal sensory awareness of and response to pain. Opioids modulate the ascending and the inhibitory descending pain pathways. The specific sites of opioids' action are opioid receptors (mu, delta, and kappa) on presynaptic and postsynaptic neurons located in the brain, in the spinal cord, and in the periphery.

Table 17-7 Opioid Analgesics: Indications, Dosing, Routes of Administration, Equianalgesic Ratios and Controlled Substance Schedules

Opioid Analgesic	Route of Administration	Starting Dose	Equianalgesic Ratio (Morphine:Drug)	Controlled Substance Schedule
Short-Acting Agonists				
Morphine sulfate	Oral	5–15 mg q 3–4 hr	1:1	II
	Parenteral	2-10 mg q 3–4 hr	3:1	
Hydrocodone	Oral	5-10 mg q 4–6 hr	1:1	II
Codeine	Oral	15-30 mg q3–4 hr	1:6.7	II
Hydromorphone	Oral	2-4 mg q 4–6 hr	4:1	II
	Parenteral	0.5-2 mg q 4–6 hr	6:1	
Oxycodone	Oral	5-10 mg q 3–4 hr	1.5:1	II
Oxymorphone	Oral	5-20 mg q 4–6 hr	3:1	II
Fentanyl	Transmucosal	200 mcg q 1–2 hr	unknown	II
	Buccal	100 mcg		
Tramadol	Oral	25–50 mg q 4–6 hr	1:4 to 1:10	
Long-Acting				
Morphine:	Oral	15 mg q 12 hr	1:1	II
(Kadian)	Oral	20 mg qd or bid		
(Avinza)	Oral	30 mg qd		
(Oramorph SR)	Oral	15 mg bid		
Oxycodone (OxyContin)	Oral	10 mg q 12 hr	1.5:1	II
Oxymorphone (Opana)	Oral	5 mg q 12 hr	3:1	II
Methadone (Dolophine)	Oral	Highly variable	3:1–10:1	II
Methadone HCl	Parenteral		Oral:parenteral 2:1	
Fentanyl (Duragesic)	Transdermal	12 mcg/h q 72 hr	25 mcg/hr = morphine 60 mg/day	II
Tramadol (Ultram ER)	Oral	100 mg qd	1:5	
Opioid Antagonists				
Naloxone (Narcan)	Parenteral	0.1–0.4 mg		
Naltrexone (ReVia)	Oral	25 mg		
Nalmefene (Revex)	Parenteral	0.25 mcg/kg		
Opioid Agonist-Antagonists				
Pentazocine (Talwin)	Parenteral	30–60 mg q 3–4 hr		IV
Butorphanol (Stadol)	Nasal	1 mg q 60–90 min		IV
	Parenteral	0.5–2 mg q 3–4 hr		
Nalbuphine (Nubain)	Parenteral	10 mg q 3–6 hr		
Buprenorphine (Buprenex)	Sublingual	2–8 mg		III
	Parenteral	0.3 mg q 6–8 hr		
Opioid Combinations with Other Analgesics (Multiple)				
Hydrocodone with acetaminophen (e.g., Lortab, Norco, Lorcet, Vicodin, Zydone)	Oral	Vary	1:1	III
Oxycodone with acetaminophen (Percocet, Endocet, Tylox, Roxicet)	Oral	Vary	1.5:1	II
Oxycodone with aspirin (Percodan, Endodan)	Oral	Vary	1.5:1	II

Effects of clinically used opioid analgesics include the following:

- CNS: Analgesia, mood alterations (euphoria/dysphoria, sedation, tranquility), depressed respiration, depressed cough, nausea and vomiting, miosis, sometimes convulsions, and neuroendocrine dysfunction, tolerance, dependence, and addiction
- Cardiovascular: Orthostatic hypotension (fainting), bradycardia
- Gastrointestinal:
  - Stomach: Decreased secretions, tone, delayed emptying
  - Intestine: Diminished secretions and peristalsis, decreased defecation
  - Biliary tract: Constriction of the sphincter of Oddi
- Smooth muscles: Increased contractions of urethra and bladder, bronchial constriction
- Skin: Pruritus, flushing, warming, sweating, urticaria (at injection site)
- Immune system: Inhibition of NK cells and lymphocyte response to mitogens

Opioid analgesics are available in a wide variety of dosage forms and can be administered by many different routes. Oral administration of opioids may result in an extensive first-pass effect. Opioids become well distributed in plasma, highly perfused tissues, muscle, and fat. The major metabolism of opioids occurs in the liver (conjugation, hydrolysis, oxidation); activities of CYP3A4 and CYP2D6 differ among individuals and can be either induced or inhibited. Opioids are excreted mainly by urine and bile.

Dose Calculations

- Titration of opioid doses: Increase by a percentage of the present 24-hour dose; increases less than 25% are meaningless.
- Equianalgesic conversions: Used to change the route of administration of the same opioid or to switch to another opioid; based on equianalgesic ratios. "Start low and go slow and steady."
- Estimation of a rescue dose for breakthrough pain:
  - For oral administration, use 10–15% of the total 24-hour dose of current opioid.
  - Administer oral rescue doses every 1–2 hours; if three or more rescue doses per day are needed, consider increasing the amount of the around-the-clock (ATC) opioid.
  - Whenever an ATC opioid is increased, the rescue dose needs to be recalculated.

Classification of Opioid Analgesics by Duration of Action

- Long-acting opioids: Fentanyl patch, methadone, modified-release morphine, oxycodone, oxymorphone.
- Short-acting opioids: Codeine, hydrocodone, hydromorphone, morphine, oxycodone, oxymorphone.
- Short-acting opioids with rapid onset: Fentanyl—transmucosal, buccal tablet, bio-erodible mucoadhesive, sublingual, liposome encapsulated.

1.3.0 Monitoring

Pharmacotherapeutic Outcomes

Complete pain relief may not be possible. The goal is optimal pain relief with minimal adverse effects and improvement of quality of life and functional status. Pain control is a process and requires multiple titrations of opioid dosing regimen and route. Rotate opioids if intolerable adverse effects occur or if the patient experiences inadequate pain relief despite dose increases.

Major Adverse Effects of Opioids

- Dysphoria
- Euphoria
- Lethargy
- Drowsiness
- Apathy
- Inability to concentrate
- Nausea
- Vomiting
- Decreased respiratory rate
- Constipation
- Biliary spasm
- Urinary retention
- Urticaria
- Pruritus
- Tolerance
- Withdrawal symptoms upon abrupt discontinuation
- Possible addiction

Safety and Efficacy Monitoring and Patient Education

In general, opioid analgesics require monitoring of pain relief, respiratory and mental status, blood pressure, and constipation. Specific-agent monitoring is as follows:

- Tramadol: Seizures, serotonin syndrome
- Meperidine: Convulsions
- Methadone: Long and variable half-life may result in cumulative toxicity

Expect and monitor development of tolerance and physical dependence. Prevent precipitation of opioid withdrawal. Be aware of the potential hazards of mixed agonists-antagonists.

Educate patients on the following points:

- Tolerance and physical dependence are expected effects of opioids.
- Addiction to opioids is very rare in patients with chronic pain.
- Constipation needs to be managed.
- Adherence is essential for optimal pain relief.

Adverse Reactions to Opioid Analgesics

- Tolerance: Physiological, predictable consequence of chronic opioid therapy; state of adaptation with diminishing desired and adverse opioid effects; develops rapidly (3–4 days, except for constipation).
- Physical dependence: Physiologic neuro-adaptation with manifested withdrawal syndrome; expected with chronic opioid therapy; not to be equated with addiction.
- Addiction: Psychological dependence; a neurobehavioral syndrome characterized by loss of control over opioid use; continuation of opioid use despite adverse consequences; preoccupation with opioids for their psychic effect; obsessive, out-of-control, compulsive opioid seeking and use.
- Opioid "pseudo-addiction": Iatrogenic syndrome; occurs when inadequate amounts of analgesics are given for pain relief; patients may display "bizarre" behaviors ("difficult patients") that resolve when pain is adequately relieved.

Pharmacotherapeutic Alternatives

Use of other therapeutic analgesic agents depends on type and intensity of pain. Adjuvant medications (NSAIDs, anticonvulsants, muscle relaxants, corticosteroids, local anesthetics) may be used in combination with opioid analgesics or as a single therapy.

ANNOTATED BIBLIOGRAPHY

Baumann TJ, Strickland J. Pain Management. In: DiPiro JT, et al., eds. *Pharmacotherapy: A Pathophysiologic Approach*, 7th ed. New York: McGraw-Hill Medical; 2008, Chapter 62, pp. 989–1004.

Gutstein HB, Akil H. Opioid analgesics. In: Brunton LL, et al., eds. *Goodman & Gillman's The Pharmacological Basis of Therapeutics*, 11th ed. New York: McGraw-Hill Medical; 2006, Chapter 21, pp 547–590.

Katzung BG, ed. *Basic and Clinical Pharmacology*, 11th ed. New York: McGraw-Hill Medical; 2009.

Koda-Kimble MA, et al., *Handbook of Applied Therapeutics*, 8th ed. Philadelphia: Lippincott Williams & Wilkins; 2007.

Lussier D, Huskey A, Beaulier P. Overview of analgesic agents. *Pain Med News Special Ed,* 5: 45–58, December 2006.

TOPIC: PARKINSON'S DISEASE

Section Coordinator: Rex S. Lott
Contributor: Christopher T. Owens

Tips Worth Tweeting

- By the time patients are diagnosed with Parkinson's disease (PD), they have already lost 50–60% of their dopaminergic neurons.
- Pseudo-Parkinsonism mimics the symptoms of PD, but may be related to use of drugs such as antipsychotics, metoclopramide, methyldopa, and certain antiemetics.
- The cardinal motor features of PD are represented by the acronym TRAP: tremor, rigidity, akinesia, and postural instability.
- Most experts agree that pharmacologic treatment for PD should be initiated when patients experience functional impairment.
- Dopamine agonists are often used as the initial drug treatment, as they can delay the need for levodopa and its dose- and duration-related adverse effects.
- Motor complications such as dyskinesias occur in as many as half of patients treated with levodopa within 6 years of initiation.

Patient Care Scenario: Ambulatory Setting

A. O. is a 65-year-old white male who was diagnosed with Parkinson's disease 6 months ago. He is currently taking selegiline 5 mg po twice daily (7:00 AM and noon).

A. O. presents to the clinic today for follow-up, complaining of stiffness, slow movement, and increasing rest tremor. He states that the selegiline "doesn't seem to be helping much" and his symptoms are beginning to adversely affect his daily activities. His physical exam findings are remarkable for itchy and scaly skin on the scalp, masked facies, tremor in the left hand while sitting, and cogwheel rigidity in the left shoulder and elbow. The patient's gait is steady and he has normal mental status. Labs are WNL.

Area 1 Competency: Assure Safe and Effective Pharmacotherapy and Optimize Therapeutic Outcomes

1.1.0 Patient Information

Parkinson's disease (PD) is the second most common neurodegenerative disorder (after Alzheimer's disease) and affects approximately 1% of the U.S. population older than the age of 60. The peak age at onset is between 55 and 65 years of age, although younger-onset cases have also been reported.

The exact cause of PD is unknown, but current theories implicate a process of neuronal toxicity, specifically affecting dopaminergic neurons in the basal ganglia and nigrostriatal pathways. While the mechanism of toxicity is not completely understood, oxidative stress as a result of environmental and other toxins likely plays a role. Interestingly, nicotine and caffeine have been identified as possibly protective against the disease.

Loss of dopaminergic neurons in the substantia nigra leads to dopamine depletion in the striatum and a loss of stimulation to the D1 and D2 receptor types. Additionally, this loss creates an imbalance between dopamine and acetylcholine. Autopsy findings show a profound loss of pigmented substantia nigra cells and the presence of Lewy bodies in remaining neurons. The threshold for appearance of clinical signs and symptoms is loss of 50–60% of dopaminergic neurons.

Medication-Induced Causes of Parkinsonism

Drug-related pseudo-Parkinsonism is a reversible condition that mimics the signs and symptoms of idiopathic PD. Agents associated with pseudo-Parkinsonism include typical antipsychotics (haloperidol, thioridazine), metoclopramide, methyldopa, and antiemetics with dopamine antagonist properties (prochloperazine, trimethobenzamide, and, occasionally, promethazine). Treatment consists of decreasing the dose or discontinuing the offending medication. If the drug cannot be safely discontinued, anticholinergic drugs may be used to lessen symptoms.

Table 17-8 Diagnostic Criteria for Parkinson's Disease

Clinically Possible
One of the following: asymmetric rest tremor, rigidity, bradykinesia
Clinically Probable
Any two of the following: asymmetric rest tremor, rigidity, bradykinesia
Clinically Definite
Criteria for clinically probable plus a definitive response to PD drugs
Exclusion Criteria
Exposure to drugs that may cause pseudo-Parkinsonism, cerebellar signs, history of encephalitis, recurrent head injury, hydrocephalus, or other structural lesions on MRI

Table 17-9 Cardinal Features of Parkinson's Disease

Tremor
• Approximately half of patients will have this sign upon presentation • Common in the hand and begins unilaterally; described as "pill rolling" • Occurs at rest and improves with intentional movement
Rigidity
• Increased resistance to passive movement • Ratchet-like, short, jerky movements; described as "cogwheel rigidity" • Diminished facial expression (masked facies), infrequent blinking, sialorrhea
Akinesia
• Absence of movement (extremely disabling); usually a late sign • Preceded by slowness of movement (bradykinesia)
Postural Instability
• Impaired balance and coordination • Related to changes in gait and movement initiation; start hesitation, freezing, festination (slow and shuffling movement)

A presumptive diagnosis of PD is based on clinical findings; a definitive diagnosis can only be made upon autopsy. The cardinal clinical features of the disease include tremor, rigidity, and bradykinesia.

In the early stages of PD, patients may experience excessive fatigue, malaise, and some shakiness or unsteadiness. Hypophonia (speaking softly), micrographia (small, cramped handwriting), and loss of sense of smell may be part of the prodrome phase as well.

Nonmotor symptoms of PD are also often present and include depression, cognitive impairment, visual hallucinations, insomnia, difficulty swallowing, orthostasis, urinary hesitancy, constipation, oily facial skin, dry and flaky scalp, and increased risk of malignant melanoma.

Instruments and Techniques Related to Patient Assessment

Once diagnosed, symptoms of PD and disease progression are assessed using two major scales: the Hoehn and Yahr Staging System and the Unified Parkinson's

Table 17-10 Hoehn and Yahr Staging System

Stage	Description	Time Frame	Comment
I	Unilateral involvement	Prodrome	Fatigue, depression, tremor
II	Bilateral involvement without balance impairment	1–2 years after onset	Triad symptoms, blank stare, social withdrawal
III	Bilateral involvement with mild postural instability	2–5 years after onset	Increased rigidity, festination
IV	Bilateral involvement with postural instability; patient is unable to live on his or her own	> 5 years	Grab rails needed in house; unable to button shirts; needs large-handle utensils
V	Fully developed disease; wheelchair or bed restricted	10 years since onset	Levodopa no longer effective; difficult to understand speech

Disease Rating Scale (UPDRS). The UPDRS is an extensive scale that includes the Hoehn and Yahr Stage in its rating. The UPDRS is much more specific, but both scales are still used in clinical practice.

There is currently no cure for PD. Thus the goals of therapy include alleviating symptoms, improving quality of life and activities of daily living (ADLs), and minimizing adverse drug effects.

As a progressive disorder, PD is characterized by symptoms that are expected to steadily worsen over the course of the disease. Patients also experience fluctuations in motor symptoms that may (or may not) be related to medication dosing. Times of increased symptoms and more severe impairment are termed "off times." Cycling between "on-off times" is also common.

Therapeutic options are continually evolving and include both nonpharmacologic (including surgical treatments) and drug therapies. Nonpharmacologic options include education and participation in support groups, exercise and physical therapy to increase or maintain flexibility and mobility, occupational therapy, nutritional support, and speech therapy. Surgical options have varying levels of success and duration of effectiveness and include pallidotomy (destruction of the globus pallidus), thalamotomy (destruction of part of the thalamus), and deep brain stimulation.

A number of antioxidant vitamins (C and E) are touted as beneficial in PD, but there is currently no conclusive evidence for their efficacy in symptomatic relief or as neuroprotectants. Coenzyme Q10 is believed to be an antioxidant essential for mitochondrial function. Doses of 1,200 mg daily are associated with slower worsening in UPDRS scores, but lower doses were no better than placebo.

1.2.0 Pharmacotherapy

Drugs, Indications, and Mechanisms of Action

Pharmacologic therapy is the mainstay of treatment for PD and may be divided into two main categories: neuroprotective and symptomatic. Neuroprotective therapies are largely theoretical and are proposed to protect populations of at-risk neurons from oxidative stress and subsequent destruction. Agents in this category include MAO-B inhibitors, coenzyme Q10, and possibly the dopamine agonists. Symptomatic therapies are designed to reduce the signs and symptoms of PD and preserve normal functioning.

In general, clinicians employ symptomatic treatments initially at low doses and titrate gradually to effect. In addition, most drug therapies must be withdrawn gradually and not abruptly discontinued. The lowest possible dose is desirable (especially with levodopa). Patient age and cognitive status are important considerations when employing certain classes of agents (e.g., anticholinergics) and treatment initiation is usually agreed to be appropriate when patients manifest functional impairment.

The major agents and drug classes used in the symptomatic management of PD include MAO-B inhibitors, amantadine, anticholinergics, dopamine agonists, levodopa, and catechol-*o*-methyltransferase (COMT) inhibitors.

MAO-B inhibitors are used predominantly as neuroprotectants in early PD, but have some mild symptomatic benefits. Agents include selegiline (Eldepryl) and rasagliline (Azilect). In addition to its standard, oral formulation, selegiline is available as an oral disintegrating tablet (Zelapar) and a transdermal patch (Emsam), although the patch is currently approved only for the treatment of major depression. MAO-B inhibitors are dosed in the morning to avoid insomnia and other common adverse effects, including nausea, dizziness, headache, and postural hypotension. Concomitant use of antidepressants should generally be avoided; concurrent use of meperidine is contraindicated. MAO-B inhibitors may increase the risk of dyskinesias in levodopa-treated patients, especially in later stages of the disease course. Patients should avoid tyramine-containing foods (e.g., wine, cheese, salami), although the risk of ingesting these dietary substances is lower than in patients receiving MAO-A inhibitors (e.g., tranylcypromine) for treatment of depression. Selegiline is metabolized to amphetamine-like compounds, which may be responsible for causing insomnia. Rasagiline does not have amphetamine-like metabolites and is associated with a lower incidence of insomnia.

Amantadine (Symmetrel) is an antiviral agent with antiparkinsonian activity. It may act via increasing dopamine release, and it may have effects on the NMDA receptor. Although often used in early stages with mild disease, this agent may be added later on to allow for decreased levodopa dosage. Its efficacy is similar to that of anticholinergics in improving tremor, but it also has effects on rigidity and bradykinesia. Adverse effects include sedation, vivid dreams, dry mouth, and livedo reticularis (edema, itching, and a mottling of the skin on the lower extremities). Dosage adjustment is required in patients with renal impairment.

Drugs with anticholinergic properties are used to help restore the balance between dopamine deficiency and acetylcholine over-activity in PD. The agents used most commonly are trihexyphenidyl (Artane) and benztropine (Cogentin). They are used most often in younger individuals with little or no cognitive impairment who manifest marked tremor and in patients who are experiencing levodopa-induced dystonias. Adverse effects of these agents include dry mouth, blurred vision, urinary retention, constipation, decreased sweating, and cognitive impairment.

Oral dopamine agonists directly stimulate D1 and D2 receptors and are commonly used as initial symptomatic therapy. They may also delay the need to start levodopa. In advanced disease, they may be added to a patient's regimen to allow for fewer fluctuations in dopamine levels, lower doses of levodopa, and decreased risk of adverse effects, such as dyskinesias. Orally available agents may be divided into two groups: ergot and non-ergot derivatives. The ergot-derived dopamine agonists include pergolide, bromocriptine, and cabergoline; however, cabergoline is not currently FDA approved for the treatment of PD. The non-ergot agents include pramipexole and ropinirole.

Rotigotine (Neupro) is a non-ergot dopamine agonist administered transdermally. A new patch is applied daily and allows for a more continuous release of the agent and receptor stimulation. The patch should be changed once daily, with the old patch being folded in half and discarded away from children and pets. Apomorphine (Apokyn) is a non-ergot agent for subcutaneous administration. It is indicated for "rescue treatment" during "off" times and has a rapid onset and short duration of action. It is associated with severe nausea and vomiting, and patients must be pretreated and continually receive trimethobenzamide as an antiemetic. Concurrent use of ondansetron is contraindicated, as it may precipitate a dangerous drop in blood pressure.

As a class, the dopamine agonists are associated with nausea, vomiting, sedation, orthostatic hypotension, confusion, and hallucinations. Obsessive–compulsive behaviors have also been reported rarely and include an excessive desire to shop, gamble, eat, or engage in sexual activity. Excessive daytime sleepiness has been reported in PD patients treated with these drugs, and sudden onset of sleep may occur in as many as 6% of patients. Patients who are still driving need to be made aware of this possibility. Apomorphine is associated with such severe nausea and vomiting that pretreatment with antiemetic agents is necessary and should be continued for at least 2 months or until tolerance develops.

Levodopa is well known as the single most effective drug for symptomatic treatment of PD. It is a precursor to dopamine and must be converted in

Table 17-11 Comparison of Oral Dopamine Agonists

Drug	Dose	Adverse Effects
Bromocriptine (Parlodel)	1.25 mg bid for 1 week; increase by 2.5 mg per day every 2–4 weeks as needed and tolerated Maintenance dose: 2.5–10 mg tid when used with levodopa	Nausea, hallucinations, postural hypotension, tachycardia, insomnia At higher doses: pleuropulmonary and/or retroperitoneal fibrosis
Pergolide (Permax)	0.05 mg/day for 2 days; increase by 0.1–0.15mg every 3 days for 12 days; if needed, can increase by 0.25 mg every 3 days as needed/tolerated Maintenance dose: usually 1 mg tid	Nausea, hallucinations, postural hypotension, tachycardia, insomnia At higher doses: Valvular heart disease, pleuropulmonary and/or retroperitoneal fibrosis
Pramipexole (Mirapex)	0.125 mg tid; increase every 5–7 days by 0.125–0.25 mg Maintenance dose: 0.5–1.5 mg tid Maximum dose: 4.5 mg/day	Nausea, hallucinations, syncope, confusion, impotence Somnolence has been reported without prior warning
Ropinirole (Requip)	Initiate at 0.25 mg tid × 1 week, then 0.5 mg tid × 1 week, then 0.75 mg tid × 1 week, then 1 mg tid May further increase by 1.5 mg weekly Maximum dose: 24 mg/day	Nausea, hallucinations, syncope, confusion, impotence

the central nervous system. It is combined with carbidopa, a dopa-decarboxylase inhibitor, to facilitate its movement into the CNS and to prevent peripheral conversion of levodopa to dopamine. Dopamine itself does not cross the blood–brain barrier into the CNS. A dose of 75–100 mg of carbidopa is required. The combination product is available as Sinemet (immediate release) and Sinemet CR (controlled release). The controlled-release product has lower bioavailability and needs to be dosed 30% higher than the IR formulation; it is often reserved for patients who are experiencing complications on the IR version. An orally disintegrating formulation (Parcopa) is available for patients with difficulty swallowing. Of note, the tablet may be dissolved in the mouth, but is not absorbed buccally and must be swallowed. Treatment with levodopa usually begins when selegiline, amantadine, and dopamine agonists are ineffective or not tolerated.

Adverse effects of levodopa include nausea, dizziness, orthostasis, sleep attacks, obsessive–compulsive behaviors, confusion, and hallucinations. The most feared adverse effect of levodopa therapy is peak-dose dyskinesia, which manifest as choreiform movements (continuous, restless, large-amplitude movements of the head, face, trunk, and upper extremities). This effect, which is dose and duration dependent, occurs in as many as 50% of levodopa-treated patients after 5 years of therapy. The treatment for dyskinesia most often consists of a decrease in the dose of levodopa. Addition of another agent such as amantadine or a dopamine agonist may also help relieve dyskinesias. MAO-B inhibitors should be discontinued in patients who are experiencing levodopa-induced dyskinesias, as they may worsen these side effects.

Catechol-*o*-methyltransferase (COMT) inhibitors act by blocking the conversion of levodopa to 3-*o*-methyldopa. The net effect is an increase in levodopa availability in the CNS, which enables the drug to be converted to dopamine. Two COMT inhibitors are currently available: tolcapone (Tasmar) and entacopone (Comtan). These agents are used with carbidopa/levodopa and have no clinical value alone. They may allow for decreased levodopa dosing and fewer motor fluctuations. There is also a combination product consisting of carbidopa, levodopa, and entacopone (Stalevo).

The adverse effects of COMT inhibitors include diarrhea, nausea, vomiting, sleepiness, orthostasis, and hallucinations. Liver toxicity has been reported with tolcapone—an effect that requires liver function test monitoring at regular intervals. Entacapone does not appear to have hepatotoxic effects.

Nonmotor symptoms of PD may respond to appropriate pharmacotherapy, but drug–drug interactions and related polypharmacy issues make treatment of orthostatic hypotension, urinary incontinence, constipation, depression, dementia, and sleep disorders difficult.

Monitoring

Pharmacotherapeutic Outcomes

Resolution of symptoms and improved quality of life and activities of daily living should be monitored throughout PD treatment. Changes should be tracked using the Hoehn and Yahr scale or the UPDRS. Patients and their caregivers should be encouraged to use a diary to track "on" and "off" times and to determine their relationship to drug dosing. As PD progresses, patients develop a tightly locked response to their medications, particularly levodopa, and experience increasing amounts of "off" time, when symptoms are less well controlled. Levodopa doses appear to last for shorter amounts of time than expected ("wearing off") or fluctuations in symptoms and severity may occur without warning ("on-off phenomenon"). End-of-dose dystonias (painful muscle cramps in the leg or foot) may also occur with increased frequency. Treatments for these effects include adjusting dosing intervals or using sustained-release carbidopa/levodopa, COMT inhibitors, transdermal rotigotine, and/or apomorphine.

Laboratory monitoring related to use of specific drug therapies should include regular renal function tests (amantadine) and liver function tests (tolcapone).

Adverse effects common to the drugs used in the treatment of PD include nausea, vomiting, orthostatic hypotension, dizziness, confusion, somnolence, and hallucinations. Vigilant monitoring of levodopa-related peak-dose dyskinesia is also essential.

ANNOTATED BIBLIOGRAPHY

Chen JJ, Swope DM. Pharmacotherapy for Parkinson's disease. *Pharmacotherapy* 2007;27(12 Pt 2): 161S–173S.

Gottwald MD, Gidal BE, Flaherty J. Parkinson's disease. In: Koda-Kimble MA, Young LY, Kradjan WA, Guglielmo BJ, eds. *Applied Therapeutics: The Clinical Use of Drugs,* 7th ed. Philadelphia: Lippincott Williams & Wilkins; 2001:51.1–51.27.

Lewitt PA. Levodopa for the treatment of Parkinson's disease. *N Engl J Med* 20084;359(23):2468–2476.

Nelson MV, Berchou RC, LeWitt PA. Parkinson's disease. In: DiPiro JT, Talbert RL, Yee GC, et al., eds. *Pharmacotherapy: A Pathophysiologic Approach,* 6th ed. Stamford: Appleton & Lange; 2005:1075–1087.

Wagner ML. Parkinson's disease. In: Chisholm-Burns MA, Wells BG, Schwinghammer TL, et al., eds. *Pharmacotherapy: Principles and Practice,* 1st ed. New York: McGraw-Hill; 2008:473–485.

TOPIC: SEIZURES

Section Coordinator: Rex S. Lott
Contributor: Rex S. Lott

Tips Worth Tweeting

- A single seizure can occur for a variety of reasons; epilepsy involves recurrent, unprovoked seizures.
- Seizures may be either partial or generalized. Partial (focal) seizures begin in a specific, isolated area of the brain, whereas generalized seizures affect both cerebral hemispheres from the outset. Secondarily-generalized seizures spread from a focal point of onset to involve the entire brain.
- The goal of pharmacotherapy of epilepsy is to completely eliminate seizure recurrences whenever possible while causing minimal adverse medication effects.
- Treatment of epilepsy with a single antiepileptic drug (AED) is preferred whenever possible.
- AEDs differ in their efficacy for certain types of seizures, and identification of a patient's seizure type is important in selection of pharmacotherapy
- Among AEDs that are effective for a specific type of seizure, there is little evidence supporting the superior efficacy of any particular drug. Instead, AEDs are often chosen on the basis of tolerability.
- Newly developed AEDs are most commonly first approved as "add-on" agents for treatment of patients who do not fully respond to other agents.
- Drug interactions between older AEDs and other AEDs or other medications are likely and require monitoring.
- Enzyme-inducing AEDs such as phenytoin, carbamazepine, and phenobarbital may reduce the effectiveness of oral contraceptives.
- Several AEDs are associated with a risk of congenital defects in children who are exposed to the drugs in utero.
- Several AEDs are associated with uncommon, idiosyncratic, but potentially important adverse effects, such as skin rashes, liver damage, and hematologic abnormalities. Patients need to be educated regarding the possible signs and symptoms of these reactions.
- Monitoring of AED serum concentrations may be helpful, but the patient's response to medication is the most important outcome.
- Phenytoin exhibits dose-dependent pharmacokinetics; small dosage changes result in large changes in serum drug concentration and pharmacologic response.
- Carbamazepine is a potent inducer of CYP450 enzymes and also induces its own hepatic metabolism.
- Carbamazepine is converted to an active epoxide metabolite, which may contribute to the therapeutic response as well as the adverse effects associated with this agent.
- Valproate is an inhibitor of hepatic metabolism of several other drugs.
- Valproate and phenytoin are highly bound to albumin, and alterations in their binding may change the relationship between total serum concentrations and clinical response.
- Lamotrigine can be associated with a risk of serious hypersensitivity reactions (skin rash) if the initial dosage is too large or if dose increases are made too aggressively.

Patient Care Scenario: Ambulatory Setting

B. T. is a 19-year-old female who was recently diagnosed with epilepsy. She experiences complex partial seizures with occasional secondarily generalized tonic–clonic seizures. Following the onset of seizures, an EEG was performed that showed focal abnormality in her right temporal lobe. An MRI showed mesial temporal sclerosis. B. T. takes citalopram 20 mg daily for depression as well as Ortho-Novum 1/35 (ethinyl estradiol 35 mcg/norethindrone 1 mg) for menstrual cycle regulation and contraception. In addition, she takes a multivitamin with minerals daily.

1.1.0 Patient Information

Diagnosis of Epilepsy

Epilepsy is diagnosed when a patient experiences more than one seizure that is not acutely provoked by some external cause (e.g., drugs, fever, illness). Epilepsy is probably not a single disorder; instead, it is most likely a group of brain disorders that are manifested by seizures.

Seizure Types and Classification

- **Partial-onset (focal) seizures** result from abnormal electrical activity beginning in a single area of the cerebral cortex.
  - **Simple** (no loss or impairment of consciousness): Motor, sensory, or psychic symptoms.
  - **Complex** (impaired consciousness): May begin as simple partial seizure with impaired consciousness occurring later. Often

associated with automatisms (purposeless behavior).
  - **Secondarily generalized**: Begin as either simple or complex partial seizures and evolve to generalized tonic–clonic seizure.
- **Generalized-onset seizures** affect both hemispheres of the cerebral cortex simultaneously from onset of the seizure.
  - **Absence:** Characterized by brief lapses of consciousness without major muscular activity; consciousness returns to normal immediately at termination of the seizure.
  - **Tonic–clonic ("grand mal")**: Initial stiffening and tonic contraction of muscles that is followed by rhythmic, alternating contraction and relaxation (clonic movements).
  - **Myoclonic**: Brief, shock-like muscular contractions.
  - **Atonic ("drop attack")**: Characterized by sudden complete loss of muscle tone, usually resulting in falls.
  - **Infantile spasms**: Seen as a component of West syndrome in young children whose seizures are characterized by massive, rapid contractions or extensions of the limbs. In addition to infantile spasms, children with West syndrome have a characteristic disorganized EEG pattern (hypsarrhthmia) and are intellectually disabled.

It is possible to identify specific epilepsy syndromes on the basis of several factors such as seizure type(s), EEG pattern, and age of onset. Specific epilepsy syndromes may also predict response to specific AEDs. Examples of commonly encountered seizure syndromes are highlighted here:

- Juvenile myoclonic epilepsy (5–10% of epilepsy cases)
  - Adolescent to young adult onset
  - Myoclonic seizures often preceding generalized tonic–clonic seizures; often precipitated by sleep deprivation or alcohol use
  - Absence seizures also occur
  - Most cases respond well to valproate (not FDA approved); levetiracetam approved as adjunctive treatment
  - Lifelong pharmacotherapy usually needed
- Childhood absence epilepsy
  - Onset usually between ages 4 and 8
  - Absence ("petit mal") seizures may occur hundreds of times daily; many patients also develop generalized tonic–clonic seizures.
  - Characteristic EEG pattern (3-Hz spike-wave)
  - Genetic component
  - Very responsive to pharmacotherapy—ethosuximide, valproate, and, probably, lamotrigine

Laboratory Testing and Physical Assessment

Physical assessment, laboratory testing, and neuroimaging (CT scan or MRI) are performed as part of the evaluation of patients with epilepsy. Often, these assessments are performed to identify possible underlying, correctable causes of seizures such as drug toxicity, metabolic abnormalities, or brain tumors. Electroencephalogram (EEG) can be very helpful in identifying the type of seizures and their origin. However, a large percentage of people with epilepsy will have a normal EEG during the period of time between active seizures (interictal period).

Disease States and Drugs Associated with Seizures or Epilepsy

By definition, seizures that result from the effects of another disease state do not represent epilepsy unless the seizures recur without provocation by the disease. Seizures may occur in association with several other disease states or conditions:

- Hypoglycemia
- Fever
- Alcohol or sedative withdrawal
- Hyponatremia
- Stroke
- Brain tumor

Seizures associated with other diseases may require treatment with AEDs to prevent recurrence if the underlying cause cannot be controlled.

A number of drugs may also be associated with precipitation of seizure activity or worsening of seizure control in patients with epilepsy. Most commonly, drug-induced seizures are associated with exposure to doses higher than those used therapeutically. The risk of drug-induced seizures may limit the doses of some medications. Drugs that may increase the risk of seizures must be used carefully in patients with epilepsy. These drugs include the following medications:

- Theophylline
- Low-potency first-generation ("typical") phenothiazine antipsychotics (chlorpromazine, thioridazine)
- Bupropion (especially at doses greater than 450 mg/day)
- Clomipramine (especially at doses greater than 200 mg/day)
- Clozapine at higher doses

1.2.0 Pharmacotherapy

Indications for Antiepileptic Drug Therapy

When no identifiable, correctable cause for recurrent, unprovoked seizures can be identified, pharmacotherapy with AEDs is the first-line approach to treatment of epilepsy. Surgical treatment may be very successful for some types of epilepsy when pharmacotherapy is not successful or is poorly tolerated. Electrical brain stimulation with vagus nerve stimulators may also be effective for improving seizure control in some patients. Some forms of epilepsy may also be responsive to high-fat, low-carbohydrate diets (ketogenic diet, modified Atkins diet). Nevertheless, nondrug therapies are often withheld until pharmacotherapy has been shown to not be effective.

The goal of AED therapy is complete prevention of recurrent seizures without production of intolerable side effects and without interference with quality of life. Although this goal cannot always be achieved, as many as 70% of patients can have their seizures prevented with adequate treatment with a single AED. It is important that adequate AED treatment be initiated as early as possible and that AED treatment be optimized. The longer epileptic seizures are allowed to recur, it is more likely that the patient may become refractory to treatment. The general principles of optimal AED treatment are as follows:

- Accurate identification of seizure and/or epilepsy syndrome. While there is little evidence that any single AED is superior to the others, AEDs are often more effective for one type of seizure. Some newer AEDs have a relatively broad spectrum of effectiveness and can be successfully used for several different types of seizures. Other AEDs have a much narrower spectrum of effectiveness and may actually worsen some types of seizures.
    - Ethosuximide is very effective for treatment of absence seizures. It has little efficacy for treatment of other generalized seizures or partial seizures with or without secondary generalization.
    - Carbamazepine is very effective for treatment of partial seizures and secondarily generalized seizures. It has little or no efficacy for absence seizures and other types of primary generalized seizures, and it may make these seizures worse.
- Selection of AED based on patient characteristics. Patient-specific factors may have a significant influence on the likelihood that treatment with a specific medication will be successful or well tolerated:
    - Ability of the specific patient to tolerate potential AED adverse side effects
    - Comorbid medical conditions
    - Age
    - Ease of medication administration
    - Cost of AED and insurance coverage

Individual AEDs: Indications, Dosing Information, and Monitoring

Owing to ethical requirements for acceptable research on new AEDs, most of these medications are originally evaluated as add-on treatment for patients with partial-onset seizures not adequately controlled by current therapy. This creates a rigorous standard for efficacy. As a result, initial FDA approval for the use of these medicines is most commonly for add-on treatment of incompletely controlled partial-onset seizures. A number of years may be required before the complete role and place of newer medications is defined.

AEDs Useful for Partial-Onset Seizures (Simple, Complex, or Secondarily Generalized)

- Carbamazepine
- Gabapentin
- Lacosamide
- Oxcarbazepine
- Phenobarbital
- Phenytoin
- Pregabalin
- Vigabatrin

AEDs Useful for Generalized-Onset Seizures

- Clobazam
- Ethosuximide (absence only)
- Ezogabine (Retigabine)
- Felbamate
- Lacosamide
- Lamotrigine
- Levetiracetam
- Rufinamide
- Topiramate
- Valproate
- Vigabatrin
- Zonisamide

AEDs with "Broad-Spectrum" Effectiveness

- Felbamate
- Lacosamide
- Lamotrigine
- Levetiracetam
- Rufinamide
- Topiramate
- Valproate
- Zonisamide

Table 17-12 Antiepileptic Drugs: Dosage Forms, Doses, and Indications by Seizure Type

AED	Dosage Forms	Dosage	Seizure Types	Comments
Carbamazepine (Tegretol, Carbatrol)	Oral immediate-release tablets and suspension Extended-release oral forms: Carbatrol and Tegretol XR	Initial: 100–200 mg bid. Weekly increases by 100–200 mg until therapeutic response. Usual target: 7–15 mg/kg/day in adults or 10–40 mg/kg/day in children.	Partial-onset seizures with or without generalized seizures.	May worsen some primary generalized seizures.
Clobazam (Onfi)	Oral immediate-release tablets	Patients ≤ 30 kg: Initiate at 5 mg/day; titrate up to 20 mg/day as tolerated. Patients > 30 kg: Initiate at 10 mg/day; titrate up to 40 mg/day as tolerated.	Lennox-Gastaut syndrome, myoclonic and akinetic seizures.	May be associated with a lower rate of tolerance than other benzodiazepines.
Clonazepam (Klonopin)	Oral immediate-release tablets	Adults: Initial 0.5 mg tid; increase every 3 days. Maximum: 20 mg/day. Children: Initially, 0.01–0.03 mg/kg/day. Increase every 3 days. Target maintenance dose in children: 0.1–0.3 mg/kg/day.	Lennox-Gastaut syndrome, myoclonic and akinetic seizures. Absence seizures not responsive to ethosuximide.	Tolerance to antiepileptic effect develops frequently (30–50% of patients).
Diazepam (Diastat)	Gel for rectal administration in 2.5 mg, 10 mg, and 20 mg prefilled syringes	2–5 years old: 0.5 mg/kg. 6–11 years old: 0.3 mg/kg. ≥ 12 years old: 0.2 mg/kg. Doses are rounded upward to the nearest 2.5 mg increment. Dosage can be repeated in 4–12 hours if necessary.	Used intermittently for bouts ("clusters") of increased seizure activity in patients on stable AED regimens.	Recommended only when caregivers can identify "clusters" of seizure activity that differ from the usual isolated seizures. Not used as a "prn" medication for each seizure. Respiration should be monitored after administration, although respiratory depression is uncommon.
Ethosuximide (Zarontin)	Oral capsules	Initially: 20 mg/kg/day or 250 mg qd or bid; then increase q 2 weeks by 250 mg/day until the therapeutic effect or target serum concentration is reached.	Absence seizures only.	
Ezogabine/ retigabine (Potiga)	Oral tablets	Initially: 100 mg tid for 1 week; then increase weekly by not more than 150 mg/day. Target doses: up to 400 mg tid (1,200 mg/day).	Partial-onset seizures with or without secondary generalization.	Unique mechanism: acts as a potassium-channel opener. Potential risk of urinary retention. May prolong the QT interval.
Felbamate (Felbatol)	Oral tablets and suspension	Initially: 400 mg tid; increase every 2 weeks by 600 mg/day. Target doses: 2,400–3,600 mg/day	Partial-onset seizures with or without generalized seizures; Lennox-Gastaut syndrome in children.	Use is limited by potential hematologic and hepatic toxicity.
Gabapentin (Neurontin)	Oral tablets, capsules, and solution	Initially: 300 mg tid. Increase to target of 1,800 mg/day over 1–2 weeks. Up to 3,600 mg/day may be necessary.	Partial seizures with or without generalized seizures as adjunctive treatment.	

Lamotrigine (Lamictal)	Oral tablets, extended-release tablets, chewable/dispersible tablets, and oral disintegrating tablets	Initial dose with enzyme-inducing agents: 50 mg/day; increase by 50 mg/day every 2 weeks to target dose of 300–500 mg/day. Initial dose with valproate: 25 mg qod; increase by 25 mg/day every 2 weeks to target dose of 200–400 mg/day.	Partial-onset seizures and generalized-onset seizures.	
Lacosamide (Vimpat)	Oral tablets, oral solution, and injection for IV administration	Initially: 50 mg bid. Increase weekly by 100 mg/day. Target dose: 200–400 mg/day. Maximum recommended dose is 400 mg/day.	Partial-onset seizures; probably generalized-onset seizures.	
Levetiracetam (Keppra)	Oral tablets, oral solution, extended-release tablets, and injection for IV administration	Initially: 250–500 mg bid. Increase every 2 weeks by 500–1,000 mg/day. Maximum dose usually 3,000 mg/day.	Partial-onset seizures and generalized-onset seizures.	
Oxcarbazepine (Trileptal)	Oral tablets and oral suspension	Initially: 300 mg bid. Increase weekly up to 1,200 mg/day.	Partial-onset seizures with or without generalized seizures.	
Phenobarbital	Oral tablets, oral solution, and injection	Initially: 1 mg/kg/day. Gradual increases every 2–3 weeks.	Partial-onset seizures with or without generalized seizures.	No longer widely used as an AED owing to tolerability.
Phenytoin (Dilantin)	Oral capsule (extended): Sodium phenytoin. Oral suspension and chewable oral tablets: Phenytoin acid. Injection: Sodium phenytoin	Initiate at a target maintenance dose of 4–5 mg/kg/day. Allow at least 3–4 weeks between dose adjustments because of slow accumulation. If used intravenously, should be admixed in normal saline solution and administered no faster than 50 mg/min to avoid cardiotoxicity.	Partial-onset seizures with or without generalized seizures.	
Fosphenytoin (Cerebyx)	Solution for injection	For treatment of status epilepticus: 15–20 PE mg/kg. May be admixed in any solution. Can be administered at up to 150 mg PE/min.	Same as phenytoin. Used for immediate treatment of status epilepticus.	Prodrug for phenytoin. Rapidly converted to phenytoin after administration.
Pregabalin (Lyrica)	Oral capsules and oral solution	Initially: 50 mg bid. Gradual titration until therapeutic response. Maximum: 600 mg/day.	Partial seizures with or without generalized seizures as adjunctive treatment.	
Rufinamide (Banzel)	Oral tablets and oral solution	Adults: Initially 400–800 mg/day given bid. Increase every 2 days by 400–800 mg/day. Target: 3,200 mg/day. Children: Initially 10 mg/kg/day given bid. Increase by 10 mg/kg/day every other day. Target dose of 45 mg/kg/day or 3,200 mg/day.	Seizures associated with Lennox-Gastaut syndrome. Partial-onset seizures; probably generalized-onset seizures.	

(*continues*)

Table 17-12 (*continued*)

AED	Dosage Forms	Dosage	Seizure Types	Comments
Tiagabine (Gabatril)	Oral tablets	Initially: 4 mg/day. Increase to 8 mg/day at 7 days, then weekly increases by 4–8 mg/day. Maximum recommended dose: 32 mg/day in adolescents or 56 mg/day in adults.	Partial-onset seizures.	
Topiramate (Topamax)	Oral tablets and oral "sprinkle" capsules	Initially: 50 mg hs. Weekly increases in daily dose by 50 mg. 200–400 mg/day recommended as target dosage range.	Partial-onset seizures and generalized-onset seizures.	
Valproic acid/divalproex (Depakene, Depakote, and Depakote ER)	Valproic acid/sodium valproate: Oral capsules and oral syrup. Divalproex sodium: Oral delayed-release tablets (Depakote), oral "sprinkle" capsules (Depakote Sprinkles), oral extended-release tablets (Depakote ER). Sodium valproate for injection (Depacon)	Children: Initially 5–10 mg/kg/day (sprinkle caps or syrup); weekly increases by 5–10 mg/kg/day to therapeutic effect or target serum concentration. Adults: Initially 15 mg/kg/day (750–1,000 mg in divided doses). Weekly increases by 500–750 mg/day until seizures are controlled. Maximum recommended dose: 60 mg/kg/day.	Partial-onset seizures and generalized-onset seizures.	Divalproex ER is only approximately 85% bioavailable compared to other valproate dosage forms. Dose adjustments may be needed when switching between the ER dosage form and other forms.
Vigabatrin (Sabril)	Oral tablets and powder for oral solution	Adults: Initially 500 mg bid; weekly increases by 500 mg/day to a target dose of 1,500 mg bid. Children (oral powder for solution): Initially: 25 mg/kg bid; increases by 25–50 mg/kg/day every 3 days. Maximum dose: 150 mg/kg/day.	Infantile spasms and refractory partial-onset seizures. Possibly for generalized-onset seizures.	Use may be limited by the potential for ocular toxicity. Patients receiving vigabatrin must be registered with a special distribution program. Only prescribers and pharmacies registered with this program can provide vigabatrin therapy.
Zonisamide (Zonegran)	Oral capsules	Initially: 100 mg qd; increase by 100 mg/day every 2 weeks. Usual maintenance dose: 200–400 mg/day. Maximum dose: 600 mg/day.	Partial-onset seizures and generalized-onset seizures.	

Biopharmaceutical Principles and Pharmaceutical Characteristics of Dosage Forms

Many AEDs are available in multiple dosage forms that provide a number of advantages over the usual tablets and capsules:

- Ease of administration (e.g., solutions, "sprinkle" capsules that can be opened and mixed with food)
- Sustained- or extended-release forms that decrease the need for frequent administration of doses and, therefore, may improve compliance
- Injectable formulations that may be substituted for oral dosage forms when necessary

In most cases, oral and injectable dosage forms are equally bioavailable. There are some significant differences for a few AEDs, however. These differences can sometimes be important for patient outcomes.

Phenytoin Dosage Forms

- Phenytoin capsules are labeled in terms of their content of sodium phenytoin (92% phenytoin acid). Phenytoin suspension and chewable tablets are labeled in terms of their content of phenytoin. When patients' dosage forms are converted, this difference must be taken into account to avoid unintended dosage changes. Because phenytoin follows Michaelis-Menten pharmacokinetics (see the chapter on pharmacokinetics), even small dosage changes may result in large changes in the patient's clinical response.
- Some phenytoin capsule dosage forms are labeled as "extended." These forms are intended to be used for once-daily dosing of phenytoin.
- Injectable fosphenytoin is labeled and prescribed in terms of "phenytoin equivalents." Phenytoin equivalents are equal to milligrams of sodium phenytoin.

Valproate Dosage Forms

- All oral dosage forms except extended-release divalproex (Depakote ER and generics) are equally available and well absorbed. Extended-release divalproex is approximately 85% bioavailable compared to the other oral dosage forms.
- Delayed-release divalproex is not an extended-release dosage form and should still be administered in divided doses. This dosage form is not absorbed until the tablet's enteric coating is dissolved in the higher pH of the intestine.

Vigabatrin Dosage Forms

- Tablet dosage forms are administered to adults.
- Children are dosed using oral powder packets for solution. The necessary number of packets should be emptied into a cup, and 10 mL of cold or room-temperature water should be added per packet. The resulting solution should be administered immediately.

Pharmacokinetic Considerations

AEDs are a group of medications for which pharmacokinetics have contributed significantly to their optimized use. An understanding of the pharmacokinetic behavior of these drugs and the relationship between serum concentrations and their clinical effect can provide important benefits to patients. Many older AEDs are extensively metabolized by hepatic CYP450 enzymes. Some of the newer agents undergo more renal excretion and may require dosage adjustments for patients with impaired renal function. Table 17-6 summarizes important pharmacokinetic characteristics of AEDs

Drug Interactions

Drug–drug interactions involving AEDs may become important. Many older AEDs (e.g., phenytoin, carbamazepine, valproate, phenobarbital) are involved in significant interactions with other medications and with AEDs. These interactions most commonly occur on the basis of their activity as inhibitors or inducers of CYP450 enzymes as well as their extensive protein binding. Many newer AEDs are less active as enzyme inducers and are less extensively bound to proteins. In addition to pharmacokinetic interactions, many AEDs may be involved in pharmacodynamic interactions. Most AEDs exert at least a small sedative effect; therefore, when they are coadministered with other sedating medicines, excessive sedation or even confusion and disorientation may result.

Pharmacokinetic drug–drug interactions involving the CYP450 enzyme system, UDP-glucuronosyltransferase (UGT), and protein binding are discussed in the chapters dealing with pharmacokinetics, drug interactions, and biopharmaceutics.

Drug Interactions Involving Enzyme Induction by AEDs

- Carbamazepine: CYP3A, CYP1A, CYP2C, and UGT
  - Also a substrate for CYP3A and, therefore, induces its own metabolism
  - Reduces the clinical effectiveness of oral contraceptives, calcium-channel blockers, and warfarin
  - Increases the clearance of phenytoin and phenobarbital
  - UGT induction increases lamotrigine clearance
- Phenobarbital: CYP2C, CYP3A, and UGT
  - Reduces the clinical effectiveness of oral contraceptives, calcium-channel blockers, and warfarin

Table 17-13 Important Pharmacokinetic Parameters for Antiepileptic Drugs

AED	$t_{1/2}$ (hr)	Target Serum Concentration (mcg/mL)	Route of Metabolism/Elimination	Dosage Modification for Impaired Renal Function
Carbamazepine	5–25	5–12	Hepatic: CYP3A4, CYP1A2, CYP2C8 Active metabolite eliminated via epoxide hydrolase	N/A
Clobazam	40–80	?	Hepatic: CYP3A4, CYP2C19, CYP2B6	N/A
Ethosuximide	30–60	40–100	Hepatic: CYP3A4	N/A
Ezogabine (Retigabine)	6–10	?	Hepatic: glucuronidation and acetylation	Yes
Felbamate	12–20	50–110	Hepatic: CYP3A4	N/A
Gabapentin	5–9	> 2 (proposed)	Renal: 100%	Yes
Lacosamide	13	?	Hepatic: CYP2C19 Renal: approximately 70%	Minimal
Lamotrigine	24 12 with enzyme inducers 60 with valproate	4–18	Hepatic: UGT	N/A
Levetiracetam	6–8	?	Non-hepatic hydrolysis Renal: 66%	Yes
Oxcarbazepine	8–13	?	Non-CYP450 hydrolysis Renal: approximately 30% for active metabolite	N/A
Phenobarbital	48–96	15–40	Hepatic: CYP2C19 Renal: approximately 25%	N/A
Phenytoin	Varies with dose > 24	10–20	Hepatic: CYP2C9/2C19 Renal: approximately 5%	N/A
Pregabalin	6	?	Renal: 100%	Yes
Rufinamide	9	?	Hepatic: non-CYP450 hydrolysis	N/A
Tiagabine	4–9	?	Hepatic: CYP3A4	N/A
Topiramate	12–24	?	Hepatic: approximately 30% via hydrolysis and glucuronidation Renal: 70%	Yes
Valproic acid/ divalproex	10–16	50–125	Hepatic: UGT, b-oxidation; can be metabolized by CYP450	N/A
Vigabatrin	8–12 (irreversible enzyme inhibitor)	N/A	Renal: 100%	Yes
Zonisamide	30–60	?	Hepatic: CYP3A4 Renal: approximately 30%	Minimal

  - UGT induction increases lamotrigine clearance
- Phenytoin: CYP3A, CYP2C, and UGT
  - Reduces the clinical effectiveness of oral contraceptives, calcium-channel blockers, and warfarin
  - UGT induction increases lamotrigine clearance
- Felbamate: CYP3A
  - Increases the production of the active epoxide metabolite of carbamazepine
  - May decrease the effectiveness of oral contraceptives
- Oxcarbazepine: CYP3A and UGT
  - Weaker inducer than carbamazepine
  - Significantly reduces the effectiveness of oral contraceptives

- Topiramate: CYP3A at high doses
  - May reduce the effectiveness of oral contraceptives at higher doses (200 mg/day or greater)

Drug Interactions Involving Enzyme Inhibition by AEDs

- Felbamate: CYP2C
  - May cause increased concentrations of phenytoin or phenobarbital
- Oxcarbazepine: CYP2C
  - May increase phenytoin concentrations at higher doses
- Topiramate: CYP2C
  - May increase phenytoin concentrations in some patients
- Valproate: CYP2C, epoxide hydrolase, and UGT
  - Can significantly increase concentrations of phenobarbital and phenytoin
  - Inhibits the metabolism of the active epoxide metabolite of carbamazepine, which may result in intoxication
  - Inhibits the metabolism of lamotrigine

AEDs are also substrates of drug-metabolizing enzymes. Induction or inhibition of these enzymes may result in significant drug interactions. Examples are listed here.

Drug Interactions Involving AEDs as Substrates for Drug Metabolizing Enzymes

- Carbamazepine: CYP3A4, CYP1A2, and CYP2C8
  - Inhibitors of these enzymes may significantly increase carbamazepine concentrations (e.g., erythromycin inhibits CYP3A4)
- Lacosamide: CYP2C19
- Lamotrigine: UGT
  - Induction of UGT by other AEDs significantly increases lamotrigine clearance
  - Valproate inhibits UGT and significantly reduces lamotrigine clearance
  - Estrogens in oral contraceptives increase UGT activity and increase lamotrigine clearance
- Phenobarbital: CYP2C9/19
  - Valproate inhibits CYP2C9/19 and reduces phenobarbital clearance
- Phenytoin: CYP2C9/2C19
  - Valproate inhibits CYP2C9/19 and reduces phenytoin clearance
- Tiagabine: CYP3A4
- Topiramate: Not known, but enzyme-inducing AEDs increase clearance of topiramate
- Valproate: UGT; also appears to be metabolized via CYP450 when these enzymes are induced
- Zonisamide: CYP3A4

Drug Interactions Involving Protein Binding of AEDs

- Phenytoin is highly protein bound and can be displaced from albumin-binding sites by valproate. The clinical results of this interaction are variable and unpredictable because phenytoin follows Michaelis-Menten kinetics and, at therapeutic doses, is often close to V_{max}. Under most circumstances, displacement from protein binding results in only transient increases in free concentration of the displaced drug, because clearance increases in proportion to the free fraction. In the case of phenytoin's displacement by valproate:
  - Phenytoin clearance may not increase in proportion to free fraction because metabolic capacity may be close to saturation.
  - Valproate inhibits the CYP450 enzymes responsible for phenytoin metabolism.
  - Clinically measured total phenytoin plasma concentrations may increase, decrease, or not change, while unbound (free) phenytoin concentrations may increase persistently.
- Valproate may be displaced from albumin binding sites by other highly protein bound substances such as aspirin and, possibly, fatty acids. The clinical results of this interaction may be difficult to predict.
  - Often, there will be only minor or no changes in unbound valproate concentrations, because valproate's clearance will increase in proportion to its free fraction.
  - High aspirin doses may inhibit the hepatic metabolism of valproate. This inhibition may prevent clearance from increasing. Under those circumstances, free concentrations of valproate may persistently increase with an increase in clinical effect of the medication.

Toxicities, Adverse Effects, and Associated Monitoring

Most AEDs cause some usually mild, dose-related adverse effects. These side effects are commonly related to depression of the central nervous system and are a direct result of the underlying mechanisms of action of these medications. Typically, these CNS-depressant effects result in sedation and possible disturbances of gait (ataxia) and vision (most commonly, diplopia). Most AEDs currently in common use do not cause significant persistent CNS-depressant side effects at therapeutic doses; these side effects may be prominent with early therapy, but tolerance often develops. At higher doses, these effects may become prominent and persistent and necessitate dosage reduction or discontinuation.

Table 17-14 Side Effects of Antiepileptic Drugs

AED	Dose-Related Adverse Effects	Idiosyncratic/Hypersensitivity Adverse Reactions and Monitoring

Carbamazepine	Nausea, vomiting, headache	• Hyponatremia:
		  ○ Monitor serum sodium if symptomatic
		• Hematologic:
		  ○ Mild leucopenia is relatively common
		  ○ Aplastic anemia and agranulocytosis are extremely rare
		  ○ Baseline and periodic CBC are recommended
		  ○ Patients should be educated to report easy bleeding or bruising, or sudden onset of severe infectious symptoms
		• Hepatotoxicity:
		  ○ Rare
		  ○ Patients should be educated to report symptoms such as abdominal pain, severe nausea and vomiting, or jaundice
		  ○ Baseline and periodic LFTs are recommended
		• Osteopenia/osteomalacia: Increased risk with long-term use
		  ○ Supplemental calcium and vitamin D may be helpful
		  ○ Monitor bone mineral density
		• Rash, possible Stevens-Johnson syndrome, toxic epidermal necrolysis:
		  ○ Rash in approximately 3–5% of patients
		  ○ Asian patients should be screened for HLA-B*1502; presence of this antigen increases the risk of Stevens-Johnson syndrome 10-fold

Clobazam	Drowsiness, sedation	• Insomnia, behavioral disinhibition (aggression)
Ethosuximide	Drowsiness, GI upset	• Mild leucopenia is common; serious blood dyscrasias are rarely seen • Possible sleep disturbances • Possible aggressive behavioral disturbances
Ezogabine (Retigabine)	Drowsiness, dizziness, confusional state, changes in attention, urinary hesitancy/retention	• May prolong the QT interval

Felbamate	Sleep disturbance (insomnia) more common than sedation	• Hematologic:
		  ○ "Black box" warning for aplastic anemia
		  ○ CBC at baseline and every 2–4 weeks is recommended
		• Hepatotoxicity:
		  ○ "Black box" warning for acute hepatic failure
		  ○ LFTs (bilirubin, AST, ALT) at baseline and every 1–2 weeks

Gabapentin	Sedation, gait disturbance, weight gain	

Lamotrigine	Blurred vision, ataxia	• Skin rash:
		  ○ 0.8–8.0% of patients
		  ○ Increased risk:
		    ▪ Rapid dosage titration
		    ▪ Valproate comedication
		  ○ Patients should be educated to self-monitor
		• Hepatotoxicity: Rare

Lacosamide	• Dizziness, ataxia, diplopia, headache, nausea • Cardiac conduction slowing	

Table 17-14 (*continued*)

AED	Dose-Related Adverse Effects	Idiosyncratic/Hypersensitivity Adverse Reactions and Monitoring
Levetiracetam	Sedation, dizziness	Psychiatric reactions: agitation, emotional lability, hostility, depression, and depersonalization

Oxcarbazepine	Dizziness, sedation, diplopia, nausea, and ataxia are commonly reported	• Hyponatremia:
		  ○ Monitor serum sodium if symptomatic
		  ○ More common than with carbamazepine
		• Anaphylaxis and angioedema
		• Dermatologic reactions:
		  ○ Approximately 25–30% cross-reactivity with carbamazepine

Phenobarbital	Sedation, cognitive impairment	• Hyperactivity in children
		• Osteopenia/osteomalacia: Increased risk with long-term use
		  ○ Supplemental calcium and vitamin D may be helpful
		  ○ Monitor bone mineral density

Phenytoin	Ataxia, nystagmus at high therapeutic doses	• Osteopenia/osteomalacia: Increased risk with long-term use
		  ○ Supplemental calcium and vitamin D may be helpful
		  ○ Monitor bone mineral density
		• Hirsutism
		• Gingival hyperplasia
		• Rash, possible Stevens-Johnson syndrome, toxic epidermal necrolysis
		  ○ Rash in approximately 3–5% of patients
		• Possible relationship to HLA-B*1502 in Asian patients
		• Hepatotoxicity is possible as part of generalized hypersensitivity syndrome
		• Cardiotoxicity:
		  ○ Related to rapid IV administration
		  ○ > 50 mg/min

Fosphenytoin	Paresthesias	• Lower risk for cardiotoxicity with IV administration • May be administered at up to 125 mg/min
Pregabalin	Dizziness, blurred vision, weight gain	Angioedema
Rufinamide	Dizziness, vomiting	Shortens QT interval
Tiagabine	Sedation, confusion, difficulty with concentration	
Topiramate	• Sedation, dizziness, difficulty concentrating, confusion • Weight loss • Metabolic acidosis	• Risk of kidney stones • Hypohidrosis and hyperthermia (especially in children) • Rare angle-closure glaucoma

Valproic acid/ divalproex	• GI upset (nausea, vomiting, heartburn)
	• Tremor
	• Thrombocytopenia
		• Alopecia (temporary, reversible)
		• Weight gain
		• Pancreatitis
		• Hepatotoxicity:
		  ○ More common in young children (younger than 2 years) receiving multiple AEDs
		  ○ Baseline and yearly LFTs recommended
		  ○ Patients should be educated regarding signs and symptoms of both acute hepatic damage and pancreatitis:
		    ■ Acute-onset nausea and severe abdominal pain
		    ■ Jaundice

(*continues*)

Table 17-14 (*continued*)

AED	Dose-Related Adverse Effects	Idiosyncratic/Hypersensitivity Adverse Reactions and Monitoring
Vigabatrin	Drowsiness, fatigue	• Progressive, permanent visual field loss (possibly dose related): o Vision testing at baseline o Repeat every 3 months o Repeat at 3–6 months after discontinuation • Weight gain • Edema
Zonisamide	Sedation, confusion, weight loss	Risk of cross-sensitive hypersensitivity reactions in patients with sulfa allergy.

Most AEDs are also associated with some risk of idiosyncratic or allergic adverse reactions. On occasion, these reactions may be life-threatening; however, for most of these drugs, such serious adverse reactions are extremely uncommon. Patients should be informed about these potential risks and educated about signs and symptoms that may be associated with them. In addition, laboratory monitoring is recommended, although the benefits of extensive laboratory monitoring may be less than those of symptomatic monitoring and vigilance.

All AEDs now carry a warning in their package inserts regarding a risk of suicidal ideation. This risk is approximately twice that associated with placebo in similar patients. Nonetheless, the actual rate of suicidal ideation or behavior is very low—approximately 0.43%. The relative contributions of AEDs and epilepsy itself (or depression, which is commonly seen in patients with epilepsy) are not clear at this time.

AED use in pregnancy may be of concern. Many AEDs are associated with some increase in the risk of congenital malformations in children exposed in utero. Several AEDs are classified into pregnancy risk Category D by the FDA: benzodiazepines, carbamazepine, phenobarbital, phenytoin, topiramate, and valproate. All other AEDs are in pregnancy risk Category C. In 2011, topiramate was reclassified into pregnancy risk Category D by the FDA based on an identified association with facial clefts in children exposed in utero. Combination AED therapy, especially involving valproate, appears to carry a higher risk. Enzyme-inducing AEDs (e.g., carbamazepine, phenytoin) cause increased hepatic metabolism of estrogens and progestins, and may decrease the effectiveness of oral contraceptives. This interaction, therefore, may increase the risk of exposure of unborn children to a potential teratogen. Women of childbearing age who take AEDs (especially those in Category D) should be counseled regarding the potential for congenital malformations. Use of 1–4 mg/day of folic acid by women who are taking AEDs is recommended to reduce the risk of congenital malformations.

Dose-related and idiosyncratic adverse effects associated with AEDs are described in Table 17-14. Both clinical and laboratory monitoring parameters are also described.

1.3.0 Monitoring

Pharmacotherapeutic Outcomes

The primary goals of pharmacotherapy in people with epilepsy are threefold:

- Full control of seizures, defined as elimination of seizure recurrence
- Absence of or minimization of drug-related adverse effects
- Maintenance of an acceptable quality of life

While these goals are sometimes not completely achievable, pharmacotherapy should be optimized until these goals are achieved or unacceptable adverse effects limit further attempts.

Patients or their caregivers should be educated to monitor seizure frequency and should be informed of signs and symptoms of both common, dose-related adverse effects and uncommon idiosyncratic adverse reactions.

ANNOTATED BIBLIOGRAPHY

McAuley J, Lott RS, Alldredge BK. Seizure disorders. In Alldredge BK, Corelli RL, Ernst ME, et al., eds. *Koda-Kimble and Young's Applied Therapeutics: The Clinical Use of Drugs,* 10th ed. Philadelphia PA: Lippincott, Williams & Wilkins; 2012: Chapter 58. pp. 1387–1419

Rogers SJ, Cavazos JE. Epilepsy. In DiPiro JT, et al., eds. *Pharmacotherapy: A Pathophysiologic Approach,* 8th ed. New York: McGraw-Hill; 2011:979–1005.

Nutrition/Fluids and Electrolytes

CHAPTER 18

TOPIC: ACID–BASE DISORDERS

Section Coordinator: Catherine M. Oliphant
Contributors: John Arross and Kristin Sampson

Tips Worth Tweeting

- Tissue oxygenation, protein binding of drugs, and certain electrolytes can be affected by patient acid–base status.
- Acid–base imbalances are not diseases in and of themselves, but rather are conditions created by disease and toxins.
- Acid–base clinical evaluation is via arterial blood gas (ABG) analysis, patient symptoms, and medical history.

Patient Care Scenario: Hospital Setting

1.1.0 Patient Information

T. A. is a 25-year-old female with a history of depression. She is found by her brother in a semi-conscious state and brought to the emergency department. The ambulance crew did a thorough job of bringing in the contents of her medicine chest.

Medicine found at the scene:

- Fluoxetine 20 mg capsules, sig: 1 cap daily #90 (20 remaining)
- Mirtazapine 30 mg tablets, sig: 1 tab at bedtime #90 (21 remaining)
- Aspirin 325 mg tablets (OTC, so no sig), bottle of 300 (10 remaining)

Patient symptoms:

- Confusion
- Lethargy
- Fever
- Tachypnea

Laboratory results:

- Na^+ = 145 mEq/L
- K^+ = 4.5 mEq/L
- Cl = 107 mEq/L
- pCO_2 = 20 mm Hg
- Bicarbonate = 19 mEq/L
- pH = 7.3
- Anion gap = 19 mEq/L

Laboratory Testing

A simple way to evaluate the cause of a pH abnormality is to visualize a see-saw and two elevators: with pH being on one side of the see-saw and pCO_2 on the other; pH on one elevator and bicarbonate on the other elevator. The see-saw evaluates the respiratory component while the elevator evaluates the metabolic component.

pH and bicarbonate must move in opposite directions on the see-saw for normal conditions to exist. If they move in the same direction, then the underlying problem is likely metabolic. To maintain a normal pH, bicarbonate moves in the opposite direction of pH. As the body becomes more acidotic, bicarbonate concentrations will increase to compensate for this imbalance. If pH is moving down (acidosis) and bicarbonate is moving down, then the acidosis is likely metabolic.

pH and pCO_2 must be trending in the same direction (riding the same elevator) for normal conditions to exist. If they are moving in opposite directions, then the problem is most likely respiratory in nature.

As pH decreases, respiratory compensation will occur in the form of hyperventilation and blowing off excess CO_2 (moving in the same direction). If pH is going down and CO_2 is going up (opposite directions), then it is likely the elevated CO_2 is causing the acidosis. If both the see-saw and the elevator are abnormal, then the anion gap is used to determine the true cause of the pH abnormality.

1. What is T. A.'s acid–base disorder?
Metabolic acidemia and respiratory alkalemia. Because both pH and pCO_2 are low (no see-saw), the primary cause cannot be respiratory. Because both pH and bicarbonate are low (riding the same elevator), the primary cause is probably metabolic. This suspicion is confirmed by an elevated anion gap. Elevated anion gap metabolic acidemias are most often caused by toxins such as aspirin and antifreeze.

Acid–Base Laboratory Values

Variables and Regulation			
Variable	**Normal Range**	**Regulated by**	**Regulation Speed and Strength**
pH	7.35–7.45	Lungs, kidney, physiological buffer	Rapid, compensation often incomplete
pCO_2	35–45 mm Hg	Lungs	Rapid. compensation often incomplete
Bicarbonate	22–26 mEq/L	Kidney	Slow, powerful, compensation can be nearly complete
Anion gap	8–12 mEq/L	Hydration, nutrition	Slow, not a compensatory action electrolyte intake, drugs/toxins, kidneys, pituitary
pO_2	80–100	Lungs and anatomical disorders	Rapid, strength highly dependent upon age and physical malady, age, and physical condition

Variables in Acid–Base Chemistry					
Variable	**Normal**	**Promotes Alkalemia**	**Promotes Acidemia**	**Compensates for Alkalemia**	**Compensates for Acidemia**
pH	7.35–7.45				
pCO_2	35–45 mm Hg	Below normal	Above normal	Above normal	Below normal
Bicarbonate	22–26 mEq/L	Above normal	Below normal	Below normal	Above normal

Directional Effects of Variables			
Variable	**pH and pCO_2 Direction**	**pH and Bicarbonate Direction**	**Results**
pH elevated, pCO_2 decreased, Bicarbonate normal	Opposite	N/A	Respiratory alkalemia with no compensation
pH decreased, pCO_2 elevated, Bicarbonate normal	Opposite	N/A	Respiratory acidemia with no compensation
pH increased, pCO_2 elevated, Bicarbonate elevated	Same	Same	Metabolic alkalemia with respiratory compensation
pH decreased, pCO_2 elevated, Bicarbonate elevated	Opposite	Opposite	Respiratory acidemia with metabolic compensation

2. Is there compensation?
There appears to be compensation, but no such compensation is actually occurring. The decrease in pCO_2 is being driven by the toxin stimulating the respiratory centers. This is confirmed by the following test for respiratory compensation in metabolic acidemia: expected $pCO_2 = (1.5 \times [\text{measured } HCO_3^-]) + 8 \pm 2$ results in an answer of 36.5. This indicates that there is no compensation. Because the pCO_2 is even lower than expected with normal respiratory compensation, a respiratory abnormality is likely contributing to the respiratory alkalemia.

3. Is the anion gap needed to complete the interpretation?
   The knowledge of the high anion gap in this case is essential to determine the cause of the disorder. It confirms that the primary disorder is metabolic. The following causes are the most likely reasons for a high anion gap: ketoacidosis, lactic acidosis, renal failure, toxic ingestions.
4. What is the likely cause of the disorder?
   Aspirin toxicity. The respiratory alkalemia is due to increased respiratory drive caused by aspirin.

1.2.0 Pharmacotherapy

5. In the case of T. A., what would be the recommended treatment?
   Activated charcoal could be administered to reduce absorption, along with alkaline diuresis to increase drug excretion (acidic drugs are eliminated more rapidly in alkaline urine). Because hypokalemia may interfere with alkaline diuresis, patients are given a solution consisting of 1 L of 5% D/W, 150 mEq of $NaHCO_3$, and 40 mEq of KCl. Serum potassium is monitored as well.
   Drugs that increase urinary HCO_3 (e.g., acetazolamide) should be avoided because they worsen metabolic acidosis. Drugs that decrease respiratory drive should be avoided if possible because they may impair hyperventilation and respiratory alkalosis, decreasing blood pH.
   Fever can be treated with physical measures such as external cooling. Seizures are treated with benzodiazepines. In patients with rhabdomyolysis, alkaline diuresis may help prevent renal failure.
   Hemodialysis may be required to enhance salicylate elimination in patients with severe neurologic impairment, renal or respiratory insufficiency, acidemia despite other measures, or very high serum salicylate levels (greater than 100 mg/dL [greater than 7.25 mmol/L] with acute overdose or greater than 60 mg/dL [greater than 4.35 mmol/L] with chronic overdose).

Patient Care Scenario: Ambulatory Setting

1.1.0 Patient Information

A 74-year-old retired shipyard laborer with a 45+ pack-years (pack-a-day for 45 years) smoking history and previous work in sandblasting and fiberglass presented with increasing dyspnea and peripheral edema.

On physical examination, he was noted to be a thin, cyanotic man in moderate pulmonary distress who was afebrile with a heart rate of 90, respiratory rate of 28, and blood pressure of 125/90. His chest showed increased A-P diameter, and the breath sounds were faint with a prolonged expiration. The liver edge was 3 cm below the right costal margin. There was digital clubbing with cyanosis and marked peripheral edema.

Blood Gases

Variable	Room Air	100% Oxygen
pO_2	43	42
pCO_2	45 mm Hg	34 mm Hg
pH	7.51	7.38
Bicarbonate	20 m Eq/L	20 m Eq/L

1. What is the acid–base disorder?
   Respiratory alkalemia due to chronic obstructive pulmonary disease (COPD). The pH is high and the pCO_2 is low (see-saw working). The pH is high and the bicarbonate is low (not taking the same elevator), so the cause is not metabolic. Therefore, the anion gap is not required for this analysis.
2. Is there compensation?
   There is incomplete compensation.

1.2.0 Pharmacotherapy

3. What would be the recommended treatment?
   Cautious treatment with oxygen. Note the response this patient has when placed on oxygen: The oxygen-induced respiratory drive decreases and the pCO_2 rises to some extent. However, the declining pH actually passes 7.4 before the pCO_2 reaches the normal level of 40 mm Hg. This is because the renal compensation is "uncovered" when the pCO_2 rises, and it cannot respond fast enough to avoid an overshoot in pH. Now the tables are turned—the kidney causes a mild metabolic acidosis (decreased pH because the bicarbonate level is too low). This will resolve over a few hours as the kidneys respond. In patients with severe COPD and severe respiratory alkalosis, a sudden treatment with pure oxygen resulting in a sudden drop in breathing rate has been known to produce dangerous levels of acidosis by this mechanism.

Patient Care Scenario: Ambulatory Setting

1.1.0 Patient Information

A 46-year-old woman with a 14-year smoking history presents with a cough and progressive dyspnea of 6 months' duration. Her symptoms have been unresponsive to antibiotic treatment.

On physical examination, she is afebrile with a heart rate of 112, respiratory rate of 20 per minute, and BP of 130/100. Decreased breath sounds over the right chest are noted. There is no peripheral edema, clubbing, or cyanosis. A chest x-ray reveals that the right hemidiaphragm is elevated.

Arterial Blood Gases

Variable	At Rest	During Exercise	At Rest/with Oxygen
pO_2	91	67	54
pCO_2	30 mm Hg	36 mm Hg	28 mm Hg
pH	7.46	7.41	7.49
Bicarbonate	24 mEq/L		

1. What is the acid–base disorder?
   Respiratory alkalemia. The pH is high and the pCO_2 is low (see-saw operational). indicating that the lung is producing the alkalemia. The pH is high and the bicarbonate level is normal, indicating no metabolic abnormality.
2. Is there compensation?
   There is no compensation; the bicarbonate level is normal.

1.2.0 Pharmacotherapy

3. What is the recommended treatment?
   This patient does not have a lowered bicarbonate level as seen in the previous case, so oxygen therapy may be instituted without worry.

Patient Care Scenario: Ambulatory Setting

1.1.0 Patient Information

An elderly woman from a nursing home is admitted because of profound weakness and areflexia. Her oral intake has been poor for a few days. Current medications: torsemide 40 mg daily and zolpidem 5 mg at bedtime as needed for insomnia. Admission biochemistry (in mmol/l): Na^+ 145, K^+ 1.9, Cl^- 86, bicarbonate 45, anion gap 14, a spot urine chloride 7 mmol/L.

Arterial Blood Gases

pH	7.58
pCO_2	49 mmHg
pO_2	Not given
Bicarbonate	44.4 mmol/L

1. What is the acid–base disorder?
   The pH is elevated, as is the pCO_2 (see-saw is not operational). Thus the problem is not respiratory in nature. The pH is elevated, as is the bicarbonate (traveling on the same elevator). This fact, coupled with the hypochloremia and severe hypokalemia, suggests a significant metabolic alkalemia.
2. Is there compensation?
   The pH is elevated, as is the pCO_2. This suggests compensation, which needs to be confirmed by the test for metabolic alkalosis compensation. The formula of expected $pCO_2 = (0.7 \times [\text{measured } HCO_3^-]) + 20 \pm 5$ results in an answer of 51. This is within range of the measured value of 49 and indicates that there is compensation.

1.2.0 Pharmacotherapy

3. What is the recommended treatment?
   There is a suggestion of a drug-related disorder. Approximately 90% of cases of metabolic alkalosis are due to diuretic therapy or loss of gastric secretions (vomiting or nasogastric suction). The areflexia could indicate a hypokalemia. There is no evidence of diarrhea, vomiting, or polyuria. The poor oral intake suggests the possibility of dehydration and may indicate lactic acidosis due to poor perfusion, but there is no indication of increased respiratory effort (as evidenced by the high pCO_2 in the face of such a high bicarbonate level). The normal urinary chloride level does not suggest a cause in the volume-resistant group (i.e., the "chloride-resistant" group). The severe hypokalemia is the cause of the weakness and requires urgent therapy. Intravenous K^+ replacement is urgently indicated. Hypokalemia can cause serious arrhythmias. It can also cause rhabdomyolysis, which can result in hyperkalemia (and malignant arrhythmias) and renal failure. Hydration with normal saline

and holding the diuretic are also important treatments.

A Note about Metabolic Alkalemia

Consider the two major groups of causes of metabolic alkalosis; these groups are differentiated by measurement of the urinary chloride level:

- Chloride-responsive group (urine chloride < 10 mmol/L). These patients have an underlying chloride deficiency. This group is typified by:
  - Loss of gastric juice (i.e., vomiting especially if pyloric obstruction, or nasogastric suction)
  - Diuretic therapy (chronic use and urine level drawn after diuretic effect has passed)
- Chloride-resistant group (urine chloride > 20 mmol/L) is generally characterized by:
  - Excess steroids
  - Current diuretic use (dosed recently)
  - Excess adrenocortical activity (e.g., primary aldosteronism, Bartter's syndrome, Cushing's syndrome, other causes of excess adrenocortical activity)
- Idiopathic group

Biphasic Action of Diuretics

Diuretics cause a high urine chloride level while they are inducing diuresis, but a low urine chloride when measured after their pharmacological action has ended. As diuretic use is common, this relationship to the timing of a dose should be known and can assist in interpretation of the urine chloride result.

4. Is the anion gap relevant in this case?
   The anion gap is 14 so there is no evidence of a coexisting high anion gap acidemia. Chloride-responsive patients will typically respond well to normal saline, whereas chloride-resistant patients will not.

ANNOTATED BIBLIOGRAPHY

Brandis K. Acid-base physiology. Available at: http://www.anaesthesiaMCQ.com.

http://www.acid-base.com/clinical.php. Accessed March 1, 2010.

http://www.anaesthesiamcq.com/AcidBaseBook/ab8_6a.php. Accessed March 1, 2010.

http://www.wrongdiagnosis.com/a/acid_base_imbalance/intro.htm.

TOPIC: COMPLEMENTARY, ALTERNATIVE, AND HERBAL MEDICINE

Section Coordinator: Catherine M. Oliphant
Contributor: Randi Lynn Griffiths

Tips Worth Tweeting

- Approximately 38% of all U.S. adults use some form of complementary and alternative medicine.
- Unlike prescription medications, herbal medications do not require collection of safety and efficacy data prior to marketing.
- Herbal medications do not undergo mandatory quality testing.
- Herbal medications can alter the levels of some prescription drugs in the body.
- Herbal medications should be held for at least 2 weeks prior to elective surgery to minimize bleeding risks.
- St. John's wort can cause serotonin syndrome if combined with other antidepressants (especially MAOIs) or foods with a high tyramine content.
- Cranberry has not been found to be effective for the treatment of urinary tract infections.
- Odorless garlic preparations are likely ineffective; the active ingredient (allicin) is also responsible for garlic's distinctive odor.
- Black cohosh may increase the risk of metastasis in patients with breast cancer.
- Saw palmetto is contraindicated in pregnant women and women of childbearing age.
- Autoimmune disorders such as rheumatoid arthritis and multiple sclerosis may be aggravated by American ginseng due to its immune-stimulating effects.
- The potency of a particular kava product depends on the extraction technique used during its production. Water extraction yields little active ingredient due to its lipophilicity.
- Kava has been banned in several countries due to its hepatotoxicity.
- Echinacea may decrease the severity and duration of colds if taken at the onset of the disease.
- Raw seeds of the ginkgo tree contain ginkgotoxin, which can cause seizures and death.
- Incorrect fermentation of rice during the production of red yeast rice can result in the production of citrinin, which can cause renal toxicity and acute renal failure.

Patient Care Scenario: Community Setting

It is a busy day in the pharmacy when you take a question from one of your patients over the phone asking your opinion regarding St. John's wort for the treatment of depression.

Age 23 y/o, F, 120 lbs, 5'2", NKA

Date	Physician	Drug	Quantity	Sig	Refills
1/2	Hunter	Lexapro	#30	Take one daily	4
1/2	Hunter	Nuvaring	#1	Use monthly	2
1/2	Hunter	Loratadine 10 mg	#30	Daily	2

Key Terms

According to the National Center for Complementary and Alternative Medicine, **complementary and alternative medicine (CAM)** is "a group of diverse medical and health care systems, practices, and products that are not generally considered part of conventional medicine. **Complementary medicine** is used together with conventional medicine, and **alternative medicine** is used in place of conventional medicine."

Natural products, commonly referred to as herbs, are defined as "a plant or plant part used for its scent, flavor or therapeutic properties." Prior to 1994, herbal medications were regulated by the Food and Drug Administration (FDA) and had to be proved safe and effective before being marketed; thus they were subject to the same regulations as prescription and over-the-counter drug products. In 1994, the Dietary Supplement Health and Education Act (DSHEA) was passed. Under DSHEA, herbal medications are no longer subject to efficacy testing but must be shown to be safe by the manufacturer. The product label cannot be false or misleading, and the manufacturer cannot make claims that the product is intended to diagnose, treat, cure, or prevent any disease. The lack of regulation on herbal medications can lead to variable quality and sometimes safety issues due to problems with the manufacturing process. Consumers should be educated to choose an herbal product that has undergone voluntary quality testing to ensure its strength and purity. Currently, several companies perform quality testing and allow their seal to be displayed on the product label; these companies include the United States Pharmacopoeia (USP), Consumer Labs, and NSF International.

Many prescription drugs marketed today are derived from natural products, and some demonstrate a narrow therapeutic index, such as digoxin, which requires a near-toxic dose to achieve therapeutic efficacy. Herbal medications, like prescription medications, can affect the absorption, distribution, function, metabolism, and excretion of other medications when taken concomitantly. They can also exacerbate certain disease states or cause complications during surgery. Finally, little or no data have been collected for CAM products related to their use in pregnancy, lactation, liver disease, or kidney disease. To avoid complications, patients should be educated to notify their doctors and pharmacists of all medications that they are taking, including herbal products.

American Ginseng

Names: *Panax quinquefolius*
Common uses: diabetes, immune stimulant, improve athletic performance
Plant part: root
Active constituent: triterpene saponins
Mechanism of action:

- Diabetes: tissue sensitization, insulin secretion
- Immune modulation: activates monocytes, TNF-alpha and others

Dose:

- DM: 3 g within 2 hours of meals
- Immune stimulant: 200 mg BID
- Athletic performance: 1,200 mg daily

Precautions/contraindications:

- Pregnancy (contraindicated): possibly teratogenic
- Lactation (avoid)

Efficacy data:

- Diabetes: possibly effective
- Immune stimulant: may reduce the severity and duration of symptoms
- Athletic performance: not effective

Adverse effects:

- GI upset
- Tachycardia
- Mania
- Stevens-Johnson syndrome
- Hepatitis

Drug/disease interactions:

- Antidiabetes drugs: hypoglycemia
- MAOIs
- Warfarin: decreased effect
- Hormone-sensitive cancers or disorders
- Surgery: hypoglycemia

Black Cohosh

Names: baneberry, black snakeroot
Common uses: menopause, dysmenorrhea
Plant parts: rhizome and root
Active constituent: triterpene glycosides
Mechanism of action:

- Largely unknown
- Possible estrogen-like effects

Dose: 20–80 mg bid
Precautions/contraindications:
- Breast cancer (contraindicated)
- Pregnancy
- Lactation

Efficacy data: conflicting evidence
Side effects:
- GI upset
- Rash
- Headache
- Dizziness
- Weight gain
- Breast tenderness
- Spotting/bleeding
- Hepatotoxicity/hepatitis (monitor LFTs)
- Thromboembolism/CV disease (theoretical)

Drug/disease interactions:
- Other hepatotoxic medications/herbals (amiodarone, statins, black cohosh, kava)
- Breast cancer and other hormone-sensitive cancers
- Liver disease
- Transplants: may increase risk of rejection
- Protein S deficiency: may increase risk of thrombosis

Cranberry

Names: *Vaccinium microcarpum*
Common use: prevention and treatment of urinary tract infections, urine deodorizer
Plant par: fruit
Active constituents: proanthocyanidins (tannins), flavanols, ascorbic acid
Mechanism of action:
- Interferes with bacterial adherence to the urinary tract epithelial cells
- Note: does not release bacteria that have already adhered to the epithelial cells

Dose: 1–10 ounces of juice daily or 300–400 mg bid
Precautions/contraindications:
- Pregnancy (contraindicated)
- Lactation
- Aspirin allergy/asthma (juice contains 7 mg salicylic acid per liter)

Efficacy data:
- Possibly effective for *prevention*
- *Not* effective for treatment
- Effective for reducing urinary odor in patients suffering from incontinence

Side effects:
- Generally well tolerated
- Bleeding (theoretical)

Drug/disease interactions:
- Anticoagulants: increased risk of bleeding (warfarin)
- CYP450 2C9 *inhibitor* (warfarin)
- Diabetes: high sugar content in cranberry cocktail
- Kidney stones: high oxalate content

Echinacea

Names: American cone flower
Common uses: treating/preventing colds and upper respiratory tract infections (URTI)
Plant parts: roots and plant
Active constituents: heteroxylan, alkylamides, echinacosides
Mechanism of action:
- Increased lymphocyte activity
- Increased production of TNF-alpha, IL-1, and interferon
- Anti-inflammatory activity

Dose:
- 2 tablets tid
- 100 mg juice extract capsules tid
- 20 gtt q2h × 1d, then tid until symptoms are resolved
- 4–5 cups of tea × 1d, then 1 cup daily

Precautions/contraindications:
- Use cautiously in first trimester of pregnancy
- Avoid in second and third trimesters of pregnancy
- Lactation
- Chrysanthemum allergy

Efficacy data: may reduce severity and duration
Adverse effects:
- Generally well tolerated
- GI upset
- Allergic reactions
- Headache
- Oral sores
- Dizziness
- Insomnia
- Impaired immune function

Drug/disease interactions:
- CYP450 1A2 and 3A4 *inhibitor*
- Immunosuppressants
- Autoimmune diseases

Garlic

Names: *Allium sativum*
Common uses: hypertension, prevention of coronary events, peripheral vascular disease, cholesterol imbalance
Plant part: bulb

Active constituents: allicin. Allicin is converted from allin by the enzyme alinase when the bulb is crushed. Allicin is responsible for the odor of the garlic; thus odorless products could be assumed to be ineffective due to the likely deficiency of active constituent.

Mechanism of action:

- Hypertension: vasodilation (nitric oxide)
- Coronary heart disease: antiplatelet and fibrinolytic activity
- Peripheral vascular disease: reduce oxidative stress, inhibit LDL oxidation, antithrombotic effects
- Cholesterol imbalance: HMG-CoA reductase inhibitor activity

Dose: 300 mg tid or 1 clove fresh garlic daily

Precautions/contraindications: in pregnancy and lactation, avoid medicinal amounts

Efficacy data:

- Hypertension: modest decrease (SBP 8% and DBP 7%)
- Coronary heart disease, peripheral vascular disease, and cholesterol imbalance: may slow development of atherosclerosis

Adverse effects:

- Breath and body odor
- GI irritation
- Bleeding
- Allergic reactions

Drug/disease interactions:

- CYP450 2E1 and 3A4 *inhibitor*
- Anticoagulants/antiplatelets: increased risk of bleeding
- Oral contraceptives: decreased effectiveness
- Hypotension
- Bleeding disorders: increased risk of bleeding
- Surgery: increased risk of bleeding

Ginkgo

Names: *Ginkgo biloba*, maidenhair tree

Common uses: dementia, memory loss

Plant parts: leaf and seed

Active constituents: flavonoids and terpenoids

Mechanism of action:

- Prevent oxidative damage: antioxidant and free-radical scavenging
- Inhibit platelet-activating factor (PAF)
- Relax vascular smooth muscle

Dose: 120–240 mg divided tid (start low and titrate to avoid adverse effects)

Precautions/contraindications:

- Pregnancy (labor-inducing and hormonal effects)
- Lactation (avoid)
- Seizure disorders (avoid)

Efficacy data: likely ineffective

Adverse effects:

- GI upset
- Headache
- Palpitations
- Muscle weakness
- Spontaneous bleeding (long term): hemorrhagic stroke
- Allergic reactions/Stevens-Johnson syndrome
- Seizures and death can occur if raw seeds are consumed due to ginkgotoxin

Drug/disease interactions:

- Anticoagulant/antiplatelet drugs: increased risk of bleeding
- CYP450 enzyme *inhibitor*
- Seizure disorder
- Diabetes: hypoglycemia
- Bleeding disorders: increased risk of bleeding
- Surgery: increased risk of bleeding

Kava

Names: Ava pepper, intoxicating pepper

Common uses: anxiety, insomnia

Plant parts: rhizome, root, and stem

Active constituent: kavalactones

Mechanism of action:

- Exact mechanism is unknown
- Increase in GABA binding sites
- Dopamine antagonism

Dose: 100 mg TID

Precautions/contraindications:

- Pregnancy
- Lactation
- Hepatitis

Efficacy data: possibly effective

Adverse effects:

- Hepatotoxicity (banned in many foreign countries, monitor LFTs)
- GI upset
- Headache
- Dizziness
- Extrapyramidal side effects
- Poor overall health (long-term/high doses)
- Dermopathy
- Parkinsonism

Drug/disease interactions:

- Other sedating drugs (e.g., benzodiazepines, narcotics)
- Ethanol: increased CNS effects and hepatotoxicity
- CYP450 enzyme *inhibitor*
- Intestinal P-glycoprotein/multidrug resistance 1 (MDR-1) drug transporter *inhibitor*

- Hepatitis or other hepatotoxic drugs
- Parkinson's disease
- Surgery

Red Yeast Rice

Names: *Monascus purpureus*
Common uses: decrease cholesterol
Plant part: rice fermented with *Monascus purpureus* yeast
Active constituent: mevinic acids (lovastatin)
Mechanism of action: inhibit HMG-CoA reductase
Dose: 1,200 mg bid with food (7.2 mg lovastatin)
Precautions/contraindications:
- Pregnancy (contraindicated)
- Lactation (contraindicated)

Efficacy data: effective at lowering total cholesterol, LDL cholesterol, and triglycerides
Adverse effects:
- Abdominal pain
- Heartburn
- Flatulence
- Anaphylaxis
- Increased LFTs (monitor LFTs)
- Myopathy
- Rhabdomyolysis
- Kidney failure (a renal toxic chemical may be produced if fermented incorrectly)

Drug/disease interactions:
- CYP450 3A4 inhibitors (grapefruit juice): increase drug concentration
- Other hepatotoxic drugs
- Statins
- Fibrates
- Niacin

Saw Palmetto

Names: American dwarf palm, cabbage palm
Common use: symptoms of BPH
Plant part: ripe fruit
Active constituent: fatty acids
Mechanism of action:
- Antiproliferative properties
- Inhibits inflammatory mediators
- Noncompetitively inhibits 5-alpha-reductase

Dose: 160 mg bid or 320 mg daily
Precautions/contraindications:
- Pregnancy (contraindicated)
- Lactation (contraindicated)
- Bleeding disorders

Efficacy data: conflicting data
Adverse effects:
- Generally well tolerated
- Dizziness
- Headache
- GI upset
- Hepatitis (case reports)
- Pancreatitis (case reports)
- Bleeding

Drug/disease interactions:
- Anticoagulants: increased risk of bleeding
- Surgery: increased risk of bleeding

St. John's Wort

Names: *Hypericum perforatum,* SJW
Common uses: depression, seasonal affective disorder (SAD), anxiety, obsessive–compulsive disorder (OCD)
Plant parts: flowers and leaves
Active constituents: hypericin and hyperforin
Mechanism of action:
- Inhibition of cortisol secretion
- Blockade of catabolic hormones (IL-6)
- Modulation of the effects of 5-HT, DA, and NE
- Mild monoamine oxidase inhibitor (MAOI) activity (questionable in vivo)

Dose: 300 mg tid (standardized to 0.3% hypericin); may take 4–6 weeks for full effects to be seen
Precautions/contraindications:
- Pregnancy (contraindicated)
- Conflicting data: some sources say that St. John's wort is safe, but animal studies suggest teratogenicity
- Lactation

Efficacy data: likely effective
Side effects: generally well tolerated
- Common: insomnia, vivid dreams, restlessness, anxiety, agitation, irritability, GI discomfort, diarrhea, fatigue, dry mouth, dizziness, headache
- Uncommon: hypertensive crisis, mania, increased liver function tests (LFTs), phototoxicity, sedation (caution with other CNS depressants), serotonin syndrome (caution with tyramine-containing foods)

Drug/disease interactions:
- Digoxin (may decrease digoxin levels by 25%)
- Other antidepressants: serotonin syndrome
- Opioids: enhance sedation
- Anesthesia: severe hypotension
- Schizophrenia: induce psychosis
- CYP3A4 *inducer*: may decrease drug concentrations of *many* medications, including oral contraceptives, calcium-channel blockers, and statins
- Intestinal P-glycoprotein/multidrug resistance 1 (MDR-1) drug transporter *inducer*: may

decrease intestinal absorption of drugs such as cyclosporine

ANNOTATED BIBLIOGRAPHY

Chung B. Natural plant extracts: export market opportunities in the USA. Rural Industries Research & Development Corporation. Available at: http://www.rirdc.gov.au/reports/EOI/00-51.pdf. Accessed August 16, 2008.

Dietary Supplement Health and Education Act of 1994. U.S. Food and Drug Administration. Available at: http://www.cfsan.fda.gov/~dms/dietsupp.html. Accessed August 16, 2008.

Natural Medicines Comprehensive Database. Available at: http://www.naturaldatabase.com/(S(ssojrcq4jgrpmmjvpnrjgxfo))/home.aspx?cs=CE&s=ND. Accessed October 16, 2008.

NCCAM. 2007 statistics on CAM use in the United States: National Health Interview Survey. Available at: http://nccam.nih.gov/news/camstats/2007/. Accessed October 28, 2009.

TOPIC: FLUIDS AND ELECTROLYTES

Section Coordinator: Catherine M. Oliphant
Contributor: Catherine M. Oliphant

Tips Worth Tweeting

- Crystalloids distribute to multiple compartments within the body, including the intracellular, interstitial, and intravascular compartments.
- Normal saline (0.9% NaCl) is considered the first-line therapy for intravascular volume expansion for most patients.
- Colloids are distributed only to the intravascular space.
- Colloids are much more expensive than crystalloids.
- For hyponatremia, serum sodium correction should not exceed 12 mEq/L per day; faster correction rates may be associated with central pontine myelinolysis.
- For hypernatremia, serum sodium correction should not lead to a fall in serum concentration of more than 10 mEq/L per day; faster rates of decline may lead to cerebral edema, convulsions, and death.
- In general, a 1 mEq/L decrease in serum potassium concentration correlates with a 100–200 mEq loss of total body potassium.
- Oral potassium doses should not exceed 40 mEq per dose to avoid gastrointestinal irritation.
- Agents to lower potassium concentrations include polystyrene sulfonate + sorbitol, loop diuretics, insulin plus dextrose, and β-agonists.
- Calcium chloride or gluconate should be administered to stabilize the myocardium in hyperkalemic patients with EKG changes.
- Magnesium oxide causes diarrhea.
- Phosphorus and calcium salts can precipitate at a calcium phosphorus product of more than 60.
- Phosphate binders include calcium carbonate, calcium acetate, aluminum-containing antacids, sevelamer, and lanthanum carbonate.
- Corrected calcium concentration = measured calcium (mg/dL) + 0.8 (4 – measured albumin).
- Concomitant administration of IV calcium products and ceftriaxone may result in precipitation in neonates younger than 28 days; in individuals older than 28 days, lines must be flushed between infusions and should not be administered at the same time via a Y-site.
- Pharmacotherapy for hypercalcemia includes hydration, loop diuretics, and bisphosphonates.

Patient Care Scenario: Hospital Setting

C. J.: 64 y/o, 5'5", F, white, 150 lbs, NKDA
PMH: Hypertension, COPD, CHF
Lab values: Na 140 mEq/L, K 7.2 mEq/L, BUN 28 mg/dL, Cr 1.3 mg/dL

C. J. presents to her primary physician with complaints of fatigue and muscle weakness. A chemistry panel is ordered and an electrocardiogram (EKG) is performed. She is admitted to the hospital for follow-up on labs and EKG.

Date	Physician	Drug	Quantity	Sig	Refills
1/3	Case	Enalapril 10 mg	#60	one bid	6
1/3	Case	Metoprolol XL 50 mg	#30	once daily	3
1/3	Case	Spironolactone 25 mg	#30	one daily	4
1/3	Case	Furosemide 40 mg	#30	one daily	3
1/3	Case	Aspirin 81 mg	#100	one daily	5
1/3	Case	Potassium chloride 20 mEq	#30	one daily	4
1/3	Case	Multivitamin	#100	one daily	4
1/3	Case	Calcium carbonate 500 mg	#60	one bid	3
1/3	Case	Tiotropium	#1	one puff daily	3
1/3	Case	Albuterol MDI	#1	1–2 puffs when needed	2
1/3	Case	Trimethoprim-sulfamethoxazole DS	#14	one bid, finished 3 days ago	

Fluids

Total body water (TBW) averages 60% of body weight in an adult male and 50% of body weight in an adult female. Approximately two-thirds of TBW is intracellular and one third is extracellular. For the extracellular fluid, one-fourth is found in the intravascular (plasma) compartment and three-fourths in the interstitial (lymphatic) compartment. Fluids are classified as crystalloid or colloid.

Key Terms

Crystalloids:

- 5% dextrose (D_5W)
- Normal saline (0.9% sodium chloride)
- 0.45% sodium chloride
- Hypertonic saline (3% sodium chloride)
- Lactated Ringer's solution

Colloids:

- Albumin
- Hetastarch
- Dextran
- Fresh frozen plasma

The advantage of using colloids is that smaller volumes can be given to achieve the same effect as occurs with much larger volumes of crystalloids. In general, there is no advantage of colloids over crystalloids; however, colloids are more expensive. Distribution of the various intravenous fluids depends on the tonicity of the crystalloids, whereas colloids remain in the intravascular space (Table 18-1).

Indications for the various intravenous fluids are listed in Table 18-2.

Hyponatremia

1.1.0 Patient Information

Sodium is the most abundant extracellular cation. Disorders of sodium are often complicated by disorders of water, as water follows sodium.

Table 18-1 Distribution of Crystalloids (based on a 132-lb male)

Fluid (1,000 mL)	Intracellular Compartment (mL)	Interstitial Compartment (mL)	Intravascular Compartment (mL)
D_5W	667	250	83
Normal saline	0	750	250
0.45% saline	333	500	167
Hypertonic	–2,600	3,000	600
Plasma (colloid)	0	0	1,000

Laboratory Testing

Hyponatremia is defined as a serum sodium concentration less than 136 mEq/L. Most patients with serum sodium greater than 125 mEq/L are asymptomatic; however, the rate of hyponatremia is also a determinant in whether symptoms appear (those who develop hyponatremia more rapidly may have more manifestations).

Classification of Hyponatremia

Hyponatremia is further classified into four categories:

- Hypotonic hyponatremia with an increased extracellular fluid (ECF) volume (Na and water retention)
- Hypotonic hyponatremia with a normal ECF volume (moderate water retention)
- Hypotonic hyponatremia with a decreased ECF volume (Na and water loss)
- Hypertonic hyponatremia (osmotic agents cause increase in water with little change in sodium)

Signs and Symptoms

Signs and symptoms of hyponatremia are usually seen with sodium concentrations of less than 125 mEq/L and include headache, confusion, lethargy, muscle cramps, nausea, vomiting, and depressed reflexes. Complications of severe hyponatremia (serum sodium less than 110 mEq/L) include seizures, coma, and death.

Medication- and Disease–State-Induced Hyponatremia

See Table 18-3.

1.2.0 Pharmacotherapy

Management of hyponatremia depends on the underlying cause. Table 18-4 lists the treatment options for the various types of hyponatremia.

1.3.0 Pharmacotherapy Monitoring

Serum sodium correction should not exceed 12 mEq/L per day. Faster correction rates may be associated with osmotic demyelination or central pontine myelinolysis.

2.1.0 Calculation

If sodium needs to be replaced, the sodium deficit can be calculated:

$$\text{NA deficit (mEq)} = (\text{TBW})(\text{desired Na concentration} - \text{observed Na concentration})$$

Approximately one-third of the sodium deficit can be replaced over the first 12 hours at a rate of less than 0.5 mEq/hr. The remaining sodium deficit can then be replaced over the next several days.

Table 18-2 IV Fluid Indications

Intravenous Fluid	Indication
Normal saline (0.9% NaCl)	• Intravascular volume expansion (first-line therapy for most patients) • Isotonic fluid (does not cause significant fluid shifts between cells and intravascular compartment) • Volume resuscitation in shock/hemorrhage/burn patients, hypotension, and hyponatremia
0.45% saline	• Hypotonic fluid (distributed to the ICF, interstitial, and intravascular compartments) that causes water to shift into cells • May be used in hypertonic patients
Hypertonic saline (3% NaCl)	• Shifts fluids back into the intravascular compartment (vascular expansion) • May be used to treat severe hyponatremia
5% dextrose (D_5W)	• Hypotonic fluid (distributed to the ICF, interstitial, and intravascular compartments) that causes water to shift into cells • May be used to treat hypernatremia
Lactated Ringer's solution	• Isotonic crystalloid • Intravascular volume expansion • Lactate metabolized to bicarbonate will increase pH • Often used in the perioperative setting • Avoid in patients with liver disease
Albumin 5% or 25%	• Intravascular volume expansion • Expensive • Adverse effects: anaphylaxis, fluid overload
Hetastarch	• Intravascular volume expansion • Contains starch and sodium chloride • Expensive • Adverse effects: hypersensitivity reactions, fluid overload, risk of bleeding • Avoid in patients with renal impairment (dose adjustment is necessary)
Dextran 40 or 70	• Intravascular volume expansion • Polysaccharide • Adverse effects: hypersensitivity reactions, fluid overload, risk of bleeding • Avoid in patients with renal impairment (dose adjustment is necessary)
Plasma	• Intravascular volume expansion • Adverse effects: anaphylaxis

ICF = intracellular fluid.

Hypernatremia

1.1.0 Patient Information

Laboratory Testing

Hypernatremia is defined as a serum sodium concentration greater than 145 mEq/L. Most patients with serum sodium less than 160 mEq/L are asymptomatic; however, the rate of hypernatremia is also a determinant in whether symptoms appear (those who develop hypernatremia more rapidly may have more manifestations).

Signs and Symptoms

Signs and symptoms of hypernatremia are usually seen with sodium concentrations greater than 160 mEq/L and include thirst, confusion, and dry mucous membranes. The level of consciousness decreases as the serum sodium concentration increases.

Medications and Disease States Associated with Hypernatremia

Causes of hypernatremia include the following conditions:

- Dehydration due to insensible losses
- Hypodipsia
- Neurogenic diabetes insipidus
- Loop diuretics
- Osmotic diuresis
- Diarrhea
- Vomiting
- Nasogastric drainage

Table 18-3 Medication- and Disease–State-Induced Hyponatremia

Type	Cause
Hypotonic hyponatremia with increased ECF	CHF, cirrhosis, nephrotic syndrome, renal failure, glucocorticoids, pregnancy
Hypotonic hyponatremia with normal ECF	Syndrome of inappropriate antidiuretic hormone (SIADH), renal failure, thiazide diuretics, hypothyroidism, adrenal insufficiency
Hypotonic hyponatremia with decreased ECF	Diuretics, adrenal insufficiency, salt-wasting nephropathy, renal tubular acidosis, diarrhea, vomiting, blood loss, excessive sweating, third spacing of fluids
Hypertonic hyponatremia	Hyperglycemia

Table 18-4 Pharmacotherapy of Hyponatremia

Type	Treatment
Hypotonic hyponatremia with increased ECF	• Na and water restriction • ± diuretics • Treatment of underlying condition
Hypotonic hyponatremia with normal ECF	• Fluid restriction • Demeclocycline for refractory SIADH
Hypotonic hyponatremia with decreased ECF	• Administration of sodium and water with 0.9%, 3%, or 5% NaCl • Most patients can be treated with normal saline • 3% or 5% NaCl is reserved for severe hyponatremia
Hypertonic hyponatremia	• Management of hyperglycemia should normalize serum sodium

- Osmotic cathartic agents
- Burns
- Impaired thirst
- Water restriction
- Excessive sweating
- NaCl-rich emetics
- Hypertonic saline infusion
- Ingestion of NaCl

1.2.0 Pharmacotherapy

Management of hypernatremia includes hypotonic fluid replacement and treatment of the underlying cause. Hypotonic fluids include 5% dextrose, 0.45% NaCl, and 0.225% NaCl.

1.3.0 Pharmacotherapy Monitoring

The rate of infusion must not lead to a fall in serum sodium of greater than 10 mEq/L per day, with a goal serum sodium of 145 mEq/L. Too great a decrease may result in cerebral edema, convulsions, and death.

2.1.0 Calculation

The total body water deficit can be calculated using the following equation:

$$\text{Water deficit (L)} = \text{TBW}\ ([\text{Serum sodium} / 140] - 1)$$

$$\text{TBW} = 0.5 \times \text{body wt (kg) for females or } 0.6 \times \text{body wt (kg) for males}$$

The fluid volume should be replaced over 2–3 days.

Hypokalemia

Potassium is the most principal cation in the intracellular fluid. Approximately 90% of the body's potassium is found in this intracellular source. Serum potassium levels are not an accurate representation of total body potassium stores, however.

1.1.0 Patient Information

Laboratory Testing

Hypokalemia is defined as a serum potassium concentration less than 3.5 mEq/L.

Signs and Symptoms

Signs and symptoms of hypokalemia are usually seen with potassium concentrations less than 3 mEq/L. Common symptoms include muscle weakness/cramps, abdominal cramps, nausea, vomiting, polyuria, polydipsia, nocturia, electrocardiogram (EKG) abnormalities, and cardiac arrhythmias. EKG changes related to hypokalemia include ST-segment depression, flattened T waves, and prominent U waves. Arrhythmias associated with hypokalemia include bradycardia, atrioventricular block, premature atrial or ventricular beats, tachycardias, and ventricular fibrillation.

Medication- and Disease–State-Induced Hypokalemia

Hypokalemia is a risk factor for digoxin toxicity. Table 18-5 lists the causes of hypokalemia.

In general, a 1 mEq/L decrease in serum potassium concentrations correlates with a 100–200 mEq loss of total body potassium. Potassium may also be shifted intracellularly without loss of total body potassium stores.

1.2.0 Pharmacotherapy

Potassium replacement can be given orally or intravenously. Potassium is available in various salt forms (e.g., chloride, acetate, gluconate, citrate, bicarbonate, and phosphate). Oral products include potassium chloride

Table 18-5 Medication- and Disease–State-Induced Hypokalemia

Renal	• Low magnesium • Hyperaldosteronism
Gastrointestinal	• Diarrhea • Vomiting or NG suctioning • Laxative abuse
Medications	• Diuretics (loop, thiazides) • β2 agonists • Insulin • Corticosteroids • Amphotericin B • Cisplatin
Decreased intake of potassium	
Alkalosis	

(available as tablet, powder, and liquid preparations) and potassium bicarbonate.

1.3.0 Pharmacotherapy Monitoring

Oral doses should not exceed 40 mEq per dose, as oral potassium products cause gastrointestinal irritation. Intravenous potassium should be administered at a rate of 10–20 mEq/hr via a peripheral or central line. If the rate exceeds 10 mEq/hr, EKG monitoring is required. The maximum infusion rate is 40 mEq/hr and must be administered through a central line with EKG monitoring. Intravenous potassium is irritating to the vein and may cause significant pain, if given via a peripheral line, at higher concentrations. Potassium for intravenous administration should be diluted in saline rather than dextrose, as glucose stimulates the release of insulin, which drives the potassium in an intracellular direction. If the patient has concurrent hypomagnesemia, the magnesium must be replaced before potassium repletion begins.

Hyperkalemia

1.1.0 Patient Information

Laboratory Testing

Hyperkalemia is defined as a serum potassium concentration greater than 5 mEq/L.

Signs and Symptoms

Signs and symptoms of hyperkalemia include fatigue, muscle weakness, paresthesias, paralysis, EKG changes, and cardiac arrhythmias. EKC changes associated with hyperkalemia include peaked T waves, shortened QT intervals, and widened QRS complexes.

Table 18-6 Medication- and Disease–State-Induced Hyperkalemia

Increased potassium intake	• Excessive dietary intake (including salt substitutes)
Decreased potassium excretion	• Acute or chronic renal failure • Hypoaldosteronism • Renal hypoperfusion
Medications	• Potassium-sparing diuretics • ACEI, ARB • Cyclosporine • Heparins • NSAIDs • Potassium supplements • Spironolactone • Trimethoprim • Pentamidine
Redistribution	• Acidosis • Tissue damage (trauma, hemolysis, rhabdomyolysis)

Medication- and Disease–State-Induced Hyperkalemia

See Table 18-6.

1.2.0 Pharmacotherapy

Management of hyperkalemia is multifactorial in nature, including discontinuation of potassium supplements or medications that increase potassium concentrations. Next, the myocardium may need to be stabilized against the arrhythmic effects of elevated potassium levels if EKG changes are present or the serum potassium level is greater than 6 mEq/L. Intravenous calcium (chloride or gluconate) is administered to stabilize the myocardium. Treatment of hyperkalemia involves two different strategies: (1) agents that drive potassium intracellularly and (2) agents that lower total body potassium. Therapies that drive potassium intracellularly include insulin plus dextrose and β-agonists such as albuterol. Treatments that reduce total body potassium include sodium polystyrene sulfonate (Kayexalate) plus sorbitol, loop diuretics, and dialysis. The sodium polystyrene sulfonate is a sodium–potassium exchange resin that binds potassium in the gastrointestinal tract in exchange for sodium. It can be given orally or as a retention enema. Loop diuretics increase the renal excretion of potassium.

Hypomagnesemia

Magnesium is the second most abundant intracellular cation. It is primarily found in bone, though approximately 1% of magnesium is located in the extracellular fluid.

Table 18-7 Medication- and Disease–State-Induced Hypomagnesemia

Gastrointestinal loss	• Malabsorption • Chronic diarrhea
Renal loss	• Acute tubular necrosis • Renal tubular acidosis • Diabetes • Hypoparathyroidism/ hyperthyroidism
Medications	• Diuretics • Cyclosporine • Aminoglycosides • Cisplatin • Amphotericin B • Laxative abuse
Hypercalcemia	
Malnutrition	• Decreased dietary intake • Alcoholism

1.1.0 Patient Information

Laboratory Testing

Hypomagnesemia is defined as a serum magnesium concentration less than 1.4 mEq/L. Many patients will be asymptomatic.

Signs and Symptoms

Signs and symptoms of hypomagnesemia include lethargy, muscle cramps, hyperactive deep tendon reflexes, tetany, altered mental status, irritability, seizures (at concentrations less than 1 mEq/L), and arrhythmias. Concurrent hypokalemia and hypocalcemia may also exist.

Medication- and Disease–State-Induced Hypomagnesemia

See Table 18-7.

1.1.0 Pharmacotherapy

Treatment of hypomagnesemia includes both oral (magnesium oxide) and intravenous (magnesium sulfate) magnesium replacement. Magnesium is usually replaced over several days, and caution must be used in patients with renal impairment—magnesium is renally eliminated. Magnesium oxide is associated with diarrhea. Magnesium sulfate dosing depends on the magnesium level; however, in general, 1 to 4 g of magnesium sulfate is given at a rate of 1 g/hr (unless the patient has severe, symptomatic hypomagnesemia); 8 mEq of magnesium sulfate is equal to 1 g. Magnesium serum levels should be monitored to avoid toxicity.

Hypermagnesemia

1.1.0 Patient Information

Laboratory Testing

Hypermagnesemia is defined as a serum magnesium level greater than 2.1 mEq/L.

Signs and Symptoms

Most patients remain asymptomatic; however, symptoms may include nausea, vomiting, weakness, decreased deep tendon reflexes, hypotension, respiratory depression, and cardiac arrest.

Disease–State-Induced Hypermagnesemia

Renal failure is the most common cause of hypermagnesemia.

1.2.0 Pharmacotherapy

Treatment consists of discontinuation of all magnesium-containing products, followed by the administration of intravenous calcium gluconate. Diuretics and dialysis may be used to increase magnesium excretion from the body.

Hypophosphatemia

Phosphorus is the most abundant intracellular anion; however, it is found primarily in bone.

1.1.0 Patient Information

Laboratory Testing

Hypophosphatemia is defined as a serum phosphorus concentration less than 2.5 mg/dL. Mild hypophosphatemia may be asymptomatic.

Signs and Symptoms

Clinical manifestations of low serum phosphorus include muscle weakness, myalgias, rhabdomyolysis, respiratory failure, impaired cardiac contractility, hemolytic anemia, confusion, seizures, and coma.

Medication- and Disease–State-Induced Hypophosphatemia

See Table 18-8.

1.2.0 Pharmacotherapy

Management of hypophosphatemia includes discontinuation of all medications that may be contributing to this condition and supplementation with oral or intravenous phosphorus. Phosphorus-containing products include Neutra Phos and K-Phos. Intravenous phosphate is available as a potassium or sodium salt; each salt contains 3 mmol phosphorus per milliliter.

Table 18-8 Medication- and Disease–State-Induced Hypophosphatemia

Intracellular shift	• Respiratory alkalosis • Diabetic ketoacidosis • Refeeding syndrome
Increased urinary excretion	• Hyperparathyroidism
Decreased intestinal absorption	• Malabsorption
Medications	• Phosphate-binding antacids • Corticosteroids • Diuretics
Decreased dietary intake	• Chronic alcoholism • Total parenteral nutrition

Mild to moderate hypophosphatemia (phosphorus concentration of 1–2.5 mg/dL) may be treated with oral phosphate products at a dose of 1.5–2 g per day. Use of oral replacement products is limited by their tendency to cause diarrhea. Intravenous phosphate is dosed based on serum phosphorus level.

Serum Phosphorus Level (mg/dL)	Phosphorus Replacement Dose
1.5–2.2	0.15 mmol/kg
1–1.5	0.3 mmol/kg
<1	0.45 mmol/kg

1.3.0 Pharmacotherapy Monitoring

Monitor the patient's phosphorus level after each phosphorus infusion, and discontinue replacement therapy when this level is greater than 2 mg/dL. Watch for hypocalcemia. Phosphorus and calcium salts can precipitate at a calcium phosphorus product (calcium × phosphorus) of greater than 60.

Hyperphosphatemia

1.1.0 Patient Information

Laboratory Testing

Hyperphosphatemia is defined as a serum phosphorus concentration greater than 5 mg/dL.

Signs and Symptoms

Signs and symptoms of hyperphosphatemia most commonly involve the central nervous and cardiovascular systems. Findings may include altered mental status, delirium, seizures, paresthesias, coma, muscle cramping, neuromuscular hyperexcitability, hypotension, heart failure, and prolongation of the QT interval.

Medication- and Disease–State-Induced Hyperphosphatemia

Most patients with hyperphosphatemia have end-stage renal disease. Other causes may include hypoparathyroidism, rhabdomyolysis, tumor lysis post chemotherapy, respiratory acidosis, lactic acidosis, diabetic ketoacidosis, and vitamin D intoxication. Medications that may cause hyperphosphatemia include phosphorus-containing laxatives or enemas, phosphorus supplements, vitamin D supplements, and bisphosphonates.

1.2.0 Pharmacotherapy

Treatment includes discontinuation of medications that contain phosphorus as well as dietary restriction of phosphorus intake. Phosphate binders reduce the GI absorption of phosphorus; they include calcium carbonate, calcium acetate (PhosLo), aluminum-containing antacids, sevelamer (Renagel), and lanthanum carbonate (Fosrenal). Intravenous calcium gluconate or chloride may be given if the patient exhibits symptoms of hypocalcemia.

Hypocalcemia

Calcium is primarily found in bone, with approximately 1% found in the extracellular fluid. Nearly 50% of the serum calcium is bound to protein (mainly albumin), with the remainder in the ionized form. Therefore, in patients with low albumin, the serum calcium concentration must be corrected using the following equation:

$$\text{Corrected calcium} = \text{Measured calcium (mg/dL)} + 0.8\,(4 - \text{measured albumin})$$

1.1.0 Patient Information

Laboratory Testing

Hypocalcemia is defined by a serum calcium concentration less than 8.5 mg/dL or an ionized calcium level less than 1 mmol/L.

Signs and Symptoms

Signs and symptoms of hypocalcemia do not usually become evident until the calcium level falls below 6.5 mg/dL. They may include muscle spasms, tetany, hypoactive reflexes, Chvostek sign, Trousseau sign, irritability, confusion, hallucinations, seizures, bradycardia, prolongation of the QT interval, and decreased cardiac contractility.

Medication- and Disease–State-Induced Hypocalcemia

See Table 18-9.

Table 18-9 Medication- and Disease-State-Induced Hypocalcemia

Inadequate intake	• Poor dietary intake • Vitamin deficiency (calcium and vitamin D) • Alcoholism
Other	• Hypoparathyroidism • Alkalosis • Renal failure • Pancreatitis • Hungry bone syndrome
Medications	• Phenobarbital • Phenytoin • Corticosteroids • Proton pump inhibitors • Loop diuretics • Phosphate replacement products • Bisphosphonates • Foscarnet
Hyperphosphatemia	
Hypoalbuminemia	
Hypomagnesemia	

1.2.0 Pharmacotherapy

Management of hypocalcemia includes both oral and intravenous calcium replacement, vitamin D supplementation, and the administration of active vitamin D (calcitriol) to patients with chronic renal failure. Oral calcium products must be given in between meals so that they will not act as a phosphate binder. Calcium gluconate and calcium chloride are intravenous calcium products. Calcium gluconate is associated with less venous irritation than calcium chloride (both should be administered via a central line), but calcium chloride provides more elemental calcium than calcium gluconate.

1.3.0 Pharmacotherapy Monitoring

Concomitant administration of intravenous calcium products and ceftriaxone may result in precipitation. According to FDA guidelines, the concomitant use of ceftriaxone and IV calcium products is contraindicated in neonates younger than 28 days of age. Ceftriaxone and IV calcium products may be administered concomitantly in individuals older than 28 days of age if the IV lines are flushed between infusions and are not administered at the same time via a Y-site.

2.1.0 Calculation

In patients with low albumin, the serum calcium concentration must be corrected using the following equation:

$$\text{Corrected calcium} = \text{Measured calcium (mg/dL)} + 0.8\,(4 - \text{measured albumin})$$

Hypercalcemia

1.1.0 Patient Information

Laboratory Testing

Hypercalcemia is defined as a serum calcium concentration greater than 10.2 mg/dL.

Signs and Symptoms

Signs and symptoms of hypercalcemia depend on the rate of calcium increase, serum calcium concentration, and underlying etiology. They may include nausea, vomiting, abdominal pain, constipation, dehydration, polyuria, lethargy, hyperreflexia, confusion, hypertension, bradycardia, QT interval alteration, and heart block.

Medication- and Disease–State-Induced Hypercalcemia

Disease-state-induced hypercalcemia may be linked to hyperparathyroidism, malignancy, granulomatous disorders, hyperthyroidism, and adrenal insufficiency. Medication-induced hypercalcemia may be associated with use of thiazide diuretics, estrogens, and lithium, as well as vitamin A, vitamin D, and calcium supplementation.

1.2.0 Pharmacotherapy

Treatment of hypercalcemia includes discontinuation of calcium-containing products, hydration, increased calcium excretion, inhibition of osteoclast activity, and identification/management of the underlying cause.

Table 18-10 Pharmacotherapy for Hypercalcemia

Hydration	Normal saline
Increased calcium excretion	Loop diuretics
Inhibition of osteoclast activity	Bisphosphonates (zolendronic acid, pamidronate)
Other	• Calcitonin • Gallium • Mithramycin • Hydrocortisone

ANNOTATED BIBLIOGRAPHY

Adrogue HJ, Madias NE. Hypernatremia. *N Engl J Med* 2000;342(20):1493–1499.

Beach CB. Hypocalcemia. Emedicine. Updated March 9, 2009. Available at: http://www.emedicine.medscape.com/article/767260-overview.

Boucher BA, Wood GC. Hypovolemic shock. In: Chisholm-Burns MA, Wells BG, Schwinghammer TL, et al., eds. *Pharmacotherapy: Principles and Practice.* New York: McGraw-Hill; 2008:201–203.

Brophy DF, Gehr TWB. Disorders of potassium and magnesium homeostasis. In: DiPiro JT, Talbert RL, Yee GC, et al., eds. *Pharmacotherapy: A Pathophysiologic Approach.* 7th ed. New York: McGraw-Hill; 2008:877–888.

Cohn JN, Kowey PR, Whelton PK, et al. New guidelines for potassium replacement in clinical practice. *Arch Intern Med* 2000;160:2429–2436.

Coyle JD, Joy MS. Disorders of sodium and water homeostasis. In: DiPiro JT, Talbert RL, Yee GC, et al., eds. *Pharmacotherapy: A Pathophysiologic Approach.* 7th ed. New York: McGraw-Hill; 2008:845–860.

Fulop T, Agraharkar M, Rondon-Berrios H, et al. Hypomagnesemia. Emedicine. Updated January 21, 2009. Available at: http://www.emedicine.medscape.com/article/246366-overview.

Fulop T, Agraharkar M, Workeneh BT, et al. Hypermagnesemia. Emedicine. Updated April 8, 2009. Available at: http://www.emedicine.medscape.com/article/246489-overview.

Garth D. Hyperkalemia. Emedicine. Updated April 2, 2010. Available at: http://www.emedicine.medscape.com/article/766479-overview.

Garth D. Hypokalemia. Emedicine. Updated April 2, 2010. Available at: http://www.emedicine.medscape.com/article/767448-overview.

Gennari FJ. Hypokalemia. *N Engl J Med* 1998;339(7): 451–458.

Hemphill RR. Hypercalcemia. Emedicine. Updated August 5, 2009. Available at: http://www.emedicine.medscape.com/article/766373-overview.

Hollander-Rodriguez JC, Calvert JF. Hyperkalemia. *Am Fam Physician* 2006;73(2):283–290.

Knochel JP. Hypophosphatemia. *West J Med* 1981; 143:15–26.

Lay AL. Fluid and electrolyte disorders. In: Koda-Kimble MA, Young LY, Kradjan WA, et al., eds. *Applied Therapeutics: The Clinical Use of Drugs.* 8th ed. Philadelphia: Lippincott Williams & Wilkens; 2005:1231–1233.

Malesker MA, Morrow LE. Fluids and electrolytes. In: Chisholm-Burns MA, Wells BG, Schwinghammer TL, et al., eds. *Pharmacotherapy: Principles and Practice.* New York: McGraw-Hill; 2008:403–417.

Moore DJ, Rosh AJ. Hypophosphatemia. Emedicine. Updated September 22, 2009. Available at: http://www.emedicine.medscape.com/article/767955-overview.

Pai AB, Rohrscheib M, Joy MS. Disorders of calcium and phosphorus homeostasis. In: DiPiro JT, Talbert RL, Yee GC, et al., eds. *Pharmacotherapy: A Pathophysiologic Approach.* 7th ed. New York: McGraw-Hill; 2008:861–876.

Patterson LA, DeBlieux PMC. Hyperphosphatemia. Emedicine. Updated December 3, 2009. Available at: http://www.emedicine.medscape.com/article/767010-overview.

U.S. Food and Drug Administration. Information for healthcare professionals: ceftriaxone. Available at: http://www.fda.gov/Drugs/DrugSafety/PostmarketDrugSafetyInformationforPatientsandProviders/ucm109103.htm

TOPIC: VITAMINS AND MINERALS

Section Coordinator: *Catherine M. Oliphant*
Contributor: *Glenda Carr*

Tips Worth Tweeting

- Vitamin C deficiency can be diagnosed when the plasma concentration of vitamin C is less than 11 micromoles per liter.
- Riboflavin can cause a yellow-orange fluorescence of the urine.
- Folic acid deficiency can be identified through a complete blood count assay. The disease is evident as megaloblastic anemia.
- Serum levels of methylmalonic acid and homocysteine are more effective at detecting vitamin B_{12} deficiency than when evaluating vitamin B_{12} serum levels.
- Vitamin A-induced xerophthalmia is a medical emergency; if not treated, it can lead to blindness.
- For light-skinned individuals, 15 minutes of sunshine exposure on the hands and face twice a week is enough sunlight for the body to make 5 mcg of cholecalciferol.
- Sunscreens with more than 8 SPF will block the ultraviolet light needed to make vitamin D.
- Newborn infants are given a dose of vitamin K immediately after birth to help prevent hemorrhage. Newborn infants are born with a sterile GI tract and cannot manufacture vitamin K until they are colonized with normal gut flora, which usually occurs within 24 hours of birth.
- Patients with vitamin C deficiency or scurvy can be given 300 mg of vitamin C daily, and body stores will be replaced in 5 days.

- Therapeutic doses of niacin for the treatment of cholesterol often cause flushing, a condition that can be prevented with a dose of aspirin (81–325 mg) or ibuprofen (200 mg) about 30 minutes before the niacin dose.
- Women of childbearing potential and pregnant women should consume at least 600 mg of folic acid each day to help prevent neural tube defects in their offspring.
- Taurine is a vitamin-like compound that is found primarily in breastmilk. Taurine is also added to infant formulas and TPN formulas.
- Individuals experiencing magnesium toxicity can be given calcium to block the effects of the magnesium.
- Municipal water supplies are fortified with fluoride to a level of approximately 1 part per million (ppm). Variable amounts are added based on regional differences in the soil concentration of fluoride and the average maximum daily air temperatures in the area. Fluoridating water has decreased dental caries in children by 50%.
- Individuals experiencing copper toxicity can be treated with penicillamine.

Patient Care Scenario: Ambulatory Setting

J. C.: 58 yo F, 5'6", 175 lbs
PMH: s/p colon resection (removal of ileum) after colon cancer; HTN, GERD, type 2 DM
Lab values: Cr 1.1 mg/dL, HgbA$_{1c}$ 6.7%

Medication Profile

Date	Physician	Medication	Sig	Quantity	Refills
5/12	Butler	Lisinopril 20 mg	one daily	30	5
5/12	Butler	Metformin 1,000 mg	one twice daily	60	5
5/12	Butler	Aspirin 81 mg	one daily	100	prn
5/15	Martin	Nexium 20 mg	one daily	30	11

1.1.0 Patient Information

Key Terms

Vitamins are organic substances that are required for the body to maintain normal metabolism, growth, and maintenance. They do not become part of structures in the body, but are required to activate enzymes to regulate and adjust metabolic processes.

Minerals are inorganic substances that become part of the body composition. The mineral content of food varies significantly depending on the soil in which the food was grown. Minerals are required for regulatory and metabolic processes in the body.

Trace minerals are similar to minerals, except they are needed in much smaller quantities.

Dietary Reference Intake (DRI) is the term used to describe the amount of a vitamin needed for optimal function. It includes four reference categories: estimated average requirements (EARs), recommended dietary allowances (RDAs), adequate intakes (AIs), and upper limits (UL).

B-complex vitamins include eight individual B vitamins: thiamin, riboflavin, niacin, vitamin B$_6$, folic acid, vitamin B$_{12}$, pantothenic acid, and biotin.

Signs and Symptoms

In general, malnutrition or low intake of nutritional sources of vitamins and minerals can precipitate signs and symptoms of disease. Symptoms may mask other deficiencies and may be common in several different disease states.

Wellness, Prevention, and Treatment

A general guideline to prevent disease is to eat a wide variety of foods, including protein sources, fruits, and vegetables. The RDAs listed in Table 18-13 are average intake recommendations for adult men and women. For infants, children, and elderly individuals, refer to the Food and Drug Administration's published list for further details.

1.2.0 Pharmacotherapy

Mechanism of Action (Function)

- Vitamin A: the metabolite is responsible for the conversion of light into electrical pulses that send the signal to the optic nerve; ensures healthy epithelial cells; slows osteoclast activity and increases osteoclast activity; maintains energy balance and heat production
- Vitamin D: promotes normal bone mineralization by (1) increasing intestinal absorption of calcium and phosphorus, (2) stimulating bone cells to use the calcium and phosphorus to build and maintain bone, and (3) stimulating the kidneys to recycle calcium to the bloodstream instead of excretion
- Vitamin E: accepts oxygen molecules to prevent oxidative damage or destruction of cellular membranes
- Vitamin K: needed to produce clotting factors II, VII, IX, and X; assists with bone metabolism through the synthesis of osteocalcin
- Vitamin C: used in the formation of collagen; has strong antioxidant properties; aids in the release

Table 18-11 Low Levels of Vitamins and Minerals

Vitamin/Mineral	Name of Disease	Signs and Symptoms	Potential Causes; People at Risk
Vitamin A	Vitamin A deficiency	Night blindness, loss of appetite, altered smell and taste, equilibrium imbalance, halting of bone growth, fetal malformations, xerophthalmia (abnormal thickening of the epithelial tissue covering the eye)	Long-lasting infectious disease, problems with fat absorption, liver disease
Vitamin D	Osteomalacia	Reflected as calcium deficiencies; softening of the bone leading to deformities primarily in the spine, pelvis, and lower extremities	Lack of sunshine, chronic liver or kidney disease, rare genetic disorders, pregnant or lactating mothers
Vitamin D	Rickets	Soft bones and deformed joints in children; bow legs, knock knees, misshapen skulls	Low intake of milk or milk products, limited exposure to sunlight
Vitamin E	Vitamin E deficiency	Neurologic symptoms, peripheral neuropathy, muscle weakness, hemolytic anemia	Premature infants, fat malabsorption syndromes
Vitamin K	Vitamin K deficiency	Prolonged bleeding time, hemorrhage	Newborn infants, adults who avoid green leafy vegetables, individuals on long-term antibiotic therapy
Vitamin C	Scurvy	Early symptoms: tender, sore gums that bleed easily Late symptoms: delayed wound healing, soft bones, fractures, loose teeth, hemorrhages around joints, stomach, and heart; may lead to death if untreated	Individuals who avoid fresh fruits and vegetables, lower socioeconomic status, people on dialysis
Thiamine (vitamin B_1)	Beriberi	Anorexia, indigestion, constipation, apathy, fatigue, muscle weakness, paralysis, muscle atrophy, cardiac failure, Wernicke-Korsakoff syndrome	Alcoholics, artificially nourished individuals, individuals in developing countries where vitamin fortification is not a standard practice
Riboflavin (vitamin B_2)	Ariboflavinosis	Lesions on lips and oral cavity, seborrheic dermatitis, normocytic anemia	Individuals who avoid all dairy products, congenital heart disease, cancer, excessive alcohol intake, women taking oral contraceptives
Niacin (vitamin B_3)	Pellagra	Three D's: dermatitis, diarrhea, and dementia; neuropathy, glossitis, stomatitis, proctitis	Alcoholism, homelessness, malabsorption disorders, GI diseases, psychiatric disorders
Vitamin B_6	Vitamin B_6 deficiency	Neurologic abnormalities, decreased immune function, mouth lesions, depression, confusion	Alcoholism, malabsorption, diarrheal syndromes, certain medications, genetic diseases
Folic acid	Folic acid deficiency	Red, smooth, swollen tongue; heartburn, diarrhea, fainting, fatigue, irritability, forgetfulness, hostile and paranoid behavior, megaloblastic anemia	Malnourished children; pregnant women, infants and young children due to increased growth; infections, malignancy, hyperthyroidism
Vitamin B_{12}	Pernicious anemia	Numbness and tingling in extremities, red blood cell changes, moodiness, confusion, depression, delusions, psychosis	Atrophic gastritis, prolonged use of medications that stop gastric acid secretions, individuals with Crohn's disease of the ileum or removal of the ileum, diets with low animal products, vegetarians
Pantothenic acid	Pantothenic acid deficiency	Somnolence, fatigue, cardiovascular instability, GI complaints, paresthesia of extremities, muscular weakness	Alcoholism, diabetes, inflammatory bowel diseases
Biotin (vitamin H)	Biotin deficiency	Rash, alopecia, muscle pain, paresthesia, depression, hallucinations	Alcoholism, gastrointestinal diseases, long-term anticonvulsant therapy, hemodialysis, long-term antibiotics
Choline	Choline deficiency	Fatty liver, cirrhosis	Growing infants, pregnant and lactating women, strict vegetarians, individuals with cirrhosis, malabsorption syndromes, people receiving TPN

Table 18-11 (*continued*)

Vitamin/Mineral	Name of Disease	Signs and Symptoms	Potential Causes; People at Risk
Carnitine	Carnitine deficiency	Muscle weakness, altered hepatic function, cardiomyopathy, high triglyceride levels, decreased ketogenesis, lipid accumulation between muscle fibers	Liver disease, infants on TPN, patients on dialysis
Taurine	Taurine deficiency	Retinal dysfunction, slow development of auditory brain stem-evoked response, limited fat absorption	Preterm infants, infants with cystic fibrosis
Phosphorus	Hypophos-phatemia	Weakness, anorexia, malaise, pain bone loss	Certain medications, malabsorption disorders, severe burns, uncontrolled diabetes
Magnesium	Magnesium deficiency	Neuroirritability, tetany, disorientation, convulsions, psychosis	Excessive excretion (major surgery, diuretic therapy, diarrhea, vomiting), chronic alcoholism, elderly with poor diets
Chromium	Chromium deficiency	Impaired glucose utilization, peripheral neuropathy, increased free fatty acids in plasma	TPN users without supplementation
Copper	Copper deficiency	Hypochromic anemia (due to impaired iron absorption), thin and fragile bone cortices, spontaneous rupture of major vessels, impaired immune function, depigmentation of skin and hair	Premature infants and infants fed cow's milk, individuals receiving TPN without copper supplementation
Fluoride	Fluoride deficiency	Potential tooth decay	Intake of nonfluoridated water
Iodine	Iodine deficiency	Goiter, myexedema in older children and adults, cretinism in infants born from hypothyroid mothers	Strict vegans who consume sea salt
Manganese	Manganese deficiency	Hypocholesterolemia, nausea, vomiting, dermatitis, pigment changes in hair	Individuals on TPN, and those deliberately trying to avoid dietary intake of manganese
Molybdenum	Molybdenum deficiency	Tachycardia, tachypnea, headache, mental changes, coma	Prolonged TPN users
Selenium	Selenium deficiency	Poor growth, muscle pain and weakness, depigmentation of skin and hair, whitening of nail beds, cardiomyopathy	Vegans, phenlykenonurics, alcoholic cirrhosis
Zinc	Zinc deficiency	Growth retardation in children, delayed wound healing, impaired smell and taste, slowed sexual maturity, hypogonadism, hypospermia, dermatitis, immunologic abnormalities, patchy alopecia	Alcoholism, chronic illness, stress, trauma, surgery, malabsorptive diseases, acrodermatitis enteropathica (genetic defect causing hypoabsorption of zinc)

of adrenaline from adrenal glands; improves iron absorption; converts folic acid into the active form

- Thiamine: coenzyme for carbohydrate metabolism; involved in nerve conduction
- Riboflavin: coenzyme responsible for protein and vitamin metabolism
- Niacin: coenzyme required for energy metabolism; aids in fatty acid synthesis
- Vitamin B_6: coenzyme needed for the synthesis and catabolism of amino acids; assists in the manufacturing of antibodies, epinephrine, dopamine, and serotonin
- Folic acid: involved in DNA and protein synthesis; required for red blood cell maturation
- Vitamin B_{12}: coenzyme required for DNA, RNA and myelin synthesis; required for normal red blood cell formation; assists with protein, fat, carbohydrate, and folate metabolism
- Pantothenic acid: precursor for coenzyme A; required for the synthesis of cholesterol, steroid, and fatty acids; required for energy production from carbohydrates
- Biotin: coenzyme needed for gluconeogenesis, fatty acid metabolism, and amino acid breakdown

Table 18-12 High Levels of Vitamins and Minerals

Vitamin/ Mineral	Name of Disease	Signs and Symptoms	Potential Causes; People at Risk
Vitamin A	Carotenemia	Yellowing of the skin, palms of hands, and feet	Infants fed too many carrots and squash
Vitamin A	Hypervitaminosis A	Headaches, blurred vision, increased intracranial pressure, joint and bone pain, dry skin, and poor appetite	Self-prescribed vitamin A supplements, eating liver multiple times per week
Vitamin E	Hypervitaminosis E	Excessive bleeding, impaired wound healing, depression	Long-term high-dose supplementation
Vitamin C	Hypervitaminosis C	Nausea, abdominal cramps, diarrhea, increased risk of urate stones	High-dose supplementation
Thiamine	Thiamine toxicity	Convulsions, cardiac arrhythmias, anaphylactic shock	Only seen with excessive doses of injectable thiamin
Niacin	Niacin toxicity	Nausea, vomiting, diarrhea, hepatotoxicity, skin lesions, tachycardia, hypertension	Excessive supplementation
Vitamin B_6	Vitamin B_6 toxicity	Neuropathies in extremities, severe ataxia, clumsiness	Excessive supplementation
Choline	Choline toxicity	Sweating, salivation, hypotension, hepatotoxicity, fishy body odor	Excessive supplementation
Carnitine	Carnitine toxicity	Increased frequency and new onset seizures	Excessive supplementation in patients at risk for seizure
Phosphorus	Hyperphosphatemia	Stomach pain, diarrhea	Excessive supplementation; infants fed cow's milk
Magnesium	Magnesium toxicity	Lethargy, sedation, hypotension, decreased pulse and respirations, loss of patellar reflex, cardiac or respiratory arrest	Decreased kidney function
Chromium	Chromium toxicity	Anemia, kidney failure, liver dysfunction, metallic taste in mouth, cognitive and perceptual dysfunction, headache, insomnia, mood changes, irritability	Excessive supplementation, absorption through skin and lungs in an industrial setting
Cobalt	Cobalt toxicity	Goiter, congestive heart failure, myxedema, cardiomyopathy	Excessive supplementation
Copper	Copper toxicity	Copper accumulation in liver, kidneys, brain, spleen, and cornea; diarrhea, nausea, vomiting, hemolysis, convulsions, GI bleeding	Wilson's disease (genetic defect), excess supplementation
Fluoride	Fluorosis	Discoloration of teeth in children up to 8 years of age, bone and kidney dysfunction	Prolonged excessive supplementation
Iodine	Iodine intoxication	Hypothyroidism, hyperthyroidism, taste changes, burning sensation in mouth and throat, soreness of teeth and gums, eye allergy symptoms (swelling, irritation, sneezing)	Excessive supplementation
Manganese	Manganese toxicity	CNS damage, muscle spasms, monotone voice	Inhalation of dust and industrial fumes over long periods of time, individuals with decreased liver function or cholestasis
Molybdenum	Molybdenum toxicity	Gout, hyperuricemia	Excessive supplementation
Selenium	Selenium toxicity	Fatigue, nausea, vomiting, halitosis, nail and hair loss	Excessive supplementation
Vanadium	Vanadium toxicity	Green tongue, GI disturbances, mental dysfunction, hypertension, renal toxicity, depressed growth, neurotoxicity	Excessive supplementation
Zinc	Zinc toxicity	Decreased HDL, decreased copper stores, suppressed immune response, vomiting, dehydration, muscle coordination difficulties, dizziness, GI irritation and abdominal pain	Excessive supplementation

Table 18-13 Vitamin and Mineral RDA and Food Sources

Vitamin/ Mineral	RDA	Common Food Sources
Vitamin A	700 RAE for women 900 RAE for men (See calculations section for a description)	Liver, kidney, egg yolk, fortified milk products, yellow and dark green leafy vegetables, carrots, sweet potatoes, apricots, cantaloupe, peaches
Vitamin D	5 mcg (measured by cholecalciferol)	Fortified milk and milk products, egg yolk, liver, salmon, tuna, sardines
Vitamin E	15 mg (alpha-tocopherol)	Vegetable oils (canola, olive), wheat germ, margarine, green leafy vegetables, milk fat, egg yolks, nuts
Vitamin K	90 mcg for women 120 mcg for men	Green leafy vegetables, vegetables from the cabbage family, liver, vegetable oils
Vitamin C	75 mg for women 90mg for men Smokers require an additional 35 mg daily	Citrus fruits, papaya, cantaloupe, broccoli, Brussels sprouts, green peppers, strawberries, white potatoes, cabbage, chard, kale, turnip greens, asparagus, berries, pineapple, guava
Thiamine	1.1 mg for women 1.2 mg for men	Pork, wheat germ, yeast, black beans, black-eyed peas, sunflower seeds, and fortified cereals
Riboflavin	1.1 mg for women 1.3 mg for men	Milk and dairy products, eggs, organ meats, legumes, fortified cereals
Niacin	14 niacin equivalents (NE) for women 16 NE for men	Meat, fish, poultry, enriched/fortified grain products
Vitamin B_6	1.3 mg for men and women	Sirloin steak, salmon, chicken breast, whole-grain products, fortified cereals and grains, vegetables, bananas, and nuts
Folic acid	400 mcg	Green leafy vegetables, lima beans, kidney beans, oranges and strawberries, liver, fortified cereals and grains
Vitamin B_{12}	2.4 mcg	Meat, milk, cheese, eggs
Pantothenic acid	5 mg*	Liver, egg yolk, legumes, whole-grain cereals, potatoes, and broccoli
Biotin	30 mcg*	Liver, egg yolk, legumes, nuts, tomatoes, cereals
Choline	425 mg* for women 550 mg* for men	Milk, eggs, liver, peanuts
Carnitine	Has not been established	Dairy products, meat
Phosphorus	700 mg for men and women	Lean animal protein, nuts, legumes, milk, egg yolks
Magnesium	310–320 mg for women 400–420 mg for men	Green vegetables, carrots, corn, seeds, nuts, legumes, seafood, chocolate, whole-grain cereals, coffee, tea, tofu
Cobalt	Not identified	Organ meats, oysters, clams, poultry, milk, cream, cheese
Fluoride	3 mg* for women 4 mg* for men	Fluoridated water, fish, fish products, tea
Copper	900 mcg for men and women	Organ meats, shellfish, nuts, seeds, chocolate, dried fruits, poultry, whole grains
Iodine	150 mcg for men and women	Saltwater fish, shellfish, seaweed, eggs, dairy products, fortified table salt
Manganese	1.8 mg* for women 2.3 mg* for men	Wheat bran, legumes, nuts, green leafy vegetables, fruits
Molybdenum	45 mcg for men and women	Legumes, meat, fish, poultry, grains, potatoes, cabbage, carrots, milk
Chromium	25 mcg* for women 35 mcg* for men	Organ meats, poultry, whole grains, cheese, mushrooms, tea, beer, wine, thyme, black pepper

(*continues*)

Table 18-13 (*continued*)

Vitamin/ Mineral	RDA	Common Food Sources
Selenium	55 mcg for men and women	Seafood, organ meats, poultry skin, eggs, nuts, fortified cereals, onions
Vanadium	Not identified	Shellfish, mushrooms, parsley, dill seed, black pepper
Zinc	8 mg for women 11 mg for men	Fortified cereals, shellfish, red meat, cheese

*RDA has not been identified; adequate intakes have been identified.

- Choline: used as a precursor to acetylcholine; assists with the movement of fats within the body
- Carnitine: required for energy production by moving long-chain fatty acids into the mitochondria
- Taurine: protects cell membranes and regulates osmolarity
- Phosphorus: structural component of bone; functional component of phospholipids, carbohydrates, DNA, RNA, and high-energy nucleotides (ADP/ATP)
- Magnesium: required for normal bone formation, transmission of nerve impulses, relaxation of skeletal muscles after contraction, protein synthesis, and carbohydrate metabolism
- Cobalt: essential component of vitamin B_{12}; see vitamin B_{12} functions
- Fluoride: required for bone mineralization; increases enamel resistance to erosion by acids and bacteria
- Copper: cofactor involved in hemoglobin and collagen formation; required for the proper function and structure of the CNS system
- Iodine: required for synthesis of T_3 and T_4
- Manganese: cofactor required in energy metabolism and bone formation
- Molybdenum: cofactor used in sulfur-containing amino acid and purine metabolism; electron transfer agent for oxidation–reduction reactions
- Chromium: potentiates insulin activity; influences cholesterol metabolism
- Selenium: protects cells against oxidation; required for iodine metabolism; protects against heavy metal poisoning; integral for sperm flagella mobility
- Vanadium: insulinomimetic effects; linked to growth and reproduction but exact mechanism is not known
- Zinc: cofactor in the synthesis of DNA and RNA; mobilizes vitamin A from the liver; enhances activity of FSH and LH; needed for immune functions; stabilizes cell membranes; required for sperm production and normal testicular function

Interaction of Drugs with Foods and Laboratory Tests

- Vitamin A: corticosteroids increase excretion of vitamin A; large doses increase the effects of warfarin; bile acid sequestrants and excessive fiber may block absorption of vitamin A; zinc deficiency impairs the conversion of carotene to vitamin A
- Vitamin D: bile acid sequestrants and excessive fiber may block absorption of vitamin D; phenytoin and barbiturates may decrease the half-life of vitamin D
- Vitamin E: bile acid sequestrants and excessive fiber may block absorption of vitamin E; increased effects of warfarin
- Vitamin K: decreases effects of warfarin; broad-spectrum antibiotics disrupt normal flora production of vitamin K; large doses of vitamin E antagonize vitamin K effects
- Vitamin C: megadoses can cause false-positive results on urine glucose tests, and false-negative results on stool guaiac tests looking for occult blood; bile acid sequestrants may block absorption
- Thiamine: alcohol impairs thiamine absorption and increases the rate of destruction of thiamine diphosphate
- Riboflavin: iron, zinc, copper, and manganese inhibit riboflavin absorption; alcohol impairs digestions and absorption of riboflavin
- Niacin: reduces effectiveness of oral hypoglycemic; inhibits uricosuric effects of sulfinpyrazone and probenecid
- Vitamin B_6: isoniazid and hydralazine antagonize pyridoxine; phenobarbital and phenytoin decrease serum levels; levodopa is less effective with supplementation of pyridoxine
- Folic acid: zinc deficiency and chronic alcohol intake decrease absorption of folic acid; methotrexate is a folic acid antagonist; aspirin displaces folic acid from its protein and increases excretion; phenytoin decreases absorption of

folic acid; trimethoprim decreases folic acid activity and effectiveness; large doses of pyrimethamine may cause megaloblastic anemia; sulfasalazine decreases folic acid absorption when the two medications are administered together

- Vitamin B_{12}: metformin, colchicine, anticonvulsants, vitamin C supplementation, antibiotics, proton pump inhibitors, and H2-blockers can decrease vitamin B_{12} absorption
- Biotin: raw egg whites contain an enzyme that blocks absorption of biotin
- Carnitine: valproic acid decreases carnitine stores
- Phosphorus: magnesium, calcium, aluminum antacids and sucralfate decrease absorption of phosphorus
- Magnesium: calcium and phosphorus can inhibit magnesium; tetracyclines and fluoroquinolones have decreased absorption when taken with magnesium antacids
- Chromium: absorption is enhanced by vitamin C; decreased absorption occurs when taken with antacids; may enhance hypoglycemic medications; NSAIDs increase absorption and retention of chromium
- Copper: high-dose vitamin C and zinc decrease the absorption and effectiveness of copper; antacids may decrease the absorption of copper
- Fluoride: decreased effects and absorption when given with magnesium, aluminum, or calcium
- Iodine: lithium may increase hypothyroid effects
- Molybdenum: antagonized by high copper intake
- Zinc: reduced absorption from fiber, phytates, oxalates, tannins, and chelating agents; iron inhibits zinc absorption; gastric alkinalizers decrease absorption of zinc; zinc taken with fluoroquinolones and tetracyclines can decrease the absorption of the antibiotic

Contraindications, Warnings, and Precautions

Niacin can cause histamine release, so it should be used with caution in patients with asthma. Also, use caution with medication in patients who have gastritis or peptic ulcer disease due to the GI side effects caused by niacin.

Physiochemical Properties, Pharmacodynamics, and Pharmacokinetic Properties

Fat-soluble vitamins are more stable and less sensitive to oxidation, heat, light and pH.

1.3.0 Pharmacotherapy Monitoring

See Table 18-15.

2.1.0 Dispensing

Calculations

Fat-soluble vitamins were once reported in International Units (IU). As this unit is still used frequently in reports and on labels, it is important to understand the measurement. IUs of fat-soluble vitamins are not equal.

Vitamin A

- Animal foods: 3.3 IU = 1 mcg of retinol activity equivalents (RAE)
- Plant foods: 10 IU = 12 mcg of beta-carotene or 24 mcg of other provitamin A carotenoids
- Supplements: 10 IU of provitamin A = 1 mcg RAE

Vitamin D

- 40 IU = 1 mcg of cholecalciferol

Vitamin E

- Natural form: 1.4 IU = 1 mg of alpha-tocopherol
- Synthetic form: 1 IU = 1 mg of alpha-tocopherol

Niacin Equivalents

- 60 mg of tryptophan = 1 mg niacin

Generic Names, Brand Names, and Dosage Forms Availability

- Vitamin D: Vitamin D_2 (ergocalciferol) is activated by sunlight in plants; vitamin D_3 (cholecalciferol) is activated by sunlight or ultraviolet light in the skin of animals and humans.
- Vitamin K: three forms. Vitamin K_1 is found in plant sources and is called phylloquinone. A synthetic water-soluble version of vitamin K_1 is available by prescription and is called phytonadione. Vitamin K_2 (menaquinone) is formed from intestinal bacteria.
- Vitamin B_6: three forms—pyridoxal, pyridoxamine, and pyridoxine. All three are found in nutritional sources, but pyridoxine is the most common form available in vitamins and supplements.
- Vitamin B_{12}: Cyanocobalamin is the most common form in supplements. Hydroxycobalamin is a longer-acting form and is equipotent to cyanocobalamin.

Iron and zinc compete for the same absorption sites. Ensure that vitamins and supplements have less than a 2:1 ratio of iron to zinc to facilitate absorption of zinc. Pregnant women consuming more than 60 mg of iron daily should be encouraged to take an additional zinc supplement. When iron and zinc are taken in as part of a meal, the absorption issues tend to be less problematic than when these nutrients are taken in a supplement.

Physical Attributes of Commercial Products

Vitamin B_{12} (cyanocobalamin) is a thick, red-colored solution that is stored in multidose or single-dose vials.

Table 18-14 Physiochemical, Pharmacodynamic, and Pharmacokinetic Properties of Vitamins and Minerals

Vitamin/ Mineral	ADME Properties	Comments
Vitamin A	70–90% absorbed when consumed with 10 g of fat	Less than 5% absorbed from raw vegetables; the body can store a years' worth of vitamin A, primarily in the liver
Vitamin D	50% of dietary intake is absorbed, most rapidly in the duodenum; greatest extent in the small intestine	Liver converts inactive vitamin D to calcitriol; absorption decreases with age; aging also decreases the skin's ability to manufacture cholecalciferol
Vitamin E	45% absorbed from normal foods along with fat; absorbed in the jejunum; excreted as bile	Maximum transfer of vitamin E across the placenta occurs just before term delivery
Vitamin K	Phylloquinone is primarily absorbed in the jejunum; menaquinone is absorbed in the distal small intestine and colon; unused vitamin K is excreted in the urine and feces	Turnover of vitamin K occurs every 2.5 hours
Vitamin C	Absorbed in the small intestine	An inverse relationship exists between consumption and absorption: as consumption increases, the amount absorbed decreases
Thiamine	Absorbed in the small intestine primarily in the jejunum; excess thiamin is excreted in the urine	Need for thiamine increases with carbohydrate intake
Riboflavin	Absorbed in the small intestine; excess is excreted by the kidneys	Excretion is enhanced by diabetes, stress, and trauma
Niacin	Liver helps convert tryptophan to niacin	Niacin found in corn cannot be absorbed by the body unless treated by lye to release the niacin; only vitamin known with an amino acid as a provitamin
Vitamin B_6	Absorbed in the small intestine, primarily in the jejunum; excretion is dominated by the kidneys	
Folic acid	50% of folate from food sources is absorbed; the jejunum is the most efficient site of absorption; excretion is through urine and bile	Folic acid is generally bound to amino acids in food and needs to be separated by an enzyme for absorption; the enzyme (folate conjugase) is found in salivary, gastric, pancreatic, and jejunal secretions; synthetic folic acid is absorbed more efficiently
Vitamin B_{12}	Absorbed in the ileum; long half-life	Absorption depends on body stores' when levels are low, more of the vitamin is absorbed; when levels are high, low amounts of vitamins are absorbed
Biotin	Absorbed in the large intestine	Gut flora can produce adequate amounts of biotin that will then be available for absorption
Phosphorus	50–70% of dietary sources is absorbed, primarily in the duodenum and jejunum; eliminated in feces; excess phosphorus is eliminated by the kidneys	Low body levels cause the liver to produce more vitamin D to help increase absorption
Magnesium	Absorbed throughout the small intestine but mostly in the distal jejunum and ileum; excess magnesium is excreted by the kidneys and is enhanced by protein, alcohol, and caffeine intakes	Absorption is better with low levels, and vice versa; may be absorbed in the colon if the small intestine is unable to handle this process
Chromium	Absorbed throughout the small intestine; excretion is dominated by the kidneys	Low bioavailability, higher absorption in lower dietary intake
Copper	Absorbed in the small intestine, primarily in the duodenum; excretion is via the liver and biliary tract into feces	Excretion increases as body stores increase, and vice versa
Fluoride	Nearly 100% of fluoridated water and toothpaste is rapidly absorbed in the stomach and small intestine; excess levels are excreted in urine primarily, followed by feces and sweat	Absorption decreases when fluoride is consumed in solid foods; gastric acid secretions increase absorption

Table 18-14 (*continued*)

Vitamin/ Mineral	ADME Properties	Comments
Iodine	Absorbed from all portions of the GI tract; excreted primarily from the kidneys, some lost in sweat	33% of absorbed iodine is used for T_3 and T_4 formation; the remainder is excreted
Manganese	Absorbed in small intestine; excretion occurs through bile	Biologic functions can sometimes be replaced by other minerals
Molybdenum	Absorbed in stomach and small intestine; excreted mainly through urine	Also excreted in feces, sweat, and hair
Selenium	Absorbed in small intestine; excreted equally in urine and feces	Urinary excretion maintains homeostasis
Zinc	Absorbed from small intestine; excreted primarily in feces but smaller amounts in exfoliated skin cells, sweat, semen, menstrual flow, and hair	Same absorption site as iron; absorption enhanced in gastric acidity

Table 18-15 Nutrient Upper Limits

Nutrient	Tolerable Upper Limit (mg/day)
Vitamin A	3
Vitamin D	0.05
Vitamin E	1,000
Vitamin C	2,000
Folic acid	1
Niacin	35
Vitamin B_6	100
Choline	3,500
Calcium	2,500
Magnesium	350
Phosphorus	4,000
Copper	10
Fluoride	10
Iodine	1.1
Manganese	11
Molybdenum	2
Selenium	0.4
Vanadium	1.8
Zinc	40

Packaging, Storage, Handling, and Disposal

- Vitamin A: Carrots packaged in plastic bags retain carotene better than bulk carrots; more beta-carotene is available to the body when lightly cooked with a small amount of fat compared to raw carrots,
- Vitamin E: Frying food sources of vitamin E can destroy this nutrient.
- Water-soluble vitamins are lost during the cooking process. Water in which vegetables were cooked contains one-third to one-half of the starting amount of the vitamin in the food source. Vitamin C is the most easily destroyed vitamin: It is sensitive to heat, oxidation, and alkaline environments.
- Frozen concentrated orange juice contains more vitamin C than ready-to-drink cartons. Concentrations of vitamin C drop quickly once the container is opened, so the juice should be consumed shortly after opening.
- Roasting coffee beans increases the niacin content by 30 times. High intake of coffee can prevent pellagra in cultures with low protein intake.

Compound Preparations and Sterile Products

Injectable phytonadione can cause anaphylaxis reactions; its use should be reserved for those patients who are hemorrhaging due to vitamin K deficiency.

ANNOTATED BIBLIOGRAPHY

http://www.fnic.nal.usda.gov/nal_display/index.php?tax_level=1&info_center=4. Accessed April 19, 2012.

http://www.ncam.nih.gov/health/vitamins?nav=rss. Accessed April 19, 2012.

Organ Transplant

CHAPTER 19

Contributor: *Michael M. Milks*

Tips Worth Tweeting

- HLA and MCH proteins are essentially equivalent and enable antigen-presenting cells to present antigen peptides to CD4 helper T cells and CD8 cytotoxic T lymphocytes.
- Most organ transplants are cost-effective in the overall management of chronic organ failure conditions.
- The biggest challenge in organ transplant is finding the appropriate balance between adequate suppression of tissue rejection and the risk of excessive immunocompromise, drug toxicity, and drug side effects.
- The main classes of drugs used to prevent rejection include glucocorticoids, antimetabolites, calcineurin inhibitors, proliferation signal inhibitors, and immunosuppressive antibodies (polyclonal or monoclonal).
- The cardinal principle in organ transplant is to combine antirejection medication classes with different pharmacologic mechanisms of action to allow the lowest possible dose of each to be used, thereby minimizing adverse drug effects.
- Aggressive immunosuppression at the outset is imperative to facilitate early engraftment success and to minimize acute rejection phenomena, while longer-term management is typically successful at substantially reduced dosages of these powerful drugs.

Organ Transplantation Immunosuppressants

Background

History of Autotransplantation and Transplantation

From the earliest reports in ancient (1000 B.C.) India of surgeons performing dermal rhinoplasty to repair certain nasal deformities by surgically attaching a flap of skin from a patient's forehead, the procedure of autotransplantation of skin from one site on a patient's body to another developed into a medical art (Tilney, 2003). As the sophistication of the surgeons' skills advanced, so, too, did the manifold applications of reconstructive surgery. Early attempts at allografts (tissue obtained from nonidentical members of the same species) and xenografts (tissue from a donor species different than that of the recipient), however, were doomed by nearly inevitable tissue rejection. Moreover, repeated attempts at performing skin allografts or xenografts were met with an accelerated rejection (Tilney, 2003).

Blood transfusions among nonrelated individuals enjoyed far greater success, providing the compatibility of donor and recipient ABO blood groups was appropriately determined according to the system described by Karl Landsteiner in 1901 (Parham, 2009). Eventually, a system of cell surface proteins, quite apart from the ABO blood group proteins, was recognized, defined, and demonstrated by Jean Dausset in the 1950s and 1960s; it was observed to profoundly determine immunogenicity and immune tolerance of transplanted tissues (Tilney, 2003).

HLA and MHC

This system of human leukocyte antigens (HLA) was subsequently realized as being equivalent to the major histocompatibility complex (MHC) proteins, which are genetically encoded in hundreds of variant alleles at multiple loci on chromosome 6. Essentially, each individual inherits a haploid set of six specific MHC gene alleles from each parent, and the exact combination of these 12 MHC genes determines that individual's immunologic "fingerprint" (Kindt et al., 2007). In fact, it is with this series of specific MHC surface proteins that antigen-presenting cells (APCs) such as macrophages, Langerhans cells, and dendritic cells bind internally processed antigens and "present" these smaller antigen peptides to the T-cell receptors (TCRs) on immunoreactive lymphocytes, particularly the CD4 helper T cells and the CD8 cytotoxic T lymphoctyes (Kindt et al., 2007).

With the advent of surgical anesthesia, advances in surgical antisepsis, and the introduction of immunosuppressant drugs (e.g., adrenocorticosteroids and cyclosporine), organ transplantation has become practically commonplace. Nearly 500,000 transplants were performed in the United States between 1988 and 2009 (OPTN, 2010), and 105,957 patients are currently waiting to receive a vital transplant (UNOS, 2010).

Despite the considerable costs involved in performing such life-sustaining surgeries, combined with the considerable expense of the ongoing immunosuppressant therapy, most organ transplants do provide long-term pharmacoeconomic advantage in the overall management of many disease states involving chronic organ failure (Cavanaugh and Martin, 2007). One particularly vexing aspect of the clinical management of transplant patients is finding the appropriate balance between adequate suppression of tissue rejection and the risk of excessive immunocompromise, drug toxicity, and other drug-associated side effects.

1.1.0 Patient Information and 1.3.0 Monitoring

Signs and Symptoms of Solid-Organ Transplant Rejection

Table 19-1 summarizes the more common signs and symptoms associated with organ rejection of the three most common solid-organ transplants—kidney, liver, and heart.

Table 19-1 Signs and Symptoms of Kidney, Liver, and Heart Transplant Rejection

Organ	Signs and Symptoms of Tissue Rejection		
Kidney	Fever Malaise Oliguria	Edema Hypertension Weight gain	Elevated BUN Elevated serum creatinine Pain and tenderness of graft
Liver	Fever Lethargy Anorexia	Back pain Ileus	Pain and tenderness of graft Elevated liver function tests: • γ-Glutamyl transpeptidase • Serum bilirubin • Alkaline phosphatase • Transaminases • Prothrombin time
Heart	Fever Lethargy Weakness	Dyspnea Tachycardia Arrhythmia	Pericardial friction rub

1.2.0 Pharmacotherapy and 1.3.0 Monitoring

Immunosuppressant Drug Classes

The commercially available immunosuppressant drugs approved by the FDA for use in organ transplant patients are typically categorized into several major pharmacological classes:

- Glucocorticoids (corticosteroids) (e.g., prednisone, methylprednisolone, dexamethasone)
- Antimetabolites (e.g., azathioprine, mycophenolate mofetil)
- Calcineurin inhibitors (e.g., cyclosporine, tacrolimus)
- Proliferation signal inhibitors (e.g., sirolimus)
- Immunosuppressive antibodies
  - Polyclonal (e.g., antithymocyte globulin)
  - Monoclonal (e.g., muromonab-CD3, basiliximab, daclizumab)

One of the cardinal pharmacotherapeutic principles of using antirejection drug therapy in managing patients who have received tissue transplants is to combine several agents, each asserting an immunosuppressive effect by a *different* pharmacological mechanism, so that synergistic effects may be developed at relatively low doses of each agent, thereby limiting the drug-specific toxicities while maximizing the overall antirejection

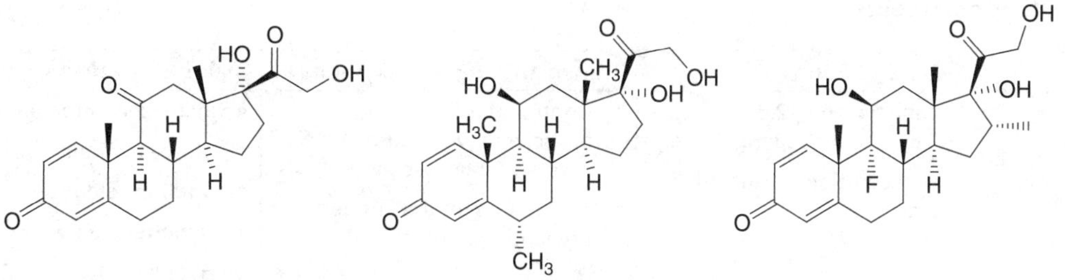

Figure 19-1 The Adrenocorticosteroid Antirejection Drugs Have a Similar Chemistry

response. Furthermore, use of aggressive immunosuppression at the outset is imperative to facilitate early engraftment success and to minimize acute rejection phenomena. Longer-term management is typically successful at substantially reduced dosages of these powerful drugs (Krensky et al., 2006). The key to therapeutic success with these "double-edged pharmacotherapeutic swords" is careful monitoring of the patient, and especially of the function of the transplanted organ or tissue, with acute vigilance for early signs of rejection or drug toxicity, and clinical acumen focused on the prevention and early treatment of infection.

Glucocorticoids

Glucocorticoids have become a mainstay of antirejection pharmacotherapeutics (Tilney, 2003). With an incredible array of pharmacological effects, glucocorticoids exert impressive anti-inflammatory and antirejection effects. After binding to cytosolic receptors, glucocorticoids are translocated to the nucleus of the cell. The drug/receptor complex then binds to and activates various "hormone response elements" at various sites along the DNA, initiating gene expression of a multitude of proteins that serve to attenuate the inflammatory response. Annexins (lipocortins) are one such group of anti-inflammatory proteins that inhibit phospholipase A_2, thereby diminishing the mobilization of arachidonic acid from cellular membranes and, in turn, decreasing the de novo synthesis of prostaglandins, leukotrienes, other eicosanoids, and even platelet-activating factor. Furthermore, glucocorticoids are known to produce a marked downregulation of the gene expression of cyclooxyengase-2 (COX-2), further diminishing any production of inflammatory prostaglandins (Smyth et al., 2006). Glucocorticoids also limit the number of lymphocytes in circulation, in part by effecting a greater degree of apoptosis in activated cells. Secretion of pro-inflammatory cytokines, such as interleukin-1 (IL-1) and interleukin-6 (IL-6), is likewise downregulated, and the phagocytic actions and chemotactic responses of neutrophils and monocytes are also diminished (Krensky et al., 2006).

The adrenocorticosteroid antirejection drugs all have a conspicuously similar chemistry (Figure 19-1) and pharmacology, differing primarily in potency, sodium-retaining propensity, duration of action, and pharmacokinetic disposition. A summary of the chemistry, therapeutic applications, and major side effects of three prominent examples of anti-inflammatory steroids appears in Table 19-2.

Antimetabolites

The antimetabolite class of immunosuppressant drugs used to manage organ rejection phenomena includes such prominent examples as azathioprine (Imuran) and mycophenolate mofetil (CellCept). Other immunosuppressant antimetabolites drugs, including methotrexate and cyclophosphamide, also have important clinical applications in a broad array of inflammatory conditions, ranging from graft-versus-host disease to rheumatoid arthritis to lupus nephritis to psoriasis. Mechanistically, all of the drugs of this class exhibit substrate-level interference with the biochemical pathways leading to the immune response, inflammation, or cytotoxicity, thereby moderating the rejection of tissue transplants.

Azathioprine, a purine antimetabolite, was first launched as an immunosuppressant drug in 1961, greatly facilitating the advance of renal allograft transplantation. Appropriately considered a "prodrug," azathioprine is metabolized to 6-mercaptopurine, which is in turn converted into several inhibitors of de novo purine biosynthesis. Additionally, the metabolic conversion of 6-mercaptopurine into 6-thio-guanosine triphosphate allows for its faulty incorporation into DNA, resulting in even more interference with DNA biosynthesis. Without DNA synthesis, lymphocyte mitogenesis is precluded and the immune rejection mediated by these important immunocytes is greatly diminished.

Although the parent drug has a typical plasma half-life of 10 minutes, its active metabolites possess half-lives as long as 5 hours, allowing for once-daily or twice-daily oral administration. Methylation by erythrocytes and hepatic metabolism by xanthine oxidase

Table 19-2 Glucocorticoids

Drug	Dosage Forms	Transplantation Applications	Major Side Effects
Prednisone	Tablets: 1 mg, 2.5 mg, 5 mg, 10 mg, 20 mg, 50 mg Oral solution: 5 mg/5 mL, 5 mg/mL	• Control of inflammation associated with acute and chronic tissue rejection • Attenuation of the antigen-presenting effect	• Increased intracranial pressure • Slowed wound healing • Sodium retention • Hypertension • Hypokalemia • Congestive heart failure • Decreased carbohydrate tolerance • Menstrual irregularities • Peptic ulcer • Muscle weakness
Methylprednisolone (Medrol)	Tablets: 2 mg, 4 mg, 8 mg, 16 mg, 24 mg, 32 mg	• Processes that perpetuate immune recognition and rejection	• Cataracts
Dexamethasone (formerly available as Decadron)	Tablets: 0.25 mg, 0.5 mg, 0.75 mg, 1 mg, 1.5 mg, 2 mg, 4 mg, 6 mg Oral elixir and oral solution: 0.5 mg/5 mL Oral solution (concentrate): 1 mg/mL		

account for the majority of 6-mercaptopurine inactivation. The xanthine oxidase pathway is critically inhibited by the antigout drug, allopurinol (Zyloprim); thus, if this xanthine oxidase inhibitor is to be coadministered with azathioprine, the dose of the latter *must* be reduced to only one fourth or one third of the typical dose.

Many of the major side effects of azathioprine are predictable consequences of its interference with DNA synthesis and cell proliferation, particularly in tissues with a typically high rate of cellular mitosis, such as bone marrow, GI mucosa, germ tissue, and fetal tissues. Thiopurine methyltransferase (TPMT) genotyping or phenotyping can help identify those patients who are at increased risk for severe, life-threatening myelosuppression due to significantly diminished TPMT activity (i.e., who are homozygous for nonfunctional alleles, especially *TPMT*2*, *TPMT*3A*, and *TPMT*3C*).

In addition to being indicated as an adjunct for the prevention of rejection in renal homotransplantation, azathioprine is indicated to reduce the signs and symptoms of active rheumatoid arthritis.

Another important antimetabolite drug utilized in the management of organ transplant patients is mycophenolate mofetil. Like azathioprine, mycophenolate is a prodrug. Subsequent to its rapid oral absorption, mycophenolate mofetil is hydrolyzed to the active metabolite, mycophenolic acid (MPA), which is a potent inhibitor of inosine monophosphate dehydrogenase (IMPDH), thereby blocking the de novo biosynthesis of guanosine nucleotides, and consequently interfering with the synthesis of DNA. Because both T lymphocytes and B lymphocytes are critically dependent on this de novo pathway for purine biosynthesis, DNA synthesis within lymphocytes is inhibited, as is proliferation and immune activity.

With an approximate plasma half-life of 18 hours, twice-daily dosing is standard for this oral immunosuppressive agent. Mycophenolate is indicated for the prophylaxis of organ rejection of allogeneic renal, cardiac, or hepatic transplants. It should be used concomitantly with cyclosporine and corticosteroids, and it has been used clinically to suppress inflammatory manifestations in such conditions as lupus nephritis, refractory uveitis, and Churg-Strauss syndrome.

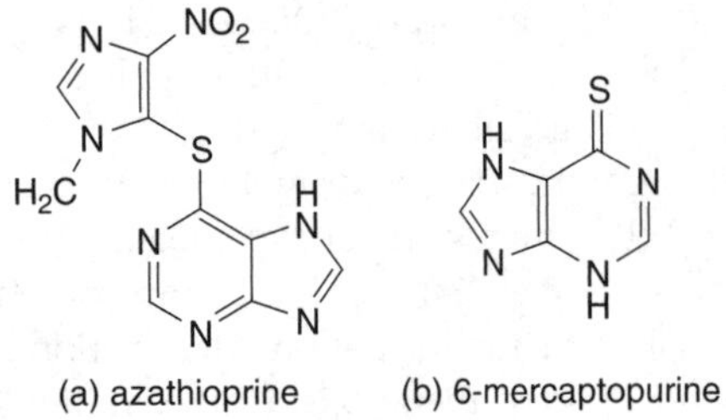

Figure 19-2 Azathioprine is Metabolized to 6-Mercaptopurine

Calcineurin Inhibitors

Some of the most potent immunosuppressant drugs used in the management of tissue and organ transplant

Table 19-3 Antimetabolites

Drug	Dosage Forms	Transplantation Applications	Major Side Effects
Azathioprine (Imuran)	Tablets: 50 mg	Adjunct for the prevention of rejection in renal transplants	• Leukopenia • Immunosuppression • Risk of severe infection • Thrombocytopenia • Macrocytic anemia • Pancytopenia • Depressed spermatogenesis • Neoplasia • Teratogenesis
Azathioprine (Azasan)	Tablets: 75 mg, 100 mg		
Azathioprine sodium	Injection: 5 mg/mL		
Mycophenolate mofetil (CellCept) Other generics	Capsules: 250 mg Tablets: 500 mg Powder for oral suspension: 200 mg/mL	For concomitant use with cyclosporine and corticosteroids to prevent organ rejections in patients receiving allogeneic renal, heart, and liver transplants	
Mycophenolate mofetil (Myfortic)	Delayed-release tablets: 180 mg, 360 mg		
Mycophenolate mofetil hydrochloride for injection (CellCept Intravenous)	Powder for reconstitution and subsequent dilution with 5% dextrose to yield 6 mg/mL for intravenous administration		

patients belong to the antibiotic class of drugs known to inhibit the activity of an important regulatory phosphatase, calcineurin. Each of these drugs binds to a separate cytoplasmic immunophilin protein: cyclosporine (Sandimmune, Neoral) binds to cyclophilin, and tacrolimus (Prograf; previously known as FK506) binds to its associated immunophilin, FK-binding protein (FKBP). The resultant drug/immunophilin complexes powerfully inhibit the action of calcineurin, a phosphatase that is critical in the dephosphorylation of the nuclear factor of activated T cells (NFAT). Only when NFAT is dephosphorylated does it become able to be translocated into the nucleus, where it is required for the transcription of interleukin-2 (previously known as T-cell growth factor [TCGF]) and other powerful lymphokines. Thus, cyclosporine (which received FDA approval in 1983) and tacrolimus (FDA approved in 1994) are potent immunosuppressive agents that have become cornerstone pharmacotherapeutic agents in managing a broad array of organ and tissue transplant patients.

For prophylaxis against organ rejection, the 11-amino acid cyclic polypeptide drug cyclosporine should be administered with adrenal corticosteroids, but *not* with other immunosuppressive agents due to the risk of increased susceptibility to infection and the possible development of lymphoma owing to profound immunosuppression. In addition to preventing and managing organ rejection in allogenic renal, heart, and liver transplants, other FDA-approved indications for cyclosporine include recalcitrant plaque psoriasis as well as rheumatoid arthritis that has not responded adequately to methotrexate. "Off-label" anti-inflammatory and immune-modulating therapeutic applications of cyclosporine include multiple sclerosis, graft-versus-host disease, aplastic anemia, and refractory leukemias.

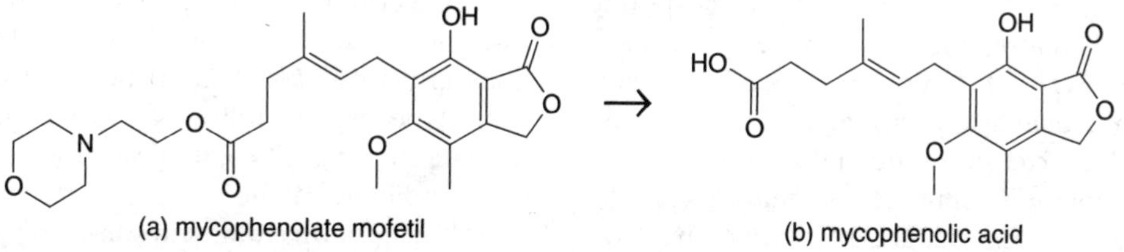

Figure 19-3 Mycophenolate Mofetil (a) is Hydrolized to the Active Metabolite, Mycophenolic Acid (b)

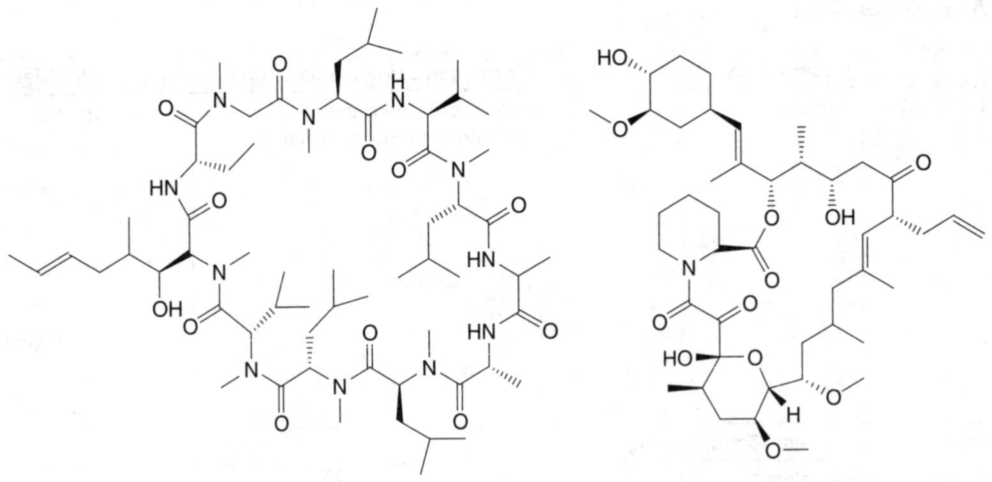

(a) cyclosporine (b) tacrolimus

Figure 19-4 Cyclosporine (a) and Tacrolimus (b) are Potent Immunosuppressive Agents

Because of the severity of certain side effects of cyclosporine, the imperative need for adequate control of rejection phenomena, and the sometimes erratic absorption of cyclosporine, routine monitoring of cyclosporine blood concentrations is an essential component of patient management. Furthermore, because cyclosporine and tacrolimus are extensively metabolized by cytochrome P-450 3A4 (CYP3A4), patients must be advised to avoid fluctuations in their ingestion of grapefruit and grapefruit juice while taking either of these two calcineurin inhibitors.

Another critical issue in the safe and effective pharmacotherapeutic management of patients receiving cyclosporine is the need to pay careful attention to the various commercial products, which may *not* always be bioequivalent. Notably, Sandimmune Soft Gelatin Capsules (cyclosporine capsules, USP) and Sandimmune Oral Solution (cyclosporine oral solution, USP) have substantially decreased bioavailability in comparison to Neoral Soft Gelatin Capsules and Gengraf capsules (cyclosporine capsules, USP [Modified]) and Neoral and Gengraf Oral Solution (cyclosporine oral solution, [Modified]). The latter "modified" products form microemulsions when dispersed in aqueous environments and yield substantially greater oral bioavailability—as much as twofold greater oral absorption than the standard cyclosporine oral solution USP preparations (e.g., Sandimmune). Clearly, such products are not bioequivalent with the standard USP versions of cyclosporine products and, therefore, they should never be used interchangeably without physician supervision. Furthermore, the microemulsion-forming cyclosporine oral liquids should be mixed in orange juice or apple juice (preferably at room temperature), but *not* milk as this combination can be unpalatable; in contrast, the standard cyclosporine USP oral solutions *may* be diluted with milk, chocolate milk, or orange juice. Both types of oral solutions should be mixed in a glass—not plastic—container.

Proliferation Signal Inhibitors

Another class of powerful immunosuppressant agents of the macrolide antibiotic class that are useful in managing renal allograft transplant patients includes sirolimus (Rapamune). Although chemically similar to tacrolimus, sirolimus (formerly known as rapamycin) also binds to the cytoplasmic immunophilin FKBP-12, but the complex does *not* inhibit the phosphatase calcineurin. Rather, the FKBP–sirolimus complex exerts powerful inhibition of the regulatory tyrosine kinase m-TOR (mammalian target of rapamycin), thereby blocking the proliferative response of T lymphocytes to antigens and to such important cytokines as interleukin -2 (IL-2), IL-4, and IL-15. The immunosuppressive effects of sirolimus not only dramatically interfere with T-lymphocyte activation and proliferation, but also potently diminish B-lymphocyte immune responses and even mononuclear cell proliferation and activation. This profound interference with biochemical pathways involved in cellular proliferation has led to the pharmacological development of a chemical analogue, everolimus (Affinitor), for the clinical management of advanced renal cell carcinoma.

Sharing similar chemistry with tacrolimus, along with powerful immunosuppressant actions, sirolimus is associated with an analogous set of adverse drug reactions and toxicities. Thus patients receiving sirolimus should be closely followed with regular therapeutic drug monitoring. The chemical structure of sirolimus is given in Figure 19-5.

The pharmacokinetic disposition of sirolimus is also quite similar to that of tacrolimus—namely,

Table 19-4 Calcineurin Inhibitors

Drug	Dosage Forms	Transplantation Applications	Major Side Effects
Cyclosporine USP (Sandimmune) Other generics	Oral capsules: 25 mg, 100 mg Oral solution: 100 mg/mL	Prophylaxis of organ rejection in kidney, liver, and heart allogeneic transplants	• Nephrotoxicity • Hypertension • Immunosuppression • Risk of severe infection • Lymphoma and other neoplasms • Tremor • Hirsuitism • Gum hyperplasia
Cyclosporine USP [modified] (Neoral, Gengraf) Other generics	Soft gelatin oral capsules: 25 mg, 100 mg		
Cyclosporine USP [modified] Other generics	Soft gelatin oral capsules: 50 mg		
Cyclosporine USP [modified] (Neoral, Gengraf) Other generics	Oral solution: 100 mg/mL		
Cyclosporine USP (Sandimmune) Other generics	Injection solution concentrate: 50 mg/mL		
Tacrolimus (Prograf) Other generics	Capsules: 0.5 mg, 1 mg, 5 mg	Prophylaxis of organ rejection in kidney, liver, and heart allogeneic transplants	• Nephrotoxicity • Hypertension • Hyperkalemia • Myocardial hypertrophy • Risk of severe infections • Lymphoma and other malignancies • Insulin-dependent post-transplant diabetes mellitus • Neurotoxicity
Tacrolimus (Prograf Injection Solution, concentrate)	Prograf solution for IV injection (5 mg/mL); must be diluted with 0.9% sodium chloride injection or 5% dextrose injection to a concentration between 0.004 mg/mL and 0.02 mg/mL prior to use		

extensive intestinal wall and hepatic metabolism by the cytochrome P-450 3A4 enzymes. In turn, sirolimus has the expected interference of metabolism by grapefruit juice and the list of drugs known to interfere with CYP3A4 activity, including the strong inducers (e.g., rifampin, rifabutin) and the strong inhibitors (e.g., ketoconazole, voriconazole, itraconazole, erythromycin, telithromycin, clarithromycin). The terminal elimination half-life ($t_{½}$) of sirolimus is about 60 hours, allowing for once-daily dosing of oral tablets or oral solution. To minimize variability in sirolimus concentrations, sirolimus should be taken consistently with or without food.

Immunosuppressive Antibodies

The use of various antisera to provide passive immunity in the medical management of a broad array of medical conditions—ranging from snakebites, to diphtheria, to rabies, to autoimmune disease—continues

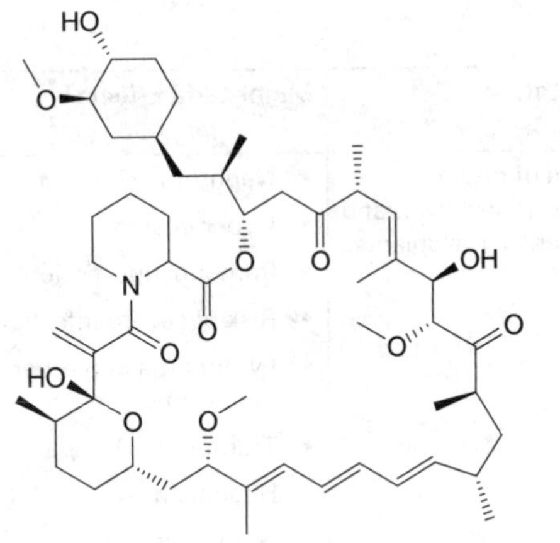

Figure 19-5 Sirolimus

to provide an immunotherapeutic approach to managing multiple medical maladies. This approach has also been applied in modulating immune rejection of various transplanted tissues and organs, and several related products are available for clinical use in managing transplant patients.

First used in 1967, the oldest and least specific of these immunosuppressive pharmaceuticals is antithymocyte globulin (equine), also known as lymphocyte immune globulin, commercially available as Atgam. This purified, concentrated, and sterile gamma globulin is obtained from the serum of horses immunized with human thymus lymphocytes. It is indicated for the management of allograft rejection in renal transplant patients and in certain cases of aplastic anemia. As a tissue transplant immunosuppressive agent, antithymocyte globulin is typically used concomitantly with azathioprine and corticosteroids, and is administered by slow intravenous infusion over 4 hours or longer. By immunologically binding to various surface antigens on human T lymphocytes, antithymocyte globulin causes profound interference with and rapid elimination of circulating lymphocytes, thereby leaving the host immune response dramatically diminished. Its use to prevent or abort acute rejection is limited by its cost, its toxicity, and the development of host antibodies to the foreign equine drug antibodies.

An analogous product is produced in rabbits (antithymocyte globulin [rabbit]; Thymoglobulin). Although this variant avoids the classic hypersensitivity to equine antibodies, a similar allergic response to rabbit immunoglobulins can develop. Like antithymocyte globulin (equine), antithymocyte globulin (rabbit) is indicated for the treatment of renal transplant acute rejection in conjunction with concomitant immunosuppression. It should be administered by slow intravenous infusion over a minimum of 6 hours for the first infusion and over at least 4 hours on subsequent days of therapy.

A similar pattern of side effects occurs with both the equine and the rabbit antithymocyte globulin preparations. In particular, these drugs are linked with cytokine release syndrome (CRS), which characteristically includes high fever (often spiking up to 107°F), chills/rigors, headache, tremor, nausea/vomiting, diarrhea, abdominal pain, malaise, muscle/joint aches and pains, and generalized weakness. Other clinical signs and symptoms of anaphylaxis should also be closely monitored, such as generalized rash, tachycardia, pulmonary edema, dyspnea, and hypotension.

Table 19-5 Proliferation Signal Inhibitors

Drug	Dosage Forms	Transplantation Applications	Major Side Effects
Sirolimus (rapamycin) (Rapamune)	Oral tablets: 0.5 mg, 1 mg, 2 mg Oral solution: 1 mg/mL (to be mixed in a glass or plastic cup containing at least 2 oz of water or orange juice)	Prophylaxis of organ rejection in kidney transplants	• Fluid accumulation • Peripheral edema • Slowed wound healing • Decline in renal function • Proteinuria • Hyperlipidemia • Hypertension • Anemia • Thrombocytopenia • Immunosuppression • Risk of severe infection • Lymphoma and other neoplasms

Table 19-6 Immunosuppressive Antibodies

Drug	Dosage Forms	Transplantation Applications	Major Side Effects
Antithymocyte globulin (equine) (lymphocyte immune globulin) (Atgam)	Intravenous solution containing 50 mg of horse gamma globulin/mL, to be diluted in a sterile vehicle; the final gamma globulin concentration should not exceed 4 mg/mL	• Indicated for the management of allograft rejection in renal transplant patients	• Anaphylaxis • Unremitting leukopenia • Thrombocytopenia • Infection • Cytokine release syndrome
Antithymocyte globulin (rabbit) (Thymoglobulin)	Each 10-mL vial contains 25 mg of sterile, lyophilized powder to be reconstituted with sterile water for injection, USP, and diluted in saline or dextrose infusion solution (final volume of 50 mL or more is recommended)		
Muromonab-CD3 (Orthoclone OKT3)	Supplied as a sterile solution in 5 mL ampules, each containing 5 mg of muromonab-CD3	• Treatment of acute allograft rejection in renal transplant patients • Treatment of steroid-resistant acute allograft rejection in cardiac and hepatic transplant patients	• Cytokine release syndrome • Pulmonary edema • Anaphylaxis • Infections • Seizures • Stiff neck • Photophobia • Encephalopathy • Cerebral edema • Cerebral herniation
Basiliximab (Simulect)	Lyophilized powder for reconstitution with sterile water to yield a 4 mg/mL solution that can be administered as a bolus intravenous injection, or diluted with normal saline or 5% dextrose and infused intravenously over 20–30 minutes	• Prophylaxis of acute organ rejection in patients receiving renal transplants, when used as part of an immunosuppressive regimen that includes cyclosporine and corticosteroids	• Gastrointestinal disorders • Local reactions, including pain • Hypertension • Headache • Tremor • Insomnia • Dyspnea • Peripheral edema • Hyperkalemia • Hypokalemia • Hypercholesterolemia • Hyperglycemia • Hyperuricemia • Hypophosphatemia
Daclizumab (Zenapax)	Discontinued product		

The development of muromonab-CD3 marked the advent of clinical therapeutics using monoclonal antibodies. A murine immunoglobulin preparation developed to recognize the epsilon chain of the CD3 transduction glycoproteins on T lymphocytes, muromonab-CD3 (Orthoclone OKT3) was introduced in 1986 as an intravenous immunosuppressant monoclonal antibody product indicated to reverse acute graft rejection of allogeneic kidney transplants. It has since become a powerful, important tool in the management of renal transplant patients. In 1993, muromonab-CD3 also received FDA approval for the treatment of steroid-resistant acute allograft rejection in cardiac and hepatic transplant patients.

In contrast to the slow intravenous infusions of the previously discussed antilymphocyte globulins, muromonab-CD3 is administered by intravenous bolus in less than 1 minute. A rapid decrease in the number of circulating CD3-positive T lymphocytes is observed in patients within minutes after administration of this product. An anticipated occurrence of CRS, attributed to the release of cytokines by activated lymphocytes or monocytes, may be attenuated by the intravenous administration of methylprednisolone sodium succinate (8 mg/kg) given 1–4 hours prior to muromonab-CD3 administration; such pretreatment is strongly recommended, particularly in conjunction with the first dose of this immunosuppressant monoclonal antibody. Also, because muromonab-CD3 is a monoclonal antibody derived from mouse hybridoma cells, signs and symptoms of anaphylaxis need to be closely monitored as well.

In 1998, two additional monoclonal antibodies were developed to provide potent immunosuppression to organ and tissue transplant patients. Basiliximab (Simulect) and daclizumab (Zenapax) are chimeric mouse/human monoclonal antibodies. Each binds to specific sites on the α-subunit (Tac), also known as CD25, of the interleukin-2 (IL-2) receptor. Because the bioengineered chimeric genes for daclizumab contain 90% human DNA sequences, this product is referred to as a humanized monoclonal antibody, and the name contains the "zu" infix designating such a preponderance of human protein code. Basiliximab, by contrast, consists of only 75% of human immunoglobulin DNA sequences; thus it is named with the typical "xi" infix designating this chimeric bioengineered combination of human and mouse antibody gene sequences that are not as extensively derived from human DNA. By binding to the CD25 subunit of the IL-2 receptor, both monoclonal antibodies interfere with the immune activation of T lymphocytes and greatly diminish immune attack and destruction of allogeneic tissue grafts.

In September 2009, the manufacturer of daclizumab announced the discontinuation of production of Zenapax, leaving basiliximab as the only commercially available IL-2 receptor antagonist. Basiliximab is administered in two separate doses (adults: 20 mg per dose; children weighing less than 35 kg: 10 mg); the first dose is given within 2 hours prior to transplantation surgery, and the second dose is administered 4 days post transplantation. Obviously, the second dose should not be administered if severe hypersensitivity reactions to basiliximab occur or if graft loss transpires. Because basiliximab is administered concomitantly with cyclosporine and corticosteroids, its causal relationship to specific adverse reactions cannot be determined. Nevertheless, its use in clinical settings does not appear to add to the usual range or intensity of adverse events experienced by renal transplant patients who receive cyclosporine and corticosteroids without basiliximab.

Summary

The field of transplantation therapeutics continues to expand and evolve, with newer and more potent immunosuppressive drugs with life-preserving activities and potentially fatal adverse effects being introduced. Carefully managing the transplant patient requires the utmost skill and attention to the pathophysiology of organ rejection, the pharmacology of immunosuppressant drugs, and the broad array of adverse drug effects that may be produced by these potent, dangerous, and yet vital drugs. Working effectively with the transplant patient regarding therapeutic expectations, proper adherence to the drug regimen, understanding of the patient's responsibilities, and open communications between the pharmacist and physician are all crucial in maximizing the safety and efficacy of these marvelous life-saving drugs.

ANNOTATED BIBLIOGRAPHY

Cavanaugh TM, Martin JE. Update on pharmacoeconomics in transplantation. *Prog. Transplant.* 2007:17(2):103–119.

Kindt TJ, Goldsby RA, Osborne, BA. The major histocompatibility complex and antigen presentation. In: *Kuby Immunology.* 6th ed. New York: Freeman; 2007:189–222.

Krensky AM, Vincenti F, Bennett WM. Immunosuppressants, tolerogens, and immunostimulants. In: Brunton LL, Lazo JS, Parker KL, eds. *Goodman & Gilman's The Pharmacological Basis of Therapeutics.* 11th ed. New York: McGraw-Hill; 2006:1405–1431.

Lake DF, Briggs AD, Akporiaye ET. Immunopharmacology. In: Katzung BG, Masters SB, Trevor AJ, eds. *Basic and Clinical Pharmacology,* 11th ed. New York: McGraw-Hill; 2009:963–986.

Lister, J. On a new method of treating compound fracture, abscesses, etc.: with observations on the conditions of suppuration. Part 1. *Lancet.* 1867:89:507–509.

Lister J. On the antiseptic principle in the practice of surgery. *Lancet.* 1867:90:353–356.

Organ Procurement and Transplantation Network. Transplant by donor type. Updated February 12, 2010. Available at: http://optn.transplant.hrsa.gov/latestData/rptData.asp. Accessed February 26, 2010.

Parham P. Over-reactions of the immune system. In: *The Immune System.* 3rd ed. New York: Garland Science; 2009:364–400.

Schonder KS, Johnson HJ. Solid-organ transplantation. In: DiPiro JT, Talbert RL, Yee GC, Matzke GR, Wells BG, Posey LM. *Pharmacotherapy: A Pathophysiologic Approach*. 7th ed. Available at: http://www.accesspharmacy.com/content.aspx?aID=3210287.

Smyth EM, Burke A, FitzGerald GA. Lipid-derived autacoids: eicosanoids and platelet-activating factor. In: Brunton LL, Lazo JS, Parker KL, eds. *Goodman & Gilman's The Pharmacological Basis of Therapeutics*. 11th ed. New York: McGraw-Hill; 2006:1405–1431.

Tilney NL. *Transplant: From Myth to Reality*. New Haven, CT: Yale University Press; 2003.

United Network for Organ Sharing. Data. Updated February 12, 2010. Available at: http://www.unos.org/data/. Accessed February 26, 2010.

Perioperative Agents

CHAPTER

20

TOPIC: ANESTHESIA

Contributor: Nathan R. Ash

Tips Worth Tweeting

- A patient history should be thoroughly reviewed before administering general anesthesia.
- Propofol is a lipid emulsion; the patient's cholesterol and triglycerides should be monitored when it is used.
- Etomidate can cause decreased cortisol production.
- Ketamine can cause postanesthetic emergence reactions (vivid dreams, hallucinations, and/or frank delirium).
- Dexmedetomidine can cause severe hypotension; the patient's blood pressure should be monitored closely during its administration.
- Thiopental, a barbiturate, can cause laryngospasm, respiratory depression, Stevens-Johnson syndrome, and bronchospasm.

Anesthesia Overview

General anesthesia involves medications that must be closely monitored. These medications can cause severe adverse reactions, and healthcare professionals must monitor patients to ensure they have safe outcomes. Pharmacists are involved in the monitoring process, and serve as a resource for other healthcare disciplines.

1.1.0 Patient Information

Patient History

A patient history should be reviewed prior to the administration of general anesthesia. Past medical history, the medication list, and family history can alert healthcare professionals to potential contraindications or warnings.

Instruments and Techniques Related to Patient Assessment

- Cardiac monitor
- Vital signs
- Transcutaneous oxygen saturation

1.2.0 Pharmacotherapy

Mechanism of Action

- Propofol: Unknown.
- Etomidate: Short-acting hypnotic that produces a rapid induction of anesthesia with minimal cardiovascular effects.
- Ketamine: Acts on the cortex and limbic system to cause the patient to dissociate from the environment. Blood pressure and heart rate are maintained due to the release of catecholamines caused by ketamine.

Table 20-1 Anesthesia Drugs: Indications, Dosing Regimens, and Routes of Administration

Drug	Indication	Dose/Route of Administration
Propofol	Induction of anesthesia in patients 3 years or older; maintenance of anesthesia in patients older than 2 months of age	Induction: 1.5–2.5 mg/kg IV Surgery: Healthy adults younger than 55 years of age, 100–200 mcg/kg/min
Etomidate	Induction and maintenance of general anesthesia	Induction: 0.2–0.4 mg/kg IV Maintenance: 5–20 mcg/kg/min IV
Ketamine	Induction and maintenance of general anesthesia	IM: 3–8 mg/kg IV: 1–2 mg/kg for induction and give approximately 33%–50% as maintenance doses Oral: IV solution can be mixed with another beverage
Dexmedetomidine	Sedation of nonintubated patients prior to and/or during surgery or other procedures; also used as an adjunct to anesthesia	Loading dose of 1 mcg/kg over 10 minutes IV, followed by a maintenance infusion of 0.2–0.7 mcg/kg/hr
Thiopental	Induction of anesthesia	Induction: 3–5 mg/kg IV Maintenance: 25–100 mg as needed IV

- Dexmedetomidine: α_2 receptor agonist.
- Thiopental: A barbiturate that depresses the sensory cortex, decreases motor activity, and alters cerebellar functions.

Food, Drug, and Laboratory Test Interactions

Lab Interactions

- Propofol: Decreased cholesterol and cortisol, increased porphyrin.

Food Interactions

- Propofol: Formulated as an oil-in-water emulsion. The emulsion contains 1.1 kcal/mL. May need to adjust caloric and nutrition requirements. The emulsion also contains EDTA, which can cause decreased zinc levels.
- Thiopental: A 1 g injection has 86.8 mg (3.8 mEq) of sodium.

Drug Interactions

- Propofol: Effects are increased by delavirdine, desipramine, fluconazole, gemfibrozil, ketoconazole, nicardipine, NSAIDs, paroxetine, sulfonamides, tolbutamide, and other inhibitors of CYP2B6 or CYP2C9. Propofol can increase the effects of substrates of CYP1A2 or CYP3A4.
- Etomidate: Verapamil can increase the effects of etomidate. Fentanyl decreases the elimination of etomidate.
- Ketamine: CYP2B6 inhibitors (e.g., desipramine and sertraline), CYP 2C9 inhibitors (e.g., fluconazole and gemfibrozil), and CYP3A4 inhibitors (e.g., azole antifungals and clarithromycin) can increase the effects of ketamine.
- Dexmedetomidine: CYP2A6 inhibitors (e.g., isoniazid) can increase this drug's effects. Dexmedetomidine can increase the effects of CYP2A6 substrates. The levels of CYP2A6 prodrugs can be decreased by dexmedetomidine.
- Thiopental: When used with other central nervous system depressants (e.g., ethanol, benzodiazepines), the sedative or respiratory depression effects may be additive. Felbamate may inhibit the metabolism of thiopental, and thiopental may increase the metabolism of felbamate.

Contraindications, Warnings, and Precautions

Propofol

- Contraindications: Hypersensitivity to propofol or any component of the formulation (which include soybean fat emulsion, egg phosphatide, and glycerol).
- Warnings/precautions: Use a slower rate of induction and avoid rapid bolus administration in the elderly, debilitated, or patients with other comorbid conditions. Use with caution in patients who are hemodynamically unstable, have a history of seizures, hyperlipidemia, severe cardiac disease, or respiratory disease.

Etomidate

- Contraindications: Hypersensitivity to etomidate or any component of its formulation.

Ketamine

- Contraindications: Hypersensitivity to ketamine or any component of its formulation, increased intracranial pressure, hypertension, aneurysms, thyrotoxicosis, congestive heart failure, angina, psychotic disorders, pregnancy.
- Warnings/precautions: Ketamine has a boxed warning that postanesthetic emergence reactions (which can manifest as vivid dreams, hallucinations, and/or

frank delirium) occur in 12% of patients; these reactions are less common in patients older than 65 years of age and when ketamine is given via the IM route. Benzodiazepines can reduce the incidence of psychosis. Dependence and tolerance can develop with prolonged use.

Dexmedetomidine

- Contraindications: Hypersensitivity to dexmedetomidine or any component of its formulation.
- Warnings/precautions: Bradycardia and sinus arrest have occurred with rapid or bolus administration. Hypotension and bradycardia can be more severe in patients with hypovolemia, diabetes mellitus, or chronic hypertension, and in the elderly. Additive pharmacodynamic effects are observed with coadministration of vasodilators or negative chronotropic agents. Transient hypertension may be observed with the loading dose.

Thiopental

- Contraindications: Hypersensitivity to thiopental or any component of its formulation, status asthmaticus, severe cardiac disease, porphyria.
- Warnings/precautions: Use with caution in patients with reactive airway disease. Patients with Addison's disease, hepatic or renal dysfunction, myxedema, increased blood urea, severe anemia, or myasthenia gravis may have prolonged hypnotic effects. Use with caution in patients with unstable aneurysms, cardiovascular disease, renal impairment, or hepatic disease. Extravasation can cause necrosis.

Physiochemical Properties, Solubility, Pharmacodynamics, and Pharmacokinetic Properties

- Propofol: Has a relatively short elimination half-life, which allows patients to recover more quickly after the dose is given or the infusion stopped.
- Ketamine: Precipitation can occur if mixed with diazepam or barbiturates.
- Dexmedetomidine: Has a rapid onset of action.
- Thiopental: Onset of action is 30–60 seconds.

1.3.0 Monitoring

Pharmacotherapeutic Outcomes

General anesthesia

Safety and Efficacy Monitoring and Patient Education

- All general anesthetics: Cardiac monitor, vital signs, transcutaneous oxygen saturation
- Propofol: Baseline triglycerides and then every 3–7 days (if propofol is continued); zinc levels (if propofol is continued)

Adverse Drug Reactions

- Propofol: Hypotension, dystonic or choreiform movement, injection-site burning, apnea, bradycardia, decreased cardiac output, tachycardia, hyperlipidemia, hypertriglyceridemia, and propofol infusion syndrome (metabolic acidosis with myocardial dysfunction).
- Etomidate: Nausea, vomiting, myoclonus, hiccups, decreased cortisol synthesis. Etomidate solution is very irritating; avoid administering it in small blood vessels.
- Ketamine: Hypertension, increased cardiac output, increased intracranial pressure, visual hallucinations, tonic–clonic movements (ketamine lowers seizure threshold), tremor, emergence reactions.
- Dexmedetomidine: Hypotension, dry mouth, nausea, bradycardia, transient hypertension (associated with loading dose).
- Thiopental: Laryngospasm, respiratory depression, Stevens-Johnson syndrome, bronchospasm.

Nonadherence, Misuse, or Abuse

- General anesthetics should be given only under careful patient monitoring and by healthcare professionals who are not participating in the procedure or surgery.
- Ketamine and thiopental have abuse potential; appropriate inventory monitoring parameters should be utilized.

2.1.0 Calculations

Caloric Content of Nutrition Sources

Propofol is formulated as an oil-in-water emulsion. The emulsion contains 1.1 kcal/mL. When this anesthetic agent is given, it may be necessary to adjust the patient's caloric and nutrition requirements.

2.2.0 Dispensing

Package, Storage, Handling, and Disposal

- Propofol: Store at room temperature. Use within 6 hours if removed from original vial. Protect from light.
- Etomidate: Store at room temperature.
- Ketamine: Store at room temperature. Protect from light.
- Dexmedetomidine: Store at room temperature.
- Thiopental: Reconstituted solutions remain stable for 3 days at room temperature and 7 days when refrigerated.

Table 20-2 Anesthesia Drugs: Generic, Brand Names, and Dosage Form Availability

Generic Name	Brand Name	Dosage Form Availability
Propofol	Diprivan	Injection: 10 mg/mL
Etomidate	Amidate	Injection, solution: 2 mg/mL
Ketamine	Ketelar	Injection, solution: 10 mg/mL, 50 mg/mL, 100 mg/mL (may be given orally)
Dexmedeto-midine	Precedex	Injection, solution: 100 mcg/mL
Thiopental	Pentothal	Injection, powder for reconstitution: 250 mg, 400 mg, 500 mg, 1 g

Medication Administration Equipment

When available, general anesthesia should be administered through an intravenous infusion pump to ensure a safe, consistent delivery.

ANNOTATED BIBLIOGRAPHY

Brunton L, Parker K, Blumenthal D, Buxton I. *Goodman and Goldman's Manual of Pharmacology and Therapeutics.* New York: McGraw-Hill; 2008.

Gerlach AT, Dasta JF. Dexmedetomidine: an updated review. *Ann Pharmacother.* 2007;41:245–254.

Ketamine. Ketalar. Anesthesia. Bedford Labs. Available at: http://www.bedfordlabs.com/products/viewProductDetails?brand=Ketalar. Accessed February 20, 2010.

Lacy CF, Armstrong LL, Goldman MP, Lance LL. *Drug Information Handbook.* 16th ed. Hudson, OH: Lexi-Comp; 2008.

Micromedex Healthcare Series. Available at: http://www.thomsonhc.com/hcs/librarian. Accessed February 20, 2010.

Precedex [Package insert]. Lake Forest, IL: Hospira; 1999.

TOPIC: NEUROMUSCULAR BLOCKING AGENTS

Contributor: Nathan R. Ash

Tips Worth Tweeting

- Neuromuscular blocking agents (NMBAs) are used to decrease muscle tone to assist with mechanical ventilation, endotracheal intubation, bronchoscopy, tracheostomy, and other conditions where muscle relaxation is needed.
- Dosing can be done based on intermittent need (intubation) or on a continuous basis (mechanical ventilation).
- Based on their mechanisms of action, NMBAs can be divided into nondepolarizing and depolarizing agents.
- NMBAs have several clinically important drug interactions that can either increase or decrease their effects.
- NMBAs are potentially very dangerous medications, and contradictions and warnings should be reviewed before these drugs are administered.
- Monitoring includes visual, tactile, and/or electronic assessment of muscle tone.
- Based on pharmacokinetic profiles, NMBAs can be classified into three groups: short, intermediate, and long duration.
- Always review storage and stability considerations when distributing NMBAs because they are often kept in intubation trays.

Neuromuscular Blocking Agent Overview

Neuromuscular blocking agents (NMBAs) are frequently used in surgery and in intensive care units (ICU). Due to safety concerns, it is important to understand the dosing, mechanism, pharmacokinetics, drug interactions, and other safety issues associated with these drugs to ensure their safe use. Pharmacists should be involved in the safe administration of NMBAs and serve as an information resource for other healthcare providers.

1.1.0 Patient Information

Laboratory Values

A baseline basic metabolic panel (BMP) and magnesium level should be reviewed before NMBAs are administered. A BMP and magnesium level can identify potentially dangerous electrolyte abnormalities when NMBAs are utilized. BMP and magnesium levels should be monitored frequently if an NMBA is used over a long period of time.

Instruments and Techniques Related to Patient Assessment

Electronic assessment utilizes a system called train of four (TOF). Four electrical stimuli are applied along a nerve, and the response of the muscle is observed. It is recommended that at least one of the stimuli should elicit a response from the muscle. If none of the stimuli elicits a response, the infusion rate should be lowered.

Table 20-3 Neuromuscular Blocking Agents: Dosing Regimens and Route of Administration

Drugs	Dose/Route of Administration
Atracurium	Initial: 0.2–0.4 mg/kg IV after initial dose of succinylcholine Surgery: 5–9 mcg/kg/min
Cisatracurium (Nimbex)	Intubation: 0.15–0.2 mg/kg IV as a component of propofol/nitrous oxide/oxygen technique; 0.1 mg/kg after initial dose of succinylcholine ICU: 0.03–0.6 mg/kg/hr IV
Doxacurium (Nuromax)	Surgery: 0.05–0.08 mg/kg IV with thiopental/narcotic; 0.025 mg/kg after initial dose of succinylcholine ICU: 0.015–0.045 mg/kg/hr IV
Mivacurium (Mivacron)	Intubation: 0.1 mg/kg IV ICU: 1–15 mcg/kg/min IV
Pancuronium (Pavulon)	Surgery: 0.05 mg/kg IV for intubation after initial dose of succinylcholine ICU: 0.05–1 mg/kg/hr IV
Rocuronium (Zemuron)	Intubation (rapid-sequence intubation): 0.6–1.2 mg/kg IV ICU: 0.6 mg/kg/hr IV
Succinylcholine	2.5–4 mg/kg IM 1–1.5 mg/kg IV, up to 150 mg total dose Continuous infusion: 10–100 mcg/kg/min IV
Vecuronium (Norcuron)	Surgery: 0.08–0.1 mg/kg or 0.04–0.06 mg/kg after initial dose of succinylcholine ICU: 0.05–0.1 mg/kg/hr IV

1.2.0 Pharmacotherapy

Drug Indications, Dosing Regimens, and Routes of Administration

NMBAs are used for the following indications:

- Facilitate mechanical ventilation
- Assist in endotracheal intubation
- Control elevations in intracranial pressure (ICP)
- Reduce muscle rigidity in tetanus
- Facilitate minor procedures such tracheostomy or bronchoscopy
- Surgeries where deep muscle relaxation is required to complete the surgery

Mechanism of Action

NMBAs are divided into two groups: nondepolarizing and depolarizing. Currently, only one depolarizing NMBA is available for clinical use in the United States—succinylcholine. Nondepolarizing neuromuscular blocking agents work by opening sodium channels associated with nicotinic receptors, causing continuous depolarization of the muscle cell. This leads to a gradual repolarization, and the sodium channel becomes resistant to depolarization. This resistance to depolarization will prevent muscle contraction.

Atracurium, cisatracurium, doxacurium, mivacurium, pancuronium, rocuronium, and vecuronium are nondepolarizing NMBAs. They work by competitively binding to and blocking the nicotinic receptors. This prevents depolarization of the muscle cell, so that the cells are not able to contract.

Food, Drug, and Lab Test Interactions

Atracurium, cisatracurium, doxacurium, mivacurium, pancuronium, rocuronium, vecuronium, aminoglycosides, beta blockers, clindamycin, calcium-channel blockers, halogenated anesthetics, imipenem, ketamine, lidocaine, loop diuretics, macrolides, magnesium sulfate, procainamide, quinidine, quinolones, tetracyclines, and vancomycin may increase NMBA effects. High-dose corticosteroids may also increase the risk of myopathy.

Atracurium, cisatracurium, doxacurium, mivacurium, pancuronium, rocuronium, vecuronium-carbamazepine, corticosteroids, phenytoin, sympathomimetics, and theophylline may decrease NMBA levels.

- Mivacurium: Acetycholinesterase inhibitors may prolong the effect of mivacurium.
- Succinylcholine: Anticholinesterase drugs, cyclophosphamide, oral contraceptives, lidocaine, thiotepa, pancuronium, lithium, magnesium salts, aprotinin, chloroquine, metoclopramide, terbutaline, and procaine can increase succinylcholine's effects. Inhaled anesthetics, local anesthetics, calcium-channel blockers, quinidine, procainamide, aminoglycosides, tetracyclines, vancomycin, clindamycin, and cyclosporine can prolong the neuromuscular blockade.

Contraindications, Warnings, and Precautions

Each NMBA is contraindicated if the patient has a hypersensitivity to any other NMBA, as cross-sensitivity may occur between agents.

- Succinylcholine contraindications: Narrow-angle glaucoma, penetrating eye injuries, disorders of pseudocholinesterase, personal or family history of malignant hyperthermia, and myopathies associated with elevated serum creatinine phosphokinase (CPK) values.
- Conditions that increase nondepolarizing NMDA effects: Severe hyponatremia, severe hypocalcemia,

severe hypokalemia, hypermagnesemia, neuromuscular diseases, acidosis, acute intermittent porphyria, renal failure, hepatic failure, myasthenia gravis, Eaton-Lambert syndrome.
- Conditions that antagonize nondepolarizing NMDA effects: Alkalosis, hypercalcemia, demyelinating lesions, peripheral neuropathies, diabetes mellitus. Resistance may be observed in patients with burns, muscle trauma, denervation, immobilization, or infections.

Warnings and precautions for succinylcholine include preexisting hyperkalemia, burns, paraplegia, denervation of skeletal muscle as a result of central nervous system injury, and degenerative or dystrophic neuromuscular disease. Succinylcholine can increase vagal tone. This agent also has a boxed warning to use it with caution in pediatric and adolescent patients secondary to undiagnosed skeletal muscle myopathy and the potential for ventricular dysrhythmias, and cardiac arrest resulting from hyperkalemia.

Nondepolarizing NMBAs have a boxed warning that they should be administered by adequately trained individuals.

Physiochemical Properties, Solubility, Pharmacodynamics, and Pharmacokinetic Properties

Nondepolarizing NMBAs can be divided into three groups based on their duration of action:

- Short duration: Mivacurium
- Intermediate duration: Atracurium, cisatracurium, rocuronium, vecuronium
- Long duration: Doxacurium, pancuronium

1.3.0 Monitoring

Pharmacotherapeutic Outcomes

The goal with NMDA use is to ensure muscle relaxation while minimizing adverse drug interactions.

Safety and Efficacy Monitoring and Patient Education

- Vital signs should be monitored closely.
- Monitoring includes visual, tactile, and/or electronic assessment of muscle tone.
- Electronic assessment utilizes a system called train of four (TOF). Four electronic stimuli are applied along a nerve, and the response of the muscle is observed. It is recommended that at least one of the stimuli should elicit a response from the muscle. If none of the stimuli elicits a response, then the infusion rate should be lowered.

Table 20-4 Neuromuscular Blocking Agents: Generic Names, Brand Names, and Dosage Form Availability

Generic Name	Brand Name	Dosage Form Availability
Atracurium	Tracrium	Injection: 10 mg/mL
Cisatracurium	Nimbex	Injection: 2 mg/mL, 10 mg/mL
Doxacurium	Nuromax	Injection: 1 mg/mL
Mivacurium	Mivacron	Injection: 2 mg/mL
Pancuronium	Pavulon	Injection: 1 mg/mL, 2 mg/mL
Rocuronium	Zemuron	Injection: 10 mg/mL
Succinylcholine	Quelicin	Injection: 20 mg/mL, 50 mg/mL, 100 mg/mL
Vecuronium	Norcuron	Injection: 10 mg, 20 mg powder for reconstitution

Adverse Drug Interactions

- Succinylcholine: Hyperkalemia, bradycardia, malignant hyperthermia, muscle rigidity, muscle soreness, hypotension, and bronchospasm (last two caused by histamine release). Malignant hyperthermia can be treated with dantrolene and techniques to cool the patient.
- Nondepolarizing NMDAs: Bradycardia, flushing, pruritus, rash, acute quadriplegic myopathy, myositis ossificans, hypotension, and bronchospasm. (Hypotension and bronchospasm are caused by histamine release).
- Pancuronium, vecuronium: Edema, circulatory collapse, and tachycardia.
- Pancuronium: Hypertension and elevated cardiac output, excessive salivation.
- Rocuronium: Hypertension, arrhythmia, hiccups, nausea, vomiting.
- Nondepolarizing NMBAs: Neostigmine can be given to reverse or antagonize neuromuscular blockade.

Nonadherence, Misuse, or Abuse

Due to safety issues, NMDAs should be used only if the benefits clearly outweigh the risk.

2.2.0 Dispensing

Package, Storage, Handling, and Disposal

- Atracurium: Store vials in refrigeration. Use vials within 14 days upon removal from the refrigerator after bringing them to room temperature.
- Cisatracurium: Store vials in refrigeration.

- Doxacurium: Stable for 24 hours at room temperature when diluted.
- Mivacurium: Store at room temperature. Protect from ultraviolet light.
- Pancuronium: Store vials in refrigeration.
- Rocuronium: Store vials in refrigeration.
- Succinylcholine: Store vials in refrigeration. Stable for 3 months or less at room temperature.
- Vecuronium: Store vials of dry powder at room temperature.

Medication Administration Equipment

When available, NMBA infusions should be administered through an intravenous infusion pump to ensure a safe, consistent delivery.

ANNOTATED BIBLIOGRAPHY

Al Harbi S, Nelson R. Neuromuscular blocking agents in the intensive care units. *Saudi Pharma J* 2007; 15(1):60–63.

Lacy CF, Armstrong LL, Goldman MP, Lance LL. *Drug Information Handbook.* 16th ed. Hudson, OH: Lexi-Comp; 2008.

Micromedex Healthcare Series. Available at: http://www.thomsonhc.com/hcs/librarian. Accessed February 20, 2010.

Reeves ST, Turcasso NM. Nondepolarizing neuromuscular blocking drugs in the intensive care unit: a clinical review. *Southern Med J* 1997;90(8): 769–774.

Psychiatry

CHAPTER

21

TOPIC: ALCOHOLISM

Section Coordinator: Rex S. Lott
Contributor: Robyn Cruz

Tips Worth Tweeting

- Benzodiazepines are used to reduce seizures, delirium, and overall symptoms of alcohol withdrawal.
- Beta blockers or $alpha_2$ agonists cannot be used as monotherapy in alcohol withdrawal.
- Lorazepam, oxazepam, and temazepam do not have active metabolites, making them superior choices in the elderly and patients with hepatic dysfunction.
- Wernicke-Korsakoff syndrome can lead to amnesia, disorientation, and impaired memory of recent events.
- Motivation to abstain from alcohol use must be present for the medications used in prevention of relapse to be efficacious.
- Patients must be free of opioid use for 5–7 days prior to initiation of naltrexone to prevent precipitation of opioid withdrawal.
- Patients taking disulfiram must be well-informed regarding its mechanism of action, other forms of alcohol to avoid while taking this medication, and its duration of effect (as long as 14 days).

Patient Care Scenario: Acute Care Setting

R. B., a 71-year-old male with a history of diabetes mellitus type 2, hypertension, gastroesophageal reflux disease, osteoarthritis, and hepatic dysfunction with a Child-Pugh score of 9, is admitted to the local hospital for acute alcohol withdrawal. He has experienced seizures during past episodes of alcohol withdrawal. What is the most appropriate medication to recommend initiating for prevention of alcohol withdrawal seizures in this patient?

1.1.0 Patient Information

Review the patient's history for medications that can lower the seizure threshold (i.e., in acute alcohol withdrawal)—for example, antipsychotics, bupropion and other antidepressants, meperidine, and tramadol.

Review the history for medications that should be used with careful consideration (i.e., in chronic alcohol abuse or dependence)—for example, benzodiazepines.

Laboratory Testing

- Urine toxicology screen: Used to determine which substances are involved in intoxication.
- Blood alcohol level (BAL): To determine the level of intoxication and tolerance.
- Gamma-glutamyltransferase (GGT): Elevated levels (more than 30 units) of this

sensitive test indicate heavy alcohol use within the past days to weeks.
- Carbohydrate-deficient transferrin (CDT): Elevated levels of this sensitive test (20 or more units) indicate 8 or more drinks on a daily basis within the past days to weeks.
- Mean corpuscular volume (MCV): High-normal values may indicate heavy drinking due to alcohol's negative effect on erythropoiesis.
- Complete blood count (CBC): To detect anemia or thrombocytopenia.
- Liver function tests (LFTs): May include alkaline phosphatase, alanine aminotransferase (ALT), and aspartate aminotransferase (AST) to determine the extent of liver damage.
- Complete metabolic panel (CMP): To determine the presence of electrolyte abnormalities.

Disease State History

Obtain a history of alcohol use:

- Amount of use
- Time since last drink
- Duration of use
- Type of alcohol consumed

Instruments and Techniques Related to Patient Assessment

- Patient history as outlined previously
- Indicators of autonomic instability (i.e., in acute alcohol withdrawal): Blood pressure, heart rate, temperature, sweating
- Clinical Institute Withdrawal Assessment for Alcohol (CIWA-Ar)

Key Terms

See Table 21-1.

Clinical Institute Withdrawal Assessment for Alcohol

Ten symptom categories:

- Sweating
- Anxiety
- Tremor
- Agitation
- Nausea and vomiting
- Auditory disturbances
- Tactile disturbances
- Visual disturbances
- Headache
- Orientation

Each category is scored 1–7 points except Orientation which is scored 1–4 points (maximum score = 67):

- Minimal–mild withdrawal: < 8
  - Usually supportive nonpharmacological therapy only
- Moderate withdrawal: 8–15
  - Usually medication given per protocol
- Severe withdrawal: > 15
  - Seizures and delirium predicted by high scores; medication should be given

Blood Alcohol Level (Concentration)

Blood alcohol level (BAL) is the most direct screen to measure alcohol consumption and tolerance.

- Example: Patients who have a BAL of 100 mg/dL without exhibiting signs of intoxication would be considered "tolerant."
- Example: Severe intoxication, including falling asleep, would be noticeable in most individuals without tolerance to alcohol at 200 mg/dL.
- Example: BAL of 300–400 mg/dL may inhibit respirations and pulse, and may lead to death.

Table 21-1 Characteristics of Acute Intoxication from Alcohol

Behavioral Changes	Signs and Symptoms
Mood lability, impaired judgment, impaired social/occupational functioning, inappropriate sexual behavior, inappropriate aggressive behavior	Slurred speech, incoordination, unsteady gait, nystagmus, impaired memory/attention, stupor/coma

Table 21-2 Characteristics and Timing of Minor Versus Major Alcohol Withdrawal

Time Since Last Drink	Clinical Scenario	Symptom Description
4–12 hours	"Minor withdrawal" symptom onset Seizures can occur any time at 7–48 hours after cessation of alcohol use	Autonomic hyperactivity (i.e., sweating, HR > 100, increased BP), hand tremor, insomnia, nausea or vomiting, hallucinations or illusions, psychomotor agitation, anxiety, grand mal seizure
24–72 hours	Symptoms peak	Same as above
48–120 hours	Symptoms begin to subside **or** "major withdrawal" symptom onset may occur (at 48–60 hours)	Same as above **or** delirium tremens with worsening of the above symptoms
3–6 months	Some symptoms may persist	Anxiety, insomnia, autonomic dysfunction

Table 21-3 Symptoms of Alcohol Abuse Associated with Each Organ System

Organ System	Symptoms
Gastrointestinal	Gastritis (dyspepsia, nausea, bloating), ulcers (stomach and duodenal), liver cirrhosis (hepatomegaly, esophageal varices, hemorrhoids) pancreatitis, esophageal and stomach cancers
Cardiovascular	Hypertension, cardiomyopathy, heart disease
Central nervous system	Cognitive deficits, severe memory impairment, degenerative changes, Wernicke-Korsakoff syndrome
Peripheral nervous system	Muscular weakness, paresthesias, neuropathy, tremor, unsteady gait, insomnia, erectile dysfunction

Wellness and Prevention

- Potential risk factors: Low educational level, unemployment, lower socioeconomic status, genetics, cultural traditions
- Average onset of abuse: Mid-teens with a peak in the 20s to mid-30s
  - Elderly: More susceptible to effects of alcohol due to factors of aging
  - Females: Higher BAL due to physiological gender differences
- Average rates in the United States according to race: Equal between Caucasians and African Americans
- Goals after diagnosis of abuse and/or dependence: Abstinence, prevention of relapse, and rehabilitation

1.2.0 Pharmacotherapy

Drug Indications, Dosing Regimens, and Routes of Administration

Medications for Use in Acute Alcohol Withdrawal

Benzodiazepines

- Benzodiazepines' efficacy is thought to be due to cross-tolerance with alcohol; these drugs reduce the incidence of seizures and delirium, and decrease the severity of withdrawal.
- Many drugs and doses have been used. All benzodiazepines appear equal in effectiveness, whether given PO or IV.
  - Example regimens: Chlordiazepoxide 50 mg q 2–4 hours, diazepam 10 mg q 2–4 hours, or lorazepam 1 mg q 2 hours.
  - Symptom-triggered therapy (i.e., using the CIWA-Ar scale) results in less drug used and shorter duration of withdrawal compared to the fixed-dose regimen. Additionally, fixed-dose regimens require less observation and assessment (i.e., consume less staffing time).
  - Considerations:
    - Longer-acting drugs may more effectively prevent seizures and result in a smoother withdrawal.
    - Shorter-acting drugs have less likelihood of oversedation, but are administered more frequently.
    - Rapid-onset drugs have higher abuse potential.
    - Lorazepam and oxazepam are better alternatives in elderly or hepatic dysfunction due to their Phase II metabolism (glucuronidation).

Beta Blockers and Alpha$_2$ Agonists

- These agents are used for control of autonomic dysfunction or hyperactivity (i.e., tremor, tachycardia, elevated blood pressure, diaphoresis) during withdrawal. They cannot be used as monotherapy due to their lack of anticonvulsant properties.
- One option is propranolol 10 mg PO q 6 hours. Atenolol has also been used.
- Clonidine in doses of 0.5 mg PO bid or tid has also been used.

Medications for Complications Related to Alcohol Use

Thiamine

- This B-vitamin can be used to treat or prevent deficiency; this deficiency, if left untreated, can lead to Wernicke-Korsakoff syndrome.
- Typically dosed as 50–100 mg PO, IM or IV; can be short term (i.e., 7–10 days) or long term depending on adequacy of nutritional intake.

Fluids and Electrolytes

- Given as needed for hydration and electrolyte imbalances.

Medications for Prevention of Relapse in Alcohol Abuse and Dependence

Naltrexone

- Opiate receptor antagonist that inhibits the euphoria and reward associated with drinking, thereby reducing cravings.
- Usual dose is 50 mg/day PO; also available as monthly IM injection.

Disulfiram

- Inhibits the enzyme aldehyde dehydrogenase, which causes a buildup of acetaldehyde

(a metabolite of alcohol). Alcohol use with disulfiram causes a toxic reaction due to the accumulation of acetaldehyde; symptoms of this toxic reaction include headache, flushing, nausea, vomiting, anxiety, hypotension, and even respiratory depression, chest pain, seizures, and death.
- Usual dose is 250 mg/day PO.

Acamprosate

- Mechanism is not fully understood; thought to restore glutamate function.
- Usual dose is 666 mg tid PO.

Drug–Drug, Drug–Food, and Drug–Lab Test Interactions

Benzodiazepines

- CNS depressants may increase the effects of these drugs. There are rare reports of respiratory depression, stupor, and/or hypotension in combination with loxapine.
    - Agents have the potential to enhance the toxic effects of clozapine.
    - CYP 3A4 inhibitors may increase the effects of chlordiazepoxide (a major substrate of 3A4).
    - CYP 3A4 inducers may decrease these effects.
- CYP 2C19 inhibitors may increase the effects of diazepam (a major substrate of 2C19).
    - CYP 2C19 inducers may decrease these effects.
- CNS stimulants such as theophylline may diminish the effectiveness of benzodiazepines.
- Valerian, St. John's wort and kava kava may increase CNS depression.
    - St. John's wort may decrease diazepam and chlordiazepoxide concentrations.
    - Diazepam concentration may increase with food; toxicity may increase with grapefruit juice.
    - There is a potential for chlordiazepoxide concentrations to increase with grapefruit juice, but negative outcomes are not well-described.

Beta Blockers and Alpha$_2$ Agonists

Propranolol

- Combination with clonidine may enhance rebound hypertension on abrupt withdrawal of clonidine.
- CYP 1A2 and 2D6 inhibitors may increase levels.
- CYP 1A2 inducers may decrease levels.
- Negative chrontropic effects may be enhanced by some drugs (e.g., acetylcholinesterase inhibitors, amiodarone, digoxin, diltiazem, dipyridamole, disopyramide, SSRIs, verapamil).
- May enhance hypoglycemic effects and mask hypoglycemic symptoms in patients using insulin and sulfonylureas.
- May increase levels of phenothiazines, lidocaine, rizatriptan, and warfarin.
- May blunt the effect of beta$_2$ agonists and theophylline.
- Multiple interactions with herbal products.

Clonidine

- Hypotensive effects may be antagonized by tricyclic antidepressants, and hypertensive rebound may be enhanced on abrupt withdrawal.
- CNS depressants may have additive effects when used in combination.
- Combination with antipsychotics, opioids, and nitroprusside may have additive hypotensive effects.
- Symptoms of hypoglycemia may be decreased in combination with insulin or oral hypoglycemic agents.
- May increase cyclosporine and tacrolimus concentrations.
- Combination with beta blockers may lead to bradycardia, and enhance rebound hypertension on abrupt withdrawal.
- Multiple interactions with herbal products.

Thiamine

- High-carbohydrate diets may require more supplementation.
- May interfere with determining serum theophylline levels. May cause false-positive test results for uric acid with some methods.

Naltrexone

- Decreases the effectiveness of opioids.
- Produces lethargy and somnolence in combination with thioridazine.
- May cause an unknown interaction with NSAIDs, leading to hepatotoxicity with doses greater than 100 mg/day.
- Potential for cross-reactivity with some opioid immunoassays.

Disulfiram

- May increase the concentrations of benzodiazepines that undergo oxidative metabolism (i.e., benzodiazepines other than lorazepam, oxazepam, and temazepam).
- May increase the concentrations of substrates of 2E1 (i.e., phenobarbital, theophylline).
- Inhibits metabolism of warfarin.
- Adverse CNS effects may occur with isoniazid, metronidazole, and MAO inhibitors.

- Potential to interact with any amount of alcohol, including that found in cough syrup and mouthwash; in foods such as vinegars, ciders, or extracts; and in topical products.

Acamprosate

- No clinically significant drug–drug or drug–food interactions have been identified.
- Each tablet contains 33 mg of elemental calcium.

Contraindications, Warnings, and Precautions

Benzodiazepines

- Contraindicated in acute narrow-angle glaucoma, central sleep apnea, severe respiratory insufficiency, and pregnancy.
- Use caution:
  - With other CNS depressants.
  - In patients with hepatic disease, renal impairment, respiratory disease, or an impaired gag reflex; the elderly; obese patients; patients with a history of drug dependence; and patients with depressive disorders or psychosis.
- Have been associated with anterograde amnesia and paradoxical reactions (hyperactive or aggressive behavior).
- All enter breastmilk and are either contraindicated or not recommended for breastfeeding women; all are classified into pregnancy Category D.

Beta Blockers and Alpha$_2$ Agonists

Propranolol

- Contraindicated in uncompensated heart failure (use with caution in compensated heart failure), cardiogenic shock, bradycardia/heart block, pulmonary edema, severe asthma or COPD (monitor closely if used in less severe disease), Raynaud's disease, and second and third trimesters of pregnancy.
- Do not abruptly discontinue.
- Use with caution:
  - In peripheral vascular disease, in diabetic patients due to masking of hypoglycemic symptoms, in myasthenia gravis, and in depression.
  - With verapamil or diltiazem (due to bradycardia/heart block).

Clonidine

- Do not abruptly discontinue.
- Use with caution: Severe coronary deficiency, conduction disturbances, recent MI or CVA, chronic renal insufficiency, or sinus node dysfunction.
- May cause CNS depression and xerostomia.
  - Use with caution in patients with CNS disease or depression, and in elderly.

Thiamine

- Monitor for hypersensitivity with parenteral routes.
- Evaluate for other possible deficiencies.
- Must administer prior to parenteral glucose to prevent complications with acute thiamine deficiency.
- Pregnancy Category A/C (if used in doses greater than the RDA).

Naltrexone

- Contraindicated with concurrent opioid use (should be opioid free for 7–10 days).
- Contraindicated in patients with acute hepatitis or liver failure; use with caution in patients with renal impairment.
- Pregnancy Category C; enters breast milk; not recommended for breastfeeding women.
- Monitor for depression and/or suicidal ideation; monitor for shortness of breath and hypoxia.

Disulfiram

- Contraindicated in patients concurrently using metronidazole, ethanol or ethanol-containing products such as cough syrup, or paraldehyde.
- Contraindicated in psychosis.
- Contraindicated in severe myocardial disease or coronary occlusion.
- Caution should be used in patients with diabetes, hypothyroidism, seizure disorders, nephritis, or hepatic cirrhosis or insufficiency.
- Pregnancy Category C; excretion in breast milk is unknown.
- Should never be administered to an acutely intoxicated patient.
- The patient must be well-informed about other forms of alcohol to avoid while taking this medication and the duration of its effects (as long as 14 days).

Acamprosate

- Contraindicated in patients with severe renal impairment (CrCl < 30 mL/min).
- Use caution in patients with moderate renal impairment (CrCl of 30–50 mL/min).
- Should be used in combination with a behavioral therapy.
- Monitor for depression and/or suicidal ideation.
- Pregnancy Category C; excretion in breast milk is unknown; caution should be used.

Table 21-4 Benzodiazepines

Drug	Peak (PO, hr)	Protein Binding (%)	Active Metabolite	Half-life (hr) (Metabolite)
Chlordiazepoxide	2–4	90–98	Yes	5–30 (24–96)
Diazepam	0.5–2	98	Yes	20–80 (50–100)
Lorazepam	1–6	88–92	No	10–20 (none)

Physiochemical Properties, Solubility, Pharmacodynamics, and Pharmacokinetic Properties

See Table 21-4.

Beta Blockers and Alpha$_2$ Agonists

Propranolol

- Onset of action is 1–2 hours; duration is approximately 6 hours; half-life is 4–6 hours
- Crosses the placenta and a small amount enters breast milk
- 93% protein bound, with extensive first-pass effect

Clonidine

- Onset of action is 0.5–1 hour; duration is 6–10 hours
- Time to peak is 2–4 hours; half-life is 6–20 hours in patients with normal renal function (18–41 hours in patients with impaired renal function)
- Undergoes enterohepatic recirculation; 20–40% protein bound, 75–95% bioavailable

Thiamine

- Highest concentrations are found in the brain, heart, kidney, and liver
- Crosses the placenta and enters breast milk
- Water-soluble vitamin, so when storage capacity is exceeded, drug is excreted in urine

Naltrexone

- Duration of action increases with dose: 50 mg = 24 hours, 100 mg = 48 hours, 150 mg = 72 hours
    - IM dose = 4 weeks
- Extensive first-pass metabolism
    - Half-life is 4 hours with oral dosage; metabolite half-life = 13 hours
    - Half-life is 5–10 days with IM dose
- Time to peak: Oral = approximately 60 minutes; IM is biphasic with first peak at 2–3 hours and second peak at 2–3 days

Disulfiram

- Full effect begins within 12 hours, so it is important that the patient has not had alcohol within 12 hours prior to taking the dose
- Lasts for up to 2 weeks after last dose

Acamprosate

- 11% bioavailable; negligible protein binding
- Half-life is 20–33 hours; excreted unchanged (not metabolized)

1.3.0 Monitoring

Pharmacotherapeutic Outcomes

- During acute withdrawal, the primary goal is to restore physiological homeostasis while controlling CNS irritation.
- To achieve the best long-term outcome, abstinence must be the primary goal of treatment.
- Medications can be used to assist with abstinence through motivation, reducing alcohol consumption, and reducing cravings and relapse rates.

Safety and Efficacy Monitoring

- Symptoms of acute withdrawal generally begin within 4–12 hours after alcohol is last consumed. Symptoms peak within 2–3 days, and usually resolve by 4–5 days.
- The CIWA-Ar may be used to monitor and evaluate symptoms and their management.
- CMP and LFTs may be monitored to assess fluid and electrolyte status and to ensure that any abnormalities in LFTs are trending back to normal.
- The laboratory tests outlined previously (i.e., AST, ALT, CMP, BAL) may be monitored longitudinally to assess abstinence also to reduce further organ dysfunction.

Adverse Drug Reactions

Benzodiazepines

- Sedation, respiratory depression, hypotension, alterations in mental status (confusion, amnesia), dizziness.

Beta Blockers and Alpha$_2$ Agonists

- Propranolol: Delirium (important to consider when using this agent in patients undergoing alcohol withdrawal), bradycardia, dizziness, fatigue, changes in glucose control, depression.
- Clonidine: Drowsiness/dizziness, dry mouth, weakness.

Thiamine

- IM/IV: Restlessness, pruritus, urticaria, nausea, weakness, diaphoresis, warmth (all at undefined frequencies).

Naltrexone

- Side effects may be similar to alcohol withdrawal symptoms, so this medication should not be started during the acute phase of withdrawal.

- Side effects are usually moderate and may include nausea/vomiting/diarrhea, abdominal pain, headache, fatigue, insomnia, anxiety, syncope, and hepatotoxicity.
  - Slow upward titration will assist in alleviating gastrointestinal distress; most other adverse effects will subside as the patient adjusts to the medication.
  - Hepatotoxicity usually occurs in obese patients on high doses; it was not observed in most clinical studies.
- Patients receiving opioids (prescription medications or street drugs) will experience withdrawal if naltrexone is initiated; efficacy of prescription opiods will be lost.
  - Must have a complete medication use history from the patient prior to initiation, and possibly a urine toxicology screen.
  - Patient should be opioid free for 5–7 days (depending on the drug's half-life) before initiation.
  - If opioid analgesia is necessary, higher than usual doses may be necessary; thus caution should be used regarding potential respiratory depression.

Disulfiram

- Multiple side effects may include drowsiness, headache, fatigue, psychosis, dermatologic reactions, metallic aftertaste, impotence, hepatitis, and peripheral neuropathy.
  - Psychosis is theorized to potentially occur due to an increase in dopamine levels through metabolism of disulfiram.
- More severe reactions may include chest pain, seizures, liver dysfunction, respiratory depression, cardiac arrhythmias, MI, and death, which are usually related to combined use with alcohol.
  - If the patient develops a severe disulfiram reaction, symptomatic/supportive management is needed for possible hypotension and hypokalemia.

Acamprosate

- Diarrhea: Primary clinically significant adverse effect; can be treated symptomatically and is usually self-limited.

Nonadherence, Misuse, or Abuse

- Ideally, adherence to medication will be increased if the patient is educated appropriately regarding possible adverse reactions and ways to avoid or remedy them, as outlined earlier.
- Patients must be motivated to quit if they are to experience efficacy from the medications used for abstinence.

Table 21-5 Pharmacotherapeutic Alternatives

Drug	Dosage Forms and Strengths Available
Chlordiazepoxide	Capsule: 5 mg, 10 mg, 25 mg Injection: 100 mg
Diazepam	Tablet: 2 mg, 5 mg, 10mg Solution: 5 mg/mL, 5 mg/5 mL Injection: 5 mg/mL
Lorazepam	Tablet: 0.5 mg, 1 mg, 2 mg Solution: 2 mg/mL Injection: 2 mg/mL, 4 mg/mL
Propranolol	Tablet: 10 mg, 20 mg, 40 mg, 60 mg, 80 mg Solution: 20 mg/5 mL, 40 mg/5 mL Injection: 1 mg/mL Capsule (long-acting): 60 mg, 80 mg, 120 mg, 160 mg
Clonidine	Tablet: 0.1 mg, 0.2 mg, 0.3 mg Injection: 100 mcg/mL, 500 mcg/mL
Thiamine	Tablet: 50 mg, 100 mg, 250 mg, 500 mg Injection: 100 mg/mL
Naltrexone	Tablet: 50 mg Injection: 380 mg/vial (long-acting depot)
Disulfiram	Tablet: 250 mg
Acamprosate	Tablet: 333 mg

- Patients must be adequately educated on the mechanism of disulfiram and which products to avoid in conjunction with its use.
- Long-term use of benzodiazepines should be approached very cautiously due to their potential for abuse by patients who abuse alcohol.
  - Medications with a rapid onset of action will have the most abuse potential (i.e., diazepam, alprazolam, lorazepam).

ANNOTATED BIBLIOGRAPHY

American Psychiatric Association. Practice guideline for the treatment of patients with substance use disorders. 2nd ed. 2006. Available at: www.psych.org.

Diagnostic and Statistical Manual of Mental Disorders. 4th ed. Text Revision (DSM-IV-TR). Washington, DC: American Psychiatric Association; 2000.

Kosten TR, O'Connor PG. Management of drug and alcohol withdrawal. *N Engl J Med* 2003;348(18): 1786–1795.

Lacy CF, Armstrong LL, Goldman MP, Lance LL. *Drug Information Handbook.* 17th ed. Hudson, OH: Lexi-Comp; 2009.

Mayo-Smith MF. Pharmacological management of alcohol withdrawal. *JAMA* 1997;278(2):144–151.

Perry PJ, Alexander B, Liskow BI, DeVane CL. *Psychotropic Drug Handbook*. 8th ed. Philadelphia, PA: Lippincott Williams and Wilkins; 2007.

TOPIC: ANXIETY

Section Coordinator: Rex S. Lott
Contributors: Sarah J. Popish and Alberto Augsten

Anxiety is a normal reaction under circumstances of real or perceived danger that threatens the safety of the individual. However, there are circumstances where anxiety is maladaptive, with symptoms of excessive worry and fear occurring that can constitute an anxiety disorder.

Anxiety disorders can be classified into five different subtypes, all of which have some symptom overlap.

- **Generalized anxiety disorder** (GAD) is classified as chronic excessive anxiety and worry accompanied by restlessness, fatigue, difficulty concentrating, irritability, muscle tension. and sleep disturbances.
- **Panic disorder** is a combination of panic attacks, which are characterized by an intense episode of fear or impending doom and anticipatory worry that the attack will reoccur resulting in significant changes in behavior.
- **Social anxiety disorder** includes symptoms of anxiety or fear about social performance and social exposure.
- **Obsessive–compulsive disorder** (OCD) consists of obsessions that are recurrent with persistent thoughts, impulses, or images that are regarded as intrusive and can cause marked anxiety. Compulsions consist of repetitive behavior (hand washing, checking), and mental acts (praying). In response to the obsession, the person is often driven to perform compulsions to relieve anxiety. It should be noted that the person often realizes that the obsessions and compulsions are excessive and/or unreasonable.
- **Post-traumatic stress disorder** (PTSD) occurs after exposure to a traumatic event that is perceived as life-threatening; later, the person reexperiences the event, avoids all things associated with the trauma, and has increased arousal and startle responses.

Anxiety disorders are treated with several different classes of medications. Selective serotonin reuptake inhibitors (SSRIs) are often considered first-line treatments, but tricyclic antidepressants (TCA), benzodiazepines, venlafaxine, monoamine oxidase inhibitors (MAOIs) and buspirone are also effective in the treatment of anxiety disorders. Some nonpharmacologic treatments (i.e., cognitive-behavioral therapy) are considered effective in the treatment of all anxiety disorders

Tips Worth Tweeting

- SSRIs are considered first-line therapy in the treatment of anxiety disorders.
- SSRIs should be started at lower doses (one-half to one-fourth of the usual dose) and escalated slowly when used in patients with anxiety disorders to prevent jitteriness.
- When using SSRIs, it may take as long as 4 weeks to see an initial response and 8–12 weeks to see the full response.
- Benzodiazepines are a safe and effective treatment in patients with no history of substance abuse.
- Lorazepam, oxazepam, and temazepam are drugs of choice for elderly patients or those with liver dysfunction—they are eliminated by glucoronidation rather than oxidation.
- Breakthrough anxiety can occur within 3–5 hours of an alprazolam dose.
- Sedation is the most common side effect of benzodiazepines but usually subsides in 1–2 weeks.
- Clomipramine is the TCA with the most evidence for the treatment of anxiety disorder; the other TCA used for this indication is imipramine.
- TCAs are given at bedtime because of their sedative effects.

Patient Care Scenario: Ambulatory Setting

S. P.: 28 yo, white male, NKDA
Chief complaint: "I went to the emergency room because I thought I was going to die, and they told me that I was just having a panic attack."
HPI: S. P., a 28-year-old male college student, was referred to a psychiatrist after presenting to the emergency department. He states that he felt like he was having a "heart attack," with intense chest pain, palpitations, sweating, shaking, and an intense feeling of losing control. He has had six similar attacks in the last 3 months with escalating frequency. Fear of another attack has limited his ability to go to crowded areas such as the grocery store and to attend his college classes. S. P. has currently withdrawn from school and is getting his groceries delivered. He denies any drug abuse but does drink occasionally. An ECG and labs were performed in the ED and found to be normal. The psychiatrist's diagnosis is panic disorder with agoraphobia.

PMH: Several ED visits with complaints of heart attack symptoms, One depressive episode when S. P. was 24 yo (successfully treated with citalopram).
VS: BP 100/65, P 68, RR 18, Wt 180 lbs, Ht 5'11"
Lab: WNL
Medication: Multivitamin 1 po qd

1.1.0 Patient Information

Secondary Causes of Anxiety Disorders

- Psychiatric: Depression, mania, schizophrenia, delirium, dementia, eating disorders
  Drugs:
  - CNS stimulants: Amphetamines, caffeine, cocaine, ephedrine, Ecstasy (MDMA), methylphenidate, PCP, pseudoephedrine
  - Antidepressants: Bupropion, buspirone, SSRIs, SNRIs, TCAs
  - Withdrawal from nicotine, barbiturates, benzodiazepines, alcohol, or opiates
  - Other medications: Albuterol, baclofen, triptans, thyroid hormone, theophylline, steroids
- Medical illness: Hyperthyroidism, hypoglycemia, electrolyte imbalances, anemia, seizure disorders, multiple sclerosis, chronic pain, traumatic brain injury, migraines, Parkinson's disease, post MI, congestive heart failure, chronic obstructive pulmonary disease, asthma, HIV infection

Instruments and Techniques Related to Patient Assessment

- *Diagnostic and Statistical Manual of Mental Disorders* (DSM-IV-TR)
- Rating scales: Hamilton Rating Scale for Anxiety (HAM-A), Zung Self-Rating Anxiety Scale (SAS), State-Trait Anxiety Inventory, Sheehan Panic and Anticipatory Anxiety Scale (SPAAS), Acute Panic Inventory (API), Yale-Brown Obsessive Compulsive Scale (Y-BOCS), Obsessive Compulsive Inventory, Clinician Administered PTSD Scale (CAPS), Liebowitz Social Anxiety Scale (LSAS)

Classification, Terminology, and Signs and Symptoms

See Table 21-6.

1.2.0 Pharmacotherapy

- It often takes 4–6 weeks to see a reduction in symptoms after initiating an antidepressant and up to 8 weeks to see the full response.
- Benzodiazepines can be added to treatment to manage anxiety symptoms while waiting for response to antidepressant and to minimize antidepressant-related jitteriness.
- With buspirone, it takes at least 2 weeks to see an effect and up to 6 weeks to see the full response. Patients who have responded to a benzodiazepine in the past may not respond to buspirone.

Mechanisms of Action

- SSRIs: Inhibit serotonin reuptake in neurons of the CNS and show little binding affinity to muscarinic, histaminergic, and alpha$_1$-adrenergic receptors.
- SNRIs: Inhibit reuptake of both serotonin and norepinephrine but show little affinity to muscarinic, histaminergic, and alpha$_1$-andernergic receptors.
- TCAs: Inhibit reuptake of both serotonin and norepinephrine and have a high affinity for muscarinic, histaminergic, and alpha$_1$-adrenergic (side effects).
- Benzodiazepines: Potentiate the inhibitory activity of GABA.
  - GABA receptors contain protein subunits arranged in a pentamer with an ion channel in the center.
  - GABA receptors control tonic inhibition and decrease neuronal excitability.
  - Benzodiazepines bind on the GABA$_A$ receptor at the alpha$_1$, alpha$_2$, alpha$_3$, and alpha$_5$ subunits; they also bind to the beta and gamma$_2$ subunits.
  - Anxiolytic effects from the alpha$_2$ subunit.
  - Sedative effects from the alpha$_1$ subunit.
- Buspirone: Anxiolytic mechanism is unknown. However, it is thought to exert its effects through 5-HT$_{1A}$ partial agonism.

Drug, Food, and Lab Interactions and Important Pharmacokinetic and Pharmacodynamic Properties

Drug Interactions

Antidepressants (SSRIs, TCAs, and SNRIs): See the "Depression" section.
Benzodiazepines:

- Glucuronidation: Temazepam, oxazepam and lorazepam are conjugated and not likely to be affected by other CYP450 inhibitors or inducers.
- CYP 3A4 substrates: Alprazolam, clonazepam, clorazepate, diazepam, estazolam, flurazepam, midazolam, prazepam, triazolam.
- CYP 2C19: Diazepam.
- Increased CNS depressant effects: Alcohol, barbiturates, antipsychotics.

Buspirone: Is a substrate of CYP3A4. Inhibitors or inducers of this enzyme may alter buspirone's effect.

Table 21-6 Treatment of Anxiety Disorders

Disorder (Adapted from DSM-IV-TR criteria)	SSRIs	TCA	Benzodiaze-pines	Buspi-rone	Other
Generalized Anxiety Disorder		X	X	X	**Venlafaxine**
• Excessive anxiety or worry more days than not for 6 or more months • Person cannot control worry • Three of the following: restlessness, irritability, easily fatigued, muscle tension, difficulty concentrating, insomnia • Worries not caused by another disorder and that cause significant distress		Clomipramine Imipramine			Duloxetine CBT
Panic Disorder	X	X	X		**MAOI**
• Recurrent panic attacks • Episode of intense fear with at least four of the following: palpitations, chest pain, sweating, shaking, choking, nausea, dizziness, depersonalization, chills, hot flashes • Fear of loss of control or dying • 1 month of worry about recurrence of attack • Symptoms are not due to another disorder					CBT
Obsessive–Compulsive Disorder	X	X			**Atypical antipsychotics**
• Obsessions: recurrent thoughts, impulses, or images that cause significant anxiety or distress • Compulsions: repetitive behavior, person is driven to perform because of the obsessions; help relieve anxiety caused by the obsession		Clomipramine			CBT
Post-traumatic Stress Disorder	X	?	**Disinhibition alters the effectiveness of CBT**		**Prazosin: Use for sleep (normalizes stage I, II, and REM)**
• Exposure to a perceived life-threatening event • More than 1 month of reexperiencing (dreams, memories, flashbacks), avoidance (thoughts, activities, conversations associated with trauma), and increased arousal (sleep disturbances, irritability, difficulty concentrating, hypervigilance)			Not an effective treatment		Venlafaxine CBT
Social Anxiety Disorder	X	X	X		**MAOI**
• Marked or persistent fear of more than one performance situation where the person is exposed to strangers • Marked anxiety in these situations that interferes with normal function		Clomipramine			CBT

X = proven effectiveness in clinical trials, MAOI = monoamine oxidase inhibitor, SSRI = selective serotonin reuptake inhibitor, TCA = tricyclic antidepressant, CBT = cognitive-behavioral therapy.

Table 21-7 Pharmacotherapy for Anxiety Disorders

Class	Drug	Initial Dose	Weekly Titration	Usual Daily Dose (mg)	Dosage Formulation
SSRIs	Citalopram (Celexa)	10	10	20–40	Tablet Liquid
	Escitalopram (Lexapro)	5	5	10–20	Tablet Liquid
	Fluoxetine (Prozac)	5	10	10–80	Capsule Liquid
	Fluvoxamine (Luvox)	50	25	150–30	Tablet CR capsule
	Paroxetine (Paxil)	10	10	10–20	Tablet CR Liquid
	Sertraline (Zoloft)	25	25	25–200	Tablet Liquid
SNRIs	Venlafaxine (Effexor)	37.5	75	37.5–225	Capsule XR capsule
	Duloxetine (Cymbalta)	30	30	30–120	Capsule
TCAs	Imipramine (Tofranil)	10	10	150–300	Capsule Tablet
	Clomipramine (Anafranil)	25	25	25–225	Capsule
Benzodiazepines	Alprazolam (Xanax)	0.25–0.5 tid	0.25–0.5 every 3–4 days	4–10	Tablet ODT XR Liquid
	Clonazepam (Klonopin)	0.25 bid	0.25 –0.5 bid every 3–4 days	1–4	Tablet ODT
	Clorazepate (Tranxene)	3.75 tid	3.75 every 3–4 days	7.5–60	Tablet
	Diazepam (Valium)	2–5 tid	2–5 every 3–4 days	2–40	Tablet Solution Injection (IV push) Rectal gel
	Lorazepam (Ativan)	0.5–1 tid	0.5 every 3–4 days	2–8	Tablet Solution Injection (IM or IV)
	Oxazepam (Serax)	10 tid	10 every 3–4 days	30–120	Capsule Tablet
Other	Buspirone (Buspar)	7.5 bid	5 mg every 2–3 days	30–60	Tablet

SSRIs = selective serotonin reuptake inhibitors, TCAs = tricyclic antidepressants, SNRIs = serotonin norepinephrine reuptake inhibitors.

Pharmacokinetic Properties

The onset of the effect depends on the rate of drug absorption (lipophilicity).

- Diazepam and clorazepate: High lipophilicity → increased rate of absorption → rapidly absorbed and distributed quickly into the CNS; onset occurs in 30–60 minutes → rapid relief of anxiety → quick redistribution to periphery (adipose tissue) resulting in shorter duration of action after a single dose .
  - Some patients may have an unpleasant feeling of drowsiness or loss of control.
  - This "rush" could be euphoric and may encourage overuse/abuse and addiction.
- Lorazepam and oxazepam: Relatively less lipophilic, slightly longer onset, smaller volume of distribution resulting in a longer duration of action.
- Clonazepam and alprazolam XR: Alternatives to immediate-release alprazolam for patients with panic disorder having breakthrough panic symptoms at the end of a dosing interval.
- IM lorazepam: Provides rapid, reliable, and complete absorption.

Contraindications, Precautions, and Warnings

Antidepressants

See the "Depression" section.

Benzodiazepines

- Avoid alcohol
- Potential for abuse and physical dependence (withdrawal): Increased in substance abusers; not significant in the general population

Table 21-8 Pharmacokinetics of Benzodiazepines

Medication	Maximum Duration of Effect (hr)	Half-life (hr)	Clinically Significant Metabolites and Their Half-Lives
Alprazolam (Xanax)	1–2	8–15	None
Clonazepam (Klonopin)	1–4	30–60	None
Clorazepate (Tranxene)	1–2		DMDZ (36–96)
Diazepam (Valium)	0.5–2	20–70	DMDZ (36–6)
Lorazepam (Ativan)	2–4	10–20	
Oxazepam (Serax)	2–4	5–15	

DMDZ = desmethyldiazepam.

- Increased risk of withdrawal symptoms with sudden discontinuation
- Withdrawal symptoms' onset, duration, and severity vary according to dose, duration, and half-life of the benzodiazepine
- Abrupt discontinuation symptoms:
  - Anxiety rebound: Return of anxiety symptoms that are often worse than before treatment
  - Withdrawal symptoms: Anxiety, insomnia, irritability, muscle aches and weakness, nausea, depression, ataxia, blurred vision, fatigue, and rarely confusion, delirium, psychosis, and seizures
- Strategies to decrease withdrawal symptoms:
  - If on a benzodiazepine with a short half-life, switch to a longer-acting agent
  - Implement a 10–25% weekly reduction in dosage until 50% of original dose is reached, and then reduce the dosage by one-eighth every 4–7 days

1.3.0 Monitoring

Pharmacotherapeutic Response

Acute and chronic relief of anxiety symptoms.

Adverse Effects

Patient education may help avoid distress and improve compliance.

ANNOTATED BIBLIOGRAPHY

American Psychiatric Association. *Diagnostic and Statistical Manual of Mental Disorders,* 4th ed. Text Revision. Arlington, VA: American Psychiatric Association; 2000:429–484.

American Psychiatric Association. Practice guideline for the treatment of patients with acute stress disorder and posttraumatic stress disorder. *Am J Psychiatry* 2004;161:1–61.

American Psychiatric Association. *Practice Guideline for the Treatment of Patients with Obsessive–Compulsive Disorder,* 2nd ed. Arlington, VA: American Psychiatric Association; 2007. Available at: http://www.psychiatryonline.com/pracGuide/pracGuideTopic_10.aspx. Accessed April 10, 2010.

American Psychiatric Association. *Practice Guideline for the Treatment of Patients with Panic Disorder,* 2nd ed. Arlington, VA: American Psychiatric Association; 2009. Available at: http://www.psychiatryonline.com/pracGuide/pracGuideTopic_9.aspx. Accessed April 10, 2010.

Baldwin DS, Polkinghorn C. Evidence-based pharmacotherapy of generalized anxiety disorder. *Int J Neuropsychopharm* 2005;8:293–302.

Table 21-9 Medications for Anxiety Disorders: Side Effects

Drug Class	Side Effect	Additional Information	Patient Counseling
Benzodiazepine	Drowsiness	Most common side effect	Tolerance to sedation often develops in 1–2 weeks, but not tolerance to anxiolytic or antipanic efficacy.
	Cognitive impairment	Confusion, problems with balance and coordination Increased CNS effects in elderly	Do not operate heavy machinery. There is a five-fold increase in motor vehicle accidents while taking benzodiazepines. Do not drink alcohol while taking benzodiazepines. Do not abruptly discontinue benzodiazepines.
	Anterograde amnesia	Impairment of the memory for events that happen after ingesting the medication	Effects are temporary and reversible.
	Paradoxical effects	Disinhibition—increased anger, hostility, and agitation	Very rare side effect.
	Respiratory depression	Clinical significance in those patients with respiratory issues and in overdose situations, especially when combined with other depressants (alcohol, opiates)	Very rare side effect.
Buspirone	Dizziness, nausea, headache, nervousness, lightheadedness, excitement	Common side effects	Increase dose slowly. May take 2 weeks to see an effect and as long as 6 weeks to see the full effect. Do not operate heavy machinery until you know how this medication affects you. Most side effects are mild and will go away in 1–2 weeks with continued therapy.
SSRIs and SNRIs	GI upset, nervousness, headache, insomnia, anorexia, weight loss, and sexual dysfunction (ejaculatory delay, anorgasmia)	Common side effects	Take in the morning to avoid insomnia. Can induce anxiety during the first few weeks of therapy. May take 4 weeks to see an initial response and as long as 12 weeks to see the full response. Take medication daily. Take with food to reduce GI upset. Do not discontinue abruptly.
TCAs	Anxiety, jitteriness, anticholinergic, sedation, orthostatic hypotension, cardiac arrhythmias, weight gain, sexual dysfunction	Common side effects	May cause drowsiness. Use sugarless candy to relieve dry mouth. May take 4 weeks to see an initial response and as long as 12 weeks to see the full response. Rise from a sitting or lying position slowly to avoid dizziness. Do not discontinue abruptly.

Bisson J. Post-traumatic stress disorder. *BMJ* 2007;334: 789–793.

Blanco C, Antia SX, Liebowitz MR. Pharmacotherapy of social anxiety disorder. *Biol Psychiatry* 2002;51:109–120.

Guthrie SK, Augustin SG. Anxiety disorders. In: Finley PR, Lee KC, eds. *Applied Therapeutics: The Clinical Use of Drugs*, 9th ed. Baltimore, MD: Lippincott Williams & Wilkins; 2009:76.1–76.41.

Kirkwood CK, Makela EH, Wells BG. Anxiety disorders II: posttraumatic stress disorder and obsessive-compulsive disorder. In Dipiro JT, Talbert RL, Yee GC, et al., eds. *Pharmacotherapy: A Pathophysiologic Approach,* 7th ed. New York, NY: McGraw-Hill Medical; 2008:1179–1189.

Kirkwood CK, Melton ST. Anxiety disorders I: generalized anxiety, panic and social anxiety disorders. In Dipiro JT, Talbert RL, Yee GC, et al., eds. *Pharmacotherapy: A Pathophysiologic Approach*, 7th ed. New York, NY: McGraw-Hill Medical; 2008:1161–1178.

Perry PJ, Alexander B, Liskow B, DaVane CL. *Psychotropic Drug Handbook*, 8th ed. Baltimore, MD: Lippincott Williams & Wilkins; 2007.

Stahl SM. *Stahl's Essential Psychopharmacology*, 3rd ed. New York, NY: Cambridge University Press; 2008.

Stein DJ, Ipser JC, Seedat S. Pharmacotherapy for posttraumatic stress disorder (Cochrane review). In: *The Cochrane Library*. Oxford: Update Software; 2007:4.

Tyer P, Baldwin D. Generalised anxiety disorder. *Lancet* 2006;386:2156–2166.

TOPIC: ATTENTION-DEFICIT HYPERACTIVITY DISORDER

Section Coordinator: *Rex S. Lott*
Contributors: *Kevin W. Cleveland and John Erramouspe*

Attention-deficit hyperactivity disorder (ADHD) requires careful understanding and evaluation of the patient and the patient's family. In addition, ADHD can be associated with comorbid conditions that can complicate treatment selection. ADHD can be effectively treated. Pharmacists can play a pivotal role in recognizing signs and symptoms of ADHD, selecting treatment regimens, and identifying adverse drug reactions and interactions.

Tips Worth Tweeting

- ADHD is the most commonly diagnosed mental disorder in children.
- ADHD is characterized by three core symptoms—hyperactivity, impulsivity, and inattention—which typically begin by age of 3 and must occur prior to 7 years of age.
- The cause of ADHD is still unknown, but dysfunctions in norepinephrine and dopamine neurotransmission are indicated as key components.
- Goals for treatment of ADHD are to improve behavior, increase attention and response inhibition, and minimize adverse effects from pharmacotherapy.
- Pharmacotherapy is superior to behavioral therapy when either is used alone. However, both pharmacotherapy and behavioral therapy should be utilized to maximize treatment outcomes.
- Stimulants are first-line agents for treatment. If the initial stimulant choice fails, then an alternative stimulant should be tried.
- Counseling patients about the controversies regarding substance abuse and growth delay is important.

Patient Care Scenario: Ambulatory Setting

B. C.: 13 y.o., 71", M, Caucasian, 156 lbs, allergic to peanuts (anaphylaxis)

PMH: ADHD (predominantly displays inattentive ADHD at present; during grade school, B. C. demonstrated combined hyperactivity-impulsivity plus inattention), depression with anxiety, primary focal hyperhidrosis (palms, soles, and gluteal crease), acne vulgaris (mostly inflammatory), emergency room visit for closed head injury secondary to football, suicidal thoughts at age 11 years following argument with father—resolved.

Vital Signs: BP 104/78 (arm sitting), HR 76.

Lab Values: Last assessed during emergency room visit 4 months ago

Na 139 mEq/L (134–144)	Hgb 13.3 g/dL (13.3–16.1)
K 4.5 mEq/L (3.6–5.2)	Hct 40.0% (39.7–48.3)
Cl 101 mEq/L (100–109)	WBC 9.5 1,000/mm^3 (3.7–10.1)
BUN 12 mg/dL (7–18)	MCV 82 µm^3 (78–102)
SCr 1.1 mg/dL (0.6–1.2)	Glu 103 mg/dL (70–110)

Medication Profile: All drugs prescribed by Dr. Jones (pediatrician) except Daytrana patch (prescribed by pediatric psychiatrist).

Date	Drug	Quantity	Sig	Refills
29-Jan	Methylphenidate ER 20 mg	180	2 tabs po q AM	0
29-Jan	Fluoxetine 20 mg	30	1 cap po q AM	3
29-Jan	Epi-Pen 2-Pak 0.3 mg/0.3 mL	2	Inject IM into thigh for severe allergic reaction, may repeat in 10 minutes prn	0
29-Jan	Benzoyl peroxide 5% gel	42	Apply q hs	prn
29-Jan	Clindamycin 1% solution	60	Apply once daily	prn
29-Jan	Oxybutynin 5 mg	45	½ tab po tid for sweating	prn
29-Oct	Methylphenidate ER 20 mg	180	2 tabs po q AM	0
29-Oct	Glycopyrrolate 1 mg	60	1 tab po bid for sweating	prn
9-Sep	FluMist	0.2	0.2 mL nasally	0
9-Sep	Drysol 20% solution	60	Apply q hs to palms, soles, and gluteal crease prn	prn

Date	Drug	Quantity	Sig	Refills
26-Jul	Methylphenidate ER 20 mg	180	2 tabs po q AM	0
28-Apr	Methylphenidate ER 20 mg	180	2 tabs po q AM	0
28-Feb	Methylphenidate ER 20 mg	180	2 tabs po q AM	0
30-Jan	Methylphenidate ER 20 mg	30	1 tabs po q AM	0
15-Jan	Daytrana patch 10 mg per 9 hr	10	Apply 1 patch daily for 9 hr, then remove	0

1.1.0 Patient Information

Diagnostic Criteria for ADHD

- Must meet *Diagnostic and Statistical Manual of Mental Health Disorders,* fourth edition, Text Revision (DSM-IV-TR) criteria for ADHD in either inattention or hyperactivity/impulsivity.
- Must exhibit symptoms after 3 years of age and prior to 7 years of age, with symptoms persisting longer than 7 months.
- Symptoms affect functioning in social situations, school, or work and are present in more than one of these settings.
- Symptoms cannot be explained by any other psychiatric disorder.

Laboratory Testing and Physical Assessment

- Baseline physical examination before starting stimulant therapy should include: blood pressure, pulse, height, and weight. An exam should also be performed yearly.
- Liver function tests (LFT): Necessary to evaluate liver function.
- Electrocardiogram (ECG): Helpful to identify cardiac conduction problems and/or underlying cardiac pathology. Recommended only if known cardiac disease exists or if the patient or family history suggests cardiac disease. ECG is required at baseline and routinely during tricyclic antidepressant therapy.

Disease States Associated with ADHD

- ADHD frequently is associated with other comorbid conditions: anxiety, depression, obsessive–compulsive disorder, tic disorders (oral, motor, Tourette syndrome), bipolar disorder, conduct disorder, oppositional defiant disorder, and learning disabilities.
- Comorbid conditions will help guide the selection of initial therapy and modification of ongoing treatment choices.

Instruments and Techniques Related to Patient Assessment

- Document ADHD core symptoms at baseline.
- Expected improvements should be individualized, including those in the following areas: family and social relationships, disruptive behavior, completing required tasks, self-motivation, appearance, and self-esteem.
- Standardized rating scales generally used in both pediatric and adult ADHD include the Conners Rating Scales—Revised, Brown Attention-Deficit Disorder Scale, and Inattentive-Overactive with Aggression (IOWA) Conners Scale. These instruments are utilized to help minimize variability in treatment assessment.
- Evaluate patients every 2–4 weeks for height, weight, pulse, and blood pressure—especially after initiation of stimulant therapy.
- Perform routine physical examination and laboratory tests (LFTs, CBC) to monitor for side effects of medications.

Key Terms

- **Three subtypes of ADHD:** (1) primarily inattentive, (2) predominately hyperactive/impulsive, and (3) combined inattentive-hyperactive/impulsive symptoms.
- **Inattention:** Difficulty paying attention to details in school, work, and social activities; difficulty completing tasks that require significant mental effort; easily distracted; forgetful.
- **Hyperactivity/impulsivity:** Difficulty sitting still, fidgety; trouble playing quietly; interrupts frequently.

Wellness and Prevention

- During grade school, ADHD has a greater incidence in males than in females.
- Symptoms can persist until adulthood; 60% of adult ADHD patients have symptoms that first became manifest during childhood.
- ADHD-related problems (social, marital, academic, career, anxiety, depression, smoking, and substance abuse) increase as patients transition into adulthood.
- Interviewing the patient and/or caregivers is important in obtaining a proper medical history, which should include family medical history, current and past prescription medications, over-the-counter medications, and diet.
- ADHD therapy can be a substantial financial burden as a result of both direct (medications, office visits, therapy monitoring) and indirect (lost school/work time and productivity) costs.

Prescription cost burden should not be the only consideration when selecting therapy; efficacy and safety should be considered foremost.

1.2.0 Pharmacotherapy

Indications for ADHD Medications

- The mechanism of ADHD pharmacotherapy is modulation of neurotransmitter function (dopamine and norepinephrine) so as to improve patient functioning.
- ADHD medications can be divided into two categories: stimulants and nonstimulants.

Drugs, Indications, Dosing, and Routes of Administration

- Stimulant medications are the most effective agents in treating ADHD and should be considered first-line therapy after a diagnosis of ADHD has been made.
- Stimulant therapy should be initiated using the lowest dose and titrated to the lowest effective dose while minimizing side effects.
- At least two stimulants should be tried prior to recommending a nonstimulant.
- Due to atomoxetine's long half-life, it can be dosed once daily.

Table 21-10 Pharmacotherapy Used in ADHD

Drug, Generic (Brand)	Typical Daily Dosing Range (Maximum Daily Dose)
Stimulants	
Short-acting	
Methylphenidate (Methylin, Ritalin)	10–60 mg in 2–3 divided doses (60 mg)
Dexmethylphenidate (Focalin)	10–20 mg in 2 divided doses (20 mg)
Dextroamphetamine (Dexedrine)	10–40 mg in 2 divided doses (40 mg)
Intermediate-acting	
Methylphenidate (Ritalin SR, Metadate ER, Methylin ER)	20–40 mg daily in the morning (60 mg)
Dextroamphetamine/amphetamine (Adderall)	10–30 mg every morning or 10–40 mg in 2 divided doses (40 mg)
Dextroamphetamine (Dexedrine Spansule)	5–30 mg daily or 10–30 mg in 2 divided doses (40 mg)
Extended-acting	
Methylphenidate	
(Concerta)	18–54 mg every morning (54 mg)
(Metadate CD)	20–40 mg daily in the morning (60 mg)
(Ritalin LA)	20–40 mg daily in the morning (60 mg)
(Daytrana transdermal patch)	10–30 mg patch once daily; remove up to 9 hours after application (30 mg)
Dextroamphetamine/ amphetamine (Adderall XR)	10–30 mg every morning or 10–60 mg in 2 divided doses (30 mg in children; 60 mg in adults)
Dexmethylphenidate (Focalin XR)	10–20 mg daily in the morning (20 mg)
Lisdexamfetamine (Vyvanse)	30–70 mg daily in the morning (70 mg)
Nonstimulants	
Atomoxetine (Strattera)	≤ 70 kg: 40–60 mg/day (1.4 mg/kg or 100 mg, whichever is less)
	> 70 kg: 40–80 mg/day divided once to twice daily (100 mg)
Imipramine (Tofranil)	Children: 1.5–3 mg/kg per day in one or two divided doses (5 mg/kg)
	Adults: 100–300 mg/day in one or two divided doses (300 mg)
Clonidine (Catapres)	0.1–0.4 mg in one to four divided doses (0.4 mg)
Guanfacine (Tenex, Intuniv)	1.5–3 mg/day divided into two or three times daily (4 mg/day). Intuniv is a sustained-release product dosed once daily.
Bupropion (Wellbutrin, Wellbutrin SR, Wellbutrin XL)	6 mg/kg per day or 400 mg/day (whichever is less)—in children; 150–450 mg/day (400 mg/day SR; 450 mg/day XL)—in adults

- Atomoxetine and bupropion can both be useful for treating ADHD with comorbid depression.
- TCAs (imipramine) will help improve comorbid depression and anxiety.
- Clonidine and guanfacine are useful as adjuncts in stimulant therapy in managing aggressive or disruptive behavior and in alleviating insomnia.

Drug, Food, and Lab Test Interactions

Stimulants

- Decreased effects of antihypertensive medications.
- Increased risk of cardiovascular effects such as hypertension and dysrhythmias when stimulants are combined with TCAs. May result from enhanced stimulant effects related to norepinephrine release. Methylphenidate may also inhibit the metabolism of TCAs.
- Methylphenidate may inhibit the hepatic metabolism of selective serotonin reuptake inhibitor (SSRI) antidepressants, resulting in elevated plasma concentrations of the antidepressant. Lower doses of SSRIs may be needed.

Atomoxetine

- Concurrent use of antidepressants (fluoxetine, paroxetine) or other cytochrome P450 2D6 inhibitors can increase atomoxetine serum levels. This will require a slower titration to an effective dose.
- In poor metabolizers of CYP2D6 (5–10% of population), the dose should be reduced to 25–50% of that used in normal metabolizers.

Contraindications, Warnings, and Precautions

- Stimulants should not be used in patients with glaucoma, hypertension, cardiovascular disease, hyperthyroidism, severe anxiety, or past/current illicit drug abuse. In addition, they should be used cautiously in patients with seizure disorders, motor tics, and Tourette syndrome.
- Atomoxetine should not be used in patients with severe hepatic insufficiency
- Atomoxetine's labeling includes a "black box" warning about suicidal ideation.
- Bupropion use is contraindicated in patients with seizure and eating disorders.
- Tricyclic antidepressants should not be used in patients with cardiovascular disease due to the risk of cardiotoxicity; they should be used cautiously in patients with seizure disorders. Due to reported fatalities, desipramine should not be considered to treat ADHD in pediatric and adolescent patients.

Biopharmaceutical Principles and Pharmaceutical Characteristics of Dosage Forms

- Stimulant medications can be divided into groups based on their onset of action.
- Short-acting formulations can have an initial response that begins within 30 minutes and lasts 4–6 hours.
- Intermediate-acting stimulants release medication in a slow, continuous manner, with an onset of action in 60–90 minutes.
- Extended-acting stimulants have been formulated to have an initial rapid release followed by a continuous or delayed pulsed release of medication. These formulations have the benefits of both quick onset of action and ability to maintain symptom control throughout the day with a single morning dose. However, the methylphenidate transdermal patches and lisdexamfetamine formulations have a slower onset of action (2 hours) than the other extended-acting formulations.

1.3.0 Monitoring

Pharmacotherapeutic Outcomes

- After initiation of therapy, patients should be evaluated every 2–4 weeks to determine treatment efficacy, height, weight, pulse, and blood pressure.
- Physical examination may be used to monitor for adverse effects. Liver function tests should be performed at baseline and routinely during atomoxetine therapy. In children being considered for ADHD pharmacotherapy, baseline electrocardiograms (ECGs) should be obtained when known or suspected cardiac disease exists or the physician judges it necessary.
- Typically, therapeutic benefits will be seen within days of initiating stimulants and within 1–2 months with atomoxetine and bupropion therapy.
- Once maintenance dosing has been achieved, schedule follow-up visits every 3 months. At these visits, assess the patient's height and weight, and screen for possible adverse drug effects.
- If a patient has failed to respond to multiple agents, reevaluate for other possible causes of behavior dysfunction.
- Typically, appropriately treated patients learn to better control their ADHD symptoms as adults.

Safety and Efficacy Monitoring

- It is important to educate the patient's parent and/or caregivers about ADHD.
- The response to stimulant therapy might take as long as 4 weeks to appear, but a trial of 3 months

Table 21-11 ADHD Pharmacotherapy Monitoring

Drug	Pharmacotherapy Monitoring
Stimulants	
Methylphenidate, dextroamphetamine, dextroamphetamine/ amphetamine, dexmethylphenidate, lisdexamfetamine	Height, weight, BP, HR, diet, and sleeping patterns; evaluate every 2–4 weeks until a stable dose is achieved, then every 3 months; obtain baseline and routine ECGs as needed if cardiac risk factors are present
Nonstimulants	
Atomoxetine	Height, weight, blood pressure, and heart rate, with baseline and routine liver function tests
Tricyclic antidepressants (imipramine)	Blood pressure, heart rate, and sleeping pattern; evaluate every 3 days until a stable dose is achieved, then evaluate every 3 months; ECG
Clonidine and guanfacine	Same as for TCAs
Bupropion	Height, weight, blood pressure, and heart rate every month until a stable dose is achieved, then every 3 months; evaluate eating and sleeping patterns to ensure there is no risk of seizures

and dose maximization should be pursued until the stimulant is considered a failure.

- The methylphenidate transdermal patch needs to be applied for no longer than 9 hours.
- Atomoxetine effects may take as long as 4 weeks to be seen.
- Sedation is typically transient with clonidine and guanfacine and subsides after 2–3 weeks.
- Growth suppression is a major concern for the caregivers of children taking stimulants. Growth delay almost always is transient, and patients generally reach their potential growth height by mid-adolescence.
- Although the diagnosis of ADHD increases the risk of substance abuse, appropriate stimulant treatment does not increase (and may actually reduce) this risk.
- Patients and their families should be counseled that treatment generally is long term.

Adverse Drug Reactions and Management

See Table 21-12.

Nonadherence, Misuse, or Abuse

- Generally, extended-release formulations of stimulants improve adherence by limiting the number of daily doses required and minimizing many potential side effects.
- Nonadherence to appropriate therapy can result in rebound or breakthrough ADHD symptoms. This can also occur when the effect of the stimulant medication wears off at the end of a dosing interval.

ANNOTATED BIBLIOGRAPHY

American Academy of Pediatrics, Subcommittee on Attention-Deficit/Hyperactivity Disorder and Committee on Quality Improvement. Clinical practice guideline: treatment of the school-aged child with attention-deficit/hyperactivity disorder. *Pediatrics* 2001;108(4):1033–1044.

American Psychiatric Association. *Diagnostic and Statistical Manual of Mental Disorders,* 4th ed. Text Revision Washington, DC: American Psychiatric Press; 2000:39–134.

Birnbaum HG, Kessler RC, Lowe SW, et al. Costs of attention deficit-hyperactivity disorder (ADHD) in the U.S.: excess costs of persons with ADHD and their family members in 2000. *Curr Med Res Opin* 2005;21(2):195–205.

Belle DJ, Ernest S, Sauer J, et al. Effect of potent CYP2D6 inhibition by paroxetine on atomoxetine pharmacokinetics. *J Clin Pharmacol* 2002;42:1219–1227.

Biederman J, Boellner SW, Childress A, et al. Lisdexamfetamine dimesylate and mixed amphetamine salts extended-release in children with ADHD: a double-blind, placebo-controlled, crossover analog classroom study. *Biol Psychiatry* 2007;62:970–976.

Biederman J, Faraone S. Attention-deficit hyperactivity disorder. *Lancet* 2005;366:237–248.

Biederman J, Heiligenstein JH, Faries DE, et al. Efficacy of atomoxetine versus placebo in school-age girls with attention-deficit/hyperactivity disorder. *Pediatrics* 2002;110(6):E75.

Boyer EW, Shannon M. Current concepts: the serotonin syndrome. *N Engl J Med* 2005;352(11):1112–1120.

Brown RT, Amler RW, Freeman WS, et al. Treatment of attention-deficit/hyperactivity disorder: overview of the evidence. *Pediatrics* 2005;115:749–757.

Centers for Disease Control and Prevention. Prevalence of diagnosis and medication treatment for

Table 21-12 Medications for ADHD: Adverse Drug Reactions and Management Techniques

Stimulants	Adverse Drug Reaction	ADR Management Techniques
	GI upset, nausea, decreased appetite, potential growth delay	Administer after meals; encourage caloric-dense meals; divide the dose; give evening snacks Change to a shorter-acting stimulant Initiate a drug holiday or use a nonstimulant if severe growth delay occurs
	Sleep disturbance	Give dose in the morning Give clonidine or guanfacine at bedtime Discontinue all doses given in the afternoon Change to a shorter-acting stimulant
	Rebound symptoms	Change to a longer-acting stimulant Shorten the dose frequency of the stimulant medication
	Mood changes	Decrease the dose or change to a longer-acting stimulant Verify diagnosis/comorbidity
	Irritability	Evaluate the time of occurrence: Early onset: Decrease the dose or switch from a shorter- to longer-acting stimulant Late onset: Switch to a longer-acting stimulant; evaluate for comorbidity
	Increased blood pressure and pulse	Decrease the dose or change to a longer-acting stimulant
	Tics	Discontinue or change to a different stimulant; give clonidine or guanfacine
Nonstimulants	**Adverse Drug Reaction**	**ADR Managegment Techniques**
Atomoxetine	Increased blood pressure and pulse, nausea, vomiting, fatigue, and insomnia	Decrease the dose or change to another medication
	Hepatotoxicity, suicidal thoughts	Discontinue or change to a another medication
Tricyclic antidepressants (imipramine)	Sedation	Administer later in the day
	Cardiac conduction delay, dizziness, increased pulse	Decrease the dose or change to another medication
	Anticholinergic effects (constipation, dry mouth, difficult urinating, blurry vision)	Decrease the dose or change to another medication
Clonidine and guanfacine	Sedation, arrhythmias, constipation, dizziness (decreased blood pressure)	Sedation: Administer in the afternoon Decrease the dose or change to another medication
Bupropion	GI upset, restlessness, sleep disturbances, rash, tics, risk of seizures	Decrease the dose or change to another medication Tics, rash, and seizures: Discontinue medication

attention-deficit/hyperactivity disorder—United States, 2003. *MMWR* 2005;54:842–847.

Collett BR, Ohan JL, Myers KM. Ten-year review of rating scales. V: scales assessing attention-deficit /hyperactivity disorder. *J Am Acad Child Adolesc Psychiatry* 2003;42(9):1015–1037

Daviss WB, Bentivoglio P, Racusin R, et al. Bupropion sustained release in adolescents with comorbid attention-deficit/hyperactivity disorder and depression. *J Am Acad Child Adolesc Psychiatry* 2001;40(3):307–314.

ECGs before stimulants in children. *Med Lett Drugs Ther* 2008;50(1291):60.

Elia J, Ambrosini PJ, Rapoport JL. Treatment of attention-deficit–hyperactivity disorder. *N Engl J Med* 1999;340(10):780–788.

Greenhill LL, Pliszka S, Dulcan MK, et al. Practice parameter for the use of stimulant medications in the treatment of children, adolescents, and adults. *J Am Acad Child Adolesc Psychiatry* 2002;41 (2 suppl):26S–49S.

Hazell PL, Stuart JE. A randomized controlled trial of clonidine added to psychostimulant medication for hyperactive and aggressive children. *J Am Acad Child Adolesc Psychiatry* 2003;42: 886-894.

Herrerias CT, Perrin JM, Stein MT. The child with ADHD: using the AAP clinical practice guideline. *Am Fam Physician* 2001;63(9):1803–1810.

Kratochvil CJ, Heiligenstein JH, Dittmann R, et al. Atomoxetine and methylphenidate treatment in children with ADHD: a prospective, randomized, open-label trial. *J Am Acad Child Adolesc Psychiatry* 2002;41(7):776–784.

Matza LS, Paramore C, Prasad M. A review of the economic burden of ADHD. *Cost Eff Resour Alloc* 2005;3:5.

Michelson D, Allen AJ, Busner J, et al. Once-daily atomoxetine treatment for children and adolescents with attention deficit hyperactivity disorder: a randomized, placebo-controlled study. *Am J Psychiatry* 2002;159:1896–1901.

Michelson D, Faries D, Wernicke J, et al. Atomoxetine in the treatment of children and adolescents with attention-deficit/hyperactivity disorder: a randomized, placebo-controlled, dose-response study. *Pediatrics* 2001;108(5):E83.

MTA Cooperative Group. A 14-month randomized clinical trial of treatment strategies for attention-deficit/hyperactivity disorder. *Arch Gen Psychiatry* 1999;56(12):1073–1086.

Perrin JM, Friedman RA, Knilans TK, et al. Cardiovascular monitoring and stimulant drugs for attention-deficit/hyperactivity disorder. *Pediatrics* 2008;122: 451–453.

Rappley MD. Attention deficit-hyperactivity disorder. *N Engl J Med* 2005;352:165–173.

Tallian K. Pharmacotherapy of ADHD. In: Schumock G, Brundage D, Chapman M, et al., eds. *Pharmacotherapy Self-Assessment Program,* 5th ed. Pediatrics II. Kansas City, MO: American College of Clinical Pharmacy; 2006:275–297.

Vetter VL, Elia J, Erickson C, et al. Cardiovascular monitoring of children and adolescents with heart disease receiving medications for attention deficit/hyperactivity disorder: a scientific statement from the American Heart Association Council on Cardiovascular Disease in the Young Congenital Cardiac Defects Committee and the Council on Cardiovascular Nursing. *Circulation* 2008;117:2407–2423.

Voeller KKS. Attention-deficit hyperactivity disorder (ADHD). *J Child Neurol* 2004;19:798–814.

Wilens TE, Faraone SV, Biederman J, et al. Does stimulant therapy of attention-deficit/hyperactivity disorder beget later substance abuse? A meta-analytic review of the literature. *Pediatrics* 2003;111: 179–185.

Wilens TE, Spencer TJ, Biederman J, et al. A controlled clinical trial of bupropion for attention deficit hyperactivity disorder in adults. *Am J Psychiatry* 2001;158:282–288.

Wolraich ML, Wibbelsman CJ, Brown TE, et al. Attention-deficit/hyperactivity disorder among adolescents: a review of the diagnosis, treatment, and clinical implications. *Pediatrics* 2005;115(6):1734–1746.

Zametkin AJ, Ernst M. Problems in the management of attention-deficit–hyperactivity disorder. *N Engl J Med* 1999;340(1):40–46.

TOPIC: BIPOLAR DISORDER

Section Coordinator: *Rex S. Lott*
Contributors: *Sarah J. Popish and Alberto Augsten*

Bipolar disorder is classified as an affective disorder; stated simply, it is a disorder that affects the mood of an individual. The different types of mood disturbances are described as major depressive disorder, hypomanic episodes, manic episodes, and mixed episodes. A person who has experienced one or more manic or mixed episodes is diagnosed as bipolar I, with or without a depressive episode. If a patient has experienced only depressive and hypomanic episodes, then the individual is diagnosed as bipolar II. Bipolar disorder affects more women than men; often women spend more time in the depressive aspect and can have several depressive episodes before they experience a manic or hypomanic episode. In addition to experiencing the manic and depressive spectra of the disorders, patients can be euthymic (normal stable mood). However, as the disease progresses, patients spend less time in a euthymic state and more time in the other spectra of the disorder. If a patient experiences four or more different mood episodes in a year, he or she is considered to be "rapid cycling."

Bipolar affective disorder is treated with mood stabilizers, with lithium being the gold standard. Other medications used are antipsychotics and antiepileptics (valproic acid, carbamazepine, lamotrigine). Often the mood stabilizers are augmented with antipsychotics to treat and shorten the manic or depressive episodes. Antidepressants are not effective in the treatment of depression in bipolar disorder and may precipitate a manic or hypomanic episode.

Tips Worth Tweeting

- Lithium is used for both acute and maintenance treatment of bipolar disorder, with 70% of patients responding to therapy.
- Lithium is the gold standard for the treatment of bipolar disorder, and its use decreases the incidence of suicide.
- Lithium levels must be monitored to avoid toxicity.
- Mania can be treated with combination therapy (mood stabilizer + antipsychotic) with good response.
- Lamotrigine must be initiated slowly to avoid Stevens-Johnson syndrome. If a patient misses a week of therapy, lamotrigine must be retitrated.
- Lamotrigine is effective in treating the depressive aspects of bipolar disorder. It should not be used in mania.
- Valproic acid can cause significant weight gain.

Patient Care Scenario: Inpatient Psychiatric Admission

Q. I. is a 23-year-old Asian female.
Chief complaint: "I've seen too much, I guess."
HPI: Q. I. was brought to the hospital by the police. According to her roommate, who called the police, Q. I. has been acting "strange" lately. She has been coming home later and later each evening, often singing disco loudly. The roommate estimates that she has been getting only 2 to 3 hours of sleep each night. Her dress and manner have changed from conservative to "racy" and "forward." Q. I. bought new living room and bedroom furniture sets even though she was recently laid off from her job as a paralegal. The roommate finally called the police when Q. I. started screaming at the roommate "be healed in the eyes of the disco goddess" and throwing books and other odds and ends.
PMH: The patient states that she has had two psychiatric hospitalizations and was treated with "tender loving care" and has never needed medications. The patient denies any medical problems
Metal status exam: The patient is dressed flamboyantly and is slightly malodorous, with a heavy application of smeared bright makeup. Since her admission, Q. I. has been pacing the halls and singing loudly. When asked how she feels, she states, "Brilliant, wonderful, sexy, I'm getting married to Frank, Henry, George, Stan! All disco kings have four names, and we are going to dance and play. Now I have to go to get ready to rule the kingdom in a big white dress like the angel on high." Her speech is pressured and loud; she often speaks in rhymes and does not finish sentences. Her affect is labile. During the interview, the patient has a difficult time sitting still and often breaks into song. Her mood is obviously elevated, but she becomes increasingly irritable throughout the interview. After being asked to spell "world" backward, she becomes angry and tearful and insists that she has to leave because she is not a "bad person": "I just have to sing the disco songs so that the earth keeps turning and we all don't die." She then starts laughing loudly and walks out of the room.
SH: The patient smokes but cannot tell how many cigarettes she smokes in a day. She denies substance abuse and does not drink because it makes her sick.
VS: BP 118/73, P 83, Wt 110 lbs, Ht 61 inches
Labs: BMP, WNL; CBC, WNL; UA, negative; urine HGC, negative; liver enzymes, WNL.
Medications: Ortho-lo 28.

1.1.0 Patient Information

Secondary Causes of Mania

- Sleep deprivation
- Medications that affect monoamine neurotransmission (antidepressants, stimulants, sympathomimetics)
- Other drugs (e.g., corticosteroids, anabolic steroids, isoniazid, and caffeine)

Instruments and Techniques Related to Patient Assessment

- *Diagnostic and Statistical Manual of Mental Disorders* (DSM IV-TR)
- Rating scales: Young Mania Rating Scale (YMRS), Clinical Global Impression (CGI), Depression and Mania Scale (SDMS-D&M), Schedule for Affective Disorders and Schizophrenia (SADS)

Signs and Symptoms

See Table 21-13.

Key Terms

- **Bipolar I:** One or more manic or mixed episodes; depression may have occurred.
- **Bipolar II:** Hypomanic and major depressive episodes.
- **Rapid cycling:** More than four episodes of mania or depression in the last 12 months.

1.20 Pharmacotherapy

See Table 21-14.

Lamotrigine Titration Schedule

- Monotherapy and no enzyme inducer present
  - Target dose = 200 mg/day; titrate over 6 weeks
  - Weeks 1 and 2: 25 mg/day; weeks 3 and 4: 50 mg/day; week 5: 100 mg/day; week 6: 200 mg/day (target dose)

Table 12-13 Diagnostic Criteria for Bipolar Disorder

Mania	Hypomania	Mixed
• Persistent irritable or elevated mood × 1 week ○ Inflated self-esteem (grandiosity) ○ Flight of ideas ○ Distractibility ○ Decreased need for sleep ○ Psychomotor agitation ○ Increased goal-directed activity ○ Increased risk taking in pleasurable activities (e.g., sex, shopping) • Causes marked social impairment or leads to hospitalization	• Irritable or elevated mood that last at least 4 days • Same symptoms as for mania but to a lesser degree • Hospitalization is not required • No marked social impairment	• Criteria for both major depressive episode and manic episode are present nearly every day for a week • Symptoms: agitation, insomnia, appetite disturbances, suicidal ideation, and psychosis • May require hospitalization

Adapted from: DSM-IV-TR.

Table 21-14 Pharmacotherapy for Bipolar Disorder

Drug	Initial Dose	Weekly Titration	Usual Daily Dose	Target Level	Dosage Formulation	Brand
Lithium carbonate Lithium citrate (liquid)	300 mg (8.1 mEq bid)	Dependent on lithium level	900–1,800 mg/day	0.9–1.2 mEq/L (acute) 0.6–0.9 meq/L (maintenance)	Capsule/tablet	Eskalith
					Tablet ER	Eskalith ER Lithobid
					Liquid	Cibalth-S
Divalproex sodium (DR) Valproic acid (IR)	500 mg bid	250–500 mg/day (dependent on level)	1,000–2,000 mg/day	50–125 mcg/mL > 94 mcg/mL correlates with decrease manic symptoms	Capsule Liquid	Depakene
					Tablet DR	Depakote
					Tablet ER	Depakote ER
Lamotrigine	See titration schedule				Tablet Chewable	Lamictal
Carbamazepine	200 mg bid	200 mg q 3 days	800–1,200 mg	4–12 mcg/mL	Tablet Liquid	Tegretol
					Tablet ER	Tegratol XR
					Capsule ER	Equetro Carbatrol
Antipsychotic medications	See the "Schizophrenia" section					

- Added to regimen containing valproate (divalproex or valproic acid)
  - Target dose = 100 mg/day; titrate over 6 weeks
  - Weeks 1 and 2: 25 mg/qod; weeks 3 and 4: 25 mg/day; week 5: 50 mg/day; week 6: 100 mg/day (target dose)
- Added to regimen containing enzyme inducer (e.g., carbamazepine) but no valproate
  - Target dose = 400 mg/day; titrate over 7 weeks
- Weeks 1 and 2: 50 mg/day; weeks 3 and 4: 100 mg/dat (divided doses); week 5: 200 mg/day (divided doses); week 6: 300 mg/day (divided doses); and week 7: up to 400 mg/day
- The initial treatment of mania usually involves a mood stabilizer or a second-generation antipsychotic (SGA); the combination of a mood stabilizer/SGA is commonly used in acute manic patients.

Mechanisms of Action

Lithium

- Modifies second-messenger system → inhibits phosphoinositide → increases inositol phosphate → membrane stabilization → decreases neuronal response

Divalproex Sodium (multiple mechanisms)

- Increases GABA
- Inhibits GABA metabolism
- Increases $GABA_B$ receptor density
- Decreases Na channel activity

Carbamazepine

- Blocks NE reuptake
- Decreases Na channel activity
- Decreases NE release
    - Decreases DA and GABA turnover
    - Blocks Ca influx

Lamotrigine

- Decreases Na channel activity
- Prolongs Na channel inactivation

Drug, Food, and Lab Test Interactions and Important Pharmacokinetic and Pharmacodynamic Properties

Drug Interactions

Antipsychotic Medications: See the "Schizophrenia" section.

Lithium: 95% renally eliminated. Thus anything affecting renal clearance will affect lithium concentrations, [Li].

- ACE inhibitors (e.g., lisinopril, fosinopril) → ≈36% ↑ [Li]
- ARBs (e.g., candesartan, losartan) → lesser extent than ACE inhibitors
- Thiazide diuretics (e.g., HCTZ, chlorthalidone) → ≈25% ↑ [Li]
- NSAID—large individual differences
    - Diclofenac → ≈26% ↑ [Li]
    - Indomethacin → ≈20–59% ↑ [Li]
    - Ibuprofen → ≈12–66% ↑ [Li]
    - Naproxen → ≈16% ↑ [Li]
    - Sulindac → minimal ↑ [Li]
    - Aspirin → minimal ↑ [Li]

Divalproex: Is a substrate of CYP 450 2C19. It is an inhibitor of 2C9, 2D6, and 3A4 as well as epoxide hydrolase. Is approximately 90% protein bound (albumin).

- Divalproex inhibits the metabolism of carbamazepine's (CBZ) active metabolite (CBZ-10, 11-epoxide).
- CBZ may induce the metabolism of divalproex.

Lamotrigine

- Divalproex inhibits the metabolism of lamotrigine.
- When combined with divalproex, lamotrigine doses must be decreased by approximately 50% to minimize the increased risk of skin rashes and potential Stevens-Johnson syndrome.
- Risk of severe rash is increased by:
    - Co-administration with valproate or any enzyme inhibitors
    - Exceeding the recommended initial dose of lamotrigine
    - Exceeding the recommended dose escalation recommendations
- Oral contraceptives decrease serum concentrations of lamotrigine, and serum lamotrigine levels rise during the placebo period.

Carbamazepine: Is a potent inducer of several CYP450 isoenzymes—especially CYP 3A4.

- Oral contraceptives' effectiveness is decreased owing to more rapid clearance of the hormones.
- Auto-induction of its own metabolism by CYP 3A4.
- Takes approximately 4 weeks for induction effects to reach their maximum.

1.3.0 Monitoring

Contraindications, Precautions, and Warnings

Antipsychotic Medications

See the "Schizophrenia" section.

Lithium Toxicity

- Mild (1.5–2.0 mEq/L): Nausea, vomiting, diarrhea, mild hand tremor, confusion, lethargy
- Moderate (2.0–2.5 mEq/L): Nausea, vomiting, diarrhea (more severe than mild toxicity), coarse hand tremor, increased confusion and lethargy, drowsiness, slurred speech, blurred vision, unsteady gait

Table 21-15 Pharmacokinetics of Mood Stabilizers

Medication	Maximum Duration (hr)	Half-life (hr)	Pb
Lithium	0.5–3 (IR), 4–12 (ER), 0.25–1 (solution)	24	0%
Valproic acid	See the "Seizure Disorders" chapter		
Carbamazepine			
Lamotrigine			

Table 21-16 Monitoring of Bipolar Disorder Pharmacotherapy

Medication	CBC	Electrolytes	LFT	Renal Function	ECG	Other
Lithium	X	X		X	X	Pregnancy, thyroid panel, weight gain, lithium levels
Carbamazepine	X	X	X		X	Pregnancy, carbamazepine level
Valproic acid	X		X			Pregnancy, weight gain, VPA level
Lamotrigine						Rash

Table 21-17 Adverse Drug Reactions with Bipolar Disorder Pharmacotherapy

Drug	Side Effect	Additional Information	Patient Education
Lithium	GI: Nausea, vomiting, diarrhea	Reduce dose or switch to ER	○ Take with food if lithium causes GI upset. ○ Maintain salt intake; changes can cause increase or decrease lithium levels. ○ Avoid large amounts of caffeine. ○ Avoid becoming dehydrated. ○ Always check with your healthcare provider before starting new medications (even OTC products). ○ Family planning is necessary when taking this medication. ○ Contact your healthcare provider if you experience confusion, coarse hand tremor, severe GI upset, or sedation. You may need to have your levels adjusted.
	Tremor (mild)	Reduce dose; add propranolol	
	Weight gain		
	Polyuria, polydipsia	Maintain adequate fluid intake	
	Hypothyroidism	Treat with levothyroxine	
	Dermatologic	Acne, rashes, exacerbation of psoriasis	
	Leukocytosis	Generally benign	
Carbamazepine	GI: Nausea, vomiting, diarrhea	Slow titration, go away with time	○ Take with food if CBZ causes GI upset. ○ Check with your healthcare provider before starting new medications ○ Do not eat or drink grapefruit while on this medication. ○ Report flu-like symptoms, because this medication can rarely cause changes in the blood cells. ○ Family planning is important while taking this medication.
	Drowsiness, dizziness, ataxia, blurred vision, confusion, headache	Slow titration, go away with time	
	Agranulocytosis, aplastic anemia	Rare	
	Leukopenia, thrombocytopenia	Mild reversible Patient should report a sore throat, easy bruising, bleeding and fever	
	Toxicity	Diplopia, cardiac changes, nystagmus, seizures, and coma	
Valproic acid	GI: Nausea, vomiting, diarrhea	Slow titration, give with food, use delayed-release formulation	○ Take with food if valproic acid causes GI upset. ○ Always consult with your healthcare provider before taking new medications, including OTC and herbal products. ○ Can cause pancreatitis or liver problems; call your healthcare provider if you experience yellowing of the skin or eyes, dark urine, nausea or vomiting, severe abdominal pain, or decreased appetite. ○ Common side effects include GI upset, drowsiness, tremors, and weight gain. Most will go away with time. Contact your healthcare provider if they become unmanageable. ○ This medication requires periodic blood work. ○ This medication may cause birth defects; family planning is advised.
	Elevation in hepatic transaminases	Usually asymptomatic	
	Tremor, sedation, ataxia	Reduce dose, tolerance develops, give at bedtime	
	Alopecia	Transient	
	Rash	Rare	
	Thrombocytopenia, platelet dysfunction	Rare, more common at higher doses	
	Weight gain	Increased appetite	
	Pancreatitis	Rare, usually occurs in the first 3 months of therapy	
	Hepatotoxicity	More common in children younger than age 2 years	

Table 21-17 (*continued*)

Drug	Side Effect	Additional Information	Patient Education
Lamotrigine	Nausea	Transient	○ Take with food if lamotrigine causes GI upset. ○ If a rash occurs, discontinue the medication and contact your healthcare provider. ○ Do not start taking any new medications without consulting your healthcare provider. ○ If you miss several doses of this medication, contact your healthcare provider because you may need to retitrate the medication.
	Headache, ataxia, dizziness, drowsiness	Slow titration, transient	
	Rashes	Stevens-Johnson syndrome/toxic epidermal necrolysis Reduced with slow dosage titration	

- Severe (> 2.5 mEq/L): Severe nausea, vomiting, diarrhea, seizures, stupor, coma, renal failure, cardiovascular collapse, and death

Pregnancy and Breastfeeding

- Lithium: Category D in pregnancy. Cardiovascular malformations (Ebstein's anomaly, tricuspid malformations) occur rarely in children exposed in utero. Contraindicated in breastfeeding.
- Carbamazepine: Dysmorphic facial features, cranial deficits, spina bifida.
- Valproic acid: Neural tube defects, minor facial defects.

ANNOTATED BIBLIOGRAPHY

Allen MH, Hirschfeld RM, Wozniak PJ, et al. Linear relationship of valproate serum concentration to response and optimal serum levels for acute mania. *Am J Psychiatry* 2006;163:272–275.

American Psychiatric Association. *Diagnostic and Statistical Manual of Mental Disorders,* 4th ed. Text Revision. Washington, DC: American Psychiatric Association; 2000:429–484.

American Psychiatric Association. Practice guidelines for the treatment of patients with bipolar disorder (revision). *Am J Psychiatry* 2002;159(4 suppl):1–50.

Bowden CL, Brugger AM, Drayton SJ, Weinstein B. Bipolar disorder. In Dipiro JT, Talbert RL, Yee GC, et al., eds. *Pharmacotherapy: A Pathophysiologic Approach,* 7th ed. New York, NY: McGraw-Hill Medical; 2008:1141–1160.

Gasper JJ, Borovicka MC, Love RC. Mood disorders II: bipolar disorder. In: Koda-Kimble MA, Young LY, Alldredge BK, et al., eds. *Applied Therapeutics: The Clinical Use of Drugs*, 9th ed. Baltimore, MD: Lippincott Williams & Wilkins; 2009:81.1–81.19.

Geddes JR, Burgess S, Hawton K, et al. Long-term lithium therapy for bipolar disorder: systematic review and meta-analysis of randomized controlled trials. *Am J Psychiatry* 2004;161:217–222.

Hurley SC. Lamotrigine update and its use in mood disorders. *Ann Pharmacother* 2002;36:860–873.

Macdonald KJ, Young LT. Newer antiepileptic drugs in bipolar disorder and the effectiveness of novel anticonvulsants. *J Clin Psychiatry* 2002;63(suppl 3): 5–9.

McElroy SL, Keck PE. Pharmacologic agents for the treatment of acute bipolar mania. *Biol Psychiatry* 2002;48:539–557.

Miklowitz DJ, Otto MW, Frank E, et al. Psychosocial treatments for bipolar depression: a 1-year randomized trial from the Systematic Treatment Enhancement Program. *Arch Gen Psychiatry* 2007;64: 419–427.

Perry PJ, Alexander B, Liskow B, DaVane CL. *Psychotropic Drug Handbook,* 8th ed. Baltimore, MD: Lippincott Williams & Wilkins; 2007.

Perucca E. Clinically relevant drug interactions with antiepileptic drugs. *Br J Clin Pharmacol* 2005;61:246–255.

Stahl SM. *Stahl's Essential Psychopharmacology,* 3rd ed. New York, NY: Cambridge University Press; 2008.

Suppes T, Dennehy E, Hirschfeld RMA, et al. The Texas implementation of medication algorithm project: update to the algorithms for the treatment of bipolar disorder. *J Clin Psychiatry* 2005;66:870–886.

Viguera AC, Cohen LS, Baldessarini RJ, Nonacs R. Managing bipolar disorder during pregnancy: weighing the risks and benefits. *Can J Psychiatry* 2002;47:426–436.

TOPIC: DEPRESSION

Section Coordinator: Rex S. Lott
Contributor: Rex S. Lott

Tips Worth Tweeting

- Depression is a common illness.
- Antidepressants have multiple possible mechanisms of action, but all currently-available

antidepressants increase activity or availability of monoamine neurotransmitters such as dopamine, norepinephrine, and/or serotonin.

- All antidepressants have a delayed onset of therapeutic effect. Continued therapy for 2–4 weeks is usually necessary before significant improvement in depressive symptoms is seen.
- SSRI antidepressants are considered first-choice agents because they are often better tolerated than other agents.
- TCAs, while effective, are poorly tolerated and less commonly used.
- TCAs are associated with significant anticholinergic, antihistaminic, and antiadrenergic side effects.
- SSRIs are associated with common gastrointestinal side effects (e.g., nausea) and sexual dysfunction.
- Several SSRIs are associated with significant inhibition of CYP450 enzymes and may interact with other drugs that are substrates of these enzymes.
- Serotonergic antidepressants that also antagonize specific subtypes of serotonin receptors may decrease the occurrence of serotonin-related side effects without decreasing the antidepressant response.
- Bupropion and mirtazapine are alternative antidepressants associated with minimal rates of sexual side effects.
- MAOIs are rarely used as antidepressants because of significant dietary restrictions and the need to avoid administration of potentially interacting drugs.
- Before MAOI therapy is initiated, other antidepressants should be stopped for a minimum of 2 weeks (5 weeks for fluoxetine).

Patient Care Scenario

R. N.: 29 y.o., 71 inch, female, Caucasian, 192 lbs
PMH: Hypertension, GERD
Vital Signs: BP 138/82 (arm sitting), HR 76
Lab Values:

Na 139 mEq/L (134–144)	Hgb 13.3 g/dL (13.3–16.1)
K 4.5 mEq/L (3.6–5.2)	Hct 40.0% (39.7–48.3)
Cl 101 mEq/L (100–109)	WBC 9.5 1,000/mm³ (3.7–10.1)
BUN 12 mg/dL (7–18)	MCV 82µm³ (78–102)
SCr 1.1 mg/dL (0.6–1.2)	Glu 103 mg/dL (70–110)

Current Medications:

- Lisinopril 10 mg/day
- Propranolol LA 120 mg/day
- Omeprazole 20 mg/day
- Docusate with Sennosides 2 capsules daily

R. N. presents to her PCP for evaluation. For the past 3–4 weeks, she has been experiencing insomnia, loss of appetite, and a feeling that "I can't get going." She describes being disinterested in her job as a salesperson at a local fabric and craft store. When she is working, R. N. has difficulty focusing her attention on the tasks at hand. Her family has noticed that she is easily irritated and become "short" with her spouse. She states, "Some days it just doesn't seem like it's worth getting out of bed in the morning and going on."

1.1.0 Patient Information

Depression has a high rate of occurrence in the United States, with 10–15 million Americans experiencing this condition in any year and a lifetime prevalence of 5–11%. As many as 15% of severely depressed people ultimately commit suicide. The peak age of onset for depression is 20–40 years, but this illness can occur at any age. Women are twice as likely as men to have major depressive disorder. First-degree relatives of people with depression are 1.5–3 times more likely to develop depression than controls. There is also an increased risk for depressive disorder the first 6 months postpartum. The etiology of major depressive disorder is unknown.

Symptoms of Major Depressive Disorder

Refer to DSM-IV for full diagnostic criteria.

Mnemonic: D-SIG-E-CAPS

D = **D**epressed mood
S = **S**leep (either insomnia or hypersomnia)
I = **I**nterest (loss of interest or pleasure)
G = **G**uilt (excessive or inappropriate guilt or feelings of worthlessness)
E = **E**nergy (loss of energy or fatigue)
C = **C**oncentration (decreased ability to concentrate and think, or indecisiveness)
A = **A**ppetite (appetite or unintended weight changes, either increased or decreased)
P = **P**sychomotor (psychomotor agitation or retardation, which is also observed by others)
S = **S**uicide (suicidal ideation or attempt)

Drug-Induced Depression

Depression or depressive symptoms have been associated with administration of several drugs. Many of these drugs (Table 21-18) alter the activity of monoamine neurotransmitters (e.g., serotonin and norepinephrine) in the central nervous system. For other agents, the mechanisms underlying their association with depression are not known. Whenever possible, these medications should be eliminated from therapy before treatment of depression is begun.

Table 21-18 Drugs that May Induce Depression

Clonidine and guanfacine	Beta-adrenergic antagonists (e.g., propranolol)
Diuretics	Oral contraceptives
Reserpine	Corticosteroids/ACTH
Hydralazine	Isotretinoin
Methyldopa	Interferon-β1a

1.2.0 Pharmacotherapy

The initial choice of therapy may be influenced by clinical (e.g., severity of symptoms) and other factors (e.g., patient preferences). Choices can include pharmacotherapy, psychotherapy, a combination of pharmacotherapy and psychotherapy, or electroconvulsive therapy (ECT). Psychotherapy or pharmacotherapy may be considered as sole initial treatment for patients with mild to moderate major depressive order (MDD). In patients with severe MDD, psychotherapy is not recommended alone for acute treatment, but is recommended in combination with pharmacotherapy or ECT.

The therapeutic efficacy of the various classes of antidepressants is roughly equivalent. Classes of antidepressants include tricyclic antidepressants (TCAs), selective serotonin reuptake inhibitors (SSRIs), dopamine-norepinephrine reuptake inhibitors (DNRIs), serotonin-norepinephrine reuptake inhibitors (SNRIs), serotonin modulators, norepinephrine-serotonin modulators, and monoamine oxidase inhibitors (MAOIs). The choice of antidepressant treatment should be based on the antidepressant's side-effect profile and the risk of the patient experiencing those side effects, patient preferences, family or patient history, and the cost of the medication. When patients fail to respond to an initial antidepressant, drugs with different proposed mechanisms or different side-effect profiles may be logical choices for additional therapeutic trials. The labels of all antidepressant drugs carry a "black box" warning regarding increased risk of suicidal thoughts and behavior for children, adolescents, and young adults taking antidepressants for major depressive disorder.

Tricyclic Antidepressants

Individual agents are placed in this class based on their chemical structure rather than on a consistently identifiable, proposed mechanism of antidepressant effect. Most TCAs act as inhibitors of neuronal reuptake of both norepinephrine and serotonin. One TCA (clomipramine) is also classified as an SSRI. TCAs were the first group of widely prescribed antidepressant drugs. They are now used predominantly as second-line agents owing to their marked side-effect profile.

TCA Side Effects

TCAs exhibit prominent sedative, anticholinergic, and hypotensive side effects. These effects result from TCAs' ability to significantly antagonize histamine (H1) receptors, muscarinic cholinergic receptors, and alpha-adrenergic (α_1) receptors respectively. These medications—particularly amitriptyline—are some of the most potent anticholinergic agents used in clinical practice. While their potency at these receptor sites varies, all TCAs are likely to cause significant side effects. The prominent antihistamine activity of TCAs is frequently exploited in practice to provide sedative effects to patients with significant sleep disturbance as part of their depressive illness.

Cardiovascular Adverse Effects

- Orthostatic hypotension, resulting in a risk for unsteady gait and falls, is relatively common with these drugs. Nortriptyline is the least problematic, although it still poses a risk.
- Slowed cardiac conduction occurs with therapeutic doses of TCAs and creates a risk of cardiac dysrhythmia or heart block; this is an especially significant risk for patients with preexisting conduction disorders or a history of myocardial infarction. TCAs should be avoided in such patients.

Toxicity in Overdose

- TCAs are associated with significant risk of fatality when taken in overdose. At doses greater than 20–35 mg/kg, there is a significant likelihood of fatal outcome, although smaller doses have resulted in death.
- Cardiac dysrhythmia is often the cause of death following TCA overdose. Supraventricular tachycardia, ventricular tachycardia or fibrillation, and multifocal PVCs may occur. ECG abnormalities with TCA overdose include prolonged PR interval, QT-interval prolongation, T-wave changes, and complete heart block.

Neurologic and Psychiatric Adverse Effects

- Tremor may occur in patients taking TCAs. It usually takes the form of a high-frequency intention tremor; resting tremor has also been described. Tremor associated with TCAs does not respond to anticholinergic antiparkinsonian therapy but may be controlled by propranolol.
- TCAs are frequently described as potentially causing seizures or increasing the risk of seizures in patients with epilepsy. This effect is generally not seen unless high therapeutic doses or overdoses are taken. People with epilepsy can be safely treated with TCAs. Clomipramine is

associated with a dose-related significant increase in seizure risk. At doses of less than 250 mg/day, approximately 0.5% of patients may experience seizures; at doses greater than 300 mg/day, the risk increases to more than 2%.

- Cognitive dysfunction and possible delirium can occur with therapeutic doses of TCAs, likely as a result of the anticholinergic activity of these agents. Associated symptoms are confusion, loss of recent memory, disorientation, and hallucinations (often visual). Resolution may not occur until 36–48 hours after TCAs are discontinued.
- Use of TCAs (or any antidepressant) without concomitant mood stabilizer treatment in patients with bipolar disorder may result in relatively rapid switching into mania or hypomania.

Table 21-19 Dosing and Pharmacokinetics for Commonly Used TCAs

Generic Name	Brand Name	Initial Dose (mg/day)	Dose Range (mg/day)	Half-Life (hr)	Cytochrome P450 Interactions	Comments
Imipramine	Tofranil Tofranil-PM	25	100–300	6–28	Substrate: CYP 1A2 and 2C19	Proposed therapeutic range of plasma concentrations: Imipramine + desipramine: 175–350 ng/mL
Desipramine	Norpramin Pertofrane	25	100–300	12–28	Substrate: CYP 2D6	Active metabolite of imipramine Proposed therapeutic range of plasma concentrations: > 115 ng/mL
Amitriptyline	Elavil	25	100–300	9–46	Substrate: CYP 1A2 and 2C19	Proposed therapeutic range of plasma concentrations: Amitriptyline + nortriptyline: 93–140 ng/mL
Nortriptyline	Pamelor Aventyl	25	50–200	18–56	Substrate: CYP 2D6	Active metabolite of amitriptyline Proposed therapeutic range of plasma concentrations: 50–150 ng/mL
Doxepin	Sinequan	25	100–300	11–23		
Clomipramine	Anafranil	25	100–250	24	Substrate: CYP 1A2 and 2C19	Only FDA-approved for treatment of obsessive–compulsive disorder; is an SSRI pharmacologically.

Table 21-20 TCA Pharmacologic and Side-Effect Profiles

TCA	5-HT Reuptake[1]	NE Reuptake[1]	Sedation	Anticholinergic	Orthostatic Hypotension	Cardiac Conduction Delays	Comments
Imipramine	+++	+	+++	+++	++++	+++	
Desipramine	++	++++	++	++	+++	+++	
Amitriptyline	+++	+	++++	++++	++++	+++	Very potent anticholinergic.
Nortriptyline	++	++	++	++	++	+++	Least problematic of TCAs for orthostasis—although still a clinical problem.
Doxepin	+	+	++++	++++	++++	+++	Very sedating. Low-dose doxepin (Silenor) is now FDA approved as a hypnotic.
Clomipramine	++++	+	+++	+++	++++	+++	Active metabolite (desmethyl clomipramine) may accumulate and is a significant norepinephrine reuptake inhibitor. This may change the pharmacologic profile in some patients. Significant risk of drug-induced seizures at doses greater than 250 mg/day.

[1]Relative activities as reuptake inhibitors should be compared in the columns for reuptake of a specific neurotransmitter. A comparison of reuptake inhibition for different neurotransmitters may be misleading.

Selective Serotonin Reuptake Inhibitors

There are currently eight SSRIs marketed in the United States: citalopram (Celexa), escitalopram (Lexapro), fluoxetine (Prozac), fluvoxamine (Luvox), paroxetine (Paxil), vilazodone (Viibryd), and sertraline (Zoloft). Clomipramine (Anafranil) is also an SSRI based on its pharmacologic activity, but is classified as a TCA based on its chemical structure. In general, all SSRIs enhance serotonin neurotransmission by blocking serotonin reuptake transporters and desensitizing serotonin receptors.

SSRIs have become the first-line antidepressant agents. They are generally as effective as TCAs and other antidepressants and are usually much better tolerated. Their prominent effects on serotonin (5-HT) neurotransmission result in a different side-effect profile from that seen with the TCAs. SSRIs are more likely to cause GI side effects, agitation, and sleep disturbance, and, probably, sexual dysfunction. They are not typically associated with anticholinergic, antihistaminic, or antiadrenergic adverse effects.

SSRI Side Effects

Gastrointestinal

- Dose-related nausea, vomiting, and diarrhea are common and usually improve after the first few weeks of therapy. These side effects can often be prevented by administering the medication with food.

Sexual Dysfunction

- Sexual side effects (erectile dysfunction or delayed ejaculation in men and anorgasmia and decreased sexual interest in both men and women) are commonly seen with SSRIs. Vilazodone may cause less sexual dysfunction.
- Management may include the following:
  - Decrease in dose of the SSRI
  - Discontinuation of the SSRI
  - Conversion to an antidepressant less likely to cause sexual dysfunction (e.g., bupropion, mirtazapine)
  - Brief drug holidays prior to sexual activity
  - Use of add-on agents to treat sexual dysfunction (e.g., sildenafil, cyproheptadine)

SSRI Withdrawal Syndrome

SSRIs (and SNRIs) may cause uncomfortable withdrawal symptoms if they are discontinued abruptly. These effects are more problematic with the SSRIs that have short half-lives (e.g., paroxetine, sertraline, citalopram). The withdrawal syndrome is characterized by the following:

- "Flu-like" symptoms (muscle aches)
- Electric shock-like sensations in the extremities and, sometimes, in the central nervous system
- Dizziness
- Sleep disturbances
- Worsened mood, crying, and irritability
- Nausea

Bleeding Tendencies

SSRIs are associated with increased risk of bleeding (inhibition of serotonin reuptake by platelets). Some studies suggest that SSRIs may be associated with

Table 21-21 SSRI Dosing, Pharmacokinetics, and FDA-Approved Indications

Generic Name	Brand Name	Starting Dose (mg/day)	Dose Range (mg/day)	Half-Life (hr)	Cytochrome P450 Interactions	FDA-Approved indications
Citalopram	Celexa	10–20	20–40	35		Major depressive disorder (MDD)
Escitalopram	Lexapro	10	10–20	27–32		Generalized anxiety disorder (GAD), MDD
Fluoxetine	Prozac	10–20	10–80	96–144	Inhibitor: CYP 2D6 and 3A4	Bulimia nervosa, MDD, obsessive–compulsive disorder (OCD), panic disorder, premenstrual dysphoric disorder
Fluvoxamine	Luvox	50–100	50–300	16–26	Inhibitor: CYP 1A2, 2C9/19, and 3A4	OCD, social phobia (not approved for treatment of depression)
Paroxetine	Paxil	20	20–60	15–21	Inhibitor: CYP 2D6 and 3A4	GAD, MDD, panic disorder, post-traumatic stress disorder (PTSD), premenstrual dysphoric disorder, social phobia
Sertraline	Zoloft	25–50	50–200	26		MDD, OCD, panic disorder, PTSD, premenstrual dysphoric disorder, social phobia
Vilazodone	Viibryd	10	40	25	Substrate: CYP3A4	MDD

increased risk of upper gastrointestinal bleeding in patients concurrently on NSAIDs. Patients should be educated to be alert for the following conditions:

- Bruising
- Ecchymoses
- Epistaxis
- Prolonged bleeding time
- Rectal bleeding

Serotonin Syndrome

This serious, potentially life-threatening condition may develop from excess serotonin effects related to SSRI use or combined use of an SSRI and other serotonergic agents. Affected patients may display the following signs and symptoms:

- Mydriasis ("belladonna eyes")
- Hypertension
- Increased bowel sounds
- Diaphorisis (excessive sweating)
- Tachycardia
- Tremor
- Fever
- Agitation/confusion
- Ataxia
- Clonus

Because of the possibility for serotonin syndrome, SSRIs are contraindicated for use in combination with monoamine oxidase inhibitors (MAOIs).

- Wait at least 2 weeks after discontinuing the MAOI to initiate an SSRI.
- Wait 2 weeks after discontinuing the SSRI before initiating therapy with a MAOI.
- Fluoxetine is an exception (long half-life); it is necessary to wait at least 5 half-lives (approximately 5 weeks) after discontinuation of fluoxetine before initiating MAOI therapy.

Table 21-22 Individual SSRI Side Effects

SSRI	Sedation	Weight Gain	Secondary Properties	Comments
Citalopram (Celexa)	Not unusual	Unusual (weight neutral overall)	*R* and *S* enantiomers (the *S* enantiomer is responsible for the therapeutic effects; the *R* enantiomer may cause antihistamine effects and CYP450 2D6 inhibition)	• Dose-related QTc prolongation. Doses should not exceed 40 mg (20 mg in elderly patients or patients taking inhibitors of citalopram metabolism). • Possibly less sexual dysfunction. • May be better tolerated and have potentially fewer CYP450 interactions than some other SSRIs.
Escitalopram (Lexapro)	Unusual	Unusual (weight neutral overall)	*S* enantiomer (minimal CYP450 2D6 inhibition and H1 antagonism caused by the *R* enantiomer in citalopram)	• May cause less sexual dysfunction than some other SSRIs. • Less QTc prolongation than with citalopram.
Fluoxetine (Prozac)	Unusual; may cause sleep disturbance and activation	Unusual (weight neutral overall)	• 5-HT_{2C} antagonist actions • The active metabolite (norfluoxetine) has a longer half-life than the parent compound	• Longest half-life (4–6 days) of all the SSRIs. • Wait 5 weeks after discontinuation of fluoxetine before initiating MAOI therapy; use caution with the addition of other serotonergic agents. • 5-HT_{2C} antagonism may cause activation (increase DA and NE) and contribute to anorexia and antibulimic effects. • Activation may be positive for patients with low energy, sedation, or fatigue. • Avoid use in agitated patients.
Fluvoxamine (Luvox)	Common	Unusual (weight neutral overall)	Inhibits multiple CYP450 isoforms	• *Not* FDA approved for depression (widely used antidepressant in other countries). • May cause less sexual dysfunction than some other SSRIs. • Potential disadvantages in patients with GI conditions, such as those with irritable bowel syndrome.

Table 21-22 (*continued*)

SSRI	Sedation	Weight Gain	Secondary Properties	Comments
Paroxetine (Paxil)	Common	More likely to cause weight gain than other SSRIs	• Mild M1 antagonist; some anticholinergic adverse effects • Mild NE reuptake inhibition • Nitric oxide synthetase (NOS) inhibitor; possibly explains more frequent sexual dysfunction	• Possibly avoid in patients with hypersomnia, fatigue, or low energy. • Higher incidence of withdrawal effects compared to other SSRIs. • More anticholinergic adverse effects compared to other SSRIs (M1 antagonism). • May be the SSRI that causes the most sexual dysfunction (NOS inhibitor).
Sertraline (Zoloft)	Unusual; may cause sleep disturbance and activation	Unusual (weight neutral overall)	Inhibits dopamine transporter (DAT); can help with energy, motivation, and concentration	• Causes more dopamine reuptake blockade than other SSRIs (minor relative to its serotonin reuptake actions). • Possibly more likely to cause GI upset (especially diarrhea) than the other SSRIs.
Vilazodone (Viibryd)	Unusual; may be somewhat activating	Unusual (weight neutral overall)	Acts as both an SSRI and a partial agonist at 5-HT_{1A} receptors; this is a pharmacologic effect shared with buspirone and may play a role in the antidepressant and antianxiety activity of vilazodone	• Appears to possibly cause less sexual dysfunction than other SSRIs. • Not available as generic (all other SSRIs are), so its cost may be an issue for some patients.

Serotonin-Norepinephrine Reuptake Inhibitors

The SNRIs are characterized by their ability to inhibit the reuptake of both serotonin and norepinephrine. Their presumed antidepressant pharmacology is, therefore, similar to that of TCAs, yet the SNRIs lack many of the other negative effects of TCAs. Currently, three SNRIs are approved by the FDA as antidepressants: venlafaxine, desvenlafaxine, and duloxetine. A fourth drug, milnacipran (Savella), is approved only for the treatment of fibromyalgia and is not used as an antidepressant in the United States.

While SNRIs do not seem to be more effective as antidepressants than SSRIs, they do appear to offer the advantage of relieving pain syndromes. Both duloxetine and milnacipran are FDA approved for pain indications. Venlafaxine and desvenlafaxine are not approved for treatment of pain conditions, but they are used for this purpose clinically. Relief of pain is believed to depend on inhibition of reuptake of both norepinephrine and serotonin. For this reason, venlafaxine is used for this purpose only at higher doses.

Norepinephrine and Dopamine Reuptake Inhibitors

Bupropion (Wellbutrin) is currently the only drug classified in this way. Therefore, it is somewhat unique. Bupropion is FDA approved for treatment of major depressive disorder, prevention of depressive episodes associated with seasonal affective disorder (XL dosage form), and smoking cessation (SR dosage form). Three different dosage forms of bupropion are available: immediate-release tablets, sustained-release (SR) tablets, and extended-release (XL) tablets. Use of the SR or XL forms is claimed to result in fewer side effects (including seizures) although this is not well established.

Bupropion Adverse Effects

- Activation or stimulation may result in insomnia or worsened anxiety. Bupropion should be administered early in the day to help avoid sleep disturbance.
- Possible neurologic side effects include tremors, seizures, and headaches.
    - The risk of seizures increases from approximately 0.4% to more than 2% when total daily doses of bupropion exceed 450 mg.
    - Bupropion is contraindicated in patients with a history of seizure disorders, in patients with eating disorders (anorexia or bulimia), and in patients undergoing abrupt discontinuation of alcohol or sedatives due to the possibility of seizures with bupropion treatment.
- There is a low risk of sexual dysfunction. The agent may be used to treat sexual dysfunction related to other antidepressants.

Table 21-23 SNRI Dosing, Pharmacokinetics, and FDA Labeled Indications

Generic Name	Brand Name	Starting Dose (mg/day)	Dose Range (mg/day)	Half-Life (hr)	Cytochrome P450 Interactions	FDA–Approved indications
Venlafaxine	Effexor Effexor-XR	IR: 75 XR: 37.5	75–375 75–225	5	Substrate: 2D6	MDD, GAD, panic disorder, and social phobia
Desvenlafaxine	Pristiq	50	50	10–11		MDD Doses greater than 50 mg/day have not been shown to be more effective than 50 mg/day
Duloxetine	Cymbalta	20	60–120	12	Substrate: 1A2, 2D6	MDD, GAD, fibromyalgia, diabetic peripheral neuropathy, chronic musculoskeletal pain

Table 21-24 Individual SNRI Side Effects

SNRI	Sedation	Weight Gain	Nausea	Comments
Venlafaxine (Effexor and Effexor-XR)	Not unusual	Unusual	Common	• Serotonin reuptake blockade at all doses; norepinephrine reuptake blockade requires higher doses (greater than approximately 150 mg/day). • Dose-related increases in blood pressure; use with caution in patients with borderline or uncontrolled hypertension. • Common side effects: nausea, insomnia, dizziness, sedation, and constipation. • Can induce sweating. • Increased risk of bleeding (similar to risk with SSRIs). • XR formulation may improve tolerability (e.g., decreased nausea).
Desvenlafaxine (Pristiq)			Common	• Active metabolite of venlafaxine. • Norepinephrine reuptake blockade at all doses. • Overall side-effect profile is similar to that of venlafaxine
Duloxetine (Cymbalta)	Not unusual	Unusual	Common	• May increase BP (may have less hypertensive effects than venlafaxine). • Use with caution in patients with hepatic insufficiency. • Off-label use for treatment of stress urinary incontinence. • Common side effects: nausea, dry mouth, and constipation. • Dizziness, insomnia, and somnolence can also occur. • Can induce sweating. • Sexual dysfunction can occur, but may be less common than with SSRIs.

- Bupropion is a potent inhibitor of CYP450 2D6. Caution should be exercised when it is added to treatment with drugs that are extensively metabolized by CYP 2D6.

Norepinephrine-Serotonin Modulators

Mirtazapine (Remeron) is the only currently approved antidepressant categorized in this way. Therefore, it is somewhat unique. Mirtazapine is not an inhibitor of monoamine reuptake. Instead, it increases both serotonergic and noradrenergic neurotransmission by antagonizing alpha$_2$-adrenergic receptors on serotonergic and noradrenergic neurons. This action decreases the inhibitory effect of these receptors relative to the release of both norepinephrine and serotonin. Thus mirtazapine is pharmacologically similar to drugs such as desvenlafaxine that increase both noradrenergic and serotonergic neurotransmission; however, it accomplishes this outcome through a different mechanism. In addition, mirtazapine antagonizes a number of other important receptors.

- Antagonist at 5-HT$_{2A}$ receptors: Believed to counteract the agitation, sleep disturbance, and sexual dysfunction often associated with serotonergic antidepressants.
- Antagonist at 5-HT$_{2C}$ receptors: May contribute to weight gain associated with mirtazapine treatment

- Antagonist at 5-HT_3 receptors: Believed to counteract GI side effects such as nausea.
- Antagonist at histamine H_1 receptors: Responsible for the prominent sedation and appetite stimulation with weight gain seen with mirtazapine treatment.

Common side effects associated with mirtazapine include sedation, dry mouth, and weight gain. The last problem is a disadvantage in patients for whom weight gain is a concern, but is a potential advantage in patients for whom weight gain is sought.

Mirtazapine is not metabolized by the CYP450 system, so it is not involved in significant pharmacokinetic drug interactions. Owing to mirtazapine's $alpha_2$ antagonism, it directly antagonizes the actions of clonidine and guanfacine.

Serotonin Modulators

Two drugs are classified as serotonin modulators: nefazodone and trazodone. Neither is widely used as an antidepressant at this time. Both of these drugs act as inhibitors of serotonin reuptake. They are also antagonists at 5-HT_{2A} receptors; this effect decreases the likelihood of their causing significant agitation, sleep disturbances, or sexual dysfunction. Both agents have significant sedative activity. Important additional points are highlighted for each drug here.

Nefazodone (Serzone)

- "Black box" warning for hepatotoxicity. Although rare, fatalities have occurred. For this reason, nefazodone is rarely used in therapy.
- Common side effects: Sedation, nausea, constipation, dry mouth, dizziness, and orthostasis.
- Rarely may cause priapism (more common with trazodone).
- Potent inhibitor of CYP450 3A4. Caution is required if nefazodone is added to therapy with drugs extensively metabolized by this enzyme.

Trazodone (Desyrel, Oleptro)

- Its original FDA-approved indication was only for depression. Commonly used at lower doses for treatment of insomnia.
- Not commonly used as antidepressant monotherapy. Many patients are unable to tolerate sedation at the doses required for antidepressant activity (400–600 mg/day).
- Recently FDA approved and relabeled as a sustained-release dosage form (Oleptro) indicated for treatment of depression.
- Can rarely cause priapism. This side effect may be more likely in at-risk populations (e.g., patients with sickle cell anemia or leukemia). Patients should be cautioned about the risk associated with prolonged erections.

Monoamine Oxidase Inhibitors

MAOIs were one of the first groups of clinically useful antidepressants. Their use has declined in recent years because better-tolerated drugs with less potential for serious drug interactions and adverse effects have become available. MAOIs may be used for patients who are unresponsive to other antidepressants. These drugs also may be preferred for patients suffering from depression with atypical features characterized by prominent anxiety, sensitivity to rejection, reduced energy with "leaden paralysis," increased sleep, and increased appetite. Patients with this form of depression may be less responsive to other antidepressants.

MAOIs used for depression increase the availability of norepinephrine, serotonin, and dopamine in neurons through irreversible inhibition of intracellular monoamine oxidase A (MAO-A) and monoamine oxidase B (MAO-B). MAO-A predominantly acts to metabolize norepinephrine and serotonin, while MAO-B is more selectively active in the metabolism of dopamine. Because MAOIs are irreversible inhibitors, their effects persist for as long as 2 weeks after their discontinuation. This time is required for synthesis of new enzymes to replace those inhibited by the drug.

MAOIs inhibit the MAO enzyme throughout the body. Inhibition of MAO in the gut wall and liver prevents first-pass metabolism of dietary tyramine. Therefore, when foods with a high tyramine content (Table 21-25) are ingested, tyramine enters the circulation in large quantities and acts as a pressor agent. Tyramine also stimulates the release of increased norepinephrine stores in adrenergic nerve-ending storage granules. These effects may result in dramatic elevations in blood pressure and are the reason for the dietary restrictions recommended for patients taking MAOIs. Sympathomimetic drugs that act by stimulating release of stored norepinephrine (e.g., pseudoephedrine) may also cause significant blood pressure elevations in patients taking MAOIs. Selegeline (EmSam transdermal) is useful for treatment of depression. In low doses, and possibly when given transdermally, it is somewhat selective for inhibition of MAO-B and may also be less likely to inhibit gastrointestinal MAO-A. Nonetheless, patients receiving higher patch strengths of transdermal selegeline should follow the dietary restrictions recommended for other MAOIs.

The following MAOIs are available for use as antidepressants in the United States:

- Phenelzine (Nardil): 15 mg tablets
    - Dose: 15–90 mg/day

- Tranylcypromine (Parnate): 10 mg tablets
  - Dose: 20–40 mg/day
- Isocarboxazid (Marplan): 10 mg tablets
  - Dose: 20–60 mg/day
- Selegeline transdermal (EmSam): 6 mg/24 hr, 9 mg/24 hr, 12 mg/24 hr
  - Dose: 6–12 mg/24 hr
  - Minimal or no dietary restrictions with 6 mg/24 hr dose
  - Tyramine-restricted diet needed with 9 mg/24 hr and 12 mg/24 hr doses

MAOI Drug–Drug Interactions

Sympathomimetic Drugs

- "Indirect-acting" agents that stimulate release of stored norepinephrine from nerve terminals may cause extreme blood pressure elevation if given with MAOIs.
- "Direct-acting" agents that stimulate adrenergic receptors may interact if they are subject to significant first-pass metabolism in the liver or gut wall.

Table 21-25 Tyramine-Containing Food Restrictions for Patients Taking MAOIs

Foods with High Tyramine Content: Avoid
• Aged cheeses and meats
• Improperly stored or spoiled meats, poultry, or fish
• Fava or broad bean *pods* (not beans)
• Yeast extract (e.g., Marmite)
• Sauerkraut
• Tap beers
• Fermented soy condiments (soy sauce is probably acceptable)
Foods with Moderate Tyramine Content: Consume in Moderation with Caution
• Bottled and micro-brew beers
• Red wines (e.g., Chianti) (may cause headache independently of MAOI interaction)
• White wines
• Avocados
Foods with Low or No Tyramine Content: May Be Consumed
• Caffeine-containing beverages
• Distilled alcoholic beverages
• Cottage cheese, cream cheese, process cheese products, and yogurt
• Freshly-packaged or processed meats
• Banana pulp (avoid peel)
• Soy sauce
• Chocolate

Modified from: Gardner DM, et al. *J Clin Psychiatry.* 1996;57:99.

Serotonergic Antidepressants (SSRIs, SNRIs, Serotonin Modulators)

- Combined use of these agents may result in serotonin syndrome secondary to release of large quantities of stored serotonin from nerve endings.
- A 2-week "washout" is necessary after discontinuation of these drugs before starting a MAOI.
- A 5-week "washout" is necessary after discontinuation of fluoxetine owing to its long half-life.

Tricyclic Antidepressants

- Combined use may result in hyperthermia and elevated blood pressure, which are believed to result from the release of large quantities of stored norepinephrine.
- Carbamazepine and cyclobenzaprine may also interact in this way
- Meperidine, tramadol, and methadone may cause reactions similar to serotonin syndrome when given with MAOIs. Opiates such as codeine and hydrocodone appear safe.

ANNOTATED BIBLIOGRAPHY

Diagnostic and Statistical Manual of Mental Disorders, 4th ed. Text Revision (DSM-IV-TR). Washington, DC: American Psychiatric Association; 2000.

Finley PR, Lee KC. Mood Disorders I: Major Depressive Disorders. In Alldredge BK, Corelli RL, Ernst ME, et al., eds. *Koda-Kimble and Young's Applied Therapeutics: The Clinical Use of Drugs,* 10th ed. Philadelphia, PA: Lippincott Williams & Wilkins, 2012:1949-1982.

Fuller MA, Sajatovic M. *Drug Information Handbook for Psychiatry,* 7th ed. Hudson, OH: Lexi-Comp; 2009.

Perry PJ, Alexander B, Liskow BI, DeVane CL. *Psychotropic Drug Handbook,* 8th ed. Philadelphia, PA: Lippincott Williams and Wilkins; 2007.

Teter CJ, Kando JC, Wells BG. Major Depressive Disorder. In DiPiro JT, Talbert RL, Yee GC, et al., eds. *Pharmacotherapy: A Pathophysiologic Approach,* 8th ed. New York, NY: McGraw-Hill Medical, 2011:1173-1190.

TOPIC: DRUG ABUSE

Section Coordinator: Rex S. Lott
Contributor: Robyn Cruz

Tips Worth Tweeting

- Obtaining a thorough history of recent use of drugs of abuse is crucial in determining initiation of the correct treatment alternatives.

- During the initial workup, it is important to consider other comorbid medical conditions for which the patient is at risk due to his or her history of drug use.
- Certain criteria must be met, and a special Drug Enforcement Agency (DEA) number assigned, prior to authorization to prescribe buprenorphine.
- Methadone can be prescribed for use in opioid detoxification and maintenance only via specially licensed programs.
- Methadone carries four boxed warnings regarding its potential for QTc prolongation, its potential for respiratory depression, the requirement that it be dispensed by a certified program, and the fact that medication is only to be used orally due to excipients in the tablet that will deter injectable use.
- Naloxone is a pure opioid antagonist used for acute reversal of opioid intoxication, whereas naltrexone is a pure opioid antagonist used in maintenance of abstinence from opioids.
- Naltrexone carries a boxed warning regarding its potential for dose-related hepatotoxicity.
- Patients must be free of opioid use for 5–7 days prior to initiation of naltrexone to prevent precipitation of opioid withdrawal.
- Motivation to abstain from drugs of abuse must be present for the medications used in prevention of relapse to be efficacious.

Patient Care Scenario: Acute Care Setting

N. D., a 29-year-old male patient, presents to your emergency department with diaphoresis, rhinorrhea, mydriasis, irritability, chills, and nausea. There is also physical evidence of previous use of injectable drugs.

1.1.0 Patient Information

Review the patient history for presence of all substances of abuse (may be multiple)—heroin, prescription opioids, cocaine, cannabis, alcohol, nicotine, benzodiazepines, and other anxiolytic or sedative-type drugs. Addition of any other substance of abuse to the primary drug of concern can complicate withdrawal and treatment.

Laboratory Testing

Tests Used During Acute Intoxication and During Relapse Prevention

- Urine toxicology screen (urinalysis) is used to determine which substances are involved in intoxication, and also helps determine whether there has been recent use of a particular substance.

Table 21-26 Urine Detection of Drugs

Drug	Detection Period
Amphetamine, methamphetamine	2–4 days
Cannabis • Occasional use • Regular use	 • 2–7 days • 30 days
Cocaine	12–72 hours
Codeine, heroin, hydromorphone, morphine	2–4 days

  - Times for detection of substances via urinalysis will vary based on individual use, metabolism, laboratory, and other factors.
- Blood concentration, by reflecting current blood levels, establishes whether there is a high tolerance to a substance, and also determines whether there has been recent substance use.

Baseline Screening for Comorbid Medical Disorders

- Complete blood count (CBC): To detect anemia or thrombocytopenia due to poor nutritional intake, and also to detect infection.
- Complete metabolic panel (CMP): To determine the presence of electrolyte abnormalities due to poor nutritional intake.
- Blood pressure: To detect hypertension related to stimulants, including nicotine, alcohol, and other substances, or hypotension related to dehydration and poor nutritional status.
- Pregnancy test: For women of childbearing age.
- Tuberculin skin test: Due to increased risk of tuberculosis (TB) exposure.
- Blood test for human immunodeficiency virus (HIV), hepatitis B virus (HBV), and hepatitis C virus (HCV): In intravenous drug users due to transmission via blood and sexual activity.
- Sexually transmitted diseases (STD) testing: Includes chlamydia, gonococcal disease, human papillomavirus, and syphilis.

Disease State History

- History of substance use
  - Type(s) of substance(s)
  - Route of administration
  - Amount of use, including quantity, frequency, and duration
  - Time since last use
  - History of previous treatment(s)
  - Readiness to change
- Medical history
  - Includes current prescription and nonprescription medication use

- Psychiatric history
  - Includes current prescription and nonprescription medication use
- Family history
  - Particularly for substance use or psychiatric diagnoses
- Social, educational, and occupational history
  - Peer and family support systems

Instruments and Techniques Related to Patient Assessment

- Patient history
- Baseline screening for substance use and comorbid conditions
- Indicators of intoxication or withdrawal

Table 21-27 Characteristics of Acute Intoxication from Cannabis

Physical Symptoms	Psychological Symptoms
Increased appetite	Euphoria
	Disinhibition
	Fatigue
	Paranoia
	Psychosis

Table 21-28 Characteristics of Withdrawal from Cannabis

Physical Symptoms	Psychological Symptoms
Appetite change/decreased appetite	Emotional and behavioral changes
Weight loss	Occasional insomnia
Physical discomfort	Occasional hyperactivity

Table 21-29 Characteristics of Acute Intoxication from Cocaine

Physical Symptoms	Psychological Symptoms
Hypertension	Agitation
Tachycardia	Excitation
Tachypnea	Insomnia
Increased body temperature	Delusions, hallucinations
Appetite suppression	Paranoid thinking
Cardiac arrhythmias	Compulsive behavior
Coronary artery vasospasm	
Myocardial infarction	
Stroke	
Seizure	

Table 21-30 Characteristics of Withdrawal from Cocaine

Physical Symptoms	Psychological Symptoms
Increased appetite	Depression
Psychomotor retardation	Anxiety
	Irritability
	Anhedonia
	Sleep disturbances
	Suicidal ideation
	Drug cravings

Table 21-31 Characteristics of Acute Intoxication from Opioids

Physical Symptoms	Psychological Symptoms
Hypotension	CNS depression
Bradycardia	
Bradypnea	
Pulmonary edema	
Extreme miosis	
Coma	

Manifestations of Intoxication and Withdrawal

Intoxication from other stimulants (i.e., amphetamines) may be expected to be similar.

Withdrawal from other stimulants (i.e., amphetamines) may be expected to be similar.

Intoxication is linked to increased levels of dopamine and norepinephrine (via blockade of reuptake and increased synthesis), so withdrawal is due to relative depletion.

Opioids include heroin and prescription pain medications. Characteristics of acute intoxication from opioids are generally the opposite of those experienced with cocaine intoxication.

- Withdrawal usually occurs if the substance is used excessively over 3 weeks or longer.
- May be due to rebound norepinephrine increase.
- Severity of symptoms varies depending on the agent: meperidine (twitching, restlessness, nervousness) > heroin/morphine = oxycodone > hydrocodone > codeine.
- Usually not fatal.

Treatment Settings

Criteria are based on many patient factors. Choose the least restrictive setting necessary that will still provide safe and effective treatment.

Table 21-32 Characteristics of Withdrawal from Opioids

Physical Symptoms	Psychological Symptoms
Nausea	Insomnia
Vomiting	Distress, panic
Anorexia	Irritability
Diarrhea	Drug cravings
Chills	
Sweating	
Muscle aches	
Lacrimation	
Rhinorrhea	
Piloerection	
Yawning	
Mydriasis	

Table 21-33 Time Course to Withdrawal from Opioids

Substance	Onset (hr)	Peak (hr)	Duration (hr)
Codeine	8–12	96–120	7–10
Heroin/morphine	8–12	36–72	7–10
Hydrocodone	24–30	72	4–5
Meperidine	4–6	8–12	4–5
Oxycodone	24–30	72	4–5

Table 21-34 Manifestations of Cocaine Use Associated with Each Organ System

Organ System	Symptoms
Respiratory	Spontaneous pneumothorax, pneumomediastinum, bronchitis; pneumonitis and bronchospasm when smoked
Cardiovascular	Ischemic heart disease, cardiac arrhythmias, cardiomyopathy, aortic dissection, myocardial infarction
Neurological	Seizures, stroke
Other	Sinusitis, nasal irritation, septal bleeding and perforation with nasal use; HIV and hepatitis with IV use; weight loss and malnutrition

Hospitalization

- Risk of severe or complicated withdrawal
  - Overdose that requires medical attention (i.e., cardiac instability)

Table 21-35 Manifestations of IV Opioid (IV Heroin) Use Associated with Each Organ System

Organ System	Symptoms
Respiratory	Treatment-resistant TB
Cardiovascular	Endocarditis
Neurological	Meningitis
Gastrointestinal	Acute and chronic viral hepatitis
Other	Cellulitis, abscesses, osteomyelitis, HIV

- Comorbid medical or psychiatric diagnoses (i.e., suicidal ideation or severe cardiac disease)
- History of noncompliance or resistance with treatment
- Acute danger to self or others

Residential Treatment

- Patient does not meet hospitalization criteria
- Patient does not have a personal support system or social or vocational skills to maintain abstinence on his or her own
- Appropriate for group therapy

Partial Hospitalization

- Patient has a better personal, social, and vocational support system and skills to maintain abstinence on his or her own than those patients in residential treatment
- May be post hospitalization or residential treatment but is at high risk for relapse
- Does not have sufficient motivation
- Severe comorbid psychiatric diagnoses
- History of relapse post hospitalization
- Poor social environment or support system
- Attempted outpatient treatment but did not do well

Outpatient

- Demonstrates motivation, and a conducive social environment and support system
- Treatment for cannabis

Wellness and Prevention

- Potential influencing factors for substance abuse and dependence: Low educational level, low wages, lower socioeconomic status, lack of family or social support system, sexual orientation.
  - May have a familial component that appears to be mostly related to the diagnosis of antisocial personality disorder.
- The 18- to 24-year-old group has the highest rate of substance *use*.

   - *Dependence* usually has initial onset in the 20s to 40s but can occur at any age.
   - Depends on the dose used, duration, and other factors.
- Educational programming in schools aids in prevention of substance use and abuse.
   - Includes discussing the consequences of substance use, ways to refuse substances, and strategies to avoid peer pressure to use substances.
- Substance use disorders are more commonly diagnosed in males than in females, but rates vary depending on the substance of abuse.

1.2.0 Pharmacotherapy

Drug Indications, Dosing Regimens, and Routes of Administration

Medications for Use in Acute Intoxication

- Cannabis
   - No specific pharmacologic treatments available.
- Cocaine
   - Usually only supportive care due to self-limited intoxication.
   - Benzodiazepines may be useful for sedation in acute agitation.
- Opioids
   - Mild–moderate: Usually no specific pharmacologic treatment.
   - Severe: May require naloxone.
- Naloxone
   - Used in suspected or known opioid overdose to rapidly reverse (partially or completely) CNS or respiratory depression.
   - Pure opioid antagonist (mu, kappa sigma) that binds to opioid receptors and displaces the opioid (e.g., heroin, morphine). No agonist activity.
   - Usual dose is 0.4–2 mg IV, repeated every 2–3 minutes. If 10 mg has been given without response, other causes of CNS depression should be examined.
   - A lower dose (0.05–0.1 mg) should be used in opioid-dependent patients to lessen the chance of precipitating withdrawal.
   - Dose is dependent on the extent of respiratory depression.
   - Depending on the duration of action of the opioid ingested, may need to repeat again at a later time (i.e., in 20–30 minutes).

Medications for Acute Withdrawal

- Cannabis
   - No specific pharmacologic treatments available.
   - Lack of data from controlled trials.
- Cocaine
   - Usually only supportive care due to a lack of efficacy data.
- Opioids
   - Methadone
      - Only available for use in withdrawal via certified programs. Other facilities have 72 hours to find an appropriate facility to which to transfer the patient.
      - Full mu agonist. Prevents opioid withdrawal by binding to opioid receptors via cross-tolerance.
      - Usual single dose is 20–30 mg/day orally; can titrate to a maximum of 40 mg/day.
         - Dosed based on the type of symptoms present
         - Less opioid-tolerant patients may require lower doses.
         - More opioid-tolerant patients may require an additional 5–10 mg if symptoms are not suppressed after 2–4 hours.
         - Renal impairment: CrCl < 10 mL/min, give 50–75% of the normal dose.
         - Hepatic impairment: Avoid in severe disease.
         - If therapy is provided on an inpatient basis, doses are often used over a course of about 7 days and tapered down by either 5 mg/day or 20%/day for long-acting opioids or 10%/day for short-acting opioids. If therapy is provided on an outpatient basis, it may take several weeks to titrate the patient off methadone.
- Buprenorphine
      - Prescriber must register for a special DEA number to prescribe buprenorphine.
      - Partial mu agonist; has agonist and antagonist activity. Binds to opioid receptors to suppress withdrawal via cross-tolerance.
      - Used during withdrawal as an induction phase to maintenance use.
      - Use at the first indication of withdrawal and titrate to effectiveness.
      - Usual dose range is 12–16 mg/day sublingually. One suggested titration schedule: 8 mg, day 1; 16 mg, day 2; induction continued for 3–4 days.
      - Tablet should be placed under the tongue to dissolve and should not be swallowed.
   - Other medications may be used to treat generalized symptoms of withdrawal such as

headache (acetaminophen) and gastrointestinal upset (histamine-2 receptor antagonists).

Medications for Prevention of Relapse of Dependence

- Cannabis
  - No specific pharmacologic treatments available.
- Cocaine
  - No FDA-approved medications.
  - Usually based on psychotherapies.
- Opioids: Maintenance medications considered if dependence has lasted for more than 1 year.
  - Methadone
    - Only available for use in maintenance via certified programs.
    - Most commonly used pharmacological option.
    - Full mu agonist. Blocks the effects of other opioids by binding to opioid receptors, and relieves withdrawal and cravings.
    - Usual target dose is 80–120 mg/day orally dosed once daily.
      - Less than 40–60 mg/day is often sufficient.
      - Must determine sufficient dose.
      - Titrate cautiously to prevent cravings, euphoric effects of other opiates, and sedative effects.
- Buprenorphine
    - Partial mu agonist; has agonist and antagonist activity. Blocks the effects of other opioids by binding to opioid receptors, and relieves withdrawal and cravings.
    - Usual dose range is 8–32 mg/day sublingually, with a target of 16 mg/day.
      - May be dosed on less than a daily basis due to its pharmacokinetics.
- Naltrexone
    - Pure opioid receptor antagonist that inhibits the euphoria and reward associated with opioid use, thereby reducing cravings.
    - Usual dose is 50 mg PO daily or 100–150 mg 3 times a week, for up to 12 weeks.
      - A test dose of 25 mg may be given initially; if it is tolerated, an additional 25 mg may be given.
      - Renal impairment: Caution advised. No adjustment in mild impairment; adjustments in moderate–severe impairment have not been adequately studied.
      - Hepatic impairment: Caution advised. No adjustment in mild–moderate impairment; adjustments in severe impairment have not been adequately studied. Area under the curve (AUC) may increase 5- to 10-fold in cirrhosis.

Drug, Food, and Lab Test Interactions

Buprenorphine

- CYP 3A4 inhibitors may increase effects (buprenorphine is a major substrate of CYP 3A4).
  - CYP 3A4 inducers may decrease effects.
- CNS depressants, including ethanol, valerian, St. John's wort, and kava kava, may increase CNS depression.
- Ammonium chloride may increase excretion of opioid analgesics.
- Amphetamines may enhance the analgesic effects of opioid analgesics.
- Antipsychotics may enhance the hypotensive effects of opioid analgesics.
- Atazanavir may increase the concentration of buprenorphine.
- Desmopressin's adverse effects and toxicity may increase in combination with opioid analgesics.
- Selective serotonin inhibitors may have increased serotonergic effects in combination with buprenorphine.
- Succinylcholine may enhance the bradycardic effect of opioid analgesics.

Methadone

- CYP 3A4 and 2D6 inhibitors may increase effects (methadone is a major substrate of CYP 3A4 and a minor substrate of CYP 2D6).
  - CYP 3A4 inducers may decrease effects.
- QTc-prolonging agents may enhance the QTc-prolonging effect of methadone (e.g., quinolones, ziprasidone).
- Ammonium chloride may increase excretion of opioid analgesics.
- Amphetamines may enhance the analgesic effects of opioid analgesics.
- Antipsychotics may enhance the hypotensive effects of opioid analgesics.
- Desmopressin's adverse effects and toxicity may increase in combination with opioid analgesics.
- Didanosine's serum concentration may decrease with methadone use.
- Selective serotonin reuptake inhibitors may have increased serotonergic effects in combination with methadone.
- Succinylcholine may enhance the bradycardic effect of opioid analgesics.

- CNS depressants, including ethanol, valerian, St. John's wort, and kava kava, may increase CNS depression.
  - St. John's wort may decrease methadone concentration.
- Consumption of grapefruit juice may increase methadone concentration.

Naloxone

- No known significant drug–drug interactions.

Naltrexone

- Decreases the effectiveness of opioids, including prescription narcotics.
- Produces lethargy and somnolence in combination with thioridazine.
- May interact with NSAIDs, leading to hepatotoxicity with doses greater than 100 mg/day.
- Potential for cross-reactivity with some opioid immunoassays.

Contraindications, Warnings, and Precautions

Buprenorphine

- Use caution in hepatic, pulmonary, or renal impairment; head injury or increased intracranial pressure (ICP); biliary tract dysfunction; hyperthyroidism; morbid obesity; adrenal insufficiency; prostatic hyperplasia; urinary stricture; CNS depression; driving or operating machinery; toxic psychosis; pancreatitis; alcoholism; delirium tremens; kyphoscoliosis; hypovolemia; cardiovascular disease; combination with drugs that may cause hypotension; history of depression or suicidal ideation; elderly or debilitated patients; and children younger than 16 years (safety and efficacy are not established in children).
- Titrate carefully to the patient's needs.
- Do no abruptly discontinue.
- Pregnancy Category C; enters breastmilk and is not recommended for breastfeeding women.

Methadone

- Contraindicated in respiratory depression in an unmonitored setting, acute bronchial asthma or hypercarbia, paralytic ileus, combination use with selegeline.
- Boxed warning regarding potential for QTc prolongation (obtain complete medical history, including medications).
  - Risk is greatest with doses greater than 100 mg/day but may happen at lower doses.
  - In patients prone to hypotension (i.e., volume depleted).
  - In patients with cardiac disease, including arrhythmias.
- Boxed warning regarding respiratory depression, especially in patients with preexisting respiratory compromise (i.e., COPD, CNS depression).
  - Incomplete cross-tolerance to other opioids may occur; titrate carefully.
- May be dispensed only by a certified program.
- Medication is only to be used orally. Excipients in tablet will deter injectable use.
- Use caution in patients with depression or suicidal ideation, driving or operating machinery, head injury or increased ICP, elderly or debilitated, biliary tract dysfunction, acute pancreatitis, severe renal or hepatic failure, hyperthyroidism or hypothyroidism, morbid obesity, adrenal insufficiency, prostatic hyperplasia, and urethral stricture, and/or in children (not an approved use).
- Do not abruptly discontinue.
- Pregnancy Category C/D (with prolonged use or at higher doses near term); enters breast milk so is not recommended for breastfeeding women (although the American Academy of Pediatrics rates it as "compatible").

Naloxone

- Use caution:
  - In patients with cardiovascular disease or on other medications that have potential cardiac ADRs (due to naloxone's association with pulmonary edema).
  - In patients with a history of seizures. Do not use for meperidine-induced seizures.
- Pregnancy Category C; excretion in breast milk is unknown, so it is not recommended for breastfeeding women.

Naltrexone

- Boxed warning: Dose-related hepatotoxicity.
- Contraindicated with concurrent opioid use (should be opioid free for 7–10 days).
- Contraindicated in patients with acute hepatitis or liver failure; use caution in patients with renal impairment.
- Pregnancy Category C; enters breast milk, so is not recommended for breastfeeding women.
- Monitor for depression and suicidal ideation; monitor for shortness of breath and hypoxia.

Physiochemical Properties, Solubility, Pharmacodynamics, and Pharmacokinetic Properties

Buprenorphine

- Peak concentration for sublingual route is at approximately 100 minutes.
- Half-life for the sublingual route is 37 hours.
  - Allows potential for doubling the daily dose to administer the medication every 48 hours

or tripling the dose to give the medication every 72 hours.
- Hepatic metabolism with extensive first-pass metabolism.

Methadone

- Peak concentration (orally) is 2–3 hours.
- Peak effect for continuous oral dosing is 3–5 days.
- Half-life is 13–55 hours; average is 25 hours.
- Hepatic metabolism via CYP 3A4, 2B6, and 2C19 to inactive metabolites.

Naloxone

- Onset of action is 2 minutes when given IV; duration is 30–120 minutes depending on route used. The IV formulation has a shorter duration than the IM formulation.
- Half-life is 0.5–1.5 hours in adults.
- Primarily metabolized via glucuronidation.

Naltrexone

- Duration of action increases with dose: 50 mg = 24 hours, 100 mg = 48 hours, 150 mg = 72 hours.
- Non-cytochrome-mediated hepatic metabolism. Extensive first-pass metabolism
  - Half-life is 4 hours with oral dose; half-life of metabolite is 13 hours.
- Time to peak for oral formulation is approximately 60 minutes.

Biopharmaceutical Principles and Pharmaceutical Characteristics of Dosage Forms

Buprenorphine

- Good parenteral bioavailability, poor oral bioavailability, fair sublingual bioavailability.
- Wide variability in sublingual absorption between patients but low individual variability. Average is 31%.
- 96% protein bound.

Methadone

- 70–85% protein bound.

Naloxone

- Crosses the placenta.

Naltrexone

- Oral dose is almost completely absorbed, with 21% protein binding.

1.3.0 Monitoring

Pharmacotherapeutic Outcomes

- During acute withdrawal, the least restrictive setting should be employed (see the "Treatment Settings" section). The primary goals are to minimize and symptomatically treat the withdrawal while considering appropriate next steps to be taken to promote abstinence.
- To achieve the best long-term outcome, sustained abstinence must be the primary goal of treatment.
  - The first step is to engage the patient in treatment.
  - A significant decrease in use may be an interim goal that will ultimately lead to complete abstinence.
  - Medications can be used, in combination with psychosocial therapies, to assist with abstinence by reducing cravings and relapse rates.
- Other goals of treatment will include treatment of comorbid medical and psychiatric diagnoses and reconciling work and personal relationships.

Safety and Efficacy Monitoring

- Times to onset of symptoms and peak of acute withdrawal vary depending on substance(s) used (see Table 21-33).
- Blood pressure, heart rate, respiratory rate, and body temperature may be monitored in acute intoxication with cocaine (or other stimulants) or opioids to ensure adequate symptomatic treatment.
- CNS status (opioids) and psychological symptoms (cocaine, stimulants) of acute withdrawal should be monitored to ensure adequate symptomatic treatment.
- Baseline screening for comorbid medical disorders should be performed to help detect and treat manifestations of substance use.
- Urine toxicology or blood concentrations may be obtained initially to detect use of substances, and monitored periodically to ensure maintenance of abstinence from substances of abuse.

Adverse Drug Reactions

Buprenorphine

- Sedation, respiratory depression (in overdose or in combination with other CNS depressants [i.e., benzodiazepines]), hypotension, dizziness, headache, nausea, vomiting, miosis, vertigo, diaphoresis.

Methadone

- Constipation, increased sweating, sexual dysfunction, respiratory depression (in overdose), arrhythmias, drowsiness, insomnia, headache, euphoria, dysphoria, depression, confusion.
- Most ADRs decrease over several weeks with continued use. Exception: sweating and constipation.

Naloxone

- ADRs are only related to precipitating withdrawal of opioids.

Naltrexone

- Side effects may be similar to alcohol withdrawal symptoms, so medication should not be started during the acute phase of withdrawal.
- Effects are usually moderate and may include nausea/vomiting/diarrhea, abdominal pain, headache, fatigue, insomnia, dysphoria, anxiety, syncope, and hepatotoxicity (especially at higher doses).
    - Slow upward titration will assist in alleviating gastrointestinal distress; most other adverse effects subside as patient adjusts to the medication.
    - Hepatotoxicity usually occurs in obese patients on high doses; it was not observed in most clinical studies.
- Patients on opioids (prescription medications or street drugs) will experience withdrawal when combined with this medication and prescriptions will lose efficacy.
    - A complete medication use history from the patient must be taken prior to initiation of therapy, and possibly a urine toxicology screen.
    - The patient should be opioid free for 5–7 days (depending on the half-life of the substance) before initiation of naltrexone therapy.
    - If opioid analgesia is necessary, higher than usual doses may be necessary; thus precautions should be taken regarding potential respiratory depression.

Nonadherence, Misuse, or Abuse

- Ideally, adherence to medication will be increased if patients are counseled appropriately regarding possible adverse reactions and ways to avoid or remedy them.
- Patients must be motivated to quit if they are to experience efficacy from the medications used for abstinence.
- The sublingual dosage form of buprenorphine is absorbed more slowly than the parenteral formulation, leading to less potential for abuse.
    - The combination of naloxone with buprenorphine in the sublingual dosage form contributes to less abuse potential.

Table 21-36 Pharmacotherapeutic Alternatives for Drug Abuse Indications

Drug	Dosage Forms and Strengths Available
Buprenorphine	Tablet (sublingual): 2 mg, 8 mg Injection: 0.3 mg/mL
Buprenorphine/naloxone	Tablet (sublingual): 2 mg/0.5 mg, 8 mg/2 mg
Methadone	Tablet: 5 mg, 10 mg Tablet (dispersible): 40 mg Solution: 5 mg/5 mL 10 mg/5 mL 10 mg/mL Injection: 10 mg/mL
Naloxone	Injection: 0.4 mg/mL (also available as preservative-free formulation), 1 mg/mL
Naltrexone	Tablet: 50 mg Injection: 380 mg extended release (only approved for alcohol dependence)

- Drug Enforcement Agency (DEA) schedule:
    - Methadone is Schedule C-II and buprenorphine is Schedule C-III.
        - Higher potential for abuse by patients.
        - Higher potential for diversion.
    - Naltrexone is not a scheduled medication.
- When treating the comorbid conditions of patients with a history of substance abuse, prescription medications with high abuse potential (i.e., benzodiazepines, opioids, stimulants) or lethality in overdose (i.e., tricyclic antidepressants) should be avoided when possible.

ANNOTATED BIBLIOGRAPHY

American Psychiatric Association. Practice guideline for the treatment of patients with substance use disorders. 2nd ed. 2006. Available at: www.psych.org.

Diagnostic and Statistical Manual of Mental Disorders, 4th ed. Text Revision (DSM-IV-TR). Washington, DC: American Psychiatric Association; 2000.

Fuller MA, Sajatovic M. *Drug Information Handbook for Psychiatry*, 7th ed. Hudson, OH: Lexi-Comp; 2009.

Kosten TR, O'Connor PG. Management of drug and alcohol withdrawal. *N Engl J Med* 2003;348(18): 1786–1795.

Perry PJ, Alexander B, Liskow BI, DeVane CL. *Psychotropic Drug Handbook*, 8th ed. Philadelphia, PA: Lippincott Williams and Wilkins; 2007.

TOPIC: INSOMNIA

Section Coordinator: Rex S. Lott
Contributor: Robyn Cruz

Tips Worth Tweeting

- A detailed patient history should be obtained prior to diagnosis and treatment of insomnia due to the many potentially contributing factors.
- The risk for developing dependence on benzodiazepines should always be considered during treatment selection and throughout treatment duration.
- The pharmacokinetic parameters of each medication, but especially benzodiazepines, are an important consideration in choosing appropriate therapy for individual patients.
- Benzodiazepines and benzodiazepine receptor agonists may work best if used short term and on an intermittently scheduled basis.
- Benzodiazepines have been associated with anterograde amnesia and paradoxical reactions.
- An FDA-approved medication guide describing the potential for performing sleep-related activities must accompany each prescription for eszopiclone, zaleplon, and zolpidem.
- Medications with a shorter half-life are best for sleep latency.
- Medications with a short or intermediate half-life are best for sleep continuity.
- Most benzodiazepines are best given 30–60 minutes prior to bedtime.
- Medications with a longer half-life have more potential for excess daytime sedation but less potential for withdrawal.
- Most manufacturers of benzodiazepines or benzodiazepine receptor agonists recommend limiting the patient supply to 30-day quantities.

Patient Care Scenario: Ambulatory Setting

B. T., a 37-year-old female patient, tells you that she has experienced a prolonged amount of time to fall asleep for the past 1 week. Her current medication list includes lisinopril, acetaminophen prn, a multivitamin, calcium/vitamin D, and Zyrtec-D 24-Hour (started 5 days ago for seasonal allergies). You inquire about her sleep history; the patient states that she does not use caffeine or nicotine and her medications are noted as previously. What is the most appropriate recommendation for this patient regarding her sleep latency?

1.1.0 Patient Information

Review the patient's medications for those that might contribute to the cause of insomnia. Examples include caffeine, theophylline, pseudoephedrine, stimulants (i.e., methylphenidate, dextroamphetamine), steroids, certain selective serotonin reuptake inhibitors, bupropion, nicotine, and diuretics (secondary to increased frequency of urination).

Disease State History

- Must determine if the patient has primary insomnia versus other causes of insomnia:
  - Difficulty initiating or maintaining sleep, or nonrestorative sleep
  - Duration for more than 1 month
  - Results in *significant* distress or impairment in social, occupational, or other areas
- Rule out other causes of insomnia:
  - Another type of sleep disorder
  - Another type of mental disorder
  - Effects of a substance abuse disorder
  - Effects of a medical condition
- Medical history and physical exam
- Sleep history and sleep log:
  - Prescription and OTC medication use
  - Drug use, including caffeine and tobacco
  - Sleep hygiene
  - Total sleep time, time to sleep onset, number of awakenings, time of awakening in morning, reports of feeling rested versus drowsy in morning

Instruments and Techniques Related to Patient Assessment

- Patient history
- Physical assessment and signs are limited, but may include fatigue, frequent headaches (especially "tension" headaches), tense muscles, and gastrointestinal upset
- Polysomnography
- Multiple sleep latency test (MSLT)

Key Terms

- **Polysomnography:** Objectively monitors electrophysiological parameters; usually performed during the normal sleep cycle (i.e., at night). Includes records of the following:
  - Electroencephalogram (EEG)
  - Electromyography (EMG)
  - Air flow (oral or nasal)

  - Respiratory effort
  - Chest/abdominal wall movement
  - Oxygenated hemoglobin saturation
  - Concentration of exhaled CO_2
- **Multiple sleep latency test (MSLT):** Objective assessment of daytime somnolence; measures time to sleep onset.
- **Characteristics of insomnia:** Terminology used to classify traits the patient experiences to determine the best treatment approach.
  - **Sleep continuity:** Balance between sleep and wakefulness.
    - Primary complaint for middle-aged to elderly adults in addition to early-morning awakening.
    - "Better": Less wakefulness.
    - "Worse": More wakefulness.
- **Sleep latency:** How many minutes it takes to fall asleep.
    - Primary complaint for young adults.
- **Sleep efficiency:** Time asleep: time in bed (higher percentage → better continuity).
  - **Acute versus chronic insomnia:**
    - Acute: Sleep disturbance lasting from one night to a few weeks.
    - Chronic: Sleep disturbance lasting at least three nights/week for 1 month minimum.
- **Gamma-aminobutyric acid (GABA):** Major inhibitory neurotransmitter. Medications that act on GABA exert their desired action through decreasing neuronal excitation.
- **Melatonin receptors:**
  - **MT1:** Induces sleepiness (i.e., decreases sleep latency).
  - **MT2:** Influences regulation of circadian rhythm.
- **Short-term treatment:** Generally defined as 7–10 days.

Wellness and Prevention

- Potential risk factors: Female gender, increasing age, alcohol or other drug abuse, shift work (i.e., graveyard shift), psychiatric and/or medical disorders
- Average onset: Young adulthood to middle age
  - Elderly: Partly due to increased rate of medical problems overall; sleep continuity and depth decrease with age
  - Approximately 1–10% of adults have primary insomnia versus 25% of elderly

Table 21-37 Other Sequelae of Insomnia

Predisposition to mental health disorders (i.e., depression, anxiety, substance abuse)
Decrease in energy, ability to concentrate, and memory
Higher rates of absence from work or school and decreased productivity
Irritability

Table 21-38 Sleep Hygiene Techniques

• Only go to bed when sleepy
• Maintain a regular schedule
• Avoid naps
• If unable to fall asleep or go back to sleep within 20 minutes, remove self from bed and return when drowsy
• Avoid watching the clock
• Avoid heavy evening meals or excess liquids

1.2.0 Pharmacotherapy

Drug Indications, Dosing Regimens, and Routes of Administration

Prescription Medications

- Benzodiazepines (BZDs)
  - Potentiate GABA by binding to the benzodiazepine receptor, thereby increasing cells' permeability to chloride ions, which leads to stabilization and a less excitable state.
  - Useful for increasing total sleep duration and may decrease sleep latency.
  - Although other BZDs are used, only five have approved indications for insomnia.
  - Considerations:
    - Efficacy and risk of developing physical dependence may be reduced by dosing "as needed" versus scheduled nightly.
      - If its half-life is more than 5 hours, the drug will accumulate if administered nightly.
    - Shorter half-life contributes less to excess daytime sedation, but has greater potential for rapid tolerance and rebound insomnia.
    - Lower doses will contribute less to adverse effects such as daytime drowsiness, anterograde amnesia, and rebound insomnia.
    - Elderly are more susceptible to adverse effects, partly due to their slowed metabolism.
      - Drugs without active metabolites, and those metabolized by Phase II (because

this metabolism is minimally affected by aging; e.g., temazepam), may be most appropriate for use in elderly patients.
    - There are no data to support efficacy of use for longer than 12 weeks.
  - Estazolam
    - Usual dose is 1–2 mg PO at bedtime.
      - Elderly patients should start at 0.5 mg.
      - Patients with hepatic impairment may require a dose adjustment.
    - Approved for short-term treatment.
  - Flurazepam
    - Usual dose is 15–30 mg PO at bedtime.
      - Elderly patients may use 15 mg, but use of flurazepam in this population should generally be avoided.
    - Approved for short-term treatment.
  - Quazepam
    - Usual dose is 15 mg PO at bedtime; it may be reduced to 7.5 mg after a few doses.
      - Caution should be used with this drug in elderly patients, and the dose should be started lower (i.e., 7.5 mg).
      - Dose reduction may also be necessary in patients with hepatic impairment.
  - Temazepam
    - Usual dose is 15–30 mg PO at bedtime.
      - Elderly or debilitated patients should use 15 mg.
    - Approved for short-term treatment.
  - Triazolam
    - Usual dose is 0.125–0.25 mg PO at bedtime; maximum dose is 0.5 mg/day.
      - Elderly patients should start at 0.125 mg, with a maximum dose of 0.25 mg/day.
      - Avoid use of triazolam or reduce the dose in patients with cirrhosis.
    - Approved for short-term treatment.
- Benzodiazepine Receptor Agonists
  - Act as benzodiazepine receptor agonists but are classified as "nonbenzodiazepines"; enhance GABA activity. More selective than BZDs, a characteristic thought to lead to fewer adverse effects because these drugs have minimal anxiolytic, myorelaxant, and anticonvulsant activity.
  - Useful for decreasing sleep latency, increasing total sleep duration (i.e., sleep maintenance), and improving overall sleep quality.
    - Exception is zaleplon; it is effective for sleep latency but does not improve sleep quality (i.e., efficiency and continuity) and duration.
  - Eszopiclone
    - Usual dose is 1 or 2 mg PO at bedtime for sleep latency or 3 mg for sleep maintenance. Maximum dose is 3 mg.
      - Dose adjustment for sleep latency in elderly patients and patients with severe hepatic impairment: Initial dose of 1 mg, with maximum dose of 2 mg.
      - Exception: Sleep maintenance in elderly patients without hepatic impairment may start at 2 mg.
  - Zaleplon
    - Usual dose is 10 mg PO at bedtime, with a range of 5–20 mg (maximum).
      - Start with 5 mg if used concurrently with cimetidine.
      - Elderly: 5 mg at bedtime, with a maximum of 10 mg.
      - Patients with hepatic impairment: 5 mg in mild to moderate impairment; not recommended in severe impairment.
    - Recommended for short-term treatment (i.e., 7–10 days) but has been studied in use as long as 5 weeks.
  - Zolpidem
    - Usual dose is 10 mg PO at bedtime (12.5 mg if controlled-release [CR] form is being used), with 10 mg being the maximum dose recommended.
      - Dose adjustment for elderly patients and patients with hepatic impairment: 5 mg regular release or 6.25 mg CR.
    - Approved for short-term treatment.
- Melatonin Receptor Agonists
  - Ramelteon
    - Useful for decreasing sleep latency and may be useful in increasing total sleep duration.
    - Selective agonist of melatonin receptors (MT1 and MT2, 8:1) with no affinity for GABA receptors.
    - Usual dose is 8 mg.
    - Not recommended in patients with severe hepatic impairment.

Nonprescription Medications

- Antihistamines
  - Block histamine-1 receptors, which causes sedation.
  - Efficacy is not well supported by current data; not shown to improve sleep. May help in sleep latency.

- Tolerance quickly develops by the third day of use.
- Use caution in elderly patients due to the potential for adverse effects.
- Diphenhydramine
  - Usual dose is 50 mg PO at bedtime.
  - Doses greater than 50 mg do not increase efficacy for insomnia but do increase CNS adverse effects.
- Doxylamine
  - Usual dose is 25 mg PO at bedtime.
  - Doses greater than 25 mg do not increase efficacy for insomnia but do increase CNS adverse effects.
- Approved for short-term treatment.

- Valerian
  - Herbal supplement.
  - Exact mechanism of action is unknown. Thought to act similarly to BZDs by binding to receptors that potentiate GABA.
  - Limited data to support its use. Same caution should be employed as with any other nutritional supplements or herbal products. Considered likely safe or possibly safe depending on quantity, dosage form, and other factors.
  - Usual dose is 200–400 mg PO at bedtime.
  - May take up to 4 weeks to achieve a therapeutic effect.
- Melatonin
  - Classified as a neutraceutical.
  - Melatonin is an endogenous hormone that regulates the sleep–wake cycle; as a supplement, it works to promote sleep. Endogenous levels decrease with age (i.e., 37% decrease between ages 20 and 70 years).
  - Limited data to support use. Same caution should be employed as with any other nutritional supplements or herbal products. Considered possibly safe when used orally for short-term therapy, and possibly unsafe in certain conditions (i.e., if driving or operating hazardous machinery).
  - Usual dose is 0.5–10 mg PO in the evening.

Drug, Food, and Lab Test Interactions

Benzodiazepines

- CNS depressants may increase the effects of these drugs.
- BZDs have the potential to enhance the toxic effects of clozapine.
- CNS stimulants such as theophylline may diminish their effectiveness.
- Valerian, St. John's wort, and kava kava may increase CNS depression.
  - St. John's wort may increase metabolism and decrease levels of quazepam, temazepam, and triazolam.
- Consumption of grapefruit juice may increase serum levels and the risk of toxicity with BZDs—an effect less likely with flurazepam due to its high oral bioavailability.
- CYP 3A4 inhibitors may increase the concentration and toxicity of BZDs.
  - CYP 3A4 inducers may decrease concentration and efficacy.
- Oral contraceptives may alter the clearance of some BZDs.
  - May decrease the clearance of estazolam, flurazepam, triazolam, and quazepam, all of which are metabolized through oxidation.
  - May increase the clearance of temazepam, which is metabolized through glucuronidation.
- Food may decrease the rate of absorption of triazolam.

Benzodiazepine Receptor Agonists

- Eszopiclone
  - CYP 3A4 inhibitors may increase this agent's concentration and toxicity.
  - CYP 3A4 inducers may decrease its concentration and efficacy.
  - Combination of eszopiclone with olanzapine may increase psychomotor slowing.
  - Eszopiclone potentiates the effects of other CNS depressants, including alcohol.
  - Valerian, St. John's wort, and kava kava may increase CNS depression.
  - Food may delay the onset of action (especially with/immediately after a heavy meal).
- Zaleplon
  - CYP 3A4 inhibitors may increase this agent's concentration and toxicity; cimetidine may decrease its metabolism by CYP 3A4 and aldehyde oxidase inhibition (the primary means of zaleplon metabolism).
  - Flumazenil and rifamycin derivatives may decrease zaleplon's efficacy.
  - Zaleplon potentiates the effects of other CNS depressants, including alcohol.
  - Valerian, St. John's wort, and kava kava may increase CNS depression.
    - St. John's wort may decrease zaleplon levels.
  - Food (high-fat meals) prolongs zaleplon's absorption and delays its onset of action.
- Zolpidem
  - CYP 3A4 inhibitors may increase this agent's concentration and toxicity.

- CYP 3A4 inducers may decrease its concentration and efficacy.
- Zolpidem potentiates the effects of other CNS depressants, including alcohol.
- Valerian, St. John's wort, and kava kava may increase CNS depression.
  - St. John's wort may decrease zolpidem levels.
- Food delays time to peak concentration (onset of action) and decreases bioavailability and maximum concentration.

Melatonin Receptor Agonists

- Ramelteon
  - CYP 1A2 inhibitors may increase this agent's concentration and toxicity; fluconazole and ketoconazole may increase its concentration and toxicity due to inhibition of CYP 1A2 (in addition to CYP 3A4, 2C9, and 2C19).
  - Rifampin may decrease the efficacy of ramelteon.
  - Ramelteon potentiates the effects of other CNS depressants, including alcohol.
  - Food (high-fat meals) increases AUC and delays T_{max}; it delays the onset of action.

Nonprescription Medications

- Diphenhydramine
  - May increase the concentration and toxicity of 2D6 substrates.
  - May decrease the effect of prodrugs that require CYP 2D6 metabolism to be converted to the active agent (e.g., tamoxifen).
  - May increase the absorption of digoxin.
  - Potentiates the effects of other agents with anticholinergic properties.
  - Antagonizes the effects of cholinergic and some neuroleptic drugs.
  - Potentiates the effects of CNS depressants, including alcohol.
  - Valerian, St. John's wort, and kava kava may increase CNS depression.
  - May suppress wheal and flare reactions to skin test antigens.
- Doxylamine
  - Potentiates the effects of other agents with anticholinergic properties.
  - Antagonizes the effects of cholinergic agents.
  - Potentiates the effects of CNS depressants, including alcohol.
  - Valerian, St. John's wort, and kava kava may increase CNS depression.
- Valerian
  - Theoretically may interact with other CNS depressants, barbiturates, antidepressants, anxiolytics, antihistamines, beta blockers, antiepileptics, loperamide, disulfiram, metronidazole, vasopressin, and alcohol.
- Melatonin
  - Theoretically:
    - May inhibit CYP 1A2.
    - May interact with CYP 2C9.
    - May interact with calcium-channel blockers.
    - May potentiate the effects of CNS depressants, including alcohol.
    - May potentiate the CNS depression associated with psychotropics.
  - May interact with immunosuppressant medications through melatonin's effect on overall immune function; concurrent use should be avoided.
  - Fluvoxamine may increase bioavailability.
  - Verapamil may increase melatonin secretion.
  - Drugs that deplete vitamin B_6 may inhibit the body's ability to endogenously synthesize melatonin—oral contraceptives/estrogen, hydralazine, loop diuretics, and theophylline.
    - Beta blockers and BZDs may also decrease melatonin concentrations through enzyme inhibition.
  - May reduce glucose tolerance and insulin sensitivity; may interact with insulin or other antidiabetic medications.
  - May cause an actual increase in human growth hormone levels.

Contraindications, Warnings, and Precautions

Benzodiazepines

- Contraindicated in acute narrow-angle glaucoma, central sleep apnea, severe respiratory insufficiency, and pregnancy.
- Use with caution:
  - With other CNS depressants.
  - In hepatic disease, renal impairment, respiratory disease, impaired gag reflex, the elderly, obese patients, patients with a history of drug dependence, and patients with depressive disorders or psychosis.
  - When patients must perform tasks requiring mental alertness.
- BZDs have been associated with anterograde amnesia and paradoxical reactions (hyperactive or aggressive behavior).
- All enter breastmilk and are either contraindicated or not recommended in breastfeeding; all BZDs listed above are pregnancy Category X.

Benzodiazepine Receptor Agonists

- Eszopiclone
  - A medication guide must accompany all outpatient prescriptions.
  - No contraindications noted by the manufacturer.
  - Use with caution:
    - With other CNS depressants or psychoactive medications.
    - In hepatic disease, respiratory disease, the elderly, patients with concomitant use of CYP 3A4 inhibitors, and patients with depression or a history of drug dependence.
    - When patients must perform tasks requiring mental alertness.
    - In withdrawing use of the medication abruptly.
  - Has been associated with abnormal thinking, behavior changes, and amnesia.
  - Excretion in breastmilk is unknown; caution is advised. Classified as pregnancy Category C.
- Zaleplon
  - A medication guide must accompany all outpatient prescriptions.
  - No contraindications other than previous hypersensitivity.
  - Use with caution:
    - With other CNS depressants or psychoactive medications.
    - In hepatic disease, respiratory disease, the elderly, and patients with depression or a history of drug dependence.
    - When patients must perform tasks requiring mental alertness.
    - In withdrawing use of the medication abruptly.
    - In patients sensitive to tartrazine (FDC-yellow #5), which is found in the capsules.
  - Has been associated with abnormal thinking, behavior changes, and amnesia.
  - Enters breastmilk; not recommended for breastfeeding women. Classified as pregnancy Category C.
- Zolpidem
  - A medication guide must accompany all outpatient prescriptions.
  - No contraindications other than previous hypersensitivity.
  - Use with caution:
    - With other CNS depressants or psychoactive medications.
    - In myasthenia gravis, hepatic disease, respiratory disease, the elderly, and patients with depression or a history of drug dependence.
    - When patients must perform tasks requiring mental alertness.
    - In withdrawing use of the medication abruptly.
  - Has been associated with abnormal thinking, behavior changes, and amnesia.
  - Enters breastmilk; not recommended for breastfeeding women (is rated "compatible" per AAP). Classified as pregnancy Category C.

Melatonin Receptor Agonists

- Ramelteon
  - Contraindicated in severe hepatic impairment, previous hypersensitivity, and concurrent use of fluvoxamine.
  - Use with caution:
    - With other CNS depressants.
    - In severe sleep apnea or COPD, moderate hepatic impairment, concomitant use of CYP 1A2 inhibitors, and patients with depression or other psychiatric diagnoses.
    - When patients must perform tasks requiring mental alertness.
  - Has been associated with abnormal thinking, behavior changes, and amnesia.
  - Excretion in breastmilk is unknown; not recommended for breastfeeding women. Classified as pregnancy Category C.

Nonprescription Medications

- Diphenhydramine
  - Contraindicated in acute asthma, previous hypersensitivity, breastfeeding, and neonates or premature infants, and for use as a local anesthetic injection.
  - Use with caution:
    - With other CNS depressants.
    - In the elderly and in patients with angle-closure glaucoma, pyloroduodenal obstruction, urinary tract obstruction, asthma, hyperthyroidism, increased intraocular pressure, cardiovascular disease, soy/peanut allergies, or phenylalanine sensitivities (only certain products).
    - In children, as excitation may occur.
    - When patients must perform tasks requiring mental alertness.
  - Enters breastmilk; contraindicated in breastfeeding women. Classified as pregnancy Category B.
- Doxylamine
  - No contraindications other than previous hypersensitivity.

- Use with caution:
  - In angle-closure glaucoma, respiratory disease, urinary tract obstruction, thyroid dysfunction, increased intraocular pressure, and cardiovascular disease.
  - With other CNS depressants.
  - When patients must perform tasks requiring mental alertness.
- Excretion in breastmilk is unknown. Classified as pregnancy Category B (approved for use in pregnancy-related nausea and vomiting).

- Valerian
  - Use with caution:
    - With other CNS depressants.
    - When patients must perform tasks requiring mental alertness.
    - In combination with hypnotics, as sleeping time may increase.
  - Products other than valepotriate and baldrinal-free products may have mutagenic properties in patients younger than age 12 years.
  - Limited data are available regarding safety in pregnancy and lactation; avoid use in pregnant and breastfeeding women.
  - The FDA does not regulate herbal and nutritional supplements; general caution is advised for use of such products due to much unknown information.
- Melatonin
  - Use with caution in patients with a history of bleeding, hemostatic disorders or drug-related hemostatic problems, or concomitant use of warfarin, aspirin/aspirin-containing products, NSAID, or antiplatelet agents, or antidiabetic agents.
  - May worsen depression.

Table 21-39 Benzodiazepines

Drug	Onset (min)	Duration (hr)	Peak (PO, hr)	Protein Binding (%)	Active Metabolite	Half-life (hr) (Metabolite)
Estazolam	60	Variable	2	93	No	10–24
Flurazepam	15–20	7–8	0.5–2	97	Yes	NS (40–114)
Quazepam	20–45	—	2	95	Yes	25–41 (25–114)
Temazepam	30–60	—	2–3	96	No	4–18
Triazolam	15–30	6–7	1	89–94	No	2–4

NS = not significant.

  - Excess doses may cause morning sedation and drowsiness.
  - Limited data are available regarding safety in pregnancy and lactation; avoid use in pregnant and breastfeeding women.
  - The FDA does not regulate herbal and nutritional supplements; general caution is advised for use of such products due to much unknown information, including long-term human studies.

Physiochemical Properties, Solubility, Pharmacodynamics, and Pharmacokinetic Properties

Benzodiazepines

Note on Aging

Absorption of benzodiazepines is not affected by aging, but changes in metabolism, increased half-life, and increased concentration of unbound drug may affect drug action.

- Aging contributes to a *reduction* in lean body mass and plasma proteins.
- Aging contributes to an *increase* in body fat.

Target Symptoms Versus Medications

- Sleep latency: BZDs with a shorter duration (half-life) are best (e.g., triazolam, zaleplon).
- Sleep continuity: BZDs with a short or intermediate duration (half-life) are best (e.g., estazolam, eszopiclone, temazepam).

Other Factors for Benzodiazepines

- The dose of zaleplon may be repeated if the patient has nocturnal awakening and has at least 4 hours remaining to sleep.
- Most BZDs are best given 1 hour before bedtime; triazolam, zolpidem, are zaleplon are best given 30 minutes or less (i.e., immediately) before bedtime.
- Drugs with a longer half-life have more potential for excess daytime somnolence, but may also have less withdrawal when discontinued.

Benzodiazepine Receptor Agonists

See Table 21-40.

Melatonin Receptor Agonists

See Table 21-41.

Nonprescription Medications

See Table 21-42.

Table 21-40 Benzodiazepine Receptor Agonists

Drug	Onset (min)	Duration (hr)	Peak (PO, hr)	Protein Binding (%)	Active Metabolite	Half-life (hr) (Metabolite)
Eszopiclone	30	–	1	52–59	Yes	6 (9 in elderly) (NS)
Zaleplon	20	6–8 (usually about 4)	1	45–75	No	0.5–1
Zolpidem	30	6–8	1.6 (2.2 with food)	93	No	1.4–4.5; 9.9 in cirrhosis; up to 32% longer in elderly

NS = not significant.

Table 21-41 Melatonin Receptor Agonists

Drug	Onset (min)	Duration (hr)	Peak (PO, hr)	Protein Binding (%)	Active Metabolite	Half-life (hr) (Metabolite)
Ramelteon	30	–	0.5–1.5	82	Yes	1–2.6 (2–5)

Table 21-42 Nonprescription Medications

Drug	Onset (min)	Duration (hr)	Peak (PO, hr)	Protein Binding (%)	Active Metabolite	Half-life (hr) (Metabolite)
Diphenhydramine	60–180	4–7	2–4	78	No	2–10 (13.5 in elderly)
Doxylamine	–	–	–	–	Yes	10–12
Valerian	–	–	–	–	–	–
Melatonin	–	–	–	–	–	0.5–1

Biopharmaceutical Principles and Pharmaceutical Characteristics of Dosage Forms

Benzodiazepines

- Estazolam: No information available
- Flurazepam: No information available
- Quazepam: Rapid absorption
- Temazepam: Slow absorption
- Triazolam: No information available

Benzodiazepine Receptor Agonists

- Eszopiclone: Rapid absorption; high-fat/heavy meal may delay absorption
- Zaleplon: Rapid and almost complete absorption; high-fat meal delays absorption
- Zolpidem: Rapid absorption; 70% bioavailable

Melatonin Receptor Agonists

- Ramelteon: Rapid absorption; high-fat meal delays T_{max} and increases AUC; absolute bioavailability 1.8%

Nonprescription Medications

- Diphenhydramine: 40–70% bioavailable
- Doxylamine: Well absorbed
- Valerian: No information available
- Melatonin: Rapid absorption

1.3.0 Monitoring

Pharmacotherapeutic Outcomes

- The goal is to achieve restorative sleep with minimal sleep-onset latency.
  - Achieving this goal may be assisted by a combination of sleep hygiene techniques, cognitive-behavioral therapy, and medications. Sleep hygiene should be incorporated so as to reduce dependency on medications for sleep induction and maintenance.
- Secondary to the goal of achieving quality sleep is the prevention of secondary complications related to insomnia, such as increased risk of developing diagnosis of other psychiatric disorders (i.e., depression, anxiety, substance abuse problems) or medical illnesses.
- Also important is the goal of decreasing compromise to such aspects of life as social, occupational, and financial roles.

Safety and Efficacy Monitoring

- Monitor and assess the patient for mental alertness and excessive daytime drowsiness; dose reduction or another alternative may need to be considered.

- Monitor for behavior changes (i.e., sleep-driving, sleep-cooking/eating).
- Monitor for changes in respiratory or cardiovascular status.
- Monitor for appropriate use of medications by the patient, especially to avoid misuse or abuse of medications.
- Obtain the patient's report of efficacy for improvement in sleep quality.
- Most medications are approved for short-term use (ranges from 7–10 days to 2–6 weeks) only. Little data support use beyond 4–6 weeks. Most studies had a duration of only 6 weeks or less.
- Eszopiclone, zolpidem CR, and ramelteon are not restricted to short-term use.
- Efficacy of medications may decrease after extended use.
- Dosing intermittently versus dosing that is scheduled nightly may alleviate this phenomenon. Examples include dosing every other or every third night versus "as needed" so as to not promote a patient focus on taking and/or relying on medications for insomnia.

Adverse Drug Reactions

Benzodiazepines

- The FDA requires all sedative-hypnotics to carry a caution regarding potential adverse effects such as anaphylaxis and angioedema. It also requires warnings regarding sleep-related behaviors such as sleep-driving and sleep-cooking/eating.
- Sedation, respiratory depression, hypotension, alterations in mental status (confusion, amnesia), dizziness, drowsiness.

Benzodiazepine Receptor Agonists

- The FDA requires all sedative-hypnotics to carry a caution regarding potential adverse effects such as anaphylaxis and angioedema. It also requires warnings regarding sleep-related behaviors such as sleep-driving and sleep-cooking/eating.
- Eszopiclone: Unpleasant taste, headache, dry mouth, dizziness, infection, somnolence, GI upset.
- Zaleplon: Headache, dizziness, somnolence, nausea, abdominal pain, weakness.
- Zolpidem: Headache, somnolence, dizziness, "hangover" feeling, nausea, parasthesias, incoordination, hallucinations, ataxia, parasomnias (e.g., sleep-walking), anterograde amnesia, falls.

Melatonin Receptor Agonists

- Ramelteon: Somnolence, dizziness, nausea, fatigue, headache, increases in serum prolactin.

Table 21-43 Pharmacotherapeutic Alternatives for Insomnia

Drug	Dosage Forms and Strengths Available
Estazolam	Tablet: 1 mg, 2 mg
Flurazepam	Capsule: 15 mg, 30 mg
Quazepam	Tablet: 7.5 mg, 15 mg
Temazepam	Capsule: 7.5 mg, 15 mg, 30 mg
Triazolam	Tablet: 0.125 mg, 0.25 mg
Eszopiclone	Tablet: 1 mg, 2 mg, 3 mg
Zaleplon	Capsule: 5 mg, 10 mg
Zolpidem	Tablet: 5 mg, 10 mg, CR 6.25 mg, CR 12.5 mg
Ramelteon	Tablet: 8 mg
Diphenhydramine	Caplet, capsule, softgel, tablet: 25 mg, 50 mg Multiple other topicals, syrups, and formulations available
Doxylamine	Tablet: 25 mg
Valerian	Tea, tincture, capsule, tablet
Melatonin	Capsule, tablet, lozenge

Nonprescription Medications

- Diphenhydramine: Drowsiness, "hangover effect," dizziness, dry mouth, constipation, increased risk of falls.
- Doxylamine: Drowsiness, "hangover effect," dizziness, dry mouth, constipation, increased risk of falls.
- Valerian: Drowsiness, dizziness, nausea, headache, GI upset, decreased alertness, uneasiness, cardiac disturbances, insomnia, excitability.
- Melatonin: Headache, daytime fatigue/drowsiness, dizziness, abdominal cramps, irritability.

Nonadherence, Misuse, or Abuse

- Benzodiazepines, eszopiclone, zaleplon, and zolpidem are DEA Schedule C-IV substances.
- Benzodiazepine receptor agonists have less abuse potential than benzodiazepines.
    - Ramelteon is the only prescription medication for insomnia that is not a DEA-scheduled medication. This suggests that it has less abuse potential than BZD receptor agonists.
- Most manufacturers recommend limiting quantities of sleep medications to a 30-day supply.
- Long-term use of benzodiazepines should be approached very cautiously due to their potential for abuse.
    - Medication with a rapid onset of action will have the most abuse potential.
    - Medication use should be assessed appropriately and often to avoid misuse and potential for abuse.

ANNOTATED BIBLIOGRAPHY

Bhat A, Shafi F, El Solh AA. Pharmacotherapy of insomnia. *Expert Opin Pharmacother* 2008;9(3): 351–362.

Diagnostic and Statistical Manual of Mental Disorders, 4th ed. Text Revision (DSM-IV-TR). Washington, DC: American Psychiatric Association; 2000.

Fuller MA, Sajatovic M. *Drug Information Handbook for Psychiatry*, 7th ed. Hudson, OH: Lexi-Comp; 2009.

Medical Letter's Natural Medicine Comprehensive Database.

Passarella S, Duong M. Diagnosis and treatment of insomnia. *Am J Health-Syst Pharm* 2008;65: 927–934.

Perry PJ, Alexander B, Liskow BI, DeVane CL. *Psychotropic Drug Handbook*, 8th ed. Philadelphia, PA: Lippincott Williams and Wilkins; 2007.

Sateia MJ, Nowell PD. Insomnia. *Lancet*. 2004;364:1959–1973.

TOPIC: SCHIZOPHRENIA

Section Coordinator: *Rex S. Lott*
Contributors: *Sarah J. Popish and Alberto Augsten*

Schizophrenia is a debilitating mental illness characterized by a mixture of symptoms that are often divided into two major categories: positive and negative. The positive signs and symptoms of schizophrenia consist of delusions and hallucinations. Delusions are defined as fixed false beliefs or misperceptions or misinterpretations of experiences or situations. Hallucinations may come by any sensory modality, although schizophrenics most often experience auditory hallucinations. Other positive symptoms include distortions in communication and language, disorganized speech, disorganized or catatonic behavior, and psychomotor agitation. The negative signs and symptoms of schizophrenia are seen as a reduction in normal function and can be defined by the "five A's": (1) alogia—poverty of speech; (2) affective flattening—restrictions in the range of emotional expression; (3) asociality—reduced social interactions and drive; (4) anhedonia—reduced ability to experience pleasure; and (5) avolition—reduced desire, drive, or motivation to pursue meaningful goals. In addition to these symptoms, patients with schizophrenia often have cognitive deficits and experience affective symptoms such as depression, dysphoria, and hopelessness.

Two groups of antipsychotics are used to treat schizophrenia: conventional (typical antipsychotics) and the newer atypical antipsychotics. The conventional antipsychotics and atypical antipsychotics are postsynaptic D2 receptor antagonists. They are thought to exert their antipsychotic effects by decreasing dopamine transmission in the mesolimbic system. Unfortunately, dopamine antagonism in other areas of the brain leads to an assortment of side effects when these drugs are prescribed. Both classes of medications are effective in the treatment of schizophrenia but differ in their side-effect profiles and their pharmacologic activity.

Tips Worth Tweeting

- Positive symptoms of schizophrenia result from dopamine overactivity in the mesolimbic system.
- Negative symptoms result from dopamine underactivity in the frontal cortex.
- Typical or conventional antipsychotic exert their antipsychotic activity through D2 receptor antagonism.
- Atypical antipsychotics are D2 and serotonin (5-HT2) receptor antagonists.
- Aripiprazole is a D2 partial agonist.
- Clozapine is the most effective antipsychotic, with a 50–60% response rate at 6–12 months after therapy is initiated.
- The patient's CBC must be monitored weekly during the first 6 months of clozapine therapy because of this drug's risk of agranulocytosis. Subsequently, the frequency of CBC measurements may be decreased.
- Clozapine decreases the seizure threshold.
- Atypical antipsychotics have a decreased incidence of extrapyramidal side effects and tardive dyskinesia as compared to the conventional antipsychotics.
- Atypical antipsychotics have an increased risk of cardiometabolic side effects (e.g., weight gain, dyslipidemia, diabetes, accelerated cardiovascular disease).

Patient Care Scenario: Hospital Setting (Acute Psychiatric)

J. B.: 28 yo Caucasian male
Chief complaint: "I'm the most sane person there is."
HPI: This is one of many psychiatric hospitalizations for this 28-year-old Caucasian male, who was admitted to the Center for Behavioral Health as a danger to himself and to others. His mother claims that J. B. has been off his medications for the last 4 months and has been increasingly agitated and unable to function in society. The patient has apparently been very delusional, claiming that aliens put

electrodes in his ears so that they can directly communicate with him. He unsuccessfully tried to squeeze a bottle of superglue in his ear "to stop the alien voices."

The patient's speech is quite tangential. When asked why he was in the hospital, he replied, "Injustice and considered to be evil. I graduated from Berkeley in 2004 and I work as a musician. This country should eliminate some of the ways we operate. We should eliminate psychiatry from life. We are human beings. We all have feelings. My mother was delivered an injustice. I hope to move to Florida to Colorado to write my book and play sports." When asked about the electrodes and aliens, the patient became guarded and suspicious.

Past psychiatric history: J. B. has had three prior hospitalizations. His first came when he was 20 years old and lasted for a total of 6 months. He is a very poor historian; when asked about past medications, he mentions only risperidone "that they forced me to take."

PMI: He denies any illnesses, injuries, or operations.

Social history: Smokes 2 ppd; occasionally drinks; has experimented with methamphetamine and cocaine, but denies any recent use.

Mental status exam: The patient is a Caucasian male, who is disheveled in appearance and slightly malodorous. His hair is unwashed and unkempt. He is extremely guarded and paranoid, and often launches into tirades about the evils of psychiatry. His thought processes are illogical with delusional thinking. His affect is blunted, with a minimal range of reactivity to his emotions. The patient denies auditory and visual hallucinations but often seems internally preoccupied. His memory is fair but difficult to assess because he is uncooperative. A & O × 3.

Vital signs: BP 135/80, P 72, Wt 190 lbs, Ht 6'2".

Labs: WNL, Urine drug screen negative.

1.1.0 Patient Information

Secondary Causes of Psychosis

Psychotic symptoms may result from utilization of a substance—for example, cocaine, methamphetamine, alcohol, sedatives, and many others.

Instruments and Techniques Related to Patient Assessment

- *Diagnostic and Statistical Manual of Mental Disorders* (DSM-IV-TR)
- Brief Psychiatric Rating Scale (BPRS), Positive and Negative Symptom Scale (PANSS), Scale for the Assessment of Negative Symptoms (SANS), Scale for the Assessment of Positive Symptoms (SAPS), Clinical Global Impressions (CGI), Global Assessment of Functioning (GAF), Barnes Akathisia Scale, Abnormal Involuntary Movement Scale (AIMS), Dyskinesia Identification System (DISCUS), and Extrapyramidal Symptom Rating Scale (ESRS)

Signs and Symptoms

To make a diagnosis of schizophrenia, the patient must have two of the following symptoms for a month and residual symptoms for at least 6 months, and the symptoms must cause marked social impairment: delusions, hallucinations, disorganized speech, negative symptoms, or unusual behavior.

Subtypes of schizophrenia include paranoid, disorganized, catatonic, undifferentiated, and residual.

1.20 Pharmacotherapy

The usual starting dose is 400–600 mg/day of chlorpromazine or its equivalent, divided into bid to qid dosing. The dosage is increased until behavior improves or side effects limit the dose. Once patient is stabilized, the total daily dose can be given at bedtime.

Conventional or Typical Antipsychotics

- Exert their antipsychotic activity through D2 receptor antagonism
- D2 receptor antagonism leads to extrapyramidal side effects (EPS) and increased prolactin release

Typical antipsychotics antagonize other receptors, producing a variety of side effects:

- Alpha adrenergic: Orthostatic hypotension
- Histaminergic (H1): Sedation, weight gain
- Muscarinic: Anticholinergic side effects (dry mouth, eyes and throat, blurred vision, mydriasis, tachycardia, constipation, urinary retention, impotence) and at higher doses can cause delirium and psychosis

Extrapyramidal Side Effects

- Normally, dopamine suppresses acetylcholine activity in the nigrostriatal pathway.
- Removal of dopamine inhibition via D2 antagonism leads to excess acetylcholine activity.
- Anticholinergic agents overcome excess acetylcholine activity, thereby reducing EPS.
- Low-potency typical antipsychotics have intrinsic anticholinergic activity.

Atypical Antipsychotics

- Exert their antipsychotic activity through D2 receptor antagonism.

Table 21-44 Typical or Conventional Antipsychotics Used for Schizophrenia Treatment

	Drug	Relative Potency	Dosage Range (mg/day)	Dosage Forms Available
Low potency	Chlorpromazine (Thorazine)	100	60–2,000	Tablet
	Thioridazine (Mellaril)	100	50–800	Tablet Liquid
	Mesoridazine (Serentil)	50	50–800	Injection Tablet Liquid
High potency	Haloperidol (Haldol)	2	1–100	Tablet Injection Long-acting injection Liquid
	Thiothixene (Navane)	5	5–60	Capsule
	Fluphenazine (Prolixin)	2	1–50	Tablet Injection Long-acting injection
	Perphenazine (Trilafon)	8	8–64	Tablet
	Trifluperazine (Stelazine)	5	2–80	Tablet
	Loxapine (Loxitane)	10	20–250	Capsule
	Pimozide (Orap)	2	2–10	Tablet

Table 21-45 Atypical Antipsychotics Used for the Treatment of Schizophrenia

Drug	Available Dosage Forms	Dosing	Maximum Dose (mg/day)	Comments
Clozapine (Clozaril, Fazaclo)	Tablet, ODT	Initiate: 12.5–25 mg/day Titrate to 300–400 mg/day Divided dosage (bid–qid)	900	○ High CM risk ○ Agranulocytosis ○ Lowers seizure threshold (dose related) ○ Anticholinergic ○ Sialorrhea ○ Sedation ○ Orthostatic hypotension
Olanzapine (Zyprexa, Zydis)	Tablet, injection, ODT	Initiate: 2.5–10 mg/day Titrate to 5–20 mg/day	20	○ High CM risk ○ Anticholinergic ○ Sedation
	Relprevv (long-acting injection)	Initiate: 210–300 mg q 2 weeks Maintain:150–300 mg q 2 weeks		
Risperidone (Risperdal)	Tablet, liquid, M-Tab (ODT)	Initiate: 0.25–2 mg/day Titrate to 2–6 mg/day 4–6 mg/day is optimal	16 Doses > 6 mg have no additional benefit and usually cause unacceptable extrapyramidal side effects	○ Low EPS with doses ≤ 6 mg/day ○ Increased prolactin ○ Orthostatic hypotension ○ Moderate to high CM risk
	Consta (long-acting injection)	25 mg q 2 weeks Maximum: 50 mg q 2 weeks Oral coverage × 3 weeks		

Table 21-45 (*continued*)

Drug	Available Dosage Forms	Dosing	Maximum Dose (mg/day)	Comments
Quetiapine (Seroquel)	Tablet, XR tablet	Initiate: 100 mg/day Titrate to 300–750 mg/day Divided dosage or qhs	800	○ Moderate to high CM risk ○ Sedation ○ Anticholinergic ○ Low risk of extrapyramidal side effects
Aripiprazole (Abilify)	Tablet, liquid, injection, Discmelt (ODT)	Initiate: 10–15 mg/day Titrate to 10–30 mg/day Dosage escalation q 2 weeks	30	○ Low CM risk ○ Akathisia
Ziprasidone (Geodon)	Capsule, injection	Initiate: 20 mg bid Titrate to 80 mg bid Give with food (500-calorie meal)	160	○ Low CM risk ○ Mild sedation at initiation ○ Initial akathisia is common ○ QTc prolongation ○ Increased absorption with food
Paliperidone (Invega)	XR tablet Sustenna (long-acting injection)	Initiate: 6 mg/day Titrate to 3 mg q 5 days Initiate: 234 mg, first week; 156 mg, second week Maintain: 117 mg q 4 weeks	SrCr > 80: 12 SrCr 50–80: 6 SrCr 10–50: 3	○ Moderate weight gain and CM risk ○ Increased prolactin ○ Increased absorption with food ○ Active metabolite of risperidone ○ Extrapyramidal side effects
Asenapine (Saphris)	SL tablet	Initiate: 5 mg bid	10 mg bid	○ Low extrapyramidal side effects ○ Orthostatic hypotension ○ Sedation ○ Low weight gain and CM risk ○ Oral hypoesthesia (numbness) ○ Avoid food or liquids 10 minutes prior to and after taking dose
Iloperidone (Fanapt)	Tablet	Initiate: 1 mg bid Titrate to 12–24 mg/day Increase by 2 mg daily	24	○ Orthostatic hypotension (slow titration) ○ Moderate weight gain and CM risk
Lurasidone (Latuda)	Tablet	40 mg once daily	160 mg	○ Some akathisia ○ Mild CM risk ○ Take with at least a 350-calorie meal ○ CYP3A4 substrate: Use lower doses in the presence of inhibitors ○ Reduce dosage in patients with renal impairment

ODT = oral disintegrating tablet, XR = extended release, SL = sublingual, CM = cardiometabolic risk (diabetes, dyslipidemia, weight gain).

Table 21-46 Mechanism of Action for Schizophrenia Pharmacotherapies

	Brain Region	Result
D2 receptor antagonism	Mesolimbic	Decrease in positive symptoms
	Mesocortical	No improvement in negative symptoms
	Nigrostriatal	EPS and tardive dyskinesia
	Tubero-infundibular	Increased prolactin secretion
$5\text{-}HT_{2A}$ receptor antagonism; stimulation of dopamine release	Mesolimbic	No effect
	Mesocortical	Reduction of negative symptoms and potential improvement in cognitive symptoms
	Nigrostriatal	Reduction in extrapyramidal symptoms
	Tubero-infundibular	Reduction in prolactin release

- $5\text{-}HT_{2A}$ antagonism makes atypical antipsychotics atypical.
- DA has a reciprocal relationship with 5-HT; that is, an increase in 5-HT decreases DA, and vice versa. Blocking $5\text{-}HT_{2A}$ receptors increases DA in the mesocortical, nigrostriatal, and tubero-infundibular pathways of the brain, which leads to the following effects:
  - Decreased EPS
  - Decreased prolactin secretion
  - Improved negative symptoms
- Aripiprazole is a D2 partial agonist, which stabilizes dopamine neurotransmission in a state between complete antagonism and full stimulation.
- Atypical antipsychotics antagonize a multitude of other receptor subtypes for both dopamine and serotonin.
- Atypical antipsychotics also antagonize alpha-adrenergic, histaminergic, and muscarinic receptors.

1.30 Monitoring

Drug, Food, and Lab Test Interactions

See Table 21-47.

Precautions and Contraindications

"Black Box" Warnings

- Thioridazine and mesoridazine: QTc prolongation; avoid inhibitors of CYP 2D6 and other drugs that can prolong QTc intervals
- Atypical and typical antipsychotics: Elderly patients with dementia-related psychosis are at increased risk of death
- Clozapine: Agranulocytosis; seizures; myocarditis—increased risk during the first month of therapy; other adverse cardiovascular and respiratory effects caused by orthostatic hypotension accompanied by respiratory or cardiac arrest

Pharmacotherapeutic Goal

Control psychotic symptoms and improve negative symptoms with the least amount of side effects.

Monitoring (per 2004 APA guidelines)

- Vital signs: Pulse, blood pressure, temperature at baseline and when clinically relevant
- Cardiometabolic: Weight, height, body mass index (BMI); obtain a baseline lipid panel; obtain fasting blood glucose and hemoglobin A_{1c} at baseline and periodically
- EPS: Assess for extrapyramidal signs and abnormal involuntary movements at each visit after starting antipsychotic therapy
- Tardive dyskinesia: Assess using AIMS (Abnormal Involuntary Movement scale) every 6 months for typical antipsychotics and yearly for atypical antipsychotics
- QTc prolongation: Obtain a baseline ECG and serum potassium measurement before treatment with thioridazine, mesoridazine, or pimozide; obtain an ECG before treatment with ziprasidone in the presence of cardiac risk factors
- Hyperprolactinemia: Screen for symptoms of hyperprolactinemia at each visit
- Pregnancy test for women of childbearing potential
- Blood chemistries: Electrolytes, renal, liver, and thyroid function tests at baseline and annually
- Hematology: CBC with differential at baseline (except for clozapine)

Clozapine CBC monitoring parameters:

- WBC > 3,500 mm^3 and ANC > 2,000
  - Weekly for 6 months
  - Every 2 weeks for 6 months
  - Every 4 weeks after 12 months of therapy if there is no substantial drop
- WBC < 2,000 mm^3 and/or ANC < 1,000: Discontinue therapy and do not rechallenge

All antipsychotics have the potential to cause movement disorders.

Table 21-47 Important Pharmacokinetic and Pharmacodynamic Properties of Schizophrenia Pharmacotherapies

Psychotropic Drug	Elimination Pathway	Increase AP Levels	Decrease AP Levels	Other
Conventional antipsychotics (chlorpromazine, haloperidol)	CYP 2D6*, CYP 3A4	CYP 2D6 inhibitors: bupropion, chloroquine, cimetidine, diphenhydramine, duloxetine, fluoxetine, fluvoxamine, haloperidol, paroxetine, propoxyphene, propranolol, ritonavir, terbinafine	Carbamazapine, barbiturates	CYP 2D6 inhibitors that can prolong QTc: amiodarone, propafenone, quindine, ranolazine. These drugs have increased plasma concentrations and prolong QTc, which could cause fatal arrhythmias.
Asenapine	CYP 1A2*	Fluvoxamine	Probably smoking	
Aripiprazole	CYP 2D6, CYP 3A4	Ketoconazole; other CYP 3A4 inhibitors Paroxetine, fluoxetine; other CYP 2D6 inhibitors	Carbamazepine	
Clozapine	CYP 1A2*, CYP 2D6	Fluvoxamine, ciprofloxacin, fluoxetine, cimetidine; other CYP 1A2 inhibitors	Smoking; carbamazepine	Carbamazepine: increased risk of bone marrow suppression.
Iloperidone	CYP 2D6, CYP 3A4	Ketoconazole; other CYP 3A4 inhibitors Fluoxetine, paroxetine; other CYP D6 inhibitors	Carbamazepine	Avoid use with other drugs that prolong QTc intervals.
Lurasidone	CYP 3A4	Diltiazem, strong CYP 3A4 inhibitors should be avoided	Carbamazepine and other strong CYP 3A4 inducers should be avoided	
Olanzapine	CYP 1A2	Fluvoxamine, ciprofloxacin Fluoxetine, cimetidine; other CYP 1A2 inhibitors	Smoking; carbamazepine	
Paliperidone	PGP, CYP 2D6, CYP 3A4 (minor)	Divalproex	Carbamazepine	
Quetiapine	CYP 3A4	Fluvoxamine, cimetidine; other CYP3A4 inhibitors	Carbamazepine, St. John's wort	
Risperidone	CYP 2D6	Fluoxetine, paroxetine; other CYP 2D6 inhibitors	Carbamazepine	
Ziprasidone (Food increases absorption)	CYP 3A4 (one-third); aldehyde oxidase		Carbamazepine	Avoid use with other drugs that prolong QTc intervals.

* = major pathway.

Table 21-48 Medications for Schizophrenia: Adverse Drug Reactions

	Medication	Anticholinergic	EPS	Sedation	Weight Gain	Orthostatic Hypotension	Increased Prolactin
FGA	High potency (haloperidol)	+	++++	+	+	+	+++
	Low potency (chlorpromazine)	+++	+++	++++	++	++++	+++
SGA	Asenapine	+/–	+	+	+	+	+/–
	Aripiprazole	+/–	+	+	+/–	+/–	+/–
	Clozapine	++++	+/–	++++	++++	++++	+/–
	Iloperidone	+/–	+	+	++	+++	+
	Lurasidone	0	+	+/–	+/–	+	
	Olanzapine	++	++	++	+++	++	+/–
	Paliperidone	+	++	+	+/–	++	++++
	Quetiapine	+	+/–	+++	+++	++	+/–
	Risperidone	+	++	+	++	++	++++
	Ziprasidone	+/–	++	+	+/–	+	+

FGA = first-generation antipsychotic, SGA = second-generation antipsychotic, +/– = insignificant, + = low, ++ = moderate, +++ = moderately high, ++++ = high.

Table 21-49 Movement Disorders Caused by Schizophrenia Pharmacotherapies

Type	Definition	Treatment
Acute dystonic reactions	• State of involuntary, abnormal tonic contraction of the skeletal muscle • Rapid onset (24–96 hours after initiation of therapy) • Risk factors: males, younger age (< 35 years old), high-potency typical antipsychotics, higher dosage	• Benztropine 1–2 mg • Diphenhydramine 25–50 mg
Pseudo-Parkinsonism	• Resembles Parkinson's disease (akinesia, bradykinesia, mask-like facial expression, slow speech, tremor, cogwheel rigidity, postural abnormalities, shuffling gait) • Appears within the first month of therapy • Risk factors: females, older age, high-potency typical antipsychotics, higher dosage	• Decrease antipsychotic dose • Benztropine 0.5–2 mg bid • Diphenhydramine 25–300 mg in divided doses • Trihexyphenidyl 5–15 mg day
Akathisia	• Inability to sit still, inner restlessness, or compulsion to move or remain in motion • Usually appears within 2–3 weeks after initiation of antipsychotic • Risk factors: females have two times greater risk than males	• Decrease antipsychotic dose • Propranolol 30–120 mg given in divided doses • Benzodiazepines
Tardive dyskinesia	• Stereotypical involuntary movements of the mouth, lips, and tongue, and choreiform movements of the extremities • Late onset, after months or years of treatment • Risk: increasing age, female gender, affective disorders, organic brain disorders, diabetes, typical antipsychotics, duration of therapy, increased dosage	• Discontinuation of treatment • Switch to clozapine

ANNOTATED BIBLIOGRAPHY

American Psychiatric Association. *Diagnostic and Statistical Manual of Mental Disorders,* 4th ed. Text Revision. Washington, DC: American Psychiatric Association; 2000.

American Psychiatric Association. Practice guidelines for the treatment of patients with schizophrenia, 2nd ed. *Am J Psychiatry* April 2004(suppl): 1–114.

Consensus Development Conference on Antipsychotic Drugs and Obesity and Diabetes. *Diabetes Care* 2004;27:596–601.

Crismon ML, Argo TR, Buckley PF. Schizophrenia. In Dipiro JT, Talbert RL, Yee GC, et al., eds. *Pharmacotherapy: A Pathophysiologic Approach,* 7th ed. New York, NY: McGraw-Hill Medical, 2008:1099–1122.

Davis JM, Chen N, Glick ID. A meta-analysis of the efficacy of second-generation antipsychotics. *Arch Gen Psychiatry* 2003;60:553–564.

Endow-Eyer RA, Mitchell MM, Lacro JP. Schizophrenia. In: Koda-Kimble MA, Young LY, Alldredge BK, et al., eds. *Applied Therapeutics: The Clinical Use of Drugs*, 9th ed. Baltimore, MD: Lippincott Williams & Wilkins; 2009:81.1–81.19.

Fuller MA, Sajatovic M. *Drug information for Mental Health,* 6th ed. Hudson, OH: Lexi-Comp: 2007.

Hanston PD, Horn JR. *The Top 100 Drug Interactions: A Guide to Patient Management.* Freeland, WA: H & H Publishing; 2009.

Leucht S, Corves C, Arbter D, et al. Second generation vs first generation antipsychotic drugs for schizophrenia: a meta-analysis. *Lancet* 2009;373: 31–41.

Perry PJ, Alexander B, Liskow B, DaVane CL. *Psychotropic Drug Handbook*, 8th ed. Baltimore, MD: Lippincott Williams & Wilkins; 2007.

Stahl SM. *Stahl's Essential Psychopharmacology*, 3rd ed. New York, NY: Cambridge University Press; 2008.

Pulmonary

CHAPTER

22

TOPIC: ASTHMA

Section Coordinator: Larry Dent
Contributor: Kendra Procacci

Tips Worth Tweeting

- Asthma is a chronic inflammatory disease of the airway.
- Inhaled corticosteroids are a mainstay of asthma treatment.
- Peak-flow meters help a patient with asthma monitor lung function.
- Patients need to be taught proper inhaler technique to optimize lung delivery of medications.
- Patients must be taught to identify and avoid environmental "triggers."

Patient Care Scenario: Ambulatory Setting

Date	Physician	Drug	Quantity	Sig	Refills
1/04	Jones	Ventolin HFA	#1	2–4 puffs prn SOB	12
1/22	Smith	Asmanex 440 mcg	#1	1 puff q day	12
1/22	Smith	Loratidine 10 mg	#30	1 po daily	12
2/16	Jones	Prilosec 20 mg	#30	1 po daily	06

1.1.0 Patient Information

Medication-Induced Causes of Asthma

Aspirin and nonsteroidal anti-inflammatory drugs can precipitate asthma in as many as 20% of patients.

Laboratory Testing

Spirometry is an objective measurement that helps determine degree of obstruction, disease severity, and reversibility of airway obstruction.

Disease States

Mast cells, eosinophils, and leukocytes are known to perpetuate the chronic inflammatory cycle associated with asthma.

Allergic rhinitis, gastroesophageal reflux disease, sinusitis, obesity, and chronic stress and depression are considered comorbidities of asthma. Treating comorbid conditions may improve asthma management.

Instruments Related to Patient Assessment

Pulmonary lung function testing with spirometry is the gold standard for asthma assessment. Peak-flow meters are hand-held devices that make lung function monitoring more practical and convenient in the outpatient setting. It is important for patients to be taught proper peak-flow monitoring techniques.

A single peak-flow reading is not a helpful value. Instead, patients should monitor such readings in the morning and again at night. The patient should sit or stand comfortably, make sure the pointer is set to 0, take a deep breath in, close the lips tightly around the mouthpiece, and blow out as hard as possible. Three consecutive readings should be taken and the best number should be recorded. The best number that is recorded over a 2-week period when a patient is feeling well is considered the personal best. Based on the patient's personal best reading, an asthma action plan can be devised to help the patient determine how and when to use asthma medications and when to seek help. Asthma action plans include medications and dosing instructions, actions to take to control environmental triggers, and to recognize and handle worsening asthma—which signs, symptoms, and peak-flow values indicate worsening symptoms; which medications to take in response; when to seek urgent care; and which emergency telephone numbers to use.

Key Terms

An **asthma action plan** is based on a zone system:

- **Green zone:** 80–100% of personal best; signals good control; patient is to take maintenance medications and possibly albuterol before exercise
- **Yellow zone:** 50–80% of personal best; signals caution; patient may be experiencing symptoms; patient is to take 2–4 puffs of rescue medication every 20 minutes for up to 1 hour or until back in the green zone
- **Red zone:** less than 50% of personal best; medical alert; patient is to use 4 puffs of albuterol and call the doctor or emergency room immediately

Signs and Symptoms

Hallmark symptoms of asthma are cough, shortness of breath (SOB), and wheezing or chest tightness. Physical exam often reveals an increased respiratory rate, reduced breath sounds, and wheeze upon expiration.

Wellness and Prevention

Activation of this chronic inflammation can be augmented upon exposure to certain inhaled triggers. Dust mites, pet dander, pollen, and mold spores are a few examples of allergen triggers.

1.2.0 Pharmacotherapy

Medications available to treat asthma come in inhaled, oral, and parenteral dosage forms. Inhaled products are most commonly used and can be delivered via metered-dose inhaler (MDI), dry-powder inhaler (DPI), or nebulizer. Inhaling medications allows for the lowest concentration of drug to be delivered directly to the site of action, thereby maximizing the benefits associated with their use while limiting systemic adverse effects. Oral agents are rarely used. Parenteral forms of medications are typically restricted to emergency room use or used during periods of hospitalization.

The proper use of inhaled devices is essential for optimal delivery of medications to the lungs and to help minimize a drug's systemic adverse effects. Pharmacists are in a unique position to train and assess patient inhaler technique. Spacers are devices that attach around the mouthpiece of metered-dose inhalers and aid in drug delivery and decrease local adverse effects. They should be used by patients who have difficulty with proper inhaler technique and by all patients using an inhaled corticosteroid. Spacers decrease the local pharyngeal adverse effects from inhaled corticosteroids, such as oral candidiasis and dysphonia.

Mechanism of Action

Medications used to treat asthma are broadly categorized into two classes: bronchodilators and anti-inflammatory agents.

Bronchodilators used for the treatment of asthma fit into one of two categories: beta$_2$ agonists or theophylline. Inhaled beta$_2$ agonists are further subdivided based on their duration of action. Beta$_2$ agonists reverse bronchospasm by causing relaxation of the smooth muscle fibers surrounding the bronchi and bronchioles of the respiratory tract. Short-acting beta$_2$ agonists have a quick onset of action, within 5–10 minutes, and a duration of action of 4–8 hours. These medications are often referred to as rescue or reliever medications. All patients with asthma should have immediate access to a short-acting beta$_2$ agonist for acute asthma exacerbations. Short-acting beta$_2$ agonists are also used to prevent exercise-induced bronchospasm when taken 15–30 minutes before exercise.

Long-acting inhaled beta$_2$ agonists have a longer duration of action, 12 hours. These medications are used to prevent symptoms and are dosed twice daily. Salmeterol has an onset of 20–30 minutes and formoterol has an onset of 5–10 minutes. Despite the quick onset of action of formoterol, patients should be counseled to never use this drug as a rescue medication or take it more than twice daily.

Theophylline is available in oral and parenteral dosage forms. This nonselective phosphodiesterase inhibitor has bronchodilator and mild anti-inflammatory properties. Its onset of action is within minutes for the parenteral form and is 15–30 minutes for the oral form. The duration of action can be up to 24 hours. Although theophylline does provide good bronchodilation, its use has fallen out of favor due to the narrow therapeutic range of blood levels. When the concentration of theophylline is not kept within this range, adverse effects can be significant and life-threatening, including cardiac flutter, tachycardia, headache, nausea, and tremor.

Bronchodilators do not work on the inflammatory component of asthma. With the exception of patients categorized as having mild intermittent asthma, all patients with asthma should have an anti-inflammatory agent prescribed. Anti-inflammatory agents are often referred to as maintenance or controller medications because they are taken daily to prevent and control symptoms. Anti-inflammatory medications for the treatment of asthma include mast cell stabilizers, leukotriene-receptor modifiers, and corticosteroids.

Mast cell stabilizers inhibit mast cell release by the inflammatory mediators histamine and leukotrienes, and stabilize mast cell membranes. These agents, which are available as inhaled products, are considered alternatives to first-line agents. However, because of their excellent safety profile, some providers prefer to prescribe these medications for pediatric patients.

Leukotriene-receptor modifiers either prevent the production of leukotrienes by inhibiting 5-lipoxygenase or bind to leukotriene receptors, thereby preventing cellular release of pro-inflammatory chemicals.

Corticosteroids block late-phase reaction to allergens, reduce airway hyperresponsiveness, and inhibit cell migration and inflammatory cell activation. Notably, they suppress generation of cytokines, recruitment of eosinophils, and release of inflammatory mediators. Corticosteroids are available as a variety of products and in numerous dosage forms. Inhaled corticosteroids are the preferred anti-inflammatory agent for the majority of asthmatics because they are the most potent and consistently effective long-term control medication for the treatment of asthma.

Omalizumab binds free IgE and IgE mast cells, which leads to decreased release of mediators in response to allergen exposure. Omalizumab is indicated for the treatment of moderate-to-severe persistent allergic asthma that is not adequately controlled with inhaled corticosteroids

Interaction of Drugs with Foods and Laboratory Tests

- Albuterol may increase the levels or effects of sympathomimetics. Albuterol's effects may be increased with atomoxetine, cannabinoids, monoamine oxidase (MAO) inhibitors, and tricyclic antidepressants; conversely, its levels may be decreased by alpha and beta blockers.
- Zafirlukast significantly increases the half-life of warfarin.
- Zileton, a P450 enzyme inhibitor, inhibits the metabolism of warfarin and theophylline.
- Omalizumab may increase the levels and effects of leflunomide and natalizumab, and may increase or decrease the levels and effects of live vaccines. Omalizumab levels may be increased by trastuzumab and decreased by echinacea.

Contraindications, Warnings, and Precautions

- Leukotriene modifiers: New FDA labeling includes neuropsychiatric events.
- Administration of omalizumab is contraindicated during acute bronchospasm and status asthmaticus. Boxed warning: anaphylaxis; administration should be under direct medical supervision with observation for 2 hours following administration.

1.3.0 Monitoring

Proper inhaler technique with MDIs and DPIs:

- MDI: remove the cap, check for foreign objects, shake 6–10 times, tilt head back and breathe out slowly, place inhaler in mouth, press down on inhaler as a slow breath is taken in, breathe in completely and slowly for 2–5 seconds, hold breath for 10 seconds
- Prime MDIs before first use and if not used for 14 days
- Maxair autohaler: breath-activated device

Adverse Reactions

- Local adverse effects of inhaled corticosteroids: oral candidiasis, dysphonia, reflex cough and bronchospasm, upper respiratory tract infection.
- Systemic adverse effects of inhaled corticosteroids: low–medium dose may have potential to decrease growth velocity in children although the effects are small and may be reversible; small dose-dependent decrease in bone mineral density may be associated with use in patients older than age 18 years; high cumulative doses may increase risk of cataracts.
- Local adverse effects of beta$_2$ agonists: headache, dizziness, vertigo, palpitations, tremor, nausea/vomiting. Hypokalemia and prolonged QTC interval may occur with overuse.
- Oral steroids: short-term: abnormalities in glucose, increased appetite, fluid retention, weight gain, mood alterations, hypertension, peptic ulcer. Long-term: adrenal axis suppression, dermal thinning, diabetes, Cushing's syndrome, muscle weakness, osteoporosis, glaucoma.
- Cromolyn: minimal adverse effects; bad taste is most common.
- Theophylline: dose related; nausea, vomiting, tremor, jitteriness, seizures, arrhythmias.
- Omalizumab: headache, local injection site reaction, upper respiratory tract infection, sinusitis, pharyngitis.

Nonadherence, Misuse, or Abuse

- Environmental trigger control measures
- Asthma action plan
- Control of comorbidities
- Patients with asthma should receive an annual influenza vaccine

Pharmacotherapeutic Outcomes

- How often the patient is using a rescue inhaler
- Number of unscheduled office visits, ER visits, or urgent care clinic visits
- Peak-flow readings
- Pulmonary function tests with spirometry
- Medication compliance and perceptions
- Night or early-morning awakenings

Safety and Efficacy Monitoring

- Inhaled corticosteroids: delay of onset, importance of taking corticosteroids daily, use of a spacer with the MDI, rinse and spit after each use to decrease oral thrush and dysphonia, when to change canister, accurate counseling and education to help with fear of steroids.
- Reporting signs and symptoms of anaphylaxis with omalizumab

Quick relief medications for all patients:

- Short-acting inhaled beta$_2$ agonist as needed for symptoms: up to 3 treatments at 20-minute intervals prn. A short course of oral systemic corticosteroids may be needed.
- Use of short-acting beta$_2$ agonist more than 2 days per week for symptom relief (not prevention of exercise-induced bronchospasm) indicates inadequate control and the need to step up treatment.

Step Down:	Step Up:
Review treatment every 1–6 months; a gradual stepwise reduction in treatment may be feasible.	If control is not maintained, consider step up after reviewing patient medication technique, adherence, and environmental control (i.e., avoidance of triggers).

These recommendations are general guidelines and are not intended to be "specific" prescriptions. Asthma is highly variable, so clinicians should tailor regimens to the patient's specific needs and circumstances.

Gain control as quickly as possible.

A rescue course of steroid may be needed at any time or at any step.

Some patients with intermittent asthma can experience life-threatening exacerbations even after long periods of normal lung functions and no symptoms.

Table 22-1 Classification of Asthma Severity in Patients 12 Years of Age and Older

Step to Initiate Therapy (Classification)	Symptoms	Nighttime Symptoms	Short-Acting Beta$_2$ Agonist Use for Symptom Control (Not for Prevention of Exercise-Induced Bronchospasm)	Lung Function	Exacerbations Requiring Oral Systemic Corticosteroids
Step 5 or 6 (severe persistent)	• Throughout the day • Normal activity extremely limited	Often 7 times per week	Several times per day	• FEV$_1$ less than 60% of predicted • FEV$_1$/FVC reduced more than 5%	≥ 2 per year
Step 3 or 4 (moderate persistent)	• Daily • Some limitation of normal activity	More than 1 time per week, but not nightly	Daily	• FEV$_1$ more than 60% but less than 80% of predicted • FEV$_1$/FVC reduced 5%	≥ 2 per year
Step 2 (mild persistent)	• More than 2 times per week, but less than 1 time per day • Minor limitation of normal activity	3–4 times per month	More than 2 days per week but not daily, and not more than once per day	• FEV$_1$ more than 80% of predicted • FEV$_1$/FVC normal	≥ 2 per year
Step 1 (intermittent)	• 2 or fewer times per week • No limitations in normal activity	2 or fewer times per month	2 or fewer times per week	• Normal FEV$_1$ between exacerbations • FEV$_1$ more than 80% of predicted • FEV$_1$/FVC normal	0–1 per year

Adapted from: NIH guidelines.

Table 22-2 Stepwise Approach for Managing Asthma in Adults and Children Older than 12 Years of Age: Treatment

Step 6 (severe persistent)	*Preferred Daily Medications* Inhaled high-dose corticosteroid + long-acting beta$_2$- agonist + oral corticosteroids **and** Consider omalizumab for patients with allergies
Step 5 (severe persistent)	*Preferred Daily Medications* Inhaled high-dose corticosteroid + long-acting inhaled beta$_2$-agonist **and** Consider omalizumab for patients with allergies
Step 4 (moderate persistent)	*Preferred Daily Medications* Inhaled medium-dose corticosteroid + long-acting inhaled beta$_2$-agonist *Alternative* Inhaled medium-dose corticosteroid + either leukotriene-receptor antagonist, theophylline, or zileuton
Step 3 (moderate persistent)	*Preferred Daily Medications* Inhaled low-dose corticosteroid + long-acting inhaled beta$_2$-agonist **or** Inhaled medium-dose corticosteroid *Alternative* Inhaled low-dose corticosteroid + either leukotriene-receptor antagonist, theophylline, or zileuton
Step 2 (mild persistent)	*Preferred Daily Medications* Inhaled low-dose corticosteroid *Alternative* Cromolyn, nedocromil, leukotriene-receptor antagonist, or theophylline (to serum concentration of 5–15 mcg/mL)
Step 1 (intermittent)	*Preferred Daily Medications* No daily medication needed

Adapted from: NIH guidelines.

This outcome may be more common when attacks are provoked by respiratory infections.

Assessment and education about environment/ allergen control should be considered for each step.

Visit http://www.nhlbi.nih.gov/guidelines/asthma/asthsumm.htm for more information.

2.2.0 Dispensing

Packaging, Storage, Handling, and Disposal

- Store HFA products at room temperature.
- Store albuterol nebulizers at room temperature.
- An albuterol nebulizer is compatible with cromolyn sodium, budesonide inhalation suspension, and ipratropium solution for nebulization.
- Store mast cell stabilizers at room temperature.
- Store dry-powder inhalers at room temperature away from humid areas. Never put a DPI in water. Wipe the mouthpiece with tissue to clean it. Never shake the DPI after the dose is loaded; never breathe into the device after the dose is loaded.
- Store omalizumab under refrigeration prior to reconstitution. Following reconstitution, it may be stored at room temperature. The reconstituted product may be stored for 8 hours under refrigeration or 4 hours at room temperature.
- Prepare omalizumab using sterile water for injection; add 1.4 mL of sterile water for injection and swirl gently for 5–10 seconds until dissolved. It may take up to 20 minutes to dissolve; the product should not be used if it takes greater than 40 minutes to dissolve.

Medication Administration Equipment

- Proper use of peak-flow monitors
- Difference between maintenance and rescue medications

Table 22-3 Asthma/COPD Medications: Typical Adult and Pediatric Dosages

Medication	Dosage Form	Adult Dose (12 years or older)	Child Dose (4–11 years)
Systemic Corticosteroids			
Methylprednisolone (Solu-Medrol) Prednisolone Prednisone		7.5–60 mg daily in a single dose in AM or qod as needed for control Short-course "burst" therapy to achieve control: 40–60 mg/day as a single dose for 3–10 days	0.25–2 mg/kg daily in a single dose in AM or qod as needed for control Short-course "burst" therapy: 1–2 mg/kg/day, maximum of 60 mg/day for 3–10 days
Inhaled Corticosteroids (Preferred medication for long-term control in asthma; indicated in stage III COPD)			
Beclomethasone (QVAR)	HFA MDI: 40 or 80 mcg/puff	160–640 mcg divided bid	40–80 mcg divided bid (5–11 years old)
Budesonide (Pulmicort)	DPI, Flexhaler: 90 or 180 mcg/puff mcg/dose Nebulizer: 0.25 mg/2 mL, 0.5 mg/2 mL	360–1,440 mcg divided bid 0.5–1 mg divided bid	360–720 mcg divided bid (6–11 years old)
Flunisolide (Aerobid)	HFA MDI: 80 mcg/puff	320–640 mcg divided bid	160 mcg divided bid (6-11 years old)
Fluticasone (Flovent)	HFA MDI: 44, 110, or 220 mcg/puff DPI: 50 mcg/dose	176–1,760 mcg divided bid 100–2,000 mcg divided bid	176 mcg divided bid (4–11 years old)
Mometasone (Asmanex)	DPI twisthaler: 110 or 220 mcg/puff	220–440 mcg once daily	110 mcg once daily (4–11 years old)
Long-Acting Inhaled Beta$_2$ Agonists (Should not be used for acute exacerbations; use with inhaled corticosteroids in patients with asthma)			
Salmeterol (Serevent)	DPI: 50 mcg/blister	1 blister q 12 hr	1 blister q 12 hr
Formeterol (Foradil)	DPI: 12 mcg/single-use capsule	1 capsule q 12 hr	1 capsule q 12 hr
Combination product: fluticasone/salmeterol (Advair)	DPI: 100 mcg/50 mcg, 250/50, or 500/50 HFA: 45/21, 115/21, or 230/21	1 inhalation bid	1 inhalation bid of 100/50mcg
Mast Cell Stabilizers (Believed by many to be the drugs of choice for children with mild asthma)			
Cromolyn (Intal)	MDI: 0.8 mg/puff Nebulizer: 20 mg/ampule	2–4 puffs tid–qid 1 ampule tid–qid	1–2 puffs tid–qid 1 ampule tid–qid
Nedrocromil (Tilade)	MDI: 1.7 5mg/puff	2–4 puffs bid–qid	1–2 puffs bid–qid
Leukotriene Inhibitors			
Montelukast (Singulair)	4 or 5 mg chew tabs 10 mg tablet	10 mg q hs	4 mg q hs (2–5 years old) 5 mg q hs (6–14 years old) 10 mg q hs (older than 14 years)
Zafirlukast (Accolate)	10 or 20 mg tabs	20 mg bid	5–11 years old: 10 mg bid
Zileuton (Zyflo)	600 mg extended-release tabs	1200 mg bid (2400 mg/day)	No indication
Methylxanthines (Serum monitoring required: 5–20 mcg/mL at Css)			
Theophylline (Theo-Dur, Slo-phyllin)	Oral solution, tablets, and capsules (immediate and extended release)	300–900 mg divided bid–tid	Weight < 45 kg: 12–20 mg/kg divided q 4–6 hr Weight > 45 kg: 300–600 mg divided tid–qid

Table 22-3 (*continued*)

Short-Acting Beta$_2$ Agonists: Quick-Relief Medications			
Albuterol HFA (Proventil, Ventolin, ProAir)	MDI: 108 mcg (equivalent to 90 mcg albuterol base) Nebulizer	2 puffs q 4–6 hr prn 2.5 mg q 4–8 hr	1–2 puffs q 4–6 hr prn Children older than 4 years can use adult doses: 1.25–2.5 mg q 4–6 hr
Levalbuterol (Xopenex)	MDI: 45 mcg/puff Nebulizer: 0.31 mg/3 mL, 0.63 mg/3 mL, 1.25 mg/mL	2–4 puffs q 4–6 hr prn 1.25–2.5 mg q 4–6 hr prn	1–2 puffs q 4–6 hr prn Children older than 4 years: 0.31–1.25 mg q 4–6 hr prn
Pirbuterol MDI (Maxair)	200 mcg/puff	2 puffs q 4–6 hr	No indication
Anticholinergics (Indicated in COPD only)			
Tiotropium (Spiriva)	DPI: 18 mcg/puff	1 puff q 24 hr	No indication
Ipratropium (Atrovent)	MDI: 17 mcg/puff Nebulizer: 500 mcg/2.5 mL	2 puffs qid (maximum 12 puffs/day) Nebulizer: 500 mcg tid to qid	1–2 puffs tid (maximum 6 puffs/24 hr) Nebulizer: 125–250 mcg tid
Combination product: ipratropium/albuterol	MDI: 0.018 mg/0.103 mg/puff Nebulizer: 0.5 mg/2.5 mg/3 mL	2 puffs qid 3 mL q 6 hr	No indication
Monoclonal Antibody			
Omalizumab (Xolair)	Powder for reconstitution; 150 mg	SubQ: based on pretreatment IgE levels and body weight 150–375 mg every 2–4 weeks Doses > 150 mg should be divided over more than one site	No indication

Adapted from: NIH guidelines

ANNOTATED BIBLIOGRAPHY

Centers for Disease Control and Prevention. Fast stats: asthma. Available at: http://www.cdc.gov/nchs/FASTATS/asthma.htm. Statistical information on public health concerns and issues.

Facts & Comparisons eAnswers. Wolters Kluwer Health, Inc.; 2010. Available at: http://online.factsandcomparisons.com/index.aspx. Accessed February 22, 2010.

Lacy CF, Armstrong LL, Goldman MR, Lance LL, eds. *Lexi-Comp's Drug Information Handbook*. 17th ed. Hudson, OH: Lexi-Comp; 2008.

McEvoy GK, ed. *AHFS Drug Information 2010*. Bethesda, MD: American Society of Health-System Pharmacists; 2010.

Micromedex Healthcare Series [Internet database]. Greenwood Village, CO: Thomson Reuters (Healthcare) Inc. Updated periodically.

National Heart, Lung, and Blood Institute. National Asthma Education and Prevention Program: Expert Panel Report 3. Guidelines for the diagnosis and management of asthma. 2007. Available at: www.nhlbi.nih.gov/guidelines/asthma/asthgdln.pdf. Evidence-based guidelines for asthma.

TOPIC: CHRONIC OBSTRUCTIVE PULMONARY DISEASE

Section Coordinator: *Larry Dent*
Contributor: *Sherril Brown*

Tips Worth Tweeting

- Chronic obstructive pulmonary disease (COPD) is a preventable and treatable disease with extrapulmonary effects.
- The most common cause of COPD is cigarette smoking.
- COPD is treated in a stepwise fashion depending on the severity of the disease.
- Bronchodilators improve FEV_1 and control symptoms.
- Inhaled corticosteroids decrease the rate of decline and decrease the frequency of exacerbations.

Patient Care Scenario: Ambulatory Setting

- L. G.: 66 y/o F, 5'2", 192 lbs, no medication allergies, no alcohol use, employed as elementary school teacher
- History of smoking ½–1 pack of cigarettes daily for 47 years, quit 6 years ago

- Medical conditions: COPD, hypertension
- BUN 9 mg/dL, Cr 0.7 mg/dL, BP 165/101
- FEV_1 = 40% predicted

Date	Physician	Drug	Quantity	Sig	Refills
5/2	Johnson	Ipratropium/albuterol 0.5/3 mg	120 vials	use one vial in nebulizer 4 times daily	6
5/2	Johnson	Budesonide 180 mcg	120 respules	use one vial in nebulizer 4 times daily	6
3/12	Johnson	Albuterol HFA	2 inhalers	2 puffs every 4–6 hr prn	6
12/30	Johnson	Atenolol/chlorthalidone 100/25 mg	30 tablets	one daily	10

1.1.0 Patient Information

Medication-Induced Causes of COPD

Bronchospasm may be caused by beta blockers and aspirin. Angiotensin-converting enzyme (ACE) inhibitors may cause cough, which is a symptom of COPD and bronchospasm. In addition, anaphylaxis to any medication may include bronchospasm as a symptom.

Laboratory Testing

Spirometry is used to diagnose and monitor COPD. Other lab tests that may be used to assess patients with COPD are arterial blood gases, chest radiography, pulmonary blood pressure, and right ventricular cardiac function. $Alpha_1$ antitrypsin deficiency screening may be done in Caucasian patients younger than age 45 years with COPD and a strong family history.

Disease States

- Chronic bronchitis
- Emphysema
- Asthma

Instruments/Techniques Related to Patient Assessment

Spirometry is used to diagnose and monitor COPD.

Key Terms

Guidelines for diagnosis, management, and prevention of COPD are available from the American Thoracic Society/European Respiratory Society and the Global Initiative for Chronic Obstructive Lung Disease (GOLD).

Signs and Symptoms

- Persistent dyspnea that worsens with exercise
- Chronic unproductive cough
- Chronic sputum production

Wellness and Prevention

Risk factors for COPD include smoking, occupational exposure and environmental pollution, recurrent bronchopulmonary infections, previous tuberculosis, poor lung growth and development, and socioeconomic status. Tobacco smoke and inhalation of other particles cause inflammation in the respiratory tract. The inflammatory response is exaggerated, leading to narrowing of the airways. Infections are also associated with inflammation of the respiratory tract. Lower socioeconomic status may increase the risk of developing COPD due to factors such as poor nutrition and increased exposure to smoking and pollution. Any factor that affects lung growth and development may increase the risk of COPD.

1.2.0 Pharmacotherapy

For drug indications, dosing regimens, and routes of administration, see Table 22-3.

Mechanisms of Action

- Beta agonists, anticholinergics, and methylxanthines: bronchodilators
- Corticosteroids: anti-inflammatory agents

Interaction of Drugs with Foods and Laboratory Tests

Caffeine should be avoided with beta agonists and methylxanthines. Most theophylline and aminophylline formulations may be taken with or without food; however, once-daily sustained-release products should not be taken with food. Avoid charcoal-broiled foods with methylxanthines. Terbutaline may be taken with or without food. Triamcinolone may decrease the uptake of radioactive iodine. Corticosteroids may suppress skin test reactions.

Specific interactions include the following:

- Levalbuterol/albuterol: beta blockers, digoxin, monoamine oxidase inhibitors, tricyclic antidepressants, non-potassium-sparing diuretics, ephedra, yohimbe, St. John's wort
- Terbutaline: beta blockers, monoamine oxidase inhibitors, tricyclic antidepressants, non-potassium-sparing diuretics, ephedra, yohimbe
- Formoterol: beta blockers, digoxin, monoamine oxidase inhibitors, tricyclic antidepressants,

atomoxetine, cannabinoids, non-potassium-sparing diuretics, methylxanthines
- Salmeterol: beta blockers, digoxin, monoamine oxidase inhibitors, tricyclic antidepressants, non-potassium-sparing diuretics, atomoxetine
- Inhaled anticholinergics: other anticholinergic medications
- Methylxanthines: propranolol, allopurinol, erythromycin, cimetidine, quinolone antibiotics, oral contraceptives, beta blockers, calcium-channel blockers, corticosteroids, influenza virus vaccine, macrolide antibiotics, thyroid hormones, carbamazepine, isoniazid, loop diuretics, phenytoin, phenobarbital, rifampin, ritonavir, barbiturates, ketoconazole, propofol
- Inhaled corticosteroids: amphotericin B, potassium-wasting diuretics, fluoroquinolones, antidiabetic medications
- Systemic corticosteroids: aprepitant, azole antifungals, calcium-channel blockers, cyclosporine, estrogens, macrolide antibiotics, amphotericin B, potassium-wasting diuretics, antidiabetic medications, isoniazid, warfarin, bile acid sequestrants, antacids, rifampin, toxoids and vaccines, aspirin and nonsteroidal anti-inflammatory drugs, St. John's wort, cat's claw, echinacea

Contraindications, Warnings, and Precautions

Beta agonists should be used with caution in patients with cardiac arrhythmias, narrow-angle glaucoma, cardiovascular disease, hyperthyroidism, or diabetes. Long-acting beta$_2$ agonists (formoterol and salmeterol) may increase the risk of asthma-related deaths and should be used only in patients on an anti-inflammatory agent, such as a corticosteroid. Long-acting beta$_2$ agonists should not be used in rapidly deteriorating COPD or in acute symptomatic COPD. Corticosteroids should be used with caution in patients at risk for osteoporosis and in patients with tuberculosis, untreated systemic infections, diabetes, glaucoma, renal or hepatic impairment, or thyroid disease. Local fungal infections may occur in patients on inhaled corticosteroids. There is a risk of GI perforation with the use of oral corticosteroids in patients with GI diseases. Hypothalamic–pituitary–adrenal axis suppression may occur with the use of inhaled or oral corticosteroids. Methylxanthines should be used with caution in patients with cardiac arrhythmias, cardiac disease, hepatic disease, hypertension, congestive heart failure, and alcoholism. Anticholinergic medications should be used with caution in patients with narrow-angle glaucoma, prostatic hyperplasia, or bladder neck obstruction.

Physiochemical Properties, Pharmacodynamics, and Pharmacokinetic Properties

See Table 22-4 – 22-6.

1.3.0 Monitoring

Pharmacotherapeutic Outcomes

- Prevent and control symptoms
- Reduce frequency and severity of COPD exacerbations

Table 22-4 Bronchodilator Bioavailability, Duration of Action, Onset of Action, and Time to Peak Effect

Drug	Bioavailability	Duration of Action	Onset of Action	Time to Peak Effect
Beta$_2$ Agonists: Short-Acting				
Albuterol (inhaled)	< 20%	3–4 hr	< 5 min	60–90 min
Albuterol (oral)	50–85%	4–6 hr, up to 12 hr for ER tablets	30 min	2–3 hr
Levalbuterol	30%	6–8 hr	10–20 min	1.5 hr
Pirbuterol	Unknown	3–4 hr	5 min	30 min
Terbutaline	10–50%	4–6 hr	60–120 min	120–180 min
Beta$_2$ Agonists: Long-Acting				
Formoterol	Plasma levels are undetectable	12 hr	3–5 min	1–3 hr
Salmeterol	Plasma levels are undetectable	12 hr	5–14 min	180 min
Anticholinergics				
Ipratropium	7%	6–8 hr	15 min	1–2 hr
Tiotropium	19.5%	24 hr	60 min	1.5–3 hr
Methylxanthines				
Aminophylline	100%	Variable, up to 24 hr	15–30 min	Up to 24 hr
Theophylline	88–100%	Variable, up to 24 hr	15–30 min	Up to 24 hr

Table 22-5 Corticosteroid Bioavailability, Duration of Action, and Time to Response

Drug	Bioavailability	Duration of Action	Time to Response
Inhaled			
Beclomethasone	NA	—	1–4 weeks
Budesonide	6–13%	12–24 hr	24 hr (inhalation) 2–8 days (nebulizer)
Flunisolide	39–40%	—	Few days
Fluticasone	13.5–30%	Several days	Variable; at least 1 week
Mometasone	< 1%	—	1–2 weeks
Systemic			
Prednisolone	92%	18–36 hr	1–2 hr
Prednisone	92%	18–36 hr	1–2 hr
Methylprednisolone	92%	30–36 hr	1–2 hr

Table 22-6 Other Drugs Used in Asthma and COPD: Bioavailability, Duration of Action, Onset of Action, and Time to Peak Effect

Drug	Bioavailability	Duration of Action	Onset of Action	Time to Peak Effect
Leukotriene-Receptor Antagonists				
Montelukast	60–78%	Up to 24 hr	3–4 hr	—
Zafirlukast	Unknown	12 hr	30 min	3.5 hr
Leukotriene-Formation Inhibitors				
Zileuton	Unknown	5–8 hr	30 min	1–5 hr
Monoclonal Antibody				
Omalizumab	62%	2–4 weeks	1 hr	1–2 hr
Mast Cell Stabilizers				
Cromolyn sodium	8%	< 2 hr	4 weeks	—
Nedocromil	2–9%	< 2 hr	1 week	—
Mucolytics				
N-acetylcysteine	6–10%	100 min	1 min	5–10 min

- Improve health status
- Improve exercise tolerance

Safety and Efficacy Monitoring

- Beta$_2$ agonists: serum potassium, spirometry, heart rate, blood pressure, arterial blood gases
- Anticholinergics: spirometry
- Methylxanthines: vital signs, serum concentration of drug, heart rate, respiratory rate, arterial blood gases, spirometry
- Corticosteroids: spirometry, signs and symptoms of adrenal suppression, blood glucose, bone mineral density (oral corticosteroids)

Adverse Drug Reactions

- Beta$_2$ agonists: sinus tachycardia, exaggerated somatic tremor in elderly patients at high doses, hypokalemia
- Anticholinergics: dry mouth, metallic taste, acute glaucoma with nebulized solutions administered with a face mask
- Methylxanthines: atrial and ventricular arrhythmias and grand mal convulsions at toxic levels; headache, insomnia, nausea, and heartburn at therapeutic levels
- Inhaled corticosteroids: oral candidiasis, dysphonia, reflex cough, bronchospasm, pneumonia, decreased bone mineral density, risk of cataracts
- Oral corticosteroids: glucose abnormalities, increased appetite, fluid retention, weight gain, mood alterations, hypertension, and peptic ulcer with short-term use; hypothalamic–pituitary–adrenal axis suppression, dermal thinning, diabetes, Cushing's syndrome, muscle weakness, osteoporosis, and glaucoma with long-term use

Nonadherence, Misuse, or Abuse

Patients are often adherent with treatment because COPD symptoms are constant. Patient education on the purpose and outcome of treatment will help improve adherence with medications as well as lifestyle modifications and proper use of medical devices.

Pharmacotherapeutic Alternatives

Step therapy is recommended based on the stage of COPD (Table 22-7).

2.2.0 Dispensing

For generic names of COPD medications, trade names, and dosage form availability, see Table 22-3.

Packaging, Storage, Handling, and Disposal

Inhalers should be stored at room temperature; avoid freezing and direct sunlight. Dry-powder inhalations should be stored at room temperature, away from direct heat and sunlight. Formoterol should be refrigerated until dispensed; it may then be stored at room temperature, away from heat and moisture. Formoterol and tiotropium capsules should be kept in the foil pack until ready to use. Vials and respules for nebulizers should be stored at room temperature.

Table 22-7 Step Therapy for COPD

Stage I: Mild	Stage II: Moderate	Stage III: Severe	Stage IV: Very Severe
$FEV_1/FVC < 0.70$	$FEV_1/FVC < 0.70$	$FEV_1/FVC < 0.70$	$FEV_1/FEV < 0.70$
$FEV_1 \geq 80\%$ predicted	$50\% \leq FEV_1 < 80\%$ predicted	$30\% \leq FEV_1 < 50\%$ predicted	$FEV_1 < 30\%$ predicted **or** $FEV_1 < 50\%$ predicted + chronic respiratory failure
Active reduction of risk factors; influenza vaccination →			
Add short-acting bronchodilator (when needed) →			
	Add scheduled treatment with one or more long-acting bronchodilators (when needed); **add** rehabilitation		
		Add inhaled corticosteroids if repeated exacerbations	
			Add long-term oxygen if chronic respiratory failure **Consider** surgical treatments

Source: Global Initiative for Chronic Obstructive Lung Disease. Global strategy for the diagnosis, management, and prevention of chronic obstructive pulmonary disease (updated 2009). Available at: http://goldcopd.com/GuidelinesResources.asp.

Medication Administration Equipment

Inhalers should be primed before first use. Formoterol capsules are placed in the chamber of the Aerolizer inhaler for use; tiotropium capsules are placed in the chamber of the HandiHaler inhaler for use. Formoterol and tiotropium capsules are not for oral administration. A spacer is not used with dry-powder inhalers, the formoterol Aerolizer, or the tiotropium HandiHaler.

ANNOTATED BIBLIOGRAPHY

American Thoracic Society/European Respiratory Society. Standards for the diagnosis and management of patients with COPD (2004). Available at: http://www.thoracic.org/clinical/copd-guidelines/index.php. Consensus statement from the American Thoracic Society and the European Respiratory Society. Contains recommendations on oxygen therapy, surgery, pulmonary rehabilitation, ventilation, sleep, air travel, end-of-life issues, and smoking.

Facts & Comparisons eAnswers. Wolters Kluwer Health, Inc.; 2010. Available at: http://online.factsandcomparisons.com/index.aspx?. Accessed February 22, 2010.

Global Initiative for Chronic Obstructive Lung Disease. Global strategy for the diagnosis, management, and prevention of chronic obstructive pulmonary disease (updated 2009). Available at: http://goldcopd.com/GuidelinesResources.asp. Evidence-based guidelines for COPD developed in collaboration by the National Heart, Lung, and Blood Institute, the National Institutes of Health, and the World Health Organization.

Lacy CF, Armstrong LL, Goldman MR, Lance LL, eds. *Lexi-Comp's Drug Information Handbook*. 17th ed. Hudson, OH: Lexi-Comp; 2008.

McEvoy GK, ed. *AHFS Drug Information 2010*. Bethesda, MD: American Society of Health-System Pharmacists; 2010.

Micromedex Healthcare Series [Internet database]. Greenwood Village, CO: Thomson Reuters (Healthcare) Inc. Updated periodically.

Raissy HH. Asthma and bronchospasm. In: Tisdale JE, Miller DA, eds. *Drug-Induced Diseases: Prevention, Detection, and Management*. Bethesda, MD: American Society of Health-System Pharmacists; 2005:249–257.

TOPIC: RHINITIS

Section Coordinator: *Larry Dent*
Contributor: *Katherine S. Hale*

Tips Worth Tweeting

- Appropriate management of rhinitis may have a significant impact on patients' quality of life, medical costs, and complicating respiratory conditions.
- Rhinitis is separated into two categories: nonallergic and allergic rhinitis syndromes.
- Congestion, rhinorrhea, sneezing, and itching are characteristic symptoms of rhinitis.
- Nonpharmacologic treatments of rhinitis include avoidance of environmental triggers, counseling, and education.
- Pharmacologic treatments of rhinitis include second-generation antihistamines, corticosteroids, leukotriene-receptor antagonists, and anticholinergics.
- Pharmacologic dosage forms for the treatment of rhinitis include oral therapies and nasal sprays.

Patient Care Scenario: Ambulatory Setting

R. D.: 58 y/o, 5'9" male, 163 lbs, allergic to penicillin, DOB 7/24/52

Chief Complaint: Complains of rhinorrhea, itchy/watery eyes, and severe nasal congestion followed by severe postnasal drip. Had used an over-the-counter nasal spray and oral diphenhydramine successfully in the past, but over the past several months these medications have stopped working. Presents to the pharmacy today to fill prescriptions for fluticasone propionate nasal spray and montelukast 10 mg tablets.

PMH: Bipolar disorder, alcoholism, hypertension, tympanostomy and adenoidectomy at age 3; allergic rhinitis × 35 years.

FH: Father died at age 96 with a history of Alzheimer's disease and allergic rhinitis; mother died at age 84 with history of Alzheimer's disease and atrial fibrillation; twin brother with moderate persistent asthma and allergic rhinitis.

SH: R. D. lives in a well-kept, two-story, four-bedroom house; married × 22 years. Spouse smokes cigarettes (½ ppd), but not in the house. He is allergic to cats, and has two short-haired dogs that sleep in the bedroom and occasionally on the bed. R. D. lives in a dry, windy region where sagebrush is prevalent; he enjoys outdoor recreational activities, such as hiking. He does all of the yard work, including mowing the lawn.

Date	Physician	Drug	Quantity	Sig	Refills
1/3	Dade	Depakote 500 mg	60	one bid	5
1/3	Rand	Fluoxetine 20 mg	30	one daily	3
12/1	Tide	Lisinopril 20vmg	30	one daily	5
11/15	Dade	Diphenhydramine 25 mg	100	one by mouth every 6 hr prn	0
11/15	Dade	Oxymetazoline nasal spray	1	one spray prn hs and post yard work 2–3 times weekly	
7/2	Tide	Aspirin 81 mg	100	one daily	5
7/2	Tide	Multivitamin	30	one daily	5
7/2	Tide	Saw palmetto	60	2 capsules daily for prostate	1

1.1.0 Patient Information

Disease State

Nonallergic rhinitis syndromes include infectious, vasomotor, nonallergic rhinitis with eosinophilia syndrome; rhinitis from food/alcohol; occupational rhinitis; hormonal rhinitis; atrophic rhinitis; and drug-induced rhinitis. Allergic rhinitis (AR) syndromes are divided into seasonal, perennial, and episodic. Notably, mixed rhinitis—a combination of allergic and nonallergic rhinitis—is more common than pure allergic or nonallergic rhinitis; it affects approximately 44% to 87% of all patients with allergic rhinitis.

Allergic rhinitis is an immune-mediated response facilitated by IgE, mast cells, and T_H2 lymphocytes, resulting from exposure to seasonal and perennial allergens such as dust mites, molds, animal allergens, occupational allergens, and pollen. The allergic reaction may vary by geographic location, climate, and length of exposure.

Risk Factors

- Family history of allergy
- Individuals born during pollen season
- Firstborn child
- Higher socioeconomic class
- Pollution
- Early introduction of foods or formula
- Cigarette smoking and exposure
- Exposure to indoor allergens (e.g., animal dander, dust mites)
- Higher serum IgE levels (greater than 100 IU/mL before age 6)
- Presence of positive allergen skin-prick tests
- Parental allergic disorders

Laboratory Testing

Laboratory confirmation of the presence of antibodies to IgE resulting from specific allergens is useful in establishing an allergic diagnosis, and is the preferred test for diagnosis of IgE-mediated sensitivity. Skin testing may be performed at any age, although children younger than 1 year may not display a positive reaction. Other tests to assess a patient with presumed allergic rhinitis include specific IgE immunoassays, fiber-optic nasal endoscopy and/or rhinomanometry, and eosinophil nasal smears.

Instruments and Techniques Related to Patient Assessment

A patient health history should be obtained to determine the pattern, chronicity, seasonality of symptoms, medication response, presence of coexisting conditions, occupational exposure, environmental history, and triggers associated with the patient's symptoms. A physical examination should be performed, and the patient's quality of life should be assessed. Pulmonary function tests may be performed to assess for the presence of asthma.

Key Terms

The American Academy of Allergy, Asthma and Immunology (AAAI) and the American College of Allergy, Asthma and Immunology (ACAAI) have established guidelines for the diagnosis and management of rhinitis.

- **Allergen:** a substance that induces an allergic reaction.
- **Eosinophil:** a white blood cell or other granulocyte with cytoplasmic inclusions readily stained by eosin.
- **IgE:** immunoglobulin E; a class of immunoglobulins, including antibodies, that function in allergic reactions by activating the release of histamines and leukotrienes in response to foreign antigens.
- **Mast cell:** a granulocyte occurring in connective tissue that has basophilic granules containing substances (e.g., histamine) that mediate allergic reactions.
- **Rhinorrhea:** excessive mucus secretion from nasal passages.
- **T_H2 lymphocyte:** a helper T cell that is essential for the development of IgE antibodies; it secretes interleukins.

Signs and Symptoms

Rhinitis is characterized by one or more of the following nasal symptoms: congestion, rhinorrhea, sneezing, and itching. Sneezing, itching, congestion, and rhinorrhea dominate the early phase, while congestion dominates the late phase.

Wellness, Prevention, and Treatment

Allergic rhinitis has been reported to affect 20 to 40 million people in the United States, indicating the high frequency of this disease state. Because population surveys typically rely on self-reporting or physician-diagnosed rhinitis for data, this methodology may result in lower reporting of rhinitis; thus the actual number of individuals affected may be much higher.

Prevention and management of allergic rhinitis should be individualized and depends on the avoidance of environmental triggers, the appropriate use of prescribed interventions, counseling and education, management of comorbid conditions, and development of a physician–patient–family partnership. In addition to environmental control, nonpharmacologic management of rhinitis includes steam, saline nasal sprays, and exercise. The use of steam increases air flow and saline acts as mild decongestant, reducing nasal blood flow. Each of these agents also helps prevent crusting of dried nasal secretions. Exercise leads to a decrease in nasal airway resistance and nasal decongestion.

1.2.0 Pharmacotherapy

Prescription medications for the treatment of allergic rhinitis are listed in Table 22-8.

Mechanism of Action

Intranasal and oral second-generation antihistamines inhibit the release of histamine from mast cells and selectively antagonize histamine (H1) receptor activity.

The mechanism by which *intranasal corticosteroids* act in the treatment of rhinitis is unknown. Corticosteroids have a range of inhibitory effects on numerous cell types and mediators involved in allergic-mediated inflammation, such as mast cells, eosinophils, neutrophils, macrophages, lymphocytes, histamine, eicosanoids, leukotrienes, and cytokines.

Montelukast is a *leukotriene-receptor antagonist* that selectively binds to cysteinyl leukotriene (CysLT) type-1 receptors found in airway smooth muscle cells and macrophages, preventing airway edema, smooth-muscle contraction, and respiratory inflammation. Cysteinyl leukotrienes are also released from the nasal mucosa after allergen exposure.

Intranasal anticholinergics exert their effect by antagonizing the action of acetylcholine. The antisecretory properties of ipratropium prevent serous and seromucous gland secretions in nasal passageways.

Drug Indications and Routes of Administration

Oral second-generation antihistamines, either alone or in a fixed combination with pseudoephedrine, may be used in children aged 6 years or older and in adults for the treatment of allergic rhinitis symptoms such as rhinorrhea, sneezing, oronasopharyngeal itching, and red, itchy, watery eyes. Azelastine and olopatadine are antihistamines nasal sprays indicated for symptomatic relief of seasonal allergic rhinitis. Azelastine may be used in adults and children 5 years of age and older; olopatadine is indicated for use in adults and children 6 years of age and older.

Intranasal corticosteroid sprays are available as solutions, aqueous suspensions, and inhalation aerosols. These medications are indicated for the treatment of nasal symptoms associated with seasonal and perennial allergic or nonallergic rhinitis. Additionally, mometasone is indicated for the prophylaxis of seasonal allergic rhinitis. Dosing of intranasal corticosteroids is described in Table 22-8; note that once symptoms are controlled, the dose should be reduced

Table 22-8 FDA-Approved Medications for the Treatment of Rhinitis

Drug Class	Drug	Dosing Regimens		Special Instructions
		Adults	Children	
Second-generation antihistamines	Fexofenadine	60 mg bid or 180 mg daily	Age 6 to < 12 years: 30 mg bid Age ≥ 12 years: same as adults	
	Desloratadine	5 mg daily	Age 6–11 months: 1 mg daily Age 12 months to 5 years: 1.25 mg daily Age 6–11 years: 2.5 mg daily Age ≥ 12 years: same as adults	May use in adults and children ≥ 6 months for treatment of perennial AR. May use in adults and children ≥ 2 years for treatment of seasonal AR.
	Levocetirazine	2.5–5 mg daily	Age 6–11 years: 2.5 mg daily Age ≥ 12 years: same as adults	
	Azelastine (Astelin NS)	*Seasonal AR:* 137 mcg/spray: 1–2 sprays in each nostril bid 0.1% and 0.15% sprays: 1–2 sprays in each nostril daily to bid *Perennial AR:* 137 mcg/spray and 0.1%: not indicated 0.15% spray: 2 sprays in each nostril bid *Vasomotor Rhinitis:* 137 mcg/spray: 2 sprays in each nostril bid 0.1% and 0.15% sprays: not indicated	*Seasonal AR:* 137 mcg/spray: Age 5–11 years: 1 spray in each nostril bid Age ≥ 12 years: same as adults 0.1% and 0.15% sprays: not indicated *Perennial AR:* not indicated (all strengths) *Vasomotor Rhinitis:* 137 mcg/spray: Age < 12 years: not indicated Age ≥ 12 years: same as adults 0.1% and 0.15% sprays: not indicated	
	Olopatadine (Patanase NS)	2 sprays in each nostril bid	Age 6–11 years: 1 spray in each nostril bid Age ≥ 12 years: same as adults	At first use, prime pump by releasing 5 sprays or until a fine mist appears. If pump has not been used within the last 7 days, reprime it by releasing 2 sprays.
Second-generation antihistamine/ decongestant combination	Acrivastine/ pseudoephedrine HCl	8 mg/60 mg (1 cap) every 4–6 hr	Age ≥ 12 years: same as adults	
	Fexofenadine/ pseudoephredrine HCl	60 mg/120 mg (1 tab) bid **or** 180 mg/120 mg (1 tab) daily	Age ≥ 12 years: same as adults	

	Desloratadine/ pseudoephedrine HCl	2.5 mg/120 mg (1 tab) bid **or** 5 mg/240 mg (1 tab) daily	Age ≥ 12 years: same as adults	
Corticosteroids	Beclomethasone dipropionate, monohydrate	42 or 84 mcg (1–2 sprays) in each nostril bid * If no response to 168 mcg daily or more severe symptoms are present, the dose may be increased to 84 mcg in each nostril bid until adequate control is achieved; then reduce dose to 84 mcg each nostril bid.	Age 6–12 years: 42 mcg (1 spray) in each nostril bid Age ≥ 12 years: same as adults	At first use, prime pump by releasing 6 sprays or until a fine mist appears. If pump has not been used within the last 7 days, reprime it until a fine mist appears.
	Budesonide	32–128 mcg (1–4 sprays) in each nostril daily	Age 6–12 years: 32–128 mcg (1–2 sprays) in each nostril daily Age ≥ 12 years: same as adults	Shake well prior to use. At first use, prime pump by releasing 8 sprays or until a fine mist appears. Repriming is required if the pump has not been used for 2 consecutive days (1 spray) or for more than 14 days (2 sprays).
	Flunisolide	50 mcg (2 sprays) in each nostril bid to tid	Age 6–14 years: 25 mcg (1 spray) in each nostril tid or 50 mcg (2 sprays) in each nostril bid Age ≥ 14 years: same as adults	Shake well prior to use. At first use, prime pump by releasing 5–6 sprays or until a fine mist appears. Repriming is required if the pump has not been used for 2 consecutive days (1 spray) or for more than 14 days (2 sprays).
	Fluticasone propionate	100 mcg (2 sprays) in each nostril daily or 50 mcg (1 spray) in each nostril bid	Age ≥ 4 years: 50 mcg (1 spray) in each nostril daily, may increase to 100 mcg (2 sprays) in each nostril daily for severe symptoms	Reduce to lowest effective dose once symptoms are controlled. Shake well before use. At first use, prime pump by releasing 5–6 sprays or until a fine mist appears. Repriming is required if the pump has not been used for 2 consecutive days (1 spray) or for more than 14 days (2 sprays).
	Fluticasone furoate	55 mcg (2 sprays) in each nostril daily (TDD 110 mcg)	Age 2–11 years: 27.5 mcg (1 spray) in each nostril daily (TDD 55 mcg); if no response, may increase to 55 mcg (2 sprays) in each nostril daily Age ≥ 12 years: same as adults	Shake well before use. At first use, prime pump by releasing 6 sprays or until a fine mist appears. If pump has not been used for more than 30 days or if cap is left off for 5 days or longer, reprime it until a fine mist appears.
	Mometasone furoate	Treatment: 100 mcg (2 sprays) in each nostril daily Prophylaxis: 100 mcg (2 sprays) in each nostril daily	Treatment: Age 2–11 years: 50 mcg (1 spray) in each nostril daily Age ≥ 12 years: same as adults Prophylaxis: Age 2–11 years: not indicated Age ≥ 12 years: same as adults	Shake well before use. At first use, prime pump by releasing 10 sprays or until a fine mist appears. If pump is unused for longer than 1 week, reprime it by releasing 2 sprays or until a fine mist appears.

(*continues*)

Table 22-8 (*continued*)

Drug Class	Drug	Dosing Regimens		Special Instructions
		Adults	Children	
Corticosteroids (*continued*)	Triamcinolone acetonide aqueous suspension spray (Nasacort AQ)	Aqueous suspension spray: 110 mcg (2 sprays) in each nostril daily (TDD 220 mcg)	Aqueous suspension spray: Age 2–5 years: 55 mcg (1 spray) in each nostril daily Age 6–12 years: 55–110 mcg (1–2 sprays) in each nostril daily (maximum TDD 220 mcg) Age ≥ 12 years: same as adults	Shake well before use. Initial priming requires 5 sprays or more; if unused for 2 weeks or more, reprime pump by actuating 1 time.
	Triamcinolone acetonide nasal inhalation aerosol (Nasacort HFA)	110–220 mcg (2–4 sprays) in each nostril daily	Age 6–11 years: 110 mcg (2 sprays) in each nostril daily (TDD 220 mcg) Age ≥ 12 years: same as adults	Shake well before use. Initial priming requires 3 sprays or more; if prime has been unused for 3 days or longer, reprime it by releasing 3 sprays.
	Ciclesonide	Seasonal and perennial allergic rhinitis: 100 mcg (2 sprays) in each nostril daily (TDD 200 mcg)	Seasonal allergic rhinitis: Age ≥ 6 years: same as adults Perennial allergic rhinitis: Age < 12 years: not indicated Age ≥ 12 years: same as adults	Shake gently before use. Initial priming requires 8 sprays or more. If pump has been unused for 4 days or longer, reprime it by releasing 1 spray or until a fine mist appears.
Glucocorticosteroids	Prednisone	5–30 mg administered as a tapering dose	0.14–2 mg/kg on day 1 in 4 divided doses, then taper	For short-term use only (e.g., 6 days).
	Methylpredn-isolone	2–60 mg daily administered as a tapering dose	0.117–1.66 mg/kg/day administered in 3–4 divided doses, tapering over time	For short-term use only (e.g., 6 days).
Leukotriene-receptor antagonists	Montelukast (Singular)	10 mg daily	Age 6–23 months: 4 mg daily Age 2–5 years: 4 mg daily Age 6–14 years: 5 mg daily Age ≥ 15 years: 10mg daily	
Intranasal anticholinergics	Ipratropium bromide	0.03%: 42 mcg (2 sprays) in each nostril bid to tid (TDD 168–252 mcg) 0.06%: 84 mcg (2 sprays) in each nostril qid (TDD 672 mcg)	0.03%: Age ≥ 6 years: same as adults 0.06%: Age ≥ 5 years: same as adults	Initial priming of both pumps requires 7 sprays. If not used for 24 hours or longer, pump will require 2 sprays or more to reprime it; if not used for 7 days or longer, it will require 7 sprays or more to reprime it.

bid = twice daily; tid = three times daily; qid = four times daily; TDD = total daily dose.

to the lowest effective dose at which rhinitis symptoms are controlled. Oral glucocorticosteroids are indicated only for the treatment of very severe or intractable nasal symptoms associated with rhinitis. Intramuscular and parenteral administration is not recommended.

The oral leukotriene-receptor antagonist montelukast is available in film-coated tablet, chewable tablet, and granule formulations. It is the only medication in this class currently approved by the FDA for the treatment of symptoms associated with seasonal or perennial allergic rhinitis. A small number of clinical trials have evaluated the effectiveness of zafirlukast in the treatment of allergic rhinitis, but it is not currently an FDA-approved indication for this agent.

Ipratropium bromide is an intranasal anticholinergic nasal spray that may be used in children and adults 6 years of age and older for the treatment of rhinorrhea associated with allergic and nonallergic perennial rhinitis.

Interaction of Drugs with Foods and Laboratory Tests

Acrivastine/Pseudoephedrine

The combination product acrivastine/pseudoephedrine is contraindicated in patients currently receiving monamine oxidase inhibitors (MAOIs) or for 2 weeks post-MAOI therapy due to the potential for MAOIs to potentiate the pressor effects of pseudoephedrine (a sympathomimetic drug). Additionally, acrivastine/pseudoephedrine may decrease the antihypertensive effects of drugs that interfere with sympathetic activity. Administration of acrivastine/pseudoephedrine with alcohol and/or other CNS depressants should be avoided due to additive effects and reduction in mental alertness and CNS impairment.

Fexofenadine and Fexofenadine/Pseudoephedrine

Antacids containing aluminum and magnesium may decrease fexofenadine absorption by 40% or more if administered within 15 minutes of fexofenadine. An increase in the bioavailability of fexofenadine is noted when this medication is administered with either ketoconazole or erythromycin. However, these changes in plasma levels are within the range achieved during clinical trials. An increase in the length of the QT_c interval or adverse events has not been observed. Combination products containing fexofenadine and pseudoephrine are contraindicated in patients currently receiving MAOIs or for 2 weeks post-MAOI therapy due to the potential for MAOIs to potentiate the pressor effects of pseudoephedrine (a sympathomimetic drug). Additionally, fruit juices, such as apple, grapefruit, and orange, may reduce the bioavailability of fexofenadine by 36% or more if taken at the same time. The clinical importance of the fruit juice interaction is currently not known.

Desloratadine and Desloratadine/Pseudoephedrine

An increase in plasma levels of desloratadine has been noted when this medication is administered with erythromycin and ketoconazole, albeit with no clinically significant changes in ECG, vital signs, or adverse effects. No formal interaction studies have been performed for this combination product, but interactions between pseudoephedrine and other medications (e.g., MAOIs) should be considered.

Levocetirazine

Coadministration of ritonovir increases levocetirazine plasma concentrations by 42%, increases the latter drug's half-life by 53%, and decreases its clearance by 29%. No drug interactions between levocetirazine and hepatic enzyme inhibitors or inducers were noted in clinical trials. Levocetirazine may have additive CNS depressant effects when coadministered with other CNS depressants (e.g., alcohol).

Azelastine

No clinically important drug interactions have been observed. Avoid coadministration with alcohol or other CNS depressants due to the potential for additive effects.

Budesonide

While systemic absorption of inhaled budesonide is minimal, concomitant administration with potent inhibitors of the cytochrome P450 (CYP) 3A4 enzyme may result in increased plasma concentrations of budesonide.

Fluticasone

Inhaled fluticasone is a substrate of the CYP3A4 enzyme. Concomitant administration of fluticasone propionate and potent CYP3A4 inhibitors (e.g., ritonovir, ketoconazole) results in increased plasma concentrations of fluticasone and a reduction in plasma cortisol AUC.

Ciclesonide

Coadministration of ciclesonide with ketoconazole (CYP3A4 inhibitor) results in a threefold increase in plasma concentrations of the active metabolite, desciclesonide, with no effect on the parent compound.

Montelukast

Coadministration of phenobarbital (a cytochrome P450 inducer) and montelukast results in as much as a 40% decrease in plasma concentrations of montelukast. Caution should be used when administering montelukast with known potent inducers of the cytochrome P450 enzyme system.

Ipratropium

Due to limited systemic absorption and low plasma drug concentrations associated with ipratropium nasal spray, drug interactions are limited. However, concomitant administration of ipratropium with other antimuscarinic agents may lead to an additive effect.

Olopatadine, Beclomethasone, Flunisolide, Mometasone, Triamcinolone, Prednisone, and Methylprednisolone

No clinically significant drug interactions have been reported.

Contraindications, Warnings, and Precautions

General precautions for the use of intranasal and oral corticosteroids relate to the following effects:

- Adrenal suppression and symptoms of hypercorticism if recommended doses are exceeded or if the patient has recently used systemic corticosteroids
- Potential immunosuppression may predispose individuals to infection
- Reduced growth velocity in pediatric patients
- Localized *Candida albicans* infections
- Nasal septum perforation
- Rare cases of wheezing, cataracts, glaucoma, and increased ocular pressure

Due to the potential for immunosuppression and infection, corticosteroids should be used cautiously if the patient has active/untreated tuberculosis (TB) infection, untreated local/systemic fungal or bacterial infection, systemic viral or parasitic infection, or ocular herpes simplex infection. Table 22-9 lists additional precautions, adverse effects, and dose adjustments of the FDA-approved medications for the treatment of rhinitis.

Physiochemical Properties, Pharmacodynamics, and Pharmacokinetic Properties

- Acrivastine: bioavailability not yet established; protein binding 50%; T_{max} 1.14 hours; $T_{1/2}$ 1.9–3.5 hours; metabolized to the active metabolite propionic acid; excretion primarily renal
- Fexofenadine: bioavailability not yet established; protein binding 60–70%; T_{max} 2.6 hours; $T_{1/2}$ 14.4 hours; administration with food delays T_{max} by 50%; approximately 5% of dose is metabolized; CYP3A4 converts 1% of dose to inactive metabolite
- Desloratadine: bioavailability not yet established; 82–87% protein binding; T_{max} 3 hours; $T_{1/2}$ adults 27 hours; $T_{1/2}$ 16.4 hours in children 2–5 years; $T_{1/2}$ 19.4 hours in children 6–11 years; metabolized extensively in liver via hydroxylation; active metabolite is 3-hydroxydesloratadine
- Levocetirazine: 85% bioavailability; T_{max} 0.5–1.5 hours; high-fat meals delay T_{max} by 1.25 hours and C_{max} by 36%; $T_{1/2}$ adults 7–9 hours; $T_{1/2}$ children 5.7 hours; protein binding 95%; metabolized in liver by aromatic oxidation, *N*- and *O*-dealkylation, and taurine conjugation; renal excretion
- Azelastine: bioavailability 40%; T_{max} 2–3 hours; $T_{1/2}$ 22 hours; primarily fecal excretion; metabolized by CYP450 enzyme system (specific enzymes not identified) to active metabolite desmethylazelastine
- Olopatadine: bioavailability 57%; T_{max} 15 minutes–2 hours; $T_{1/2}$ 8–12 hours; protein binding 55%; not extensively metabolized
- Beclomethasone: absolute bioavailability unknown; up to 43% of each dose is deposited on nasal mucosa; protein binding 87%; $T_{1/2}$ 3 hours; extensively metabolized by lung, partially by liver; primarily renal and fecal excretion
- Budesonide: bioavailability 21%; protein binding 85–90%; T_{max} 0.6 hour; $T_{1/2}$ 2–3 hours; primarily renal excretion; extensive hepatic metabolism by CYP3A4
- Flunisolide: bioavailability 50%; T_{max} 10–30 minutes; $T_{1/2}$ 1–2 hours; rapidly metabolized in liver to a 6-beta-hydroxylated active metabolite; renal and biliary excretion
- Fluticasone propionate: poorly absorbed from nasal tract; bioavailability < 2%; protein binding 91%; T_{max} 0.5–6 hours; $T_{1/2}$ 3 hours; rapidly metabolized by CYP3A4; fecal excretion
- Fluticasone furoate: bioavailability 0.5%; protein binding 99%; $T_{1/2}$ 15.1 hours; hepatic metabolism by CYP3A4 to inactive metabolite; fecal excretion
- Triamcinolone: T_{max} 1.5 hours; $T_{1/2}$ 3.1 minutes; minimal systemic absorption
- Ciclesonide: bioavailability < 1%; protein binding ≥ 99%; metabolism to active metabolite desciclesonide via hepatic enzyme CYP3A4 and 2D6; $T_{1/2}$ 2.7 hours (parent) and 5.9 hours (metabolite); biliary excretion
- Prednisone: bioavailability 92%; protein binding 70%; $T_{1/2}$ 2.6–3 hours; extensive hepatic metabolism
- Methylprednisolone: hepatic metabolism via reversible oxidation of the 11-hydroxyl group; $T_{1/2}$ 2–3 hours; primarily renal excretion
- Montelukast: bioavailability 64–73%; protein binding 99%; T_{max} 3–4 hours; $T_{1/2}$ 2.7–5.5 hours; fecal elimination; extensively metabolized by CYP3A4 and 2C9
- Ipratropium: poorly absorbed via nasal administration (less than 20% of each dose); bioavailability up to 9%; $T_{1/2}$ 1.6 hours; partially metabolized to esther hydrolysis products, tropic acid, and tropane

Table 22-9 Additional Precautions, Adverse Effects, and Dose Adjustments of FDA-Approved Medications for the Treatment of Rhinitis

Product	Precautions	Adverse Effects	Dose Adjustments
Acrivastine/ pseudoephedrine	• Contraindicated for use in the following patient populations: ○ Severe hypertension ○ Severe coronary artery disease ○ Concurrent use of MAOIs or within 14 days of stopping an MAOI • Use cautiously in patients with arrhythmias, diabetes mellitus, geriatric patients, glaucoma, hyperthyroidism, ischemic heart disease, prostatic hypertrophy, and renal failure. • Pregnancy category B. • Excreted in breastmilk; use cautiously in nursing women.	• Dry mouth • Somnolence • Insomnia • Nervousness • Agitation	Renal impairment (CrCl < 48 mL/min): Contraindicated. Hepatic impairment: No dose adjustment needed.
Fexofenadine and fexofenadine/ pseudoephedrine	• Associated with increased QT_c interval, syncope, and ventricular arrhythmia. • Oral disintegrating tablets contain phenylalanine. • Monitor renal function; if renal impairment is present, start at the lowest initial dose and titrate. • Pregnancy category C. • Excreted in breastmilk; use cautiously in nursing women.	• Headache • Back pain • Stomach discomfort • Dizziness • Cough • Upper respiratory tract infections • Pyrexia • Otitis media • Vomiting • Diarrhea • Somnolence/fatigue • Rhinorrhea	Hepatic impairment: No dose adjustment necessary. Renal impairment: Age ≥ 12 years: initial dose of 60 mg daily (may be given in combination with 120 mg pseudoephedrine) Age 6–11 years: initial dose of 30mg daily Combination of 180 mg fexofenadine and 240 mg pseudoephedrine should be avoided in renal impairment and hemodialysis due to pseudoephedrine accumulation.
Desloratadine and desloratadine/ pseudoephedrine	• Pregnancy category C. • Excreted in breastmilk; use cautiously in nursing women. • Oral disintegrating tablet formulation contains aspartame, which is metabolized to phenylalanine—avoid in patients with phenylketonuria.	• Pharyngitis • Dry mouth • Myalgia • Somnolence/fatigue • Dysmenorrhea • Dizziness • Headache • Nausea	Renal and hepatic impairment: Begin with 5 mg every other day and titrate to effective dose. No recommendations exist for pediatrics due to lack of data.
Levocetirazine	• Contraindicated in patients with ESRD or undergoing hemodialysis. • Contraindicated in patients aged 6–11 years with renal impairment. • Prolongation of QT_c interval when given with potent CYP3A4 inhibitors. • Additive CNS side effects—caution required when performing hazardous activities requiring mental alertness or physical coordination. • Pregnancy category B. • Excreted in breastmilk—not recommended for use in nursing women.	• Somnolence • Fatigue • Nasopharyngitis • Pyrexia • Cough • Epistaxis • Dry mouth • Pharyngitis	Adjust dose based on degree of renal impairment: CrCl 50–80 mL/min = 2.5 mg daily CrCl 30–50 mL/min = 2.5mg every other day CrCl 10–30 mL/min = 2.5mg twice weekly (every 3–4 days) CrCl < 10 mL/min = contraindicated Hepatic impairment: No dose adjustment needed.

(continues)

Table 22-9 (*continued*)

Product	Precautions	Adverse Effects	Dose Adjustments
Azelastine	• May reduce mental alertness—use caution when operating heavy machinery or participating in activities requiring mental alertness. • Potential additive CNS depressant side effects—avoid alcohol use and coadministration with other CNS depressant medications.	• Bitter taste • Dyesthesia • Nasal burning • Pharyngitis • Paroxysmal sneezing • Somnolence • Headache • Rhinitis • Sinusitis • Epistaxis	No dose adjustments needed.
Olopatadine	• Nasal exam prior to initiation of olopatadine and periodic reassessments are recommended due to reports of epistaxis, nasal ulceration, and nasal septum perforation. • Potential additive CNS depressant side effects—avoid alcohol use and coadministration with other CNS depressant medications. • Pregnancy category C. • Unknown if excreted in breastmilk—use cautiously in nursing mothers.	• Bitter taste • Headache • Epistaxis • Pharyngolaryngeal pain • Postnasal drip • Cough • CPK elevation • Dry mouth • Urinary tract infection • Fatigue/somnolence	No dose adjustments needed.
Beclomethasone	• Pregnancy category C. • Unknown if excreted in breastmilk—use cautiously in nursing mothers.	• Nasopharyngeal irritation • Epistaxis • Sneezing attacks • Headache • Nausea • Lightheadedness • Nasal stuffiness • Tearing eyes • Rhinorrhea • Nasal dryness	No dose adjustments needed.
Budesonide	• Pregnancy category B. • Unknown if excreted in breastmilk—use cautiously in nursing mothers.	• Epistaxis • Cough • Pharyngitis • Bronchospasm • Nasal irritation	No dose adjustments needed.
Flunisolide	• Pregnancy category C. • Unknown if excreted in breastmilk—use cautiously in nursing mothers.	• Nasal burning/stinging • Epistaxis • Nasal dryness • Pharyngitis • Cough • Nausea • Aftertaste • Hoarseness • Abnormal sense of smell	No dose adjustments needed.

Table 22-9 (*continued*)

Product	Precautions	Adverse Effects	Dose Adjustments
Fluticasone	• Pregnancy category B. • Unknown if excreted in breastmilk—use cautiously in nursing mothers.	• Headache • Pharyngitis • Epistaxis • Nasal burning/irritation • Nausea/vomiting • Asthma symptoms • Cough • Alteration in senses of taste and smell	No dose adjustments needed.
Mometasone	• Pregnancy category C. • Unknown if excreted in breastmilk—use cautiously in nursing mothers.	• Headache • Pharyngitis • Epistaxis • Nausea/vomiting • URI • Viral infection • Cough • Sinusitis • Dysmenorrhea	
Triamcinolone	• Pregnancy category C. • Unknown if excreted in breastmilk—use cautiously in nursing mothers.	• Pharyngitis • Epistaxis • Flu-like symptoms • Increased cough • Bronchitis • Dyspepsia • Tooth disorder • Headache • Pharyngolaryngeal pain • Nasopharyngitis • Abdominal pain • Diarrhea • Excoriation	
Ciclesonide	• Pregnancy category C. • Unknown if excreted in breastmilk—use cautiously in nursing mothers.	• Headache • Epistaxis • Nasopharyngitis • Nasal discomfort • Pharyngolaryngeal pain • Ear pain	
Prednisone and methylprednis-olone	• Use cautiously in individuals with the following conditions: cirrhosis, diverticulitis, hypothyroidism, hypertension, myasthenia gravis, osteoporosis, peptic ulcer, psychotic tendencies, renal insufficiency, and ulcerative colitis. • Pregnancy category A.	• Indigestion • Increased appetite • Trouble sleeping • Irritability • Confusion • Depression • Euphoria	Hepatic or renal impairment: No dose adjustments needed. Dose may need to be increased in patients with hyperthyroidism.

(*continues*)

Table 22-9 (*continued*)

Product	Precautions	Adverse Effects	Dose Adjustments
Prednisone and methylprednis-olone *(cont'd)*	• Negligible amounts found in breastmilk—may use in nursing mothers.	• Retention of body fluids • Hypernatremia	
Montelukast	• Use cautiously in patients with underlying liver disease, hepatitis, and alcohol use. • Not indicated for reversal of acute bronchospasm. • If known aspirin sensitivity—continue avoidance of aspirin and NSAIDs while taking montelukast. • Neuropsychiatric events (e.g., agitation, aggressive behavior, suicidal ideation, depression, dream abnormalities) have been reported; patients should be carefully monitored and treatment should be reevaluated if such an event occurs. • Monitor for the presence of eosinophilia, vasculitic rash, pulmonary symptoms, cardiac complications, and/or neuropathy. • Chewable tablets contain aspartame, which is metabolized to phenylalanine—avoid in patients with phenylketonuria. • Pregnancy category B. • Unknown if excreted in breastmilk—use cautiously in nursing mothers.	• Headache • Influenza • Abdominal pain • Cough • Increased serum ALT or AST concentration • Dyspepsia • Dizziness • Asthenia/fatigue • Dental pain • Nasal congestion • Rash • Fever • Infectious gastroenteritis • Pyuria • Otitis • Sinusitis	Renal impairment: No dose adjustment needed. Hepatic impairment: No dose adjustment needed in mild-to-moderate impairment; not recommended for use in severe hepatic impairment.
Ipratropium	• Use with caution in narrow-angle glaucoma, prostatic hyperplasia, bladder neck obstruction, renal insufficiency, and hepatic insufficiency. • Pregnancy category B. • Unknown if excreted in breastmilk—use cautiously in nursing mothers.	• Epistaxis • Nasal dryness • Dry mouth/throat • Nasal congestion • Pharyngitis • URI • Abnormal taste • Sinusitis	No studies performed to evaluate use in patients with renal or hepatic insufficiency—use with caution.

ESRD = end-stage renal disease (creatinine clearance < 10 mL/min); URI = upper respiratory tract infection.

1.3.0 Monitoring

Pharmacotherapeutic Outcomes

Monitor improvement of symptoms, symptom prevention or aggravation, changes in patient quality of life, efficacy and tolerability of treatment, and patient satisfaction. Therapy response ranges from 24 hours to 3 weeks depending on the agent used. If an inadequate response occurs, consider therapy nonadherence, substitution with another medication class, addition of another medication class, allergen immunotherapy, surgery (if the patient has structural/mechanical issues or comorbid conditions, such as nasal polyps), and/or diagnosis change.

Safety and Efficacy

Antihistamine and Antihistamine/Decongestant Combinations

Patients with hypertension should monitor for significant changes in blood pressure while taking combination products. Avoid use of combination products in patients with severe hypertension. Monitor renal and hepatic function to guide dose adjustments as necessary.

Intranasal and Oral Corticosteroids

Patients using intranasal and oral corticosteroids at high doses and/or for long-term therapy should be monitored for signs and symptoms of systemic corticosteroid effects (e.g., adrenal suppression, hypercorticism) and changes in bone mineral density. Because of the effect of corticosteroids on growth, children and adolescents should be monitored for changes in growth and development. Additionally, an ACTH stimulation test, AM plasma cortisol test, and urinary free cortisol test may be performed. Blood pressure, electrolytes, glucose levels, and mental status should also be monitored in patients on long-term oral corticosteroid therapy.

Leukotriene Receptor Antagonists

Monitor for suicidal ideation, changes in behavior/mood, neuropsychiatric changes, and changes in liver function tests.

Intranasal Anticholinergics

Monitor for nasal dryness and epistaxis.

Table 22-10 Generic Names, Brand Names, and Dosage Form Availability for FDA-Approved Treatments for Rhinitis

Generic	Trade Name	Dosage Form Availability (How Supplied)
Acrivastine/pseudoephedrine HCl	Semprex-D	Oral capsules: 8 mg/60 mg
Fexofenadine	Allegra	Oral capsules: 60 mg Oral tablets: 30 mg, 60 mg, 180 mg
Fexofenadine/pseudoephdrine HCl	Allegra D	Oral tablets: 60 mg/180 mg, 180 mg/240 mg
Desloratadine	Clarinex	Oral solution: 0.5 mg/mL Oral tablets: 5 mg Tablets, orally disintegrating: 2.5 mg, 5 mg
Desloratadine/pseudoephedrine sulfate	Clarinex D	Oral tablets: 5 mg/120 mg
Levocetirazine	Xyzal	Oral tablets: 5 mg
Azelastine	Astelin Ready Spray Astepro Nasal Spray	Nasal spray: 137 mcg/actuation Nasal spray: 205.5 mcg/actuation
Olopatadine	Patanase	Nasal spray: 0.06%
Beclomethasone dipropionate, monohydrate	Beconase Vancenase	Nasal aerosol powder: 0.042 mg/actuation
Budesonide	Rhinocort Rhinocort Aqua	Nasal aerosol powder: 0.032 mg/actuation Nasal spray: 0.032 mg/actuation
Flunisolide	Nasalide Nasarel	Nasal spray: 0.025 mg/actuation
Fluticasone propionate	Flonase Novaplus fluticasone propionate	Nasal spray: 0.05 mg/actuation
Fluticasone furoate	Veramyst	Nasal spray: 27.5 mcg/actuation
Mometasone furoate	Nasonex	Nasal spray: 0.05 mg/actuation
Triamcinolone acetonide aqueous suspension	Nasacort AQ	Nasal spray: 55 mcg/actuation
Triamcinolone acetonide nasal inhalation aerosol	Nasacort HFA	Nasal aerosol: 55 mcg/actuation
Ciclesonide	Omnaris	Nasal spray: 50 mcg/actuation
Prednisone	Prednisone Prednisone intensol	Oral tablets: 1 mg, 2.5 mg, 5 mg, 10 mg, 20 mg, 50 mg Oral solution: 5 mg/mL
Methylprednisolone	Medrol	Oral tablets: 2 mg, 4 mg, 8 mg, 16 mg, 32 mg
Montelukast	Singulair	Oral granules: 4 mg/packet Oral tablets: 10 mg Oral tablets, chewable: 4 mg, 5 mg
Ipratropium bromide	Atrovent	Nasal spray: 0.3% (21 mcg/actuation), 0.6% (42 mcg/actuation)

Adverse Drug Reactions

Common adverse drug reactions (ADRs) to antihistamines include somnolence/fatigue, dizziness, dry mouth, and headache. Common ADRs related to all nasal sprays include nasal irritation, nasal dryness, epistaxis, pharyngitis, changes in taste, cough, and headache. Common ADRs related to leukotriene-receptor antagonists include headache, cough, dizziness, and dyspepsia. A detailed list of ADRs is presented in Table 22-8.

Nonadherence, Misuse, or Abuse

Nonadherence may occur when symptoms of rhinitis improve or are completely resolved. Appropriate counseling emphasizes the appropriate use of drug therapy and avoidance of triggers during exacerbations of rhinitis. If the patient is using mometasone for rhinitis prophylaxis, appropriate counseling addresses continued therapy to reduce the potential for a rhinitis exacerbation.

Pharmacotherapeutic Alternatives

Medications in a similar class may be substituted for one another. For example, levocetirazine may be substituted for fexofenadine or mometasone nasal spray for fluticasone, with the appropriate dose adjustments.

2.2.0 Dispensing

Generic, Trade Name, and Dosage Form Availability

Packaging, Storage, Handling, and Disposal

Store all medications listed in Table 22-10 at room temperature (20–25°C), avoid freezing. Nasal spray applicators may be cleansed using lukewarm water as needed following the manufacturer's instructions.

Medication Administration Equipment

All nasal sprays require pump priming.

ANNOTATED BIBLIOGRAPHY

Druce HM. Allergic and nonallergic rhinitis. In: Middleton E, Ellis EF, Ynginger JW, Reed CE, Adkinson NF, Busse WW, eds. *Allergy: Principles and Practice*. 5th ed. St. Louis, MO; Mosby-Year Book; 1998: 1005–1016.

Joint Task Force on Practice Parameters. The diagnosis and management of rhinitis: an updated practice parameter. *J Allergy Clin Immunol* 2008;122:S1–S84.

McEvoy GK, ed. *AHFS Drug Information 2009*. Bethesda, MD: American Society of Health-System Pharmacists; 2009.

Skoner DP. Allergic rhinitis: definition, epidemiology, pathophysiology, detection, and diagnosis. *J Allergy Clin Immunol* 2001;108:S2–S8.

Wickersham RM, ed. *Drug Facts and Comparisons*. St. Louis, MO: Wolters Kluwer Health, Inc.; 2010.

Wright AL, Holberg CJ, Martinez FD, Halonen M, Morgan W, Taussig LM. Epidemiology of physician-diagnosed allergic rhinitis in childhood. *Pediatrics* 1994;94:895–901.

TOPIC: SMOKING CESSATION

Section Coordinator: *Larry Dent*
Contributor: *Larry Dent*

Tips Worth Tweeting

- The *U.S. Clinical Practice Guideline for Treating Tobacco Use and Dependence* recommends that all clinicians, including pharmacists, should provide every tobacco user with at least a minimal intervention using the five A's: Ask, Advise, Assess, Assist, and Arrange.
- Medication and counseling are important strategies to counter the physical and psychological components of nicotine addiction.
- All patients who are attempting to quit smoking should be encouraged to use pharmacotherapy unless contraindicated.
- Behavioral and cognitive counseling when combined with medication increases the likelihood of successful smoking cessation and should be offered to all patients who are attempting to quit.

Patient Care Scenario: Ambulatory Setting

V. L.: 36 y/o, 5'6", F, white, 154 lbs, no known allergies, PMH unknown, labs not available.

V. L. visited your pharmacy presenting a new prescription for Ortho-Novum 1/35 po once daily. She has a history of smoking about 1 pack/day since she was 14 years of age. V. L. stated that she has made multiple attempts to quit smoking without success. Her most recent attempt at quitting, in which she used Commit lozenges, lasted about 2 weeks. She mentioned that she is concerned about gaining weight if she quits smoking. Her triggers were identified as having a cigarette with her morning coffee, while driving, and while socializing with her friends and coworkers.

1.1.0 Patient Information

Medications, Laboratory Testing, and Disease State

Smoking is a known cause of multiple cancers, heart disease, stroke, complications of pregnancy, chronic obstructive pulmonary disease, and many other diseases.

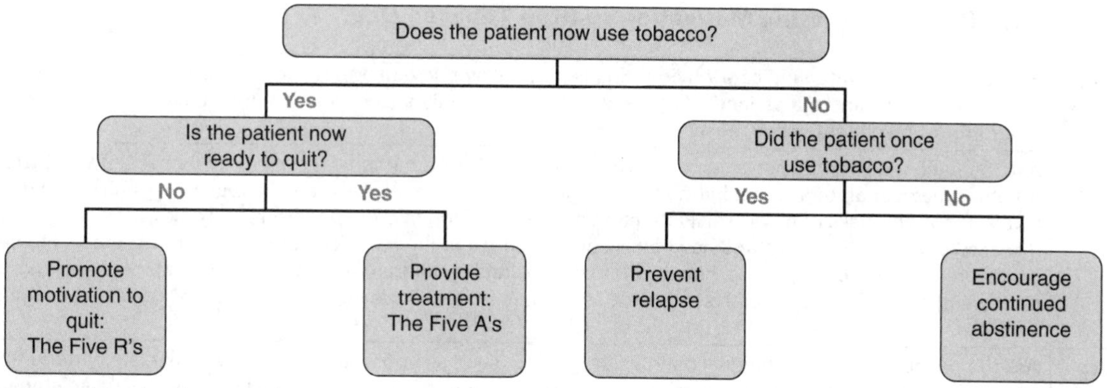

Figure 22-1 Algorithm for Treating Tobacco Use
Data from: Fiore MC, Jaen CR, Baker TB, et al. Treating Tobacco Use and Dependence: 2008 Update. Clinical Practice Guideline. Rockville, MD: Department of Health and Human Services. Public Health Service; 2008.

In addition, involuntary exposure to tobacco smoke has been documented as a substantial health risk leading to premature death and disease in nonsmokers The prevalence of smoking varies by sociodemographic factors, including sex, race-ethnicity, education level, age, and socioeconomic status.

Instruments and Techniques Related to Patient Assessment

The *U.S. Clinical Practice Guideline for Treating Tobacco Use and Dependence* recommends that all clinicians, including pharmacists, provide every tobacco user with at least a minimal tobacco intervention.[4] Further, it recommends that all patients who are attempting to quit smoking should be encouraged to use pharmacotherapy, except in those cases where contraindications exist. Once a tobacco user is identified and advised to quit, the pharmacist should assess the patient's willingness to quit, as outlined in Figure 22-1.[4]

If the patient is *willing* to make a quit attempt at this time, deliver the five A's (Table 22-11).[4]

Table 22-11 Five A's for Brief Smoking-Cessation Intervention

Ask about tobacco use.	Identify and document tobacco use status for every patient.
Advise to quit.	Advise every tobacco user to quit.
Assess willingness to make a quit attempt.	Determine whether the tobacco user is willing to make a quit attempt at this time.
Assist in the quit attempt.	Offer counseling and pharmacotherapy to assist with quitting.
Arrange for follow-up.	Make arrangements to follow up with the patient within the first week after the quit date.

Adapted from: *U.S. Clinical Practice Guideline for Treating Tobacco Use and Dependence.*

If the patient is *unwilling* to quit at this time, a motivational intervention should be provided, utilizing the five R's (Table 22-12).[4]

Key Terms

Nicotine addiction is a two-component problem that involves both physical dependence and psychological addiction. **Physical dependence** is created by physiologic changes in brain chemistry; nicotine stimulates dopamine release, creating a pleasurable feeling that reinforces repeat administration. **Psychological addiction** is a strong habit pattern that becomes established over time. To successfully treat both the physical and psychological components of nicotine dependence, medication in combination with counseling is more effective than either alone. **Medication** is used to treat the physical dependence to nicotine, while **counseling** targets the psychological addiction associated with tobacco use.

Wellness and Prevention

The health benefits associated with smoking cessation over time are listed in Table 22-13.

1.2.0 Pharmacotherapy

Drugs and Indications

All patients attempting to quit smoking should be encouraged to use effective pharmacotherapies for smoking cessation except in presence of contraindications or in special populations for whom there is insufficient evidence of effectiveness, such as pregnant women, smokeless-tobacco users, light smokers, and adolescents. Seven FDA-approved first-line agents are available for smoking cessation—bupropion, varenicline, and five formulations of nicotine replacement therapy (NRT), which include gum, lozenge, transdermal patch, oral inhaler, and nasal spray (Table 22-14). The nicotine gum, lozenge, and transdermal patch are available without a prescription; all other therapies require a prescription.

Table 22-12 Five R's for Promoting Motivation to Stop Tobacco Use

Relevance	Encourage the patient to indicate why quitting is personally relevant. Motivational information has the greatest impact if it is relevant to a patient's disease status or risk, family social situation, health concerns, age, sex, and other important patient characteristics.
Risks	Ask the patient to identify potential negative consequences of tobacco use, such as acute risks of shortness of breath, exacerbation of asthma, harm to pregnancy, impotence, infertility, and increased serum carbon monoxide levels; long-term risks of myocardial infarction and stroke, lung and other cancers, chronic obstructive pulmonary disease, long-term disability, and need for extended care; and environmental risks of increased risk of lung cancer, heart disease in spouses, higher rates of smoking by children of tobacco users, and increased risk for low birth weight, sudden infant death syndrome, asthma, middle ear disease, and respiratory infections in children of smokers.
Rewards	Ask the patient to identify potential benefits of quitting, such as improved health; food will taste better; improved sense of smell; save money; feel better about yourself; home, car, and clothing will smell better; can stop worrying about quitting; set a good example for children; have healthier babies and children; not worry about exposing others to smoke; feel better physically; perform better in physical activities; and reduced wrinkling/aging of skin.
Roadblocks	Ask the patient to identify barriers to quitting and note elements of treatment that could address those barriers. Typical barriers might include withdrawal symptoms, fear of failure, weight gain, lack of support, depression, and enjoyment of tobacco.
Repetition	Repeat the motivational intervention every time an unmotivated patient visits the clinical setting. Reassure tobacco users who have failed in previous quit attempts that most people must make repeated quit attempts before they are successful.

Adapted from: *U.S. Clinical Practice Guideline for Treating Tobacco Use and Dependence.*

Table 22-13 Benefits of Smoking Cessation

At 20 minutes after quitting	Blood pressure drops to a level close to that before the last cigarette. Temperature of hands and feet increases to normal.
8 hours after quitting	Blood levels of carbon monoxide level drop to normal.
24 hours after quitting	Chance of having a heart attack decreases.
2 weeks to 3 months after quitting	Circulation improves and lung function improves by as much as 30%.
1 to 9 months after quitting	Coughing, sinus congestion, fatigue, and shortness of breath decrease, and cilia regain normal function in the lungs, increasing the ability to handle mucus, clear the lungs, and reduce infection.
1 year after quitting	Excess risk of coronary heart disease is decreased to half that of a smoker.
5 years after quitting	Risk of stroke is reduced to that of a nonsmoker 5 to 15 years after quitting.
10 years after quitting	The lung cancer death rate is about half that of continuing smokers. The risk of cancer of the mouth, throat, esophagus, bladder, kidney, and pancreas is also lower than that of continuing smokers.
15 years after quitting	Risk of coronary heart disease is similar to that of a nonsmoker.

Adapted from: *The Health Consequences Of Smoking: A Report of the Surgeon General.*

There are no well-accepted algorithms to guide optimal selection among the first-line medications. The choice of a specific agent should be guided by clinician familiarity with the medications and patient factors, such as contraindications, preference, previous experience, and individual characteristics (e.g., depression or concerns about weight gain).

Use of a long-acting formulation of NRT (transdermal patch) or bupropion SR can be combined with a short-acting self-administered formulation of NRT such as gum, inhaler, or nasal spray for patients unable to quit using a single type of first-line pharmacotherapy. The nicotine lozenge has not been sufficiently studied as part of combination therapy. A disadvantage of combination therapy is the possibility of side effects such as nicotine toxicity and increased cost. Varenicline is not recommended for use in combination with NRT because of its nicotine antagonist properties.

Mechanism of Action

NRT medications work by replacing nicotine obtained from cigarettes to reduce the severity of nicotine withdrawal symptoms. When the physical withdrawal symptoms associated with quitting are diminished, individuals are able to focus on changing their smoking behaviors. As behaviors are changed, the strength of the various NRT products is gradually decreased over time until they are no longer needed.

Bupropion is believed to promote tobacco cessation by blocking neural reuptake of dopamine and norepinephrine and by blocking nicotinic acetylcholinergic receptors in the brain, thereby decreasing cravings and withdrawal symptoms. It also acts as an antidepressant, which is beneficial for tobacco users, who are more likely to have a history of depression than nonusers.

Varenicline is a selective $\alpha_4\beta_2$ nicotinic acetylcholine-receptor partial agonist. It has dual agonist and antagonist activities, resulting in the release of a lesser amount of dopamine than nicotine from the ventral tegmental area at the nucleus accumbens of the mesolimbic system of the brain; it also physically prevents nicotine from binding at the receptor site. These acetylcholine receptors are responsible for causing some of the pleasure/reward feelings associated with smoking. The inhibition of nicotine binding prevents activation of these receptors and helps take the pleasure out of smoking. Table 22-14 shows the product/formulation, dosing, and special instructions for the FDA-approved first-line medications for smoking cessation.

Interaction of Drugs with Foods and Laboratory Tests

Many clinically significant interactions between tobacco smoke and medications have been identified. Tobacco smoke interacts with medications through pharmacokinetic or pharmacodynamic mechanisms that may lead to reduced therapeutic efficacy or increased toxicity.

The polycyclic aromatic hydrocarbons in tobacco smoke are metabolic inducers of some isoforms of the hepatic cytochrome P450, primarily CYP1A2. Thus, when smokers quit and the P450 system returns to its basal level of functioning, the concentration of drugs metabolized by these particular CYP isoforms may increase. As a result, smokers who quit can experience side effects from supratherapeutic drug levels of certain drugs such as caffeine, theophylline, warfarin, fluvoxamine, olanzapine, and clozapine.

A significant pharmacodynamic interaction occurs with tobacco smoke and oral combined contraceptives. Research indicates that cigarette smoking substantially increases the risk of serious adverse cardiovascular events such as stroke, myocardial infarction, and thromboembolism in women using oral combined contraceptives. This risk is markedly increased in women who are aged 35 years or older and smoke 15 or more cigarettes per day. Accordingly, all oral combined contraceptives are contraindicated in this population and an alternative form of contraception should be used.

Nicotine is metabolized by CYP2A6, but does not appear to induce CYP enzymes. Thus, when a smoker switches from cigarettes to a nicotine replacement product, changes in drug metabolism are similar to those seen when quitting without NRT.

Nicotine produces sympathetic activation that may reduce the sedative effects of benzodiazepines. The vasoconstrictive effects of nicotine may decrease subcutaneous absorption of insulin. Nicotine also may attenuate the ability of beta blockers to lower blood pressure and heart rate, and may lessen opioid analgesia. When nicotine replacement products are withdrawn, adjustments in these types of medications may be necessary.

Bupropion and its metabolites inhibit CYP2D6 and could affect the impact of agents metabolized by this enzyme, such as tricyclic antidepressants, antipsychotics, type 1c antiarrhythmics, or certain beta blockers. Due to the extensive metabolism of bupropion, enzyme inducers such as carbamazepine, phenobarbital, and phenytoin and inhibitors such as valproate and cimetidine may alter its plasma concentration. Bupropion should be used with caution in conjunction with medications that can also lower seizure threshold. Specifically, use of bupropion within 14 days of discontinuation of therapy with any MAOI is contraindicated.

Varenicline is eliminated unchanged by kidney excretion and, therefore, is believed to pose no metabolic effects. No significant drug–drug interactions are known.

Contraindications, Warnings, and Precautions

All seven FDA-approved first-line medications for treatment of smoking cessation have specific contraindications, warnings, precautions, side effects, and other concerns, which are listed in Table 22-15.

1.3.0 Monitoring

Pharmacotherapeutic Outcomes

Tobacco dependence is a chronic disease that often requires repeated intervention and multiple attempts to quit tobacco use. It is essential that pharmacists consistently identify and document tobacco use status and attempt to treat every tobacco user. Clinicians should encourage every patient willing to make a quit attempt to use counseling and medications as recommended in the *U.S. Clinical Practice Guideline,* as these interventions are effective across a broad range of populations.

Safety and Efficacy Monitoring

First-line pharmacotherapies have been found to be safe and effective for tobacco dependence treatment. The relative safety of the tobacco dependence treatments versus the hazards of continued tobacco use is well established.

Adverse Drug Reactions

The adverse reactions to the seven FDA-approved first-line medications for treatment of smoking cessation are listed in Table 22-15.

Table 22-14 FDA-Approved Medications for Smoking Cessation

Product	Brand Name	Dosing	Special Instructions
Nicotine Polacrilex Gum, 2 mg, 4 mg OTC	Nicorette	25 or more cigarettes/day: 4 mg Fewer than 25 cigarettes/day: 2 mg Weeks 1–6: 1 piece a 1–2 hr Weeks 7–9: 1 piece q 2–4 hr Weeks 10–12: 1 piece q 4–8 hr	• Maximum: 24 pieces/day. • Chew each piece slowly. • Park between the cheek and gum when peppery or tingling sensation appears (15–30 chews). • Resume chewing when the taste or tingle fades. • Repeat the chew/park steps until most of the nicotine is gone (taste or tingle does not return; generally 30 minutes). • Park in different areas of the mouth. • Avoid food or beverages 15 minutes before or during use. • Duration: up to 12 weeks.
Nicotine Polacrilex Lozenge, 2 mg, 4 mg OTC	Commit	First cigarette ≤ 30 min after waking: 4 mg First cigarette > 30 min after waking: 2 mg Weeks 1–6: 1 lozenge q 1–2 hr Weeks 7–9: 1 lozenge q 2–4 hr Weeks 10–12: 1 lozenge q 4–8 hr	• Maximum: 20 lozenges/day. • Allow to dissolve slowly (20–30 minutes). • Nicotine release may cause a warm, tingling sensation. • Do not chew or swallow. • Occasionally rotate to different areas of the mouth. • Avoid food or beverages 15 minutes before or during use. • Duration: up to 12 weeks;
Nicotine Transdermal Patch, 7 mg, 14 mg, 21 mg OTC	NicoDerm CQ	10 or more cigarettes/day: 21 mg/day × 4–6 weeks, 14 mg/day × 2 weeks, 7 mg/day × 2 weeks Fewer than 10 cigarettes/day: 14 mg/day × 6 weeks 7 mg/day × 2 weeks	• May wear patch for 16 hours if the patient experiences sleep disturbances (remove at bedtime). • Duration: 8–10 weeks.
Nicotine Nasal Spray, 0.5 mg nicotine in 50 mcL aqueous nicotine solution Rx 10 mg/ml	Nicotrol NS	1–2 doses/hr (8–40 doses/day) One dose = 2 sprays (one in each nostril); each spray delivers 0.5 mg of nicotine to the nasal mucosa	• Maximum: 5 doses/hr or 40 doses/day. • For best results, initially use at least 8 doses/day. • Patients should not sniff, swallow, or inhale through the nose as the spray is being administered. • Duration: 3–6 months.
Nicotine Oral Inhaler, 10 mg cartridge (delivers 4 mg inhaled nicotine vapor) Rx	Nicotrol Inhaler	6–16 cartridges/day Individualize dosing; initially use 1 cartridge q 1–2 hr	• Best effects are achieved with continuous puffing for 20 minutes. • Initially use at least 6 cartridges/day. • Nicotine in cartridge is depleted after 20 minutes of active puffing. • Patient should inhale into the back of the throat or puff in short breaths. • Do *not* inhale into the lungs (like a cigarette) but "puff" as if lighting a pipe. • Open cartridge retains potency for 24 hours. • Duration: 3–6 months.

Table 22-14 (*continued*)

Product	Brand Name	Dosing	Special Instructions
Bupropion SR, 150 mg sustained-release tablet Rx	Zyban	150 mg po q AM × 3 days, then 150 mg po bid	• Do not exceed 300 mg/day. • Patients should begin therapy 1–2 weeks prior to the anticipated quit date. • Allow at least 8 hours between doses. • Avoid bedtime dosing to minimize insomnia. • Dose tapering is not necessary. • Can be used safely with nicotine replacement therapy. • Duration: 7–12 weeks, with maintenance up to 6 months in selected patients.
Varenicline, 0.5 mg, 1 mg tablet Rx	Chantix	Days 1–3: 0.5 mg po q AM Days 4–7: 0.5 mg po bid Weeks 2–12: 1 mg po bid	• Begin therapy 1 week prior to the anticipated quit date. • Take the dose after eating with a full glass of water. • Dose tapering is not necessary. • Nausea and insomnia are side effects that are usually temporary. • Duration: 12 weeks; an additional 12-week course may be used in selected patients.

AM = every morning; q = every; bid = twice daily; po = orally.

Nonadherence, Misuse, or Abuse

Adherence to treatment—both medication and counseling—is important for optimal outcomes. Patients frequently do not use cessation medications as recommended; for example, they do not use them at recommended doses or for recommended durations, which may reduce these medications' effectiveness.

Tobacco dependence medications may be used on a long-term basis, up to 6 months. This approach may be helpful with smokers who report persistent withdrawal symptoms during the course of medications, who have relapsed in the past after stopping medication, or who desire long-term therapy. A minority of individuals who successfully quit smoking use as-needed NRT medications (gum, lozenge, nasal spray, inhaler) on a long-term basis. The use of these medications for up to 6 months does not present a known health risk, and developing dependence on medications is uncommon. Additionally, the FDA has approved the use of bupropion SR, varenicline, and some NRT medications for 6-month use

Pharmacotherapeutic Alternatives

There is a strong correlation between the number of sessions of counseling when combined with medication and the likelihood of successful smoking cessation. Therefore, multiple counseling sessions in addition to medication are recommended, if possible.

Two types of counseling and behavioral therapies result in higher abstinence rates: (1) providing smokers with practical counseling (problem-solving skills/skills training) and (2) providing support and encouragement as part of treatment. These types of counseling elements should be included in smoking cessation interventions.

The best philosophy for preparing individuals to quit tobacco use is to offer an assortment of tools, techniques, and strategies in helping them individually tailor a quit plan. Behavioral strategies involve specific actions that the patient can take to disrupt habits or situations associated with tobacco use over the period leading up to and immediately following the quit date. Cognitive strategies focus on retraining the way a patient thinks and may include review of commitment to quit, distractive thinking, positive self-talks, relaxation through imagery, and mental rehearsal and visualization. Patients who receive social support and encouragement are more successful in quitting and should be encouraged to seek support from family, friends, and coworkers. The decision to use tobacco is prompted by internal cues such as anger, boredom, and stress, and by external cues such as time of day, certain people, places, or situations. If a patient can learn which feelings and situations trigger tobacco use, methods can be developed to alter routines.

Pharmacists can take advantage of telephone quitlines by implementing referral systems for patients identified as tobacco users. Telephone quitlines have

Table 22-15 Precautions, Adverse Effects, and Advantages and Disadvantages of FDA-Approved Medications for Smoking Cessation

Product	Precautions	Adverse Effects	Advantages	Disadvantages
Nicotine Polacrilex gum	• Recent (≤ 2 weeks) myocardial infarction • Serious underlying arrhythmias • Serious or worsening angina pectoris • Temporomandibular joint disease • Pregnancy (category D) and breastfeeding • Adolescents (< 18 years)	• Mouth/jaw soreness • Hiccups • Dyspepsia • Hypersalivation • Effects associated with incorrect chewing technique: lightheadedness, nausea/vomiting, throat and mouth irritation	• Might satisfy oral cravings. • Might delay weight gain. • Patients can titrate therapy to manage withdrawal symptoms. • Variety of flavors are available.	• Need for frequent dosing can compromise compliance. • Might be problematic for patients with significant dental work. • Patients must use proper chewing technique to minimize adverse effects. • Gum chewing may not be socially acceptable.
Nicotine Polacrilex lozenge	• Recent (≤ 2 weeks) myocardial infarction • Serious underlying arrhythmias • Serious or worsening angina pectoris • Pregnancy (category not assigned) and breastfeeding • Adolescents (< 18 years)	• Nausea • Hiccups • Cough • Heartburn • Headache • Flatulence • Insomnia	• Might satisfy oral cravings. • Might delay weight gain. • Easy to use and conceal. • Patients can titrate therapy to manage withdrawal symptoms. • Variety of flavors are available.	• Need for frequent dosing can compromise compliance. • Gastrointestinal side effects (nausea, hiccups, heartburn) might be bothersome.
Nicotine transde-rmal patch	• Recent (≤ 2 weeks) myocardial infarction • Serious underlying arrhythmias • Serious or worsening angina pectoris • Pregnancy (category D) and breastfeeding • Adolescents (< 18 years)	• Local skin reactions (erythema, pruritus, burning) • Headache • Sleep disturbances (insomnia, abnormal/vivid dreams); associated with nocturnal nicotine absorption	• Provides consistent nicotine levels over 24 hours. • Easy to use and conceal. • Once-daily dosing associated with fewer compliance problems.	• Patients cannot titrate the dose to acutely manage withdrawal symptoms. • Allergic reactions to adhesive might occur. • Patients with dermatologic conditions should not use the patch.
Nicotine nasal spray	• Recent (≤ 2 weeks) myocardial infarction • Serious underlying arrhythmias • Serious or worsening angina pectoris • Underlying chronic nasal disorders (rhinitis, nasal polyps, sinusitis) • Pregnancy (category D) and breastfeeding • Adolescents (< 18 years)	• Nasal and/or throat irritation (hot, peppery, or burning sensation) • Rhinitis • Tearing • Sneezing • Cough • Headache	• Patients can titrate therapy to rapidly manage withdrawal symptoms. • Mimics hand-to-mouth ritual of smoking (could also be perceived as a disadvantage).	• Need for frequent dosing can compromise compliance. • Nasal/throat irritation may be bothersome. • Patients must wait 5 minutes before driving or operating heavy machinery. • Patients with chronic nasal disorders or severe reactive airway disease should not use the spray.

Table 22-15 (*continued*)

Product	Precautions	Adverse Effects	Advantages	Disadvantages
Nicotine oral inhaler *(cont'd)*	• Recent (≤ 2 weeks) myocardial infarction • Serious underlying arrhythmias • Serious or worsening angina pectoris • Bronchospastic disease • Pregnancy (category D) and breastfeeding • Adolescents (< 18 years)	• Mouth and/or throat irritation • Cough • Headache • Rhinitis • Dyspepsia • Hiccups	• Patients can titrate therapy to rapidly manage withdrawal symptoms. • Mimics hand-to-mouth ritual of smoking (could also be perceived as a disadvantage).	• Need for frequent dosing can compromise compliance. • Initial throat or mouth irritation can be bothersome. • Cartridges should not be stored in very warm conditions or used in very cold conditions. • Patients with underlying bronchospastic disease must use with caution.
Bupropion SR tablet	• Concomitant therapy with medications or medical conditions known to lower the seizure threshold • Severe hepatic cirrhosis • Pregnancy (category C) and breastfeeding • Adolescents (< 18 years) Warnings: • "Black box" warning for neuropsychiatric symptoms Contraindications: • Seizure disorder • Concomitant bupropion (e.g., Wellbutrin) therapy • Current or prior diagnosis of bulimia or anorexia nervosa • Simultaneous abrupt discontinuation of alcohol or sedatives/benzodiazepines • MAOI therapy in previous 14 days	• Insomnia • Dry mouth • Nervous/difficulty concentrating • Rash • Constipation • Seizures	• Easy to use; oral formulation might be associated with fewer compliance problems. • Might delay weight gain. • Can be used with NRT. • Might be beneficial in patients with depression.	• Seizure risk is increased. • Several contraindications and precautions preclude use in some patients.
Varenicline tablet	• Severe renal impairment (dosage adjustment is necessary) • Pregnancy (category C) and breast feeding • Adolescents (< 18 years) Warnings: • "Black box" warning for neuropsychiatric symptoms • Safety and efficacy have not been established in patients with serious psychiatric illness	• Nausea • Sleep disturbances (insomnia, abnormal/vivid dreams) • Constipation • Flatulence • Vomiting • Neuropsychiatric symptoms: behavior change, hostility, agitation, depression, suicidality, and worsening of preexisting psychiatric illness	• Easy to use; oral formulation might be associated with fewer compliance problems. • Offers a new mechanism of action for patients who have failed other agents.	• May induce nausea in up to one-third of patients. • Postmarketing surveillance data indicate potential for neuropsychiatric symptoms.

Table 22-16 Pharmacokinetic Properties of Smoking and Smoking Deterrents

Drug	Bioavailability (%)	Half-life (hours)	Peak Plasma Level (ng/mL)	Time to Peak Levels (hours)
Smoking	NA	15–20 (cotinine)	44	No data
Nicotine Polacrilex gum	Depends on pH of mouth and chewing	3–4	5–10	0.25–0.5
Nicotine lozenge	Depends on pH of mouth and dissolution	3–4	5–10	0.25–0.5
Nicotine patch	68	3–4	5–17	2–12
Nicotine oral inhaler	< 5	No data	6	0.25
Nicotine nasal spray	53	1–2	12	0.25
Bupropion SR	No data	21	91–143	3
Varenicline	100	24	No data	3–4

been shown to significantly increase abstinence rates in those who use them. The Internet is another resource that pharmacists can utilize for patients seeking help in quitting. There are numerous websites that individuals can access for basic information or assistance in developing a quit plan. The advantages of off-site programs include around-the-clock availability and access from home.

ANNOTATED BIBLIOGRAPHY

1. U.S. Department of Health and Human Services. *The Health Consequences of Smoking: A Report of the Surgeon General.* Atlanta, GA: U.S. Department of Health and Human Services, Public Health Service, Centers for Disease Control and Prevention, National Center for Chronic Disease Prevention and Health Promotion, Office on Smoking and Health; 2004.
2. Centers for Disease Control and Prevention. *Best Practices for Comprehensive Tobacco Control Programs—2007.* 2007.
3. Centers for Disease Control and Prevention. Cigarette smoking among adults—United States, 2006. *Morbid Mortal Weekly Rep* 2007;56:1157–1161.
4. Fiore MC, Jaen CR, Baker TB, et.al. *Treating Tobacco Use and Dependence: 2008 Update. Clinical Practice Guideline.* Rockville, MD: Department of Health and Human Services, Public Health Service; 2008.
5. Smoking deterrents: drug facts and comparisons 4.0. Wolters Kluwer Health Inc.; 2007. Available at: http://online.factsandcomparison.com/index.aspx. Accessed February 26, 2010.
6. Fiore MC, Novotny TE, Pierce JP, et al. Methods used to quit smoking in the United States. Do cessation programs help? *JAMA* 1990;263:2760–2765.

Renal Disorders

CHAPTER

23

TOPIC: ASSESSMENT OF RENAL DISORDERS

Contributor: Bradley W. Shinn

Introduction

Because many of the drugs that pharmacists recommend are eliminated from the body primarily by renal mechanisms, it is critical for pharmacists to understand how to estimate a patient's renal function and adjust drug doses appropriately. Patients with compromised renal function who receive "usual" doses of renally eliminated medications risk suffering significant drug toxicities. Several methods of estimating a patient's renal function, or glomerular filtration rate (GFR), exist, but all of them primarily rely on measurement of the serum creatinine (SCr) concentration. It is important to understand that no method of estimating a patient's renal function is completely accurate; therefore, the pharmacist practitioner must become familiar with clinical situations in which renal elimination equations are less reliable if medications are to be dosed effectively and safely in patients with renal dysfunction. Even if a renal function estimation equation is correctly calculated, if it is used in an inappropriate clinical situation, erroneous dosage adjustment decisions may be made. In many clinical settings, pharmacists are given the primary responsibility for adjusting drug doses in patients with renal dysfunction. Thus, it is critical for pharmacists to fully understand and to correctly interpret renal function estimation methods.

Tips Worth Tweeting

- The nephron is the functional unit of the kidney and produces urine via processes of filtration, active and passive reabsorption, and active secretion.
- The rate of excretion of a substance through the kidney is calculated as follows: [rate of filtration + rate of secretion] – [rate of reabsorption].
- The blood urea nitrogen (BUN) is not a very good measure of renal function because the reabsorption rate is variable and dependent on the degree of water reabsorption.
- Because creatinine (a waste product of muscle metabolism) is completely filtered, very minimally secreted, and not reabsorbed, the serum creatinine concentration (SCr) is a much more accurate indication of renal function (creatinine clearance [CrCl]) and drug clearance than is the BUN.
- In general, the rate of creatinine production equals its rate of excretion; therefore the SCr concentration shows very little day-to-day variation in persons with healthy kidneys.
- A "normal" SCr does *not* necessarily indicate a "normal" CrCl.
- Many clinical factors may cause the commonly utilized renal function estimation equations to either overestimate or underestimate a patient's true renal function.
- The most commonly utilized method to estimate a patient's renal function for the purposes of drug dosing is the Cockcroft-Gault

(C-G) equation, which incorporates a patient's age, body weight, and SCr concentration.

- A newer renal function estimation method—the modification of diet in renal disease (MDRD) equation—has been proposed as a method that is more accurate than the C-G equation.
- It is possible to measure a patient's CrCl by performing a 12- or 24-hour urine creatinine collection; however, this method is labor intensive, time consuming, expensive, and subject to collection errors.
- The urinalysis (U/A) is a convenient, commonly ordered test that can aid in the diagnosis of a wide variety of disorders in both outpatient and inpatient settings.

Patient Care Scenario: Hospital Pharmacy

A. B.: 77 yo, 5'4", 50 110 lbs, F, Caucasian
HPI: Admitted directly to general medicine service from nursing home with acute mental status changes, two vomiting episodes, and a suspected urinary tract infection.
Allergies: NKDA.
PMH: Type 2 diabetes mellitus, HTN, osteoporosis, stage III COPD.
Social Hx: Resident of nursing home. Approximately 50-year smoking history; quit 10 years ago when COPD worsened. No current alcohol use.
ROS/PE: Slight fever, occasional chills. Costovertebral angle (CVA) tenderness and flank pain.
Vitals: BP = 115/70; P = 104; RR = 22; T = 99.1°F
Lab Values:

Na: 146 mEq/L	Hgb: 11.6 g/dL
K: 4.3 mEq/L	Hct: 35%
Cl: 110 mEq/L	Platelets: 150 × 10^3/mcL
CO_2: 28 mEq/L	WBCs: 16.1 × 10^3/mcL
BUN: 25 mg/dL	Protein: 5.7 g/dL
SCr : 0.7 mg/dL	Albumin: 2.5 g/dL
Glu: 160 mg/dL	Hemoglobin A_{1c}: 8.6%

Urinalysis: Macroscopic: cloudy. Microscopic/Biochemical: WBCs > 5–10/hpf, bacteria > 100 cfu/mL, (+) red blood cells, 2+ protein, (+) nitrite, (+) leukocyte esterase.

Hospital Medication Profile

Drug	Route	Sig
Lisinopril 20 mg	PO	Once daily
Metformin 500 mg	PO	bid (with breakfast and dinner)
Byetta 10 mcg	SQ	bid (30 minutes before breakfast and dinner)
Flovent HFA 220 mcg	INH	bid
DuoNeb	Nebulizer	q 4–6 hr prn (SOB, bronchospasm)
Theophylline 300 mg	PO	q 12 hr
Levofloxacin 500 mg	IVPB	q 24 hr
Calcium 500 mg	PO	bid (with meals)
Heparin 5,000 units	SQ	q 8 hr
Tylenol 325–650 mg	PO	q 4–6 hr prn (pain, fever)
Lorazepam 1–2 mg	IVP	q 4–6 hr prn (anxiety, agitation)
Regular insulin: per sliding scale	SQ	AC and HS

1.1.0 Patient Information

Background

Generally, medications that are renally eliminated have fairly precise guidelines as to how they should be dosed in patients with varying degrees of renal dysfunction. These guidelines are usually noted in FDA-approved prescribing information and are based on an estimation of the patient's renal function, or glomerular filtration rate (GFR). The parameter estimated is commonly referred to as the creatinine clearance (CrCl) because it is the patient's serum creatinine (SCr) concentration on which this estimation is usually based. Published guidelines most commonly recommend that, as a patient's renal function worsens, the dosage interval be lengthened so that the drug is dosed less frequently. This is based on the fact that a drug's elimination half-life increases as a patient's renal function declines; it is primarily the half-life that determines a drug's recommended dosing interval. In many cases, a lower dose of the drug may also be recommended, although this is not true for all drugs. An example of recommended dosage adjustment guidelines for the antibiotic levofloxacin is shown in Table 23-1.

Renal Assessment Instruments

The real challenge for the clinical pharmacist practitioner is to accurately estimate the patient's renal function so that the published dosing guideline is properly used to adjust the patient's drug dose. The two most commonly used laboratory parameters to assess a patient's renal function are the blood urea nitrogen (BUN) and SCr concentrations. Both of these laboratory tests are part of a basic metabolic panel, which means they are easily obtained and readily available.

Table 23-1 Recommended Dosage Guidelines for Levofloxacin

Dosage in Normal Renal Function Every 24 Hours	Creatinine Clearance: 20–49 mL/min	Creatinine Clearance: 10–19 mL/min	Hemodialysis or Continuous Ambulatory Peritoneal Dialysis (CAPD)
750 mg	750 mg every 48 hours	750 mg initial dose, then 500 mg every 48 hours	750 mg initial dose, then 500 mg every 48 hours
500 mg	500 mg initial dose, then 250 mg every 24 hours	500 mg initial dose, then 250 mg every 48 hours	500 mg initial dose, then 250 mg every 48 hours
250 mg	No dosage adjustment required	250 mg every 48 hours	No information available

Term	Definition
Glomerular filtration rate (GFR)	The volume of fluid filtered from the renal glomerular capillaries into the Bowman's capsule per unit time.
Azotemia	A higher than normal concentration of blood urea nitrogen (BUN).
Prerenal azotemia	An elevated BUN due to extrarenal causes that reduce renal blood flow and GFR.
Hyponatremia	A decreased serum sodium concentration.
Anuria	The complete suppression of urine formation and excretion (less than 50 mL/day).
Oliguria	A diminished urine production and excretion in relation to fluid intake (50-400 mL/day).
Urinary casts	Cylindrical masses of glycoproteins that form in the renal tubules in many pathologic conditions.
Bacteriuria	The presence of bacteria in the urine.
Hematuria	The presence of red blood cells in the urine.
Proteinuria	The presence of protein in the urine.
Pyuria	The presence of white blood cells in the urine.

Table 23-2 Factors Affecting BUN Concentration

Increased BUN (Azotemia)	Decreased BUN
Renal dysfunction	Liver disease
High protein intake	Malnutrition especially an insufficient dietary protein intake
Upper GI bleed	Decreased muscle mass (emaciated state)
Intravascular fluid depletion/dehydration	Overhydration from IV fluids
Heart failure	

BUN is produced in the liver via the urea cycle and is a waste product of the digestion of proteins. Although it does increase in a patient with renal dysfunction, this marker is not an ideal measure of a patient's GFR because the serum concentration depends on many factors other than renal function. The reabsorption rate of BUN in the renal tubules is quite variable and depends, to a great extent, on the amount of water reabsorbed in the kidney. Thus the reabsorption of BUN in the kidney will be increased in any clinical situation in which the kidney is stimulated to increase water reabsorption, such as dehydration. The BUN concentration also depends on the rate of production of urea in the liver as well as the amount of protein breakdown in the body. The BUN concentration is most clinically useful when it is interpreted in conjunction with the patient's SCr concentration. For example, a BUN/SCr ratio that is greater than 20:1 is consistent with a patient who has intravascular fluid depletion with decreased renal perfusion (prerenal azotemia).

Many factors may affect a patient's BUN concentration (normal = 8–20 mg/dL), as outlined in Table 23-2.

Because creatinine, which is a breakdown product of muscle metabolism, is completely filtered, very minimally secreted, and not reabsorbed, it is a much more accurate indication of a patient's renal function than is the BUN. The normal range for the SCr concentration is 0.7–1.3 mg/dL, with a mean value of 1 mg/dL. Commonly used estimations of renal function, which form the basis for most pharmacokinetic and drug-dosing recommendations, use the SCr as the primary parameter for estimating a patient's GFR. It is critical for pharmacists to understand how the SCr is evaluated and how to properly use CrCl estimation equations to make appropriate dosing decisions. To understand how to best use and interpret CrCl equations, it is important to note the following points about the pharmacokinetics of creatinine in the body:

- The daily production of creatinine remains relatively stable if muscle mass does not change substantially.
- In normal patients, the daily rate of creatinine production equals the daily rate of its excretion; therefore, the SCr concentration varies little from day to day in a patient with healthy kidneys.
- As patients age, their muscle mass (i.e., rate of creatinine production) and renal function (i.e., rate

of creatinine excretion) decline in similar ratios. Thus the SCr concentration remains relatively constant even though renal function declines as patients age.

- The time for the serum creatinine concentration to reach 95% of steady state in patients with 10% of normal renal function is approximately 4 days; therefore, when a patient develops acute renal failure, the SCr will not fully reflect the functional disability for several days.
- Unlike the BUN, an elevated SCr almost always indicates worsening renal function. The SCr concentration is not significantly influenced by changes in diet, hydration status, or urine flow.
- Some tubular secretion of creatinine does occur (approximately 10% with normal renal function):
  - Tubular secretion of creatinine may lead to slight overestimation of GFR; however, this is clinically insignificant in most patients with moderate to normal renal function.
  - As renal function declines, proportionally more secretion occurs compared to the filtration rate; thus the SCr becomes a less reliable indicator of GFR as the renal function worsens. Most estimation equations tend to overestimate a patient's' GFR as renal function declines.
  - Several drugs inhibit the tubular secretion of creatinine, which leads to an elevated SCr concentration that is not due to a decreased GFR. This factor leads to an underestimation of renal function when using SCr-based estimation equations. These drugs include the following agents:
    - Aspirin
    - Cimetidine
    - Methyldopa
    - Probenecid
    - Potassium-sparing diuretics (spironolactone, amiloride, triamterene)
    - Pyrimethamine
    - Trimethoprim (an ingredient in Bactrim)
    - Some cephalosporins

Urinalysis

The urinalysis (U/A) is a convenient, commonly ordered test that can aid in the diagnosis and evaluation of a wide variety of disorders, both renal and nonrenal. For this test to be most useful, it is important to ensure a clean, midstream urine collection, which is often referred to as a "clean catch." The U/A consists of three different types of tests: macroscopic, microscopic, and biochemical.

Table 23-3 Drugs That Alter Urine Color

Urine Color	Implicated Drugs
Red to orange	Rifampin, phenazopyridine, daunorubicin, doxorubicin, phenolphthalein, phenothiazines, chlorzoxazone
Blue to green	Amitriptyline, methylene blue, Clorets abuse, mitoxantrone, triamterene, resorcinol
Brown to black	Cascara, chloroquine, clofazimine, senna, methocarbamol, metronidazole, nitrofurantoin, sulfonamides

Macroscopic analysis is done by looking at the urine sample and consists of examining the color and character (e.g., clear, turbid, foamy) of the urine. The color of normal urine varies greatly depending on the concentration of solutes, with a darker yellow, or even amber, color being associated with more concentrated urine. A urine sample may also be red to orange, or even black, in some pathologic conditions. Several drugs can also cause the urine to take on characteristic colors.

Normal fresh urine should not be hazy or cloudy. However, urine may appear turbid, or cloudy, if large numbers of red blood cells or white blood cells are present (as may occur in a urinary tract infection). An unusual amount of foaming in the urine is associated with large amounts of protein in the urine.

Microscopic analysis involves examining a centrifuged sample of urine under 400–455 × magnification, which is commonly described as a high power field (hpf). Some laboratories perform a microscopic analysis selectively, based on the results of the macroscopic and biochemical screenings. Three important components may be found during a microscopic analysis of the urine: cells, casts, and crystals.

Biochemical analyses of the urine include a group of semi-quantitative tests performed quickly using dipsticks containing reagent-impregnated pads. Commonly reported results include protein, pH, specific gravity, bilirubin, bile, urobilinogen, blood, hemoglobin, leukocyte esterase, nitrite, glucose, and ketones. Monitoring for the presence of protein in the urine (proteinuria) is recommended for several disease states, including diabetes mellitus and chronic kidney disease. Common causes are noted in Table 23-5.

pH

Because it generally reflects the ability of the kidneys to regulate blood pH, the pH of the urine can vary widely under normal circumstances (4.5–8), although the average urine pH is approximately 6. An alkaline pH may be associated with infection secondary to

Table 23-4 Etiologies of Microscopic Urinalysis Findings

Microscopic U/A Finding	Possible Etiology
Microorganisms Significant bacteriuria: $\geq$ 100,000 cfu/mL (cfu = colony-forming units)	Urinary tract colonization Urinary tract infection (UTI)
Red blood cells (RBCs) Hematuria Gross hematuria: urine is red or pink	Glomerulonephritis Infection (e.g., pyelonephritis) Renal infarction/papillary necrosis Tumors Stones Coagulopathies
White blood cells (WBCs) Pyuria	Bacterial UTI General inflammation of the urinary tract (e.g., interstitial nephritis)
Tubular epithelial cells	Acute tubular necrosis (ATN) Nephrotic syndrome
Hyaline casts (clear)	Concentrated urine Prerenal condition (e.g., CHF, dehydration) Strenuous exercise Not indicative of intrinsic renal disease
Cellular casts (cells in casts originate from within the kidney)	Intrinsic renal disease RBC casts: glomerulonephritis, ischemic injury to the kidney WBC casts: intrarenal inflammation, upper UTI Epithelial cell casts: tubular destruction
Granular ("muddy brown") casts (older, degenerated form of other casts)	ATN: usually associated with renal damage secondary to ischemic or toxic insults (e.g., shock, sepsis, liver failure, aminoglycoside toxicity, contrast media toxicity)
Urate crystals	Uric acid uropathy
Phosphate crystals	UTIs due to urea-splitting bacteria (e.g., *Proteus*) Persistently alkaline urine

a urea-splitting organism (e.g., *Proteus mirabilis*), renal tubular acidosis (RTA), or several drugs (e.g., acetazolamide, bicarbonate or acetate salts, thiazide diuretics). Highly acidic urine usually reflects the presence of a metabolic acidosis (e.g. diabetic ketoacidosis or lactic acidosis), or the use of certain drugs (e.g., ammonium chloride, high-dose ascorbic acid).

Table 23-5 Causes of Proteinuria

Minor Proteinuria (< 0.5 g/day)
Hemoglobinuria (hemolysis)
High blood pressure
Lower UTI
Renal tubular damage
Fever
Exercise
Moderate Proteinuria (0.5–3 g/day)
Diabetic nephropathy (may be major in severe cases)
Glomerulonephritis (may be major in severe cases)
CHF (usually severe)
Pyelonephritis
Preeclampsia of pregnancy
Multiple myeloma (high globulins)
Major Proteinuria (> 3 g/day)
Membranous glomerulonephritis
Focal glomerulosclerosis (AIDS or heroin abuse)
Minimal change disease
Lupus nephritis
Amyloidosis

Specific Gravity

An elevated specific gravity (normal: 1.01–1.025) is associated with a concentrated urine, SIADH, or exogenous agents in the urine (e.g., toxins, drugs). A low specific gravity (SG) suggests very dilute urine, such as occurs in a patient with diabetes insipidus. The urinary SG should be considered abnormal if it is the opposite of what one would expect given the patient's clinical condition.

Urinary Bilirubin

Urinary bilirubin, which may turn the urine dark yellow or brown, may occur in patients with liver disease or internal bleeding. Urobilinogen, which is formed in the intestine by bacterial conversion of conjugated bilirubin, increases in the urine when the turnover of heme pigments is abnormally rapid (e.g., hemolytic anemia, viral hepatitis, drug-induced hepatotoxicity).

Blood/Hemoglobin

Blood and/or hemoglobin (consistent with lysed red blood cells) may be present when the urinary tract is damaged or red blood cell hemolysis is present. Due to structural similarities, the test for hemoglobin may also be positive when significant myoglobin is found in the urine, which may occur with muscle trauma, infarction, or significant infection.

Leukocyte Esterase

Leukocyte esterase (LE) indicates the presence of white blood cells in the urine and is consistent with presence of a urinary tract infection. This test is commonly used in the office or clinic setting to help determine whether empiric antimicrobial therapy should be initiated.

Nitrite

The nitrite test is positive if an infection is present secondary to the presence of a gram-negative bacterial organism. A positive nitrite test is often associated with a positive LE test in a patient with a urinary tract infection. However, the nitrite test may also be negative in a patient with a urinary tract infection if the UTI is caused by a bacterium that is unable to reduce nitrates to nitrites (e.g., gram-positive bacteria).

Urinary Electrolytes

Tests for urinary electrolytes are obtained much less commonly than are urinalyses and are rarely definitive for any diagnosis. These tests must be interpreted in context of the clinical situation, serum electrolyte concentrations, and dietary intake. Although urinary potassium and chloride are occasionally evaluated, sodium is the urinary electrolyte that is most commonly ordered and clinically useful. The primary clinical utility of a urinary sodium concentration is to assist in the differential diagnosis of volume depletion, acute oliguria, and hyponatremia, and may be interpreted as shown in Table 23-6.

Because diuretic therapy inhibits the body's ability to retain sodium and increases the loss of sodium in the urine, this test may be useful to monitor a patient's compliance with a diuretic regimen. Compliant patients should have a sodium concentration in the range of 1–20 mEq/L in their urine. Another test, the percent fractional excretion of sodium (%FE_{Na}), is occasionally ordered in a patient who develops acute azotemia or oliguria to help distinguish prerenal (e.g., dehydration, CHF) from intrarenal causes (e.g., ATN). If the result is less than 1%, the cause is probably prerenal; if it is greater than 1–2%, the patient probably has acute tubular necrosis.

Table 23-6 Interpretation of Urinary Electrolytes Findings

Medical Problem	Urinary Sodium Value → Likely Diagnosis
Volume depletion	0–10 mEq/L → Extrarenal sodium loss
	> 10 mEq/L → Renal sodium wasting or adrenal insufficiency
Acute oliguria	0–10 mEq/L → Prerenal azotemia
	> 30 mEq/L → Acute tubular necrosis
Hyponatremia	0–10 mEq/L → Volume depletion or edematous disease
	Greater than dietary intake → SIADH or adrenal insufficiency

2.1.0 Calculations

The Cockcroft-Gault Equation

Many equations are available to estimate a patient's renal function based on a SCr determination. Historically, the most commonly used equation in clinical practice has been the Cockcroft-Gault (C-G) equation, which was first published in 1976 (Cockcroft and Gault, 1976). The C-G equation is very easy to calculate, has been successfully used for many years, and is the equation on which most dosing recommendations are based. Unfortunately, this equation is less accurate in some clinical situations. Thus, pharmacists must recognize both those situations in which the C-G equation is generally reliable as well as those in which it is less reliable.

The original C-G equation was based on a population of patients who were relatively "normally proportioned" for their age and who had stable renal function. Thus, this equation is most accurate in patients who meet these criteria and is less clinically useful in patients who are very overweight or underweight, who have a reduced muscle mass *for their age*, and who have a SCr concentration that is changing rapidly (i.e., not at steady state). It is often stated that the C-G equation is less accurate in patients who are older than 65 years. Because age is one of the parameters included in the equation, it is not necessarily true that this equation is less reliable in older patients. However, if the patient has a reduced muscle mass compared to normal patients of the same age, or is very underweight or overweight, the equation will not provide an accurate reflection of the patient's actual GFR. The CrCl is calculated via the C-G equation as follows:

$$\text{CrCl(mL/min)} = \frac{[(140\text{-age}) \times (\text{IBW})\ (\times 0.85 \text{ if female})]}{\text{SCr} \times 72}$$

The original C-G equation recommended using a patient's actual body weight (ABW) in this equation. However, subsequent studies have generally demonstrated that using a patient's ideal body weight (IBW) is more accurate, especially for patients who are more than 30% above their IBW. Thus, the recommended clinical practice is to use a patient's IBW if the ABW is greater

Table 23-7 Factors Affecting Estimation of Renal Function

Overestimation of CrCl	Underestimation of CrCl
Secretion of creatinine in renal tubules—this effect is greater as the SCr increases	Concurrent use of inhibitors of creatinine secretion in renal tubules
Decreased muscle mass or activity level (for a given age)	Acute muscle damage or unusually elevated muscle metabolism
Decreased dietary protein intake (e.g., vegetarians)	Rapidly decreasing SCr concentration (SCr not at a steady state)
Significant liver dysfunction/cirrhosis	
Rapidly increasing SCr concentration (SCr not at a steady state)	

than the IBW, and to use the ABW if it is less than a patient's IBW. It should be appreciated, however, that the C-G equation is a less reliable indicator of a patient's renal function if that individual's ABW varies significantly from his or her IBW (either above or below). Several other clinical factors may lead to either an overestimation or underestimation of a patient's renal function using the C-G equation, as described in Table 23-7.

A common problem with use of the C-G equation in clinical practice occurs in patients who have a decreased muscle mass compared to other patients of a similar age. This factor should be suspected to play a role in very old patients, emaciated patients, patients who are bedridden, and patients whose ABW is less than their IBW. These patients often demonstrate a SCr concentration that is very low (0.3–0.6 mg/dL). If these very low SCr values are used in the C-G equation, the calculated CrCl will be inappropriately high. Many clinicians choose to use a SCr of 1.0 mg/dL in the C-G equation in these situations; however, it has also been suggested that this practice may lead to an underestimation of renal function in many patients. More importantly, it should be understood that the C-G equation is less reliable in these patients and it is not possible to know precisely what a patient's SCr would be if a normal muscle mass were present.

A "normal" CrCl for a male is 120–140 mL/min; for a female, it is 100–120 mL/min. These values hold until about the age of 40 years, after which the CrCl decreases by approximately 1 mL/min/year. This method may provide a reasonable estimation of renal function for patients in whom a SCr determination is not available and/or in those patients for whom the use of an estimation equation may be unreliable.

The MDRD Equation

More recently, a new equation has been proposed to estimate a patient's renal function in the clinical setting (Coresh J, Astor BC, McQuillan G, et al., 1999). This equation is based on a multiple regression analysis of data obtained from the Modification of Diet in Renal Disease (MDRD) Study, which evaluated the effect of dietary protein restriction and strict blood pressure control on the progression of renal disease. The original equation included six variables; however, a modified four-variable equation seems to perform as well as the original equation and is now the version most commonly used. In the patient population studied, who had a mean CrCl of approximately 40 mL/min, the MDRD equation provided a more precise estimate of GFR than did either the measured CrCl or a value calculated via the C-G equation. The MDRD equation is believed to underestimate a patient's GFR, especially at higher values.

In 2009, the Chronic Kidney Disease Epidemiology Collaboration (CKD-EPI) equation was proposed as a more precise and accurate replacement for the MDRD equation, especially at higher GFRs. Using this new equation could potentially decrease false-positive results—that is, the mislabeling of people with a high GFR as having poor kidney function (Levey AS, Stevens LA, Schmid CH, et al., 2009). The MDRD (four-variable) equation is calculated as follows:

$$\text{GFR} = 186 \times [\text{Scr}]^{-1.154} \times [\text{age}]^{-0.203} \times [0.742 \text{ if female}] \times [1.212 \text{ if African American}]$$

Automatic calculators for both the MDRD and CKD-EPI equations can be found at www.nephron.org/MDRD_GFR.cgi.

It should be noted that neither the MDRD equation nor the CKD-EPI equation was originally developed for the purpose of making drug dosage adjustments. Furthermore, most recommendations for drug dosage adjustments in the FDA-approved labeling are based on the C-G equation. As a consequence, many practicing pharmacists continue to use the C-G equation for adjusting drug doses in renally impaired patients and have questioned whether the MDRD equation should be used for this purpose (Jennings S, de Lemos ML, Levin A, et al., 2008; Greenberg E, Saad N, Abraham T, Balmir E, 2009; Moranville MP and Jennings HR, 2009). It should also be noted that because both the MDRD and CKD-EPI equations rely on the SCr as the primary indicator of GFR, both are subject to the same factors that can lead to either an overestimation or underestimation of renal function as noted in the C-G equation discussion (e.g., reduced muscle mass, SCr concentration not at a steady state). Regardless of which method is used, it is important that the practicing pharmacist clearly understand the advantages and disadvantages of all of these equations and be able to use them appropriately to make drug dosage recommendations.

Urine Collection Method

The CrCl can also be determined via a 12- or 24-hour urine collection, which is often referred to as a "creatinine catch." This method is labor intensive, expensive, time consuming, and prone to collection errors. Consequently, this test is not ordered very commonly in clinical practice, but it may be useful for those patients for whom SCr-based estimation equations may be unreliable. The major complication associated with this test is incomplete urine collection, which will greatly affect the accuracy of the test. Thus, if this test is to be interpreted correctly, it is very important for the pharmacist to ensure that a complete urine collection was made. This can be done by calculating the total creatinine collected in a 24-hour period. If the total collection is less than 10 mg/kg/24 hrs, then an incomplete collection should be suspected; in such a case, the result is invalid and should not be used to make clinical decisions. This test also requires that a SCr determination be made at some point during the period of the urine collection, often at the midpoint of the urine collection period. The CrCl is calculated as follows:

$$\text{CrC1(mL/min)} = \frac{(\text{Ucr})}{(\text{Scr})} \times \frac{(\text{V})}{(\text{T})}$$

Ucr = urine creatinine concentration (mg/dL)
V = volume of urine collected (mL)
SCr = serum creatinine concentration (mg/dL)
T = time of urine collection (min)

ANNOTATED BIBLIOGRAPHY

Cockcroft DW, Gault MH. Prediction of creatinine clearance from serum creatinine. *Nephron* 1976;16:31–41.

Comstock TJ, Whitley KV. The kidneys. In: Lee M, ed. *Basic Skills in Interpreting Laboratory Data.* 3rd ed. American Society of Health-System Pharmacists; 2004:233–262.

Dowling TC. Quantification of renal function. In: Dipiro JT, Talbert RL, Yee GC, et al., eds. *Pharmacotherapy: A Pathophysiologic Approach.* 7th ed. China: McGraw-Hill; 2008:705–722.

Golik MV, Lawrence KR. Comparison of dosing recommendations for antimicrobial drugs based on two methods for assessing kidney function: Cockcroft-Gault and modification of diet in renal disease. *Pharmacotherapy* 2008;28:1125–1132.

Greenberg E, Saad N, Abraham T, Balmir E. Drug dosage adjustments using renal estimation equations: a review of the literature. *Hosp Pharm* 2009;44:577–583, 603.

Levey AS, Bosch JP, Lewis JB, et al. A more accurate method to estimate glomerular filtration rate from serum creatinine: a new prediction equation. *Ann Intern Med* 1999;130:461–470.

Levey AS, Stevens LA, Schmid CH, et al. A new equation to estimate glomerular filtration rate. *Ann Intern Med* 2009;150:604–612.

Moranville MP, Jennings HR. Implications of using modification of diet in renal disease versus Cockcroft-Gault equations for renal dosing adjustments. *Am J Health-Syst Pharm* 2009;66:154–161.

TOPIC: ACUTE KIDNEY INJURY

Contributor: Bradley W. Shinn

Introduction

Acute kidney injury (AKI), formerly referred to as acute renal failure, occurs most commonly in hospitalized patients. It is associated with significant morbidity and mortality and adds a very large service and cost burden to the U.S. healthcare system. For example, sepsis-associated AKI carries a mortality rate of almost 75% and the average total cost for a patient who requires renal replacement therapy is approximately $50,000.

This disorder is of particular importance to pharmacists for at least two reasons. First, many cases of AKI are directly associated with the use of renally toxic drugs. Second, even if the precipitating cause is not drug related, some medications will need to be discontinued to avoid worsening the acute renal dysfunction, and most renally eliminated drugs will require dose reduction to avoid toxicities of other organ systems. Thus, a complete medication review by a pharmacist is critically important when a patient develops signs of AKI.

Strategies to prevent episodes of AKI, especially in hospitalized patients, are particularly important because no proven treatment exists for a patient with established AKI and the outcomes are often poor. It is much better for patient care, and much more cost-effective, to prevent an episode of AKI than to treat an established case. Pharmacists are often intimately involved with developing and implementing these preventive programs.

Tips Worth Tweeting

- Acute kidney injury (AKI) occurs most commonly in hospitalized patients. When it presents in an outpatient setting, it is most commonly medication related.
- An episode of AKI may be classified as either non-oliguric (urine output > 450 mL/day) or oliguric (urine output < 450 mL/day).
- AKI is defined by an increase in baseline SCr, a decrease in GFR, or an acute decrease in urine output.
- Etiologies associated with AKI may be broadly classified as prerenal, functional, intrinsic, or postrenal.
- A medical history and complete medication review are absolutely essential and should be done as quickly as possible once a patient is identified with AKI.
- Important labs to identify the cause of AKI include BUN, SCr, urinalysis, and serum and urinary electrolytes.
- Prevention of an episode of AKI is a very important component of the care of hospitalized patients, especially those who are critically ill.
- Many commonly used medications, including radiocontrast dye, are the cause of many episodes of AKI in both inpatient and outpatient settings.
- No drug therapies have been proven to accelerate recovery from an episode of AKI; therefore, supportive therapies are critical.
- Renal replacement therapy (RRT) is often required on a temporary basis to maintain fluid and electrolyte balance and to remove accumulating waste products while renal recovery takes place.
- Early therapeutic strategies often focus on converting oliguria to non-oliguria (i.e., increasing urine output) with the use of aggressive loop diuretic regimens.
- Many important changes in pharmacokinetic parameters take place in a patient with AKI and must be considered if appropriate dosing recommendations are to be made.

Patient Care Scenario: Hospital General Medicine Service

C. S.: 56 yo, 5'11", 209 lbs (baseline ~ 90 kg), M, Caucasian
Chief Complaint: "I haven't been able to pee for the last couple of days."
HPI: Approximately 3 weeks ago, C. S. underwent root canal surgery. He was prescribed levofloxacin for an oral infection and advised to purchase ibuprofen and take it as needed for pain relief. Subsequently, C. S. required two follow-up dental procedures and received one dose of ketorolac (60 mg) each time. Throughout this period, he continued to self-administer ibuprofen (at least 2,400 mg per day and "more than that" during periods of acute pain) and, occasionally, acetaminophen. Over the past several days he has noticed a significant decrease in urine production and states that his "urine is darker than usual." He also complains of feeling "very tired" and reports feeling "chilled" the last couple of nights.

Medication List Prior to Admission (PTA)

Drug	Route	Dose	Sig
Lisinopril/ hydrochlorothiazide	PO	10 mg/25 mg	Once daily
Digoxin	PO	0.25 mg	Once daily
Glyburide	PO	10 mg	Once daily
Aspirin	PO	325 mg	Once daily
Levofloxacin	PO	500 mg	Once daily (× 5 more days)
Recent ibuprofen and acetaminophen (as detailed above)			

Allergies: NKDA.
PMH: Type 2 diabetes mellitus, HTN, h/o AMI (5 years ago), CHF (stage 2), recent dental infection (detailed above).
Social Hx: Negative for smoking (quit 5 years ago at time of AMI); social alcohol use (no more than 2 days per week); married and lives at home with wife.
ROS/PE: Ill-appearing; (+) JVD; basilar rales; (+) abdominal distention; 2+ LE edema; neuro—grossly intact, very lethargic, answers questions very slowly.
Vitals: BP = 140/90; P = 88; RR = 24; T = 100.5°F.
Lab Values:

Na: 127 mEq/L	Hgb: 10.8 g/dL
K: 5.8 mEq/L	Hct: 32%
Cl: 85 mEq/L	Platelets: 90 × 10^3/mcL
CO_2: 20 mEq/L	WBCs: 15.5 × 10^3/mcL
BUN: 105 mg/dL	Protein: 5.9 g/dL
SCr : 7.3 mg/dL	Albumin: 3.0 g/dL
Glu: 220 mg/dL	Total bilirubin: 4.4 mg/dL
Calcium: 8.5 mg/dL	Magnesium: 2.3 mg/dL
Phosphate: 5.5 mg/dL	

Urinalysis: Macroscopic: dark yellow, cloudy. Microscopic/Biochemical: specific gravity = 1.020, pH = 5.0, protein = 130 mg/dL, 2–5 RBCs/hpf, 5–10 granular casts/hpf, 5–10 WBCs/hpf, few bacteria, (–) nitrite, (+) leukocyte esterase, 1+ glucose, (–) ketones.

Other Information:

- Total urine output first 6 hours in hospital: 100 mL
- Renal ultrasound: Kidneys normal in size, shape, and position; no evidence of urinary obstruction; small amount of abdominal ascites noted
- Foley catheter placement: Negligible urine return; slightly traumatic placement
- Nephrologist report of visual examination of urinary sediment: "Many fine granular casts with degenerating cellular casts, coarse granular casts, and red blood cells"
- % FE_{Na} = 3.5%
- Blood and urine cultures: Pending

1.1.0 Patient Information

Assessment of Patient Information

Acute kidney injury (AKI) is a common complication that occurs in hospitalized patients; the highest incidence rate is seen in ICU patients (6–23%). AKI often occurs secondary to the use of nephrotoxic medications. When this condition occurs in an outpatient setting, it is most commonly due to medications. For example, nonprescription NSAIDs are estimated to cause more than 1 million cases of nephrotoxicity each year in the United States. When reviewing the preceding case scenario, the following points should be carefully assessed in designing a pharmaceutical care plan:

- Signs and symptoms that indicate C. S. is suffering from AKI. All available information should be examined, including the chief complaint, HPI, physical examination, and laboratory findings, including both the urinalysis and other specific renal lab tests and measurements.
- Previous medical conditions that may have predisposed C. S. to suffering a bout of AKI.
- A complete medication review—is critically important. Medications that may either precipitate or worsen an episode of AKI should be discontinued, if at all possible. The following medications should receive particular focus:
  - Diuretics
  - NSAIDs
  - Antihypertensive agents (e.g., ACEIs, ARBs)
  - Several antibiotics (e.g., aminoglycosides, Bactrim, acyclovir)
  - Any new medications
  - Any medications for which the dose has recently been increased
- Medications eliminated via renal mechanisms will generally require dosage reductions to avoid the occurrence of drug toxicities affecting multiple organ systems.

Table 23-8 Classification of Acute Kidney Injury: RIFLE System

Disease Stage	GFR/SCr Criteria	Urine Output (UOP) Criteria
Risk	SCr ↑ 50% **or** GFR ↓ 25%	UOP < 0.5 mL/kg/hr × 6 hr
Injury	SCr ↑ 100% **or** GFR ↓ 50%	UOP < 0.5 mL/kg/hr × 12 hr
Failure	SCr ↑ 200% **or** GFR ↓ 75% **or** SCr > 4 mg/dL	UOP < 0.3 mL/kg/hr × 24 hr **or** Anuria × 12 hr

Disease Identification/Diagnosis

AKI is usually identified by a combination of an acute increase in SCr concentration and/or an acute decrease in urine output. In many cases, both may be present. When a patient's renal function is changing rapidly, the SCr concentration will lag behind the event that initiated the renal compromise by as much as several days. Thus an acute decrease in urine output may provide an earlier indication of renal function compromise than an increase in the SCr concentration.

A consensus-derived classification system for AKI, known as the RIFLE system, makes use of both GFR and urine output to define an episode of acute renal insufficiency within one of the following stages: risk, injury, or failure (Bellomo R, 2005).

Etiologies/Clinical Findings

AKI may be classified in several other ways, including a system based on urine output and suspected etiology.

Clinical outcomes associated with each of these etiologies vary widely. Prerenal, or functional AKI, generally develops secondary to either decreased renal perfusion (e.g., dehydration, CHF, cirrhosis with ascites)

Table 23-9 Classification of Acute Kidney Injury: Urine Output (UOP)

Classification	Criteria	Comments
Oliguric AKI	UOP < 400 mL/day	Most patients who develop AKI also have a decreased urine output. One of the goals of therapy is to increase urine output with diuretic therapy (see the "Pharmacotherapy" section).
Non-oliguric AKI	UOP > 400 mL/day	Non-oliguric patients are easier to manage clinically compared to patients with oliguria; they also have a better prognosis.

Table 23-10 Classification of Acute Kidney Injury: Etiology

Classification	Clinical Signs	Comments
Prerenal AKI	↓ BP ↓ UOP ↓ $\%FE_{Na}$	Associated with decreased renal perfusion. May or may not be associated with systemic hypotension. *Prompt* correction of volume depletion may restore renal function because no structural damage to the kidney has occurred.
Functional AKI	Urinary indices consistent with prerenal azotemia	Hemodynamic changes at the level of the glomerulus → ↓ glomerular hydrostatic pressure → ↓ filtration rate. Associated with: • ↓ EABV conditions (e.g., CHF, cirrhosis with ascites, hypoalbuminemia) • Renovascular disease (e.g., renal artery stenosis) • Drug therapies (e.g., cyclosporine, NSAIDs, ACEIs, ARBs)—rapid discontinuation of suspected medication allows renal function to return to normal
Intrinsic AKI	↑ Urine protein ↑ RBCs Tubular cells or casts ↑ % FE_{Na} Urine eosinophils	Structural damage to the kidney: • Small blood vessel damage (e.g., vasculitis) • Glomerulonephritis • Renal tubule damage (e.g., ATN) • Acute interstitial nephritis • Cortical necrosis (very high mortality)
Postrenal AKI	Urinary indices relatively normal	Obstruction of urine flow that occurs in the urinary tract below the level of the kidney. Suggested by onset of acute anuria in absence of other signs and symptoms of AKI. Often identified clinically by insertion of a urinary catheter: if doing so yields a large volume of urine, obstruction is present.

or the use of drugs that lead to a decrease perfusion pressure across the glomerulus (e.g., NSAIDs, ACEIs). If recognized quickly, and if appropriate steps are taken to perfuse the kidney or to restore glomerular pressure, the AKI will resolve quickly and no permanent damage ensues—an outcome that highlights the importance of a prompt and complete medication review. This scenario most likely represents the "risk" level in the RIFLE classification.

However, if appropriate fluid therapy is delayed or if timely drug discontinuation does not occur, then prerenal or functional AKI can develop into intrinsic AKI (e.g., ATN)—a serious complication associated with a higher morbidity and mortality rate. This would represent either the "injury" or "failure" level in the RIFLE classification. In these cases, direct damage to the tubules commonly leads to the presence of tubular cells and casts upon urinalysis. These patients also lose urine-concentrating ability, which causes the $\%FE_{Na}$ to increase to levels greater than 1%.

Other causes of intrinsic renal failure include vasculitis, malignant hypertension, autoimmune disorders (e.g., SLE), many toxins (e.g., radiocontrast agents, heavy metals, aminoglycoside antibiotics, myoglobin), crystal deposition within the renal tubules (e.g., uric acid, sulfonamides, acyclovir), and allergic reactions (e.g., interstitial nephritis). Postrenal obstruction rarely

Table 23-11 Clinical and Laboratory Findings Associated with Acute Kidney Injury

Signs/Symptoms/ Physical Exam	Laboratory Findings
Peripheral edema/ weight gain Hypertension JVD Shortness of breath/ rales Nausea/vomiting Mental status changes Fatigue Volume depletion (prerenal AKI) Hypotension/ orthostasis (prerenal AKI) Rash (acute interstitial nephritis) Bladder distention (postrenal bladder outlet obstruction)	↑ Serum creatinine ↑ BUN ↓ CrCl Hyperkalemia Metabolic acidosis BUN/SCr ratio > 20:1 (prerenal AKI) Urinalysis: • Minimal or no sediment (prerenal or postrenal AKI) • Muddy granular casts (ATN) • Proteinuria (glomerulonephritis, allergic interstitial nephritis) • Eosinophiluria (allergic interstitial nephritis) • Hematuria/RBC casts (glomerular disease or active bleeding) • WBCs or casts (interstitial nephritis, severe pyelonephritis)

results in any serious renal complications and is usually resolved acutely by insertion of a urinary catheter.

Common clinical and laboratory findings associated with AKI are summarized in Table 23-11.

Prevention of AKI

Because very few definitive therapies exist for established AKI, and because it is so frequently associated with a bleak outcome, prevention strategies related to such injury are of paramount importance, especially in hospitalized patients. It is much preferred to prevent an episode of AKI than to treat an established case. Also, because medications are an important cause of many episodes of AKI, pharmacists often play an integral role in developing and implementing AKI-prevention strategies. One of the most important causes of AKI in hospitalized patients is the use of radiocontrast dye (Rabb H, Colvin RB, 2008). Several factors predispose a patient to developing contrast-induced nephropathy (CIN), many of which are risk factors for drug-induced nephrotoxicity in general. The CIN-prevention strategies in Table 23-12 should be recommended for patients with these risk factors.

Although several other agents have been studied for the prevention of CIN, there is no evidence of preventive efficacy with use of any of the following and they should not be recommended: fenoldopam (Corlopam), "low-dose" dopamine, theophylline, loop diuretics, mannitol, and calcium-channel blockers.

Several other medications are commonly associated with drug-induced AKI, some of which are listed in Table 23-13. Pharmacists should be especially vigilant for the use of these agents in patients with developing or established renal dysfunction and should be prepared to offer rational patient-care recommendations to avoid or attenuate the worsening renal dysfunction.

1.2.0 Pharmacotherapy

Supportive Measures

Because no drug therapies have been proven to accelerate recovery from AKI, supportive measures are critical. The usual recovery time from an episode of ATN is approximately 10–14 days. The kidney has an impressive capacity to heal itself if appropriate supportive care is provided. Most patients who initially survive an episode of AKI in the hospital do recover adequate renal function by the time of discharge; however, some

Table 23-12 Contrast-Induced Nephropathy: Risk Factors and Prevention Strategies

Risk Factors for CIN	Prevention of CIN
History of CKD/elevated Scr Diabetic nephropathy Dehydration/↓ intravascular volume Higher doses of contrast dye Use of ionic contrast agents	Sodium loading: infuse 0.9% NaCl at 1 mL/kg/hr beginning at least 6 hr before dye (± sodium bicarbonate) *N*-acetylcysteine (Muco-Myst): 600 mg (PO) bid × 1–2 doses before and 2–3 doses after procedure (4 total doses)

Table 23-13 Medications That Induce Acute Kidney Injury

Nephrotoxic Agent	Preventive Strategies
Aminoglycoside antibiotics	Avoid administering to high-risk patients—other antibiotic options are usually available: • Elderly patients • Patients with preexisting renal disease • Patients taking concurrent nephrotoxic agents Avoid prolonged or repeated courses Use extended-interval dosing (e.g., Harford nomogram)
Amphotericin B	Sodium loading Liposomal formulation for high-risk patients Alternative antifungal agent
ACEIs/ARBs	May lead to acute, rapid rise in SCr if compromised renal blood flow—recognize high-risk patients: • Preexisting renal disease • Volume depletion • ↓ EABV conditions (e.g. CHF, cirrhosis) • Renal artery stenosis Initiate at low dose and titrate dose slowly in high-risk patients Monitor SCr closely after initiating therapy Monitor serum potassium concentration closely, especially in patients who develop renal dysfunction
NSAIDs	Common cause of AKI due to OTC availability Counsel high-risk patients (e.g., those with CHF or preexisting renal insufficiency) to use other methods of pain control
Acyclovir/ trimethoprim-sulfamethoxazole (Bactrim)	May crystallize in renal tubules, especially in conjunction with decreased urine flow Decrease doses in patients with preexisting renal dysfunction Ensure adequate patient hydration

Table 23-14 Supportive Care Strategies for Acute Kidney Injury

Supportive Strategy	Comments
Discontinue and/or decrease dose of appropriate medications	Critical role for the pharmacist
Fluid management	Prerenal etiology: aggressive fluid therapy is often needed to optimize renal perfusion Administration of an acute fluid bolus (250–500 mL) may help determine the etiology Anuria or oliguria: edema may develop rapidly and fluids will need to be restricted Often a fine "balancing act" between too much and too little (i.e., ↓ tissue perfusion) fluid; careful monitoring of patient weight and "ins and outs" ("I's & O's") is usually necessary Recommendations to decrease the overall fluid burden in patients with oliguria/edema should be offered: • Maximally concentrate IV medications • Discontinue unnecessary IV agents • Change to oral therapy, if possible
Electrolyte management	Monitor closely for accumulation: • Potassium • Phosphate • Magnesium
Nutrition management	Preexisting nutritional status is a strong predictor of outcomes in AKI Forced enteral nutrition may lead to improved outcomes in ICU patients with AKI (a similar effect is not shown with TPN) Dietary restrictions may be important (e.g., protein, sodium, potassium, phosphate)
Renal replacement therapy (RRT)	Often needed on temporary basis to maintain F/E balance and to remove waste products while recovery takes place Indications for RRT: • Fluid overload (e.g., pulmonary edema) • Hyperkalemia • Metabolic acidosis • Uremia (↑ BUN + symptoms) Mortality is higher in patients who require RRT than in those who do not

will demonstrate varying degrees of chronic insufficiency. To maximize the opportunity for a successful outcome, it is critical for the healthcare team, including pharmacists, to rapidly ensure an environment that best allows for renal recovery. If the initial insult is allowed to continue, such as an inappropriate drug therapy, and/or if appropriate supportive care is delayed, the recovery period and hospitalization will be longer, the mortality rate higher, and the likelihood of chronic kidney disease higher. Specific supportive strategies are listed in Table 23-14.

Treatment of Edema

The use of loop diuretics, although quite common in patients with AKI, is controversial. These agents should not be expected to hasten renal recovery or improve survival and, in some cases, may actually worsen renal function. However, they have been shown to increase urine output in approximately 25% of patients with oliguric AKI, which may simplify patient management by decreasing complications associated with fluid overload. Thus loop diuretics should be administered in AKI only to those patients who are experiencing volume overload and edema; they should never be administered to patients who are hypovolemic or demonstrating signs of prerenal azotemia. These agents are equally effective when administered in equivalent doses. Ethacrynic acid is an older product with a high incidence of ototoxicity and is rarely used. The more commonly used loop diuretics are compared in Table 23-15.

Because the urinary excretion of loop diuretics correlates directly with diuretic response, higher doses are generally required as a patient's renal function declines. In patients with AKI, therapy is usually initiated with a lower dose, as noted in Table 23-15. If urine output does not increase adequately over 1–2 hours, then the dose is customarily doubled until

Table 23-15 Loop Diuretics

Parameter	Furosemide (Lasix)	Bumetanide (Bumex)	Torsemide (Demadex)
Bioavailability	60%	85%	85%
Onset of action (min)	40 (PO) 5 (IV)	40 (PO) 5 (IV)	40 (PO) 10 (IV)
Equivalent dose	40 mg	1 mg	20 mg
Initial dose in AKI	40–80 mg/day	1–2 mg/day	20–40 mg/day
Maximum dose in AKI	IV: 200 mg PO: 400 mg	10 mg	100 mg

the maximum recommended dose is reached. Dosage titration should stop once a urine output of 1 mL/kg/hr or a euvolemic state is achieved. This total dose should then be continued, usually divided into a once- or twice-daily dosing schedule.

Patients who do not respond satisfactorily to higher doses of loop diuretics may have developed "diuretic resistance." If this occurs, additional interventions may increase the effectiveness of diuretic therapy:

- Aggressive fluid and/or sodium restriction
- Change to IV route (if PO therapy was initiated)
- Decrease dosage interval (e.g., q 12 hr to q 6 hr)
- Add hydrochlorothiazide or metolazone (Zaroxolyn); generally, these agents are administered 30–60 minutes prior to the loop diuretic
- Switch to a continuous infusion loop diuretic and titrate upward to the desired response; usual starting doses:
  - Furosemide: 10–20 mg/hr
  - Bumetanide: 0.5–1 mg/hr

When high doses of loop diuretics are administered, especially in combination with metolazone, the hemodynamic and fluid status of the patient must be monitored very closely. In addition, electrolytes should be monitored daily to prevent life-threatening electrolyte disorders, especially hypokalemia. Ultimately, if hypervolemia persists after maximal diuretic therapy, RRT will need to be initiated.

Pharmacokinetic Considerations

Several important clinical changes occur in patients with AKI that alter normal pharmacokinetic parameters. It is critical to have an understanding of these changes because they significantly influence the dosage recommendations for many drugs:

- Edema/ hypervolemia → ↑ volume of distribution for many drugs:
  - Especially influences drugs with small Vds and/or ↑ water solubility
  - Acute fluid shifts (e.g., dialysis) may alter dosing recommendations
- Decreased renal clearance:
  - ↓ Dose of renally eliminated medications
- Initiation of RRT:
  - Drug clearances attained by various types of RRT differ significantly
  - Well-proven dosing guidelines for most types of RRT are lacking
- Protein binding parameters may be altered in AKI/uremic patients (e.g., phenytoin)
- Altered cytochrome P-450 activity has been documented in AKI → ↓ clearance of some hepatically cleared drugs
- Therapeutic drug concentration monitoring may need to be performed more frequently than usual due to altered pharmacokinetic parameters and imprecise dosage guidelines

ANNOTATED BIBLIOGRAPHY

Bellomo R. Defining, quantifying, and classifying acute renal failure. *Crit Care Clin* 2005;21:223-237.

Dager W, Spencer AP. Acute renal failure. In: Dipiro JT, Talbert RL, Yee GC, et al., eds. *Pharmacotherapy: A Pathophysiologic Approach*. 7th ed. China: McGraw-Hill; 2008:723-743.

Massicotte A. Contrast medium-induced nephropathy: strategies for prevention. *Pharmacotherapy* 2008; 28:1140–1150.

Rabb H, Colvin RB. Case 31-2007: a 41-year-old man with abdominal pain and elevated serum creatinine. *N Engl J Med* 2007;357:1531–1541.

Stamatakis MK. Acute kidney injury. In: Chisholm-Burns MA, Schwinghammer TL, Wells BG, et al., eds. *Pharmacotherapy: Principles and Practice*. 2nd ed. New York: McGraw-Hill; 2010:431–444.

TOPIC: CHRONIC KIDNEY DISEASE

Contributor: Bradley W. Shinn

Introduction

Chronic kidney disease (CKD) is defined as the presence of kidney damage, or a decreased GFR, for 3 months or more. It generally portends a progressive decline in kidney function that occurs over several months to years. This functional decline is usually irreversible and ultimately results in end-stage renal disease (ESRD), at which point the patient requires a renal transplant or dialysis therapy. Early kidney disease has no symptoms and, if left undetected, it can progress to kidney failure with little or no warning. It is estimated that approximately 8 million people in the United States suffer from stage 3 or worse CKD and more than 500,000 have ESRD. The prevalence of ESRD has increased more than fivefold since 1980.

CKD is a debilitating disease associated with high healthcare utilization and attendant costs. Public and private spending to treat patients with kidney failure in the United States in 2003 amounted to $27.3 billion. Clinical manifestations secondary to CKD eventually affect almost every organ system in the body and lead to premature mortality.

In general, treatment strategies are subdivided into two major groups: (1) those that slow the rate of progression of CKD to ESRD and (2) those that manage disease complications and alleviate symptoms. Patients with CKD are prescribed a large number of medications, which result in very complicated and costly drug regimens that are difficult to manage. For this reason, pharmacists are routinely involved in the care of these patients. Studies have documented that pharmacist interventions decrease medication errors, result in more consistent achievement of therapeutic goals, and decrease the cost of care.

Tips Worth Tweeting

- Chronic kidney disease (CKD) is a progressive decline in renal function that is generally irreversible.
- CKD is classified into five stages; however, symptoms are usually not apparent until stage 3.
- Stage 5 CKD is synonymous with end-stage renal disease (ESRD), the point at which the patient requires renal replacement therapy (renal transplantation or dialysis).
- Risk factors for the development of CKD are subdivided into susceptibility factors, initiation factors, and progression factors.
- Clinical manifestations associated with CKD ultimately affect almost every organ system and lead to significant patient morbidity.
- The goal of some therapeutic initiatives is to decrease the rate of progression to ESRD; the goal of other initiatives is to manage disease complications and reduce patient morbidity.
- Therapeutic interventions that slow the progression of kidney disease include reduction of dietary protein intake, intensive blood glucose control, optimal blood pressure control, reduction of proteinuria, treatment of hyperlipidemia, and smoking cessation.
- The anemia associated with CKD can be effectively treated with erythropoietin-stimulating agents; however, controversy exists over how aggressively these agents should be dosed and whether they should be recommended for all patients with CKD.
- Maintaining fluid and electrolyte homeostasis becomes increasingly difficult as renal function worsens; it is often these imbalances that lead to the initiation of dialysis.
- Phosphate accumulation disrupts calcium–phosphate homeostasis and leads to secondary hyperparathyroidism and renal osteodystrophy.
- Patients with CKD require a large number of therapeutic interventions and benefit from patient-focused pharmaceutical care programs.
- As patients progress toward ESRD, renal transplantation, hemodialysis (HD), and peritoneal dialysis (PD) become therapeutic options.
- HD removes a large amount of fluid and solutes over a short period of time, whereas PD removes fluid and solutes in a continuous, more physiologic manner.
- Important complications associated with HD include hypotension, muscle cramps, and catheter-related problems including thrombosis and infection.
- Important complications associated with PD include mechanical and catheter-related problems, peritoneal damage, infections, and patient burnout.

Patient Care Scenario: Ambulatory Nephrology Clinic

F. L.: 45 yo, 5'6", 209 lbs, F, African American

Chief Complaint: "I've been sent to your clinic by my regular doctor because of my kidneys."

HPI/ROS: F. L. has been referred to the nephrology clinic by her primary care physician, who has been seeing her intermittently at the town's "low-income" clinic, due to worsening renal function. It is hoped that a nephrologist might provide recommendations to slow the progression of her renal dysfunction. Upon presentation at the clinic, F. L. complains of increasing fatigue over the past few months and states that "It is getting more difficult to breathe, especially when I have to climb stairs." She also notes that she is more intolerant of cold weather, her skin is quite "itchy," and her urine is very foamy. She also notes that her rings no longer fit on her fingers and that her hands and feet seem to swell more when she "eats a lot of potato chips." Information from the general medicine clinic reveals that her fasting blood sugars have been elevated recently (averaging 180–250 mg/dL), that she has a history of medication noncompliance, and that she often misses clinic appointments.

Medication List Prior to Admission (PTA)

Drug	Route	Dose	Sig
Procardia XL	PO	60 mg	Once daily
Hydrochlorothiazide	PO	25 mg	Once daily
Glyburide	PO	10 mg	Once daily
Advil prn for headaches			
Maalox prn for "upset stomach"			

Allergies: Penicillin (thinks she gets a rash, but is not really sure).
PMH: Type 2 diabetes mellitus (× 8 years), HTN (× 5 years).
Social Hx: (+) smoking (about ½ pack per day, but admits to more when "stressed"), no alcohol, does not work (on disability), sedentary life style, questionable compliance with medications.
PE: Appears older than her stated age, A&O × 3 (but speaks very slowly; lethargic), red and weeping eyes, (+) JVD, bilateral basilar crackles/rales, (+) abdominal distention, (+) shifting dullness, 2(+) LE edema (to knees), swollen hands, ↓ sensation in feet to light touch, (+) dry skin.
Vitals: BP = 150/95; P = 85; RR = 22; T = 98.8°F.
Lab Values:

Na: 126 mEq/L	Hgb: 9.6 g/dL
K: 4.8 mEq/L	Hct: 28%
Cl: 88 mEq/L	Platelets: 150 × 10^3/mcL
CO_2: 18 mEq/L	WBCs: 9.7 × 10^3/mcL
BUN: 60 mg/dL	Protein: 5.6 g/dL
SCr : 3.4 mg/dL	Albumin: 2.8 g/dL
Glu: 220 mg/dL	Hgb A_{1c}: 8.6%
Calcium: 7.9 mg/dL	Total cholesterol: 230 mg/dL
Phosphate: 6.4 mg/dL	MCV: 82.0 μm3
Magnesium: 3.2 mg/dL	Transferrin saturation (T_{Sat}): 25%
iPTH: 100 pg/mL	Ferritin: 150 ng/mL

Other Information:

- Urine albumin-to-creatinine ratio (UACR): 500 mg/g
- Chest x-ray: haziness in both lower bases; (+) LV hypertrophy

1.1.0 Patient Information

Patient Assessment and Diagnosis

Chronic kidney disease (CKD) is categorized into five stages (stage 1–5) as defined by the National Kidney Foundation based upon estimated GFR (as defined via the MDRD equation—see the "Assessment of Renal Disorders" section) and the presence of specific symptoms. Patients are generally asymptomatic until they reach stage 3 (GFR = 30–59 mL/min). At stage 4 (15–29 mL/min), many of the more common signs and symptoms of CKD become evident. Stage 5 (< 15 mL/min) is also referred to as end-stage renal disease (ESRD) and is generally the point at which dialysis is initiated. Specific clinical findings associated with stages 3–5 are noted in Table 23-16.

Table 23-16 Findings Associated with Chronic Kidney Disease, Stages 3–5

CKD Stage	Clinical Finding
3	• Nocturia • Hypertension • Anemia
4	• Fatigue • Cold intolerance • Abnormal taste/anorexia • Hyperphosphatemia • Hypocalcemia • Hyperkalemia • Metabolic acidosis • Worsening anemia • Inability to adjust to changes in sodium intake
5	• Malaise/lack of energy • Pruritus • Intractable nausea/vomiting • Leg cramps/myoclonus • Clouded sensorium/asterixis/seizures • Worsening laboratory parameters

When assessing and staging a patient with CKD, it is important to consider all components of the patient's medical record, including history, ROS, physical examination, and laboratory findings. In the previously described patient encounter, F.L. appears to have advanced to stage 4 CKD. This assessment is supported by the following findings:

- Fatigue
- Cold intolerance
- Several electrolyte abnormalities
- Metabolic acidosis
- Worsening anemia (Hgb < 10 g/dL)
- Fluid overload (+ JVD, rales, abdominal distention, LE edema, swollen hands)
- Inability to adjust to changes in sodium intake (↑ edema after eating potato chips)

Table 23-17 Clinical Manifestations of Chronic Kidney Disease

Organ System	Clinical Manifestation of CKD
Cardiovascular	• Edema/hypertension • Dyslipidemia • LV hypertrophy/worsening of CHF • ECG abnormalities
Musculoskeletal	• Cramping • Myoclonus
Neuropsychiatric	• Anxiety • Depression • ↓ Mental cognition
Gastrointestinal	• GERD • Abdominal distention • ↑ Risk of GI bleeding
Genitourinary	• Changes in urine volume and consistency • Foaming of urine (indicative of proteinuria) • Sexual dysfunction
Hematologic	• Anemia of CKD (↓ Hgb, Hct, RBC count)
Metabolic	• Many electrolyte imbalances • Metabolic acidosis • ↑ PTH, ↓ vitamin D • Hypoalbuminemia (also indicative of poor nutrition, which is also a complication of CKD)

Later-stage CKD is a debilitating disease that leads to significant patient morbidity and disability. In Table 23-17, note the wide variety of clinical manifestations that may be found in a patient with CKD. See how many of these you can find in patient encounter described earlier.

Risk Factors

CKD occurs as a complication of several common disease states, which helps to explain the worldwide prevalence of this disorder. Risk factors for the development of CKD are divided into three categories. Susceptibility factors are associated with an increased risk of developing CKD, but are considered nonmodifiable by pharmacologic therapy. Initiation factors lead directly to CKD and are modifiable by pharmacologic therapy. Progression factors result in a more rapid decline of kidney function and lead to a worsening of already established CKD. The most common causes of kidney failure are diabetes and hypertension, which together account for approximately 70% of new cases. Additional risk factors are detailed in Table 23-18.

Table 23-18 Risk Factors for Chronic Kidney Disease

Classification	Risk Factor
Susceptibility factors	• Advanced age • Low birth weight • ↓ Kidney mass • Racial/ethnic minority • Family history of kidney disease • Low-income status • Systemic inflammation
Initiation factors	• Diabetes mellitus • Hypertension • Autoimmune disease (e.g., glomerulonephritis) • Polycystic kidney disease • Drug toxicities • Urinary tract pathology (e.g., infection, obstructions, stones)
Progression factors	• Hyperglycemia/poor blood glucose control • Hypertension/poor BP control • Hyperlipidemia • Proteinuria • Tobacco smoking • Anemia

1.2.0 Pharmacotherapy

Therapies to Slow Progression

Several therapeutic interventions that are recommended for a patient with CKD are intended to slow the rate of progression to ESRD. One of the primary goals of current diagnostic strategies in kidney disease, including use of the MDRD equation, is to define patients in earlier stages of CKD, before symptoms become readily apparent, so that effective interventions can be initiated as early as possible in the disease process. Delaying dialysis has great societal benefits, both in reducing patient morbidity and disability and in controlling healthcare costs, most of which are covered by government programs. These patients are also at high risk to develop cardiovascular disease, which further contributes to the high morbidity and mortality in CKD. Goals for the treatment of high blood pressure and hyperlipidemia are similar to those for patients with established cardiovascular disease. High blood pressure is often a very difficult problem in patients with CKD, especially when significant fluid and sodium retention develops. Many of these patients will require multiple medications from several different drug classes to adequately control blood pressure. Recommended interventions and therapy goals are noted in Table 23-19.

Table 23-19 Chronic Kidney Disease: Therapeutic Strategies

Therapeutic Strategy	Comments
Restriction of dietary protein intake	NKF recommendations: • Pre-dialysis patients (GFR < 25 mL/min/1.73 m^2): 0.6–0.8 g/kg/day • Dialysis patients: 1.2–1.3 g/kg/day Must balance against risk of malnutrition; consultation with dieticians should be recommended
Intensive blood glucose control for diabetics	Therapy goals: • Preprandial glucose: 70–120 mg/dL • Postprandial glucose: < 180 mg/dL • Hgb A_{1c}: < 7% Treatment with metformin is acceptable in stage 1, 2, and 3 CKD Glipizide or repaglinide is preferred over glyburide in patients with GFR < 30 mL/min/m^2 Insulin may require dose adjustment

Optimal blood pressure control	NKF BP goal: < 130/80 mm Hg
	Therapeutic options:
	• ACEI or ARB preferred—especially if the patient has significant proteinuria (UACR ≥ 300 mg/g)
	• Diuretic is usually needed due to fluid retention:
	  ○ CrCl ≥ 30 mL/min: consider a thiazide agent
	  ○ CrCl < 30 mL/min: a loop diuretic is required
	• Long-acting calcium-channel blocker and/or β-blocker: choice may depend on other indications
	• Often require multiple agents to control blood pressure, especially as fluid accumulation worsens

Reduction of proteinuria	ACEIs/ARBs:
	• ↓ Amount of protein filtered through glomerulus (up to 35–40%); the effect is independent of any reduction in BP
	• Indicated in the following patients regardless of BP:
	  ○ Documented proteinuria (UACR > 300 mg/g)
	  ○ Diabetes mellitus
	• Initiate with a low dose and titrate upward to the maximum tolerated dose
	• Consider dose reduction or discontinuation in the following circumstances:
	  ○ Sudden ↑ in SCr > 30%
	  ○ Hyperkalemia
	  ○ Symptomatic hypotension

Treatment of hyperlipidemia	NKF LDL goal: < 100 mg/dL Decreases proteinuria and slows decline in GFR Statin therapy recommended Renal impairment may increase risk of myopathies
Smoking cessation	Strongly recommended

Anemia of Chronic Kidney Disease

The anemia associated with CKD occurs primarily due to a decreased renal production of erythropoietin (EPO), which stimulates red blood cell production in the bone marrow. Effective treatment of anemia improves patient exercise capacity and tolerance, reduces morbidity and mortality associated with negative cardiovascular effects of anemia (e.g., LV hypertrophy), and slows the progression of renal disease (*J Am Soc Nephrol* 2003;14:S173–S177). The presence of anemia, which is defined by NKF guidelines as a hemoglobin concentration less than 11 g/dL, correlates directly with the degree of renal dysfunction. It is present in approximately 75% of patients with a GFR less than 15 mL/ min. It should be noted that patients with CKD are predisposed to develop anemia associated with other etiologies, which may occur in combination with an EPO deficiency:

- Nutritional deficiency: Iron, folate, vitamin B_{12}
- RBC hemolysis: Secondary to hemodialysis
- Blood loss: Multiple blood draws, hemodialysis
- Uremia: Decreases the life span of RBCs
- Infection/chronic inflammation: Anemia of chronic disease

Effective treatment of anemia in CKD involves repletion and maintenance of adequate iron stores, the correction of any other correctable cause of anemia, and administration of an erythropoietin-stimulating agent (ESA). Recently, concerns have been raised about the risk of cardiovascular complications (e.g., hypertension, acute coronary syndrome, stroke) in patients whose hemoglobin is corrected too aggressively with an ESA (National Kidney Foundation, 2007). Prescribing information now recommends that a patient's hemoglobin concentration be corrected to no more than 12 mg/dL, and many practitioners are targeting even lower concentrations if the patient remains asymptomatic. For an ESA to be effective, adequate iron stores must be maintained, which is best reflected by the serum ferritin concentration. Guidelines for provision of iron therapy in a patient with CKD are presented in Table 23-20.

Four IV iron products are currently available in the United States, which are summarized in Table 23-21. Adverse effects associated with IV iron administration include severe hypersensitivity reactions (e.g., anaphylaxis), infusion-related hypotension, flushing, nausea, injection-site reactions, and iron overload. While severe hypersensitivity reactions can occur with any of these agents, they are much more likely to occur with the use of iron dextran, which is why a test dose (25 mg) is required before initiating therapy with this product. In addition, anaphylactic reactions have been reported in patients who previously received doses of iron dextran without a problem. Primarily for this reason, the use of iron dextran has greatly decreased in favor of newer iron preparations. Ferumoxytol is the newest product available and may be administered most rapidly (over less than a minute); however, it is approved only as a two-dose regimen intended to replete iron stores, not as a maintenance therapy.

Table 23-20 Chronic Kidney Disease: Recommendations for Iron Therapy

Ferritin Concentration	Recommended Iron Therapy
< 100 ng/mL	1 g IV iron (divided doses): may be divided over 8–10 hemodialysis (HD) sessions or given in larger doses over a prolonged infusion time
100–500 ng/mL (at goal)	Maintenance iron therapy: • PO iron: 200 mg elemental iron per day; change to IV therapy if not effective • IV iron once weekly (maintenance dose): usually needed once ESA therapy is initiated
> 800 ng/mL	Hold IV iron doses until below 500 ng/mL

Table 23-21 Intravenous Iron Medications

Product	Test Dose Required	Approved Routes	Usual Maintenance Dose (Weekly)	Maximum Recommended Single Dose
Iron dextran (INFeD, Dexferrum)	Yes	IV, IM	50 mg	500 mg*
Sodium ferric gluconate (Ferrlecit)	No	IV	62.5 mg	250 mg
Iron sucrose (Venofer)	No	IV	50 mg	300 mg
Ferumoxytol (Feraheme)	No	IV (may be given more rapidly)	Not approved	510 mg (may repeat the dose 3–8 days later)

* Iron dextran may be given as a total dose infusion (TDI) in which the total calculated iron deficit is given as a single infusion over 4–6 hours (diluted in 500 mL of 0.9% NaCl).

Primary Treatment for Anemia with CKD

The primary treatment for anemia associated with CKD is administration of an ESA. ESAs are synthetic formulations of EPO produced by recombinant DNA technology. Therapy with an ESA should be considered if a patient's hemoglobin remains below 11 g/dL after correcting for other causes of anemia, including iron deficiency. Prior to initiation of ESA therapy, the patient's transferrin saturation (TSat) should be at least 20% and the serum ferritin concentration at least 100 ng/mL.

Two ESAs are currently available in the United States: epoetin alfa (Epogen, Procrit) and darbepoetin alfa (Aranesp). Epoetin alfa has the same biological activity as endogenous EPO; darbepoetin has a longer half-life, which allows for less frequent dosing. These agents are equally efficacious and have similar adverse effects, of which the most important is increased blood pressure. The patient's blood pressure should be well controlled at the initiation of ESA therapy and must be monitored closely during therapy. Either initiation or escalation of antihypertensive therapy is frequently required in patients receiving ESAs.

ESAs may be administered either subcutaneously (SC) or by the IV route. Subcutaneous administration is preferred because it provides a more predictable and sustained response; however, the IV route is often utilized in patients who have established IV access or are receiving hemodialysis.

Table 23-22 Erythropoietin-Stimulating Agents: Dosage and Adjustment Strategies

Product	Recommended Initial Dose	Dose Adjustment Strategies
Epoetin alfa (Epogen, Procrit)	50–100 units/kg 2–3 times per week	Increase the dose by 25% if: • Hgb is less than 10 g/dL and has not increased by 1 g/dL after 4 weeks of therapy • Hgb decreases to less than 10 g/dL Reduce the dose by 25% if: • Hgb approaches 12 g/dL • Hgb increases by more than 1 g/dL in any 2-week period If Hgb continues to increase after the dosage reduction, temporarily withhold the dose until Hgb begins to decrease; then reinitiate therapy at a dose 25% below the previous dose
Darbepoetin alfa (Aranesp)	0.45 mcg/kg once weekly **or** 0.75 mcg/kg every 2 weeks (if not on dialysis)	Increase the dose by 25% if: • Increase in Hgb is less than 1 g/dL over 4 weeks and iron stores are adequate Reduce the dose by 25% if: • Hgb approaches 12 g/dL • Hgb ↑ by more than 1 g/dL in any 2-week period If Hgb continues to increase after dosage reduction, temporarily withhold dose until Hgb begins to decrease; then reinitiate at a dose 25% below the previous dose

As noted earlier, it is critical to maintain adequate iron stores after ESAs are initiated or they will not achieve optimal effectiveness. Most patients will require maintenance IV iron therapy to maintain adequate stores after initiation of an ESA. Although the starting dose of an ESA depends on many factors (e.g., patient hemoglobin concentration, target hemoglobin concentration, the rate of hemoglobin increase), recommended initial doses are noted in Table 23-22. However, these initial doses will need to be carefully titrated to achieve and maintain a hemoglobin concentration between 10 and 12 g/dL. Dosage increases should not be made more frequently than once a month. Individual patients may require a wide variety of doses to maintain recommended hemoglobin concentrations.

When converting a patient from epoetin alfa therapy, the starting weekly dose of darbepoetin should be estimated on the basis of the weekly epoetin alfa dose at the time of substitution. A chart is available in the prescribing information to assist with this conversion. For example, if a patient is receiving between 5,000 and 10,999 units of epoetin alfa per week, the recommended initial dose of darbepoetin is 25 mcg per week. Due to the longer serum half-life, darbepoetin should be administered less frequently than epoetin alfa.

Therapies to Manage Complications

Several therapeutic interventions recommended for the patient with CKD are intended to manage disease complications. Unlike therapies designed to slow progression of renal dysfunction, these therapies are not usually initiated until the patient becomes symptomatic, which generally does not occur until the patient's CrCl is less than 60 mL/min. Many of these complications result in significant morbidity and mortality and ultimately lead to the initiation of renal replacement therapy. These complications include impaired sodium and water homeostasis, resulting in fluid overload, hyperkalemia, hyperphosphatemia, secondary hyperparathyroidism, renal osteodystrophy (ROD), metabolic acidosis, an increased risk of bleeding, and pruritus.

As the nephron mass declines, sodium load overwhelms the remaining nephrons and a decrease in total sodium excretion occurs. This increases fluid retention, leading to peripheral edema, worsening hypertension, and breathing difficulties secondary to pulmonary edema. In the earlier stages of CKD, fluid restriction is generally unnecessary as long as the patient's sodium intake is controlled. Fluid intake should be maintained to equal the rate of urine output. If free water intake is increased, volume overload and dilutional hyponatremia will develop. As a patient's renal function worsens, fluid overload becomes more of a clinical problem, which may hasten the need for dialysis. The therapeutic recommendations in Table 23-23

Table 23-23 Strategies to Minimize Sodium and Fluid Overload in Patients with Worsening Renal Function

- Limit sodium intake to less than 2.4 g (approximately 100 mEq) per day
- Use saline-containing IV fluids cautiously—they may precipitate fluid overload
- Diuretic therapy:
  - Thiazide diuretic if CrCl > 30 mL/min
  - Loop diuretic if CrCl < 30 mL/min; will require increasing doses as renal failure worsens
  - Combination therapy: loop diuretic + thiazide diuretic (e.g., metolazone)
  - Acute care situation: consider continuous infusion of a loop diuretic

Table 23-24 Signs and Symptoms of Secondary Hyperparathyroidism/Renal Osteodystrophy

- ↑ BP, ↑ HR, ↑ stroke index
- Bone pain
- Muscle weakness
- Pruritus of the skin
- ↑ Serum phosphorus concentration, low or normal serum calcium concentration, ↑ Ca-P product, ↑ iPTH, ↓ vitamin D concentration
- Radiographic studies may show calcium–phosphate deposits in joints and/or the cardiovascular system

may be implemented to minimize sodium and fluid overload as the patient's renal function worsens.

The decreased nephron mass also leads to a decrease in the tubular secretion of potassium, predisposing patients to hyperkalemia, which affects more than 50% of patients with stage 5 CKD. Dietary potassium intake should be restricted to 2–3 g (50–80 mEq) per day. Because an increasing proportion of potassium excretion takes place via the GI tract as renal function worsens, it is also helpful to minimize episodes of constipation. For patients with mild to moderate hyperkalemia (serum concentration less than 6.5 mEq/L and no EKG changes), sodium polystyrene sulfonate (SPS, Kayexalate) may be recommended at a dose of 15–30 g. A loop diuretic may be used in patients with adequate urine output to reduce potassium levels. Severe hyperkalemia may be managed by acute calcium gluconate (1 g IV) to stabilize the heart, an insulin plus glucose infusion and/or nebulized albuterol to shift potassium intracellularly, and initiation of hemodialysis.

The impairment in phosphorus excretion that occurs in CKD leads to hyperphosphatemia and hypocalcemia and is the initial step in the development of secondary hyperparathyroidism and renal osteodystrophy (ROD). A decrease in vitamin D activation in the kidney also decreases calcium absorption in the GI tract, which further contributes to this problem. The parathyroid glands release parathyroid hormone (PTH) in response to the decreased serum calcium and increased serum phosphorus concentrations, leading to secondary hyperparathyroidism, increased calcium reabsorption from bone, and ROD. In addition, soft-tissue deposition of hydroxyapatite crystals ("soft tissue calcification"), which primarily affects the coronary arteries, lungs, and vascular tissue, is associated with a Ca-P product greater than 55 mg^2/dL^2. This complication leads to increased cardiovascular mortality. The presence of metabolic acidosis also aggravates these metabolic and bone disorders via several mechanisms. The onset of secondary hyperparathyroidism and ROD is often very subtle and may not be associated with significant symptoms.

The first step in the treatment of these CKD complications is to control hyperphosphatemia. This goal is accomplished by use of a dietary phosphorus restriction (800–1,000 mg/day) and administration of a phosphate-binding agent. Foods high in phosphate also tend to be foods high in protein, which may make it difficult to provide enough protein to avoid malnutrition. In addition, phosphorus-containing food additives are increasingly being included in processed and fast foods. A recent study suggests that educating ESRD patients to avoid phosphorus-containing food additives may result in modest improvements in hyperphosphatemia (Sullivan C, Sayre SS, Leon JB, et al., 2009). Several phosphate-binding agents, which lead to a decreased absorption of dietary phosphorus, are available in the United States. These agents should be administered with each meal (usually 1–2 tablets initially), with dose adjustments as necessary based on serum phosphorus concentrations. Neither hemodialysis nor peritoneal dialysis removes enough phosphorus to control hyperphosphatemia; therefore, pharmacologic therapy must continue even after initiating dialysis. Dietary phosphate binders include calcium-containing agents (calcium carbonate and acetate) and non-calcium-containing agents (sevelamer, lanthanum). The calcium-containing products are best recommended for patients who have a low or low-to-normal serum calcium concentration, and the non-calcium-containing products are best utilized for patients with higher serum calcium concentrations and/or an elevated Ca-P product, as these patients are at risk for soft-tissue calcification. Selected products are summarized in Table 23-25.

When the reduction of serum phosphorus does not sufficiently reduce PTH levels, then a vitamin D analog or calcimimetic agent should be considered. Exogenous vitamin D compounds act directly on the

Table 23-25 Phosphate-Binding Agents

Calcium-Containing Products	Comments
Calcium carbonate (Tums, Oscal 500) Calcium acetate (Phos-Lo)	Dissolution characteristics and phosphorus-binding effect may vary between calcium carbonate products Calcium acetate is generally considered the first-line agent; it has comparable efficacy to calcium carbonate with one-half the dose of elemental calcium May aid in the treatment of metabolic acidosis Inexpensive Avoid in patients with high-to-normal or high serum calcium concentrations Limit intake of elemental calcium to 2,000 mg per day ADRs: • Constipation • Hypercalcemia
Non-Calcium-Containing Products	
Sevelamer HCl (Renagel) Sevelamer carbonate (Renvela) Lanthanum carbonate (Fosrenol)	May be preferred in patients with ↑ serum calcium concentration and/or vascular or soft-tissue calcification Sevelamer: also may be preferred in patients with ↓ LDL-C and ↑ HDL-C Sevelamer: may decrease mortality in hemodialysis patients compared to calcium-based products due to decreased calcifications in coronary arteries Sevelamer carbonate: does not lower serum bicarbonate concentrations more than sevelamer HCl; may help control metabolic acidosis More expensive ADRs: • Nausea, diarrhea, constipation • Peripheral edema, myalgias (lanthanum)
Aluminum-Containing Products	
Aluminum hydroxide (AlternaGel, Amphojel) Aluminum carbonate (Basaljel)	These agents are no longer recommended for chronic use due to the risk of aluminum toxicity: • Weakened bone structures • Encephalopathy, dementia

parathyroid gland to decrease PTH synthesis and secretion. However, these agents also increase calcium and phosphorus absorption in the GI tract, which increases the risk of hyperphosphatemia and hypercalcemia. The Ca-P product should be less than 55 mg^2/dL^2 before initiating vitamin D therapy. Ergocalciferol (vitamin D_2) may be used in stage 3 CKD; however, stage 4 or 5 CKD will require use of one of the vitamin D analogs noted in Table 23-26. In general, higher doses are required in stage 5 CKD (compared to stage 4) and in patients with higher serum PTH concentrations. After vitamin D therapy is initiated, it is important to monitor the patient carefully to make sure that PTH secretion is not overly suppressed, as this condition can lead to adynamic bone disease, decreased bone formation, and low bone turnover. Although vitamin D therapy is routinely used in patients with CKD, a recent meta-analysis questioned whether this therapy has beneficial effects on patient outcomes and concluded that the value of vitamin D treatment in CKD is uncertain (Palmer SC, McGregor DO, Macaskill P, et al., 2007).

Cinacalcet (Sensipar) is a calcimimetic agent that increases the sensitivity of parathyroid gland receptors to serum calcium concentrations. This agent decreases both serum calcium and serum phosphorus concentrations and is particularly beneficial for patients who may not be able to receive vitamin D therapy due to an elevated Ca-P product. However, because cinacalcet lowers serum calcium concentrations, it should not be initiated in a patient who is hypocalcemic (< 8.4 mg/dL). Thus, for patients whose PTH concentrations are not adequately controlled by the reduction of serum phosphorus concentrations, either a vitamin D analog or cinacalcet may be considered. Cinacalcet is probably a better choice for patients who have adequate serum calcium concentrations and/or a Ca-P product approaching or greater than 55 mg^2/dL^2, whereas a vitamin D analog is preferred for patients

Table 23-26 Vitamin D Analogs

Product	Route	Comments
Calcitriol (Rocaltrol: PO; Calcijex: IV)	PO, IV	Same biologic activity as endogenous calcitriol Dosage range: 0.25–0.5 mcg daily to 3–5 mcg per HD session
Paricalcitol (Zemplar)	PO, IV	Less effect on vitamin D receptors in the GI tract; more useful for patients with ↑ Ca-P product Not recommended for patients on peritoneal dialysis Dosage range: 1–2 mcg daily to 10–15 mcg per HD session
Doxercalciferol (Hectoral)	PO, IV	Has similar effects as calcitriol on receptors in the parathyroid gland and intestines Dosage range: 2.5 mcg 3×/week to 10–20 mcg per HD session

who have a low serum calcium concentration and/or a lower Ca-P product. It is very important to closely monitor patients with the metabolic and bone disorders associated with CKD, especially those who are receiving aggressive treatment. The serum calcium, phosphorus, and iPTH concentrations should be monitored every 1–4 weeks while initiating or titrating therapies, and every 3 months once target levels are achieved. If patients continue to demonstrate an iPTH concentration greater than 800 pg/mL that is refractory to medical therapy, a parathyroidectomy will be considered. After this procedure, bone production will suddenly outweigh bone resorption, which may lead to acute hypocalcemia, hypophosphatemia, and hypomagnesemia ("hungry bone syndrome"). These electrolytes need to be monitored very frequently for the first 48–72 hours after a parathyroidectomy is performed.

Because the renal excretion of hydrogen ions is increasingly compromised as renal function declines, most patients with stage 4 or 5 CKD will develop an elevated anion gap (AG) metabolic acidosis (AG > 17 mEq/L). This complication contributes to many negative effects associated with CKD, including increased protein catabolism and muscle wasting, increased bone dissolution and bone resorption, impaired glucose tolerance, aggravation of cardiac disease, and impaired thyroid and growth hormone function. The goal of therapy is to return the serum bicarbonate concentration to 22–24 mEq/L. As noted earlier, the use of a calcium-containing phosphate binder or sevelamer carbonate (versus sevelamer HCl) may help in the control

Table 23-27 Treatments for Metabolic Acidosis

Product	Comments
Sodium bicarbonate tablets	650 mg = 7.7 mEq each of sodium and bicarbonate Sodium load may lead to volume overload, HTN, and worsening CHF
Sodium citrate/ citric acid (Shohl's solution, Bicitra)	Provide 1 mEq/L each of sodium and bicarbonate The citrate portion is metabolized in the liver to bicarbonate Citrate may promote aluminum toxicity by ↑ GI absorption
Sodium/ potassium citrate/ citric acid	Provides 2 mEq/L of bicarbonate and 1 mEq/L of both sodium and potassium May worsen hyperkalemia

of metabolic acidosis. More definitive treatments are noted in Table 23-27.

Other complications that may occur in a patient with CKD include uremic bleeding and uremic pruritus. Patients with CKD have an increased risk of bleeding owing to decreased production of thromboxane, which alters platelet function and aggregation; decreased activity of von Willebrand factor (vWf) which impairs platelet–vessel wall interactions; and use of anticoagulants to prevent or treat clotting complications in hemodialysis patients. Most of these bleeding complications are relatively mild; however, the steady loss of red blood cells can contribute to chronic iron loss and make the anemia of CKD more difficult to correct. Patients with CKD/ESRD who are admitted to an ICU should receive stress-related mucosal damage (SRMD) prophylaxis to prevent serious GI bleeding. The initiation of dialysis will improve platelet function in a patient with stage 5 CKD and decrease bleeding time. Patients with CKD who undergo surgical procedures may be prescribed desmopressin (DDAVP), which increases the release of vWf from endothelial tissue and decreases the risk of bleeding for 4–8 hours. This agent may be administered by IV, SC, or intranasal routes. Estrogens may also be prescribed to decrease bleeding time. The onset of action of these agents is slower than that of DDAVP, but more sustained (for up to 2 weeks after stopping therapy). These agents may be given by IV, PO, or transdermal routes.

The prevalence of uremic pruritus (UP) has declined in the past 10 years as a result of improvements in dialysis and the development of biocomparable dialysis membranes. However, this complication continues to affect 42–52% of adults with CKD (Dialysis Outcomes and Practice Patterns Study [DOPPS]), Pisoni RL, Wikstrom B, Elder SJ, 2006). The cause of the pruritus associated with CKD is unknown, and this adverse effect is difficult to alleviate. UP has a substantial effect on quality of life, as it causes serious discomfort, anxiety, depression, and sleeping disorders, which lead to chronic fatigue and have a negative effect on mental and physical abilities. UP often leads to considerable mechanical skin damage due to continuous scratching, with excoriations, superimposed infections, and chronic lesions. It remains an underappreciated complication that adversely affects the quality of life of many patients with CKD. Treatment strategies for UP include both nonpharmacologic and pharmacologic interventions. No single therapy is considered the first-line option for the treatment of UP, and usually a combination of approaches will be tried to find the ideal regimen for an individual patient. Treatment options are noted in Table 23-28.

Renal Replacement Therapy

As patients progress to stage 5 (end-stage) renal disease, renal replacement therapy (RRT) becomes necessary. This treatment includes initiation of dialysis, including both hemodialysis (HD) and peritoneal dialysis (PD), and kidney transplantation. HD is initiated in approximately 65% of the patients in the United States who require dialysis. Planning for dialysis should begin when a patient's CrCl falls to less than 30 mL/min, which allows time to educate both the patient and the family on the various modalities available. The initiation of dialysis is a major, life-changing event, and it is best if the patient is well educated and prepared, regardless of which modality is chosen. Specific indications for initiation of dialysis are as follows:

- Persistent anorexia, N/V, fatigue, pruritus
- Poor nutritional status/low serum albumin concentrations
- Volume overload → uncontrolled HTN, pulmonary edema, CHF
- Uncontrolled hyperkalemia
- Uncontrolled metabolic acidosis
- Elevated BUN → uremia (especially CNS confusion, ↓ mental acuity, coma)

Table 23-28 Treatments for Uremic Pruritus

Nonpharmacologic Treatments	
Optimize dialysis efficacy and biocompatible membranes	
Improve nutritional status—especially in terms of restriction of dietary phosphorus and protein	
Control calcium and phosphate concentrations—minimize the Ca-P product	
Treat secondary hyperparathyroidism effectively	
Ultraviolet B phototherapy: 8–10 total sessions	
Pharmacologic Treatments	**Comments**
Skin emollients with a high water content	Hydrates the stratum corneum
Capsaicin 0.025% cream	Impractical for large areas or generalized pruritus
Tacrolimus ointment (Protopic)	Not recommended for prolonged periods or as first-line therapy
Gabapentin (Vila T, Gommer J, Scates A, 2008)	Administer after each dialysis session (100–300 mg)
Antihistamines (e.g., diphenhydramine, hydroxyzine)	Limited beneficial effect in UP; may help by promoting sleep
Cholestyramine	5 g twice daily
Activated charcoal therapy	Well tolerated and effective in many cases; 1–1.5 g qid in therapy-resistant UP
Naltrexone	Trial results have been conflicting
Ondansetron	Trial results have been conflicting

Hemodialysis

Hemodialysis (HD) involves the exposure of blood to a semipermeable membrane (dialyzer) against which a physiologic solution (dialysate) is flowing. Different dialyzers may be used and affect which substances are removed and how efficiently each is removed. For example, a high-flux dialyzer has larger pores than a conventional membrane and will remove higher-molecular-weight substances (e.g., many drugs) more efficiently. The dialysate is composed of purified water and electrolytes, and the type and quantity of substances removed from the blood may be altered by adjusting the electrolyte and chemical makeup of the dialysate solution. HD requires vascular access, which is usually achieved by surgical placement of an arteriovenous fistula or graft in the patient's forearm. Advantages and disadvantages associated with HD are noted in Table 23-29.

The most important complication associated with HD is hypotension, which occurs in 10–50% of patients. Significant hypotension is defined as a sudden decrease of more than 30 mm Hg in MAP or SBP and/or the development of the following symptoms: dizziness, N/V, sweating, and chest pain. The primary cause is too-rapid or too-aggressive removal of fluid from the intravascular space. It is often the development of hypotension that limits the length and overall efficacy of a dialysis session, especially in critically ill patients who are already showing signs of compromised organ perfusion. Management of HD-associated hypotension may include the following measures:

- Place the patient in the Trendelenburg position (head lower than feet)
- Decrease the ultrafiltration rate: leads to the removal of less fluid

- Fluid administration: must be done cautiously in patients with ESRD
- Mannitol administration: 12.5–25 g × 1–2 doses
- Midodrine (Proamatine): an α-adrenergic agonist; may be especially useful for patients with autonomic dysfunction:
  - 2.5–10 mg × 1 dose prior to each HD session
  - 5 mg bid-tid for chronic hypotension
- Levocarnitine: indicated for patients with documented low levocarnitine levels
  - Expensive: should not be used as first-line therapy
  - 20 mg/kg (IV) following each HD session

Other complications associated with HD include muscle cramps, thrombotic events, infections, and water-soluble vitamin deficiencies. The development of muscle cramps, which often occur at the conclusion of an HD session, is thought to be due to muscle hypoperfusion secondary to excessive ultrafiltration. Thus decreasing the ultrafiltration rate may help control this complication. Vitamin E therapy (400 IU once daily) may also help control muscle cramps.

Thrombosis is the most common cause of catheter failure. The need to replace the catheter may be prevented by local administration of a thrombolytic agent, which is placed into the clotted port and allowed to dwell for 30–60 minutes. Both alteplase (TPA, Cathflo) at a dose of 2 mg per port or reteplase at a dose of 0.5 unit per port may be used.

A variety of infections are an important cause of morbidity and mortality in patients undergoing HD. The greatest risk is the development of bacteremia, which can develop very quickly into sepsis. Blood cultures should be obtained in any HD patient who develops a fever. Because skin organisms are frequently implicated in these infections, antimicrobial therapy for an HD patient who develops a fever should always provide adequate coverage of gram-positive organisms (e.g., *Staphylococcus, Streptococcus*). Broader empiric antimicrobial regimens may be indicated for patients with other predisposing conditions, such as diabetes mellitus, and those who are receiving immunosuppressive therapy. Antibiotics for catheter-related infections usually need to be continued for 2–4 weeks.

Finally, because water-soluble vitamins and folic acid are small molecules that are lost during HD, patients should be supplemented with a vitamin product that supplies vitamins B and C, and folic acid (e.g., Nephrocap, Rena-Vite). These supplements should not include fat-soluble vitamins, which can accumulate in patients with kidney failure.

Table 23-29 Advantages and Disadvantages of Hemodialysis

Advantages
Higher solute clearance allows intermittent treatment
Underdialysis is easily detected
Low failure rate
Clotting parameters are better corrected with HD versus PD
Regular contact with the healthcare system enables closer patient monitoring
Disadvantages
Perceived "loss of control" by the patient due to multiple visits to the HD center
May take several months for patients to tolerate HD; disequilibrium, hypotension, and muscle cramps are common
The necessary vascular access is commonly associated with thrombosis and infection
Decline of residual renal function is usually more rapid than occurs with PD

Peritoneal Dialysis

Peritoneal dialysis (PD) makes use of similar principles as in HD; however, in this case the patient's own peritoneal membrane is used as the semipermeable membrane. The blood vessels that supply the abdominal organs, muscles, and mesentery serve as the blood component of the system. A sterile, pre-warmed dialysate solution is then instilled into the peritoneal cavity, via use of an indwelling catheter, where it dwells for a specified length of time (1 to several hours), allowing waste products to diffuse into the dialysate from the blood. At the end of the dwell time, the old dialysate, which contains toxins and waste products that have diffused from the blood, is drained and replaced with fresh dialysate. Various concentrations of glucose (1.5%, 2.5%, 4.25%) are added to the dialysate solutions to create an osmotic gradient between the dialysate and the blood, which causes fluid to move from the blood into the peritoneal cavity. Increasing the concentration of glucose in the dialysate solution allows for increased removal of fluid from the patient. Because of the continuous nature of PD, it provides a more physiologic removal of waste products than does HD and better mimics endogenous renal function. Advantages and disadvantages associated with PD are noted in Table 23-30.

Important complications associated with PD include mechanical complications with the indwelling catheter, pain, peritoneal damage, and both catheter-related infections and peritonitis. Abdominal pain often occurs when the catheter tip impinges on visceral organs. Pain can also occur secondary to the rapid inflow of the dialysate solution, chemical irritation from dialysate additives (e.g., antibiotics), and a low dialysate temperature. After several episodes of peritonitis, sclerosis of the peritoneal membrane may occur,

Table 23-30 Advantages and Disadvantages of Peritoneal Dialysis

Advantages of PD
Improved hemodyanamic stability versus HD due to slower ultrafiltration rates
Improved clearance of larger solutes
Improved preservation of residual renal function versus HD
Provides a convenient intraperitoneal route for administration of many drugs (e.g., antibiotics, insulin)
Less blood loss versus HD: • Lower risk of iron deficiency and possibly easier management of anemia of CKD • Lower requirements for ESAs and parenteral iron
No systemic heparinization requirements
Freedom from a machine gives the patient a sense of independence and makes it easier to carry out a "normal" work schedule and other daily activities
Disadvantages of PD
Predisposes patients to malnutrition: • ↑ Protein and amino acid losses via the peritoneum versus HD • Continuous glucose load leads to a sense of abdominal fullness and ↓ appetite
Excessive glucose absorption may predispose to obesity and worsen diabetic control
Risk of peritonitis; may preclude use of PD after several episodes due to peritoneal membrane compromise
Inadequate ultrafiltration and solute removal, especially in larger patients
Catheter malfunction or mechanical problems may occur
Patient burnout and high rate of technique failure

decreasing the efficacy of PD. Once the peritoneal membrane can no longer function as an effective semipermeable membrane, the patient may have to convert to HD.

Catheter-related infections include exit-site infections and tunnel infections. If the patient is exhibiting minimal symptoms, antimicrobial therapy may be delayed until culture and sensitivity results are available. Oral antibiotics may be effective for these infections, but usually at least 2 weeks of therapy is necessary to ensure complete eradication. Treatment should continue until the exit site appears normal, with no erythema or drainage present. If these infections do not resolve adequately, it may be necessary to replace the PD catheter.

Peritonitis, however, is an infectious complication that is usually more serious and is the leading cause of morbidity and hospital admission in PD patients. The use of improper or nonsterile technique during exchanges is the most common cause of peritonitis. Signs of developing peritonitis in a PD patient include a cloudy dialysate drainage and abdominal pain and distention. Peritonitis is a systemic infection that can quickly develop into sepsis and septic shock. Therefore, antibiotics should be administered immediately upon suspicion of this infection. Empiric antibiotics should cover both gram-positive and gram-negative organisms and are best based on protocols and sensitivity patterns of organisms known to commonly cause peritonitis in the area where the patient lives. Because many PD patients have a history of multiple infections, the infection history of an individual patient should also be considered when choosing an empiric antimicrobial regimen. Once a causative organism is identified, then the empiric antimicrobial regimen should be changed to the most cost-effective, focused therapy that will treat the identified pathogen. If multiple pathogens are identified in the dialysate sample, then the patient should be evaluated for other intra-abdominal pathologies, such as a bowel perforation.

ANNOTATED BIBLIOGRAPHY

Abboud H, Henrich WL. Stage IV chronic kidney disease. *N Engl J Med* 2010;362:56–65.

Bailie GR. Calcium and phosphorus management in chronic kidney disease: challenges and trends. *Formulary* 2004;39:358–365.

Hudson JQ. Chronic kidney disease: management of complications. In: Dipiro JT, Talbert RL, Yee GC, et al., eds. *Pharmacotherapy: A Pathophysiologic Approach*. 7th ed. China: McGraw-Hill; 2008: 765–791.

Joy MS, Kshirsagar A, Franceschini N. Chronic kidney disease: progression-modifying therapies. In: Dipiro JT, Talbert RL, Yee GC, et al., eds. *Pharmacotherapy: A Pathophysiologic Approach*. 7th ed. China: McGraw-Hill; 2008:745–763.

National Kidney Foundation. KDOQI clinical practice guideline and clinical practice recommendations for anemia in chronic kidney disease: 2007 update of hemoglobin target. *Am J Kidney Disease* 2007;50:471–530.

Pedrini MT, Levey AS, Lau J, et al. The effect of dietary protein restriction on the progression of diabetic and nondiabetic renal diseases: a meta-analysis. *Ann Intern Med* 1996;124:627–632.

Schonder KS. Chronic and end-stage kidney disease. In: Chisholm-Burns MA, Schwinghammer TL, Wells BG, et al., eds. *Pharmacotherapy: Principles and Practice*. 2nd ed. New York: McGraw-Hill; 2010: 445–478.

Snively CS, Gutierrez C. Chronic kidney disease: Prevention and treatment of common complications. *Am Fam Physician* 2004;70:1921–1928.

Self-Care

CHAPTER

24

TOPIC: CONSTIPATION AND DIARRHEA

Section Coordinator: James R. Clem
Contributor: Jaclynn Chin

Tips Worth Tweeting

Constipation

- Constipation is a decrease in stool frequency characterized by difficult passage of hard, dry stool.
- Always gather pertinent patient information and medication history to determine if self-treatment is appropriate. Look for signs of laxative abuse.
- To prevent constipation, do not ignore the urge to defecate and maintain a healthy diet, regular exercise routine, and adequate intake of fluids.
- Over-the-counter laxative agents are meant only for short-term or acute treatment (less than 1 week) of constipation. Otherwise, prompt referral to a physician is warranted.
- Avoid taking laxatives within 2 hours of other medications to avoid drug interactions.
- Most laxative agents are not recommended for children younger than 6 years of age, except for glycerin suppositories.

Diarrhea

- Diarrhea is an abnormal increase in stool frequency, liquidity, or weight.
- Avoiding dehydration is key to treatment of diarrhea. Self-treatment with over-the-counter antidiarrheal agents is limited to patients with minimal, mild, or moderate dehydration only.
- Loperamide is not recommended for children younger than 6 years of age except under medical supervision. Bismuth subsalicylate is not recommended for children younger than 12 years of age.
- If symptoms do not improve within 48 hours with self-treatment and oral rehydration, prompt referral to a physician is warranted.

Patient Care Scenario: Ambulatory Pharmacy Setting

A. B.: 57 y/o, M, walks into the pharmacy seeking advice on an over-the-counter product for constipation and diarrhea.

Allergies: none

Date	Physician	Drug	Quantity	Sig	Refills
7/1	Stieg	Acetaminophen 325 mg	#120	two qid prn	3
6/2	Stieg	Lisinopril 40 mg	#30	one daily	3
5/2	Stieg	Simvastatin 20 mg	#30	one daily	
4/2	Stieg	Aspirin 325 mg	#30	one daily	
4/2	Stieg	Hydrochlorthiazide 25 mg	#30	one daily	

Table 24-1 Constipation and Diarrhea: Medication-Induced Causes and Associated Disease States

	Medication-Induced Causes	Associated Disease States
Constipation	Analgesics, antidepressants, antacids, anticholinergics, antihistamines, ACE inhibitors, calcium-channel blockers, calcium supplements, diuretics, iron, opiates (morphine, codeine)	Hypercalcemia, hypothyroidism, dementia, pregnancy, irritable bowel syndrome, diabetes, Parkinson's disease, multiple sclerosis, depression, colon cancer, stroke
Diarrhea	Antibiotics, antacids containing magnesium, cytotoxic agents, laxative abuse	Bacterial infections, viral infections, inflammatory bowel disease, Crohn's disease, ulcerative colitis

PMH: hypertension, dyslipidemia, coronary artery disease, osteoarthritis

1.1.0 Patient Information

Laboratory Testing

Routine labs are appropriate to evaluate significant medical conditions but generally are not essential for the diagnosis or management of common outpatient gastrointestinal (GI) disorders like constipation and diarrhea.

Instruments and Techniques Related to Patient Assessment

- A patient interview including medication history
- General health status (for recurrent conditions)
- Duration of use of self-treatment agents
- Location of the pain, onset, and duration
- Associated symptoms (e.g., fever, nausea, vomiting)
- Exacerbating or alleviating factors

Key Terms

- **Constipation:** decrease in stool frequency characterized by difficult passage of hard, dry stool
- **Diarrhea:** abnormal increase in stool frequency, liquidity, or weight

Signs and Symptoms

- Constipation: straining to have a stool, passage of hard and dry stool, passage of small stools, feelings of incomplete bowel evacuation, bloating
- Diarrhea: cramping, bloating, abdominal pain, nausea, urgent need to defecate, watery stools

Wellness and Prevention

In most cases, common GI disorders can be prevented by different lifestyle measures. The following are some steps that could be taken:

Table 24-2 Drugs for Constipation: Mechanisms of Action and Dosage

Type	Mechanism of Action	Drug	Common Daily Doses for Adults
Bulk-forming laxatives	Dissolve and swell in the intestines, forming emollient gels and stimulating peristalsis	Methylcellulose	4–6 g
		Polycarbophil	1–6 g
		Psyllium	2.5–30 g
Emollient laxatives (stool softeners)	Anionic surfactant that increases wetting efficiency	Docusate sodium/docusate calcium	50–360 mg
Lubricant laxatives	Emulsify contents, prevent absorption of fecal water	Mineral oil	14–45 mL
Saline laxatives	Highly osmotic ions in the intestine draw in water, causing an increase in intraluminal pressure and motility	Magnesium hydroxide	30–60 mL
		Magnesium citrate	150–300 mL
		Magnesium sulfate	10–30 g
		Monobasic sodium phosphate; dibasic sodium phosphate	8.3–16.6 g;1.9–3.8 g
Hyperosmotic laxatives	Osmotic effect and local irritant effect to stimulate bowel movement.	Polyethylene glycol 3350 (PEG)	17 g in 8 oz of water
		Glycerin	3 g daily (solid); 5–15 mL daily (liquid)
Stimulant laxatives	Irritate localized mucosa and stimulate bowel movement; increase secretion of fluids into bowel	Bisacodyl	10–30 mg
		Sennosides (senna)	8.6–15 mg
		Castor oil 95%	15–60 mL

Table 24-3 Drugs for Diarrhea: Indications, Mechanisms of Action, and Common Doses for Adults

Drug	Mechanism of Action	Common Daily Doses for Adults
Loperamide	Slows gastrointestinal motility	4 mg initially, then 2 mg after each loose stool without exceeding 8 mg/day
Bismuth subsalicylate	Improves stool consistency and provides direct antimicrobial effect	525 mg every 30–60 minutes, maximum of 8 doses per day

- Constipation: Increase intake in fiber and liquids, maintain a regular exercise routine, follow the urge to defecate when needed
- Diarrhea: Avoid foods that are raw and not served at the right temperature; avoid unpasteurized milk and drinking tap water

1.2.0 Pharmacotherapy

Interaction of Drugs with Foods and Laboratory Tests

Bulk-forming laxatives may reduce the effectiveness of other medications when used together. Concurrent use of mineral oil and docusate should be avoided due to an increased risk of systemic absorption. Mineral oil may decrease absorption of fat-soluble vitamins. It may also reduce the absorption of oral anticoagulants and oral contraceptives. Saline laxatives may interact with phenothiazines, digoxin, and oral anticoagulants. Avoid administering bisacodyl tablets within an hour of histamine-2-receptor antagonists, antacids, or proton pump inhibitors, as erosion of the tablets' enteric coating may occur.

There are no significant drug–drug interactions with loperamide. However, bismuth subsalicylate (BSS) can interact with medications that interact with aspirin due to its salicylate moiety. These medications include warfarin, valproic acid, methotrexate, probenecid, tetracyclines, and quinolones.

Contraindications, Warnings, and Precautions

Use of bulk-forming and saline laxatives is inappropriate in patients with renal disorders and patients who are fluid restricted (e.g., patients with congestive heart failure, hypertension, or edema). Docusate sodium and mineral oil should not be used concurrently. Mineral oil is contraindicated in children and the elderly. Bisacodyl is compatible with breastfeeding, whereas senna is contraindicated with breastfeeding. Castor oil is contraindicated in pregnancy. Stimulants should not be used in patients with rectal bleeding, intestinal obstruction, or appendicitis. Toxicity may result when saline laxatives are taken in patients with severe renal impairment due to an increased absorption of magnesium ion. Bulk-forming, emollient, lubricant, and oral saline laxative agents and loperamide are not recommended for use in children younger than 6 years of age.

BSS is not recommended for children younger than 12 years of age; it is also contraindicated in nursing and pregnant women. In addition, it contraindicated in patients with aspirin allergy and in children with viral illnesses (Reye's syndrome).

Physiochemical Properties, Solubility, Pharmacodynamics, and Pharmacokinetic Properties

Bulk-forming agents have an approximate onset of action of 12–72 hours. No systemic absorption of these agents occurs. Emollient agents have an approximate onset of action of 24–72 hours, but their effectiveness is mostly achieved within 48 hours. Saline laxatives have an onset of action of 0.5–3 hours for oral dosing, and 2–5 minutes for rectal dosing. Glycerin has an onset of action of 0.25–1 hour, while polyethylene glycol has a longer onset of 24–72 hours. Senna and bisacodyl have an onset of action of 6–10 hours, while castor oil has an onset of 2–6 hours.

1.3.0 Monitoring

Pharmacotherapeutic Outcomes

The goals of therapy are to improve signs and symptoms of acute constipation and diarrhea.

Safety and Efficacy Monitoring/Patient Education

Constipation

- Monitor for improvements of signs and symptoms within 1 week of use. If symptoms are unrelieved, refer to primary care provider for further evaluation.
- Avoid routine or extended use of laxatives, as it can alter the functioning of a normal bowel movement and lead to dependence.
- Monitor for drug–drug interactions, and use precaution in patients with conditions requiring electrolyte or fluid restriction.

Diarrhea

- Improvements of symptoms with acute diarrhea usually occurs within 48 hours.
- Preventing dehydration is the most important factor, and patients should be monitored by assessing body weight, vital signs, and mental alertness.
- Referral to a primary care provider is necessary if the patient presents with high fever, bloody

stools, diarrhea lasting for more than 48 hours, or signs of worsening dehydration.

Adverse Drug Reactions

- Bulk forming agents: cramping, flatulence, esophageal obstruction in older adults
- Emollients: mild abdominal cramping, diarrhea, nausea, bitter taste
- Lubricants: pneumonitis due to aspiration, anal irritation, pruritus, rectal discharge
- Saline agents: abdominal cramping, nausea/vomiting, diarrhea, dehydration, hypermagnesemia
- Hyperosmotic agents; minimal side effects with glycerin suppositories; PEG 3350 may cause bloating, abdominal discomfort, cramping and flatulence
- Stimulants: severe cramping, diarrhea, abdominal pain
- Loperamide: hyperglycemia, abdominal pain, nausea/vomiting, dizziness, dry mouth
- BSS: tinnitus, gout, black-staining stool, Reye's syndrome

Nonadherence, Misuse, or Abuse

Misuse or abuse is highly unlikely with these products if they are used to treat acute symptoms. Laxative abuse may occur in patients with chronic constipation or in younger adults for the use of weight control. Excessive use of laxatives can also lead to severe chronic watery diarrhea and vomiting.

Pharmacotherapeutic Alternatives

- Constipation: misoprostol, lubiprostone (severe constipation), botulinum toxin
- Diarrhea: empiric antibiotic therapy (for community-acquired acute diarrhea), diphenoxylate, probiotics

ANNOTATED BIBLIOGRAPHY

Curry CE, Butler DM. Constipation. In: Berardi RR, Ferreri SP, Hume AL, et al. *Handbook of Nonprescription Drugs*. 16th ed. Washington, DC: American Pharmacists Association; 2009:263–288.

Locke GR 3rd, Pemberton JH, Phillips SF. American Gastroenterological Association Medical position statement: guidelines on constipation. *Gastroenterology* 2000;119:1761.

Monaghan MS. Gastrointestinal system. In: Jones RM, Rospond RM. *Patient Assessment in Pharmacy Practice*. Baltimore, MD: Lippincott Williams and Wilkins; 2003:261–285.

Wald A. Treatment of constipation in adults. *UpToDate, online 17.3*. Last updated June 20, 2009. Available at: http://www.uptodate.com/index. Accessed February 17, 2010.

Walker PC. Diarrhea. In: Berardi RR, Ferreri SP, Hume AL, et al. *Handbook of Nonprescription Drugs*. 16th ed. Washington, DC: American Pharmacists Association; 2009:289–308.

Wanke CA. Approach to the adult with acute diarrhea in developed countries. *UpToDate, online 17.3*. Last updated October 1, 2009. Available at: http://www.uptodate.com/index. Accessed February 17, 2010.

TOPIC: COUGH, COLD, AND ALLERGIC RHINITIS

Section Coordinator: James R. Clem
Contributor: Kimberly Messerschmidt

Tips Worth Tweeting

- Coughing is a natural defense mechanism designed to expel secretions from the lower airways. Because a cough may be a symptom of several different disease states, some of which may be serious, it is always important to identify the underlying cause of a chronic cough rather than just suppress it.
- Dextromethorphan and codeine are the antitussives of choice to treat a nonproductive (dry), tickling cough; diphenhydramine is a second-line alternative. Few data support the efficacy of any of these agents in the treatment of a cough associated with the common cold. Instead, a first-generation antihistamine plus an oral decongestant may be used to dry up secretions that can cause postnasal drip.
- Camphor and menthol are topical antitussives that are available in creams, ointments, lozenges, and inhalant solutions; few data support their efficacy as cough suppressants.
- When treating a cold, first-generation (sedating) antihistamines are moderately effective at reducing sneezing and nasal discharge due to their anticholinergic (drying) effects, but many individuals do not tolerate their side effects.
- Expectorants are designed to thin out and help expel thick respiratory secretions, but there are few data to support their efficacy.
- According to the FDA, OTC cough and cold products should not be recommended for use in children younger than 2 years of age due to their lack of efficacy and potential for harm; manufacturers have broadened this advisory to include children younger than 4 years of age.
- When treating allergic rhinitis, talk to the patient to find out what the most bothersome symptoms

are, and initiate monotherapy targeted at these symptoms; additional drugs may be added later as needed.
- Second-generation (nonsedating) antihistamines are recommended as first-line treatment for most patients with mild to moderate intermittent allergic rhinitis symptoms; decongestants may be added for patients with significant nasal congestion.
- Antihistamines and mast cell stabilizers are most effective when taken on a regularly scheduled basis, and ideally should be started 1 to 2 weeks prior to the anticipated allergy season.

Patient Care Scenario: Ambulatory Pharmacy Setting

D. K. is a 46-year-old white female who comes to your pharmacy seeking advice for the treatment of nasal congestion and drainage. She is wondering if these symptoms could be related to allergies. She is 5'4", 185 lbs, and has no known drug allergies.

PMH: Hypertension

Medication Profile

Date	Physician	Drug	Quantity	Sig	Refills
1/10	Jones	Hydrochlorothiazide 12.5 mg	#30	one PO daily	6 refills

1.1.0 Patient Information

Medication-Induced Causes of Cough

ACE inhibitors are the most frequent cause of a drug-induced cough. Other commonly used medications that may cause a dry cough or bronchospasm in susceptible individuals include beta blockers (both oral and ophthalmic), inhaled medications, and NSAIDs.

Disease States Associated with Cough

- Upper and lower respiratory tract infections (e.g., sinusitis, colds, pneumonia, TB, bronchitis)
- Tobacco smoke
- Allergic rhinitis
- Postnasal drip
- GERD
- Heart failure
- Aspiration
- Pulmonary malignancies
- Asthma and COPD

Disease States Associated with Allergic Rhinitis

Allergic rhinitis has a strong genetic predisposition and is especially common in individuals who have, or have family members with, allergies, atopic dermatitis, and asthma.

Instruments and Techniques Related to Patient Assessment and Diagnosis of Cough, Colds, and Allergic Rhinitis

The diagnosis of a cough, cold, or allergic rhinitis relies primarily on a thorough history and physical examination. Further diagnostic testing (e.g., CBC, sinus or chest x-ray, spirometry) may be warranted to rule out a more serious cause of a chronic cough. Allergy testing may be helpful in identifying triggering allergens.

Key Terms

Classification of cough:

- **Productive:** a cough associated with the expectoration of secretions from the lower respiratory tract
- **Nonproductive:** a dry, hacking cough that does not produce secretions and serves no useful purpose
- **Acute:** a cough lasting less than 3 weeks (most commonly due to an upper respiratory infection)
- **Chronic:** a cough lasting more than 8 weeks (most commonly due to chronic conditions such as postnasal drip, asthma, or GERD)

Classification of allergic rhinitis:

- **Intermittent allergic rhinitis** (seasonal allergic rhinitis, hayfever) is usually due to airborne pollens from trees, grasses, and weeds that are released during the spring or fall blooming seasons
- **Persistent allergic rhinitis** (perennial allergic rhinitis) is caused by year-round allergens found in the home environment (e.g., dust mites, mold, pet dander, cockroaches).

Wellness and Prevention

Preventing the common cold involves frequent hand washing and the use of hand sanitizers. It is also advisable to keep hands away from the nose and eyes, avoid close contact with individuals with a cold, cover the mouth and nose when coughing or sneezing, and take basic measures to keep the immune system functioning at an optimal level (e.g., healthy diet, exercise, adequate sleep, avoidance of tobacco smoke). The use of nonmedicated throat lozenges, saline gargles, and humidifiers may help sooth irritated airways associated with a dry cough.

One of the first, and most important, steps in the treatment of allergic rhinitis is allergen avoidance. Unfortunately, this can be very difficult and impractical, and is often insufficient to treat symptoms. Some of the more common avoidance strategies include

Table 24-4 Signs and Symptoms of the Common Cold and Allergic Rhinitis

Symptom	Common Cold	Intermittent Allergic Rhinitis	Persistent Allergic Rhinitis
Fever	Rare, low-grade	Absent	Absent
Headache	Mild or absent	Variable	May be a result of chronic sinusitis
Myalgias/arthralgias	Mild or absent	Absent	Absent
Fatigue	Mild or absent	Common	Common
Rhinorrhea, sneezing	Common	Common	Common
Nasal congestion	Common	Common	More common; tends to be more severe
Sore throat	Common during first few days	May occur due to postnasal drip	May occur due to postnasal drip
Cough (usually nonproductive)	Less common; usually mild, hacking	May occur due to postnasal drip	May occur due to postnasal drip
Ocular	Watery eyes	More common; watery, itchy, red puffy eyes	Watery, itchy, red, puffy eyes
Itching	Absent	Common	Common
Usual duration of symptoms	Seven days	Less than 4 days per week, or less than 4 weeks in total	More than 4 days per week **and** longer than 4 weeks

reducing household humidity to less than 40% (to reduce molds and dust mites), encasing the mattress and pillows in fabric that is impervious to dust mites, washing bedding in hot water at least weekly (for dust mites), removing pets from sleeping areas, using high-efficiency air filters, and remaining indoors during peak pollen days.

1.2.0 Pharmacotherapy

Mechanism of Action

- Decongestants: alpha-adrenergic activity produces vasoconstriction in the nasal and sinus mucosa
- Antihistamines: anticholinergic activity causes a drying effect (common cold); blocks histamine from binding to receptors (allergic rhinitis)
- Expectorants: stimulates the production of respiratory secretions, thereby thinning them out and making them easier to expectorate
- Antitussives: depresses the cough center in the brain
- Mast cell stabilizers: prevents mast cell degranulation and release of inflammatory mediators

Interaction of Drugs with Foods and Laboratory Tests

Oral decongestants are contraindicated in patients who are currently on monoamine oxidase inhibitors (MAOIs), or who have taken MAOIs within the past 14 days, as their use may result in a hypertensive crisis. Dextromethorphan is also contraindicated in these patients because concurrent use may lead to serotonin syndrome. Loratadine should be used with caution in patients receiving amiodarone due to the potential for QT prolongation.

Contraindications, Warnings, and Precautions

Decongestants may aggravate hypertension, heart disease, diabetes, BPH, closed-angle glaucoma, bladder-neck obstruction, and hyperthyroidism. Avoid use of these medications in the first trimester of pregnancy (pregnancy category C). Oral decongestants may decrease breastmilk production when used during lactation.

Avoid using first-generation antihistamines during tasks that require mental alertness (e.g., driving, using heavy machinery). These agents should also be used with caution in patients with a history of urinary retention/symptomatic BPH, stenosing peptic ulcer, pyloroduodenal obstruction, narrow-angle glaucoma, hyperthyroidism, and cardiovascular disease (pregnancy categories B and C).

Avoid the use of guaifenesin during the first trimester of pregnancy due to the increased risk of neural tube defects (pregnancy category C).

Antitussives should be avoided or used with caution when treating a productive cough, as they may cause retention of secretions in the lower respiratory tract and predispose the patient to complications (e.g., pneumonia, airway obstruction). Both codeine and dextromethorphan should be used with caution in combination with other CNS depressants, and in persons with underlying respiratory conditions (pregnancy category C).

Intranasal cromolyn is the preferred agent in pregnancy and lactation due to its low systemic absorption (pregnancy category B).

Physiochemical Properties, Pharmacodynamics, and Pharmacokinetic Properties

- Nasal decongestants have a more rapid onset of action and fewer systemic side effects than

Table 24-5 Cough, Cold, and Allergic Rhinitis: Drug Indications and Common Doses

Drug Class	Indications (Symptoms Treated)	Examples of Common Drugs, Adults Doses, and Routes of Administration
Decongestants	Nasal and/or eustachian tube congestion, and to a lesser degree, nasal discharge/postnasal drip	Nasal: • Phenylephrine (Neo-Synephrine): 2–3 sprays in each nostril up to every 4 hours as needed • Oxymetazoline (Afrin): 2–3 sprays in each nostril every 10–12 hours as needed Oral: • Phenylephrine (Sudafed PE): 10 mg PO every 4 hours as needed • Pseudoephedrine (Sudafed): 30–60 mg po every 4–5 hours as needed *or* 120 mg SR po every 12 hours as needed
First-generation antihistamines	Sneezing and rhinorrhea associated with allergies and the common cold (only moderately effective for cold symptoms)	Chlorpheniramine (Chlor-Trimeton): 4 mg po every 4–6 hours *or* 12 mg SR po every 12 hours as needed Diphenhydramine (Benadryl): 25–50 mg po every 4–6 hours as needed Triprolidine (Actifed): 2.5 mg po every 4–6 hours as needed
Second-generation antihistamines	Allergic rhinitis (rhinorrhea, sneezing, itching, ocular symptoms)	Cetirizine (Zyrtec): 5–10 mg po daily Loratadine (Claritin): 10 mg po daily
Ocular antihistamines	Ocular symptoms of allergic rhinitis	Ketotifen fumarate (Zaditor): 1 drop in each eye every 8–12 hours
Expectorants	Facilitates removal of thick respiratory secretions	Guaifenesin (Robitussin Chest Congestion, Mucinex): 200–400 mg po every 4 hours *or* 600–1200 mg ER tablet po every 12 hours as needed
Antitussives	Suppression of a nonproductive cough	Codeine: 10–20 mg po every 4–6 hours as needed Dextromethorphan (Delsym): 10–20 mg po every 4 hours *or* 30 mg po every 6–8 hours *or* 60 mg ER po every 12 hours as needed Diphenhydramine: 25 mg po every 4 hours as needed
Mast cell stabilizers	Mild allergy symptoms (itching, sneezing, rhinorrhea)	Cromolyn sodium (Nasalcrom): 1 spray in each nostril tid to qid at regular intervals, starting 2–4 weeks prior to the anticipated allergy season

oral decongestants. Sprays cover more mucosal surface area than drops and, therefore, are the preferred product in adults.

- Phenylephrine has a low oral bioavailability (38%), making it less effective than oral pseudoephedrine.
- Increasing the dose of dextromethorphan does not increase its efficacy, but will increase its duration of action.
- First- and second-generation antihistamines are similar in efficacy when used to treat allergic rhinitis. First-generation agents are highly lipophilic, however, which enables them to easily cross the blood–brain barrier and cause CNS side effects.

1.3.0 Monitoring Pharmacotherapeutic Outcomes

- Cough: minimize coughing episodes, resolve underlying condition, prevent complications
- Cold: minimize symptoms, prevent potential complications, reduce transmission to others
- Allergic rhinitis: minimize symptoms, improved quality of life

Safety and Efficacy Monitoring and Patient Education

Cough

Consult a physician for a cough that fails to improve after 7 days or worsens with self-treatment. Patients with the following symptoms or conditions should be referred to their physician for further evaluation: purulent respiratory secretions, fever, hemoptysis, a history of unintentional weight loss or chronic pulmonary disease, night sweats, or suspected aspiration. Camphor- and menthol-containing creams, ointments, and inhalant solutions may be toxic if taken orally.

Cold

Cold medications do not shorten the duration of or cure the common cold; they simply decrease the severity of symptoms. Because colds are caused by viral infections, antibiotics are not indicated and should be avoided in most circumstances. Patients should be instructed to contact their physician if symptoms worsen or if they indicate a possible bacterial infection (e.g., fever, shortness of breath, chest pain, wheezing, purulent respiratory secretions, persistent headache, ear pain, a sore throat lasting longer than a couple days, a cough that lasts longer than 1 week). Patients who are frail, elderly, immunosuppressed, or younger than 9 months of age, or who have chronic underlying cardiac or pulmonary conditions, should be referred to their physician. Consult a physician for a cough that persists for more than 1 week, is recurrent, or is accompanied by a fever, rash, or persistent headache. OTC cough and cold products should be avoided in children younger than 4 years of age due to a lack of efficacy data regarding their use and increased risk of adverse effects.

Allergic Rhinitis

Patients who should be referred to their physician include children younger than 12 years of age (due to concerns regarding undiagnosed asthma), patients with uncontrolled asthma, patients who are unresponsive or intolerant of OTC treatment, pregnant or lactating women, and patients with symptoms of potential complications (e.g., otitis media, sinusitis, bronchitis, or other infection). Cromolyn nasal spray may take as long as 4 weeks of regular use to achieve maximal benefits.

Adverse Drug Reactions

- Decongestants: Topical nasal decongestants may cause rebound nasal congestion (rhinitis medicamentosa) when used for longer than 3–5 days, or at doses higher than recommended. These agents may also cause local irritation (e.g., stinging, burning). Oral decongestants are more likely to cause CNS side effects (e.g., insomnia, restlessness, anxiety, tremors) and cardiac stimulation (e.g., increased blood pressure and heart rate, palpitations).
- Antihistamines: First-generation agents may cause sedation; dryness of the eyes, mouth, and nose; blurred vision; urinary retention; and impaired mental and physical performance. They may also cause a paradoxical reaction (nervousness, irritability, confusion, and restlessness) in the very young and the elderly. Cetirizine may be more sedating than other second-generation antihistamines. Ocular antihistamine side effects include burning, stinging, and dryness of the eyes.
- Expectorants: Side effects are minimal but may include nausea, vomiting, and dizziness.
- Antitussives: Codeine may cause nausea, drowsiness, lightheadedness, and constipation. Dextromethorphan is usually well tolerated, but may cause drowsiness, dizziness, stomach upset, and constipation.
- Mast cell stabilizers: Side effects are mostly limited to local nasal irritation (burning, stinging, sneezing).

Nonadherence, Misuse, or Abuse

Nasal decongestants may cause rebound congestion when used for longer than recommended, or when used at higher doses than recommended.

Codeine has a low potential for dependence when used as directed, but may cause problems with prolonged use. Dextromethorphan also has potential for abuse; when used in larger doses than recommended, it can produce intoxication, euphoria, respiratory depression, hallucinations, ataxia, nystagmus, vomiting, altered mental status, psychosis, mania, and seizures. Pharmacists should be suspicious when this product is purchased in large quantities.

Large doses of pseudoephedrine have been used to illegally manufacture methamphetamines. For this reason, federal and state regulations require this product to be stored in secure areas of the pharmacy and sold in limited quantities.

Pharmacotherapeutic Alternatives

Many dietary supplement products claim to reduce the incidence and severity of the common cold, with high-dose vitamin C, echinacea, and zinc being the most common. Few data support the use of vitamin C for the prevention of the common cold, but some studies show it may be effective in decreasing the severity and duration of cold symptoms once a person has a cold. Similarly, few data support the use of echinacea in preventing a cold, but it may be useful in reducing the severity and duration of cold symptoms. The data on zinc are also controversial. Intranasal zinc should be avoided due to concerns regarding loss of smell.

ANNOTATED BIBLIOGRAPHY

Abramowicz M, ed. Treatment guidelines from the *Medical Letter:* drugs for allergic disorders. *The Medical Letter, Inc.* (New Rochelle, NY); February 2010.

Scolaro KL. Disorders related to colds and allergy. In: Berardi RR, Ferreri SP, Hume AL, et al. *Handbook of Nonprescription Drugs*. 16th ed. Washington, DC: American Pharmacists Association; 2009:177–202.

Simasek M, Blandino DA. Treatment of the common cold. *Am Fam Physician* 2007;75:515–520.

Tietze KJ. Cough. In: Berardi RR, Ferreri SP, Hume AL, et al. *Handbook of Nonprescription Drugs*. 16th ed. Washington, DC: American Pharmacists Association; 2009:203–212.

Young SS. Appropriate use of common OTC analgesics and cough and cold medications. Available at: http://www.aafp.org/online/etc/medialib/aafp_org/documents/news_pubs/mono/otc.Par.0001.File.tmp/OTCmonograph.pdf.

TOPIC: FEVER AND PAIN

Section Coordinator: James R. Clem
Contributor: Kimberly Messerschmidt

Tips Worth Tweeting

- The main indication for the use of antipyretics is patient discomfort. Because a fever may serve a beneficial purpose, the decision of whether to treat should be made on an individual basis.
- Hyperpyrexia is a medical emergency in which the body temperature exceeds 106°F; it may be associated with seizures, dehydration, or changes in mental status.
- Aspirin, acetaminophen, and NSAIDs all have similar efficacy in regard to fever reduction, although NSAIDs have a slightly longer duration of action.
- Combining or alternating antipyretics in an effort to increase efficacy should not be recommended.
- For children, acetaminophen and ibuprofen dosing should be based on body weight rather than age.
- The use of cool baths and sponging (with water or alcohol) is not recommended for bringing down a fever.
- Avoid using aspirin in children younger than 15 years with viral illnesses due to the potential association with Reye's syndrome.
- NSAIDs tend to work very well for inflammatory pain (e.g., strains, sprains, dysmenorrhea).
- Dosage formulations come in several strengths; it is imperative to know which product the patient is using when making recommendations to avoid serious medication errors.
- Concern regarding acetaminophen—a leading cause of drug-induced liver toxicity—is the most common reason for contacting a poison control center. Inadvertent overdosing is common, and may occur as a result of measurement or calculation errors.
- Always recommend using appropriate measuring devices (not kitchen utensils) for liquid products.
- Patients should be aware that acetaminophen is a hidden ingredient in many OTC and prescription products; watch for unintentional duplication that may result in overdosing.
- Capsaicin products need to be applied three to four times daily, on a daily basis, to achieve maximum effectiveness.
- Normal body temperature is best defined as a range, most commonly being anywhere from 96°F to 100°F.
- There is no universally accepted temperature that defines a fever, but most clinicians would agree that a body temperature greater than 100.4°F qualifies as a fever.
- Most nonprescription topical analgesics are classified as counterirritants; they produce their analgesic effect by creating a less severe, superficial "irritation" to mask a more intense, deeper pain.
- Due to toxicity concerns, several manufacturers have reduced their maximum recommended daily dose of acetaminophen to 3,000 mg per day instead of 4,000 mg; daily doses greater than 4,000 mg have been associated with increased risk of hepatotoxicity.

Patient Care Scenario: Ambulatory Pharmacy Setting

G. D. is a 4 y/o M who comes to your pharmacy accompanied by his mother. Since yesterday, he has been running a low-grade fever (100.8°F) that is causing him some mild discomfort. His mother states that she kept him home from his daycare program, and although G. D. has not been eating much, she feels he is staying well hydrated. His activity level has been low and she would like a medication to lower his temperature and allow him to rest more comfortably.

PMH: No chronic illnesses or medications; vaccinations are up-to-date. No known drug allergies.

1.1.0 Patient Information

Medication-Induced Fever

A variety of drug classes have been implicated in drug-induced fever (e.g., anti-infectives, antineoplastics, anticonvulsants, antidepressants, vaccinations). Malignant hyperthermia and neuroleptic malignant syndrome are two rare, but potentially life-threatening drug reactions that require immediate intervention.

Disease States Associated with Fever

Most fevers are the result of a systemic infection (i.e., bacterial, viral, fungal), but fever can also be caused by a variety of other conditions (e.g., malignancy, heat stroke, tissue damage, hyperthyroidism, allergic reactions).

Table 24-6 Fever and Pain: Drug Indications and Common Doses

	Indications	Examples of Common Drugs and Doses
Oral Medications		
Acetaminophen	Mild to moderate pain; fever; (no anti-inflammatory or antiplatelet effects)	Adults: 325–1,000 mg every 4–6 hours as needed (maximum: 4,000 mg per day; some manufacturers have reduced to 3,000 mg per day) Children: 10–15 mg/kg per dose every 4–6 hours as needed (maximum: 5 doses or 60 mg/kg per day)
Salicylates (aspirin, magnesium salicylate, sodium salicylate)	Mild to moderate pain; fever; (limited anti-inflammatory activity with OTC dosing; aspirin has antiplatelet activity)	Adult aspirin dose: 325–1,000 mg every 4–6 hours as needed (maximum: 4,000 mg per day)
NSAIDs (ibuprofen, naproxen)	Mild to moderate pain; fever; (limited anti-inflammatory activity with OTC dosing)	Adult ibuprofen (Advil, Motrin) dose: 200–400 mg every 4–6 hours as needed (maximum: 1,200 mg per day) Children older than 6 months: 5–10 mg/kg per dose every 6–8 hours (maximum: 4 doses or 30 mg/kg per day) Adults and children 12 and older, naproxen (Aleve) dose: 220 mg every 8–12 hours as needed (may take 440 mg for first dose; maximum: 660 mg per day)
Topical Medications		
Counterirritants (methylsalicylate, camphor, menthol) Capsaicin	Minor muscle and joint pain Minor muscle and joint pain; neuralgias	Methylsalicylate, menthol, and camphor (Ultra Strength Bengay Cream): apply topically to affected area up to 4 times daily Capsaicin (Zostrix): apply topically to affected area 3–4 times daily on a regular basis

Instruments and Techniques Related to Patient Assessment and Diagnosis

Measurement of body temperature may be done by the oral, rectal, axillary, temporal, or otic route. Rectal measurement is often considered the standard of care due to its accurate reflection of core body temperature, but this method is limited by poor patient acceptance. Axillary measurement tends to be less reliable.

1.2.0 Pharmacotherapy

Mechanism of Action

- Acetaminophen: inhibits central prostaglandin synthesis
- Salicylates and NSAIDs: inhibit peripheral prostaglandin synthesis
- Counterirritants: stimulate cutaneous receptors by causing a mild irritation or inflammation of the skin, which masks perception of deeper pain
- Capsaicin: depletes substance P, a neurochemical that facilitates transmission of pain impulses

Interaction of Drugs with Foods and Laboratory Tests

- Although acetaminophen is the OTC analgesic of choice for patients on warfarin, doses greater than 2,275 mg per week may increase these individuals' INR.
- Concurrent use of salicylates may increase the risk of toxicity with valproic acid, methotrexate (also occurs with some NSAIDs), and sulfonylureas; ibuprofen may increase free levels of phenytoin.
- NSAIDs and salicylates can decrease the efficacy of antihypertensives, and increase the risk of bleeding when used together, or with anticoagulants or alcohol.
- Aspirin use may produce a false-positive fecal occult blood test; discontinue for at least 3 days prior to testing.

Contraindications, Warnings, and Precautions

Exclusions for self-treatment of a fever:

- Children younger than 6 months with a rectal temperature of 101°F or greater, and children older than 6 months with a rectal temperature of 104°F or greater
- Any child who is vomiting or refusing to take fluids, has a history of seizures, or is sleepy and difficult to rouse
- Any fever that lasts more than 3 days or is accompanied by significant infection, rash, or respiratory impairment
- Any patient with CNS impairment (e.g., history of head trauma, stroke), or immunocompromise (e.g., malignancy, HIV, immunosuppressive drugs)

Exclusions for self-treatment of pain:

- Moderate to severe pain
- Pain that persists for more than 10 days, or for more than 1 week after treatment initiation
- Pain that originates in the pelvis (except for dysmenorrhea) or abdomen, or is accompanied by nausea, vomiting, fever, or other signs of infection
- Third trimester of pregnancy
- Children younger than 2 years of age

Some manufacturers now recommend not to exceed 3,000 mg (rather than the 4,000 mg) of acetaminophen within a 24-hour period; consider limiting the total dose to less than 2,000 mg per 24-hour period in individuals with an increased risk for hepatotoxicity (e.g., preexisting liver disease, malnutrition, chronic intake of three or more alcoholic drinks per day, concurrent use of other potentially hepatotoxic drugs). Doses exceeding 4,000 mg per day may increase the risk of liver toxicity.

Avoid using NSAIDs in patients who are allergic to salicylates (less cross-reactivity with sodium or magnesium salicylate). Also, use salicylates and NSAIDs with caution in patients with asthma or nasal polyps due to increased risk of hypersensitivity. Avoid salicylates and NSAIDs if the patient has a history of stomach problems, ulcers, chronic kidney disease, or bleeding problems. Absence of GI symptoms does not rule out GI toxicity. Patients who are taking prescription medications for diabetes, gout, and arthritis, and those on chronic anticoagulation should consult their physician prior to taking salicylates. Aspirin should generally be discontinued at least 1 week prior to major surgical procedures. Effervescent formulations should be used with caution in people who need to limit their sodium intake (e.g., patients with hypertension, heart failure, or renal disease). Avoid using aspirin and NSAID products during pregnancy and lactation unless directed by a physician (pregnancy category C; category D in third trimester).

Patients who consume three or more alcoholic beverages per day on a regular basis should consult their physician prior to using any OTC pain reliever.

Most topical analgesics are indicated for use in adults and children older than 12 years of age (capsaicin products should be used only in adults). Keep all topical analgesics out of reach of children, as oral ingestion is potentially lethal.

Physiochemical Properties, Pharmacodynamics, and Pharmacokinetic Properties

Aspirin and acetaminophen suppositories are erratically absorbed, resulting in unpredictable results with their use. Enteric coatings may significantly reduce the rate and extent of absorption of aspirin, but controversy exists as to whether such coatings help reduce GI toxicity. Effervescent formulations are rapidly absorbed, but do not have a faster onset of action or improved efficacy. Peak antipyretic efficacy for all of the OTC agents usually occurs around 2 hours. Capsaicin generally takes at least 2 weeks to start working. The use of buffered aspirin does not significantly reduce GI toxicity.

1.3.0 Monitoring

Pharmacotherapeutic Outcomes

- Fever: alleviate discomfort, identify and treat underlying cause
- Pain: decrease severity and duration of pain

Safety and Efficacy Monitoring and Patient Education

Patients with fever should increase their fluid intake to replace insensible losses and prevent dehydration.

Although OTC analgesics are generally safe and effective when used as directed, they can cause significant toxicity when used inappropriately. These products should be used to self-treat pain for only 10 days in adults and 5 days in children (only 3 days for ibuprofen).

Patients should be advised to consult their physician if their pain increases, or if any of the following occurs: redness, swelling, abnormal bleeding, change in stool color or consistency, persistent GI pain, persistent change in frequency or quality of urination, swelling of the lower extremities, abnormal weight gain, ringing in the ears, hearing loss, or symptoms of liver dysfunction (e.g., jaundice, RUQ pain, nausea, pruritus, fatigue, lethargy).

Take each dose of aspirin or NSAID with a full glass of water; take with food or milk if stomach upset occurs. The chronic use of ibuprofen has been associated with an increased risk of cardiovascular complications (e.g., heart failure, hypertension, stroke, myocardial infarction).

Acetaminophen is considered safe for use in pregnancy and lactation (pregnancy category B). Ibuprofen is considered to be compatible with breastfeeding.

Avoid using external analgesics on open wounds or damaged skin, with heating pads, or under tight bandages or occlusive dressings. Do not use these products more than three to four times daily, or for more than 7 days without consulting a physician. Discontinue use if irritation, rash, burning or stinging (except capsaicin), swelling, or signs of infection occur. Avoid getting topical products in the eyes or other sensitive areas of the body, and always wash hands thoroughly after use.

Adverse Drug Reactions

- Acetaminophen rarely causes side effects when used at recommended OTC doses.
- The most common side effects associated with salicylates and NSAIDs involve the GI tract (e.g., bleeding, dyspepsia, nausea, stomach pain); bleeding, fluid retention, and renal toxicity may occur with higher doses or longer duration of use. Aspirin and NSAID hypersensitivity may result in angioedema, urticaria, bronchospasm, and respiratory distress.
- The topical use of capsaicin may cause burning, stinging, and redness at the application site; these side effects usually decrease within 72 hours of consistent use.

Nonadherence, Misuse, or Abuse

It is extremely important to refer all acetaminophen overdoses to a poison control center, even if no signs or symptoms of toxicity are apparent at the time, as serious clinical manifestations may not become apparent for 2–4 days after the ingestion

Pharmacotherapeutic Alternatives

Chondroitin sulfate, glucosamine sulfate, methyl-sulfonyl-methane (MSM), and *S*-adenosyl-l-methionine (SAMe) have all been used as alternative therapies for pain and discomfort associated with osteoarthritis.

ANNOTATED BIBLIOGRAPHY

Feret B. Fever. In: Berardi RR, Ferreri SP, Hume AL, et al. *Handbook of Nonprescription Drugs*. 16th ed. Washington, DC: American Pharmacists Association; 2009:83–94.

Remington TL. Headache. In: Berardi RR, Ferreri SP, Hume AL, et al. *Handbook of Nonprescription Drugs*. 16th ed. Washington, DC: American Pharmacists Association; 2009:68–82.

Wright E. Musculoskeletal injuries and disorders. In: Berardi RR, Ferreri SP, Hume AL, et al. *Handbook of Nonprescription Drugs*. 16th ed. Washington, DC: American Pharmacists Association; 2009:100–106.

TOPIC: HEMORRHOIDS AND HEARTBURN

Section Coordinator: James R. Clem
Contributor: Jaclynn Chin

Tips Worth Tweeting

Hemorrhoids:

- Hemorrhoids are swollen or inflamed veins around the lower rectum or anus.
- A patients should only self-treat hemorrhoids when symptoms are limited to burning, itching, discomfort, swelling, and irritation.
- Prompt referral to a physician is key if symptoms do not improve within 7 days or if patients are younger than 12 years of age.
- Use only external products (except for protectants) in patients who are pregnant or breastfeeding.
- Avoid nonprescription hemorrhoid products in patients with diabetes, hypertension, or cardiovascular disorders.

Heartburn:

- Heartburn is a burning sensation at the substernal area due to irritation of the esophagus caused by stomach acidity.
- Avoid concurrent administration of antacids and oral medications.
- Prompt referral to a physician is key if symptoms do not improve within 2 weeks with self-treatment or if patients are younger than 12 years of age.
- Antacids provide the most immediate relief, followed by H2RAs and then PPIs. The duration of action also correlates with the onset of action, with antacids having the shortest duration of action and PPIs the longest.
- Combining an antacid with an H2RA provides both immediate relief and a longer duration of action.

Patient Care Scenario: Ambulatory Pharmacy Setting

C. D., 64 y/o M, 5'9", 181 lbs, walks into the pharmacy seeking advice on over-the-counter products for hemorrhoids and for heartburn.

NKA

PMH: diabetes, hypertriglyceridemia, hypertension, chronic constipation

Date	Physician	Drug	Quantity	Sig	Refills
8/5	Smith	Aspirin 325 mg	#100	one daily	5
8/5	Smith	Gemfibrozil 600 mg	#60	one BID	3
8/6	Smith	Lisinopril 10 mg	#30	one daily	4
8/6	Smith	Hydrochlorothiazide 25 mg	#30	one daily	4
8/6	Smith	Psyllium	1 canister	one teaspoonful in water daily	2

Table 24-7 Hemorrhoids and Heartburn: Medication-Induced Causes and Associated Disease States

	Medication-Induced Causes	Associated Disease States
Hemorrhoids	None	Persistent diarrhea or constipation, pregnancy, overweight
Heartburn	Aspirin/NSAIDs, iron, anticholinergics, alpha-adrenergic antagonists, $beta_2$-adrenergic agonists, benzodiazepines, narcotic analgesics, cytotoxic agents	Obesity, pregnancy, smoking, stress, motility disorders (gastroparesis)

1.1.0 Patient Information

Laboratory Testing

Routine labs are appropriate to evaluate significant medical conditions but generally are not essential for the diagnosis or management of common outpatient gastrointestinal disorders such as hemorrhoids and heartburn.

Instruments and Techniques Related to Patient Assessment

The patient interview should include medication history; general health status (for recurrent conditions); location of the pain, as well as its onset and duration; associated symptoms (e.g., fever, nausea, vomiting), and exacerbating or alleviating factors.

Key Terms

- **Heartburn:** burning sensation at the substernal area due to irritation of the esophagus caused by stomach acidity
- **Hemorrhoids:** swollen or inflamed veins around the lower rectum or anus

Signs and Symptoms

- Hemorrhoids: bleeding during bowel movements, anal itching or burning, discomfort, inflammation, or swelling
- Heartburn: burning pain in the chest that occurs after eating and worsens when lying down, dysphagia, chronic cough, sore throat, and chronic hoarseness

Wellness and Prevention

In most cases, common GI disorders can be prevented by different lifestyle measures. The following are some steps that could be taken:

- Hemorrhoids: preventing constipation, avoiding use of dry toilet paper, keeping a clean anal area
- Heartburn: maintaining a healthy weight, eating smaller meals, smoking cessation, elevating the head of the bed, avoiding tight-fitting clothes, avoiding triggers (food and drinks) that exacerbate the condition

Table 24-8 Hemorrhoids: Drug Indications, Mechanism of Action, and Common Doses for Adults

Type	Mechanism of Action	Drug/Active Ingredients	Maximum Frequency of Application
Local anesthetics	Reversibly blocks transmission of nerve impulses and temporarily relieves symptoms of itching, irritation, burning, or pain	Benzocaine, benzyl alcohol, dibucaine, dyclonine, lidocaine, pramoxine, tetracaine	Up to 4–6 times daily
Vasoconstrictors	Reduce swelling and relieve itching and discomfort; slight anesthetic effect	Ephedrine, epinephrine, phenylephrine	Up to 4 times daily
Protectants	Form a physical barrier on the skin and decrease water loss	Aluminum hydroxide gel, cocoa butter, glycerin, kaolin, lanolin, mineral oil, white petrolatum, petrolatum, zinc oxide, calamine	Up to 6 times daily; no maximum frequency of use for petrolatum and white petrolatum
Astringents	Coagulate skin cells, decrease secretions, and decrease anal itching, burning, and irritation	Calamine, zinc oxide, witch hazel	Up to 6 times daily
Keratolytics	Debride epidermal cells and expose underlying tissue; reduce itching and discomfort	Alcloxa, resorcinol, menthol, juniper tar, camphor	Up to 6 times daily
Corticosteroids	Anti-inflammatory, antipruritic, vasoconstrictive agents	Hydrocortisone	Up to 3–4 times daily

Table 24-9 Heartburn: Drug Indications, Mechanism of Action, and Common Doses for Adults

Type	Mechanism of Action	Drug	Maximum Daily Dose for Adults
Antacids	Neutralize stomach acid	Magnesium (hydroxide, carbonate)	Varies depending on ingredients, acid-neutralizing capacity (ANC), and formulation; do not exceed more than 4 times daily dosing
		Aluminum (hydroxide, phosphate)	
		Calcium carbonate	
		Sodium bicarbonate	
Histamine-2-receptor antagonists (H2RAs)	Decrease gastric acid secretion	Ranitidine	75 mg, 150 mg (2 tablets)
		Cimetidine	200 mg (2 tablets)
		Nizatidine	75 mg (2 tablets)
		Famotidine	10 mg, 20 mg (2 tablets)
Proton pump inhibitors (PPIs)	Decreases gastric acid secretion	Omeprazole	20 mg

1.2.0 Pharmacotherapy

Interaction of Drugs with Foods and Laboratory Tests

Protectants such as aluminum gel and kaolin should not be administered with greasy substances, as they interfere with the medication's ability to adhere to the skin. These substances include cocoa butter, cod liver oil, lanolin, mineral oil, shark liver oil, petrolatum, and white petrolatum. Vasoconstrictors that are administered rectally may increase blood pressure when administered concomitantly with an oral antihypertensive, so concurrent use should occur only under supervision of a primary care provider.

In general, antacids should not be administered together with oral medications, as this combination can affect absorption levels. Cimetidine and ranitidine bind to cytochrome P450 and interact with medications that share the same metabolism pathway (e.g., phenytoin, warfarin, theophylline, amiodarone). However, ranitidine binds to a lesser extent, so interactions are uncommon with over-the-counter dosing. Omeprazole may interact with medications that depend on CYP 2C19 for metabolism, and patients taking medications such as phenytoin, warfarin, and diazepam should be cautioned about this interaction. Medications that depend on an acidic environment, such as ketoconazole, itraconazole, and iron, may have a decreased absorption when administered concurrently with antacids, H2RAs, or PPIs.

Contraindications, Warnings, and Precautions

Use of vasoconstrictors should be avoided in patients with diabetes, cardiac disorders, and hypertension without a physician's approval due to an increased risk for systemic adverse effects. This is also true when using local anesthetics internally or when using keratolytics in open wounds.

Antacid use should be avoided in patients with renal failure, as the risk for electrolyte toxicity (aluminum, magnesium, and calcium) are increased in these patients. Patients who require sodium restriction (e.g., those with hypertension, congestive heart failure, or edema) should avoid use of sodium bicarbonate.

Physiochemical Properties, Solubility, Pharmacodynamics, and Pharmacokinetic Properties

Hemorrhoidal symptom relief should occur within the first few days of self-treatment. Corticosteroids, in particular, may have an onset of action up to 12 hours but exhibit a longer duration of action than most other agents.

Antacids in general have an onset of action of less than 5 minutes and provide relief for approximately 20–30 minutes. H2RAs take a little longer to work, and patients usually feel the relief within 30–45 minutes. The duration of relief, however, can last up to 4–10 hours. When antacids and H2RAs are used in combination, they provide immediate relief and a longer duration of action. PPIs, in contrast, have the slowest onset of relief (approximately 2–3 hours) but the longest duration of action (12–24 hours).

1.2.0 Monitoring

Pharmacotherapeutic Outcomes

The goal of treatment is to improve signs and symptoms of self-treatable hemorrhoids and heartburn.

Safety and Efficacy Monitoring and Patient Education

Hemorrhoids

Use only selected internal agents, such as astringents (calamine and zinc oxide), vasoconstrictors (ephedrine and phenylephrine), and protectants (except glycerin), for application inside the rectum. Pregnant or breastfeeding women should use only products recommended for external use except for the use of protectants. In general, vasoconstrictors should be avoided in patients with cardiovascular disorders, hypertension, or diabetes due to an increased risk of systemic adverse effects.

If symptoms do not improve within 7 days, a primary care provider should be consulted immediately. Also, if patient experiences pain, increased/unusual bleeding, seepage, or changes in bowel pattern, prompt medical referral is required, as these conditions may be a sign of a nonhemorrhoidal or more serious anorectal disorder.

Heartburn

Patients with renal impairment should consult their primary care provider before using any antacids. It is recommended to separate antacids within 2 hours of taking any oral medications to avoid any drug interactions. Patients with symptoms lasting more than 2 weeks despite self-treatment with either an antacid, PPI, or H2RA should be referred to a primary care provider.

Omeprazole should be taken with a full glass of water 30 minutes before breakfast for a total of 14 days. Complete resolution of symptoms should be seen within 4 days of treatment with omeprazole.

Adverse Drug Reactions

- Local anesthetics: potential systemic effects; contact dermatitis
- Vasoconstrictors: nervousness, nausea, tremor, rebound vasodilation with prolong use
- Protectants: lanolin allergy
- Astringents: prolonged use may cause systemic zinc toxicity; witch hazel causes a slight stinging sensation and possible contact dermatitis
- Keratolytics: tinnitus, increased pulse rate, sweating
- Corticosteroids: mask symptoms of bacterial and fungal infections
- Antacids: diarrhea (magnesium), constipation (aluminum), belching and flatulence (calcium and sodium carbonate)
- H2RAs: headache, diarrhea, dizziness, constipation
- PPIs: diarrhea, constipation, headache

Nonadherence, Misuse, or Abuse

Misuse or abuse is highly unlikely with these products if used for short-term self-treatment.

Pharmacotherapeutic Alternatives

Prescription formulations for the treatment of heartburn are alternatives for over-the-counter medications:

- H2RAs: ranitidine, cimetidine, nizatidine, famotidine
- PPIs: pantoprazole, lansoprazole, rabeprazole, esomeprazole
- Promotility agents: metoclopramide, bethanechol and cisapride

ANNOTATED BIBLIOGRAPHY

American Gastroenterological Association Institute technical review on the management of gastroesophageal reflux disease. *Gastroenterology* 2008;135:1392–1413.

American Gastroenterological Association medical position statement: diagnosis and treatment of hemorrhoids. *Gastroenterology* 2004;126:1461.

Bleday R, Breen E. Treatment of hemorrhoids. *UpToDate, online 17.3*. Last updated April 14, 2009. Available at: http://www.uptodate.com/index. Accessed February 17, 2010.

Chan J, Berardi RR. Anorectal disorders. In: Berardi RR, Ferreri SP, Hume AL, et al. *Handbook of Nonprescription Drugs*. 16th ed. Washington, DC: American Pharmacists Association; 2009:209–324.

Kahrilas PJ. Medical management of gastroesophageal reflux diseases in adults. *UpToDate, online 17.3*. Last updated June 9, 2009. Available at: http://wwwuptodate.com/index. Accessed February 17, 2010.

Monaghan MS. Gastrointestinal system. In: Jones RM, Rospond RM. *Patient Assessment in Pharmacy Practice*. Baltimore, MD: Lippincott Williams and Wilkins; 2003:261–285.

Zweber A, Berardi RR. Heartburn and dyspepsia. In: Berardi RR, Ferreri SP, Hume AL, et al. *Handbook of Nonprescription Drugs*. 16th ed. Washington, DC: American Pharmacists Association; 2009:231–246.

TOPIC: OTIC, DENTAL, AND OPHTHALMIC

Section Coordinator: *James R. Clem*
Contributor: *Thaddaus R. Hellwig*

Tips Worth Tweeting

- Common otic disorders include impacted cerumen and water-clogged ears.
- Impaired hearing may be secondary to impacted cerumen.
- Simple irrigation with saline or warm water may aid in the removal of impacted cerumen.
- Use of cotton swabs may increase impaction and lead to perforated tympanic membranes.
- A physician evaluation should be done before treatment of water-clogged ears is undertaken to differentiate this condition from swimmer's ear, which may require antibiotic therapy.

- Overuse of alcohol-containing products for water-clogged ears may lead to overdrying.
- Avoid artificial tear products that contain preservatives if the patient requires application more than four times per day.
- Gel products are best for nighttime administration because they may cause blurry vision.
- Dry eyes may be related to other chronic medical conditions and require consultation with a physician.
- Medications are a common cause of dry eyes.
- Decongestants are contraindicated in patients with narrow-angle glaucoma and should be used with precautions in patients with hypertension, cardiovascular disease, and prostatic hypertrophy.
- Naphazoline and tetrahydrozoline may cause fewer rebound symptoms.
- Recurrent aphthous stomatitis (RAS) may occur secondary to increased stress, trauma, food allergies, and nutritional deficiencies.
- Herpes simplex labialis (HSL), or cold sores, may be expressed secondary to other immunosuppressive disease states.
- Apply therapy for HSL only to the lips and face, not to genital areas.

Patient Care Scenario: Ambulatory Pharmacy Setting

T. W.: 66 y/o with complaints of excessive ear wax that has possibly led to some hearing problems.

Allergies: NKDA.

PMH: hypertension, type I diabetes, hyperlipidemia, osteoarthritis

Date	Physician	Drug	Quantity	Sig	Refills
9/3	Cart	Lisinopril 40 mg	#30	one daily	5
9/2	Cart	Hydrochlorothiazide 50 mg	#30	one daily	5
8/1	Cart	Metformin 500 mg	#60	one bid	4
7/1	Cart	Glyburide 5 mg	#30	one bid	4
8/1	Cart	Simvastatin 20 mg	#30	one daily	4
8/1	Cart	Acetaminophen 325 mg	#120	one qid	5

1.1.0 Patient Information

Laboratory Testing

Routine labs may be necessary to evaluate medical conditions that could lead to cerumen impaction, but the physical exam is the main diagnostic tool.

Instruments and Techniques Related to Patient Assessment

A physician evaluation may be needed to exclude possible otitis externa, eardrum perforation, foreign bodies, or infection as causes of the patient's symptoms before attempting cerumen removal.

Key Terms

Cerumen impaction is an excessive buildup of cerumen in the ear canal that can lead to obstruction or total occlusion of the ear canal.

Signs and Symptoms

- Pain
- Itching
- Impaired hearing
- Tinnitus
- Dizziness
- Vertigo
- Social withdrawal (secondary to hearing loss)
- Chronic cough

Wellness and Prevention

- Irrigation of the ear canal may be able to remove impacted cerumen. Irrigating the ear with warm water or saline may be enough to soften and remove the buildup of cerumen.
- Avoid use of cotton swabs because they can worsen impaction.

1.2.0 Pharmacotherapy

Mechanism of Action

- 3% hydrogen peroxide: releases oxygen, causing effervescence that leads to loosening or breakup of cerumen
- Carbamide peroxide: releases oxygen, causing effervescence that leads to loosening or breakup of cerumen
- Olive oil: emollient used to soften cerumen

Contraindications, Warnings, and Precautions

Carbamide peroxide contraindications include age less than 3 years, dizziness, ear drainage or discharge seen, ear perforation, ear pain/irritation, and hypersensitivity to carbamide peroxide.

1.3.0 Monitoring

Monitor for buildup of cerumen.

Pharmacotherapeutic Outcomes

The therapeutic goal is to prevent and/or remove cerumen impaction.

Table 24-10 Cerumen Impaction: Specific Uses and Indications of Medications

Drug	Dosing
3% Hydrogen peroxide	Fill affected ear canal before irrigation
Carbamide peroxide	5–10 drops into affected ear bid for up to 4 days Allow to sit for at least 15 minutes
Olive oil	3–4 drops into affected ear at bedtime for 3–4 days

Safety and Efficacy Monitoring and Patient Education

- Use caution with cotton swabs, as they may increase impaction or perforate the tympanic membrane.
- Use caution when applying irrigation; remove all of the liquid to prevent infection or water-clogged ears.
- If the patient develops severe pain, vertigo, or severe swelling, a physician referral is needed.
- Do not attempt self-treatment if there are signs of infection, bleeding, or recent ear surgery.
- Ear candles may cause injuries without improving impacted cerumen.

2.2.0 Dispensing

Carbamide peroxide is the active ingredient in the following products: Debrox, Auro Ear Drops, Murine Earwax Removal System, Otix Drops, Audiologist's Choice, E-R-O, and Dent's Ear Wax Drops.

1.1.0 Patient Information

Laboratory Testing

Routine labs may be appropriate to distinguish water-clogged ears from differential diagnosis of external otitis or swimmer's ear, and to detect the presence of (possible) infection.

Disease States Associated with Water-Clogged Ears

A physician referral should be made before any treatment is started for water-clogged ears to check for possible ruptured tympanic membranes or infection.

Key Terms

Water-clogged ears happen when water becomes trapped in the ear canal and may occur secondary to excessive cerumen or anatomical abnormalities.

Signs and Symptoms

- A feeling of wetness or water trapped in the ear
- Possible hearing loss

Table 24-11 External Otitis: Specific Uses and Indications of Medications

Drug	Dosing
Isopropyl alcohol 95% in glycerin 5%	Apply 4–5 drops in affected ear

- Development of infection
- Itching
- Pain
- Inflammation

Wellness and Prevention

- Avoid swimming, hot humid climates, and sweating, and use caution when bathing.
- Tilting the affected ear downward may expel some excess water
- Gently drying the ear following swimming/bathing may prevent complications.
- Use of earplugs during swimming is recommended.

1.2.0 Pharmacotherapy

Mechanism of Action

Alcohol evaporates faster than water, so when isopropyl alcohol mixes with water it acts as a drying agent. Isopropyl alcohol also may act as an anti-infective agent.

Contraindications, Warnings, and Precautions

Do not use isopropyl alcohol if you have drainage or discharge from the ear.

1.3.0 Monitoring

- Amount of water in the eyes
- Frequency of water-clogged ears
- Conditions that lead to water-clogged ears (avoid these conditions)
- Development of signs of infection

Pharmacotherapeutic Outcomes

- Expel water from water-clogged ears
- Decrease in frequency of water-clogged ears

Safety and Efficacy Monitoring and Patient Education

- Overuse of alcohol-containing products may lead to overdrying of the ear canal.
- If there is an open wound, stinging may occur.
- Physician referral is needed for swimmer's ear, as it may also have an infectious component and needs treatment with antibiotics and/or steroids.
- Avoid contact with the eyes.

Adverse Drug Reactions

Isopropyl alcohol may cause burning on exposed skin or excessive drying with overuse.

Pharmacotherapeutic Alternatives

Upon physician diagnosis, topical antibiotics and steroids may be prescribed for external otitis or swimmer's ear.

2.2.0 Dispensing

Isopropyl alcohol 95% is available as a generic product. Anhydrous glycerin products include Auro-Dri Drops and Swim Ear Drops.

1.1.0 Patient Information

Medication-Induced Causes

Recurrent aphthous stomatitis (RAS) may be caused by some chemotherapeutic agents.

Laboratory Testing

Routine labs may be appropriate to evaluate medical conditions that could lead to RAS but generally are not needed for the management of this condition.

Disease States Associated with RAS

- Behcet's disease
- SLE
- Allergens
- Nutritional deficiencies
- HIV/AIDS
- Inflammatory bowel disease

Instruments and Techniques Related to Patient Assessment

A physician visit may be the first step to determine whether a patient's RAS is secondary to a systemic disease or nutritional deficiency, especially if the patient has lesions present for longer than 14 days, the lesions frequently recur, or the patient has failed to respond to outpatient therapy.

Key Terms

Recurrent aphthous stomatitis (RAS) is an epithelial ulceration that presents in the mouth or upper throat; it is also known as a canker sore.

Signs and Symptoms

Patients may have complaints of a tingling or burning sensation at the site of the ulcer. Other symptoms include pain that may increase during eating or drinking, discomfort, and decreased oral intake.

Wellness and Prevention

- Avoid increased stress.
- Avoid local trauma (toothbrush abrasions).
- Avoid any possible food allergies (e.g., spicy foods, acidic foods).
- Increase consumption of iron, folate, or vitamin B_{12} if a nutritional deficit exists.
- Ice compressions may help decrease pain.
- Ensure regular use of a nonalcoholic mouthwash.
- Use warm saltwater rinses to soothe ulcers.

1.2.0 Pharmacotherapy

Mechanism of Action

Oral debriding/wound cleansing agents have antiseptic properties due to their oxygenating effects. They also promote natural wound healing and help with wound cleaning. These agents include carbamide peroxide and hydrogen peroxide.

Topical anesthetics decrease sodium ion permeability through stabilization of neuronal membranes, thereby blocking nerve impulses. The most common agent is benzocaine.

Interaction of Drugs with Foods and Laboratory Tests

Eating and swallowing may be difficult following application of mouth rinses containing anesthetic agents.

1.3.0 Monitoring

Assess for improved ulcer pain.

Pharmacotherapeutic Outcomes

- Improvement in oral ulcers
- Decreased pain
- Prevention of infection

Safety and Efficacy Monitoring and Patient Education

- Do not swallow medications.
- Allow gel formulations to sit for 1 minute.

Table 24-12 Recurrent Aphthous Stomatitis: Specific Uses and Indications of Medications

Active Ingredient	Dosing
Debriding/cleansing agents • Carbamide peroxide • Hydrogen peroxide	• Up to 4 times daily after meals and at bedtime • Rinse with ½ capful for 1 minute and then spit
Topical anesthetics: benzocaine	Apply to affected area up to 4 times daily

- Swish oral rinses for at least 1 minute and then spit them out.
- Most agents are to be used for only 7 days.

Adverse Drug Reactions

Skin irritation

Pharmacotherapeutic Alternatives

Prescription therapy may consist of corticosteroids, antiviral medications, or debacterol.

2.2.0 Dispensing

- Carboxamide peroxide: Gly-Oxide Oral Cleanser Liquid
- Hydrogen peroxide: Orajel Antiseptic Mouth Sore Rinse
- Benzocaine: Anbesol Regular Strength Gel, Orabase Maximum Strength Gel

1.1.0 Patient Information

Medication-Induced Causes

Herpes simplex labialis (HSL) may be caused by certain chemotherapies or other immunosuppressive medications.

Laboratory Testing

Routine labs may be appropriate to evaluate medical conditions that can lead to activation or reactivation of HSL.

Disease States Associated with HSL

Immunosuppressive diseases

Instruments and Techniques Related to Patient Assessment

A physician evaluation may be needed to determine whether a patient has any other disease state that would predispose him or her to an infection.

Key Terms

Herpes simplex labialis (HSL) is a disorder caused by the herpes simplex virus-1 (HSV-1), which typically causes oral or labial lesions, also known as cold sores.

Signs and Symptoms

- Pain
- Fever
- Bleeding

Wellness and Prevention

Avoid triggers of HSL, such as ultraviolet light, fatigue, stress, and immunosuppression.

Table 24-13 Herpes Simplex Labialis: Specific Uses and Indications of Medications

Drug	Common Doses
Docosanol	Apply topically 5 times per day

1.2.0 Pharmacotherapy

Mechanism of Action

Docosanol reduces viral replication.

Contraindications, Warnings, and Precautions

Use docosanol only on the lips and face.

Physiochemical Properties, Solubility, Pharmacodynamics, and Pharmacokinetic Properties

There is minimal systemic absorption of docosanol.

1.3.0 Monitoring

Assess for improvement in lesions.

Pharmacotherapeutic Outcomes

Quicker resolution of sores

Safety and Efficacy Monitoring and Patient Education

- Medication is for face and lips only.
- Do not use docosanol on genital herpes.
- Avoid contact with the eyes.

Adverse Drug Reactions

- Headache
- Application-site reactions

Pharmacotherapeutic Alternatives

Acyclovir, valacyclovir, and penciclovir may also be prescribed for HSL.

1.1.0 Patient Information

Medication-Induced Causes

- Antidepressants
- Antihistamines
- Beta blockers
- Decongestants
- Diuretics
- Oral contraceptives
- Phenylephrine
- Parkinson's medications
- Pain medications

Laboratory Testing

Routine labs are appropriate to evaluate medical conditions that can lead to dry eyes but generally are not essential for the diagnosis or management of dry eyes.

Disease States Associated with Dry Eyes

Dry eyes have been linked to Sjogren's syndrome, lupus, rheumatoid arthritis, diabetes, the normal aging process, Parkinson's disease, lacrimal gland deficiency, and sarcoidosis. Patients may also experience dry eyes for several weeks to months following LASIK eye surgery.

Instruments and Techniques Related to Patient Assessment

A physician's appointment may be an initial step to determine whether a patient's dry eyes are secondary to a chronic medical condition, especially in patients with a long history of dry eyes.

Key Terms

The **tear film** is a layer of substances secreted by glands to prevent the eyes from becoming dry. The tear film consists of lipids, mucins, and a liquid/watery component.

Signs and Symptoms

Patients may have complaints of blurred vision, discharge from the eyes, eye discomfort, eye burning, eye redness, increased sensitivity to light, a feeling of objects in the eye, eye fatigue, uncomfortable contact lenses, decreased tolerance of reading or working on a computer, inability to cry, and pain in the eyes.

Wellness and Prevention

Patients may need a physician evaluation to determine other medical causes of dry eyes.

- Avoid dry environments and possible use of humidifiers.
- Avoid dusty environments.
- Avoid prolonged reading or work on a computer.
- Avoid any allergen triggers.
- Avoid wearing contact lenses if they lead to dry eyes.
- Substitute or avoid medications that can cause dry eyes.

1.2.0 Pharmacotherapy

Mechanism of Action

- Methylcellulose and other cellulose ethers are ocular lubricants used to stabilize the tear film and prevent tear evaporation, thereby preventing dry eyes.
- Glycerin may produce an osmotic effect that prevents the eyes from drying out.

Table 24-14 Dry Eyes: Specific Uses and Indications of Medications

Active Ingredient	Doses
Methylcellulose	Apply 1–2 drops into affected eye as needed
Propylene glycol and glycerin	Apply 1–2 drops into affected eye as needed
Povidone and polyvinyl alcohol	Apply 1–2 drops into affected eye as needed
Gels	Apply 1–2 drops into affected eye as needed
Emollients	Apply ¼ inch onto the inside of the eyelid one or more times daily
Ointments	Apply ¼ inch onto the inside of the eyelid one or more times daily

- Povidone and polyvinyl alcohol act like cellulose ethers, in that they form a hydrophilic layer on the eye and lead to wetting of the eye.
- Ointments typically contain petrolatum, mineral oil, or lanolin, which can help enhance the tear film.
- Benzalkonium chloride (BAK) is a preservative used in ophthalmic products because of its ability to prevent microbial growth.

1.3.0 Monitoring

Assess for eye pain and redness.

Pharmacotherapeutic Outcomes

The goal of treatment is to improve symptoms of dry eyes.

Safety and Efficacy Monitoring and Patient Education

- Monitor for symptom improvement of dry eyes.
- Remove contact lenses before administering medication.
- See your physician if you experience eye pain, changes in vision, or continued redness or irritation for more than 72 hours.

Adverse Drug Reactions

Benzalkonium chloride (BAK) is a preservative that is found in some ophthalmic products and may lead to allergy, fibrosis, worsening dry eyes, or glaucoma surgery failure by possibly damaging the corneal epithelium. Patients who require multiple daily doses of a product should avoid agents with BAK as a preservative.

Pharmacotherapeutic Alternatives

Alternatives to over-the-counter products include prescription medication, which may be needed in certain circumstances. Physician referral may be needed to determine whether dry eyes are secondary to a chronic medical condition.

2.2.0 Dispensing

- Methylcellulose-like products: Bion Tears, Genteal Mild, Optive, Refresh Tears, Thera Tears, Visine Tears
- Propylene glycol and glycerin agents: Advanced Eye Relief, Oasis Tears, Optive, Systane
- Povidone and polyvinyl alcohol agents: Dakrina, Hypotears, Nutra Tear, Refresh Lubricant Eye Drops
- Gels: Genteal Gel, Systane Free
- Emollients: Soothe

1.1.0 Patient Information

Laboratory Testing

Routine labs may be appropriate to determine the cause of the conjunctivitis and to evaluate whether a bacterial component is present. White blood cell counts and eosinophil counts may be obtained. Allergy tests may be done to determine the cause of recurrent allergic conjunctivitis.

Disease States Associated with Allergic Conjunctivitis

- Seasonal allergies
- Hayfever
- Asthma

Instruments and Techniques Related to Patient Assessment

A physician's visit may be warranted to determine whether a patient's conjunctivitis is secondary to a bacterial or allergic component.

Key Terms

Conjunctivitis is an inflammation of the tissue lining of the eyelids secondary to a reaction with an allergy-causing substance.

Signs and Symptoms

- Bilateral red eyes
- Dilated vessels in the clear tissue of the eyes
- Intense itching
- Burning eyes
- Puffy eyelids
- Excessive tearing

Wellness and Prevention

Patients may need a physician evaluation to determine whether there is a bacterial component to the conjunctivitis.

Table 24-15 Conjunctivitis: Specific Uses and Indications of Medications

Drug	Indications/ Nonprescription Concentration	Common Doses
Decongestants	Allergic conjunctivitis: short-term	
Phenylephrine	0.12%	1–2 drops up to qid
Naphazoline	0.03–0.1%	1–2 drops up to qid
Oxymetazoline	0.025%	1–2 drops qid
Tetrahydrozoline	0.05%	1–2 drops qid
Antihistamine/ Mast Cell Stabilizers	Allergic conjunctivitis: short-term	
Ketotifen	0.025%	1 drop bid–tid
Antihistamines	Allergic conjunctivitis: short-term	
Pheniramine	0.3%	1–2 drops tid–qid
Antazoline	0.5%	1–2 drops tid–qid

- Avoid the allergen trigger if it is known (e.g., pollen, animal dander, or topical eye products).
- Avoid going outdoors if the pollen count is high.
- Use air filters on air conditioners.
- Cold compresses to the eyes several times a day may reduce symptoms.

1.2.0 Pharmacotherapy

Mechanism of Action

Decongestants primarily act on the alpha-adrenergic receptors of the ophthalmic system, leading to vasoconstriction. This ophthalmic vessel vasoconstriction leads to decreased eye redness.

Ketotifen is a combination antihistamine and mast cell stabilizer. It possesses properties of a selective noncompetitive antagonist on the histamine-1 (H1) receptor, inhibits the release of inflammatory mediators from cells involved in hypersensitivity reactions, and inhibits the activation of eosinophils.

Antihistamines act as H1-receptor antagonists.

Drug Interactions of Medical Therapy

Decongestants may interact with MAOIs and tricyclic antidepressants.

Contraindications, Warnings, and Precautions

- Decongestants: Contraindications include anatomical narrow angle, hypersensitivity to adrenergic agents, and narrow-angle glaucoma. Precautions are warranted in case of bronchial asthma, cardiovascular

disease, diabetes, hypertension, prostatic hypertrophy, rebound miosis, and rebound vasodilation.
- Ketotifen: Hypersensitivity to benzoate compounds is a contraindication.
- Antihistamines: Contraindications include angle-closure glaucoma. Precautions are warranted in case of angle-closure glaucoma, asthma/COPD, bladder-neck obstruction, cardiovascular disease, hypertension, and history of urinary retention.

1.3.0 Monitoring

- Symptomatic improvement
- Reduction in ocular itching and irritation

Pharmacotherapeutic Outcomes

- Improvement in allergic conjunctivitis symptoms is the therapeutic goal.
- Naphazoline and tetrahydrozoline may be less likely to cause rebound symptoms.

Safety and Efficacy Monitoring and Patient Education

- Limit use of medications to 3–5 days.
- Advise patients not to wear contact lenses while taking these medications.
- Ocular decongestants should be used cautiously by patients with hypertension or history of cardiovascular disease.
- Referral to a physician should be recommended if the patient has foggy vision, haloes around light sources, photophobia, extreme pain, or presence of a foreign body.

Adverse Drug Reactions

- Decongestants: erythema, mydriasis, pain in eye, increased intraocular pressure, epithelial xerosis, potentially tachycardia and aggravation of arrhythmias if absorbed systemically
- Ketotifen: headache, dry eyes, eye irritation, pain in eye, pupil dilation
- Antihistamines: burning or stinging in the eyes, pupil dilation

Nonadherence, Misuse, or Abuse

Ocular decongestants may have the potential to produce rebound hyperemia.

Pharmacotherapeutic Alternatives

Alternatives to over-the-counter products include prescription medications, which may be needed in certain circumstances. Physician referral may be needed to determine whether symptoms are due to bacterial conjunctivitis or other disease states.

2.2.0 Dispensing

Decongestants

- All Clear (naphazoline 0.012%)
- Clear Eyes (naphazoline 0.012%)
- Naphcon (naphazoline 0.012%)
- Murine Tears Plus (tetrahydrozoline 0.05%)
- Relief (phenylephrine)
- Visine L.R. (oxymetazoline 0.025%)
- Visine Clear (tetrahydrozoline 0.05%)

Antihistamine/Mast Cell Stabilizers

- Zaditor (ketotifen 0.025%)
- Alaway (ketotifen 0.025%)

Antihistamine/Decongestants

- Naphcon-A (pheniramine 0.3% and naphazoline 0.025%)
- Opcon-A (pheniramine 0.315% and naphazoline 0.02675%)
- Vasocon-A (antazoline 0.5% and naphazoline 0.05%)

ANNOTATED BIBLIOGRAPHY

Otic Medications

Burton MJ, Doree C. Ear drops for the removal of ear wax. *Cochrane Database of Systemic Reviews* 2009;1:CD004326. doi: 10.1002/14651858.CD004326.pub2.

Krypel L. Otic disorders. In: Berardi RR, Ferreri SP, Hume AL, et al. *Handbook of Nonprescription Drugs*. 16th ed. Washington, DC:, American Pharmacists Association; 2009: 633–648.

McCarter DF, Courtney AU, Pollart SM. Cerumen impaction. *Am Fam Physician* 2007;75:1523–1528.

Dental Medications

Gonsalves WC, Chi AC, Neville BW. Common oral lesions: Part I. Superficial mucosal lesions. American Family Physician. 2007;75: 501–507.

Marciniak MW. Oral pain and discomfort. In: Berardi RR, Ferreri SP, Hume AL, et al. *Handbook of Nonprescription Drugs*. 16th ed. Washington, DC: American Pharmacists Association; 2009;601–623.

Scully C, Gorsky M, Lozada-Nur F. The diagnosis and management of recurrent aphthous stomatitis. *J Am Dental Assoc* 2003;134:200–207.

Ophthalmic Medications

Bielory L, Friedlaender MH. Allergic conjunctivitis. *Immunol Allergy Clin N Am* 2008;28:43–58.

Giscella RG, Jensen MK. Ophthalmic disorders. In: Berardi RR, Ferreri SP, Hume AL, et al. *Handbook of Nonprescription Drugs*. 16th ed. Washington,

DC: American Pharmacists Association; 2009; 519–543.

TOPIC: INSOMNIA

Section Coordinator: James R. Clem
Contributor: Debra K. Farver

Tips Worth Tweeting

- Insomnia is a very common complaint from patients; it can be related to situations, medical diseases, psychiatric disorders, and medications.
- Diphenhydramine can be used for short-term treatment (fewer than 14 consecutive days) of insomnia.
- Diphenhydramine has significant adverse effects (i.e., residual daytime sedation, anticholinergic effects) and potential drug–drug interactions that can limit its use, especially in the elderly.
- Many over-the-counter antihistamine sleep aids may contain additional medications such as aspirin, acetaminophen, or ibuprofen.
- Limited evidence has been gathered to support the effectiveness of melatonin, valerian, and kava in inducing sleep.
- Kava should be avoided due to its risk of hepatotoxicity.

Patient Care Scenario: Ambulatory Pharmacy Setting

T. T: 66 y/o M, 5'3", has been having problems going to sleep for the past 2–3 weeks.

Allergies: none

PMH: hyperlipidemia, migraines, occasional pain

Date	Physician	Drug	Quantity	Sig	Refills
1/7	Tag	Propranolol 20 mg	#60	one bid	4
2/9	Tag	Fluoxetine 20 mg	#30	one bid	3
3/2	Tag	Atorvastatin 20 mg	#30	one hs	4
3/2	Tag	Acetaminophen 325 mg	#100	one qid	3

1.1.0 Patient Information

Medication-Induced Causes

- Amphetamines
- Atomoxetine
- Antidepressants (SSRIs, SNRIs, bupropion)
- Beta blockers
- Corticosteroids
- Anabolic steroids
- Diuretics
- Modafinil
- Theophylline
- Thyroid supplements
- Phenylephrine
- Pseudoephedrine
- Ephedrine
- Alcohol
- Nicotine
- Caffeine

Laboratory Testing

Routine labs are appropriate to evaluate medical conditions but generally are not essential for the diagnosis or management of insomnia.

Disease States Associated with Insomnia

- Cancer
- Chronic pain
- Diabetes mellitus
- Gastroesophageal reflux disease
- Heart disease
- Menopause
- Obesity
- Pulmonary disease
- Sleep apnea
- Narcolepsy
- Restless legs syndrome
- Urinary incontinence
- Psychiatric disorders

Instruments and Techniques Related to Patient Assessment

A patient interview concerning sleep patterns, along with a history and physical, is warranted to determine whether the insomnia is due to situational problems (e.g., loss of a loved one, shift work, jet lag), medical diseases, psychiatric disorders, or medications.

Key Terms

- **Primary insomnia:** difficulty falling asleep, intermittent wakefulness during sleep, and/or nonrestorative sleep (poor-quality sleep) for at least 1 month resulting in significant impairment of one's functioning (e.g., social, occupational)
- **Chronic insomnia:** insomnia that lasts for more than 1 month

Signs and Symptoms

- Difficulty falling asleep, intermittent wakefulness during sleep, and/or nonrestorative sleep (poor-quality sleep)

- Daytime-related effects of fatigue, drowsiness, decreased attention, decreased energy, lack of motivation, and deteriorated mood

Wellness and Prevention

Avoidance or minimization of alcohol, nicotine, and caffeine may help to improve sleep. Education about good sleep hygiene is a major factor in both preventing and treating insomnia. Nonpharmacologic methods to manage insomnia can benefit 50–80% of patients.

Common sleep hygiene recommendations follow:

- Have consistent times for waking up and going to bed every day.
- Use the bedroom for sleep or intimacy—not for reading or watching television.
- Exercise regularly but not immediately before bedtime.
- Use relaxation techniques at bedtime.
- Keep the bedroom quiet and cool.
- Avoid napping.

1.2.0 Pharmacotherapy

Mechanism of Action

Diphenhydramine and doxylamine are over-the-counter first-generation histamine-1 antagonists. Their ability to affect sleep is related to blocking histamine-1 and muscarinic receptors. Clinical trials report subjective sleep improvement with antihistamines, but the evidence is based on small numbers of patients over a short period of time. The sustained improvement in sleep is not confirmed. Tolerance appears to develop after 3 days of use. Antihistamines are not recommended for chronic insomnia. Diphenhydramine is commonly used in many over-the-counter sleep aids, with some products including other medications such as aspirin, acetaminophen, or ibuprofen. The addition of these analgesics has not been proved to enhance the sedative properties of antihistamines. Doxylamine is less commonly used.

Melatonin, valerian, and kava have been marketed as alternative and complementary products to induce sleep. Melatonin's action is unknown but may be related to stimulation of melatonin receptors, which regulate sedation and the sleep–wake cycle (circadian rhythms). Valerian's mechanism of action is unknown but is reported to be related to increasing concentrations of gamma aminobutyric acid (GABA). Evidence from clinical studies is conflicting as to the efficacy of melatonin, valerian, and kava for insomnia.

Table 24-16 Insomnia: Drug Indications and Common Doses

Drug	Indications for Adults or Children Older Than 12 Years	Common Doses
Diphenhydramine HCl or citrate	Insomnia: short-term and transient sleep difficulty	25–75 mg (commonly recommended: 50 mg) orally 30 minutes prior to bedtime for fewer than 14 consecutive nights
Doxylamine	Insomnia: short-term and transient sleep difficulty	25 mg orally 30 minutes prior to bedtime for fewer than 14 consecutive nights
Melatonin	Sleep difficulty	0.3 mg orally 30–120 minutes prior to bedtime; maximum dose: 5 mg
Valerian	Sleep difficulty	400–900 mg orally of aqueous extract 30–60 minutes prior to bedtime; 2–3 g dried valerian root soaked in one cup of hot water for 20–25 minutes prior to bedtime

Interaction of Drugs with Foods and Laboratory Tests

Diphenhydramine is a potent and competitive inhibitor of CYP2D6; thus its use can result in decreased metabolism of medications such as tricyclic antidepressants, antiarrhythmics, beta blockers, codeine, risperidone, and tramadol. Avoid use of diphenhydramine with alcohol, other sleep-inducing medications, and CNS depressants.

Doxylamine has interactions with pramlintide, anticholinergics, alcohol, CNS depressants, and acetylcholinesterase inhibitors.

Melatonin is metabolized by CYP1A2 and CYP2C19; caution in its use is warranted with warfarin and antiplatelet agents.

Contraindications, Warnings, and Precautions

Diphenhydramine is contraindicated in newborns, premature infants, nursing mothers, and persons with a hypersensitivity reaction. Doxylamine is also contraindicated in individuals with a hypersensitivity reaction. Precautions with the use of diphenhydramine and doxylamine are related to these medications' anticholinergic activity—it is essential to exercise care in the setting of urinary tract obstruction, decrease in mental alertness, elderly age, asthma, narrow-angle glaucoma, increased intraocular pressure, hyperthyroidism, cardiovascular disease (hypertension, tachycardia), and prostatic hypertrophy. Diphenhydramine is on the Beers list of medications to avoid in the elderly due to its propensity to cause mental confusion, cognitive impairment, urinary retention, constipation, and increased risk of falls. Over-the-counter diphenhydramine is not recommended for use in children younger than 6 years of age, and doxylamine is not recommended in children younger than 12 years of age.

Valerian and kava are contraindicated in patients with liver dysfunction.

Physiochemical Properties, Solubility, Pharmacodynamics, and Pharmacokinetic Properties

Diphenhydramine is well absorbed from the gastrointestinal tract. Its time to maximum plasma concentration is 1–4 hours, protein binding is 80–85%, elimination half-life is 2.4–9.3 hours, bioavailability is 40–60%, and metabolism is by *N*-demethylation. Diphenhydramine has lipophilic properties that enable it to cross the blood–brain barrier, resulting in 3–6 hours of sedation. There is not a linear increase in sedative effect as the dose is increased.

Doxylamine is well absorbed from the gastrointestinal tract. Its time to maximum plasma concentration is 2–4 hours, elimination half-life is 10 hours, and duration of sedation is 3–6 hours.

Melatonin has an elimination half-life of 60 minutes.

The parent drug for valerian contains more than 150 individual compounds. It has a high first-pass effect and a large volume of distribution (brain, blood, liver, heart, lung, intestines).

1.3.0 Monitoring

Pharmacotherapeutic Outcomes

The goal of therapy is to improve insomnia symptoms with short-term use (fewer than 14 days).

Safety and Efficacy Monitoring and Patient Education

Monitor for improvement in insomnia symptoms but recognize that long-term use of these medications is unlikely to sustain the sedative effect. Recommend using the medications for fewer than 14 days consecutive days. Educate the patient on appropriate sleep hygiene. Evaluate the potential for drug-induced insomnia. If the medication proves ineffective, the patient should consult his or her physician.

Safety monitoring concerns include daytime sedation and its impact on the patient's life. Monitor for anticholinergic adverse effects with diphenhydramine and doxylamine, and avoid use of these medications in the elderly. Perform a drug–drug interaction check for diphenhydramine. Avoid use of these agents with alcohol and other sleep-inducing medications. Counsel the patient on use of aspirin and acetaminophen. Monitor for adverse effects with melatonin and valerian. Discourage all use of kava due to its hepatotoxicity.

Adverse Drug Reactions

Diphenhydramine and doxylamine:

- Residual effect of daytime sedation (10–25%)
- Anticholinergic adverse effects, especially in the elderly: dry mouth, urinary retention, constipation, blurred vision, delirium
- Orthostatic hypotension
- Dizziness, which may affect driving
- Lower seizure threshold
- May produce excitation in children

Melatonin:

- Fatigue, dizziness, headache, irritability, drowsiness
- Less common: mood changes, hypotension, hyperglycemia, gastrointestinal distress, fluctuations in reproductive and thyroid hormones

Valerian:

- Unpleasant odor due to isovaleric acid component of valerian
- Dizziness, hangover effect, headache, insomnia, excitability, ataxia
- Less common: withdrawal tachycardia, questionable hepatotoxicity

Kava:

- Hepatotoxicity—avoid use

Nonadherence, Misuse, or Abuse

Misuse and abuse are unlikely with these medications due to their potential to induce tolerance with long-term use. Increasing the dose may not result in improved sleep but may lead to more pronounced adverse effects.

Pharmacotherapeutic Alternatives

Alternatives to over-the-counter medications for insomnia include prescription medications such as zolpidem, eszopiclone, ramelteon, and benzodiazepines.

2.2.0 Dispensing

Antihistamines

- Compoz Nighttime Sleep Aid (diphenhydramine HCl 50 mg tablets and gelcaps)
- Nytol Quick Caps (diphenhydramine HCl 25 mg caplets)
- Sominex Maximum Strength (diphenhydramine HCl 50 mg caplets)
- Sominex Nighttime Sleep Aid (diphenhydramine HCl 25 mg tablets)
- Unisom Sleepgels (diphenhydramine HCl 50 mg gelcaps)

- Unisom Nighttime Sleep Aid (doxylamine succinate 25 mg tablets)

Antihistamine–Analgesic Combination Products

- Advil PM (diphenhydramine citrate 38 mg/ibuprofen 200 mg caplets)
- Bayer PM Extra Strength (diphenhydramine citrate 38.3 mg/aspirin 500 mg caplets)
- Excedrin PM (diphenhydramine citrate 38 mg/acetaminophen 500 mg geltabs, caplets, and tablets)
- Tylenol PM Extra Strength (diphenhydramine HCl 25 mg/acetaminophen 500 mg geltabs, caplets, and gelcaps)

ANNOTATED BIBLIOGRAPHY

American Psychiatric Association. Sleep disorders. In: *Diagnostic and Statistical Manual of Mental Disorders, Fourth Edition, Text Revision*. Washington, DC: American Psychiatric Publishing; 2000.

Armstrong SC, Cozza KL. Antihistamines: med-psych drug–drug interactions update. *Psychosomatics* 2003;44:430–434.

Bain KT. Management of chronic insomnia in elderly patients. *Am J Ger Pharmacother* 2006;4(2):168–192.

Kirkwood CK, Melton ST. Insomnia. In: Berardi RR, Kroon LA, McDermott, JH, et al. *Handbook of Nonprescription Drugs*. 16th ed. Washington, DC: American Pharmacists Association; 2009:869–881.

Meoli AL, Rosen C, Kristo D, et al. Oral nonprescription treatment for insomnia: an evaluation of products with limited evidence. *J Clin Sleep Med* 2005;1(2):173–187.

Micromedex DrugDex. Diphenhydramine, doxylamine. Available at: http://www.thomsonhc.com. Accessed January 20, 2010.

Morin AK, Jarvis, CI, Lynch AM. Therapeutic options for sleep-maintenance and sleep-onset insomnia. *Pharmacotherapy* 2007:27(1):89–110.

Passarella S, Duong MT. Diagnosis and treatment of insomnia. *Am J Health-Syst Pharm* 2008;65:927–934.

TOPIC: SMOKING CESSATION

Section Coordinator: James R. Clem
Contributor: James R. Clem

Tips Worth Tweeting

- Do not smoke or use any forms of tobacco when using nicotine replacement therapy.
- When using nicotine gum, remind patients to activate (chew) the gum a few times and then park the gum between the cheek and gum of the mouth. This should be repeated every 1 to 2 minutes for 30 minutes.
- When using nicotine lozenges, let the lozenge dissolve slowly and rotate the lozenge to different areas of the mouth.
- The location for placement of nicotine replacement patches should be rotated, and a site should be used only once a week.
- Close patient counseling and follow-up are important for successful smoking cessation.
- Nicotine transdermal patches should be disposed of properly by folding the adhesive side onto itself before throwing it away.

Patient Care Scenario: Community Pharmacy Setting

E. H. is a 58 y/o M truck driver who recently became a grandfather. He comes into your pharmacy because he has been a smoker for 35 years. He is interested in quitting smoking to allow him to feel better and interact with his grandson.

Allergies: none

PMH: hypertension, back injury, obesity

Date	Physician	Drug	Quantity	Sig	Refills
6/26	Oliver	Hydrochlorothiazide 25 mg	#30	one daily	4
4/2	Oliver	Lisinopril 20 mg	#30	one daily	3
5/1	Oliver	Acetaminophen 325 mg	#120	one qid	3

1.1.0 Patient Information

Medication-Related Issues with Smoking Cessation Therapy

There are a number of known interactions between tobacco smoke and medications. These interactions can have continued significance once a smoker is successful with smoking cessation; thus adjustment in medication doses may be required once someone has been successful with smoking cessation.

Medications that are known to interact with tobacco smoke include benzodiazepines, bendamustine, beta blockers, caffeine, chlorpromazine, inhaled corticosteroids, erlotinib, flecainide, fluvoxamine, haloperidol, heparin, subcutaneous insulin, irinotecan, mexilitine, olanzapine, opioids, hormonal contraceptives, ropinirole, tacrine, theophylline, and tinzanidine.

Laboratory Testing

No routine labs are required for initiating smoking cessation therapy with nicotine replacement products.

Disease States History

Identification of smoking history and number of cigarettes smoked per day are data needed to determine the initial dosing of nicotine replacement therapy. In addition, how soon a patient smokes a cigarette after waking from sleep is needed for dosing nicotine lozenges.

Instruments and Techniques Related to Patient Assessment

A patient interview, including discussion of smoking habits and behaviors, is important in assisting a patient in smoking cessation. Identifying the reason for wanting to quit helps in developing strategies for successful smoking cessation. The five A's represent an important smoking cessation strategy:

- Ask (determine smoking status)
- Advise (encourage smokers to quit)
- Assess (determine willingness to quit)
- Assist (start pharmacotherapy and provide cessation counseling)
- Arrange (set up a follow-up visit or phone call)

Key Terms

Nicotine addiction is defined as multiple failed attempts to stop tobacco use before successful cessation occurs.

Wellness and Prevention

Smoking cessation carries several significant health benefits. A reduction in mortality is the most noteworthy benefit that has been demonstrated. Additionally, lower blood pressure, reduced risk of stroke, reduction in heart attack risk, decrease in breathing difficulty, and decrease in fatigue occur with smoking cessation. A downside to quitting smoking is the potential for weight gain. Although smoking neither reduces weight nor increases metabolism, once smoking cessation is successful, patients often replace their smoking habit with an increase in food intake, resulting in weight gain. It is important to remember that any increase in weight gain carries a much lower health risk in comparison to smoking.

1.2.0 Pharmacotherapy

Mechanism of Action

Nicotine replacement therapy maintains a therapeutic nicotine level in the body and is utilized in smoking cessation to prevent nicotine withdrawal from occurring once a smoker stops using tobacco. Nicotine withdrawal typically occurs for 3 days after quitting smoking. Because successful smoking cessation involves changing behaviors and habits associated with smoking, nicotine replacement therapy prevents nicotine withdrawal from occurring while patients work to change their habits and behaviors, thereby increasing the likelihood of successful smoking cessation.

Table 24-17 Smoking Cessation: Drug Indications and Common Doses

Drug	Indications for Adults	Common Doses
Nicotine Polacrilex gum	Nicotine replacement therapy for smoking cessation	2 mg if smoke < 25 cigarettes/day 4 mg if smoke ≥ 25 cigarettes/day Weeks 1–6: 1 piece every 1–2 hours Weeks 7–9: 1 piece every 2–4 hours Weeks 10–12: 1 piece every 4–8 hours
Nicotine Polacrilex lozenge	Nicotine replacement therapy for smoking cessation	2 mg if have first cigarette > 30 minutes after waking up 4 mg if have first cigarette ≤ 30 minutes after waking up Weeks 1–6: 1 lozenge every 1–2 hours Weeks 7–9: 1 lozenge every 2–4 hours Weeks 10–12: 1 lozenge every 4–8 hours
Nicotine transdermal systems (NicoDerm CQ and generic patches)	Nicotine replacement therapy for smoking cessation	> 10 cigarettes per day: • 21 mg/day for 6 weeks, then • 14 mg/day for 2 weeks, then • 7 mg/day for 2 weeks ≤ 10 cigarettes per day: • 14 mg/day for 6 weeks, then • 7 mg/day for 2 weeks

Interaction of Drugs with Foods and Laboratory Tests

No significant drug, food, or lab interactions exist with nicotine replacement therapy, although changes in drug metabolism may occur when a patient's smoking status changes.

Contraindications, Warnings, and Precautions

Nicotine replacement therapy is typically not required when a patient smokes fewer than 10 cigarettes per day. It should be used with caution in patients who are immediately post myocardial infarction (within the last 2 weeks), patients with life-threatening arrhythmias, and patients with severe or worsening angina pectoris.

Nicotine replacement therapy may cause fetal harm when used by pregnant women. Smoking cessation therapy in pregnant and breastfeeding women should be referred to a physician.

Physiochemical Properties, Solubility, Pharmacodynamics, and Pharmacokinetic Properties

Nicotine is absorbed well through the lungs, as well as through skin, buccal, and nasal surfaces. These routes of administration are effective in maintaining therapeutic serum nicotine levels in smokers who are in the process of smoking cessation. Nicotine from cigarette smoke produces a high peak serum concentration of nicotine, which leads to the pleasurable effects that occur from smoking and using tobacco. Nicotine replacement products maintain a minimum steady serum concentration of nicotine to prevent nicotine withdrawal symptoms; as a consequence, they do not produce the higher peak concentrations that reinforce the pleasurable effects of nicotine, yet help prevent nicotine withdrawal symptoms from occurring.

1.3.0 Monitoring

Pharmacotherapeutic Outcomes

The goal of treatment is successful smoking cessation without relapse.

Safety and Efficacy Monitoring and Patient Education

Appropriate monitoring of a patient who has started nicotine replacement therapy for smoking cessation includes follow-up counseling.

- Closely monitor a patient's cessation during the entire quit attempt.
- Assess the various aspects of the quit attempt for proper counseling;
  - Slips (smokes just one cigarette)
  - Relapses (starts smoking regularly again)
  - Adherence to nicotine replacement therapy
  - Adverse reactions to nicotine replacement therapy
  - Any triggers—provide information on how to deal with triggers and slips in the future
  - Positive reinforcement
- Do not smoke or use any forms of tobacco when using nicotine replacement therapy.
- When using nicotine gum, remind patients to activate (chew) the gum a few times and then park it between the cheek and gum of the mouth. This should be repeated every 1 to 2 minutes for 30 minutes.
- When using nicotine lozenges, let the lozenge dissolve slowly and rotate it to different areas of the mouth.
- The location for placement of nicotine replacement patches should be rotated, and a site should be used only once a week.
- If patients complain of vivid dreams while on nicotine patch therapy, advise them to remove the patch at bedtime and place a new one on in the morning.
- Nicotine transdermal patches should be disposed of properly by folding the adhesive side onto itself before throwing it away.

Adverse Drug Reactions

Nicotine gum:

- Unpleasant taste
- Mouth irritation
- Muscle soreness of the jaw
- Jaw fatigue
- Increased salivation
- Hiccups
- Dyspepsia

Nicotine lozenge:

- Mouth irritation
- Nausea
- Hiccups
- Cough
- Headache
- Heartburn

Nicotine transdermal system:

- Local skin irritation
- Vivid dreams
- Headache
- Insomnia

Nonadherence, Misuse, or Abuse

Patients should be instructed to not smoke or use other tobacco products when using nicotine replacement therapy. Nicotine replacement products—specifically, nicotine transdermal patches—should be disposed of appropriately (fold the adhesive edge onto itself before placing the patch in the trash). Patients should be told to keep nicotine replacement products out of the reach of children and pets.

Pharmacotherapeutic Alternatives

Alternatives to over-the-counter nicotine replacement products consist of prescription medications that reduce the craving for tobacco. Prescription medications for smoking cessation include other nicotine replacement delivery products, bupropion, varenicline, nortriptyline, and clonidine. The prescription non-nicotine products can be utilized in combination with over-the-counter nicotine replacement products to further increase the rates of successful smoking cessation.

2.2.0 Dispensing

Gum:

- Nicorette and generic 2 mg (regular, mint, orange)
- Nicorette and generic 4 mg (regular, mint, orange)

Lozenge:

- Commit 2 mg (regular, mint, cherry)
- Commit 4 mg (regular, mint, cherry)

Transdermal delivery (patches):

- NicoDerm CQ 21 mg (24 hour)
- NicoDerm CQ 14 mg (24 hour)
- NicoDerm CQ 7 mg (24 hour)
- Generic 21 mg (24 hour)
- Generic 14 mg (24 hour)
- Generic 7 mg (24 hour)

ANNOTATED BIBLIOGRAPHY

Kroon LA, Suchanek Hudmon K, Corelli RL. Smoking cessation. In: Berardi RR, Kroon LA, McDermott, JH, et al. *Handbook of Nonprescription Drugs.* 16th ed. Washington, DC: American Pharmacists Association; 2009:893–913.

Fiore MC, Jaen CR, Baker TB, et al. Treating Tobacco Use and Dependence: 2008 Update. Clinical Practice Guideline. Rockville, MD: U.S. Department of Health and Human Services. Public Health Service. May 2008.

TOPIC: SUNSCREENS AND ACNE

Section Coordinator: James R. Clem
Contributor: Stacy J. Peters

Sunscreens

Tips Worth Tweeting

- Ultraviolet radiation (UVR, including both UVA and UVB) is responsible for a variety of photodermatoses, sunburn, photosensitivity, skin cancer, premature skin aging, and ocular damage such as cataracts.
- A sunscreen product with an SPF rating of 30+ provides maximum protection from UV radiation.
- Broad-spectrum sunscreens, due to their added UVA protection, are best at preventing long-term effects secondary to UVR exposure regardless of a patient's history.
- Commonly used sunscreen ingredients include octinoxate for UVB protection and avobenzone for broad-spectrum UVA protection.
- Counsel patients on product selection, proper application of such products, and the importance of sun avoidance.

Patient Care Scenario: Community Pharmacy Setting

S. S. is a 26 y/o F who presents to your pharmacy with an antibiotic prescription. She mentions that she is taking a tropical cruise and hopes this antibiotic clears up her sinus infection. You offer to help her select a sunscreen.

Allergies: none

PMH: seasonal allergies, recurrent sinusitis

Date	Physician	Drug	Quantity	Sig	Refills
3/17	Irish	Loratidine	#30	one daily	5
4/1	Irish	Sulfamethoxazole-trimethoprim	#14	one bid	0

1.1.0 Patient Information

Medications Associated with Increased Photosensitivity

Medications that are sun sensitizers include, but are not limited to, fluoroquinolones, nonsteroidal anti-inflammatory agents, phenothiazines, antihistamines, estrogens, progestins, sulfonamides, sulfonylureas, thiazide diuretics, and tricyclic antidepressants.

Disease States and Risk Factors Associated with Increased Risk for the Development of UVR-Induced Problems

In general, patients who have multiple risk factors for UVR-induced problems—for example, previous growths on the skin or lips caused by UV exposure, current use of an immunosuppressive drug, history of an autoimmune disease, current use of photosensitizing drugs, or existing UV-induced disorder—should significantly limit their sun exposure or use extensive sun protection. Those who should avoid the sun altogether include infants younger than 6 months of age, people with allergies to all sun protectant ingredients, and patients with the rare condition xeroderma pigmentosum.

Risk factors for the development of UVR-induced problems:

- Fair skin that always burns and never tans
- A history of one or more serious or blistering burns
- Blonde or red hair
- Blue, green, or gray eyes
- A history of freckling
- A previous growth on the skin or lips caused by UVR exposure
- The existence of a UVR-induced disorder
- A family history of melanoma
- Current use of an immunosuppressive drug
- Current use of a photosensitizing drug
- Excessive lifetime exposure to UVR, including tanning beds and booths
- History of an autoimmune disease

Instruments and Techniques Related to Patient Assessment

- A patient interview assessing risk factors for the development of UVR-induced problems
- Age of patient
- Current medications
- Medication and nonmedication allergies
- Type of sun protection needed (waterproof, sweat resistant, area of body to be protected)
- Preferred product formulation (e.g., lotions, sprays, sticks)

Key Terms

- **UVR (ultraviolet radiation):** consists of three major bands—UVA, UVB, and UVC.
- **UVA (ultraviolet A):** longest wavelength (320–400 nm). Can be subdivided further into UVA I (340–400 nm) and UVA II (320–340 nm). Penetrates deeper into the skin than UVB. Greater effect on the dermis than on epidermis, causing tissue and vascular damage. Contributes to premature aging of the skin. May augment carcinogenic effects of UVB. Responsible for photosensitizing reactions with medications. May also suppress immune system and damage DNA. Can trigger herpes simplex labialis.
- **UVB (ultraviolet B):** wavelength between 290 and 320 nm. Most active UV wavelength for producing erythema or sunburn. Most intense from 10 AM to 4 PM. Primarily responsible for skin cancer and premature aging. Only beneficial effect is vitamin D_3 synthesis.
- **UVC (ultraviolet C):** wavelength between 200 and 290 nm. Little UVC radiation reaches earth from the sun due to filtering by the ozone layer.
- **Photodermatoses:** examples include, but are not limited to, actinic prurigo, solar urticaria, atopic dermatitis, drug-induced photosensitivity, pemphigus, pellagra, rosacea, and herpes simplex labialis.
- **Drug photoallergy:** relatively uncommon immunologic response consisting of chemically induced reactivity of the skin to UVR that results in an antigenic skin reaction.
- **Drug phototoxicity:** increased, chemically induced reactivity of the skin to UVR but not immunologic in nature.
- **MED (minimum erythema dose):** the minimum UVR dose that produces clearly marginated erythema on the irradiated site, given a single exposure. Used to calculate SPF.
- **SPF (sun protection factor):** calculated by dividing the MED on unprotected skin by the MED on protected skin. Products with higher SPF ratings have better sunburn protection.
- **Substantivity:** ability of a sunscreen to adhere and remain active during prolonged exercising, sweating, and swimming.
- **Broad spectrum:** term used to describe sunscreens that have both UVA and UVB protection.

Table 24-18 Sunburn and Tanning History

Skin Type	Sunburn/Tanning History
I	Always burns easily; never tans (sensitive)
II	Always burns easily; tans minimally (sensitive)
III	Burns moderately; tans gradually (normal)
IV	Burns minimally; always tans well (normal)
V	Rarely burns; tans profusely (insensitive)
VI	Never burns; deeply pigmented (insensitive)

Adapted from: U.S. Food and Drug Administration. Sunscreen drug products for over-the-counter human use: Code of Federal Regulations. 21CFR352.72.

Signs and Symptoms of UVR-Induced Skin Disorders

- Sunburn: Usually superficial burn ranging from mild erythema to tenderness, pain, and edema. Severe reactions may produce a second-degree burn, which may include development of vesicles, bullae, fever, chills, weakness: and shock in extreme situations.
- Drug photosensitivity:
  - Phototoxicity most commonly appears as an exaggerated sunburn with pruritus.
  - Photoallergy typically appears similarly to allergic contact dermatitis and is characterized by pruritus with erythamatous papules, vesicles, bullae, and/or urticaria.

- Photodermatoses: Numerous types are possible, and the presentation will vary.
- Skin cancer:
  - Basal cell carcinoma: translucent nodule with a smooth surface. Usually firm to the touch and may be ulcerated or crusted. Typically found as a lesion on the nose or other parts of the face.
  - Squamous cell carcinoma: slow-growing, isolated papule or plaque on sun-exposed areas of the body.
  - Melanoma. Five factors are used for evaluation of moles, known as ABCDE: Asymmetric shape, Border irregular, Color variation, and Diameter larger than 6 mm, Evolving in shape, size, color, or symptoms such as itching, bleeding, or crusting. A mole with these characteristics or any new growth on the skin or lips should be evaluated by a dermatologist.

Wellness, Prevention, and Treatment

UVR-induced skin disorders can be prevented by minimizing UVR exposure and using sunscreens and protective clothing. The more risk factors a patient has for developing UVR-induced skin disorders, the greater the need to minimize or avoid UVR exposure. Simple steps can be taken to minimize UVR exposure and protect the skin when UVR exposure is unavoidable:

- Avoid sun exposure between 10 AM to 4 PM to avoid peak UVR intensity.
- Wear protective clothing, including a hat with a 4-inch brim, long pants, long-sleeved shirts, and protective eyewear.
- If sun exposure is unavoidable, use a broad-spectrum sunscreen with at least a 30 SPF. Be sure to cover all sun-exposed areas, including lips, ears, nose, scalp/hair parts/hairline, tops of feet, and eye area.

1.2.0 Pharmacotherapy

Drug Indications

FDA Regulations

Most standard sunscreens are regulated as an OTC product by the FDA. The FDA has proposed new regulations (*Federal Register of June 17, 2011 {76 FR 35620}* for a sunscreen drug products final monograph (FM).

Proposed changes include:

- Inclusion of a standard OTC "Drug Facts" label complete with active ingredients, directions for use, warnings, etc.
- Products can only state "Broad Spectrum" if it has proportional UVA to UVB protection and meets FDA testing standards.
- Products labeled as Broad Spectrum with SPF values 15 or higher may claim to reduce the risk of skin cancer and early skin againg.
- Products with SPF between 2 and 14 may be labeled as Broad Spectrum after passing FDA testing, but may not claim to reduce the risk of skin cancer or early skin aging.
- Products not passing Broad Spectrum testing and have SPF less than 15 will be required to carry a warning stating the product has not been shown to reduce skin cancer or early skin aging.
- New rules will limit maximum labeled SPF to 50 + as there is insufficient data to show that SPF values greater than 50 provide additional benefit.
- Products may no longer use terms such as Waterproof, Sweatproof, or Sunblock as they overstate efficacy.

Sunscreen Efficacy

The SPF is determined by dividing the MED on protected skin by the MED on unprotected skin. To explain, if a person requires 50 mJ/cm^2 of UVB radiation to experience 1 MED on unprotected skin and requires 500 mJ/cm^2 of radiation to produce 1 MED after applying a given sunscreen, the product would be assigned an SPF of 10. Thus, if it normally takes a person 1 hour to develop 1 MED, a sunscreen with an SPF rating of 8 would extend the time to 8 hours for the same person to develop the same 1 MED (assuming correct application and reapplication). Of note, doubling the SPF does not mean twice as much UVB protection. A product with an SPF of 15 blocks 93% of UVB, a product with an SPF of 30 blocks 96.7%, and a product with an SPF of 40 blocks 97.5%. As the SPF increases, so do the number and amount of sunscreen ingredients, which could increase the risk for adverse skin reactions as well as the product cost. Padimate O is the most potent UVB absorber of the chemical sunscreens.

UVA protection is of growing concern. However, UVA is much less potent than UVB at producing erythema. Although higher-SPF products are likely to block significant amounts of UVA, the amount of UVA blockage may vary considerably among products with the same SPF values. This difference arises because to achieve a high SPF (UVB coverage), the sunscreen product often will contain many ingredients that *may* or *may not* confer UVA protection. After the new FDA regulations are implemented, products that state Broad Spectrum will have proportional amounts of UVA and UVB.

A broad-spectrum product must contain ingredients that absorb or reflect UVB and absorb UVA up to 360 nm. Most such sunscreens contain a minimum of two ingredients, and some have four or more. To ensure good UVA coverage, look for products that contain avobenzone and have a minimum SPF rating of

15 or a "broad-spectrum" sunscreen with an SPF rating of 30 or higher.

Substantivity also determines the efficacy of the sunscreen. The substantivity of a sunscreen can be related to the active ingredient, vehicle, or both. In general, products with a cream-based (water-in-oil) vehicle appear to be more resistant to water removal than those with alcohol bases. Oil-based products are typically more popular and easy to apply, but they may offer lower SPF values. The FDA's FM requires labeling of sunscreen substantivity as follows:

- Water resistant: Product retains its SPF for at least 40 minutes.
- Very water resistant: Product retains its SPF for at least 80 minutes.

Sunscreens are divided into two major classifications: chemical and physical sunscreens. They are listed according to class in Table 24-19.

Table 24-19 Sunscreen Products: Active Ingredient Concentration and Absorbance

Sunscreen Agent	Concentration	Absorbance
ABA and Derivatives		
Aminobenzoic acid (PABA)	Up to 15%	UVB
Padimate O	Up to 8%	UVB
Anthranilates		
Menthyl anthranilate (meradimate)	Up to 5%	UVA II
Benzophenones		
Dioxybenzone	Up to 3%	UVB, UVA II
Oxybenzone	Up to 6%	UVB, UVA II
Sulisobenzone	Up to 10%	UVB, UVA II
Cinnamates		
Cinoxate	Up to 3%	UVB
Octocrylene	Up to 10%	UVB
Octyl methoxycinnamate (octinoxate)	Up to 7.5%	UVB
Dibenzoylmethane Derivatives		
Avobenzone	2–3%	UVA I
Salicylates		
Homosalate	Up to 15%	UVB
Octyl salicylate (octisalate)	Up to 5%	UVB
Trolamine salicylate	Up to 12%	UVB
Miscellaneous		
Phenyl benzimidazole sulfonic acid (ensulizole)	Up to 4%	UVB
Terephthalyidene dicamphor sulfonic acid (ecamsule)	2%	UVA II
Titanium dioxide	2–25%	Physical
Zinc oxide	2–20%	Physical

Adapted from: Crosby KM. Prevention of sun-induced skin disorders. In: Berardi RR, Kroon LA, McDermott, JH, et al. *Handbook of Nonprescription Drugs.* 16th ed. Washington, DC: American Pharmacists Association; 2009:719–734; Levy SB. Sunscreens and photoprotection. *eMedicine.* Updated January 13, 2009. Available at: www.emedicine.com/derm/topic510.htm. Accessed February 9, 2010.

Application and Dosage Guidelines

Two primary causes of inadequate sun protection with sunscreen are insufficient amounts and infrequent reapplication. Sunscreen needs to be applied liberally to all exposed areas of skin. Reapplication must be performed at least as often as label recommendations state, and more frequently if swimming or sweating. Recommend the following for application amounts and frequency:

- Apply sunscreen 15 to 30 minutes prior to UV exposure. Sunscreen has to bind to various skin constituents before it becomes effective; the time required for such binding ranges from 15 to 30 minutes.
- Apply sunscreen at least as frequently as directed by label recommendations or at a minimum of every 2 hours.
- Reapply sunscreen after every episode of swimming, toweling dry, or excessive sweating even if product states it is *very water resistant* or *water resistant*.
- The average adult should apply nine portions of sunscreen of approximately one-half teaspoon each or roughly 22.5 mL (approximately one ounce or shot glass) to adequately cover the entire body. Distribution should be as follows:
  - Face and neck: one-half teaspoon
  - Arms and shoulders: one-half teaspoon to each side of body
  - Torso: one-half teaspoon to front and back
  - Legs and top of feet: one teaspoon to each side of body

Factors to consider when selecting a sunscreen include the patient's risk factors for UVR-induced skin disorders, photosensitizing medications, skin type, the skin area to be protected, and the activity the individual will be doing while wearing sunscreen. If the patient has risk factors or a skin type that burns easily, recommend a product with a high SPF rating. Consider the area of the body to be protected when recommending a formulation. Sunscreen sticks or chapsticks work well for the lips and nose, and often have higher substantivity. Sunscreen sprays are more expensive but offer a good formulation for scalp application. Lotions are preferred for covering the majority of skin areas and typically are the least expensive. Ask the patient which activities he or she will be doing outdoors. If excessive sweating or swimming is expected, recommend a product that is very water resistant.

Avoid recommending combination sunscreen/insect repellent products, as these products may result in decreased sunscreen efficacy and increased DEET (*N,N*,-diethyl-*m*-toluamide) absorption.

Mechanism of Action

Two major classes of sunscreens are distinguished based on their mechanisms of action: chemical sunscreens and physical sunscreens. *Chemical sunscreens* include an active ingredient that absorbs at least 85% of UV radiation at wavelengths from 290 to 320 nm, but may or may not allow transmission of radiation to the skin at wavelengths longer than 320 nm. *Physical sunscreens* include an active ingredient that reflects or scatters all UV light and visible light at wavelengths from 290 to 777 nm, thereby preventing or minimizing suntan and sunburn.

Contraindications, Warnings, and Precautions

Avoid use of sunscreens in infants younger than 6 months of age.

Aminobenzoic acid (formerly known as para-aminobenzoic acid [PABA]) has been widely replaced by other agents due to its role as a major sensitizer. It is commonly found in an alcoholic base, which increases the risk of contact dermatitis, photosensitivity, stinging and drying of the skin, and yellow staining of clothing on exposure to the sun. Patients who have had a photosensitivity reaction to aminobenzoic acid should avoid products containing it and related derivatives.

Benzophenones as a group are found in many sunscreen products owing to the possibility of allergic reactions to aminobenzoic acid and its derivatives. However, oxybenzone has been shown to be a significant sensitizing agent among sunscreens. As the frequency of use of benzophenones has increased, so has the reported incidence of sensitivity to these agents.

Physical sunscreens may discolor clothing. They also may occlude the skin and result in miliaria (prickly heat) and folliculitis.

Biopharmaceutical and Pharmaceutical Characteristics of Dosage Forms

The vehicle type is a large determinant of a sunscreen's substantivity. Most sunscreen ingredients are lipid soluble and are incorporated into the oil phase of the emulsion. Higher-SPF products may contain as much as 20–40% sunscreen oil, which accounts for the greasy feel of many sunscreens. Sports formulations are often formulated as "dry lotions" or "ultra sheer" products and may rely on silica as a major vehicle component. Water- and alcohol-based vehicles provide a less greasy feel, but fewer active sunscreen ingredients are water soluble; in addition, these formulations have less substantivity.

In general, the various sunscreen ingredients have differing physiochemical properties, which in turn may contribute to a particular sunscreen's substantivity and stability. Here are a few physicochemical properties of interest:

- Para-aminobenzoic acid (PABA) requires an alcoholic vehicle, which increases its side-effect profile.
- Octocrylene may be used in combination with other UV absorbers, including avobenzone, to achieve a higher SPF and add to the overall stability of a given formula.
- Ensulizole is water soluble and is used in products formulated to feel lighter and less oily.
- Avobenzone is used frequently for its good UVA coverage. However, concerns have arisen regarding its photostability and its potential to degrade other sunscreen ingredients.
- Ecamsule is water soluble, which makes it less water resistant. It may also demonstrate photoinstability; it is often combined with octocrylene to increase photostability.
- Titanium dioxide and zinc oxide are physical blockers and often leave a white residue on the skin. With advanced technology, newer micronized products with added skin tone pigments have been developed to improve their cosmetic appearance. There is concern that the user may not apply such products liberally enough and, therefore, end up with lower UV protection.

1.3.0 Monitoring

Pharmacotherapeutic Outcomes

The goal of sunscreens is to prevent UVR-induced skin disorders including, but not limited to, sunburn, photodermatoses, premature aging, skin cancers, and phototoxic and photoallergic skin reactions.

Safety and Efficacy Monitoring and Patient Education

Monitor for effective UV protection. If sunburn or undesired suntan develops, consider using a sunscreen with a higher SPF or a *very water-resistant* formulation. Also, question the patient's application technique to ensure that an adequate amount is being used, the sunscreen is being applied prior to sun exposure, and it is being reapplied as directed by label instructions or more frequently if the patient is swimming, sweating, or toweling dry. Also, recommend that the patient throw away sunscreen that is more than 2 years old or that has not been stored properly (out of direct light, heat, and temperature extremes).

Monitor for any adverse reactions, including, but not limited to, rash, redness, itching, and photosensitivity. If such a reaction occurs, document the name of the product and ingredients to avoid in the future.

Educate the patient on general principles of sun avoidance and protection as previously discussed. Help the patient with product selection based on patient risk factors, skin type, intended use (e.g., exercise, beach, golf, work), and area of skin to be protected.

Adverse Drug Reactions

If rash, vesicles, hives, or exaggerated sunburn develops, it is most likely a photosensitivity or allergic reaction. The patient should stop use of the product and refer to the primary care provider for evaluation. Any prior reactions to sunscreen products should be documented, along with the active ingredients, to avoid future use of sunscreens containing the same products or their derivatives.

Nonadherence, Misuse, or Abuse

Proper application and reapplication are the most common causes of sunscreen failure. Educate the patient on the risks of UV exposure and on ways to minimize exposure and protect the skin with clothing and sunscreen.

Pharmacotherapeutic Alternatives

There are no prescription-strength sunscreens. Utilize nonpharmacologic alternatives if sunscreen is not an option. These include avoiding sun during peak hours of 10 AM to 4 PM and wearing protective clothing, a wide-brimmed hat, and sunglasses.

ANNOTATED BIBLIOGRAPHY

American Cancer Society. Skin cancer prevention and early detection. Updated May 21, 2009. Available at: http://www.cancer.org/docroot/PED/content/ped_7_1_Skin_Cancer_Detection_What_You_Can_Do.asp?sitearea=PED.

Acne

Tips Worth Tweeting

- Acne may be controlled enough to improve cosmetic appearance and reduce scarring.
- Prescription topical retinoids are the gold standard treatment for acne.
- Benzoyl peroxide is the most effective nonprescription medication treatment for acne.
- Utilizing nonpharmacologic and pharmacologic measures consistently is important in achieving acne control.
- Individual patient characteristics should be taken into consideration when recommending a nonprescription acne treatment plan.

Patient Care Scenario: Community Pharmacy Setting

T. J., a 17 y/o M, presents to your pharmacy. He has mild acne and is looking for something to "get rid of it."

Allergies: none

PMH: occasional headaches

Date	Physician	Drug	Quantity	Sig	Refills
11/2	Riger	Multivitamin	#100	one daily	3
11/2	Riger	Ibuprofen 400 mg	#120	one qid	3

1.1.0 Patient Information

Medication-Induced Causes of Acne

Drugs known to exacerbate acne include, but are not limited to, phenytoin, isoniazid, moisturizers, phenobarbital, lithium, ethionamide, and steroids (think PIMPLES).

Disease States Associated with Acne

Stress and emotions may play a role in acne by increasing the release of neuroendocrine modulators, which in turn may stress the sebaceous glands and potentially contribute to progression of acne. Medical conditions or medications that increase androgen production and pregnancy may also be an underlying cause of acne or may exacerbate preexisting acne.

Instruments and Techniques Related to Patient Assessment

Underlying risk factors for acne, cleansing habits, cosmetic usage, and previous acne medications tried, including duration of use, are important factors to address in a patient interview when assessing an acne patient and recommending a product.

Assessing the type of acne and severity of acne is also critical. It is necessary to determine whether the acne is self-treatable or should be referred to a practitioner before recommending treatment. Only patients with Grade I acne should self-treat with nonprescription products unless the practitioner recommends their use.

Signs and Symptoms of Acne

- Noninflammatory lesions (open or closed comedones) are often the first to appear during the early stages of puberty and frequently appear on the forehead.
- With increased age and progression of puberty, lesions may start to appear on other parts of the body such as the chest and back.

Wellness and Prevention

- Eliminate any exacerbating factors such as dirt, dust, petroleum products, cooking oils, or chemical irritants.
- To prevent friction or irritation, avoid wearing tight-fitting clothes, headbands, or helmets; avoid resting the chin on the hand.
- Avoid using oil-based cosmetics and shampoos.
- Avoid wearing nonbreathable clothing that results in excessive hydration of skin.
- Avoid stressful situations when possible, and practice stress-management techniques.
- Do not pick or squeeze pimples. This may further irritate skin, and possibly worsen acne and lead to scarring.
- Cleanse skin twice daily with a mild soap or nonsoap cleanser.
- Avoid use of abrasive products and overcleansing, as this may worsen acne.
- Stay well hydrated. Dehydration may increase release of inflammatory mediators and cause dysfunction in the natural desquamation process of the stratum corneum.

1.2.0 Pharmacotherapy

Drug Indications and Common Doses

Topical retinoids are the gold standard treatment for all types of acne. These medications are available by prescription only, however, and referral should be made to the patient's practitioner for treatment of moderate-to-severe acne. For Grade I comedonal acne, treatment with over-the-counter products is appropriate. These products include benzoyl peroxide, salicylic acid, alpha- and beta-hydroxy acids, sulfur, sulfur/resorcinol, and sulfur/sodium sulfacetamide products. These medications come in a variety of strengths and formulations ranging from cleansers to creams.

- Benzoyl peroxide: Most effective and widely used nonprescription medication for acne. Nonprescription formulations are available in concentrations ranging from 2.5% to 10%. Recommend starting with a 2.5% solution and applying it daily or every other day for the first few weeks. The initial application should be left on for only 15 minutes and then washed off. If tolerated, continue to increase the time left on the skin until the product is tolerated for 2 hours; at that point, it may be left on overnight. After the initial 1–2 weeks of treatment, application may be increased to twice or thrice daily. If treatment is tolerated but desired improvement is not seen, consider increasing the concentration strength to 5% for 1 week and then up to 10% if needed. Continue the treatment regimen after lesions are cleared to prevent new lesions from developing.
- Salicylic acid: Available in nonprescription strengths of 0.5% to 2%. This medication represents a milder and less effective alternative to prescription topical retinoid products. It is generally considered less effective than benzoyl peroxide. It can be used once or twice daily as a cleanser or topical gel. Gel formulations should be applied only to the affected area.
- Alpha- and beta-hydroxy acids: Typically considered less potent and used mainly when patients cannot tolerate other topical acne treatments. Beta-hydroxy acids, such as salicylic acid, are commonly used for hypertrophic conditions. Alpha-hydroxy acids (AHAs) include glycolic, lactic, and citric acids. AHAs are available in several nonprescription formulations in concentrations ranging from 4% to 10%, or through dermatologists at higher concentrations. A study comparing AHAs to benzoyl peroxide found benzoyl peroxide to be superior at 8 weeks of treatment. Currently, there are not enough data to support the regular use of AHAs in acne. Once acne is controlled, however, chemical peels utilizing AHAs may be helpful to reduce scarring and hyperpigmentation.
- Sulfur: Over-the-counter strengths ranging from 3% to 10%. Sulfur-containing products should be applied as a thin film to the affected area one to three times per day. Sulfur is not as effective as benzoyl peroxide.
- Sulfur/resorcinol: Sulfur 3% to 8% combined with resorcinol 2% to 3% products are available in nonprescription strength.
- Sulfur/sodium sulfacetamide: Combinations of sulfur with sodium sulfacetamide are available in nonprescription strength.
- Triclosan: Recently determined by the FDA to be eligible for inclusion in the OTC topical acne drug products monograph. Dosages likely to be available include 0.2% to 0.5% formulations for leave-on treatments and 0.3% to 1.0% formulations for rinse-off dosage forms.

Interaction of Drugs with Foods and Laboratory Tests

Salicylic acid, if used over large areas for long periods of time, may result in salicylate toxicity, which may be potentiated by intake of oral salicylates.

Contraindications, Warnings, and Precautions

Benzoyl peroxide:

- Classified as a Category III drug by the FDA, which means more data are needed to determine its safety and use for nonmonograph conditions due to the concerns about its tumorigenic potential.
- Pregnancy category C medication. The decision to continue or start acne treatments during pregnancy should be discussed with the patient's physician.
- May bleach hair, clothing, and bedding.
- May cause sun sensitivity.

Salicylic acid:

- May cause sun sensitivity.
- Widespread and prolonged use may result in salicylate toxicity.

Biopharmaceutical and Pharmaceutical Characteristics of Dosage Forms

Topical acne agents are minimally absorbed into the systemic circulation. Salicylic acid, when used over a large treatment area and for prolonged time periods, may be absorbed systemically and result in salicylate toxicity.

Nonprescription acne medications come in a variety of formulations, with the formulation affecting their efficacy and side-effect profiles:

- Medicated cleansing products are of little value and leave little active ingredient residue on the skin.
- Gels are typically most effective because they remain on the skin for the longest period of time.
- Gels and solutions are more drying and may increase side effects.
- Gels may be more beneficial for patients with oily skin.
- Creams and lotions are less irritating than gels or solutions.
- Creams and lotions are intended to counteract drying and peeling.
- Creams and lotions should be recommended for patients with dry or sensitive skin.
- Ointments are not used due to their occlusive properties, which may worsen acne.

1.3.0 Monitoring

Pharmacotherapeutic Outcomes

- Monitor for improvement in acne lesions. The goal is to control or prevent lesions. Look for decreases in the number and severity of lesions.
- Prevent or minimize scarring.
- Minimize morbidity associated with acne (such as lower self-esteem, psychological and social impact).

Safety and Efficacy Monitoring and Patient Education

Monitor for improvement in acne lesions. Initial improvement in acne may be seen in 1–2 weeks; however, acne may worsen before it improves. The maximum benefit from most topical agents will take up to 6 weeks to be achieved. If no improvement is seen after 6 weeks, consider an alternative treatment and refer the patient to the primary care practitioner.

Educate the patient on causes of acne, correct any misconceptions regarding acne, and explain the rationale for the recommended treatment. Review nonpharmacologic measures to prevent and control acne. Advise patients of adverse effects, including recommending sun protection with benzoyl peroxide and salicylic acid.

Adverse Drug Reactions

Benzoyl peroxide and salicylic acid:

- Erythema, and scaling of skin, especially during first several days of treatment. Scaling typically will subside after 1 to 2 weeks of treatment.
- Increased sun sensitivity.
- Salicylate toxicity—rare but may be associated with widespread and prolonged salicylic acid use. Symptoms include nausea, vomiting, dizziness, loss of hearing, tinnitus, lethargy, hyperpnea, diarrhea, and psychic disturbances.

Sulfur:

- Noticeable color and odor associated with product use.

Sulfur/resorcinol:

- Dark brown scale may appear on some darker-skinned individuals.

Nonadherence, Misuse, or Abuse

Nonadherence may be a factor due to the adverse effects of acne treatment and long treatment periods needed to see results.

Pharmacotherapeutic Alternatives

Many prescription treatments for acne are available. Topical retinoids are the gold standard of care. Other effective treatment options include, but are not limited to, topical antibiotics, oral antibiotics, oral contraceptives, and isotretinoin.

2.2.0 Dispensing

Benzoyl Peroxide Products

- Stridex Power pads (benzoyl peroxide 2.5%)
- Clean & Clear Gel (benzoyl peroxide 10%)
- Oxy Maximum Strength Acne Wash (benzoyl peroxide 10%)

Salicylic Acid Products

- Neutrogena Rapid Defense (salicylic acid 2%)
- Nature's Cure Body Acne spray (salicylic acid 2%)

Benzoyl Peroxide/Salicylic Acid Products

- University Medical Acne Free Spot Treatment (salicylic acid 1.5%/benzoyl peroxide 1.5%)

Alpha-Hydroxy Acid Products

- Gly Derm (glycolic acid)
- M.D. Forte (glycolic acid)

Alpha/Beta-Hydroxy Acid Products

- Neutrogena Pore Refining Lotion (glycolic and salicylic acids)

Sulfur Product

- Bye Bye Blemish (sulfur 10%)

Triclosan Product

- Clearasil Daily Face Wash (triclosan 0.3%)

Combination Product

- Clearasil Acne Control (resorcinol 2%/sulfur 8%)

ANNOTATED BIBLIOGRAPHY

American Cancer Society. Skin cancer prevention and early detection. Updated May 21, 2009. Available at: http://www.cancer.org/docroot/PED/content/ped_7_1_Skin_Cancer_Detection_What_You_Can_Do.asp?sitearea=PED. Accessed February 9, 2010.

Cheigh NH. Dermatologic drug reactions and self-treatable skin disorders. In: DiPiro JT, Talbert RL, Yee GC, et al. *Pharmacotherapy: A Pathophysiologic Approach*. 7th ed. 2008:1577–1590.

Crosby KM. Prevention of sun-induced skin disorders. In: Berardi RR, Kroon LA, McDermott, JH, et al. *Handbook of Nonprescription Drugs*. 16th ed. Washington DC: American Pharmacists Association; 2009:719–734.

FDA Sheds Light on Sunscreens: FDA consumer health information. May 2012. Available at: http://www.fda.gov/ForConsumers/ConsumerUpdates/ucm258416.htm on 6/21/12.

Hexsel CL, Bangert SD, Hebert AA, Lim HW. Current sunscreen issues: 2007 Food and Drug Administration sunscreen labeling recommendations and combination sunscreen/insect repellent products. *J Am Acad Dermatol* 2008;59(2):316–323.

Levy SB. Sunscreens and photoprotection. *eMedicine*. Updated January 13, 2009. Available at: www.emedicine.com/derm/topic510.htm. Accessed February 9, 2010.

Quairoli K, Foster KT. Acne. In: Berardi RR, Kroon LA, McDermott JH, et al. *Handbook of Nonprescription Drugs*. 16th ed. Washington, DC: American Pharmacists Association; 2009:707–717.

Schwartz RN, Corporon LJ. Skin cancer. In: DiPiro JT, Talbert RL, Yee GC, et al. *Pharmacotherapy: A Pathophysiologic Approach*. 7th ed. 2008:2311–2330.

Strauss JS, Krowchuk DP, Leyden JJ, Lucky AW, Shalita AR, Siegried EC, Thiboutot DM, et al. Guidelines of care for acne vulgaris management. *J Am Acad Dermatol* 2007;56:651–663.

TOPIC: VAGINAL DISORDERS

Section Coordinator: *James R. Clem*
Contributor: *Kelley Oehlke*

Tips Worth Tweeting

- The majority of women who experience vaginal symptoms have a vaginal infection caused by vulvovaginal candidiasis (VVC), bacterial vaginosis (BV), or trichomoniasis.
- Accurately distinguishing VVC from BV and trichomoniasis is important because of the availability of nonprescription antifungal therapy.
- The symptom most apt to differentiate a candidal vaginal infection from bacterial vaginosis and trichomoniasis is the absence of a malodorous vaginal discharge.
- Self-treatment for a vaginal candidal infection is most appropriate when the woman's symptoms are mild to moderate, no predisposing illnesses or medications are present, and symptoms are not recurrent.
- All of the over-the-counter imidazole antifungals are equally effective. Selection includes dosage form or length of regimen and is determined by patient preference.
- Atrophic vaginitis—inflammation of the vagina secondary to decreased estrogen levels—can occur after menopause, postpartum, during breastfeeding, or as a result of antiestrogenic medications.
- Vaginal dryness can be relieved by use of topical personal lubricant products.

- If symptoms do not improve within a week, medical evaluation is necessary.
- Douching is not necessary for vaginal cleansing, and adverse consequences may occur if douches are used.

Patient Care Scenario: Ambulatory Pharmacy Setting

J. W.: 23 y/o F. She is experiencing vulvar redness and itching with a noticeable white, thick discharge.

Allergies: NKA

PMH: diagnosed with VVC infection twice, last infection 3 years ago

Date	Physician	Drug	Quantity	Sig	Refills
4/24	Jager	Yasmin	30	one daily	5
4/23	Jager	Multivitamin	30	one daily	4
4/1	Jager	Calcium carbonate 500 mg	120	one qid	4

1.1.0 Patient Information

Medication-Induced Causes of Vulvovaginal Candidiasis

- Broad-spectrum antibiotics
- Immunosuppressants
- Antineoplastics
- Systemic corticosteroids
- High-dose estrogen oral contraceptives
- Intrauterine or vaginal sponge contraceptives
- Estrogen replacement therapy

Laboratory Testing

Routine labs are appropriate to evaluate medical conditions but generally are not essential for the diagnosis or management of vulvovaginal candidiasis (VVC). Routine culture is not recommended as the initial diagnostic test because it is costly, delays the time to diagnosis, and may give positive results due to asymptomatic colonization (10–20% of women are colonized with *Candida* species and other yeasts). Vaginal pH testing devices assist patients in distinguishing between candidal vaginal infections that can be self-treated and infections requiring medical evaluation and prescription drug therapy. Fungal vaginal infections typically do not affect vaginal pH, whereas a pH greater than 4.5 indicates a bacterial or trichomonal vaginal infection.

Disease States Associated with Vulvovaginal Candidiasis

- Pregnancy
- Menopause
- Menstruation
- Diabetes mellitus
- Organ transplant
- HIV
- Sexual activity

Instruments and Techniques Related to Patient Assessment

Self-treatment of VVC with nonprescription antifungal therapy can be appropriate for patients with uncomplicated disease (infrequent episodes, mild-to-moderate symptoms), whereas women with complicated (more severe symptoms or concurrent predisposing illness or medications) or recurrent infections should be referred

Table 24-20 Vulvovaginal Candidiasis: Drug Indications and Dosage

Drug	Indication	Dosage*
Butoconazole Products		
Butoconazole 2% cream	Uncomplicated vulvovaginal candidiasis ("yeast infection")	Insert cream into vagina until gone
Clotrimazole Products		
Clotrimazole 1% cream	Uncomplicated vulvovaginal candidiasis ("yeast infection")	Insert cream into vagina until gone
Clotrimazole 2% cream		
Clotrimazole 100 mg tablet		Insert tablet into vagina as directed until gone
Miconazole Products		
Miconazole 2% cream	Uncomplicated vulvovaginal candidiasis ("yeast infection")	Insert cream into vagina until gone
Miconazole 4% cream		
Miconazole 100 mg suppository		Insert suppository into vagina until gone
Miconazole 200 mg suppository		
Miconazole 1,200 mg suppository		
Tioconazole Products		
Tioconazole 6.5%	Uncomplicated vulvovaginal candidiasis ("yeast infection")	Insert ointment into vagina until gone

*Refer patient to product instructions for specific directions and duration of use.

for assessment and treatment by a medical provider. Recurrent infections are defined as four or more infections within a 12-month period and symptoms occurring within 2 months of previous vaginal symptoms.

Key Terms

Candidiasis (yeast infection, moniliasis): Classic symptoms include thick, white ("cottage cheese") discharge with no odor and a normal vaginal pH. The most common causative organism is *Candida albicans*.

Signs and Symptoms

- Vaginal itching, burning, rash, and a clumpy, white discharge with no odor.
- Yellow/green vaginal discharge with an unpleasant odor is not a symptom of a vaginal yeast infection and warrants examination by a medical provider.

Wellness and Prevention

- Decrease consumption of sucrose and refined carbohydrates
- Increase consumption of yogurt containing live cultures

1.2.0 Pharmacotherapy

Mechanism of Action

Imidazoles (butoconazole, clotrimazole, miconazole, tioconazole) increase the membrane permeability of various intracellular substances by permeating the chitin of the fungal cell wall. This causes the death of the fungal cell. These medications are effective in vaginal yeast infections caused by an overgrowth of *Candida albicans*.

Interaction of Drugs with Foods and Laboratory Tests

Because of the limited systemic absorption of topical antifungals, drug, food, and laboratory test interactions are unlikely.

Contraindications, Warnings, and Precautions

Reserve OTC products for use in females with past vaginal fungal infections when the symptoms are identical. Do not use in the presence of a fever; pain in the lower abdomen, back, or either shoulder; or a vaginal discharge with an unpleasant odor. Do not use in children younger than the age of 12 years. If therapy is not successful, consult a medical provider. Intractable candidiasis may be a symptom of unrecognized diabetes mellitus or HIV.

Physiochemical Properties, Solubility, Pharmacodynamics, and Pharmacokinetic Properties

Topical vaginal imidazole preparations are not absorbed to any appreciable extent. Systemic absorption rates for butoconazole, clotrimazole, miconazole, and tioconazole are approximately 1.7%, between 3% and 10%, 1.4%, and negligible amounts of a vaginal dose, respectively. Fungicidal clotrimazole concentrations are detectable in the vaginal fluid for as long as 3 days after a single 500-mg dose.

1.3.0 Monitoring

Pharmacotherapeutic Outcomes

Studies have shown the imidazoles to be equally effective in VVC, with effectiveness rates of approximately 80–90%. Different treatment durations have been studied with similar overall cure rates. Symptoms should improve within 2–3 days after application of a vaginal antifungal and the infection should be resolved within a week.

Safety and Efficacy Monitoring and Patient Education

Symptoms that return within 2 months or infections that do not clear up easily with proper treatment require medical evaluation. Inappropriate use of vaginal antifungal products does carry some risk, including unnecessary use of the antifungal agent, delay in effective treatment, and possible delay in treatment of a serious condition. The risk of exposure to the vaginal antifungals is minor—primarily local irritations and the cost of the therapy.

Patient Education

- Complete the full course of therapy.
- Products may stain clothing; take appropriate precautions.
- Avoid sexual intercourse during therapy.
- Do not use tampons concurrently, as they may absorb the medication.
- Contact a medical provider if symptoms persist.
- Closely follow the enclosed directions for application of the product.

Adverse Drug Reactions

Side effects from topical imidazoles are minimal and include vulvovaginal burning, itching, and irritation in 3–7% of patients.

Pharmacotherapeutic Alternatives

An alternative to intravaginal over-the-counter medications is the oral prescription medication fluconazole.

2.2.0 Dispensing

- Mycelex-3 Cream (butoconazole 2% cream)
- Gyne-Lotrimin 3 Cream (clotrimazole 2% cream)

- Gyne-Lotrimin 7 Cream (clotrimazole 1% cream)
- Myclelex-7 Cream (clotrimazole 1% cream)
- Mycelex-7 Combination Pack (clotrimazole 100 mg tablet, 1% cream)
- Monistat 1 Combination Pack (miconazole 1,200 mg suppository, 2% cream)
- Monistat 1 Daytime Ovule (miconazole 1,200 mg suppository)
- Monistat 3 Combination Pack (miconazole 200 mg suppository, 2% cream)
- Monistat 3 Cream (miconazole 4% cream)
- Monistat 7 Suppository (miconazole 100 mg suppository)
- Monistat 7 Cream (miconazole 2% cream)
- Monistat 7 Combination Pack (miconazole 100 mg suppository, 2% cream)
- Monistat 1 Ointment (tioconazole 6.5% ointment)

ANNOTATED BIBLIOGRAPHY

Anderson MR, Klink K, Cohrssen A, et al. Evaluation of vaginal complaints. *JAMA* 2004;291:1368–1379.

Lodise NM, Shimp LA. Vaginal and vulvovaginal disorders. In: Berardi RR, Ferreri SP, Hume AL, et al. *Handbook of Nonprescription Drugs.* 16th ed. Washington, DC: American Pharmacists Association; 2009:117–135.

TOPIC: WEIGHT LOSS

Section Coordinator: James R. Clem
Contributor: Annette M. Johnson

Tips Worth Tweeting

- Obesity is a growing concern worldwide, and especially in the United States.
- Diet and exercise are the cornerstones of weight loss.
- Maintaining a healthy diet and exercise are vital to prevention of weight gain.
- The over-the-counter version of orlistat (Alli) is the only nonprescription medication that the FDA has approved for weight loss.
- Orlistat should be used in combination with healthy diet and exercise to attain the full benefit.
- Numerous dietary supplements on the market advertise efficacy in weight loss but none of the claims made by these supplements has proof of efficacy. Moreover, in some instances, there are definite safety issues.

Patient Care Scenario: Ambulatory Pharmacy Setting

S. P. is a 33-year-old female who asks for your recommendation about medication to help her lose weight. She is not on any other medications. She weighs 200 pounds and is 5'5" tall, making her BMI 33.3 kg/m^2.

Allergies: None.

1.1.0 Patient Information

Medication-Induced Causes of Weight Gain

- Insulin
- Sulfonylureas
- Thiazolidinediones
- Many atypical antipsychotics

Laboratory Testing

No lab tests are routinely performed to assess obesity.

Disease States Associated with Obesity

- Hypertension
- Left ventricular hypertrophy
- Congestive heart failure
- Coronary artery disease
- Stroke
- Obstructive airway disease
- Sleep apnea
- Pulmonary hypertension
- Dyslipidemia
- Diabetes
- Polycystic ovary syndrome
- Osteoarthritis
- Gastroesophageal reflux disease
- Depression
- Breast cancer
- Colon cancer

Instruments and Techniques Related to Patient Assessment

A scale to measure weight and a way to measure height are needed to calculate a body mass index (BMI). Body mass index is calculated with the following equation:

$$\text{BMI} = \frac{\text{weight (kg)}}{[\text{height (m)}]^2}$$

The Heart, Lung, and Blood Institute (NHLBI) 1998 expert report developed the classification of overweight and obesity shown in Table 24-21.

Table 24-21 Classification of Overweight and Obesity

Classification	BMI (kg/m²)
Underweight	< 18.5
Normal weight	18.5–24.9
Overweight	25.0–29.9
Obese—Class I	30.0–34.9
Obese—Class II	35–39.9
Obese—Class III (extreme obesity)	> 40.0

Wellness and Prevention

- Eat a healthy, balanced diet containing no more than 30% of total calories from fat (8–10% calories from saturated fat) and at least 55% of calories from carbohydrates.
- Maintain an active lifestyle including at least 30 minutes of aerobic exercise on most days of the week.

1.2.0 Pharmacotherapy

Mechanism of Action

Orlistat works by decreasing dietary fat absorption, thereby aiding in weight loss. It also generates activity relative to gastric and pancreatic lipases, causing inhibition of their production, and hinders triglycerides from undergoing hydrolysis.

Interaction of Drugs with Foods and Laboratory Tests

Orlistat has the potential to decrease the absorption of fat-soluble vitamins (A, D, E, K), so patients should take a daily multivitamin separated by at least 2 hours from any orlistat dose.

Because minimal absorption of orlistat occurs, drug interactions are not common.

There is a theoretical interaction of orlistat with warfarin, which has the potential to block vitamin K–containing foods. Thus it is important to monitor the patient's INR closely when on orlistat.

Caution is warranted with use of orlistat in patients also on cyclosporine, as orlistat may potentially decrease plasma concentrations of cyclosporine.

Table 24-22 Drug Indications and Common Doses of OTC Weight-Loss Medications

Drug	Indications for Adults Older Than 18 Years	Common Doses
Orlistat	Adjunct to diet and exercise for additional weight loss	60 mg three times daily before a fat-containing meal.
	Indicated for obese patients with BMI of 30.0 kg/m² or higher **or** for overweight patients with BMI of 27.0 kg/m² or higher with risk factors such as diabetes, hypertension, or dyslipidemia.	Orlistat is also available as a prescription medication at higher doses: 120 mg three times daily.
Numerous dietary supplement ingredients	No dietary supplement has been proved both safe and effective for weight loss.	

Contraindications, Warnings, and Precautions

Orlistat is contraindicated in patients with malabsorption disorders. Before taking orlistat, patients with a history of thyroid disease, cholelithiasis, nephrolithiasis, or pancreatitis should contact their primary care provider.

Physiochemical Properties, Solubility, Pharmacodynamics, and Pharmacokinetic Properties

Systemic absorption of orlistat is minimal. Metabolism is thought to occur in the gastrointestinal wall. Fecal excretion of the unchanged drug is the primary route of elimination.

1.3.0 Monitoring

Pharmacotherapeutic Outcomes

- Depends on the patient's clinical situation
- Weight loss goal varies with each patient's situation
- Preventing weight gain after losing weight

Safety and Efficacy Monitoring and Patient Education

Patients on orlistat should be counseled to monitor their weight as a measure of efficacy. Patients also need to be educated that orlistat should be used in combination with a reduced-calorie, low-fat diet and exercise to achieve the most benefit. Adverse effects related to the GI tract are more likely to occur in patients who consume a high-fat, low-carbohydrate diet.

Adverse Drug Reactions

Common GI effects of orlistat:

- Flatulence with oily spotting
- Loose stools
- Frequent stools
- Fatty stools
- Fecal urgency and incontinence

These GI effects are not as common in the over-the-counter dosing and tend to improve within a few weeks of beginning to take orlistat.

Nonadherence, Misuse, or Abuse

Orlistat has an unlikely potential for abuse.

Pharmacotherapeutic Alternatives

The alternatives to over-the-counter orlistat are all prescription agents: orlistat (higher dose), sibutramine, phentermine, diethylpropion, and phendimetrazine.

2.2.0 Dispensing

- Alli Starter Pack: orlistat 60 mg capsules plus Alli Shuttle carrying case and reference booklets for the patient
- Alli Refill Pack: orlistat 60 mg capsules plus the *Read Me First Guide* and the *Companion Guide*

ANNOTATED BIBLIOGRAPHY

Miller SJ, Bartels CL. Overweight and obesity. In: Berardi RR, Kroon LA, McDermott, JH, et al. *Handbook of Nonprescription Drugs*. 16th ed. Washington, DC: American Pharmacists Association; 2009:497–515.

National Institutes of Health, National Heart, Lung, and Blood Institute. Clinical guidelines on the identification, evaluation, and treatment of overweight and obesity in adults: the evidence report. 1998. Available at: http://www.nhlbi.nih.gov/guidelines/obesity/ob_gdlns.pdf. Accessed February 19, 2010.

Special Populations

CHAPTER

25

TOPIC: BENIGN PROSTATE HYPERTROPHY

Section Coordinator: Sandra Hrometz
Contributor: Sandra Hrometz

1.1.0 Patient Information

Patient History

Testosterone (which is metabolized to the more potent hormone dihydrotestosterone) stimulates prostate hyperplasia. Alpha$_1$-adrenergic receptor (AR) agonists (pseudoephedrine, phenylephrine) can cause contraction of prostatic smooth muscle and worsen urinary symptoms. Medications (anticholinergics, antihistamines, antidepressants, antipsychotics, sedative-hypnotics, narcotics, alcohol, calcium-channel blockers) that can cause overflow incontinence may worsen urinary symptoms of benign prostate hypertrophy (BPH).

Laboratory Testing

A diagnosis of BPH is based on a physical examination (digital rectal exam), symptom evaluation, and blood tests to determine the presence of elevated levels of prostate-specific antigen (PSA).

Disease States That Can Mimic Urinary Symptoms of BPH

The following disease states produce urinary symptoms similar to those associated with BPH: urinary incontinence, stricture disease, hypotonic bladder, neurogenic bladder, prostatitis, prostate cancer, urinary tract infection, and renal failure.

Instruments/Techniques for Patient Assessment and Diagnosis

Diagnostic tools commonly used for BPH include the American Urological Association (AUA) Symptom Score Index (SSI) questionnaire (Table 25-1), the International Prostate Symptom Score (I-PSS), and the presence of lower urinary tract symptoms (LUTS; Table 25-2). The urinary symptom questions on the AUA SSI and I-PSS focus on issues such as incomplete emptying, frequency, intermittency, urgency, weak stream, straining, and nocturia.

When a patient presents with LUTS, these symptoms must be differentiated from other disease states such as prostatitis, prostate cancer, and urinary tract infection.

The first seven questions of the I-PSS are identical to the questions appearing on the AUA SSI. The one additional question on the I-PSS refers to the patient's perceived quality of life.

Signs and Symptoms of BPH

The prostate encircles the neck of the bladder and urethra. Hyperplasia of the stromal and epithelial cells of the prostate results in the formation of large nodules in the periurethral region. As these cells begin to undergo hyperplasia, the nodules compress and narrow the lumen of the urethra to cause partial to complete obstruction and resulting LUTS. Histologic evidence of nodular hyperplasia can be seen in 70% of men

Table 25-1 American Urological Association Symptom Score Index Questionnaire

Purpose: Determine baseline BPH symptom severity and efficacy of treatment
Points: 0 = Not at all 1 = Less than 1 time in 5 2 = Less than half of the time 3 = About half of the time 4 = More than half of the time 5 = Almost always A score of 0 to 7 is termed mild; 8 to 19, moderate; 20 or greater, severe.
1. Throughout the past month, how often have you had the sensation of not emptying your bladder completely after you finished urinating?
2. Throughout the past month, how often have you had to urinate again less than 2 hours after you finished urinating?
3. Throughout the past month, how often have you found that you stopped and started again several times after you started urinating?
4. Throughout the past month, how often have you found it difficult to postpone urination?
5. Throughout the past month, how often have you had a weak or diminished stream?
6. Throughout the past month, how often do you feel you had to push or strain to begin urination?
7. Throughout the past month, how many times did you most typically get up to urinate from the time you went to bed at night until the time you got up in the morning?

Adapted from: AUA Guideline on Management of Benign Prostatic Hyperplasia. *J of Urol* 2003;170:530–547.

by age 60 and in 90% of men by the age of 70. There is, however, no direct correlation between histological changes and clinical symptoms. Only 50% of those patients with microscopic evidence of nodular hyperplasia have clinically detectable enlargement of the prostate; of these, only 50% develop clinical symptoms. By age 70, 80% of men have some degree of BPH.

In addition to the enlarged size of the prostate due to hyperplasia, urinary symptoms of BPH are caused by smooth muscle-mediated contraction of the prostate. LUTS can be further characterized as obstructive or irritative symptoms (Table 25-2). Downstream effects of urethra obstruction secondary to BPH include urine retention with subsequent distention and hypertrophy of the bladder, microbial growth in stagnant urine, and the development of cystitis and renal infections.

Maintenance of Wellness and Prevention/Treatment of BPH

Due to the effects of cumulative testosterone (and dihydrotestosterone) exposure, age is the predominant risk factor for BPH.

Table 25-2 Lower Urinary Tract Symptoms

Obstructive Symptoms	Irritative Symptoms
Weak/diminished urine stream Incomplete emptying of the bladder	Nocturia Polyuria (daytime frequency) Urinary urgency
Difficulty commencing urination	Dysuria
Stopping and starting again during urination	
Dribbling at the end of urination	
Hematuria Urinary tract infection	

Treatment Goals

The goal of treatment is to improve or relieve symptoms and halt disease progression to prevent complications. The decision to treat BPH depends on how the patient's urinary symptoms are affecting his quality of life. If urinary symptoms are not adversely affecting quality of life, it is recommended that pharmacologic therapy not be initiated. This practice, "watchful waiting," includes lifestyle changes (limiting fluid intake close to bedtime, avoiding caffeine-containing beverages close to bedtime, taking diuretics in the morning rather than at night) as well as monitoring (annual digital rectal exam, symptom evaluation, and PSA levels). Pharmacologic treatment is reserved for patients with symptoms that affect quality of life. Symptoms are classified as mild, moderate, or severe.

Urinary symptoms of BPH occur when the urethra undergoes some degree of occlusion. Urethral occlusion can be caused by both smooth muscle-mediated contraction of the prostate as well as enlarged size of the prostate due to hyperplasia. Because of the two mechanisms of urethral occlusion, treatment can target the contractile state of the prostate or the hyperplasia of the prostate. The contractile state of prostatic smooth muscle is controlled by α_1-AR located in the gland. Alpha$_1$-AR antagonists (terazosin, doxazosin, alfuzosin, tamsulosin, and silodosin) are first-line agents for BPH due to their rapid onset of action and proven safety and efficacy. AR antagonists do not reduce prostate size; they simply relax prostatic smooth muscle to lessen urethral occlusion.

The predominant cause of prostatic hyperplasia is dihydrotestosterone (DHT), a metabolite of testosterone. DHT is synthesized in the stromal cells of the prostate from circulating testosterone by the action of 5-α-reductase (type 2). 5-α-Reductase inhibitors (RI) such as finasteride and dutasteride inhibit the conversion of testosterone to DHT, thereby providing symptomatic relief and potentially reversing the hyperplastic process. Because they can reduce prostate hyperplasia, the 5-α-RI agents are most useful in men with enlarged prostates, and they are considered superior to α_1-AR blockers in preventing the long-term progression of BPH and decreasing the need for surgery. The α_1-AR antagonists and 5-α-RI agents can each be initiated as monotherapy or used in combination. The rationale for combination drug therapy includes targeting the two causes of BPH symptoms, taking advantage of the immediate effects with α_1-AR antagonists while waiting for the delayed effects of the 5-α-RI.

For patients with moderate to severe BPH that is resistant to pharmacologic treatment, a variety of invasive procedures exist. These procedures—which range from destroying obstructive prostate tissue using heat or radiofrequency energy to surgically removing a portion or the entire gland—are effective in reducing symptoms, improving flow rates, and decreasing post-void residual urine. Potential drawbacks of these procedures include increased cost, recovery time, and side effects such as urinary incontinence and impotence.

1.2.0 Pharmacotherapy

Uses and Indications for Drug Products

The α_1-AR antagonists (terazosin, doxazosin, alfuzosin, tamsulosin, and silodosin) are indicated for treatment of symptomatic BPH. Alpha$_1$-AR antagonists decrease the tone of the prostate to rapidly decrease LUTS. Alpha-1α-RIs (finasteride and dutasteride) decrease the amount of plasma DHT to halt and potentially reverse hyperplasia and growth of the prostate gland. The 5-α-RI agents are indicated for symptomatic BPH in men with an enlarged prostate to improve symptoms, reduce the risk of acute urinary retention, and/or reduce the need for BPH-related surgery. Although anticholinergic medications may increase the risk of urinary retention, they are also commonly used to treat urge incontinence and may be beneficial for urinary symptoms of BPH, especially in men with good urinary flow rates. These agents include oxybutynin (Ditropan), tolterodine (Detrol), darifenacin (Enablex), solifenacin (Vesicare), fesoterodine (Toviaz), flavoxate (Urispas), and trospium (Sanctura). These anticholinergic medications can be used as second-line options if urinary symptoms do not improve with α_1-AR blockers and/or 5-α-RIs.

Mechanisms of Action

Smooth muscle tone in the prostate and bladder neck is mediated by sympathetic nervous stimulation of α_1-ARs, which are abundant in the prostate, prostatic capsule, and bladder neck. Specific α_1-AR antagonists that have received FDA approval for the treatment of BPH (terazosin, doxazosin, alfuzosin, tamsulosin, and silodosin) block norepinephrine receptor binding to prevent smooth-muscle contraction and subsequently decrease tone in the prostate. These agents relax prostatic smooth muscle; they do not reduce prostate size. Terazosin (Hytrin) and doxazosin (Cardura) are α_1-AR selective but not subtype specific. Their original use and indication were for hypertension; thus they have more generalized and vasodilatory side effects. The newer α_1-AR antagonists—alfuzosin (Uroxatral), tamsulosin (Flomax), and silodosin (Rapaflo)—are considered "uroselective" and have minimal effects on the systemic vasculature. Both tamsulosin and silodosin are selective antagonists at the α_{1A}-AR. Alfuzosin is not α_1-AR subtype selective; however, it has high selectivity for the lower urinary tract and is considered "uroselective." Alfuzosin is the only α_1-AR blocker that has been reported to significantly decrease post-void residual volume, which may decrease the incidence of urinary tract infections.

The 5-α-RI agents (finasteride, dutasteride) inhibit the conversion of testosterone to the more potent DHT. These agents not only provide symptomatic relief by decreasing the size of the prostate and lessening urethral occlusion, but may also reverse the hyperplastic process. Therapeutic effects are not seen until endogenous levels of DHT are chronically lowered. Finasteride is solely a type 2 inhibitor, whereas dutasteride inhibits both types of 5-α-reductase.

Interactions with Drugs, Food, and Lab Tests

Use of concurrent antihypertensive medications or vasodilators can result in additive hypotension with the α_1-AR antagonists (especially the agents that are not uroselective). Alfuzosin and silodosin should be taken with a meal, while all of the other agents can be taken without regard to meals.

Concurrent use of potent CYP3A4 inhibitors is contraindicated with alfuzosin and silodosin. Use of mild and moderate CYP3A4 inhibitors should be used with caution. Use caution with tamsulosin (especially at doses greater than 0.4 mg) in combination with cimetidine and warfarin. Finasteride has no drug interactions of clinical importance.

Contraindications, Warnings, and Precautions

Use of these agents is contraindicated in those patients with a known sensitivity to any of the active or inert ingredients. Because of the similarity in urinary symptoms, prostate cancer must be ruled out before treating BPH.

Risk of postural hypotension and syncope exists with the α_1-AR antagonists (especially doxazosin and terazosin) especially if these medications are coadministered with other drugs that cause hypotension. Marked orthostatic effects are most common with the first dose, but can also occur when a dosage increase occurs, or if therapy is interrupted for more than a few days. Warn patients of the possible occurrence of such events, and caution them to avoid situations in which syncope could result in injury.

Doxazosin should be administered with caution to patients with evidence of impaired hepatic function or to patients receiving drugs known to influence hepatic metabolism. Alfuzosin is contraindicated in patients with moderate to severe hepatic impairment and administration with potent CYP3A4 inhibitors.

Silodosin is contraindicated in patients with severe renal impairment (CrCl < 30 mL/min), severe hepatic impairment (Child-Pugh score > 10), or who are taking any strong CYP3A4 inhibitors.

Caution should be exercised when alfuzosin is administered to patients with severe renal insufficiency and those with acquired or congenital QT prolongation or who are taking medications that prolong the QT interval. Caution should be exercised with silodosin in those patients with renal and hepatic impairment. Tamsulosin (particularly at doses more than 0.4 mg) should be used with caution in combination with cimetidine and warfarin. Use caution in the administration of finasteride to patients with liver function abnormalities.

Due to the risk of birth defects to the male fetus, both dutasteride and finasteride are FDA Pregnancy Category X drugs. Because of the potential for absorption of the medication across skin, women who are pregnant or may become pregnant should avoid contact with dutasteride and finasteride tablets/capsules and the semen of a man taking a 5-α-RI. If contact does occur, the area should be washed immediately with soap and water. It is recommended that men taking 5-α-RIs refrain from donating blood until 6 months after their last dose (in case the blood recipient is a pregnant female).

1.3.0 Monitoring

Pharmacotherapeutic Outcomes and Endpoints

The goal of treatment is to improve or relieve symptoms, halt disease progression, and prevent complications. Therefore, assessments of baseline symptom severity are necessary to determine efficacy of treatment. Other outcomes to measure include stabilization or a decrease in PSA, increased maximal urinary flow rate, and decreased prostate size.

Evaluation of Patient Signs and Symptoms and Results of Monitoring Tests and Procedures to Determine the Safety and Effectiveness of Pharmacotherapy

Improvements in symptoms can be evaluated using the AUA SSI (Table 25-1). Progress can also be evaluated by measuring prostate size and post-void urine retention. Men with BPH should have annual follow-up (even if they are not actively treating their BPH) that includes a digital rectal exam, AUA SSI, and PSA to monitor for changes.

Mechanism of Adverse Reactions, Allergies, Side Effects, and Iatrogenic or Drug-Induced Illness and Remedies

Side effects of the nonspecific α_1-AR antagonists doxazosin and terazosin are due to dilation of the systemic vasculature. These effects include dizziness, asthenia (lack or loss of strength and energy), postural hypotension, syncope, headache, and sexual dysfunction (which may include both erectile and ejaculatory components). These side effects can be lessened by starting with a lower dose and slowly titrating the dose upward for several weeks. Dosing at bedtime and staggering the doses with other antihypertensive medications the patient may be taking will also help reduce side effects.

Subtype-selective α_1-AR antagonists have minimal effects on the systemic vasculature. Therefore, side effects are less common with these agents than with the non-"uroselective" agents, but still include dizziness, headache, and fatigue. Additionally, tamsulosin and silodosin are reported to be the most likely of the alpha blockers to cause ejaculatory disorders. Alfuzosin is the least likely of the AR antagonists to cause ejaculatory problems. Along with the general side effects of the other uroselective agents, alfuzosin has been associated with increased incidence of upper respiratory tract infection.

Side effects of the 5-α -RI agents include decreased ejaculate volume, decreased libido, impotence, and breast tenderness and/or enlargement. Pregnant women should avoid contact with the tablets and the semen of a man taking a 5-α-RI due to the risk of birth defects.

Prevention of Medication Nonadherence, Misuse, and Abuse

Providers should stress that daily/chronic use of RIs is necessary to keep DHT levels suppressed. The AR antagonist effects are immediate. Titrate the dose of AR antagonists (especially nonselective agents) slowly to minimize vascular side effects. Extended-release products and capsules should be swallowed whole; they must not be chewed, divided, cut, crushed, or opened.

Pharmacotherapeutic Alternatives

Mild cases of BPH can be managed by nonpharmacologic treatments, which include lifestyle changes such as avoiding caffeine- and alcohol-containing beverages

Table 25-3 Medications for Benign Prostate Hypertrophy: Generic Names, Brand Names, and Dosage Forms

Generic	Brand Name	Dosage Forms
Nonspecific Alpha-Adrenergic Antagonists		
Doxazosin	Cardura	Oral tablets: 1, 2, 4 and 8 mg
	Cardura XL	Oral tablets, extended release: 4 and 8 mg XL
Terazosin	Hytrin	Oral tablets and capsules: 1, 2, 5 and 10 mg
Specific (Uroselective) Alpha-Adrenergic Antagonists		
Alfuzosin	Uroxatral	Oral tablets, extended release: 10 mg
Silodosin	Rapaflo	Oral capsules: 4 and 8 mg
Tamsulosin	Flomax	Oral capsules: 0.4 mg
5-Alpha Reductase Inhibitors		
Dutasteride	Avodart	Oral capsules: 0.5 mg
Finasteride	Proscar	Oral tablets: 5 mg

close to bedtime, following timed voiding schedules, and taking diuretics in the morning instead of at night. For moderate to severe cases that are resistant to pharmacologic treatment, a variety of invasive procedures exist. These procedures, which range from destroying obstructive prostate tissue using heat or radiofrequency energy to surgically removing a portion or the entire gland, are effective in reducing symptoms, improving flow rates, and decreasing post-void residual urine. Drawbacks of these procedures include increased cost, recovery time, and side effects such as urinary incontinence and impotence.

Packaging, Storage, Handling, and Disposal

In general, oral incontinence medications are best stored at room temperature and protected from moisture and humidity. Alfuzosin, silodosin and finasteride should be protected from light.

Access, Evaluate, and Apply Information to Promote Optimal Health Care

The AUA website provides guidelines and diagnostic tools for BPH (http://www.auanet.org). I-PSS is available at http://www.usli.net/uro/Forms/ipss.pdf.

Educate the Public and Healthcare Professionals Regarding Medical Conditions, Wellness, Dietary Supplements, and Medical Devices

A number of dietary supplements are used to decrease symptoms of BPH. These products are not regulated by the FDA, so their efficacy is suspect. The most commonly used agents include saw palmetto, African plum, South African star grass, and Cernilton.

ANNOTATED BIBLIOGRAPHY

Andersson KE. α-Adrenoceptors and benign prostatic hyperplasia: basic principles for treatment with α-adrenoceptor antagonists. *World J Urol* 2002;19:390–396.

AUA guideline on management of benign prostatic hyperplasia. *J Urol* 2003;170:530–547.

Brunton L, Parker K, Blumenthal D, Buxton I. *Goodman & Gilman's The Pharmacological Basis of Therapeutics.* 11th ed. New York: McGraw-Hill; 2008;183–200.

Chapple C, Anderson K-E. Tamsulosin: an overview. *World J Urol* 2002;19:397–404.

Giuliana F. Impact of medical treatments for benign prostatic hyperplasia on sexual function. *BJU Intl* 2006;97:34–38.

Facts & Comparisons. Available at: http://www.efactsonline.com. Accessed June 2010.

Höfner K, Jonas U. Alfuzosin: a clinically uroselective α_1-blocker. *World J Urol* 2002;19:405–412.

Kumar V, Abbas AK, Fausto N. *Robbins and Cotran's Pathologic Basis of Disease.* 7th ed. Philadelphia: Elsevier Saunders; 2005;1023–1058.

McNeill SA, Hargreave TB, Geffriaud-Ricouard C, et al. Post void residual urine in patients with lower urinary tract symptoms suggestive of benign prostatic hyperplasia: pooled analysis of eleven controlled studies with alfuzosin. *Urology* 2001;57:459–465.

Neal RH, Keister D. What's best for your patient with BPH? Let symptom scores and patient preferences guide your level of work-up and your treatment approach. *J Fam Pract* 2009;58:241–247.

Roehrborn CG, Kerrebroeck PV, Nordling J. Safety and efficacy of alfuzosin 10 mg once-daily in the treatment of lower urinary tract symptoms and clinical benign prostatic hyperplasia: a pooled analysis of three double-blind, placebo-controlled studies. *BJU Intl* 2003;92:257–261.

Roehrborn CG, McConnell JD, Barry MJ, et al., for the AUA BPH Guideline Update Panel. *Guidelines on the Management of Benign Prostatic Hyperplasia (BPH).* American Urological Association; 2006.

Thiyagarajan M. α-Adrenoceptor antagonists in the treatment of benign prostate hyperplasia. *Pharmacology* 2002;65:119–128.

Van Dijk MM, de la Rosette JJ, Michel MC. Effects of α_1-adrenoceptor antagonists on male sexual function. *Drugs* 2006;66:287–301.

TOPIC: GLAUCOMA

Section Coordinator: Sandra Hrometz
Contributor: Sandra Hrometz

1.1.0 Patient Information

Patient History

Risk factors for glaucoma include advancing age, family history of glaucoma, high intraocular pressure (IOP), African or Asian descent, diabetes mellitus, myopia (nearsightedness), regular or long-term corticosteroid use, previous eye injury, and hypertension. Glaucoma usually manifests itself in individuals after age 35, and prevalence increases with age.

Medication-Induced Glaucoma

Corticosteroids increase IOP by decreasing the outflow of aqueous humor. The corticosteroids with more potent anti-inflammatory effects (dexamethasone, betamethasone) have the greatest effect on IOP. Anticholinergic agents dilate the pupil, which can precipitate an episode of ACG. The most likely anticholinergic agents to worsen glaucoma are those with a prolonged duration of action (atropine and scopolamine); although they worsen angle-closure glaucoma (ACG), they are unlikely to have an effect on primary open-angle glaucoma (POAG).

Laboratory Testing

General eye exams for glaucoma include visual acuity test, IOP measurement, and visual inspection of the retina, optic nerve, and blood vessels.

Patient Assessment and Diagnosis: Instruments and Techniques

Initial tests should include direct ophthalmoscopy, tonometry, perimetry, and gonioscopy. Direct ophthalmoscopy is used to examine the optic nerve head, cornea, anterior chamber, iris, and vitreous. IOP is measured by tonometry. Perimetry measures defects in the visual field. Gonioscopy measures the angle of the anterior chamber (to determine if the aqueous humor drainage angles are closed or open).

Key Terms

Glaucoma is defined as damage to the optic nerve and ganglion cells, which leads to peripheral vision decline and later loss of central vision. Glaucoma is usually classified as **open-angle glaucoma** (primary open-angle glaucoma) or **angle-closure glaucoma**, based on the mechanism of obstruction of outflow of aqueous humor. **Aqueous humor** is the clear fluid (produced by the ciliary body) that nourishes and circulates around the lens and cornea. Aqueous humor flows out of the anterior chamber through the pupil into the trabecular meshwork and canal of Schlemm before it enters the venous system. This is the primary pathway, accounting for 80–95% of the total outflow. An alternative pathway for aqueous humor outflow is via the uveoscleral route, which is through the ciliary muscles.

IOP is determined by the balance in aqueous humor production and elimination. Increased IOP is the most important risk factor for developing glaucoma. Normal IOP is 10–20 mm Hg. In general, pressures of 20–30 mm Hg cause damage over several years, whereas pressures of 40–50 mm Hg can cause rapid vision loss. Those persons with an IOP exceeding 21 mm Hg who do not develop glaucoma are referred to as having **ocular hypertension**.

In POAG, a physical blockage occurs in the trabecular meshwork that slows elimination of aqueous humor. In ACG, increased IOP is caused by papillary blockage of aqueous humor outflow and is usually severe. POAG occurs in 80–90% of cases and is characterized by an insidious onset, while ACG tends to be more acute.

Signs and Symptoms of Glaucoma

POAG and ACG are both characterized by increased IOP. The increase in IOP in POAG is gradual and asymptomatic early on. The loss of peripheral vision and other damage occurs over a period of months to years. Acute ACG onset is very sudden and is considered a medical emergency. Initial signs and symptoms of acute ACG include sudden onset of blurred vision (usually with rainbow-colored rings or halos perceived as lights), cloudy cornea, visual field loss, and severe ocular pain. Additional clinical presentations due to rapid buildup of IOP include nausea and vomiting, headaches, photophobia, blepharospasm (involuntary blinking or spasm of eyelids), strabismus (misalignment of the eyes), epiphoria (excessive tearing), and amblyopia (lazy eye). Complete blindness can occur in 2–5 days if not treated. Chronic ACG is less severe than acute ACG. Symptoms may range from none to intermittent and severe ocular pain, halo formation. and ocular congestion.

Maintenance of Wellness and Prevention/Treatment of Glaucoma: Treatment Goals

Nonpharmacologic treatment includes ruling out concurrent use of medications that may exacerbate glaucoma. There is currently no cure for glaucoma. However, medications, laser therapy, and incisional surgeries aid in maintaining normal IOP and decreasing further risk of optic nerve damage and vision loss. Treatment of glaucoma is focused on reducing IOP by improving aqueous humor outflow, decreasing aqueous humor production, or a combination of the two.

1.2.0 Pharmacotherapy

Uses and Indications for Drug Products

Agents that improve aqueous humor outflow include prostaglandin agonists (bimatoprost, latanoprost, travoprost) and miotics (direct-acting cholinergic miotics such as ascarbachol and pilocarpine, and cholinesterase inhibitor miotics such as echothiophate). Agents that decrease aqueous humor production include nonselective β-adrenergic receptor (AR) antagonists (carteolol, levobunolol, metipranolol, timolol); selective β_1-AR antagonists (betaxolol); selective α_2-AR agonists (apraclonidine, brimonidine); and carbonic anhydrase inhibitors (acetazolamide, brinzolamide, dorzolamide, methazolamide). In general, all of these agents are indicated for the treatment of elevated IOP in POAG and intraocular hypertension. This chapter focuses on only those agents used for chronic treatment.

Initial treatment of POAG typically consists of a topical medication. The efficacy of treatment can be evaluated at least 2 weeks after initiating or changing therapy. For POAG, it is recommended to initiate therapy with a sole agent. If the target IOP is not reached with a single agent, other agent(s) should be added to the therapeutic regimen. Beta-AR antagonists (beta blockers) and prostaglandin agonists are usually considered first because of their convenient dosing (once to twice daily); in addition, they have few ophthalmic adverse effects and do not constrict the pupil (which can cause blurred vision and accommodation). Second-line medications include α_2-AR agonists and topical carbonic anhydrase inhibitors (CAI). These medications have few systemic side effects, but must be administered two to three times daily. Miotics (direct-acting cholinergics and cholinesterase inhibitors) cause pupil constriction, which leads to accommodation and blurred vision. These side effects have caused the miotics to be regarded as third-line treatment options. Systemic CAIs may be added to the course of therapy if the IOP is still uncontrolled after using maximal tolerated topical medications.

Pharmacologic treatment for ACG is to reopen the angle to aid in dropping IOP. This requires constricting the pupil with a miotic agent. Miotics need not be the sole therapy for ACG. Patients receiving such treatment will also benefit from concomitant use of agents that further decrease IOP. However, for ACG, a miotic must be part of the treatment regimen.

Mechanisms of Action

Topical beta blockers reduce IOP by blocking sympathetic nerve endings in the ciliary epithelium, causing a decrease in aqueous humor production. Nonselective agents block both β_1- and β_2-ARs, while cardioselective agents block only β_1-ARs. Prostaglandin agonists reduce IOP by increasing aqueous outflow from the eye through the uveoscleral pathway.

Miotics (direct-acting cholinergics and cholinesterase inhibitors) cause pupil constriction and ciliary muscle contraction, which leads to aqueous humor outflow. However, this mechanism leads to blurred vision. Cholinesterase inhibitor miotics prolong the activity of endogenous acetylcholine. These agents are more potent and longer acting than the direct-acting cholinergic agents, therefore side effects and systemic toxicity are more common and of greater significance.

Carbonic anhydrase inhibitors decrease the formation of bicarbonate in the ciliary body. The decreased bicarbonate formation means less sodium and water enter the ciliary body, resulting in decreased aqueous humor production and a subsequent decrease in IOP. Both oral (acetazolamide, methazolamide) and topical products (brinzolamide, dorzolamide) are available. Alpha$_2$ selective agents (apraclonidine, brimonidine) stimulate the trabecular meshwork to increase aqueous humor outflow. Apraclonidine is not recommended as long-term therapy due to its high incidence of local adverse reactions and tachyphylaxis.

Interactions with Drugs, Food, and Lab Tests

Although minimal, some degree of systemic absorption occurs with the topical products used to treat glaucoma. Therefore, there is always a chance of systemic drug interactions, albeit only a small risk. Topical α_2-AR agonists and β-AR antagonists may cause additive hypotension and bradycardia in those individuals being treated for hypertension. Both apraclonidine and brimonidine interact with monoamine oxidase inhibitors (MAOIs). Brimonidine interacts with tricyclic antidepressants (TCAs) and has additive effects with CNS depressants (e.g., alcohol, barbiturates, opiates, sedatives or anesthetics). Other reported drug interactions with topical beta blockers include interactions with digitalis, which can lead to prolonged AV conduction time; quinidine, which specifically interacts with timolol to decrease heart rate; and phenothiazines.

Echothiophate may have additive effects with other cholinesterase inhibitors, such as succinylcholine and organophosphate and carbamate insecticides. Those persons who are routinely exposed to carbamate or organophosphate-type insecticides and pesticides (e.g., professional gardeners, farmers, workers in plants manufacturing or formulating such products) should be warned of the additive systemic effects possible from absorption of the pesticide through the respiratory tract or skin. This risk merits wearing respiratory masks, and frequent washing and clothing changes during periods of exposure to such insecticides/pesticides.

Contraindications, Warnings, and Precautions

General Contraindications

With all of these agents, hypersensitivity to active ingredients or any other components of the medication is a contraindication for its use. Beta blockers are contraindicated in those patients with a history of bronchial asthma or severe chronic obstructive pulmonary disease; sinus bradycardia; second-degree and third-degree AV block; overt cardiac failure; and cardiogenic shock. Cholinergic miotics are contraindicated in any situation where pupil constriction is undesirable (e.g., acute iritis, acute or anterior uveitis, some forms of secondary glaucoma, pupillary block glaucoma, acute inflammatory disease of the anterior chamber). Contraindications for echothiophate include active uveal inflammation and most cases of angle-closure glaucoma, due to the possibility of increasing angle block. $Alpha_2$-AR agonists are contraindicated with concomitant use of MAOIs and concomitant use of oral clonidine with apraclonidine.

General Warnings and Precautions with Topical Eye Medications

Bacterial keratitis is a potential issue with the use of multiple-dose containers of topical ophthalmic products, as they may inadvertently become contaminated. The incidence is greater in those patients with concurrent corneal disease or a disruption of the ocular epithelial surface. Patients should be advised that many eye drops contain benzalkonium chloride, which may be absorbed by soft contact lenses. Contact lenses should be removed prior to administration of the solution. Lenses may be reinserted 15 minutes following eye drop administration. Be aware of potential systemic reactions to topical products, as such effects could interfere with or potentiate ongoing therapy for a separate condition, exacerbate a concurrent illness, or interact with systemic medications.

Beta-AR Antagonists: Warnings and Precautions

Beta-AR agents may be absorbed systemically. The same adverse reactions found with systemic beta blockers may occur with topical use of such medications—namely, severe respiratory reactions and cardiac reactions, including death due to bronchospasm in asthmatics, and (rarely) death associated with cardiac failure. Use these agents with caution in patients with cerebrovascular insufficiency due to the potential for beta blockers to decrease heart rate and blood pressure. Administer them with caution in patients subject to spontaneous hypoglycemia and in diabetic patients (especially labile diabetics), as signs and symptoms of acute hypoglycemia may be masked. Beta blockers may also mask clinical signs of hyperthyroidism (e.g., tachycardia). Abrupt withdrawal may precipitate thyroid storm in those individuals with thyrotoxicosis. Beta blockade may potentiate muscle weakness consistent with certain myasthenic symptoms (e.g., diplopia, ptosis, generalized weakness). Products containing sulfites may cause allergic-type reactions (e.g., hives, itching, wheezing, anaphylaxis).

Prostaglandin Agonists: Warnings and Precautions

Patients who are expected to receive treatment (especially if only in one eye) should be informed about the potential for increased brown pigmentation of the iris, periorbital, or eyelid tissue and, therefore, the risk of heterochromia between the eyes. They should also be advised of the potential for a disparity between the eyelashes in length, thickness, or number. Use these products with caution in patients with macular edema. Use bimatoprost with caution in patients with active intraocular inflammation (e.g., uveitis) because the inflammation may be exacerbated.

Cholinergic Miotics: Warnings and Precautions

Caution is advised when cholinergic miotics are used by patients with marked vagotonia, acute cardiac failure, bronchial asthma, peptic ulcer, hyperthyroidism, GI spasm, urinary tract obstruction, Parkinson's disease, bradycardia, recent MI, epilepsy, or hypotension. Retinal detachment has been caused by miotics in susceptible individuals, in individuals with preexisting retinal disease, and in those who are predisposed to retinal tears. Fundus examination is advised for all patients prior to initiation of therapy. Temporary discontinuance of medication is necessary if cardiac irregularities, excessive salivation, urinary incontinence, diarrhea, profuse sweating, muscle weakness, or respiratory difficulties occur. Miosis usually causes difficulty in dark adaptation, so advise patients to use caution while driving at night or performing hazardous tasks in poor light. Miotics can occasionally precipitate angle closure by increasing resistance to aqueous flow from the posterior to anterior chamber. Patients with darkly pigmented irides may require higher strengths of pilocarpine. Avoid or use cholinesterase inhibitors cautiously in those patients with quiescent uveitis or a history of this condition, as intense and persistent miosis and ciliary muscle contraction may occur. Echothiophate iodide should be used with great caution, if at all, where there is a prior history of retinal detachment.

Carbonic Anhydrase Inhibitors: Warnings and Precautions

Concomitant administration of ophthalmic and oral CAIs is not recommended because of the potential for additive effects. CAIs are sulfonamides, so there is a potential for serious reactions in those patients with sulfonamide allergies.

Alpha$_2$-AR Agonists: Warnings and Precautions

Tachyphylaxis is a concern with apraclonidine and brimonidine. This loss of the IOP-lowering effect appears with a variable time of onset in each patient and should be closely monitored. Because these agents can cause dizziness and somnolence, warn patients who engage in hazardous activities requiring mental alertness of the potential for a decrease in mental alertness while using these agents. Use of apraclonidine can lead to an allergic-like reaction (hyperemia, pruritus, discomfort, tearing, foreign body sensation, and edema of the lids and conjunctiva). If this effect occurs, discontinue the medication. Use alpha$_2$-AR agonists with caution in patients with severe cardiovascular disease (including hypertension, coronary insufficiency, recent myocardial infarction, and cerebrovascular disease), orthostatic hypotension, chronic renal failure, Raynaud's disease, or thromboangiitis obliterans.

1.3.0 Monitoring

Once treatment is initiated, the only way to assess efficacy is to monitor the visual field and optic disk. It is assumed that the more the IOP is lowered, the lower the probability of progressive glaucoma damage. However, the IOP value should not be substituted for assessing visual function. Additional monitoring includes checking medication compliance, reviewing adverse effects of treatment, and monitoring for indications that therapy is not effective (worsening or no improvement in symptoms).

Pharmacotherapeutic Outcomes and Endpoints

The therapeutic goal is to decrease IOP and minimize risk of optic nerve damage and vision loss.

Mechanism of Adverse Reactions, Allergies, Side Effects, and Iatrogenic or Drug-Induced Illness and Remedies

Ophthalmic β-AR Antagonists

Although multiple systemic adverse reactions are listed here, the most commonly experienced side effects will be localized to the eye.

- Cardiovascular: Arrhythmia; syncope; bradycardia; heart block; hypotension; cerebral vascular accident; cerebral ischemia; congestive heart failure; palpitations
- CNS: Headache; depression, dizziness, lethargy, worsening of symptoms for patients with myasthenia gravis
- Dermatologic: Hypersensitivity, including localized and generalized rash
- Endocrine: Masked symptoms of hypoglycemia in insulin-dependent diabetics
- GI: Nausea
- Respiratory: Bronchospasm (predominantly in patients with preexisting bronchospastic disease); pulmonary distress characterized by dyspnea, bronchospasm, thickened bronchial secretions, asthma, and respiratory failure
- Ophthalmic: Transient local discomfort following instillation; keratitis; blepharoptosis; visual disturbances (blurred/cloudy vision, refractive changes, diplopia, decreased night vision), edema, ptosis

Prostaglandin Agonists

The most frequent ophthalmic adverse reactions associated with the prostaglandin agonists are conjunctival hyperemia, growth of eyelashes, ocular pruritus, and increased pigmentation of the iris, periorbital tissue (eyelid), and eyelashes (which also increase in length, thickness, and number). Pigmentation is expected to increase for as long as the product is administered. After discontinuation of the medication, pigmentation of the iris is likely to be permanent, while pigmentation of the periorbital tissue and eyelash changes have been reported to be reversible in some patients. Predominant systemic effects that have been reported include upper respiratory tract infection/cold, chest pain, muscle pain, headache, and rash.

Cholinergic Miotics

Carbachol:

- Ophthalmic: Transient stinging and burning; corneal clouding; persistent bullous keratopathy; postoperative iritis following cataract extraction with intraocular use; retinal detachment; transient ciliary and conjunctival injection; ciliary spasm with resultant temporary decrease of visual acuity.
- Systemic: Headache; salivation; GI cramps; vomiting; diarrhea; asthma; syncope; cardiac arrhythmia; flushing; sweating; epigastric distress; tightness in bladder; hypotension; frequent urge to urinate.

Pilocarpine:

- Ophthalmic: Transient stinging and burning; tearing; ciliary spasm; conjunctival vascular congestion; temporal, peri- or supra-orbital headache; superficial keratitis; induced myopia (especially in younger individuals who have recently started administration); blurred vision; poor dark adaptation; reduced visual acuity in poor illumination in older individuals and in individuals with lens opacity. A subtle corneal granularity has occurred with pilocarpine gel.

- Systemic: Hypertension, tachycardia, bronchiolar spasm, pulmonary edema, salivation, sweating, nausea, vomiting, diarrhea (rare).

Echothiophate:

- Ophthalmic: Stinging, burning, lacrimation, lid muscle twitching, conjunctival and ciliary redness, brow ache, and induced myopia with visual blurring may occur. Lens opacities have been reported. Activation of latent iritis or uveitis may occur. Iris cysts may form; if treatment is continued, the cysts may enlarge and obscure vision. This occurrence is more frequent in children. The cysts usually shrink upon discontinuation of the medication, reduction in strength of the drops, or reduction in frequency of instillation. Rarely, they may rupture or break free into the aqueous. Prolonged use may cause conjunctival thickening and obstruction of nasolacrimal canals. A paradoxical increase in intraocular pressure may follow echothiophate instillation.
- Systemic: Cardiac irregularities.

Carbonic Anhydrase Inhibitors

- Dorzolamide and brinzolamide (higher incidence with dorzolamide): Ocular burning, stinging, or discomfort, and bitter taste disturbances (bitter, sour, or unusual) immediately following administration; superficial punctate keratitis; signs and symptoms of ocular allergic reaction (conjunctivitis and lid reactions that resolved upon discontinuation of the medication); blurred vision, tearing, dryness, photophobia.
- Acetazolamide and methazolamide: Adverse reactions, occurring most often early in therapy, include paresthesias, particularly a "tingling" feeling in the extremities; hearing dysfunction or tinnitus; loss of appetite; taste alteration; GI disturbances (nausea, vomiting, and diarrhea); polyuria; metabolic acidosis; electrolyte imbalance; transient myopia (subsides upon diminution or discontinuance of the medication); and occasional instances of drowsiness and confusion. These products carry a boxed warning regarding sulfonamide allergies and concomitant use of high-dose aspirin.

Alpha$_2$ Selective Agonists

0.5% Apraclonidine:

- Hyperemia, pruritus, tearing, discomfort, lid edema, dry mouth, and foreign body sensation
- Ophthalmic discomfort, hyperemia, and pruritus
- Blanching, blurred vision, conjunctivitis, discharge, dry eye, foreign body sensation, lid edema, and tearing
- Abnormal vision, blepharitis, blepharoconjunctivitis, conjunctival edema, conjunctival follicles, corneal erosion, corneal infiltrate, corneal staining, edema, irritation, keratitis, keratopathy, lid disorder, lid erythema, lid margin crusting, lid retraction, lid scales, pain, photophobia
- Abnormal coordination, asthenia, arrhythmia, asthma, chest pain, constipation, contact dermatitis, depression, dermatitis, dizziness, dry nose, dyspnea, facial edema, headache, insomnia, malaise, myalgia, nausea, nervousness, paresthesias, parosmia, peripheral edema, pharyngitis, rhinitis, somnolence, and taste perversion

0.15% Brimonidine:

- Allergic conjunctivitis, conjunctival hyperemia, and eye pruritus
- Burning sensation, conjunctival folliculosis, hypertension, oral dryness, and visual disturbance
- Allergic ocular reaction, asthenia, blepharitis, bronchitis, conjunctival edema, conjunctival hemorrhage, conjunctivitis, cough, dizziness, dyspepsia, dyspnea, epiphora, eye discharge, eye dryness, eye irritation, eye pain, eyelid edema, eyelid erythema, flu syndrome, follicular conjunctivitis, foreign body sensation, headache, pharyngitis, photophobia, rash, rhinitis, sinus infection, sinusitis, superficial punctate keratopathy, visual field defect, vitreous floaters, and worsened visual acuity
- Corneal erosion, insomnia, nasal dryness, somnolence, and taste perversion

0.2% Brimonidine:

- Adverse events are the same as at lower concentrations but potentially more severe
- Fatigue/drowsiness, corneal staining/erosion, ocular ache/pain, tearing, gastrointestinal symptoms, asthenia, conjunctival blanching, muscular pain, lid crusting, conjunctival discharge, depression, anxiety, palpitations and syncope

Prevention of Medication Nonadherence, Misuse, and Abuse

Counsel the patient on the following:

- With respect to all eye drops, do not touch the dropper tip to any surface, as this may contaminate the contents.
- Ensure appropriate storage and handling.
- Discard expired products.
- Compliance is key to effective therapy.

Pharmacotherapeutic Alternatives

Iridectomy (surgical excision of a peripheral piece of the iris to ensure free flow of aqueous humor)

Table 25-4 Medications for Glaucoma: Classes, Generic Names, Brand Names, Formulations, and Dosing

Class	Brand	Dose
Nonselective beta-adrenergic antagonists	Betagan Liquifilm (levobunolol solution 0.25% and 0.5%)	0.25% = 1–2 drops in the affected eye(s) bid 0.5% = 1–2 drops in the affected eye(s) qd to bid for more severe cases
	Ocupress (carteolol solution, 1%)	One drop in the affected eye(s) bid
	OptiPranolol (metipranolol solution, 0.3%)	One drop in the affected eye(s) bid
	Timoptic, Betimol (timolol solution, 0.25%) Timoptic, Betimol, Istalol (timolol solution, 0.5%)	One drop in the affected eye(s) bid One drop in the affected eye(s) bid Starting dose for Istalol is 1 drop in the affected eye(s) once daily in the morning
	Timoptic-XE (timolol gel-forming solution, 0.25% and 0.5%)	One drop in the affected eye(s) qd
	Timolol GFS (timolol gel-forming solution, 0.25% and 0.5%)	One drop qd (usually in the morning)
Selective beta$_1$-adrenergic antagonists	Betoptic (betaxolol solution, 0.5%) and Betoptic-S (betaxolol suspension, 0.25%)	One to two drops in the affected eye(s) bid
Selective alpha$_2$-adrenergic agonists	Iopidine (apraclonidine, 0.5%)	0.5% = one to two drops into the affected eye(s) tid
	Alphagan P (brimonidine solution, 0.1%, 0.15%, and 0.2%)	One drop tid
Carbonic anhydrase inhibitors	Diamox (acetazolamide 500 mg sequels, 125 mg and 250 mg tablets)	Up to 1,000 mg daily in divided doses
	Neptazane (methazolamide 25 and 50 mg tablets)	Maximum dose: 50–100 mg bid–tid
	Trusopt (dorazmide solution, 0.25%)	One drop tid
	Azopt (brinzolamide suspension, 1%)	One drop tid
Direct-acting cholinergic miotics	Isopto-carbachol (carbachol 0.75%, 1.5%, 2.25%, and 3%)	One drop tid
	Pilocar (pilocarpine solution, 0.5%, 1–4%, and 6%)	One drop up to 6 times daily
	Pilocarpine HS gel (pilocarpine gel, 4%)	Into eye at bedtime
Cholinesterase inhibitor miotics	Phospholine iodide (echothiophate iodide, 0.03%)	One drop bid
Prostaglandin agonists	Lumigan (bimatoprost solution, 0.03%)	One drop qd
	Xalatan (latanoprost solution, 0.005%)	One drop qd
	Travatan (travoprost solution, 0.004%)	One drop qd

is a procedure for ACG that should be reserved for those patients who have not responded adequately to pharmacologic therapy. Argon laser trabeculoplasty is a surgical procedure for POAG that has not responded adequately to pharmacological therapy. Argon laser trabeculoplasty makes small burns in the trabecular meshwork to reduce its resistance to the outflow of aqueous humor, thereby lowering IOP.

Inhaled, oral, or intravenous marijuana has been shown to decrease IOP; topical administration is not effective, however. The use of medical marijuana is controversial due to its potential for addiction and misuse for recreational purposes. It does not have FDA approval for the management of glaucoma.

Storage and Handling

See Table 23-5.

Patient education must stress the importance of compliance with the medication regimen. This may be a challenge due to the asymptomatic nature of glaucoma, coupled with the uncomfortable side effects and cost of the medications. Patients should be repeatedly counseled on proper eye drop administration technique, including hand washing, checking

Table 25-5 Storage and Handling of Glaucoma Medications

Class	Agent	Storage and Handling
Nonselective beta-adrenergic antagonists	Levobunolol solution	Store at 15–30°C (59–86°F). Protect from light.
	Carteolol solution	Store at 15–25°C (59–77°F). Protect from light.
	Metipranolol solution	Store at 15–30°C (59– 86°F). Replace cap immediately after use.
	Timolol solution Timolol gel-forming solution	Store at 15–30°C (59–86°F). Protect from freezing. Protect from light. Because evaporation can occur through the unprotected polyethylene unit dose container of the preservative-free solution and prolonged exposure to direct light can modify the product, keep the unit dose container in the protective foil overwrap and use within 1 month after the foil package has been opened. Istalol: Store at 15–25°C (59–77°F).
Selective $beta_1$-adrenergic antagonists	Betaxolol solution and suspension	Store at room temperature.
Selective $alpha_2$-adrenergic agonists	Apraclonidine solution	Store at 2–25°C (36–77°F). Protect from freezing and light.
	Brimonidine solution	Store at 15–25°C (59–77°F).
Carbonic anhydrase inhibitors	Dorzolamide solution	Store at 15–30°C (59–86°F). Protect from light.
	Brinzolamide suspension	Store at 4–30°C (39–86°F).
Direct-acting cholinergic miotics	Carbachol solution	Store at 15–30°C (59–86°F).
	Pilocarpine solution and gel	Store at 2–27°C (36–80°F). Avoid excessive heat. Do not freeze.
Miotics: cholinesterase inhibitors	Echothiophate solution	Store under refrigeration (2–8°C). The reconstituted product may be stored at room temperature (approximately 25°C) for up to 4 weeks. Preparation for administration: Tear off the aluminum seals and remove and discard the rubber plugs from both the drug and diluent containers. Pour the diluent into the drug container. Remove the dropper assembly from its sterile wrapping. Holding the dropper assembly by the screw cap and without compressing rubber bulb, insert it into the drug container and screw down tightly. Shake for several seconds to ensure mixing.
Prostaglandin agonists	Bimatoprost solution	Store in the original container at 2–25°C (36–77°F).
	Latanoprost solution	Store unopened bottle under refrigeration at 2–8°C (36–46°F). During shipment to the patient, the bottle may be maintained at temperatures up to 40°C (104°F) for a period not exceeding 8 days. Once a bottle is opened for use, it may be stored at room temperature, up to 25°C (77°F) for 6 weeks. Protect from light.
	Travoprost solution	Store at 2–25°C (36–77°F). Discard the container within 6 weeks of removing it from the sealed pouch.

the solution for discoloration, appropriate storage and handling, checking the expiration date, avoiding touching the dropper to the eye surface, and ways to minimize systemic absorption. Advise the patient to either close the eye or to place an index finger over the tear duct for 3–5 minutes (nasolacrimal occlusion) to minimize systemic absorption. Instruct patients to stagger administration of different eye drops by 10 minutes to allow complete absorption of each eye drop and avoid washout of the previous medication. Patients should also be instructed to immediately contact their physician if they experience any changes in (or the development of) symptoms.

ANNOTATED BIBLIOGRAPHY

Alexander CL. Prostaglandin analog treatment of glaucoma and ocular hypertension. *Ann Pharmacother* 2002;36:504–511.

Brunton L, Lazo J, Parker K. Good*man & Gilman's The Pharmacological Basis of Therapeutics*. 11th ed. New York: McGraw-Hill; 2008;1707–1737.

Brunton L, Parker K, Blumenthal D, Buxton I. *Goodman & Gilman's Manual of Pharmacology and Therapeutics.* New York: McGraw-Hill; 2008;1095–1114.

Facts & Comparisons. Available at: http://www.efactsonline.com. Accessed February 22, 2012.

Lee DA, Higginbotham EJ. Glaucoma and its treatment: a review. *Am J Health Syst Pharm* 2005;62:691–699.

Wurtzbacker JD, Gourley DR. Glaucoma. In: Helms RA, Quan DJ, Herfindal ET, et al., eds. *Textbook of Therapeutics: Drug and Disease Management.* 8th ed. Philadelphia: Lippincott Williams and Wilkins; 2006.

TOPIC: URINARY INCONTINENCE

Section Coordinator: Sandra Hrometz
Contributor: Sandra Hrometz

1.1.0 Patient Information

Patient History

Urinary incontinence (UI) is more prevalent with increasing age. UI incidence is stable until age 50, and then it increases through age 70 so that almost 50% of women 70 and older have some form of urinary leakage. With the exception of overflow incontinence due to enlarged prostate, UI is much more common in women than in men.

General and common risk factors for UI include increased body mass index, current cigarette smoking, menopause, hysterectomy, parity, and chronic medical conditions such as diabetes mellitus, multiple sclerosis, and Parkinson's disease. Specific risk factors for stress incontinence include conditions associated with pelvic floor injury (vaginal childbirth, surgery), intrinsic urethral sphincter deficiency, and deficient estrogen levels. Specific risk factors for urge incontinence include neurologic disorders (stroke, multiple sclerosis, Parkinson's disease, and spinal cord lesions), enlarged prostate, and bladder stones. Specific risk factors for overflow incontinence include diabetic neuropathy, low spinal cord injury, radical pelvic surgery, multiple sclerosis, previous anti-incontinence surgery and enlarged prostate.

Medication-Induced Incontinence

Several classes of medicines affect bladder contraction and sphincter tone. Depending on the situation, the same medication may act to cause either a desirable or an unwanted change in bladder control. Therefore, medications that may cause incontinence may also be prescribed to treat incontinence.

Table 25-6 Medications Causing Incontinence

Medications Causing Overflow Incontinence	Mechanism
Anticholinergics, antidepressants, antihistamines, antipsychotics, sedative-hypnotics, narcotics, alcohol, calcium-channel blockers	Relaxation of bladder causes decreased contractions, and the resulting urine retention or increased bladder sphincter resistance causes outflow obstruction
Sedatives	Lack of appreciation or concern for bladder events
Antihistamines, alpha-adrenergic agonists	Increased bladder sphincter resistance causes outflow obstruction
Medications Causing Stress Incontinence	
Alpha-adrenergic antagonists	Relaxation of bladder sphincter resistance causes urinary leakage
Medications Causing Urge Incontinence	
Diuretics	Increased urine flow stimulates bladder contractions
Caffeine	Diuretic effect
Sedative-hypnotics	Lack of appreciation or concern of bladder events and depressed central inhibition of micturation
Alcohol	Diuretic effect, lack of appreciation or concern of bladder events, and depressed central inhibition of micturation

Instruments and Techniques for Patient Assessment and Diagnosis

Patient assessment includes urodynamic and imaging tests of the genitourinary tract; a medical, neurological, and genitourinary history; pertinent laboratory testing; a medication review (including nonprescription items); and a review of urinary symptoms. Urinalysis is used to determine the presence of factors that contribute to incontinence, such as infection, kidney stones, renal function, and diabetes. Renal function is evaluated by measuring blood urea nitrogen and creatinine levels. A post-void residual (PVR) volume should be determined by catheterization or pelvic ultrasound. A PVR volume greater than 100 mL is considered abnormal; one that is greater than 200 mL is considered inadequate emptying. If stress incontinence is suspected, the urethra is visualized for urine loss as the patient alternates between relaxing and coughing vigorously. Patient questionnaires and a voiding diary are also valuable in evaluating urinary symptoms.

Key Terms

Urinary incontinence is the involuntary or unintentional leakage of urine. UI is most common in women and the incidence increases with age. The predominant types of UI are stress, urge, mixed, and overflow incontinence.

Stress incontinence is caused by malfunction of the urethral sphincter and occurs secondary to increases in intra-abdominal pressure such as occurs with exertion, laughing, sneezing, or coughing. Stress UI is often related to pelvic floor changes that occur with pregnancy and childbirth. Specifically, this type of incontinence is caused by poor intrinsic urethral sphincter function and urethral hypermobility secondary to failure of the normal anatomic supports of the bladder neck. Symptoms of stress incontinence include leakage (dribbling) with physical activity.

Urge incontinence (also known as "overactive bladder") results from uncontrolled bladder contractions (detrusor overactivity due to instability or hyperreflexia) that overwhelm the central nervous system centers that control voiding. Symptoms include urine loss accompanied by or immediately preceded by a robust sensation of bladder fullness and urge to void (urgency). Although a strong urge is present, the bladder may not actually be full. The patient experiences symptoms during the day and throughout the night (**nocturia**) in addition to increased frequency and potentially copious urine loss (or variable urine loss if the frequency is present).

Mixed incontinence is the combination of both stress incontinence and overactive bladder. With mixed incontinence, the patient has involuntary leakage associated with urgency and also with exertion, sneezing, or coughing.

Overflow incontinence occurs when the bladder over-distends and can be caused by an obstruction or neurological condition. In this situation, the chronic retention of urine occurs and urine is leaked when the bladder cannot fully empty. An enlarged prostate is a very common cause of overflow incontinence secondary to urethral obstruction as it passes through the prostate gland. Symptoms of overflow incontinence include constant dribbling, dribbling after voiding and/or incomplete bladder emptying.

Maintenance of Wellness and Prevention/Treatment of Incontinence

Prevention

- Maintain a healthy weight (obesity is a risk factor for incontinence).
- Completely empty the bladder every 2 to 4 hours.
- Regularly perform pelvic muscle exercises to strengthen the muscles that support pelvic organs.
- Stop smoking (coughing can contribute to stress incontinence).
- Limit alcohol use (diuretic effect).
- Have regular bowel routine (constipation may makes it difficult to empty the bladder).
- Keep a dietary and voiding diary if a problem is suspected.
- Determine whether current medications may affect bladder control.

Treatment

Management of UI includes medications, physical therapy, behavioral therapy, surgery, and the use of protective undergarments. Pharmacologic agents used for UI are specific for the type of UI. Anticholinergic medications—oxybutynin (Ditropan), tolterodine (Detrol), darifenacin (Enablex), solifenacin (Vesicare), fesoterodine (Toviaz), flavoxate (Urispas), and trospium (Sanctura)—are the only agents FDA approved for UI (specifically overactive bladder or urge incontinence).

Other agents have, however, been shown to be beneficial for different types of UI. These medications include alpha$_1$-adrenergic agonists (phenylephrine, pseudoephedrine) and duloxetine for stress incontinence; topical estrogen therapy for stress and urge incontinence in postmenopausal women with vaginal atrophy; alpha$_1$-adrenergic antagonists (terazosin, alfuzosin) for overflow incontinence in men with enlarged prostates; and imipramine for mixed incontinence.

The physical therapy techniques used in women include pelvic floor muscle training (i.e., Kegel exercises, weighted vaginal cones, and electrical stimulation). Behavioral therapy is useful in men and women; it consists of planned voiding at regular intervals, bladder retraining with the aim of increasing the time interval between voiding, and fluid and diet management. Surgery is beneficial in situations of damaged anatomy (e.g., sphincters, urethra, bladder, pelvic floor) or to clear an obstruction.

1.2.0 Pharmacotherapy

Uses and Indications for Drug Products

Anticholinergic medications that are FDA approved for overactive bladder or urge incontinence include oxybutynin (Ditropan), tolterodine (Detrol), darifenacin (Enablex) solifenacin (Vesicare), and trospium (Sanctura). Although there are no other agents with FDA approval for the treatment of UI, many other agents are also used for treating UI. Both alpha-adrenergic agonists (pseudoephedrine, phenylephrine) and topical

Table 25-7 Medications for Urinary Incontinence: Generic Names, Brand Names, and Indications

Generic	Brand Name	Indications
Oxybutynin	Ditropan Ditropan XL Oxytrol Gelnique	Tablets and syrup: For the relief of symptoms of bladder instability associated with voiding in patients with uninhibited neurogenic or reflex neurogenic bladder (i.e., urgency, frequency, urinary leakage, urge incontinence, dysuria) Extended-release tablets: For the treatment of overactive bladder with symptoms of urge urinary incontinence, urgency, and frequency Transdermal and topical: For the treatment of overactive bladder with symptoms of urge urinary incontinence, urgency, and frequency
Tolterodine	Detrol Detrol LA	For the treatment of patients with an overactive bladder with symptoms of urge urinary incontinence, urgency, and frequency
Darifenacin	Enablex	For the treatment of overactive bladder with symptoms of urge urinary incontinence, urgency, and frequency
Solifenacin	Vesicare	For the treatment of overactive bladder with symptoms of urge urinary incontinence, urgency, and urinary frequency
Trospium	Sanctura Sanctura XR	For the treatment of overactive bladder with symptoms of urge urinary incontinence, urgency, and urinary frequency
Fesoterodine	Toviaz	For the treatment of overactive bladder with symptoms of urge urinary incontinence, urgency, and frequency
Flavoxate	Urispas	For symptomatic relief of dysuria, urgency, nocturia, suprapubic pain, frequency, and incontinence as may occur in cystitis, prostatitis, urethritis, and urethrocystitis/urethrotrigonitis

low-dose estrogen therapy have been shown to have some value in treating stress incontinence. Localized low-dose estrogen therapy may be beneficial in menopausal women with stress and urge incontinence. For mixed incontinence, treat the type of incontinence for which symptoms predominate (i.e., stress or urge incontinence).

Alpha-adrenergic receptor antagonists are indicated for incontinence secondary to enlarged prostate. All of the alpha blockers are indicated for the treatment of signs and symptomatic of benign prostate hyperplasia (BPH). Although urge incontinence is a major symptom of BPH, these agents do not have FDA approval for the specific treatment of UI. Imipramine, a tricyclic antidepressant with both anticholinergic and alpha-adrenergic effects, is thought to be beneficial for the treatment of stress and urge UI.

Mechanisms of Action

By blocking the effects of acetylcholine on muscarinic receptors in the bladder, anticholinergics increase the bladder capacity (the volume threshold for initiation of involuntary contractions that lead to voiding) and decrease the strength and frequency of involuntary contractions. These agents are beneficial for urge incontinence (overactive bladder). In addition to anticholinergic effects, some agents have antispasmodic properties (trospium, oxybutynin, flavoxate), whereas others have direct smooth-muscle relaxing effects (oxybutynin), which depress bladder tone.

Alpha-adrenergic agonists (pseudoephedrine, phenylephrine) increase resting urethral tone, which may increase bladder outlet resistance. They can be used for stress incontinence, as they increase resting urethral tone and thereby increase bladder outlet resistance.

Because the bladder and urethral tissue is sensitive to estrogen, vaginal application of low-dose estrogen in menopausal women may reduce some of the symptoms of stress and urge incontinence in this population. Topical estrogen is commonly used in perimenopausal women to treat vaginal atrophy, but the beneficial effects of this regimen for UI are unknown. Nevertheless, vaginal use of estrogen is reported to improve periurethral blood flow, enhance nerve function, and improve urethral function. Local low-dose estrogen also enhances nerve function by increasing alpha-adrenergic responsiveness of urethral muscle. No estrogen products have FDA approval for the treatment of incontinence.

Alpha-adrenergic receptor antagonists are indicated for incontinence secondary to enlarged prostate. The alpha-adrenergic blockers function to relax smooth muscle of the prostate gland, which applies pressure on the urethra when it becomes enlarged. The nonspecific alpha blockers (terazosin and doxazosin) are indicated for UI. The uroselective agents—tamsulosin (Flomax), silodosin (Rapaflo), and alfuzosin (Uroxatral)—have fewer systemic side effects than the nonspecific alpha blockers.

Interactions with Drugs, Food, and Lab Tests

In general, anticholinergic agents may potentially alter the absorption of some concomitantly administered drugs due to their anticholinergic effects on gastrointestinal motility. This tendency may raise concerns with drugs having a narrow therapeutic index.

Darifenacin metabolism is primarily mediated by the cytochrome P450 enzymes CYP2D6 and CYP3A4. The metabolism of darifenacin may be decreased by moderate (diltiazem, erythromycin, fluconazole, verapamil) and potent (clarithromycin, itraconazole, ketoconazole, nefazodone, protease inhibitors) CYP3A4 inhibitors. No dosage adjustment is needed with moderate CYP3A4 inhibitors, but the dosage should not exceed 7.5 mg with potent CYP3A4 inhibitors. A drug interaction occurs with other medications that are metabolized by CYP2D6 (predominantly) and have a narrow therapeutic window (flecainide, thioridazine, tricyclic antidepressants), as their levels will increase when darifenacin is used. Concomitant use of digoxin leads to increased digoxin levels.

Coadministration of CYP3A4 inducers (rifampin) increases levels of fesoterodine, but no dosing adjustments are recommended. Coadministration of potent CYP3A4 inhibitors (clarithromycin, itraconazole, ketoconazole, nefazodone, protease inhibitors) with fesoterodine may increase levels of the latter medication. Doses of fesoterodine of more than 4 mg are not recommended in patients taking potent CYP3A4 inhibitors.

For patients receiving ketoconazole, other potent CYP3A4 inhibitors, macrolide antibiotics, cyclosporine, or vinblastine, the recommended dose is 1 mg twice daily of immediate-release tolterodine or 2 mg/day of extended-release tolterodine. Administer trospium at least 1 hour before meals or on an empty stomach.

Although studies to assess drug–drug interactions with trospium have not been conducted, trospium has the potential to generate pharmacokinetic interactions with other drugs that are eliminated by active tubular secretion (e.g., digoxin, procainamide, pancuronium, morphine, vancomycin, metformin, tenofovir). Coadministration of trospium with drugs that are eliminated by active renal tubular secretion may increase the serum concentration of trospium and/or the coadministered drug due to competition for this elimination pathway. Carefully monitor patients receiving such drugs.

Contraindications, Warnings, and Precautions

With all of these agents, hypersensitivity to active ingredients or any other components of the medication is a contraindication for its use. Contraindications for anticholinergic medications include the following: urinary retention, gastric retention and other severe decreased GI motility conditions, uncontrolled narrow-angle glaucoma, and at-risk status for any of these conditions. General warnings and precautions with anticholinergic medications include cautious administration in patients with clinically significant bladder outflow obstruction because of the risk of urinary retention; patients with gastrointestinal obstructive disorders (severe constipation, ulcerative colitis, and myasthenia gravis) because of the risk of gastric retention; those with controlled narrow-angle glaucoma; those with renal/hepatic function impairment; and the elderly due to risk of dementia, urinary retention, sedation and blurred vision.

Specific warnings and precautions with tolterodine and solifenacin include renal and/or hepatic function impairment. Solifenacin is also labeled with a precaution regarding its use in persons with congenital or acquired QT prolongation. Trospium should be used cautiously in individuals with renal function impairment.

Pharmacodynamic and Pharmacokinetic Properties

- Solifenacin and tolterodine require dose adjustments in patients with renal and/or hepatic impairment.
- Solifenacin (Vesicare): The tablet must be swallowed whole (not crushed) with liquid. A daily dose greater than 5 mg is not recommended in patients with severe renal impairment (defined as creatinine clearance less than 30 mL/min) and/or moderate hepatic impairment (Child-Pugh B). Use is not recommended in those patients with severe hepatic impairment (Child-Pugh C).
- Tolterodine: For patients with significantly reduced renal or hepatic function, the recommended dose is 2 mg daily for extended-release capsules or 1 mg twice daily for immediate-release tablets.
- Trospium: Dosage reduction is required in patients with renal impairment and patients 75 years of age and older. Extended-release capsules are not recommended for use in patients with severe renal impairment (creatinine clearance [CrCl] less than 30 mL/minute). Instead, use immediate-release tablets, 20 mg, taken once daily at bedtime.

1.3.0 Monitoring

Pharmacotherapeutic Outcomes and Endpoints

A standard definition for a successful outcome with incontinence therapy (other than a complete cure) does not exist. Therapeutic impact can be determined by multiple methods that grade symptomatic responses to treatment. Objective criteria for assessing treatment efficacy include physical examination, the pad test, and urodynamic evaluation. Subjective criteria include voiding diaries and quality-of-life instruments. Positive outcomes include lowered incidence of incontinent episodes, decreased symptoms, and increased quality of life.

Mechanism of Adverse Reactions, Allergies, Side Effects, and Iatrogenic or Drug-Induced Illness and Remedies

- Common anticholinergic adverse effects include dry mouth, constipation, dry eyes, blurred vision, orthostasis, and increased heart rate.
- Adverse reactions reported with darifenacin use include urinary tract infection as well as serious constipation and acute urinary retention that require treatment.
- The transdermal oxybutynin (Oxytrol) is associated with a lower incidence of side effects than oral immediate- or extended-release formulations.

Pharmacotherapeutic Alternatives

Behavioral therapy and surgery are alternatives for pharmacotherapy. Behavioral therapy will improve medication efficacy and is typically used in tandem with pharmacologic interventions. Surgery is usually the last resort for patients who do not respond well to behavioral therapy and/or UI medications.

Packaging, Storage, Disposal, and Handling

In general, oral incontinence medications are best stored at room temperature and protected from moisture and humidity. Protect extended-release tolterodine capsules from light.

The Oxytrol (oxybutynin) transdermal system should be applied immediately after removal from the protective pouch. Do not store transdermal patches (oxybutynin) outside the sealed pouch. Apply to dry, intact skin on the abdomen, hip, or buttock, avoiding the waistline area. A new application site should be selected with each new system to avoid reapplication to the same site within 7 days. The patch should not be exposed to sunlight; thus it should be worn underneath clothing.

Protect extended-release tolterodine capsules from light.

Table 23-8 Anticholinergic Agents Indicated for Urinary Incontinence: Generic Names, Brand Names, and Dosage Forms

Generic	Brand Names	Dosage Forms
Oxybutynin	Ditropan Ditropan XL Oxytrol Gelnique	Oral tablets: 5 mg Oral tablets, extended release: 5, 10, and 15 mg Oral syrup: 5 mg/5 mL Transdermal patch: 3.9 mg/24 hr Gel, topical: 10%
Tolterodine	Detrol Detrol LA	Oral tablets: 1 and 2 mg Oral capsules, extended release: 2 and 4 mg
Darifenacin	Enablex	Oral tablets, extended release: 7.5 mg Oral tablets: 15 mg
Solifenacin	Vesicare	Oral tablets: 5 and 10 mg
Trospium	Sanctura Sanctura XR	Oral tablets: 20 mg Oral capsules, extended release: 60 mg
Fesoterodine	Toviaz	Oral tablets, extended release: 4 mg Oral tablets: 8 mg
Flavoxate	Urispas	Oral tablets: 100 mg

Access, Evaluate, and Apply Information to Promote Optimal Health Care

Although UI is overlooked by many primary care providers, it has been shown to be more widespread than diabetes mellitus and hypertension. UI is often listed as the primary reason for admittance into a long-term care facility. It is important to encourage primary care health providers to question their patients about bladder function. Additionally, patient surveys can facilitate diagnosis and treatment efficiency. Numerous patient questionnaires dealing with the signs and symptoms of incontinence have been published.

Educate the Public and Healthcare Professionals Regarding Medical Conditions, Wellness, Dietary Supplements, and Medical Devices

The Society of Urologic Nurses and Associates (SUNA) created the "Bladder Health Awareness Initiative & Presentation" task force. This task force has partnered with the National Association for Continence (NAFC) and the Simon Foundation for Continence to develop a resource that any healthcare professional can use to educate both patients (in the form of patient education fact sheets) and members of the community (in the form of PowerPoint presentations).

ANNOTATED BIBLIOGRAPHY

Bhatia NN, Bergman A, Karram MM. Effects of estrogen on urethral function in women with urinary incontinence. *Am J Obstet Gynecol* 1989;160: 176–181.

Brunton L, Parker K, Blumenthal D, Buxton I. *Goodman & Gilman's The Pharmacological Basis of*

Therapeutics. 11th ed. New York: McGraw-Hill; 2008;183–200.

Culligan PJ, Heit M. Urinary incontinence in women: evaluation and management. *Am Fam Physician* 2000;62:2433–2344.

Dmochowski R. Evaluating the effectiveness of therapies for urinary incontinence. *Rev Urol* 2001;3: S7–S14.

Herbruck LF. Stress urinary incontinence: prevention, management, and provider education. *Urol Nurs* 2008;28:200–206.

Holroyd-Leduc JM, Straus SE. Management of urinary incontinence in women. *JAMA* 2004;291:986–995.

National Association for Continence (NAFC). Available at: http://www.nafc.org. Accessed June 2010.

Quinn SD, Domoney C. The effects of hormones on urinary incontinence in postmenopausal women. *Climacteric* 2009;12:106–113.

Sampselle C, Palmer M, Boyington A, et al. Prevention of urinary continence in adults; population-based strategies. *Nurs Res* 2004;53:S61–S67.

Society of Urologic Nurses and Associates (SUNA). Available at: http://www.suna.org. Accessed June 2010.

Spencer J. Summary of current policy to address urinary incontinence. *Urol Nurs* 2009;29:149–153.

SUNA Bladder Health Awareness Initiative & Presentation. Available at: http://www.suna.org/cgi-bin/WebObjects/SUNAMain.woa/wa/viewSection?s_id=1073743840&ss_id=536873615. Accessed June 2010.

Weiss BD. Diagnostic evaluation of urinary incontinence in geriatric patients. *Am Fam Physician* 1998;57:2675–2684, 2688–2690.

TOPIC: OSTEOPOROSIS

Section Coordinator: Sandra Hrometz
Contributor: Sandra Hrometz

1.1.0 Patient Information

Patient History

Medication-Induced Osteoporosis

The following medications may induce osteoporosis: anticonvulsants (phenytoin and phenobarbital), glucocorticoids, lithium, methotrexate, loop diuretics, excess thyroid hormone, and chronic use of phosphate binding antacids.

Secondary Causes of Osteoporosis

Secondary cause of osteoporosis include hyperthyroidism, hyperparathyroidism, Paget's disease, GI dysfunction, rheumatoid arthritis, anorexia and/or bulimia, dietary vitamin D and/or calcium deficiency, corticosteroid use, Cushing's syndrome, hypogonadism (in both men and women), estrogen deficiency, and renal failure.

Risk Factors Associated with Osteoporosis

- Increased age
- Female gender
- Caucasian or Asian ancestry
- Thin body frame
- Early menopause (before 45 years old) or postmenopausal (early or surgically induced)
- Late menarche (after 16 years old), amenorrhea, or irregular menses
- Family history of osteoporosis
- Calcium- and vitamin D–deficient diet
- Sedentary lifestyle or immobilization
- Cigarette smoking
- Heavy alcohol use

Disease States That Can Mimic Osteoporosis

Osteoporosis has symptoms similar to those of Paget's disease, bone metastases, estrogen deficiency, and, to a lesser extent, testosterone deficiency.

Patient Assessment and Diagnosis

Instruments/Techniques

Bone mineral density (BMD) is most commonly measured using dual x-ray absorptimetry (DXA or DEXA). DEXA is used to measure BMD in the spine, hip, or wrist and is expressed as the amount of mineralized tissue in the area scanned. BMD values are inversely related to the risk of fracture. The difference between the patient's score and the norm is expressed as the standard deviation above or below the mean for a "young normal" adult (a 20-year-old healthy female).

BMD is a static parameter that gives the current risk of fracture; it does not give insight into the rate of bone turnover, however. Specific biochemical markers are used to look at the rate of bone turnover. Alkaline or acid phosphatase levels can be measured to determine osteoblast (bone building) activity, while osteocalcin is measured as a product of bone matrix breakdown.

Key Terms

Osteoporosis is a systemic disease characterized by low bone mass and microarchitecture deterioration (more porous bone) with a consequential increase in bone fragility and susceptibility to fracture. Osteoporosis is defined by the World Health Organization (WHO) in women as a BMD that is 2.5 standard deviations or more below that of a "young normal" adult. The term "osteoporosis" also includes the presence of a fragility fracture, which is where a fracture occurs as a result of a fall from standing height or less (or an event of minimal impact or physical stress).

Osteopenia is low bone mass, where BMD is between 1 and 2.5 standard deviations below that of a "young normal" adult. Those persons with osteopenia are at risk of developing osteoporosis.

Laboratory Testing

Osteoporosis is diagnosed with a DEXA scan; however, multiple lab tests can be run to determine the cause of osteoporosis. A standard complete blood count (CBC), chemistry panels, and a thyroid test are standard tests. In more complicated cases, other lab tests may include a parathyroid hormone test, a kidney function test, a measurement of male or female hormones, a measurement of calcium in the urine, and a vitamin D test.

Signs and Symptoms of Osteoporosis

There are no overt signs or symptoms of early osteoporosis, so early screening for those at risk of this disease is imperative. Osteoporosis may exacerbate itself, as weakened bones can result in a fragility fracture, loss of height (due to spinal compression), or curvature of the spine (hunched appearance).

Maintenance of Wellness and Prevention/Treatment of Osteoporosis

Methods to prevent bone loss include the following:

- Ensuring adequate calcium and vitamin D intake
- Smoking cessation
- Limiting alcohol intake
- Exercising regularly (weight-bearing exercise to strengthen bone)
- Minimizing sedentary lifestyle
- Managing conditions that lead to secondary osteoporosis

Treatment Goals

Treatment of osteoporosis includes preventing or slowing existing bone loss and/or building up existing bone. Calcium and vitamin D supplementation should occur with all osteoporosis medications, as such supplements replace the calcium that is vital for bone structure. Vitamin D is necessary for absorption of oral calcium from the small intestine. The specific agents indicated for the treatment of osteoporosis include the bisphosphonates (alendronate, risedronate, ibandronate, zoledronic acid), calcitonin (Miacalcin), and teriparatide (Forteo). Estrogen, selective estrogen receptor modulators (Raloxifene), and testosterone can be used to treat osteoporosis when it occurs secondary to low levels of estrogen or testosterone, respectively.

1.2.0 Pharmacotherapy

Uses and Indications for Drug Products

Calcium and vitamin D are dietary supplements. They are used for the prevention of calcium and vitamin D deficiency. Additionally, vitamin D is necessary for intestinal calcium absorption. Calcium and vitamin D should be used as an adjunct for all other osteoporosis treatments.

Bisphosphonates and raloxifene are indicated for the treatment and prevention of osteoporosis. Except for alendronate (Fosamax), the same dose of bisphosphonate is used for both the prevention and the treatment of osteoporosis. The osteoporosis prevention dose for alendronate is 5 mg/day or 35 mg in a once-weekly tablet, while the dose for treatment of osteoporosis is 10 mg/day or 70 mg in a once-weekly tablet.

Calcitonin is indicated for the treatment of postmenopausal osteoporosis in females more than 5 years postmenopausal with low bone mass relative to healthy premenopausal females. Calcitonin is less efficacious than bisphosphonates and estrogens; its use should be reserved for those patients who refuse or are unable to take these other medications. Due to its analgesic effect, calcitonin is the first drug to consider for osteoporotic patients who have acute or chronic bone pain (i.e., fracture).

Estrogens are commonly used as hormone replacement therapy in postmenopausal women due to their ability to relieve moderate to severe vasomotor symptoms and to decrease the risk of osteoporosis. Due to estrogen's serious side effects, its use has dramatically decreased in the last decade. None of the available estrogen products are indicated for the treatment of osteoporosis, and only some have specific indications for the prevention of osteoporosis. Nevertheless, as a class, estrogens are beneficial in both the prevention and the treatment of osteoporosis. In 2004, the U.S. Surgeon General's position statement on the use of estrogen for osteoporosis was that it should be considered for the treatment of postmenopausal osteoporosis only in women at a significant risk for osteoporosis or in women who cannot tolerate nonestrogen treatments.

Teriparatide (Forteo) is indicated to increase bone mass in men and women who are at high risk for a fracture. These individuals include those with a history of osteoporotic fracture, those who have multiple risk factors for fracture, and those who have failed or are intolerant to previous osteoporosis therapy.

Mechanisms of Action

Bisphosphonates bind to active sites of bone remodeling to inhibit osteoclasts and suppress their resorptive effects. Calcitonin reduces osteoclastic bone resorption via many mechanisms, including decreasing cell number, shrinking cells, reducing resorptive activity, and shortening osteoclast life span. Estrogen directly inhibits osteoclast activity and stimulates osteoblast activity. It indirectly influences calcium homeostasis by antagonizing the bone-resorbing action of parathyroid hormone and by affecting calcium absorption and excretion. The selective estrogen receptor modulator, raloxifene (Evista), is an estrogen agonist on bone. Teriparatide acetate (Forteo) predominantly stimulates osteoblast activity.

Interactions with Drugs, Food, and Lab Tests

Oral bisphosphonates must be administered after an overnight fast and at least 30 minutes (60 minutes for ibandronate) prior to the first food or drink (other than water). They should be taken with a full glass (6 to 8 oz) of plain water.

Many calcium salts are available as over-the-counter products (carbonate, glubionate, gluconate, lactate, citrate, tricalcium phosphate). With the exception of calcium citrate and lactate, calcium supplements should be taken with food to ensure appropriate absorption.

Contraindications, Warnings, and Precautions

With all of these agents, hypersensitivity to active ingredients or any other components of the medication is a contraindication for its use.

Bisphosphonates

- Contraindications: Hypocalcemia; severe renal insufficiency; abnormalities of the esophagus that delay esophageal emptying such as stricture or achalasia (alendronate, oral ibandronate, risedronate); inability to stand or sit upright for at least 30 minutes for alendronate and risedronate or at least 60 minutes for ibandronate; increased risk of aspiration (alendronate solution).
- Warnings and precautions
    - GI irritation/disorders: Instruct patients to alert their healthcare providers to any signs or symptoms signaling a possible esophageal reaction, and instruct patients to discontinue bisphosphonates and seek medical attention if they have or develop dysphagia, esophageal disease, gastritis, ulcers, odynophagia, retrosternal pain, or new or worsening heartburn. The risk of severe esophageal adverse experiences appears to be greater in patients who lie down after taking bisphosphonates, who fail to swallow it with a full glass of water, or who continue to take bisphosphonates after developing symptoms suggestive of esophageal irritation.
    - Jaw osteonecrosis: Most reported cases with bisphosphonates have been in cancer patients undergoing dental procedures. Known risk factors for osteonecrosis include a diagnosis of cancer, concomitant therapies (i.e., chemotherapy, radiotherapy, corticosteroids), and comorbid disorders (i.e., anemia, coagulopathy, infection, preexisting dental disease). Most reported cases have been in patients treated with parenteral bisphosphonates, but some have been in patients treated orally.
    - Musculoskeletal pain: Severe and occasionally incapacitating bone, joint, and/or muscle pain has been reported in patients taking bisphosphonates. The time to onset of symptoms varies from 1 day to several months after starting the medication.
    - Bronchoconstriction in aspirin-sensitive asthmatic patients: This side effect is associated with oral bisphosphonates, but not with the parenteral bisphosphonate, zoledronic acid (Reclast).
    - Hypocalcemia/mineral metabolism: Treat hypocalcemia and other disturbances of bone and mineral metabolism before starting bisphosphonate therapy. Adequate intake of calcium and vitamin D is important in all patients to prevent hypocalcemia.
    - Renal function impairment: Use of oral bisphosphonates is not recommended for patients with severe renal failure. In general, no dosage adjustment is needed when CrCl is greater than 30 mL/min.
- Warnings and precautions with Reclast (zoledronic acid): Patients must be appropriately hydrated prior to administration of zoledronic acid. For patients with a CrCl of 35 mL/min or more, zoledronic acid is administered as a single dose (5 mg) infused for no less than 15 minutes through a separate vented infusion line. Use zoledronic acid with caution with other nephrotoxic drugs.

Calcitonin

- Contraindications: Clinical allergy to calcitonin-salmon.
- Warnings and precautions: Perform a nasal examination (with visualization of the nasal mucosa, turbinates, septum, and mucosal blood vessel status) prior to the start of treatment with nasal calcitonin and whenever nasal complaints occur. The most commonly reported nasal adverse reactions include rhinitis, epistaxis, and sinusitis. Because this medication is a polypeptide, the possibility of a systemic allergic reaction exists with calcitonin.

Estrogens

- Contraindications: Known or suspected breast cancer, except in appropriately selected patients being treated for metastatic disease; known or suspected estrogen-dependent neoplasia; undiagnosed abnormal vaginal bleeding; active deep vein thrombosis (DVT), pulmonary embolism (PE), or a history of these conditions; active or recent (i.e., within past year) arterial thromboembolic disease (i.e., stroke, myocardial infarction); active thrombophlebitis or thromboembolic disorders; history of thrombophlebitis, thrombosis, or thromboembolic disorders associated with previous estrogen use (except when used in treatment of breast or prostatic malignancy); known or suspected pregnancy.
- Warnings and precautions: Estrogen use may induce malignant neoplasms of the endometrium, ovaries, and breast. Increased risk of gallbladder disease; cardiovascular events such as myocardial infarction (MI), stroke, venous thromboembolism (VTE), and pulmonary embolism (PE); elevations of plasma triglycerides; hypercoagulability (primarily related to decreased antithrombin activity); endometrial hyperplasia.

Selective Estrogen Receptor Modulators

- Contraindications: Women who are pregnant or may become pregnant; breastfeeding women; individuals with an active VTE or a history of VTE or PE (deep vein thrombosis or pulmonary embolism), and retinal vein thrombosis.
- Warnings and precautions: VTE (greatest risk within first 4 months). In a situation of prolonged immobilization (i.e., surgery), discontinue raloxifene at least 72 hours prior to and during prolonged immobilization. Resume raloxifene only after the patient is fully ambulatory. Advise women taking raloxifene to move about periodically during prolonged travel. Breast exams and mammograms should be performed before starting and while taking raloxifene. Monitor serum triglycerides in individuals with elevated levels.

Forteo

- Contraindications: None.
- Black box warning: This drug caused osteosarcoma (malignant bone tumor) in rats given 3–60 times the human dose. Because of the uncertain relevance of the rat osteosarcoma finding to humans, prescribe teriparatide only to those patients for whom the potential benefits are considered to outweigh the potential risk. Teriparatide should not be prescribed for patients at an increased baseline risk for osteosarcoma (i.e., those with Paget's disease or unexplained elevations of alkaline phosphatase, children and young adult patients with open epiphyses, and patients with prior external-beam or implant radiation therapy involving the skeleton).
- Warnings and precautions: Do not use in patients with bone metastases, a history of skeletal malignancies, or metabolic bone diseases other than osteoporosis. Teriparatide has not been studied in patients with preexisting hypercalcemia. Do not treat these patients with teriparatide because of the possibility of exacerbating hypercalcemia. Do not use teriparatide in individuals with an underlying hypercalcemic disorder, such as primary hyperparathyroidism.

Physiochemical Properties, Solubility, Pharmacodynamics, and Pharmacokinetic Properties

Calcium must be in a soluble, ionized form for absorption to occur. For most calcium salts (except the citrate and lactate salts), ionization of calcium occurs when it is exposed to an acidic pH. Therefore, oral calcium absorption is increased when this supplement is taken with food. Adequate absorption of calcium citrate and lactate will occur at higher pH levels, such as when taken on an empty stomach, in those persons with achlorhydria, and in those individuals taking acid-reducing medications (H2 antagonists, proton pump inhibitors). Although there is no need to take calcium lactate or citrate with food, taking these medications with food will not adversely affect their absorption.

Bisphosphonates have very low oral bioavailability (less than 1%). To maximize absorption, they must be administered after an overnight fast and at least 30 minutes (60 minutes for ibandronate) prior to the first food or drink (other than water).

1.3.0 Monitoring

Pharmacotherapeutic Outcomes and Endpoints

The DEXA scan should show less bone loss or increased BMD. Endpoints also include fewer initial fractures or refractures. Bone turnover markers can be used as an adjunct to BMD to monitor the response to therapy.

Mechanism of Adverse Reactions, Allergies, Side Effects, and Iatrogenic or Drug-Induced Illness and Remedies

Bisphosphonates

Side effects of oral bisphosphonates are gastrointestinal in nature, and include abdominal pain, flatulence, abdominal distension, esophageal ulcer/esophagitis, and dysphagia. Other side effects include severe bone, joint, and muscle pain and headache. Side effects of Reclast (parenteral zoledronic acid) are the same as those for oral bisphosphonate agents, but also include hypocalcemia redness and swelling at the infusion site and flu-like acute-phase reactions (fever, myalgia, headache, arthalgia). The majority of acute-phase reaction symptoms occur within the first 3 days following the dose of zoledronic acid and usually resolves within 3 days of onset. Taking the standard oral dose of acetaminophen (unless contraindicated) following zoledronic acid administration may reduce the incidence of acute-phase reaction symptoms.

Calcitonin

Side effects include nausea with or without vomiting, irritation at the injection site/nasal irritation, and flushing.

Estrogens

Side effects include nausea and vomiting, headache, fluid retention, and thromboembolism.

Raloxifene

Side effects include hot flashes, leg cramps, and a low risk of thromboembolism.

Forteo

The most common side effects are leg cramps and dizziness.

Prevention of Medication Nonadherence, Misuse, and Abuse

Oral Bisphosphonate Administration

All oral bisphosphonates are absorbed very poorly from the intestines. As a consequence, they must be administered after an overnight fast and at least 30 minutes (60 minutes for ibandronate) prior to the first food or drink (other than water). To facilitate delivery to the stomach, and thus reduce the potential for esophageal irritation, swallow tablets whole with a full glass of plain water while standing or sitting in an upright position. Bisphosphonates should be taken only with a full glass of plain water (some mineral waters may have a higher concentration of calcium, so they should not be used). To avoid or minimize esophageal side effects, remain sitting or standing upright for 30 minutes after oral bisphosphonate administration. Due to their inconvenient dosing (i.e., the requirement for an overnight fast and having to be upright for at least 30 minutes), many preparations are now available in extended-release preparations (i.e., once weekly), which eliminates the need for once-daily dosing.

Special Instructions for Missing Doses

- Once weekly: Take the product on the same day of each week. If a dose of the once-weekly bisphosphonate is missed, take that dose the morning after it is remembered and return to taking a dose once a week, as originally scheduled. Do not take two doses on the same day.
- Twice monthly (risedronate 75 mg on 2 consecutive days per month): Take the product on the same 2 consecutive days each month. If both doses are missed and the next month's scheduled doses are more than 7 days away, take one risedronate 75 mg tablet in the morning after it is remembered and then the other tablet on the next consecutive morning. Do not take more than two 75 mg tablets within 7 days. If only one tablet is missed and the next month's scheduled doses are more than 7 days away, take the missed tablet in the morning after it is remembered. Continue taking the risedronate 75 mg dose on two consecutive mornings per month as originally scheduled. If one or both tablets are missed and the next month's scheduled doses are within 7 days, wait until the next month's scheduled doses and then continue taking risedronate 75 mg on two consecutive mornings per month as originally scheduled.
- Once monthly: Take the once-monthly tablet on the same day of each month. If the once-monthly bisphosphonate dose is missed and the next scheduled dose is more than 7 days away, take one tablet in the morning after it is remembered. Return to taking the next once-monthly tablet on the original treatment day. Do not take two of the once-monthly bisphosphonate tablets within the same week. If the once-monthly bisphosphonate dose is missed and the next scheduled dose is less than 7 days away, wait until the next scheduled treatment day to take the tablet. Maintain the original treatment day for all subsequent once-monthly doses.

Pharmacotherapeutic Alternatives

Expose hands, arms, and feet to UV light (sunlight) 10–15 minutes twice weekly without a sunscreen to synthesize adequate vitamin D. Weight-bearing exercises help build bone.

2.2.0 Dispensing

Calcium salts do not have a uniform amount of elemental calcium. Be sure to check the label for the actual amount of elemental calcium present.

Table 23-9 Medications for Osteoporosis: Generic Names, Brand Names, and Dosage Forms

Generic	Brand Name	Dosage Forms
Alendronate	Fosamax	Oral tablets: 5, 10, and 40 mg tablets daily
	Fosamax Plus D	Oral tablets, extended release: 35 mg tablet/week and 70 mg tablet/week
		Oral solution: 70 mg/75 mL once weekly
		Oral tablets: 70 mg alendronate and 70 mcg vitamin D tablet/week (equivalent to 2,800 IU vitamin D/week)
		Oral tablets: 70 mg alendronate and 140 mcg vitamin D tablet/week (equivalent to 5,600 IU vitamin D/week)
Risedronate	Actonel	Oral tablets: 5 and 30 mg daily
	Actonel with Calcium	Oral tablets, extended release: 30 mg tablet/week and 35 mg tablet/week
		Oral tablets, extended release: 75 mg tablet on 2 consecutive days/month and 150 mg tablet/month
		Oral tablets: 35 mg risedronate and 1,250 mg calcium carbonate tablet/week
Ibandronate	Boniva	Oral tablets: 2.5 mg tablet daily
		Oral tablets, extended release: 150 mg tablet /month
Zoledronic acid	Reclast	5 mg per 100 mL injection once yearly
Calcitonin-salmon injection	Miacalcin	Injection: 200 units/mL (supplied as 2 mL vials)
Calcitonin-salmon nasal spray	Miacalcin	Nasal spray: 200 units per 0.09 mL
	Fortical	
Teriparatide	Forteo	Injection: 250 mcg/mL (2.4 mL vial)
Estrogen	Various	Various
Raloxifene	Evista	Oral tablets: 60 mg

Medication Administration Equipment

Zoledronic acid (Reclast) administration: 5 mg administered IV once yearly. Infuse over no less than 15 minutes through a separate vented infusion line.

Educate the Public and Healthcare Professionals Regarding Medical Conditions, Wellness, Dietary Supplements, and Medical Devices

Information about osteoporosis for clinicians and the general public is available through the National Osteoporosis Foundation (NOF; www.nof.org). NOF offers health professionals, their patients, and the general public free publications and services including awareness handouts for patients, materials for community events and health fairs, PowerPoint presentations for grand rounds and peer-to-peer health professional meetings, brochures and handouts for people of varying ages and backgrounds (e.g. English and Spanish), and osteoporosis support group information.

Pharmacists and physicians should educate patients concerning over-the-counter supplements:

- Over-the-counter calcium supplements will have differing amounts of elemental calcium depending on which salt form they contain; therefore, the user must read labels carefully.
- With the exception of calcium citrate and calcium lactate, all calcium supplements must be taken with food for appropriate absorption.
- Calcium citrate and lactate are the best options for those persons who cannot take their medication with food, those who have achlorhydria (low stomach acid, a condition more common in the elderly compared to young patients), and those who chronically take stomach acid–reducing medications.
- Adequate levels of vitamin D are necessary for calcium absorption; therefore, the best option is to take a combination calcium and vitamin D product.

ANNOTATED BIBLIOGRAPHY

Brunton L, Parker K, Blumenthal D, Buxton I. *Goodman & Gilman's The Pharmacological Basis of Therapeutics.* 11th ed. New York: McGraw-Hill; 2008;1647–1678.

Favus MJ, et al. *Primer on the Metabolic Bone Diseases and Disorders of Mineral Metabolism* (4th ed.). Philadelphia: Lippincott Williams & Wilkins; 1999;257–288.

Heaney RP, Dowell MS, Barger-Lux MJ. Absorption of calcium as the carbonate and citrate salts, with some observations on method. *Osteoporos Intl* 1999;9:19–23.

National Osteoporosis Foundation. *Clinician's Guide to Prevention and Treatment of Osteoporosis.* Washington, DC: Author; 2010. Available at: http://www.nof.org/professionals/pdfs/NOF_ClinicianGuide2009_v7.pdf. Accessed July 2010.

TOPIC: SPECIAL CONSIDERATIONS FOR THE GERIATRIC PATIENT

Section Coordinator: *Sandra Hrometz*
Contributor: *Sandra Hrometz*

Introduction

Aging is characterized by a progressive reduction in the homeostatic reserve of organ systems. As a result of this trend, basal function may remain intact but the ability of organ systems to compensate or handle increased demands may not be sufficient. Compared to younger patients, the elderly (defined as persons 65 years of age and older) have an increased likelihood of suffering from disease, disability, and medication side effects.

From a medical standpoint, the aging population is unique due to the physical, pharmacokinetic, and pharmacodynamic changes that occur with the aging process. This altered physiology not only leads to changes in function but also alters how a patient will respond to drug therapy. The elderly tend to have multiple concomitant disease states (which may mask or exacerbate each other), have an increased susceptibility to disease, and generally present with atypical signs and symptoms. Because the brain, musculoskeletal, and cardiovascular systems are the least capable of compensating for increased stress, the dominant presenting symptoms of acute changes in disease or medications with this population include acute confusion, acute delirium, depression, incontinence, falls, and syncope.

Lastly, older patients are at an increased risk for adverse drug reactions compared to the young. This higher risk is due to a number of factors: increased sensitivity to medications and side effects; increased drug interactions due to an increased number of chronic diseases and medications; decreased medication compliance due to excessive numbers of medications; cognitive impairment (which may decrease compliance, especially with complicated dosing regimens); medication toxicity due to age-related changes in metabolism and excretion; and atypical presentation of an adverse drug reaction that may go undetected.

There is little that can be done to modify the aging process itself; however, an understanding of what is happening will allow drugs to be used appropriately and with minimal complications in the elderly population.

Important Physiological Changes in the Elderly

Cardiovascular System

Aging-related changes in the cardiovascular system include decreases in heart rate, pumping efficiency, vascular elasticity, baroreceptor responsiveness, and increased incidence of dehydration (hypovolemia). These changes may culminate in cardiovascular disease, heart failure, dizziness, and an increased susceptibility to medication side effects such as hypotension and syncope. Complications of dizziness and hypotension include falls, fractures secondary to falls, and confusion. Additionally, systemic organ perfusion decreases as a result of reduced cardiac output and increases in peripheral vascular resistance. Decreased renal and hepatic perfusion leads to a reduced capability for drug metabolism and excretion.

Respiratory System

Aging-related changes in the respiratory system include decreases in the cough reflex, lung elasticity, and maximal expiratory flow. Aging-related decreases in immune system function also increase the risk of respiratory infection. Increased patency of the esophageal sphincter leads to an increased risk of aspirating stomach contents. Geriatric patients are at a much higher risk of death due to influenza and pneumonia.

Central Nervous System

Aging-related changes in the CNS include decreased cerebral blood flow, which may lead to confusion and even impair cognition; decreased dopamine and acetylcholine content in the brain, which can lead to Parkinson's disease or Parkinson's symptoms and increased adverse effects with antipsychotics and anticholinergic medications; increased blood–brain barrier permeability, which increases susceptibility to CNS side effects; decreases in the righting reflex, which contributes to falls; and changes in autonomic function, which lead to bradycardia, decreased thermoregulation (hypothermia), decreased thirst reflex (dehydration), decreased cough reflex (pulmonary infection), and decreased baroreceptor sensitivity (hypotension, syncope).

Gastrointestinal System

Aging-related changes in the GI system include relaxation of the lower esophageal sphincter and achlorhydria (decreased stomach acid production). Relaxation of the esophageal sphincter leads to increased incidence of heartburn and gastroesophageal reflux disease (GERD).

Achlorhydria, which allows for more microbes to grow in the stomach, in combination with GERD dramatically increases the risk of aspiration pneumonia. Geriatric patients also have a higher risk for dysphagia, choking, and aspiration due to decreased saliva production. Lastly, GI motility is slowed. The predominant effect associated with decreased motility is constipation—a widespread complaint among elderly patients.

Pharmacokinetic Changes

Many of the physiologic changes that occur in the elderly affect the pharmacokinetics (absorption, distribution, metabolism and elimination) of medications. Of the four pharmacokinetic parameters, absorption is affected the least and elimination is affected the most. These changes and their results are outlined in Table 25-10.

Pharmacodynamic Changes

Pharmacodynamic changes in the elderly are not characterized nearly as well as pharmacokinetic changes. Homeostatic regulation is compromised in the elderly and the tight integration of peripheral and central feedback mechanisms is lacking. The pharmacodynamic effect of a given medication may be increased or

Table 25-10 Pharmacokinetic Changes in the Elderly

Parameter	Change	Result
Absorption	Decreased GI motility, delayed stomach emptying, increased transit time through gut. Achlorhydria. Reduced saliva production.	Rate of drug absorption (but usually not extent) from the GI tract may be slowed, leading to a delayed onset of action. Usually not an issue except for GI absorption of most calcium salts (excluding lactate and citrate). Increased risk of choking on food and subsequent aspiration.
Distribution	Body composition changes include an approximate 15% decrease in total body water, a 13–40% increase in body fat, and a 12–19% decline in lean body mass (muscle). The effect of these changes on drug distribution depends largely on a drug's lipid or water solubility. Decreased plasma albumin levels. Changes in drug distribution secondary to decreases in cardiac output and systemic organ perfusion.	Decreased fluid V_d. Drugs that are distributed through the fluid V_d (water-soluble drugs) may become more concentrated. Such drugs include gentamicin, ethanol, digoxin, caffeine, lithium, theophylline, and cimetidine. Increased fat V_d. Drugs that are distributed through the fat V_d (lipid-soluble drugs) have an increased half-life. These changes affect most psychotropic agents. Increased plasma concentration of drugs that are highly protein bound, including nonsteroidal anti-inflammatory drugs (NSAIDs), tricyclic antidepressants (TCAs), phenytoin, and quinidine. Difficult to predict.
Metabolism	Overall, hepatic metabolism of medications is decreased secondary to decreases in liver perfusion, metabolic capacity and albumin synthesis. Decreased liver perfusion. Decreased metabolic capacity. Phase I reactions (oxidation, reduction, hydroxylation) are reduced or slowed. Decreased activity of some cytochrome P450 enzymes. Decreased plasma protein synthesis (predominantly albumin).	A significant decrease in the amount of drug delivered to the liver for metabolism and first-pass effect results in major alterations in bioavailability. Hepatic metabolism decreases, which can mean decreased activation of prodrugs to active drugs and/or decreased inactivation of active drugs. Drugs metabolized by phase I reactions (e.g., nortriptyline, theophylline, diazepam) will accumulate and should be given in lower doses. Increased activity of warfarin, phenytoin, and theophylline. Increased free fraction of medications that are usually highly bound to albumin.
Elimination	Renal function declines at an estimated 10% every decade starting at age 30 or 7% per decade. There are also decreases in the glomerular filtration rate and creatinine clearance. Renal function cannot be estimated by serum creatinine alone due to reduced muscle mass in the elderly.	Reduced drug excretion may result in increased half-life, increased duration of action, and drug accumulation. Drugs that are eliminated unchanged solely or mainly by renal excretion should be dosed based on renal function (gentamicin, digoxin). Must use the Cockcroft-Gault equation to estimate creatinine clearance for renal dosing in the elderly. Cockcroft-Gault equation: ClCr = (140 – age) × ideal body weight (in kg)/72 × SCr in mg/dL (multiply the answer by 0.85 for women) If the person weighs less than his or her ideal body weight, use the actual body weight (in kilograms).

Table 25-11 Age-Related Pharmacodynamic Changes

Pharmacodynamic Change	End Result
Decreased beta receptor sensitivity	Diminished response to beta agonist and antagonist medications
Decreased baroreceptor responsiveness	Increased risk of postural hypotension and syncope with antihypertensive medications, including diuretics Decreased reflex tachycardia
Renal changes affecting pharmacodynamics include decreases in the ability to concentrate urine (regulate water and electrolyte balance), renin and aldosterone activity, and sodium conservation	Increased incidence of orthostasis, dehydration, hyponatremia, and incontinence with diuretics
Decreased glucose tolerance, insulin secretion, and insulin sensitivity	Increased risk of hypoglycemia with anti-diabetic medications
Increased sensitivity to the anticoagulant effects of warfarin	Excessive bleeding with warfarin
Increased sensitivity to the anticholinergic effects of medications	Potentially profound constipation, urinary retention (obstructive bladder incontinence), sedation, mental confusion, dizziness, and xerostoma
Increased CNS sensitivity to centrally acting medications such as sedatives, benzodiazepines, antipsychotics, antidepressants, anticonvulsants, $alpha_2$ agonists, narcotic analgesics, corticosteroids, and antihistamines	Increased sensitivity to side effects (such as sedation and dry mouth) in addition to more severe side effects such as agitation, mental confusion, and delirium
Decreased dopaminergic content in the brain	Higher incidence of tardive dyskinesia, akathesia, and Parkinson's syndrome with use of long-term antipsychotics
Decreased acetylcholine content in the brain	Increased susceptibility to the anticholinergic effects of antipsychotics and TCAs

Table 25-12 Medications Associated with Severe Adverse Reactions in the Elderly

Medication	Concern
Indomethacin (Indocin, Indocin SR)	Of all available NSAIDs, this drug produces the most CNS adverse effects.
Pentazocine (Talwin)	Narcotic analgesic with more CNS adverse effects, including confusion and hallucinations than other narcotic drugs. Additionally, it is a mixed agonist and antagonist.
Trimethobenzamide (Tigan)	Extrapyramidal effects are possible; drug is less effective than other antiemetics.
Amitriptyline (Elavil) Doxepin (Sinequan)	Strong anticholinergic and sedation properties.
Meprobamate (Miltown)	Highly addictive and sedating.
Disopyramide (Norpace)	Strong anticholinergic effects and the most negative inotrope of all antiarrhythmics. May induce heart failure in elderly patients.
Methyldopa	May cause bradycardia and exacerbate depression in elderly patients.
Chlorpropamide	Long half-life in elderly patients, which can cause prolonged hypoglycemia. The only oral hypoglycemic agent that can cause syndrome of inappropriate antidiuretic hormone secretion (SIADH).
All barbiturates (except phenobarbital for seizures)	Highly addictive and higher incidence of adverse effects than most other sedative or hypnotic drugs in elderly patients.
Meperidine (Demerol)	Not an effective oral analgesic with the doses most commonly used. May cause confusion.
Ticlopidine (Ticlid)	Has been shown to be no better than aspirin in preventing clotting and may be considerably more toxic.
Ketorolac	Immediate and long-term use should be avoided in the elderly because a significant number of the elderly have asymptomatic GI pathologic conditions.
Amphetamines (excluding methylphenidate and anorexics)	Excess CNS stimulant effects.

Table 25-12 (*continued*)

Medication	Concern
Amphetamines and anorexics	Potential for causing dependence, hypertension, angina, and myocardial infarction.
Muscle relaxants, muscle antispasmodics, and GI antispasmodics	Poorly tolerated due to anticholinergic adverse effects, sedation, and weakness. Orphenadrine (Norflex) is especially severe. Effectiveness at doses tolerated by elderly patients is questionable.
Higher doses of short-acting benzodiazepines: • Lorazepam (Ativan) 3 mg • Oxazepam 60 mg • Alprazolam (Xanax) 2 mg • Temazepam (Restoril) 15 mg • Triazolam (Halcion) 0.25 mg	Smaller doses of benzodiazepines may be effective as well as safer due to increased sensitivity to benzodiazepines in the elderly. The total daily doses should rarely exceed the suggested maximums.
Long-acting benzodiazepines: • Flurazepam • Chlordiazepoxide • Diazepam (Valium) • Chlorazepate (Tranxene-T)	Long half-life in the elderly, which leads to prolonged sedation and increased risk of falls and fractures. Short- and intermediate-acting benzodiazepines are preferred if a benzodiazepine is required.
Anticholinergics and antihistamines	Anticholinergic properties (both OTC and prescription products). Non-anticholinergic antihistamines are preferred.
Long-term use of full-dose, longer half-life, non-COX-selective NSAIDs (naproxen, oxaprozin, piroxicam)	GI bleeding, renal failure, hypertension, and heart failure.
Fluoxetine (Prozac) daily	Long half-life and risk of producing excessive CNS stimulation, sleep disturbances, and increasing agitation.
Long-term stimulant laxatives (unless taking narcotics)	Dehydration; may exacerbate bowel dysfunction.
Amiodarone (Cordarone)	Associated with prolonged QT interval and risk of inducing torsades de pointes. Lack of efficacy in older adults.
Nitrofurantoin (Macrodantin)	Potential for renal impairment.
Methyltestosterone	Potential for prostatic hypertrophy and cardiac problems.
Thioridazine	CNS and extrapyramidal adverse effects.
Short-acting nifedipine (Procardia, Adalat)	Potential for hypotension and constipation.
Mineral oil	Potential for aspiration and adverse effects.
Desiccated thyroid (Armour Thyroid)	Concerns about cardiac effects. Safer alternatives are available.

decreased in elderly persons. Examples of pharmacodynamic changes and their consequences in the elderly are listed in Table 25-11. The extent of the pharmacodynamic change and the end result are very individualized.

Medication Use in the Elderly

Due to changes in pharmacokinetics and pharmacodynamics in the elderly, many medications' side effects are amplified. The "Beers List" was developed by a panel of experts to identify medications that are not appropriate for use in the elderly. This list was initially published in 1993, then revised and updated in both 1997 and 2003. The medications that are considered inappropriate are divided into two categories: (1) specific medications or medication classes that are either ineffective or pose an unnecessary high risk of adverse effects and (2) medications that are harmful in those persons with specific disease states. In most cases, alternative medications (many times in the same class as the inappropriate drug) are acceptable for use in the elderly.

Table 25-13 Medications Inappropriate for Use in Elderly with Specific Disease States

Disease or Condition	Drug	Concern
Heart failure	Disopyramide	Negative inotropic effect. Potential to promote fluid retention and exacerbation of heart failure.
GI ulcer	NSAIDs, aspirin (more than 325 mg/day)	May exacerbate existing ulcers or produce new/additional ulcers.
Syncope/falls	Short- to intermediate-acting benzodiazepines and TCAs	Additional falls due to ataxia, impaired psychomotor function, sedation, and syncope.
Epilepsy	Clozapine (Clozaril), chlorpromazine, thioridazine, thiothixene (Navane)	May lower seizure thresholds.
Hypertension	Amphetamines	May elevate blood pressure.
Clotting disorders	Aspirin, NSAIDs, clopidogrel (Plavix), ticlopidine (Ticlid), dipyridamole (Persantine)	Increased bleeding, as these agents may prolong clotting time, elevate INR values, and inhibit platelet aggregation.
Arrhythmias	TCAs	Concern due to proarrhythmic effects and ability to produce QT interval changes.
Stress incontinence	Alpha blockers, TCAs, anticholinergics, long-acting benzodiazepines	May produce polyuria and worsening of incontinence.
Bladder outflow obstruction	Anticholinergics, muscle relaxants, antihistamines, GI antispasmodics, oxybutynin (Ditropan XL)	Urinary retention secondary to decreased urinary flow.
Insomnia	Decongestants, theophylline, monoamine oxidase inhibitors, methylphenidate (Ritalin), amphetamines	Concern due to CNS stimulant effects.
Parkinson's disease	Metoclopramide (Reglan), tacrine (Cognex), conventional antipsychotics	Concern due to cholinergic agonist and antidopaminergic effects.
Cognitive impairment	Barbiturates, muscle relaxants, anticholinergics, antispasmodics, CNS stimulants	Concern due to CNS-altering effects.
Depression	Sympatholytics, long-term benzodiazepines, methyldopa	May produce or exacerbate depression.
Anorexia and malnutrition	Methylphenidate, fluoxetine	Concern due to appetite-suppressing effects.
COPD	Long-acting benzodiazepines, propranolol (Inderal LA)	CNS adverse effects. May induce, exacerbate, or cause respiratory depression.

Table 25-14 Criteria of the Medication Appropriateness Index

1. Is there an indication for the medication?
2. Is the medication effective for the condition?
3. Is the dosage correct?
4. Are the directions correct?
5. Are the directions practical?
6. Are there clinically significant drug–drug interactions?
7. Are there clinically significant drug–disease interactions?
8. Is there unnecessary duplication with other medication(s)?
9. Is the duration of therapy acceptable?
10. Is this drug the least expensive alternative compared to others of equal utility?

Medications that are inappropriate in the elderly (category 1) typically have strong anticholinergic or sedative properties or have adverse effects that are significant in elderly populations. The medications with the most severe adverse reactions and the specific concerns that arise with their use are listed in Table 25-12. The medications considered to be inappropriate when used in those persons with a specific disease state are listed in Table 25-13.

The Medication Appropriateness Index (MAI) is a rating scale that evaluates 10 key elements of medication prescribing in the elderly. Table 25-14 lists the specific questions or criteria of the MAI. The MAI serves as a guideline for questions to pose when evaluating the medication profile of a geriatric patient. Ideally, the answer to each of the listed questions (except questions six, seven, and eight) should be "yes."

ANNOTATED BIBLIOGRAPHY

Beers MH. Explicit criteria for determining potentially inappropriate medication use by the elderly. *Arch Intern Med* 1997;157:1531–1536.

Cusack BJ. Pharmacokinetics in older persons. *Am J Geriatr Pharmacother* 2004;2:274–302.

Fick DM, Cooper JW, Wade WE, et al. Updating the Beers criteria for potentially inappropriate medication use in older adults: results of a US consensus panel of experts. *Arch Intern Med* 2003;163(22):2716–2724.

Hanlon JT, Schmader KE, Samsa GP, et al. A method of assessing drug therapy appropriateness. *J Clin Epidemiol* 1992;45:1045–1051.

Hutchison LC, Sleeper RB. *Fundamentals of Geriatric Pharmacotherapy: An Evidence-Based Approach.* Bethesda, MD: American Society of Health-System Pharmacists; 2010.

Kane RL, Ouslander JG, Abrass IB. *Essentials of Clinical Geriatrics.* 4th ed. New York: McGraw-Hill; 1999.

TOPIC: SPECIAL CONSIDERATIONS IN PEDIATRIC POPULATIONS

Section Coordinator: Sandra Hrometz
Contributor: Vinita B. Pai

Introduction

Children are not miniature adults. Most efficacy, safety, pharmacokinetic, and pharmacodynamic trials for new drugs are initially conducted in adults and may never be extended to the pediatric population; even so, these drugs may be used in children despite the lack of pediatric-specific labeling. Adult doses scaled down based on body weight may not be safe and effective in children. Body water, body fat, plasma proteins, hormonal composition, and renal and hepatic function all change as the human body grows from a newborn to an adolescent into an adult. Pharmacists taking care of pediatric patients need to recognize the effect of these changes on drug dosing and disposition to provide safe and effective pharmaceutical care to these patients.

Tips Worth Tweeting

- Children are grouped by age, and drug dosing changes by age group.
- Within the pediatric population, newborns (especially premature infants) differ greatly from the rest of the age groups in terms of body composition and organ function.
- Oral, intramuscular, and percutaneous drug absorption in children varies with physical and physiologic growth and maturation.
- Body water, body fat, and differences in plasma protein binding determine differences in drug distribution between pediatric and adult patients.
- Age-dependent differences in the activity of important Phase I and Phase II drug-metabolizing hepatic enzymes are observed.
- Glomerular filtration rate, tubular secretion, and reabsorption affecting drug elimination undergo significant anatomical and functional maturation as a premature newborn grows into an adolescent.
- Use of over-the-counter medications—cough and cold medications, in general—is not recommended for the pediatric population.
- Infants and children 5 years of age or younger are unable to swallow medications administered as tablets and capsules, and may need these drugs to be extemporaneously compounded into a liquid dosage form.

Table 25-15 Classification of Different Age Groups in the Pediatric Population

Terminology	Definition
Neonate	Birth to 4 weeks (28 days) of age
Premature neonate	Newborn of gestational age 37 weeks or younger at birth
Full-term neonate	Newborn of gestational age between 38 and 41 weeks at birth
Post-term neonate	Newborn of gestational age 42 weeks or older at birth
Infant	Child between 1 and less than 12 months of age
Child	1 to 12 years of age
Adolescent	13 to 16 years of age
Pediatric	Birth to 18 years of age
Gestational age (GA)	Number of weeks from the mother's first day of the last normal menstrual period to the birth of the child
Postnatal (chronologic) age (PNA)	Age since birth
Postconceptional (PCA) age/ postmenstrual age/corrected age/ adjusted age	PCA = Chronologic age in months – [(40 – GA at birth in weeks) ÷ 4 weeks] Example: Baby boy A. B. is a 35-day-old, premature baby born at 36 weeks' gestational age = 1.25 – [(40 – 36) ÷ 4 weeks] = 1.25 – 1 = 0.25 months × 4 weeks = 1 week Gestational age in weeks + postnatal age in weeks = 36 + 5 = 41 weeks (40 weeks can be considered average GA; 41 weeks would make the child 1 week old after reaching the normal gestation)

Patient Care Scenario

A.B. is a 35-day-old, premature baby boy born at 36 weeks' gestational age. To determine correct drug dosing for A. B., the baby's GA, PNA, and PCA must be determined.

1.1.0 Patient Information

The pediatric patient population age range is from birth to 17 years of age. In the United States in 2008, nearly 74 million individuals were classified as members of the pediatric age group, and 25 million were 5 years of age or younger. In the newborn pediatric population, age may be reported in days, weeks, or months (Table 25-15).

Of the 3.6 billion retail prescriptions filled in the United States in 2008, 280 million were for children, resulting in a rate of 3.8 prescriptions/child/year. To provide safe and effective drug therapy to pediatric patients, a pharmacist should know the effects of physical and physiologic maturation on the pharmacokinetics and pharmacodynamics of the drug administered. Drug dosing in the pediatric population depends not only on age, but also on body size and the disease being treated. Pediatric drug doses are usually calculated in units of mg/kg/dose or mg/kg/day. Based on patient weight, the mg/day dose for a child might seem to exceed the mg/day dose for an adult patient. Hence, use of pediatric drug dosing guides is recommended to determine safe doses for children.

Anthropometric and Vital Signs Changes with Growth and Development

Anthropometric measurements such as weight, length or height or stature, and head circumference are used to assess a child's overall health and nutritional status, and to predict performance and survival as the child grows into an infant, a child, an adolescent, and finally a young adult. The Centers for Disease Control and Prevention publishes growth charts on its website (http://www.cdc.gov/growthcharts/). These growth charts are segmented by gender and age (birth to 36 months and 2 to 20 years of age) and include weight-for-age, length-for-age, weight-for-length, and head circumference-for-age (birth to 36 months) measurements. The CDC also publishes BMI-for-age charts for children between 2 and 20 years of age. These growth charts are used by pediatricians to document a child's growth and attainment of certain physical milestones with age.

At birth, a term newborn is expected to weigh between 3.23 kg (female) and 3.27 kg (male) (50th percentile weight for age) and measure between 19 and 20 inches in length (50th percentile length for age). After that point, infants can be expected to double their birth weight at 4 to 5 months of age and triple their birth weight by 12 months of age.

Vital signs such as heart rate, blood pressure, respiratory rate, and body temperature vary based on age. Heart rates are highest in neonates and infants, ranging from 95–180 beats per minute, decreasing to adult values of 60–80 beats per minute by 10 years of age. Blood pressure in pediatric patients varies based on gender, age, and height percentile. Tables listing the 50th, 90th, 95th, and 99th percentiles for systolic blood pressure (SBP) and diastolic blood pressure (DBP) according to height, gender, and age are provided at the National Heart, Lung, and Blood Institute's website (http://www.nhlbi.nih.gov/guidelines/hypertension/child_tbl.htm). The 50th percentile SBP/DBP provides the clinician with the BP level at the midpoint of the normal range. Although the 95th percentile provides a BP level that defines hypertension, management decisions about children with hypertension should be determined by the degree or severity of hypertension. Neonates and infants breathe at a faster rate (24–38 breaths per minute), with respiratory rates falling to adult values (12–20 breaths per minute) around the age of 15 years. Body temperature can be measured rectally in children 4 years of age or younger. For older children, axillary or oral temperature measurements are more appropriate. Rectal temperature is generally 0.6 °C (1°F) higher than the oral temperature, which is generally 0.6 (1°F) higher than the axillary temperature.

Maturational Factors Affecting Drug Absorption

Factors such as gastric pH, gastric and intestinal motility, blood flow to the gastrointestinal tract, and the surface area of absorption affect the rate and extent of GI absorption and undergo considerable maturational changes as a neonate grows into an adult. The amount of gastric acid produced increases and the pH decreases in a newborn with age. Newborns of 32 weeks' or less gestational age rarely have any gastric acid production; in a term newborn, the gastric acid is alkaline (pH 6–8) at birth but becomes acidic within 24 hours (pH 1.5–3) of birth. The gastric acid volume and concentration approach the lower extremes of adult values by 3 months of age and reach adult values around the age of 2 years. These maturational changes may affect the rate and extent of absorption of oral drugs that are weak acids or weak bases, depending on their partition coefficients (pK_a) and the gastric and intestinal pH. Increased bioavailability of orally administered acid labile drugs such as penicillin G, ampicillin, and nafcillin has been observed in neonates and infants when compared to adults. Decreased bioavailability of weak organic acids such as phenobarbital can be expected. There are no recommendations for drug dosing changes based on acid production and pH of the GI tract. However, close monitoring for efficacy and safety is required; lack of drug absorption should be considered a likely cause of subtherapeutic efficacy despite use of optimal/maximal drug doses.

The gastric emptying rate is delayed in infants, but reaches the adult capacity by 6–8 months of age. In infancy and beyond, differences in GI maturation and absorption between different age groups may not be significant enough to affect dosing recommendations for most drugs.

Drug absorption after intramuscular administration may vary in premature newborns due to their smaller volume of skeletal muscle mass and subcutaneous fat compared to older infants, children, and adults. Drugs administered by the intramuscular route are generally well absorbed in infants and children, although painful. This route is more commonly used for vaccine administration, and occasionally when oral and intravenous routes are unavailable.

Percutaneous drug absorption is significantly more pronounced in premature neonates due to immature development of the epidermal barrier when compared to term infants, older children, and adults. In general, percutaneous drug absorption is greater in pediatric patients when compared to adults due to children's greater skin hydration, thinner or immature stratum corneum, and greater body surface area to weight ratio; it is increased when skin is damaged, such as in a diaper rash. Topical drugs with limited safety information should be applied cautiously. Application of high-potency steroid creams or ointments to diaper rash can lead to systemic absorption and should be avoided. Toxic effects have been reported with topical agents such as EMLA (eutectic mixture of lidocaine and prilocaine) and hexachlorophene solution. EMLA should be used with caution in patients younger than 3 months of age. This product is used in children for numbing of an area before insertion of a needle for establishing an intravenous line or drawing blood for laboratory measurements. Use of this product can increase the risk of methemoglobinemia from increased percutaneous absorption of prilocaine and decreased methemoglobin reductase, especially in combination with other methemoglobinemia-inducing agents.

Maturational Factors Affecting Drug Distribution

Differences in body composition of water, fat, and plasma proteins determine the differences in drug distribution between infants and adults. A premature infant has the highest proportion of total body water at 80–90% (60% extracellular water and 25% intracellular water), which decreases to 71–83% in a full-term newborn (45% extracellular water and 34% intracellular water), falls to 60% by 1 year of age (25% extracellular water and 35% intracellular water), and approaches adult values of 50–60% (20% extracellular water and 40% intracellular water) by 12–13 years of age. The proportion of extracellular water decreases and the proportion of intracellular water increases as the infant matures into an adult. Drugs such as aminoglycosides, digoxin, and linezolid—all of which are extensively distributed in the extracellular fluid—have large volumes of distribution in neonates compared to older infants and children. Larger volumes of distribution require larger milligram-per-kilogram doses in neonates compared to infants and older children and even adults to achieve similar serum drug concentrations.

Total body fat increases from 12–16% of body weight at birth to 20–25% at 1 year of age and continues to increase until puberty. At puberty, females experience a rapid increase in body fat compared to males. Owing to the differences in body fat, lipophilic drugs have a lower volume of distribution in children compared to adults. For example, the mean apparent volume of distribution (V_d) for the lipophilic drug diazepam is lower in infants (1.3–2.6 L/kg) compared to adults (1.6–3.2 L/kg).

The rates at which drugs bind to various plasma proteins also differ between pediatric patients and adults. Total protein composition, including albumin and alpha$_1$ acid glycoprotein, is decreased in neonates and approaches adult values by the first year of age. The binding capacity of these proteins to various drugs is also lower. Endogenous substances such as bilirubin and free fatty acids compete with the drugs for albumin binding sites. Drugs such as ceftriaxone and sulfonamides should be used with caution in newborns, as these drugs are highly protein (albumin) bound and will easily displace albumin-bound bilirubin to cause kernicterus.

Maturational Factors Affecting Drug Metabolism

Phase I reactions (oxidation, reduction, hydrolysis, and hydroxylation) and Phase II reactions (conjugation) are involved in drug biotransformation. The hepatic enzymes that catalyze these reactions are not well developed at birth in full-term infants compared to older children and adults. This development is further delayed in premature neonates. For example, premature and term infants show prolonged elimination of drugs such as phenytoin and diazepam because oxidizing enzymes necessary for metabolism of phenytoin and diazepam are not well developed in this population. The development of cytochrome P450 enzymes is also delayed in newborns; these enzymes reach adult values between 6 months and 1 year of age.

In Phase II reactions, endogenous agents such as sulfate, acetate, glucuronic acid, glutathione, and glycine conjugate with the drug substrate and convert it to a more water-soluble compound that can be easily excreted. The activity of these enzymes is greatly decreased in premature and term neonates and may attain adult values by 3–6 months of age. For example, in premature and term neonates, acetaminophen is primarily metabolized by sulfation because the enzyme system glucuronyl transferase, which is necessary for the glucuronidation of acetaminophen, is still immature. As the newborn grows, however, glucuronidation becomes the primary pathway of acetaminophen's metabolism. The ratio of glucuronide conjugate to sulfate conjugate of acetaminophen increases from 0.34 in a newborn to 0.8 in a child between 3 and 10 years of age, to 1.61 in an adolescent, and then to 1.8–2.3 in an adult. Hence, acetaminophen is one of the safest drugs in newborns when administered appropriately.

Immaturity of metabolic pathways may also expose premature neonates to morbidity and mortality due to the commonly used preservatives in drugs. For example, neonatal deaths have been linked to benzyl alcohol, a preservative used in some intravascular solutions. Benzyl alcohol is normally oxidized to benzoic acid, conjugated with glycine in the liver, and excreted as hippuric acid; however, the glycation pathway is not well developed in premature neonates. Benzyl alcohol exposure in this population is minimized by using benzyl alcohol–free drugs when available; when benzyl alcohol–free drugs are unavailable, the intravenous preparation may be diluted to decrease the amount of benzyl alcohol being administered.

Maturational Factors Affecting Drug Elimination

Drugs may be eliminated from the body unchanged or as metabolites via the kidneys or in the feces. Glomerular filtration, tubular secretion, and reabsorption affect renal elimination of drugs. The glomerular filtration rate (GFR) increases in a pediatric patient from the time of birth and approaches adult values by 3–5 months of age. A positive correlation between GA and GFR is observed between 27 and 43 weeks of GA. Thus, the lower the GA age, the lower the GFR and the renal function. The GFR increases from 10–15 mL/min/m^2 at birth and reaches adult values of 73–127 mL/min/m^2 by 3 months of age. Low GFR or decreased renal function has a significant effect on drug dosing. Serum creatinine and urine output are parameters commonly used to evaluate renal function or GFR in pediatric patients. Serum creatinine can be used to determine creatinine clearance using the Bedside Schwartz equation:

$$\text{CrC1} = (0.413 \times L)/\text{SCr}$$

where CrCl is creatinine clearance in mL/min/1.73m^2; L is body length in centimeters; and SCr is serum creatinine in mg/dL. The serum creatinine value used in this equation should be measured using an enzymatic assay with an isotope dilution mass spectrometry (IDMS)–traceable international standard. The use of this assay is advocated by the National Kidney Foundation and the National Kidney Disease Education Program to ensure an accurate estimate of GFR in patients. All laboratories throughout the U.S. have switched to using this assay.

A urine output of 1–2 mL/kg/hr is considered adequate. Creatinine clearance may not be the most accurate assessment of renal function, however, especially in premature or term neonates and when renal function is decreased. In these cases, creatinine is excreted not only by glomerular filtration but also by renal tubular secretion, which may result in normal SCr levels despite the decrease in GFR and renal function. Newborns and premature neonates also have lower muscle mass, resulting in lower SCr values, which may lead to a falsely high CrCl value. Urine output may be influenced by fluid intake, hydration status, renal solute load, urine concentration capabilities, and use of diuretics. The effects of these factors should be evaluated when using urine output as an assessment of renal function.

1.2.0 Pharmacotherapy

Over-the-Counter Medications in the Pediatric Population

Community pharmacists serve as a first-line drug information resource for parents of infants and children seeking an over-the-counter remedy for their child's malady. When parents seek dosing recommendations regarding OTC mediations, they should always be directed to the active ingredient medication label and the manufacturer's recommendations. If parents request recommendations for OTC medications not indicated in pediatric patients due to the child's age or lack of dosing information, the parents should be directed to contact their pediatrician for a prescription for an appropriate drug.

Key concepts regarding use of OTC medications in children to be reviewed during parent and caregiver education include the following:

- Always read and follow the medication label exactly. Also, use the measuring device that comes with the medicine to administer the medication.
- Do not give a medication intended for an adult to a child.
- Read the label carefully to identify the active ingredients.

- Never give a child two medications at the same time that contain the same active ingredient.
- Do not use an OTC medication to make a child sleepy.
- Do not give aspirin-containing products to a child for cold and flu symptoms unless instructed to do so by a doctor.
- Talk to a doctor, pharmacist, or other healthcare provider if any questions arise regarding the child's OTC medication.

The most recent controversy regarding OTC medications in children involves the use of cough and cold medications. Pursuant to an investigation initiated by the FDA in March 2007 regarding the safety and efficacy of cough and cold medications in children, a public health advisory was released stating that giving more than the recommended amount of OTC cough and cold products can be harmful to children. Serious injuries and death have been reported in infants and children who received OTC cough and cold medications, but most adverse events have been related to overdoses and unsupervised ingestions. In October 2008, the Consumer Healthcare Products Association announced that the leading manufacturers of pediatric OTC cough and cold medications would voluntarily modify the labels on these products to state that they should not be used in children younger than age 4 years. Previous product labels stated that these medicines should not be used in children younger than age 2 years.

Another common OTC medication use controversy in pediatric patients relates to the practice of alternating acetaminophen doses with ibuprofen to treat high fevers. This practice is not endorsed by the American Academy of Pediatrics, the FDA, or pharmaceutical companies. Such practice enhances the toxicity of acetaminophen due to ibuprofen-induced decreased renal blood flow and a subsequent decrease in the excretion of acetaminophen metabolites. This synergy can result in increased renal and hepatic toxicity. Recent labeling changes for acetaminophen highlight the potential for hepatotoxicity, draw attention to this drug's presence in combination products, and include doses for children younger than 2 years of age. Recent labeling changes for ibuprofen highlight the potential for stomach bleeding and require the word "NSAID" to be prominently displayed on the label with the active ingredient.

Extemporaneous Formulations

Nearly 75% of the drugs marketed for adults in the United States are not labeled (FDA approved) for use in the pediatric population, yet have been commonly used to treat childhood diseases. Thus, these drugs are typically not available in a dosage form suitable for administration to infants and children. Because most drugs administered to pediatric patients are based on body weight (mg/kg) or body surface area (mg/m^2), the available fixed-dose solid forms (tablets or capsules) are not practical for use in infants and young children. Infants and children 5 years of age and younger are usually unable to swallow a solid dosage form. For drugs requiring therapeutic serum concentration measurements, dose adjustments required to achieve these concentrations may be limited by the availability of a particular strength of the dosage form. In these cases, drugs can be made available by extemporaneously formulating liquid dosage forms from their commercially available solid dosage form (e.g., amlodipine and enalapril).

An extemporaneous formulation should be physically and chemically stable for the duration of and the temperature at which the label recommends storage; it should also be palatable and easy to compound. Information regarding the compounding formula and the stability and storage conditions can be obtained through numerous resources, including the United States Pharmacopeia, which publishes official monographs of compounded preparations with valid stability data to establish beyond-use dates. Books and peer-reviewed publications are also reliable sources of information for compounding extemporaneous formulations. On rare occasions, manufacturers of the solid dosage form may include the extemporaneous formulation in their package insert.

Community pharmacists often face greater challenges in providing extemporaneous formulations to their patients due to the limited resources available for compounding as well as issues with reimbursement. A list of pharmacies capable of extemporaneous compounding should be maintained and provided to the parents and caregivers when needed.

ANNOTATED BIBILIOGRAPHY

Phan H, Pai VB, Nahata MC. "Pediatrics." In *Pharmacotherapy: Principles and Practice*. 2 ed. Edited by Chisholm-Burns MA, Schwinghammer TL, Wells BG, Malone PM, Kolesan JM, DiPiro JT. 23–33. New York: The McGraw-Hill Companies, Inc., 2010.

Pai VB, Nahata MC. "Drug Dosing in Pediatric Patients." In *Clinical Pharmacokinetics*. 5 ed. Edited by Murphy John E. 30-38. Bethesda: American Society of Health-System Pharmacists, 2012.

Kearns GL, Abdel-Rahman SM, Alander SW, Blowey DL, Leeder JS, Kauffman RE. Developmental pharmacology–drug disposition, action, and therapy in infants and children. N Engl J Med. 2003;349:1157–67.

Nahata MC, Pai VB. *Pediatric Drug Formulations.* 6 ed. Cincinnati: Harvey Whitney Books Company, 2011.

TOPIC: CONTRACEPTION

Section Coordinator: *Sandra Hrometz*
Contributor: *Joy K. Lehman*

Introduction

More than 200 million women worldwide use hormonal contraception to prevent unwanted pregnancies. Patients often choose these agents based on the benefits to the menstrual cycle and other health conditions. In the United States, hormones and contraception rank in the top five therapeutic categories for number of prescriptions dispensed. Contraception differs from other medications in that many patients are young and otherwise healthy. In addition, women may continue to take these agents for decades. The pharmacist must understand how these agents interact with the body's natural hormonal regulation and which adverse effects may lead to their discontinuation or improper use. Pharmacists are uniquely positioned to provide patients with information to help them to optimize contraception, to effectively deal with side effects, and to handle contraception emergencies.

Tips Worth Tweeting

- There are many noncontraceptive benefits to consider when selecting a hormonal contraceptive.
- Progestin agents have both progestin and androgen activity.
- Side effects of estrogen excess will decrease over time.
- Breakthrough bleeding can be an estrogen or progestin side effect, depending on when the bleeding takes place during the menstrual cycle.
- Patients who are older than age 35 and smoke should use a progestin-only product.
- Newer dosage forms, such as the contraceptive patch or vaginal ring, may improve patient adherence with contraceptives.
- Medications that induce the cytochrome P450 3A4 enzyme may clinically decrease the effectiveness of combined oral contraceptives (COCs).
- Emergency contraception will prevent pregnancy if taken within 72 hours of unprotected intercourse.

Patient Care Scenario: Outpatient Community Pharmacy Setting

L.C. is a 20-year-old female who recently became sexually active. She is 5'4", 123 lbs; NKDA; nonsmoker; no other medications except fexofenadine 180 mg as needed for seasonal allergies. Her medication history is as follows (in the table below).

L.C. returns to the pharmacy in May and states that she is very frustrated. The OrthoNovum 1/35 she was prescribed caused breast tenderness, bloating, and nausea. Those symptoms have now resolved, but she is having late-cycle breakthrough bleeding that is very bothersome. L. C. wants to know if the pharmacist can recommend something else that will not make her "fat" or cause breakthrough bleeding.

Date	Physician	Drug	Quantity	Sig	Refills
2/2/10	Dr. Jones	OrthoNovum 1/35	1 pack	1 tab po qd	11
3/1/10	Dr. Jones	Ortho TriCyclen Lo	1 pack	1 tab po qd	11

1.1.0 Patient Information

Patient Assessment

Prior to starting hormonal contraception, especially combined oral contraception (COC), patients should have a complete history and physical exam. This exam should include, at a minimum, height, weight, blood pressure, lipid profile, and blood glucose. A Pap smear should also be completed to rule out cervical cancer. The clinician should discuss the patient's and family's history of cancer, cardiovascular disease, and thromboembolic events. In addition, the patient's smoking history should be reviewed. After the history and physical exam is completed, the clinician should discuss the patient's menstrual history, including amount and duration of flow.

1.2.0 Pharmacotherapy

Mechanism of Action

Contraception works in one of two ways: (1) by preventing sperm from coming in contact with the mature egg or (2) by preventing the fertilized ovum from being implanted in the endometrium. All hormonal contraception contains progestin, which both thickens cervical secretions to decrease sperm motility and causes endometrial atrophy. Estrogens suppress the release of follicle-stimulating hormone, which prevents ovulation.

Ethinyl estradiol (EE) is the most commonly used estrogen for hormonal contraception; multiple progestins are also used in combined oral contraceptives (COCs). The potency and effect of these medications

Table 25-16 Combined Oral Contraceptives

Product	Estrogen (mcg), Progestin (mg)	Estrogen Activity	Progestin Activity	Androgen Activity
Ovcon-50	EE 50, norethindrone 1	High	Intermediate	Intermediate
Demulen 1/50	EE 50, ethynodiol diacetate 1	High	High	High
Ovral	EE 50, norgestrel 0.5	High	High	High
Ortho Novum 1/35	EE 35, norethindrone 1	Intermediate	Intermediate	Intermediate
Ortho Cyclen	EE 35, norgestimate 0.25	Intermediate	Low	Low
Demulen 1/35	EE 35, ethynodiol diacetate	Intermediate	High	Low
Yasmin	EE 30, drospirenone 3	Low	Intermediate	No effect
Desogen	EE 30, desogestrel 0.15	Low	High	Low
Lo/Ovral	EE 30, norgestrel 0.3	Low	Intermediate	Intermediate
Aless	EE 20, levonorgestrel 0.1	Very low	Low	Low
Micronor	Norethindrone 0.35	None	Very low	Very low
Triphasic Contraceptives				
Ortho Novum 7/7/7	EE 35, norethindrone 0.5, 0.75, 1	Intermediate	Intermediate	Low
Ortho Tri-Cyclen	EE 30 × 6, 40 × 5, 30 × 10	Intermediate	Low	Low
Ortho Tri-Cyclen Lo	EE 25, norgestimate 0.18, 0.215, 0.25	Low	Low	Low
Biphasic Contraceptives				
Mircette	EE 20 × 21, 0 × 2, 10 × 5	Very low	High	Low

depend on the dose. Table 25-16 shows various COCs and their relative activity.

Adverse Effects

Most adverse effects from hormonal contraception involve imbalances of circulating estrogen or progestin. Signs and symptoms of estrogen excess include the following:

- Nausea
- Breast tenderness and breast enlargement
- Headache
- Edema and bloating
- Hypermenorrhea

These symptoms typically decrease over time and usually disappear 2 to 3 months after starting the agent. In contrast, signs and symptoms of estrogen deficiency tend to increase over time:

- Early-cycle breakthrough bleeding
- Hypomenorrhea
- Vaginal dryness
- Hot flashes

Progestins have both progestin and androgen (A) effects based on the type of progestin. Symptoms of progestin excess tend to increase over time and include the following:

- Weight gain (P/A)
- Decreased flow length (P)
- Decreased libido (P); increased libido (A)
- Decreased breast size (P)
- Acne/oily skin (A)
- Hirsuitism (A)

Acne and weight gain are common concerns for women. Choosing a progestin with low androgen activity (see Table 25-16) or drosperinone, which has no androgen activity, will help decrease or prevent these side effects.

Progestin deficiency, like estrogen excess, will decrease over time. Symptoms of this imbalance include the following:

- Late-cycle breakthrough bleeding
- Delayed withdrawal bleeding
- Heavy flow with clots

Serious adverse effects happen only rarely, but include venous thrombosis, pulmonary embolism, MI, arterial thromboembolism, and cerebral thrombosis. Patients should be counseled to watch for severe headache, leg pain, chest pain, abdominal pain, or acute vision changes. If any of these problems occur, use of the contraceptive should be stopped immediately and a physician should be contacted.

Risks

A great deal of research has examined the actual and theoretical risks of COCs. One of the most concerning issues was the risk of breast cancer in women who take oral contraceptives. However, a large study in 1996 found only a slight increase in relative risk (1.24) in women who take COCs compared to nonusers. The authors also concluded that this increase in risk disappeared after 10 years. Cardiovascular risk associated with COCs has also been studied, with WHO concluding that the risk of MI is increased only in current COC users who are also smokers. The total relative risk was 1–1.1 for MI, ischemic stroke, and hemorrhagic stroke for users versus nonusers.

The most common cardiovascular event among COC users is venous thromboembolism (VTE), but mortality in COC users due to this use is very low. The risk of VTE is up to 4 times higher in patients who take COCs. This is primarily an estrogen dose-related phenomenon. Recent surgery, obesity, malignancy, and coagulation disorders also increase the risk of VTE. This risk may also be slightly increased in women who take a COC containing desogestrel and in those who use the contraceptive patch.

Contraindications

Contraindications to COCs are commonly, but not exclusively, related to the estrogen component. Absolute contraindications include the following:

- Known or suspected pregnancy
- History of CVA or MI, or multiple risk factors for coronary artery disease (older, smoker, hypertension, DM)
- Thrombophilia or thromboembolic disorder
- Severe congenital hyperlipidemia
- History or current diagnosis of breast cancer or any estrogen-dependent cancer
- Severe liver dysfunction
- Abnormal uterine bleeding
- Heavy smoker who is 35 years or older
- Breastfeeding

Benefits

Many positive noncontraceptive benefits are associated with use of COCs. Most importantly, these medications have been linked to decreased risk of endometrial, ovarian, and (possibly) colon cancer. They also bring about a reduction in benign breast disease, blood loss, anemia, and dysmenorrhea. Many women choose contraception based on the ability to control and regulate menstrual flow. Recently, some contraceptives have been FDA approved to treat mild to moderate acne. Any contraceptive containing a low-androgenic-potency progestin will decrease the incidence of acne.

Dosage Forms

The most common form of hormonal contraception is the combined oral contraceptive pill (see Table 25-16).

Table 25-17 Extended-Interval Combined Oral Contraceptives

Product	Estrogen (mcg), Progestin (mg)	Cycle Length
Lybrel	EE 20, levonorgestrel 0.09	Continuous cycle, no placebo
Seasonale	EE 30 × 84 days, levonorgestrel 0.15	91-day cycle: on 84 days, off 7 days
Seasonique	EE 30 × 84 days, EE 10 × 4; levonorgestrel 0.1	91-day cycle: on 84 days, off 7 days
LoEstrin-24Fe	EE 20 × 24, off 4 days; norethindrone 1	28-day cycle: on 24 days, off 4 days
Yaz	EE 20 × 24 days, off 4 days; drospirenone 3	28-day cycle: on 24 days, off 4 days

Most recently added to the COC roster is the category of extended-interval pills (Table 25-17). These formulations allow women to decrease or eliminate their monthly menstrual flow.

Progestin-only formulations and the "mini-pill" are available for those women who are breastfeeding or have an absolute contraindication to estrogen. These formulations are less effective than COCs and require increased compliance. Missing a dose by even a few hours can decrease effectiveness and increase the incidence of breakthrough bleeding.

Several other progesterone formulations are available for long-term contraceptive needs. These products generally cause breakthrough bleeding initially (3–6 months), which is then followed by amenorrhea. All of the non-oral progesterone products have increased progestin and androgen potency as compared to their oral counterparts. Most often women who use these products will experience increased breakthrough bleeding and irregular periods, followed by lighter periods or amenorrhea.

Medroxyprogesterone acetate (Depo-Provera) is given as a quarterly IM or subcutaneous injection. Its package insert carries a "boxed warning" stating that there is a risk of decreased calcium deposition in bones while patients are taking the medication. Studies have shown, however, that bone health will clinically return to baseline once the medication is stopped, and there should be no age restrictions when prescribing Depo-Provera.

Etonogestrel (Implanon) is available as an implant that provides effective contraception for as long as 3 years. Implanon is a flexible, 4-cm rod that is placed subdermally in the upper arm. It can be removed at any time, and fertility will return to baseline within one or two menstrual cycles.

Levonorgestrel (Mirena) is available as an intrauterine device (IUD) that provides as long as 5 years of effective contraception. In addition to the side effects mentioned previously, abdominal cramping is a frequent side effect with this contraceptive and the most common reason why patients stop using the product.

Paraguard is a copper IUD that contains no hormones. It is thought that the copper itself acts as a spermacide. Paraguard can be used for as long as 10 years, and its side-effect profile is similar to that of levonorgestrel (Mirena).

Recently, new routes of administration have improved compliance with combined hormonal contraception. The Ortho Evra patch is a once-weekly transdermal contraceptive system containing ethinyl estradiol and norelgestromin. The patient places a new patch on once weekly for 3 weeks and then has a hormone-free week. Ortho Evra has been shown effective in any type of daily activity, including bathing and swimming. The amount of estrogen delivery is higher when compared to a COC containing 35 mcg of ethinyl estradiol. Therefore, women who have an increased risk of thromboembolism, and particularly women who are older than age 35 and smoke, should not use the patch. The effectiveness of the patch is decreased in women who weigh more than 198 lbs.

Nuva Ring is a once-monthly vaginal ring that contains ethinyl estradiol and etonogestrel. This vaginal ring delivers very low consistent levels of hormones and has much lower progestin and androgen potency when compared to COCs. Increased patient weight does not decrease its effectiveness.

Emergency Contraception

Plan B One Step (levonorgestrel 150 mcg) is available as emergency contraception with a prescription or as an OTC product for women 17 years of age and older. It should be taken within 72 hours of unprotected intercourse or contraceptive failure. Levonorgestrel (LNG) halts ovulation and prevents fertilization by thickening the cervical mucus and decreasing sperm motility. Rarely, if fertilization has occurred, LNG will prevent implantation in the uterine wall. This progestin will not affect the outcome of pregnancy once the gestational sac has implanted in the uterine wall. If a patient does not have access to emergency contraceptive, she may use her own birth control if it contains levonorgestrel or norgestrel as the progestin component. A total of 1 mg levonorgestrel or 2 mg norgestrel should be taken in two divided doses 12 hours apart within 72 hours of unprotected intercourse. The patient should be counseled that an antiemetic may be necessary due to the large estrogen dose.

For patients taking oral contraceptives, missed doses can be a frequent and stressful problem depending on patient compliance. If doses are missed, patients can be counseled as shown in Table 25-18.

Table 25-18 Management of Missed COC Doses

Missed Dose	Makeup	Backup
Missed 1 pill anytime	Take as soon as possible (if next day, take 2 pills at once)	No backup necessary
Missed 2 pills in a row during first 2 weeks	Take 2 pills as soon as possible and 2 pills the next day	Use backup for 7 days
Missed 2 pills in a row during third week or 3 or more pills at any time	Take 1 pill every day until Sunday or the usual starting day, then start a new pack	Use backup for 7 days (may miss period)

1.3.0 Monitoring

Drug Interactions

Oral ethinyl estradiol is metabolized via the cytochrome P450 3A4 enzyme. Medications that induce the 3A4 enzyme will increase the metabolism of estrogen and potentially decrease the effectiveness of the COC. A list of cytochrome P450 3A4 enzyme inducers appears in Table 25-19. If a patient is taking one of these medications, then she should switch to a progestin-only product or take a non-oral formulation (e.g., transdermal patch, vaginal ring). If she is taking a CYP3A4 inducer for a short period of time, the patient may choose to use backup contraceptive during the course of this medication. Most anti-infective agents (other than those listed in Table 25-19) will not clinically decrease the effectiveness of COCs; however, patients should be counseled to expect an increase in breakthrough bleeding. Combined oral contraceptives may also cause decreased levels of the interacting medications, such as lamotrigine.

Patient Counseling

In the patient care scenario that appears at the beginning of this section, it is important to highlight several important counseling points:

- Symptoms of estrogen excess and progestin deficiency will usually decrease over 2–3 months.

Table 25-19 Cytochrome P450 Inducers: Agents That Decrease the Effectiveness of COCs

Anticonvulsants		
• Carbemazepine	• Oxcarbemazepine	• Phenytoin
• Phenobarbital	• Topiramate (high dose only)	• Felbamate (high dose only)
• Primidone		
Antibiotics		
• Rifampin	• Tetracylines	
• Griseofulvin	• Sulfonamides	

- Breakthrough bleeding and change in menstrual flow is common when initiating a new contraceptive.
  - Noncompliance is the most common reason for breakthrough bleeding.
  - If compliance is assured, the patient should note when the bleeding is occurring to help the clinician determine if it is an estrogen- or progestin-related effect.
- Weight gain is a highly publicized side effect of hormonal contraceptives. However, only those products with a high dose and/or high-potency progestin have been shown to cause a clinically significant change in weight.
- Patients should be counseled regarding the signs and symptoms of VTE, stroke, and MI.
- Information regarding emergency contraception and steps to take if a dose is missed should be given with the initial prescription.

TOPIC: DRUG THERAPY IN PREGNANCY AND LACTATION

Section Coordinator: Sandra Hrometz
Contributor: Debra K. Gardner

Introduction

Unnecessary drug exposure should be avoided in pregnant women; however, chronic medical disorders, acute medical conditions, or pregnancy complications may develop during pregnancy, necessitating drug therapy to preserve the health of the mother and the baby. Evaluation of the risk the disease presents to the mother and fetus must be weighed against the benefit and risks of pharmacotherapy. It is important for pharmacists to understand which medications are safe in pregnancy and under which circumstances they can be used. It is equally important to know which drugs may cause harm to the developing embryo or fetus so that use of these medications can be avoided at critical stages during pregnancy.

Drug therapy concerns during lactation differ from those noted during pregnancy. Medications taken by the lactating mother becomes distributed throughout her body, so that only a small fraction appears in breastmilk. Lactation can be safely continued during drug treatment for most conditions as long as the medication is wisely chosen.

Tips Worth Tweeting

- Although the risk of drug-induced anomalies is of concern, the actual risk of birth defects from most drug exposures is small.
- Exposure to a potential teratogen poses the greatest risk during organogenesis, which occurs during the first 8 weeks of pregnancy.
- Most maternal conditions or diseases that require pharmacotherapy during pregnancy present more risk to the fetus than the drugs used to treat them.
- Women of childbearing age should take folic acid, 400 mcg daily, to reduce the risk of neural tube defects.
- During lactation, most conditions can be treated adequately by selecting drug therapy with a low risk to the baby.

Patient Care Scenario: Outpatient Community Pharmacy Setting

J.P. a 35-year-old, single black female who states she has not had a period in 8 weeks. She has been taking a low-dose oral contraceptive for 5 years and normally has very light periods, but she is concerned she may be pregnant. J. P. has hypertension, which is controlled with lisinopril 20 mg daily. A pregnancy test confirms she is pregnant.

Date	Physician	Drug	Quantity	Sig	Refills
2/28/10	Dr. Spencer	Ortho TryCyclen Lo	#28	1 daily	12
2/28/10	Dr. Fey	Lisinopril 20 mg	#30	1 daily	6

1.1.0 Patient Information

Epidemiology and Background: Drug Therapy in Pregnancy

The background incidence of birth defects in populations without any known risk factors is approximately 3% at birth, but increases to 5–6% at 1 year of age as time allows discovery of those defects not evident at birth. Birth defects can be caused by dominant or recessive genes, by chromosomal abnormalities, and by environmental agents such as radiation, chemicals, and toxins. Drugs also fall under the "environmental agents" category but contribute to only a small fraction of anomalies. Drugs known to be harmful during pregnancy are listed in Table 25-20. The majority of birth defects are multifactorial in nature, resulting from a combination of genetic and environmental factors. Another important contributor to birth defects and pregnancy complications is untreated maternal diseases such as diabetes and infection.

Table 25-20 Drugs Known to Have Harmful Effects During Pregnancy

Drug or Drug Class	Examples (Not Inclusive)	Comment
ACE inhibitors	Captopril Enalapril Lisinopril	Drug class effect; renal anomalies in second and third trimesters
Angiotensin II receptor antagonists	Candesartan	
Vitamin A derivatives	Isotretinoin (Accutane) Etretinate Acetretin Vitamin A doses > 18,000 units daily	Drug class effect; teratogenic in first trimester
Antineoplastics	Busulfan Chlorambucil Cyclophosphamide Methotrexate	Teratogenic in first trimester
Androgens	Methyltestosterone Oxandrolone Oxymetholone Testosterone	Masculinization of female fetus
Antibiotics	Fluconazole (high-dose, 800 mg daily)	Lower doses may be used in pregnancy
	Kanamycin Streptomycin	Eighth cranial nerve toxicity
	Tetracycline	Weakens and discolors bones and teeth
	Trimethoprim	Folic acid antagonist; avoid in first trimester
Abortifacient	Misoprostol	Misoprostol has many obstetrical uses, including induction of labor and treatment of postpartum hemorrhage
	Miifepristone	Only use in pregnancy is for pregnancy termination
Antiepileptics	Valproic acid Depakote	Neural tube defects (NTD); folic acid 4 mg daily prior to conception decreases the risk of NTD
Antivirals	Efavirenz (HIV drug)	May cause neural tube defects
Diethylstilbestrol	DES Dienestrol	First-trimester effects: cervical cancer, uterine anomalies, infertility in female offspring
Lithium	Eskalith Lithobid	First-trimester heart defect, Ebstein's anomaly (low risk)
NSAIDs	Ibuprofen Naprosyn Sulindac Indomethacin	Class effect; first-trimester effects: abortion, heart defects, oral cleft; third-trimester effects (after 32 weeks): premature closure of the ductus arteriosus; NSAIDs used for preterm labor weeks 24–32
Substances of abuse	Cocaine	Abortion, growth restriction, preterm labor, abruption
	Alcohol	Fetal alcohol syndrome, mental retardation
HMG-CoA reductase inhibitors (statins)	Atorvastatin Fluvastatin Lovastatin	Risks of drug exposure outweigh benefits of lipid lowering in pregnancy
Thalidomide	Thalomid	First-trimester teratogen; causes limb, skeletal, and craniofacial defects
Warfarin	Coumadin	Warfarin embryopathy: bone stippling

Table 25-21 FDA Pregnancy Categories

Category A	Adequate, well-controlled studies in pregnant women have not shown an increased risk of fetal abnormalities.
Category B	Animal studies have revealed no evidence of harm to the fetus, but there are no well-controlled studies in pregnant women; or animal studies have shown an adverse effect, but adequate, well-controlled studies in pregnant women have failed to demonstrate a risk to the fetus.
Category C	Animal studies have shown an adverse effect, but there are no adequate and well-controlled studies in pregnant women; or no animal studies have been conducted and there are no adequate, well-controlled studies in pregnant women.
Category D	Adequate, well-controlled, or observational studies in pregnant women have demonstrated a risk to the fetus, but the benefits of therapy may outweigh the potential risk.
Category X	Adequate, well-controlled, or observational studies in animals or pregnant women have demonstrated positive evidence of fetal abnormalities. The use of the product is contraindicated in women who are or may become pregnant.

Source: Food and Drug Administration Center for Drug Evaluation and Research. Pregnancy labeling subcommittee of the advisory committee for reproductive health drugs. Available at: http://www.fda.gov/ohrms/dockets/ac/00/transcripts/3601t1.rtf. Accessed March 26, 2011.

1.2.0 Pharmacotherapy

Mechanism of Action

Although the risk of drug-induced teratogenicity is concerning, the actual risk of birth defects from most drug exposure is small. Organogenesis occurs in the first 8 weeks of pregnancy (10 weeks from the last menstrual cycle); during this phase, the risk of structural anomalies reaches its highest point. However, exposure to a teratogen at this time does not always result in a birth defect. The risk of an anomaly occurring increases with increasing medication doses and duration of exposure. Developmental toxicity that occurs after the first trimester can manifest as functional abnormalities, growth restriction, and neurodevelopmental deficits as well as complications of pregnancy. The dose of the agent, timing, and duration of exposure also are important considerations. Even a known teratogen has a dose at which no effect will occur, called the NOEL (no observable effect level). This value is particularly important in animal studies, but the value for humans is rarely known. The NOEL for some drugs has been determined for humans through observational studies—for example, 50 mg/day for the cardioselective beta blocker atenolol and 25 mg/day for the SSRI paroxetine.

In 1979, the FDA developed the Pregnancy Category System (Table 25-21), which was intended to be a simple and quick guide for the prescriber to assess safety of drugs in pregnancy. Unfortunately, this goal was not achieved. The system provides little actual drug data, is overly simplistic, and is rarely updated. A common misconception among clinicians is the notion that drugs in Category B are safer than Category C drugs; in reality, no information may be known for drugs in both categories with regard to human pregnancy. Therefore, the system does not always provide a gradation in reproductive risk. The FDA has recognized these shortcomings and has adopted an improved system that provides information on fertility, pregnancy, and lactation. Information about risk assessment, clinical management, and published data is provided. This new system is being phased in gradually, and has been introduced on a voluntary basis for new drugs for the past several years.

Physiology of Medication Transfer

When determining drug safety during pregnancy, the pharmacist should understand the determinants of placental drug transfer. The physical and chemical properties of the drug, including molecular weight and lipid solubility, as well as the drug's pharmacokinetic properties such as half-life and protein binding, determine the amount and extent of drug transfer. Large molecules with high molecular weights have limited placental transfer. Heparin and low-molecular-weight heparins are examples of large molecules that do not reach the fetus. Drugs that are highly protein bound and have relatively short half-lives also have limited placental transfer.

3.1.0 Access, Evaluate, and Apply Information to Promote Optimal Health Care

Drug Information

Several reliable sources of information for prescribing drugs in pregnancy and lactation exist (Table 25-22). In general, the package insert is the least informative place to find information on drug safety in pregnancy and lactation, because its content is often litigation driven. The Reprotox section of Micromedex (the online drug information service) provides a summary of the published literature and is updated frequently. Pregnancy exposure registries that collect and maintain data on the effects of drugs that are prescribed to and used by pregnant women are another excellent source of information and are available for many classes of drugs, including antiepileptic medications, transplant drugs, and migraine medications. A list of pregnancy registries can be found on the FDA website (www.fda.gov).

Table 25-22 Sources of Reliable Information for Drug Use in Pregnancy and Lactation

Briggs GG, Freeman RK, Yaffe SJ. *Drugs in Pregnancy and Lactation.* 8th ed. Philadelphia: Lippincott Williams & Wilkins; 2008.
Hale TW. *Medications in Mother's Milk.* 14th ed. Amarillo, TX: Pharmacroft; 2010.
LactMed. National Library of Medicine. Available at: www.toxnet.nlm.nih.gov.
Organization of Teratology Information Services (OTIS). Available at: www.otispregnancy.org.
Pregnancy Registries. See www.FDA.gov for the current listing.
ReproRISK: part of Micromedex, Inc.; includes the Reprotox, Shepards, and Teris databases.

One of the best ways to provide pregnant women with correct information about the risks related to therapy in pregnancy is to consult a teratology information service such as the Organization of Teratology Information Specialists (OTIS). OTIS experts include physicians with pediatric, obstetric, or genetic backgrounds who are trained in embryology, teratology, and clinical pharmacology. They are available to counsel women and clinicians when an exposure has taken place already or when pharmacotherapy is intended.

Patient Information and Counseling

Pregnant women often contact their doctors and pharmacists and search the Internet to determine whether they should be concerned about a brief drug exposure that took place before a pregnancy was determined. Misinformation regarding the danger of drug exposure during pregnancy may result in unnecessary termination of pregnancy. For example, the estrogens and progestins found in oral contraceptives are classified as belonging in Pregnancy Category X, indicating they are contraindicated in pregnancy. However, if a woman becomes pregnant while taking oral contraceptives, this drug exposure presents very little risk if it is discontinued when the pregnancy is discovered. Pharmacists can play an important role by counseling and reassuring women in such a situation. Table 25-23 lists drugs the American College of Obstetrics and Gynecology (ACOG) considers nonteratogenic with brief exposure.

Prevention of Potential Drug-Induced Teratogenicity

Untreated Disease

Untreated disease during pregnancy can be a cause of birth defects and pregnancy complications. Inadequately treated diabetes is one major contributor to this problem. The higher the HbA_{1c} level is at the time of conception and during the first trimester, the greater the risk of birth defects. Strict control of blood glucose must begin months before pregnancy to lower this risk and must continue throughout pregnancy to prevent complications such as macrosomia, birth trauma, stillbirth, and neonatal hypoglycemia.

Table 25-23 Drugs Considered Safe with Brief Exposure During Pregnancy

Acetaminophen	Safe at any time during pregnancy
Acyclovir	Safe at any time during pregnancy
Antiemetics	Metoclopramide, promethazine, prochlorperazine, ondansetron
Antihistamines	Doxylamine, diphenhydramine, dimenhydrinate, meclizine, hydroxyzine
Artificial sweeteners	Aspartame
Benzodiazepines	Lorazepam, diazepam, midazolam, alprazolam (prolonged use may cause neonatal withdrawal)
Caffeine	Large amounts in first trimester may be harmful
Marijuana	If combined with alcohol, may potentiate alcohol's harmful effects
Oral contraceptives	Discontinue once pregnancy is diagnosed
Vaginal spermacide nonoxyl-9	Discontinue once pregnancy is diagnosed

Source: ACOG Educational Bulletin #236, *Teratology*, 1997.

Changes in the immune system that prevent rejection of the fetus may also put the pregnant woman at increased risk of complications when mother and fetus become infected. Early and aggressive treatment of infections is imperative to prevent preterm labor and maternal complications. Most antibiotics are safe to use during pregnancy, including penicillins, cephalosporins, and macrolides. Cotrimoxazole should be avoided in the first trimester because the trimethoprim in this medication is a folic acid antagonist. Its use in the second and third trimesters is acceptable and will not cause kernicterus in the newborn. Tetracyclines, including tigecycline, are the only truly contraindicated antibiotics in pregnancy. Although the quinolone antibiotics are generally not used during pregnancy in the United States because of animal teratogenic data, they are commonly used in many parts of the world and evidence for human harm is lacking. The aminoglycosides gentamicin and tobramycin are listed in Pregnancy Category D, but are often used in pregnancy to treat gram-negative urinary tract infections because the benefit outweighs the risk.

Drug Selection for Treatment of Chronic Conditions

All clinicians should consider the childbearing potential of their patients when selecting drug therapy for chronic conditions such as hypertension and epilepsy, as drugs commonly used to treat these conditions can be teratogenic. Daily folic acid intake of at least 0.4 mg has been shown to decrease the risk of neural tube defects and other malformations and should be recommended to all women who plan to eventually have a family.

The benefit-to-risk ratio must always be considered when treating any condition during pregnancy. In general, if drug therapy improves maternal health, it will also be healthful for the pregnancy and the baby. This is particularly true in life-threatening conditions. As long as the drugs in Table 25-20 are avoided, most diseases, conditions, and pregnancy complications pose more risk to the fetus and pregnancy than the medications used to treat them.

Patient Scenario Follow-up

In the patient care scenario that appears at the beginning of this section, J.P.'s treatment for hypertension will have to be changed from lisinopril—an ACE inhibitor known to cause renal defects in the fetus—to a safer drug. Diuretics can cause dehydration and electrolyte disturbances, and beta blockers can cause fetal growth restriction and, therefore, are not the first choice of antihypertensive agents in pregnancy. However, a calcium-channel blocker such as nifedipine would be a good choice for J.P. Now that she knows she is pregnant, she can stop the oral contraceptive and be reassured that they have not caused harm to her baby.

Lactation

Background

Human breastmilk is the most complete and digestible form of nutrition for babies, and breastfeeding offers numerous benefits to both the infant and the mother. Breastfeeding provides important behavioral and psychological benefits by improving bonding between mother and infant. The many health benefits to the infant from breastfeeding include the following:

- Provides secretory IgA
- Decreased illness: otitis media, upper respiratory infections, diarrhea
- Less childhood and adult obesity
- Less diabetes

The mother who breastfeeds also receives health benefits:

- More rapid uterine involution
- Less postpartum blood loss
- Decreased breast cancer risk
- Decreased ovarian cancer risk

When a mother has made the decision to breastfeed, her healthcare providers should support her and do everything to help her continue breastfeeding even in the face of obstacles such as illness. This is especially true when drug therapy is required. Many women are told to discontinue breastfeeding unnecessarily because of inaccurate information in package inserts regarding safety of drugs during lactation. Many computer systems used in pharmacies also derive their information on drug safety in lactation from package inserts. The lactation section in package inserts is litigation driven and makes breastfeeding sound risky when it is rarely based on actual published information. Table 25-22 identifies sources of pertinent information on drugs in breastfeeding.

Equally problematic is extrapolating the pregnancy categories or information on drug safety in pregnancy to drug safety during lactation. The issues with drug safety during pregnancy are completely different than those that arise during lactation. Teratogenicity is no longer an issue, and the extent of drug exposure is more than 10 times greater for the fetus in pregnancy than it is for the infant during breastfeeding. Even though most drugs gain access into breastmilk, in most cases the amount is small and clinically insignificant and does not present a danger to the infant.

1.1.0 Patient Information

Physiology of Lactation

The rapid drop in estrogen, progestin, and other hormones after the delivery of the placenta, plus the infant suckling at the breast, causes release of prolactin and oxytocin from the pituitary gland, which ensures that milk synthesis and release occur to fulfill the infant's needs. Milk generally comes in by postpartum day 3 and the infant achieves full feedings of 150 mL/kg/day by 5 to 7 days of life. Most breastfed babies eat about every 3 hours around the clock. By 6 months of age, most infants begin eating solid foods and milk consumption starts to decrease.

1.2.0 Pharmacotherapy

Determinants of Drug Transfer into Breastmilk

- Molecular weight
- Protein binding
- Degree of ionization
- Lipid solubility

Most drugs gain access to breastmilk by passive diffusion down a concentration gradient. Small lipid-soluble molecules diffuse more easily than larger hydrophilic molecules. Most drugs have some degree of protein binding to albumin in the mother's blood, such that only the unbound drug will freely diffuse into breastmilk. Drugs that are highly protein bound tend to have lower milk concentrations. Examples of highly protein-bound drugs that are safe during lactation include the following medications:

- Nafcillin
- Glipizide
- Furosemide
- Ibuprofen
- Nifedipine
- Propranolol
- Warfarin

Most drugs are weak acids or bases; because breastmilk is more acidic than serum, the degree of drug ionization becomes a determinant of the extent of drug transfer into milk. Weak acids are more ionized at plasma pH; given that only the un-ionized drug easily passes through cell membranes, their passage into milk is not favored. The following acidic drugs achieve low breastmilk concentrations:

- Aspirin (low to moderate doses)
- Cephalexin
- Naproxen
- Valproic acid
- Warfarin

Basic drugs, in contrast, are more un-ionized in the higher pH of the serum and readily diffuse into the more acidic milk. There they become ionized and trapped, causing drug concentrations in breastmilk to exceed serum concentrations. The following are basic drugs that may accumulate in breastmilk:

- Atenolol
- Cocaine
- Diazepam
- Hydralazine
- Meperidine

Determining the Clinical Significance of Drug Concentrations in Breastmilk

The relative infant dose is the percentage of the maternal dose that is excreted into breastmilk and consumed by the infant, which is then adjusted for the infant's weight, assuming the infant consumes an average of 150 mL/kg/day of breastmilk. If this value is less than 10%, it is considered clinically insignificant and probably safe for the baby. This value has been calculated for drugs that have published information on maternal serum and breastmilk levels. The Thomas Hale reference, *Medications in Mother's Milk*, often has this information.

1.3.0 Monitoring

Patient Counseling

A certain amount of information about the baby and its eating habits must be obtained before the answer to a question regarding a drug's safety in breastfeeding can be determined:

- Gestational age
- Chronologic age
- Drug exposure during pregnancy
- Weight
- Frequency of feedings
- Amount of milk consumed

A common question is whether a drug that was taken during pregnancy is safe to continue during lactation after the baby's birth. In general, this practice does not pose additional threat and, in some cases, should be encouraged. For example, for a mother on methadone maintenance during pregnancy, her infant will have developed a tolerance to the drug and will experience opiate withdrawal after delivery. Breastfeeding in this situation will provide a small amount of methadone that can reduce neonatal abstinence syndrome (NAS) symptoms and decrease hospital length of stay.

For infants who have not been exposed to drugs in utero, the medications that are most likely to cause adverse effects through breastmilk are central nervous system depressants, particularly long-acting sedatives and high doses of narcotic analgesics. Medications that have been associated with adverse effects in breastfeeding infants include the following:

- Atenolol
- Cocaine
- Codeine
- Diazepam
- Doxepin
- Ergotamine
- Lithium
- Sotolol

Serious side effects in infants of mothers who have taken medications during lactation are rare. Of the case reports published on adverse effects of medications via breastmilk, very few required any intervention and many were clearly not caused by the maternal medication. Withholding breastfeeding is necessary only for the most toxic drugs, such as certain cancer chemotherapeutic agents and radiopharmaceuticals.

TOPIC: MENOPAUSE

Section Coordinator: Sandra Hrometz
Contributor: Joy K. Lehman

Introduction

Hormone replacement therapy (HRT) has been the mainstay of treating menopausal symptoms for more than a half century. Today, women in industrialized countries may spend one-third of their lives in the postmenopausal period. In addition to having decreasing hormone levels, as women age, there is an increased probability that they will experience comorbidities. These conditions must be taken into consideration when starting or changing hormonal therapy. Some confusion remains among both patients and clinicians regarding which patients are eligible to receive HRT, which products should be used, and which doses are appropriate to prescribe. Pharmacists should be aware of these issues as well as the normal physiology of perimenopause and menopause. This knowledge will allow the pharmacist to provide appropriate counseling to both patients and physicians.

Tips Worth Tweeting

- Vasomotor and genitourinary symptoms affect 80% of all women during perimenopause and may greatly diminish quality of life.
- Estrogen is the most effective therapy for all symptoms of menopause.
- Progestin therapy should be added to estrogen replacement in women who have an intact uterus or those who have had a hysterectomy and suffered from endometriosis.
- Lower-dose products have been shown to be equally efficacious without increasing side effects.
- Low-dose, short-term use of estrogen should not increase the risk of coronary heart disease.
- Many treatment options are available for women who have a contraindication to estrogen therapy.

Patient Care Scenario: Outpatient Community Pharmacy Setting

L.W. is a 47-year-old female who comes into the pharmacy wondering if any of her medications could cause her to have hot flashes. She states that she has been very bothered by hot flashes that seem to come from "out of nowhere." She also states that she often wakes up at night with her pillow soaked in sweat. L.W. has been talking to her friends, who have told her she should look into bio-identical hormones; however, she states, "I know this is not menopause because I am still having a period."

L.W. is 5'2", 176 lbs. Allergies: Penicillin. SH: Occasional glass of wine with dinner. PMH: Depression, hypertension.

Date	Physician	Drug	Quantity	Sig	Refills
09/20	Dr. Johnson	Zoloft	30	1 tab po qd	11
08/15	Dr. Johnson	Lisinopril	30	1 tab po qd	11

1.1.0 Patient Information

Patient Information and Assessment

The clinician needs to consider many factors when a woman is showing signs and symptoms of menopause. A complete history and physical exam should be completed, including, at a minimum, height, weight, blood pressure, lipid profile, and blood glucose. Thyroid function tests may also be included. Similar to the case when initiating a contraceptive, the past medical history should include family history of cancer, cardiovascular disease, and thromboembolic events. The clinician should also discuss menstrual history, including the timing of the last menstrual period occurrence and the amount and duration of flow. A mammogram and pelvic exam should be performed yearly and a DEXA (bone density) exam should be performed every 2–5 years.

Physiology

Perimenopause is defined as the "menopause transition." This phase of the life cycle generally begins 3–5 years prior to menopause and is initiated with sporadic failure of the ovarian follicles. Subsequently, the estrogen levels can be abnormally low or high at different times. Menopause is defined as beginning 1 year after the last menstrual period. The production of estradiol (E2 active estrogen) declines at this time, and estrone (E1) instead predominates. Estrone has one-third the physiologic activity of estradiol. As hormone levels fluctuate and then decline, women can be at risk for a variety of health concerns.

Eighty percent of women will experience vasomotor symptoms. These symptoms typically begin in the perimenopausal period and can last from a few months to several years. In fact, hot flashes and night sweats are the most common reason women seek treatment. Urogenital symptoms may also greatly affect quality of life, although some women are reluctant to discuss these problems. Unfortunately, many of the health concerns related to menopause do not have obvious signs and symptoms. Most of these conditions, including cognition issues and declining bone density, will worsen over time. Therefore, women should be encouraged to have yearly check-ups with a physician starting at the age of 50 or at the first signs of perimenopause.

Wellness and Prevention

Obesity, sedentary lifestyle, and smoking all can increase a woman's risk of vasomotor symptoms. Women entering the perimenopausal period should be encouraged to maintain a healthy diet and exercise regimen. Smoking cessation should also be encouraged. Several nonpharmacologic suggestions may also help

Table 25-24 Health Concerns Linked to Menopause

CNS	Cardiovascular	Cancer	Urogenital	Bone and Joint
Cognitive function	Cardiovascular disease	Breast	Sexual dysfunction	Arthritis
• Memory problems			• Painful intercourse	
Vasomotor symptoms		Colorectal	Vaginal dryness	Osteoporosis
• Hot flashes			• Burning	
• Night sweats			• Itching	
Fatigue		Ovarian	Urogenital atrophy	
			• Atrophy of bladder epithelium	
Depression			Stress incontinence	

reduce the severity of vasomotor symptoms. For example, women should avoid or decrease intake of hot beverages, soups, and spicy foods, all of which may trigger hot flashes. Also, patients should be counseled to dress in layers and, if possible, to keep a fan at their desk and bedside. Keeping the ambient air temperature lower, especially at night, may also help reduce the incidence of hot flashes. The use of vaginal lubricants and moisturizers may help with vaginal dryness and painful intercourse.

1.2.0 Pharmacotherapy

Mechanism of Action

Estrogen is the primary treatment for menopausal symptoms. Conjugated estrogens have been the most extensively studied medications for this indication and are effective in reducing all menopausal symptoms. Conjugated estrogens, as well as the other forms of estrogen found in HRT products, are converted to the active hormone, estradiol, in the body. Progestin is added to estrogen therapy only if the patient has an intact uterus or in women who have had a hysterectomy but have been diagnosed with or have a history of endometriosis. The addition of progestin prevents endometrial hyperplasia and adenocarcinoma. The common progestins used in HRT are medroxyprogesterone, micronized progesterone, norethindrone acetate, and norgestimate. As with contraceptive therapies, the progestin and androgen effects depend on the type of progestin and dose.

Adverse Effects

The dose of estrogen used in HRT is much lower than the dose of estrogen used to prevent pregnancy in contraceptives. Table 25-25 shows the equivalent potency. Because the dose is lower in HRT, patients rarely complain of symptoms of estrogen excess. Other side effects are similar to those seen in contraceptives:

- Nausea
- Headache
- Breast tenderness
- Edema and bloating
- Cholestasis

Recently, several low-dose estrogen products have been introduced. Studies have shown that these products have equal efficacy with lower incidence of side effects than the traditional higher-dose products. Regardless of the product, as a woman ages, she faces a greater risk of developing certain comorbidities. Estrogen therapy can exacerbate these conditions, so close monitoring is required. These conditions include the following problems:

- Thromboembolism (usually occurs in first year of therapy)
- Hypertriglyceridemia (may need to discontinue HRT)
- Gallbladder disease (increased risk with increased duration of therapy)

Side effects of progestins are the similar to those seen with combined oral contraceptives:

- Headache
- Depression
- Irritability
- Weight gain

Table 25-25 Equivalent Estrogen Doses

Estrogen	Approximate Dose Equivalent
Conjugated estrogens (CEE)	0.625 mg
Micronized estradiol (E2)	1 mg
Ethinyl estradiol (EE)	5 mcg
Estradiol patch (E2)	50 mcg

Risks

Hormone replacement therapy is generally well tolerated. Women who are 60 years of age and older do have a slightly higher risk of developing coronary heart disease (CHD) while on HRT. If a patient is more than 10 years past menopause and has risk factors for CHD, the prescriber should weigh the risks versus the benefits prior to initiating or continuing hormone therapy. Other risks include a slightly increased risk in occurrence of stroke, breast cancer, and gallbladder disease. Estrogen use may also exacerbate diabetes (glucose intolerance) and hypertriglyceridemia. A woman suffering from hypothyroidism may require an increase in her thyroid medication dose when estrogen therapy is initiated.

Contraindications

Contraindications to hormone replacement therapy are most commonly linked to the estrogen (estradiol) component. Absolute contraindications include the following:

- Pregnancy
- Current or history of breast cancer
- Current or history of estrogen-dependent neoplasia

Table 25-26 Hormone Replacement Products

Product	Available Doses (mg)	Dosage Form
Estrogens		
Conjugate equine estrogen (Premarin)	0.3, 0.45, 0.625, 0.9, 1.25, 2.5	Oral tablet, taken once daily
Synthetic CE (Cenestin)	0.3, 0.45, 0.625, 0.9, 1.25	Oral tablet, taken once daily
Estropipate (Ogen)	0.625, 0.9, 1.25, 2.5, 5	Oral tablet, taken once daily
Micronized Estradiol (Estrace)	0.5, 1, 1.5, 2	Oral tablet, taken once daily
Transdermal Products		
17β estradiol (Climara, Vivelle Dot)	0.025, 0.0375, 0.05, 0.075, 0.1	Once- or twice-weekly patch
Estradiol + levonorgestrel (Climara Pro)	0.45/0.15	Once-weekly patch
Estradiol + norethindrone (CombiPatch)	0.05/0.14, 0.05/0.25	Twice-weekly patch continuous Twice-weekly patch cyclic
Estradiol (Estrasorb)	0.05	Topical lotion
Estradiol (Estrogel)	0.06% (metered-dose applicator)	Topical gel
Divigel	0.25, 0.5, 0.1	Topical gel
Combination Products		
CEE + medroxyprogesterone (MPA) (Premphase)	CEE 0.625 × 28 days, MPA 5 mg × 14 days	Daily oral tablet, cyclic
CEE + MPA (Prempro)	CEE 0.625/MPA 2.5, CEE 0.3/MPA 1.5, 0.45/MPA 1.5	Continuous
Estradiol 5 mcg + norethindrone (FemHRT)	5 mcg/1 mg	Continuous
Estradiol + norgestimate (Ortho-Prefest)	Estradiol 1 mg, estradiol 1 mg/0.09	E2 3 days alternating with E2/norgestimate × 3days
Estradiol/norethindrone (Activella)	1/0.1, 0.5/0.1	Continuous
Vaginal Estrogens		
E2, CEE, or estropipate	Various	Vaginal cream
Estradiol (Vagifem)	25 mcg	Vaginal tablet
Estradiol (Estring)	7.5 mcg/day	Vaginal ring for urogenital symptoms only
Estradiol acetate (Femring)	0.05, 0.1 mg/day	Vaginal ring: provides systemic hormone levels

- Undiagnosed abnormal genital bleeding
- Current or history of stroke
- Thromboembolism associated with previous estrogen use
- Recent myocardial infarction

Dosage Forms

Estrogen replacement comes in many different forms:

- Oral tablet
- Transdermal patch
- Topical cream or gel
- Vaginal ring, cream, or tablet

Combination estrogen and progestin products are also available as either oral tablets or patches. Hormone replacement products are listed in Table 25-26. If a patient has an intact uterus, a combination product should be prescribed or a separate progestin (e.g., Micronor norethindrone 0.35 mg) should be added to an estrogen-only regimen to decrease the risk of endometrial cancer. Likewise, women who have had a hysterectomy but have suffered from endometriosis should also take a progestin.

Patient compliance should also be considered when choosing a product. The oral tablets are taken daily, while the patches are changed once or twice weekly and the vaginal ring is changed every 3 months. Currently, however, the transdermal systems and vaginal rings are significantly higher in cost than many of the oral formulations. Patients should generally start on the lowest dose of a product and then increase the dose only if symptoms are not relieved.

Recently, there has been an increased demand for "bio-identical" hormones. Many of these products are advertised as being "safe" alternatives to traditional HRT products. The bio-identical products are not FDA approved. They contain plant-derived hormones similar or identical to those produced in the ovary and body. The hormones found in bio-identical products are the same as the hormones found in FDA-approved formulations and, therefore, carry the same risks. Pharmacists should counsel patients receiving bio-identical hormone products in the same manner they would patients taking FDA-approved products.

For women with a contraindication to HRT, several prescription and over-the-counter products are available to help with symptoms of menopause. Table 25-27 lists several nonhormonal prescription medications (along with their doses and side effects) that may be used to treat vasomotor symptoms in those patients for whom HRT is contraindicated. These products can be used alone or together based on the severity of symptoms.

Table 25-27 Nonhormonal Prescription Medications

Medication	Dose	Common Side Effects
Clonidine	0.1 mg/day (weekly transdermal patch)	Dry mouth, drowsiness
Paroxetine	10–20 mg/day	Headache, nausea, sexual dysfunction
Venlafaxine	Extended release, 37.5–75 mg/day	Dry mouth, nausea, insomnia
Gabapentin	300 mg once daily; 300 mg three times daily	Fatigue, dizziness, rash, peripheral edema

Patients for whom the primary complaint is urogenital symptoms (e.g., vaginal dryness and pain with intercourse), some vaginal estrogen products are available that do not achieve significant systemic concentration. Nonprescription medications that may be effective in relieving vasomotor symptoms include the following options:

- Isoflavone supplements
- Soy products
- Black cohosh
- Vitamin E

There is little scientific evidence substantiating the effectiveness of herbal products as compared to placebo.

1.3.0 Monitoring

Monitoring and Drug Interactions

Estrogen is metabolized via the cytochrome P450 3A4 enzyme. Medications that induce release of this enzyme will cause a decrease in the circulating level of estrogen. It is difficult to predict whether the interaction will cause a clinical return of menopausal symptoms. A dose adjustment or product switch may be necessary if the patient's symptoms were previously controlled when the interacting medication is started. Medications that induce the cytochrome P450 3A4 enzyme include the following agents:

- Phenobarbital
- Carbamazepine
- Rifampin
- St. John's wort
- Phenytoin
- Topiramate

Patient Counseling

The patient care scenario at the beginning of this section highlights several important counseling points:

- Vasomotor symptoms (hot flashes and night sweats) occur in as many as 80% of women going through perimenopause.
- Vasomotor symptoms improve over time, but other symptoms of menopause, such as declines in cognition and decreasing bone density, worsen over time.
- Estrogen is the most effective treatment for symptoms of menopause.
- Side effects of progestin therapy include depression, headache, irritability, and weight gain. Patients who are already suffering from depression should be aware that therapy may need to be adjusted even if symptoms were previously under control.
- Bio-identical hormones are not FDA-approved but contain plant-derived hormones that are the same as those found in FDA-approved products. Patients should be counseled that these products are not regulated and carry the same risks as the FDA-approved products.

Toxicology

CHAPTER

26

TOPIC: TOXICOLOGY

Contributor: B. Shane Martin

1.1.0 Patient Information

General Approach to Medical Toxicology

When dealing with an apparent toxic situation, the following steps in treatment should be taken in order:

- Assess and manage the ABCs (airway, breathing, and circulation).
- Obtain vital signs and manage any symptomatic or life-threatening abnormalities.
- Treat convulsive seizures, cardiac dysrhythmias, or severe metabolic abnormalities, if present.
- Consider administration of dextrose, thiamine, and naloxone for unstable, unresponsive patients.
- Obtain a rapid history and perform a rapid physical examination.
- If a specific toxic syndrome can be identified, treat it.
- Obtain a thorough history and perform a thorough physical examination.
- Obtain pertinent lab tests.
- Consider gastric decontamination if indicated.
- Consider enhanced elimination if indicated.
- Consider administration of antidote if indicated.
- Continue with supportive care and monitoring as indicated.

Initial Evaluation of the Poisoned Patient

Vital signs (BP, HR, RR, and temperature), along with findings involving the ophthalmic, gastrointestinal, dermatological, genitourinary, and central nervous systems, provide essential information. Initial and continued monitoring provides guidance as to the cause of intoxication (based on a characteristic toxic syndrome), severity of illness, and need for and patient response to supportive care and/or antidotes.

Laboratory Testing

Lab tests are not always required in the poisoned patient. The following labs are most useful in medical toxicology: basic metabolic panel (BMP); liver function tests (LFTs); O_2 saturation; and qualitative urine toxicology screen for drugs of abuse (commonly includes amphetamines, barbiturates, benzodiazepines, cannabinoids, cocaine, opioids, and phencyclidine; the results of screening rarely alter management); quantitative toxicology assays for identifying and/or managing certain toxins (i.e., acetaminophen, alcohols, digoxin, iron, lithium, phenobarbital, salicylates, theophylline); and anion gap, osmolal gap, and oxygen saturation gap calculations.

Table 26-1 Common Toxic Syndromes

	BP	HR	RR	Temp	Mental Status	Pupil Size	Peristalsis	Diaphoresis	Other
Anticholinergics	0/↑	↑	↑↓	↑	Delirium	↑	↓	↓	Dry mucous membranes, flushing, urinary retention
Cholinergics	↑↓	↑↓	0/↑	0	Normal to depressed	↑↓	↑	↑	Salivation, lacrimation, urination, diarrhea, bronchorrhea, fasciculations, paralysis
EtOH or sedative-hypnotic intoxication	↓	↓	↓	0/↓	Depressed	↑↓	↓	0	Hyporeflexia
EtOH or sedative-hypnotic withdrawal	↑	↑	↑	↑	Agitated, disoriented	↑	↑	↑	Tremor, seizure
Opioid intoxication	↓	↓	↓	↓	Depressed	↓	↓	0	Hyporeflexia
Opioid withdrawal	↑	↑	0	0	Normal, anxious	↑	↑	↑	Vomiting, rhinorrhea, piloerection, diarrhea
Sympathomimetics	↑	↑	↑	↑	Agitated	↑	0/↑	↑	Tremor, seizure
Serotonin syndrome	↑	↑	↑	↑	Agitated, coma	↑	↑	↑	Increased muscle tone, hyperreflexia, clonus
Neuroleptic malignant syndrome (NMS)	↑	↑	↑	↑	Stupor, alert, mutism, coma	0	0/↓	↑	"Leap-pipe" rigidity, bradyreflexia

↑ = increase; ↓ = decrease; ↑↓ = variable; 0 = no change

Other Tests

ECG is commonly used to monitor for cardiac toxicity and response to therapy.

Terminology and Signs and Symptoms

Toxic syndromes overlap and are less specific when multiple substances are involved. See the descriptions of select acute medication poisonings later in this chapter.

Anion gap (mEq/L) = Na+ – [Cl^- + HCO_3^-]

- Normal range = 3–12 mEq/L
- Toxic ingestions associated with an elevated anion gap metabolic acidosis include, but are not limited to, the following: cyanide, ethylene glycol, iron, isoniazid, metformin, methanol, paraldehyde, phenformin, protease inhibitors, and salicylate.
- Concurrent ethanol use delays the development of elevated anion gap metabolic acidosis in ethylene glycol and methanol intoxication.

Osmolal gap (mOsm/L) = $\text{Osmolality}_{\text{measured}}$ – $\text{Osmolality}_{\text{calculated}}$

- Normal $\text{Osmolality}_{\text{measured}}$ = 285–295 mOsm/L.
- $\text{Osmolality}_{\text{calculated}}$ (mOsm/L) = 2Na+ + BUN /2.8 + glucose/1.8 + ethanol/4.6.
- Freezing-point depression osmometry is the preferred method of measurement. Vapor pressure osmometry does not detect volatile alcohols such as ethanol and methanol.
- Toxic ingestions associated with an elevated osmolal gap include, but are not limited to, the following: ethanol, ethylene glycol, isopropanol, methanol, and propylene glycol.

Oxygen saturation gap = O_2 $\text{saturation}_{\text{calculated (arterial blood gas)}}$ – O_2 $\text{saturation}_{\text{measured (co-oximetry)}}$

- An O_2 saturation gap exists when the difference is greater than 5%.
- This measurement is helpful in the identification and management of toxins (e.g., carbon monoxide, cyanide, hydrogen sulfide) and conditions associated with an elevated oxygen saturation gap.

1.2.0 Pharmacotherapy

Uses/Indications for Drug Products

Products for gastric decontamination, specific antidotes, and supportive care are frequently used in medical toxicology. Please see the tables later in this section for more information.

Mechanism of Action

Gastric decontaminants and specific antidotes work by several different mechanisms. Please see the tables later in this section for more information.

Interaction of Drugs with Foods and Laboratory Tests

Please see the tables later in this section for any pertinent details.

Table 26-2 Gastric Decontamination

	Use	Dosing	Contraindications	Miscellaneous
Activated charcoal	Preferred means of GI decontamination; should be considered following ingestion of a potentially toxic amount of a substance that can be adsorbed to activated charcoal.	Administer within 60 minutes of ingestion. Dose recommended: 1–2 g/kg is a rough guideline (10:1 charcoal to intoxicant ratio); should be mixed with water (30 g per 240 mL). Adult: 30–100 g Child: 15–30 g	Bowel obstruction or perforation; risk for GI bleeding or perforation. Decreased level of consciousness.	Do not use for substances with low affinity for binding to activated charcoal; may obscure visualization of gastroesophageal lesions by endoscopy.
Cathartics	Single dose used as an adjunct to activated charcoal to enhance rectal elimination of a poison-activated charcoal complex.	Sorbitol 1–2 g/kg	Unprotected airway; bowel obstruction or perforation. Volume depletion or electrolyte abnormalities.	Only administered with the first dose of a multidose charcoal regimen used to enhance elimination.
Gastric lavage	Situations involving a potentially toxic amount of a substance not readily adsorbed to activated charcoal (see the list in the "whole-bowel irrigation" entry).			
Ipecac syrup	*No role* in healthcare setting; *not* recommended for routine home use.	Give 240 mL (adult) or 120 mL (child) of water prior to administering. Administer within 30–90 minutes of ingestion. Adults and adolescents: 15–30 mL Child (1–12 years): 15 mL Child (6–12 months): 5–10 mL	Ingestion of following substances: those that may compromise airway reflexes (e.g., CNS depressants); corrosives; substances with high aspiration potential (e.g., hydrocarbons); seizure-inducing substances (e.g., Wellbutrin). Medical condition that could be compromised by emesis.	Should *only* be used when there is no contraindication; there is high risk for substantial toxicity from substance ingested; and there is no available alternative for GI decontamination; or there will be a delay of greater than 1 hour before the patient can be seen in an emergency facility. Can affect the administration of an oral antidote.
Whole-bowel irrigation	Consider for poisonings involving sustained-release and enteric-coated formulations; substances not adsorbed by activated charcoal [heavy metals (e.g., iron), inorganic ions (e.g., lithium), corrosives, hydrocarbons, alcohols (e.g., ethylene glycol)]; substances known to form bezoars (e.g., iron).	Polyethylene glycol solution may be administered via NG tube or by having the patient drink it; give until rectal effluent is clear. Adults and adolescents: 1,500–2,000 mL/hr Child (6–12 years): 1,000 mL/hr Child (9 months–6 years): 500 mL/hr	Unprotected airway; bowel obstruction, bowel perforation; ileus; uncontrolled GI bleed or emesis; hemodynamic instability.	Drug "packers" and "stuffers."

Table 26-3 Common Antidotes

	Use	Adult Dose	Contraindications	Miscellaneous
Atropine: antimuscarinic agent	Treatment of muscarinic effects of carbamoylate acetylcholinesterase and organophosphate poisoning.	1–5 mg IV, doubled every 3–5 minutes until bronchorrhea resolves.	Narrow-angle glaucoma, paralytic ileus, myasthenia gravis, Mobitz type II heart block.	
N-acetylcysteine: prevents NAPQI-induced hepatotoxicity by promoting acetaminophen metabolism through nontoxic pathways	Acute acetaminophen toxicity.	Oral: 140 mg/kg loading dose, followed by 70 mg/kg every 4 hours for 17 doses. IV: 140 mg/kg loading dose infused over 15 minutes, followed by 50 mg/kg infusion over 4 hours, followed by 100 mg/kg infusion over 16 hours.		Obtain an APAP plasma level no sooner than 4 hours post ingestion and plot the value on the Rumack-Matthew nomogram. If the value plots below the "possible hepatic toxicity" line, no treatment is needed. The Rumack-Matthew nomogram is valid after 4 hours and up to 24 hours after an acute ingestion.
Cyanide antidote kit (2 ampules sodium nitrite, 2 ampules sodium thiosulfate, 12 aspirols of amyl nitrite) Amyl nitrite and sodium nitrite cause methemoglobinemia as they oxidize iron in Hgb from ferrous ($Fe^{2}+$) to ferric ($Fe^{3}+$); $Fe^{3}+$ removes cyanide from cytochrome oxidase to form cyanomethemoglobin and restore cellular respiration; cyanomethemoglobin reacts with sodium thiosulfate to form thiocyanate; thiocyanate is renally eliminated and methemoglobin is left free to bind more cyanide	Significantly symptomatic cyanide toxicity associated with sodium nitroprusside.	Sodium nitrite: 300 mg (10 mL of 3% conc.) IV over 20 minutes. Sodium thiosulfate: 12.5 g (50 mL of 25% concentration) IV over several minutes. Amyl nitrite: break and inhale for 30 seconds every minute; new ampule every 3 minutes.		
Cyproheptadine Nonspecific serotonin receptor antagonist blocks the effects of increased intrasynaptic serotonin concentrations	Serotonin syndrome.	Initial dose: 12 mg, then 2 mg every 2 hours if patient is still symptomatic. Maintenance: 8 mg every 6 hours; up to 32 mg in 24 hours.	Narrow-angle glaucoma, bladder neck obstruction, GI tract obstruction.	Slight to moderate drowsiness.
Deferoxamine High affinity and specificity for ferric iron ($Fe^{3}+$); binds to free iron and iron transported between transferrin and ferritin	Chelating agent used for iron poisoning.	5–15 mg/kg/hr IV titrated as tolerated, with total dose of 6–8 g/day. Treat severe toxicity (major GI hemorrhage, metabolic acidosis, hypotension), mild to moderate toxicity (if serum iron > 350 mcg/dL).	Severe renal disease or anuria, primary hemochromatosis.	Dosing adjustments are required in patients with renal insufficiency. Urine discoloration (vin-rose color); can exacerbate aluminum-related encephalopathy.

Digoxin immune antibody-binding fragment or Fab Fab fragments rapidly bind to digoxin in the serum and extracellular fluid, causing redistribution of digoxin out of tissue and away from Na-K ATPase	Cardiac glycoside (digoxin, digitoxin) toxicity.	Empiric dosing is as follows: Acute ingestion: 10 vials Chronic toxicity: 5 vials If digoxin steady-state concentration is known (~ 4–6 hours post ingestion), can calculate the dose using this equation: Vials = (digoxin serum concentration [ng/mL]) × 5 L/kg ÷ patient weight (kg)÷ (1,000 × 0.5 mg/vial)		Indicated: Ventricular dysrhythmias; bradydysrhythmias unresponsive to atropine; serum digoxin 10–15 ng/mL in acute ingestion. Infuse over 30 minutes with 0.22-micron filter. Digoxin levels are greatly increased with Fab use; misleading until Fab is eliminated from body.
Dimercaprol Contains two sulfhydryl groups and forms a nontoxic chelate five-membered ring with heavy metals; metals are kept inert until excreted	Chelating agent use for acute arsenic, gold, lead, and mercury poisoning.	Dose is different for each type of poisoning. Range of 2.5–5 mg IM per dose, 1–4 doses per day, continued for 7–10 days or until recovery (see the package insert).	Hepatic insufficiency (unless due to arsenic poisoning); iron, cadmium, or selenium poisoning.	When used for lead poisoning, administer at a different site from $CaNa_2EDTA$.
Edetate calcium disodium ($CaNa_2EDTA$)	Used in combination with chelating agents; reduces blood concentrations and depot stores of lead.	Dosing depends on the lead level; range is 1,000–1,500 mg/m²/day to threshold level or clinical improvement endpoint (see the package insert).	Active renal disease or anuria; hepatitis.	Dosing adjustments are required in patients with renal insufficiency. Do not administer with a loading dose of dimercaprol; begin with the second dose.
Fomepizole Prevents metabolism of parent compound to toxic metabolite (methanol to formic acid; ethylene glycol to oxalic acid) by inhibition of alcohol dehydrogenase	Methanol and ethylene glycol poisoning.	15 mg/kg IV loading dose; 4 maintenance doses of 10 mg/kg. Peak (within 30–60 minutes) ethylene glycol concentration < 20 mg/dL is considered nontoxic; treat when ethylene glycol concentration > 20 mg/dL, or there is a metabolic acidosis, or history suggesting potentially toxic ingestion and ethylene glycol concentration is not rapidly available. Treat when peak (within 30–60 minutes) methanol concentration > 20 mg/dL or history suggesting ingesting toxic amounts of methanol and osmolal gap greater than 10 mOsm/L or strong clinical suspicion of methanol ingestion with two or more of the following: arterial pH < 7.3; serum bicarbonate < 20 mEq/L; osmolal gap > 10 mOsm/L.		Dosing adjustments are required in patients undergoing dialysis. Fomepizole levels ≥ 0.8 mg/dL provide for continuous inhibition of alcohol dehydrogenase.
Sodium bicarbonate	Salicylates—moderate poisoning; salicylate level (adult) 600–800 mg/L,	1 L D_5W + 3 ampules of sodium bicarbonate (150 mEq $NaHCO_3$) + 40 mEq KCl; administer at 2–3 mL/kg/hr to produce urine flow of 2–3 mL/kg/hr; maintain urine pH 7.5–8 and arterial pH 7.45–7.55.		

(*continues*)

Table 26-3 (*continued*)

	Use	Adult Dose	Contraindications	Miscellaneous
Sodium bicarbonate	Tricyclic antidepressant poisoning (for dysrhythmias).	If QRS > 0.1 second, administer 1–2 mEq/kg IV bolus as needed to achieve arterial pH of 7.45–7.55.		
Glucagon Binds to a specific cell membrane receptor that stimulates conversion of ATP to cAMP	Beta blocker poisoning; calcium-channel blocker poisoning; hypoglycemia.	5–10 mg IV bolus, followed by 1–10 mg/hr IV infusion.	Insulinoma, pheochromocytoma.	Bolus may be associated with nausea and vomiting.
Methylene blue	Reversal of drug-induced methemoglobinemia.	1–2 mg/kg IV over 5 minutes; repeat at 1 mg/kg IV after 30 minutes if needed.	Methemoglobinemia in cyanide poisoning.	
Naloxone Opioid receptor antagonist	Reversal of opioid-induced apnea.	0.2–0.4 mg IV; if no clinical response after 2–3 minutes, give 1–2 mg IV; titrate to effect, up to 10 mg total.		
Pralidoxime (2-PAM) AChE reactivator; cleaves OP-AChE complex, allowing AChE to metabolize Ach; reverses both the muscarinic and nicotinic effects of OP intoxication	Reversal of organophosphate (OP) toxicity; used adjunctively with atropine.	1–2 g IV over 15–30 minutes; repeat the initial dose within 1 hour if muscle fasciculations or weakness persists.	Poisonings due to phosphorus, inorganic phosphates, or organic phosphates without anticholinesterase activity; poisonings due to pesticides of the carbamate class.	Dosing adjustments are required in patients with renal insufficiency.
Pyridoxine Replenishes depleted pyridoxine and pyridoxal-5-phosphate stores to reverse the CNS excitatory (seizure) and inhibitory (coma) effects of isoniazid (INH)	Treatment of isoniazid-induced seizures and coma.	Amount of INH ingested: Unknown: 5 g or 70 mg/kg Known: 1 g of pyridoxine per g of INH Repeat every 20 minutes until desired effect is achieved.		Burning may occur at the injection site of an IM or SC dose; seizures have been reported following administration of large IV doses.
Flumazenil Competitive antagonist at the benzodiazepine binding site on the GABA-A receptor complex	Reversal of benzodiazepine toxicity.	0.2 mg IV initially; if no response, give 0.3–0.5 mg doses every minute, titrated to effect, up to 3 mg total.	Patients displaying signs of severe cyclic antidepressant overdosage; patients given benzodiazepines for control of potentially life-threatening conditions.	
Physostigmine Reversible AChEI	Reversal of antimuscarinic symptoms.	1–2 mg IV over 5 minutes, titrated to effect, up to 4 mg total.	GI or GU obstruction, asthma, gangrene, any vagotonic state, coadministration of choline esters and depolarizing neuromuscular-blocking agents.	Infuse slowly over 5 minutes; rapid administration can cause bradycardia and hypersalivation leading to respiratory distress and seizures.

Table 26-4 Common Antidotes: Brand Names and Dosage Forms

	Brand Names	Dosage Forms
Atropine	Various	Injection solution: 0.05 mg/mL, 0.1 mg/mL, 0.4 mg/mL, 1 mg/mL
N-acetylcysteine	Acetadote (injection), Mucomyst (oral/inhalation)	Inhalation solution: 4 mL and 10 mL vials (10% and 20%) Injection solution: 30 mL vial (200 mg/mL)
Cyanide antidote kit (2 ampules sodium nitrite, 2 ampules sodium thiosulfate, 12 aspirols of amyl nitrite)	Cyanide Antidote Kit	Sodium nitrite: 300 mg in 10 mL Sodium thiosulfate: 12.5 g in 50 mL Amyl nitrite inhalants: 0.3 mL
Cyproheptadine	Periactin	4 mg tablet 2 mg/5 mL syrup
Deferoxamine	Desferal	500 mg and 2 g vials for reconstitution
Digoxin immune antibody-binding fragment or Fab	Digibind, DigiFab	Injection solution: 4 mL vial (10 mg/mL)
Dimercaprol	BAL in Oil	Intramuscular oil: 3 mL ampules (100 mg/mL)
Edetate calcium disodium ($CaNa_2EDTA$)	Calcium Disodium Versenate	5 mL vial (200 mg/mL)
Flumazenil	Romazicon	5 and 10 mL vials (0.1 mg/mL)
Fomepizole	Antizol	1.5 mL vial (1 g/mL)
Glucagon	GlucaGen, Glucagon Emergency Kit	1 unit = 1 mg
Methylene blue	Urolene Blue	1, 5, and 10 mL vials (10 mg/mL)
Naloxone	Narcan	0.4 mg/mL, 1 mg/mL
Physostigmine	Antilirium	2 mL vial (1 mg/mL)
Pralidoxime (2-PAM)	Protopam	2 mL vial (300 mg/mL), 1 g vial for reconstitution
Pyridoxine	Various	1 mL vial (100 mg/mL)

Contraindications, Warnings, and Precautions

Gastric decontaminants and specific antidotes can do more harm than good when used incorrectly and when administered to an inappropriate patient.

Pharmaceutical Characteristics of Dosage Forms

Benefits may outweigh risks associated with contraindications in cases of severe intoxications.

2.1.0 Dispensing

Regional Poison Control Centers provide information and poison management advice over the phone to both the general public and other healthcare professionals. Poison centers are staffed by nurses and pharmacists who are trained to answer questions and provide advice regarding poisonings. Poison centers also provide consultation with board-certified medical toxicologists and education to the public (e.g., literature and presentations with school-aged children) regarding poison prevention. All poison centers can be reached at the following phone number: 1-800-222-1222.

ANNOTATED BIBLIOGRAPHY

Alapat PM, et al. Toxicology in the critical care unit. *Chest* 2008;133:1006–1013.

Betten DP, et al. Antidote use in the critically ill poisoned patient. *J Intensive Care Med* 2006;21(5): 255–277.

Frithsen IL, et al. Recognition and management of acute medication poisoning. *Am Fam Physician* 2010; 81(3):316–323.

Lacy CF, Armstrong LA, Goldman MP, Lance LL, eds. *Drug Information Handbook,* 18th ed. Hudson, OH: Lexi-Comp; 2009.

Micromedex [Internet database]. Greenwood Village, CO: Thomson Reuters (Healthcare); updated periodically.

Mokhlesi B, et al. Adult toxicology in critical care: Part I: general approach to the intoxicated patient. *Chest* 2003;123:577–592.

Mokhlesi B, et al. Adult toxicology in critical care: Part II: specific poisonings. *Chest* 2003;123: 897–922.

Poisindex System [Internet database]. Greenwood Village, CO: Thomson Reuters (Healthcare); updated periodically.

Wonsiewicz MJ, Edmonson KG, Boyle PJ, eds. *Goldfrank's Toxicologic Emergencies,* 8th ed. New York: McGraw-Hill; 2006.

NAPLEX Competency 3—Healthcare Information That Promotes Public Health

SECTION

4

Home Diagnostic Equipment, Supplies, and Medical Devices

CHAPTER

27

Contributor: Karen L. Kier

The sale of home diagnostic equipment has steadily increased over the years, to the point that sales in the United States now exceed $3 billion annually. Growth in this market is driven by several factors, including increased interest in health and self-care by consumers. These tests afford consumers an opportunity to be more active in their own health and to seek treatment earlier in the disease process. Home diagnostic kits provide either early diagnosis/identification (e.g., pregnancy) or a means of self-monitoring of a disease (e.g., diabetes mellitus). A recently released kit even enables consumers to collect DNA to be sent off for confidential results of paternity.

Factors that need to be taken into consideration with the various tests include the ease of use, the complexity of the kit, the cost, and the ability to have anonymity. Pharmacists can play an integral role in helping patients select the most appropriate tests and can provide patient counseling on the proper use and interpretation of the kits.

The ability to self-monitor is an essential component of patients taking responsibility for their diseases; it may also allow patients to self-control their therapy. Accurate and complete results when reported back to the healthcare professional can really allow patients, with their healthcare providers' guidance, to select the best therapies as well as to understand which therapies may not be working for them. The feedback from these tests can be invaluable in helping patients manage their diseases. Patients need to understand how to use the devices correctly and why the data are so important to the practitioner. A major limitation for some patients is the cost of the testing device and the continuous need for supplies. Pharmacists need to work with patients, providers, and insurers to find solutions to encourage self-monitoring.

Tips Worth Tweeting

- Pharmacists should check expiration dates on kits.
- Pharmacists should understand the directions (steps) for each test they recommend.
- Appropriate storage of the tests is critical.
- Timing for tests is an important factor in determining accuracy of results.
- Make sure patients know the timing of each step.
- Let consumers know they can contact a pharmacist or a toll-free number for help.
- Assist consumers in choosing products that are user friendly.

TOPIC: HOME BLOOD PRESSURE MONITORING

Studies continue to show the benefits of tightly managed blood pressure (BP) and the importance of getting patients to hit target goals. The overall risk of cardiovascular complications is reduced with each reduction in both systolic and diastolic pressure. Evidence-based medicine guidelines are recommending lower blood pressure targets. Recent studies have also shown the benefit of home blood pressure monitoring (HBPM). Many patients suffer from "white coat hypertension" (stress-induced increases in BP based on being in the healthcare setting), or their BP may not accurately be reflected when it is measured only once every 6 months to a year during office visits. Educating patients on the proper technique and the need for continuous monitoring is essential. Advantages of HBPM include the ability to detect patterns in BP over time to aid in patient treatment as well as to encourage compliance with lifestyle modifications or drug therapy. HBPM can be an essential component in pharmacist-directed medication therapy management (MTM). Problems can arise, however, when patients perform the tests incorrectly or they misinterpret the results. Patients may alter their prescribed regimens based on HBPM numbers rather than understanding the constant need for medication and lifestyle modifications.

There are two basic types of HBPM devices. The most traditional is the aneroid meter, which depends on the use of a stethoscope to detect Korotkoff sounds. These traditional meters and the use of stethoscope are the most accurate when used properly and are less expensive than their electronic alternatives. However, this method requires skill and training to be used properly. The second type is the electronic device, which requires cuff placement and turning on the device; thus very little skill and training are involved. These monitors can also be helpful in that many have some memory ability and can keep track of measurements prior to recording in a log. Some units have extra-large displays as well as printing options.

Tips Worth Tweeting

- Proper cuff size is important when selecting a BP monitor (especially with very large adults or very small adults).
- Avoid finger products because of issues with inaccuracy.
- Follow all of the manufacturer's directions.
- Consult the American Heart Association (AHA) website for recommended products.
- Patients should avoid exercising 15 minutes prior to testing BP.
- Patients should avoid caffeine and nicotine intake 30 minutes prior to testing BP.
- Patients should sit with their arm resting comfortably and relaxed when performing HBPM.
- Patients should not monitor BP while wearing tight-fitting shirts or clothes that restrict blood flow.
- The patient's arm should not be above the level of the heart when BP measurement is taken.
- Patients should have both feet firmly on the floor and be relaxed prior to taking BP measurement.
- Avoid nonprescription medications that can increase BP, such as pseudoephedrine or NSAIDs.
- Avoid herbal products that can increase BP (e.g. licorice).
- Additional BP readings should be taken at least 2 minutes apart.
- Patients should take both morning and evening readings.
- Wait 10 to 15 minutes after a bath or 30 minutes after eating before using HBPM.
- Empty the bladder prior to measuring BP.
- Equipment should be calibrated once per year.
- Patients with irregular heart rhythms may not be suitable candidates for HBPM.

TOPIC: FECAL OCCULT BLOOD TESTING

Fecal occult blood testing kits are devices used for screening purposes to help identify patients who may have an increased risk of lower intestinal bleeding. These products screen for occult blood in the stool, which may indicate blood in the feces that is not visually detectable but can be an early warning sign of a more serious gastrointestinal disorder. The kits are most commonly used to screen for colorectal cancer—the second most common form of cancer in the United States. Early detection has many benefits, including early management and potential cure of the cancer. Some other conditions can also cause blood to be found in the stool, including Crohn's disease, colitis, diverticulitis, hemorrhoids, and ulcers.

The kits for ambulatory, in-home use rely on chromogenic dyes to detect occult blood. The heme portion of hemoglobin acts as an oxidizing agent, catalyzing the oxidation of the test reagent. The chemically treated paper is floated in the toilet after a bowel movement. If blood has been released from the stool, then the test pad will turn a blue-green color. These kits include three separate tests to be conducted on three consecutive bowel movements to help prevent false-positive and false-negative results.

Tips Worth Tweeting

- Fecal occult blood tests require proper color vision (color blindness in the blue-green spectrum is a problem).

- Toilet bowel cleaners, disinfectants, and deodorizers can interfere with the test.
- Recent ingestion of rare beef can interfere with some tests.
- Recent ingestion of medications that can cause some GI irritation—such as aspirin, NSAIDs, iron, corticosteroids, and dipyridamole—may cause occult blood to be present.
- Vitamin C in large doses (more than 250 mg/day) can interfere with the test, resulting in a false-negative result.
- Rectally administered products such as suppositories or enemas may cause false-positive results.
- Test pads should be placed in the toilet within 5 minutes of the bowel movement.
- Some kits provide a quality control measure, so following directions is critical.
- Increasing dietary fiber may facilitate stool production for consecutive testing.
- Avoid alcohol for at least 2 days prior to testing due to alcohol's propensity to cause GI irritation.
- Hemorrhoid or menstrual bleeding may cause false-positive results.
- Urinate and flush prior to testing a bowel movement, as the presence of large amounts of urine can interfere with test.
- Avoid throwing toilet paper into toilet prior to testing due to its potential to interfere with the test.
- Hold the test pad by the corners; do not touch the middle of the pad prior to testing.
- Negative test results do not rule out the possibility of a GI disorder.

TOPIC: HOME HEPATITIS C SCREENING

Hepatitis C is estimated by the Centers for Disease Control and Prevention (CDC) to affect more than 4 million people within the United States. The highest incidence of hepatitis C is found in the age group of 20- to 39-year-olds. One of the problems with hepatitis C is that it often develops into a chronic form of viral hepatitis; this chronic condition puts patients at risk for developing chronic liver failure as well as hepatocellular carcinoma. Chronic hepatitis C is the most common reason for liver transplantation in the United States today.

Hepatitis C is diagnosed by direct detection of hepatitis C virus RNA in the serum. The RNA can be detected by two different types of testing. The less specific one is known as enzyme immunoassay (EIA), while the more specific test is done using recombinant immunoblot supplemental assay (RIBA). The home screening kits use both of these methods; they have been found to be 99% accurate. Accurate results depend on proper use of the kit and proper sample collection and handling.

Pharmacists can play an integral role in determining good candidates for screening. Keep in mind that the incubation period is approximately 2 months after exposure, but only one-third of exposed patients will actually develop the disease. Symptoms of the acute infection are fairly nonspecific and may include malaise, anorexia, and weakness. Jaundice develops in only 25% of patients, so it is not considered a good indicator of the presence of disease. Some patients may be positive for long periods (20–30 years) before developing acute signs of liver damage such as jaundice and liver enzyme elevations. Risk factors for developing hepatitis C include blood or blood product transfusions prior to 1992; drug abuse involving injectable drugs; healthcare workers with known history of blood, needlestick, or mucosal exposure; long-term hemodialysis; tattoos or body piercings from an unregulated setting; and sexual contact with a person known to be infected with hepatitis C.

Tips Worth Tweeting

- Results could be negative to antibody testing if the exposure occurred less than 6 months before the time of testing.
- Each test kit is assigned a personal identification number (PIN) used to register the patient via a toll-free telephone number.
- Wash the hands, and clean the side of the finger with an alcohol swab.
- Use a lancet to obtain a large drop of blood, and place it within circle on the card until it fills the circle completely and soaks to the back of the card.
- Blood is collected and must dry for 30 minutes prior to shipping the card in the return pouch and envelope.
- Results are available within 10 business days by calling the toll-free number and using the patient's PIN.
- The manufacturer provides counseling and physician referral information.

TOPIC: HOME HIV TESTING

The CDC has indicated that as many as 25% of people who are HIV infected may be unaware of their HIV status. Home testing is a means to screen for an early diagnosis prior to the development of full-blown AIDS. HIV infection is spread by sexual contact, sharing needles or syringes, or blood transfusions (prior to 1985). HIV-infected mothers can pass the infection to their children via the birth canal or through breastfeeding.

Home HIV testing can determine the presence of antibodies to HIV-1 but does not detect antibodies to HIV-2 or HIV-3. Antibody formation may take from 3 weeks to 6 months after exposure to develop to a degree that would result in a positive test.

Home testing kits require a blood specimen that is sent to a laboratory, where enzyme-linked immunoabsorbant assay (ELISA) testing is performed. All positive samples are retested twice via ELISA. If positive results still occur, the sample is then tested using immunofluorescent assay (IFA) for confirmation. The results can take 3–7 business days to become available. The manufacturer offers counseling and help lines to patients who have positive results. Overall accuracy rates are 99.99%.

Tips Worth Tweeting

- The Food and Drug Administration (FDA) has warned consumers about some Internet-based companies that sell unreliable kits.
- The kits known as Home Access and Home Access Express have been approved by the FDA for home HIV testing.
- An anonymous code number in each kit allows the patient to register with the company and to get results.
- Patients use a lancet to prick a finger to get two to four large droplets of blood, which are then placed on a card.
- Home Access results are available in 7 days, while Home Access Express provides results in 3 days.

TOPIC: HOME DRUG TESTING KITS

These kits are designed to test for illegal drug use, and are marketed to parents who want to test their children in cases of suspected abuse. The kits facilitate collection of samples, which are then sent to the kit manufacturer for analysis. Some kits require urine samples, whereas others use hair samples for testing.

Urine testing must be done within 2–3 days of drug exposure and is subject to false-positive results from dietary exposures such as poppy seed ingestion. The urine sample is tested by the company to determine whether alterations have occurred, such as adding household chemicals. One screen is the pH of the urine. The company also measures creatinine in the sample to determine whether attempts have been made to dilute the sample. The urine is initially screened using a standard enzyme multiplied immunoassay technique (EMIT). If a foreign substance is identified via EMIT, the sample is then run though gas chromatography–mass spectrometry (GC-MS) testing, which identifies the specific substances present. The urine testing is not quantitative; it shows only the presence or absence of the substance.

The hair testing kits identify drugs that get into the hair core and then remain in the hair as it grows. The drug residue remains in the hair and is very stable over time, so hair samples can detect drug use within the last 90 days. A 1½-inch sample starting at the scalp is sent in to obtain results. As with urine testing, the hair test procedure done by the company involves two separate tests. The first test is a RIA test that looks for the presence of the drugs, with all positive results being confirmed for specific substances using GC-MS.

These tests should be done in conjunction with the knowledge of the person involved. When positive results are confirmed, it is important to be prepared to provide counseling.

Tips Worth Tweeting

- Samples can be taken from hairbrushes, but this approach is usually not recommended because there is no guarantee that the sample is from the person and that it was taken during the right time frame.
- Some foods, such as poppy seeds, can interfere with test results.
- Some medications can produce false-positive results, including cough and cold products, codeine-containing medications, decongestants, ADHD medications, and antidiarrheal agents.
- Herbal medications may also interfere with drug testing results.
- Ideally, urine should be collected within a few hours of exposure to the drug, while hair is best collected 5–7 days after exposure.
- Store urine after collection as directed by the manufacturer; do not set the sample in hot or warm places prior to mailing it for testing.
- The kit contains temperature strips that ensure the sample is in the body temperature range (90°F to 100°F) and has not been altered.
- The kits come with codes that are required when calling for results.
- Urine results are available in 2–3 days, while hair results are available in approximately 5 days.
- Check the kits carefully to determine what they test for—not all kits test for the same drugs.
- Negative results do not guarantee a lack of abuse.
- Positive results may be false-positives or result from poor sample collections—be careful in drawing conclusions.

TOPIC: OVULATION DETECTION

Ovulation detection kits provide couples with a method for identifying the time of ovulation so as to improve their chances of contraception. The kits are meant to be an adjuvant for couples who are having trouble conceiving and are not for the sole purpose of ovulation prediction. They are based on monoclonal or polyclonal antibodies that are specific for luteinizing hormone (LH) in the urine. The LH level surges just prior to ovulation, with the egg usually being released 24–36 hours after the surge. These urine-based kits use a change in color to indicate the presence of LH. More intense color in the urine is associated with higher levels of LH.

Saliva kits are also available that look for hormonal changes as an indicator of ovulation. The saliva will actually form a fern-like pattern or crystal pattern when viewed under the microscope; this finding can be used to predict ovulation.

Tips Worth Tweeting

- These kits are not intended to be used for birth control.
- Medications such as anticonvulsants, anti-Parkinson agents, and antipsychotics can interfere with test results.
- Color defects in vision can affect the ability to accurately read the test.
- Not all women ovulate mid-cycle; thus some women may require more than the number of tests available in one kit (five to nine, depending on kit) to detect ovulation.
- Women may not ovulate with every cycle.
- Certain conditions can increase LH levels in the urine, such as endometriosis, ovarian cysts, menopause, recent pregnancy, and hyperthyroidism.
- Excess protein or blood in the urine may interfere with test results.
- Saliva-based tests should be used first thing in the morning before eating, drinking, smoking, or brushing teeth.
- Saliva samples obtained under the tongue may yield the most accurate results.
- Urine testing can usually be done any time during the day *but* must be consistently done at the same time every day in that cycle of testing (check the manufacturer's directions).
- With urine testing, once an LH surge has been detected by intense color change, stop testing and save kits for the next cycle.

TOPIC: HOME PREGNANCY TESTING

Home pregnancy testing is one of the longest-standing home-based diagnostic tests. Several generations of tests have been developed, with today's products being especially easy to use and more accurate than their predecessors. The early detection of pregnancy provides the opportunity for early prenatal care, which can reduce the risk of birth defects as well as allow the mother to provide optimal nutrition for growth and development.

Home pregnancy tests simply measure human chorionic gonadotropin (hCG) in the urine. This hormone is present immediately after fertilization, and its level peaks at 60–70 days after conception. Current tests use monoclonal antibodies to bind to hCG present in the urine of a pregnant female. This binding results in a color change in the testing device. If the patient is not pregnant, then there will be no color change on the testing device. Home pregnancy tests are reported to be 95–99% accurate when used correctly. Some tests can detect hCG within days of fertilization. Reading the package information is very important in selecting the right test. Most tests are simple to use and require only one to two steps.

Tips Worth Tweeting

- Most medications do not interfere with pregnancy testing.
- Drugs used during infertility treatment that contain LH or hCG will cause false-positive results.
- Ectopic pregnancy, abortions, and miscarriages may lead to positive results as well.
- Most products are best used on the first day of expected menstruation.
- Women who have an irregular menstrual schedule or those who are breastfeeding can perform the test 14 days after they believe fertilization may have occurred.
- Check the expiration date on the box.
- Avoid exposing the test to extreme cold or heat.
- Although most kits allow users to test anytime during the day, hCG is most concentrated in the first morning urine.
- Some kits are highly sensitive and provide very early results (4 days before a missed period).
- Collect urine as instructed on the package. Use of wax cups or cups washed in detergent may interfere with the test.
- Urine may be stored in the refrigerator until testing *but* must be brought to room temperature before using the kit.

- If a test produces negative results and menstruation has not started, perform a second test a few days later.
- Color-vision impairment may affect the ability to accurately read some tests. Those products that give a yes or no or a plus sign versus a negative sign as a result may be a good option in such cases.

TOPIC: HOME CHOLESTEROL TESTING

Cholesterol screening has become an important aspect of understanding cardiovascular risk in the general population. Both adult and pediatric guidelines for screening cholesterol have been established. The single-use kits for cholesterol testing can be useful for a general screen of cholesterol level. These kits have been reported to be 97% accurate when reporting total cholesterol values. The limitation of these systems is the inability to test total cholesterol in conjunction with levels of LDL, HDL, and triglycerides, which give the pharmacist a better picture of the overall lipid profile. Many pharmacists are doing cholesterol screening that can be more valuable in reflecting all parameters than the home testing kits. Consideration should be given to the value of using machines that measure more than one parameter at a time.

Tips Worth Tweeting

- Proper finger stick technique is essential with home cholesterol tests.
- Excessive squeezing of the finger can change the quality of the sample.
- Vitamin C (more than 500 mg/dose) should be avoided for at least 4 hours before performing the test.
- Acetaminophen (325–500 mg doses) may interfere with results if taken within 4 hours of the test.
- Use a lancet to prick the finger, wipe off the first sign of blood, and then fill the test cassette from the finger.
- Obtaining test results requires numerous steps and as long as 30 minutes to read.
- The patient needs to sit and relax for 10 minutes prior to testing.
- The patient can test the cholesterol level at any time during the day.

TOPIC: HOME URINARY TRACT INFECTION TESTS

Urinary tract infections (UTIs) are the result of bacteria infecting the urethra, the bladder, or even the kidney. Many patients who suffer from frequent UTIs are aware of the tell-tale signs of an infection. The home kits are really designed to just identify the presence of bacteria and are used for simple screenings. They do not replace the methods used in the practitioner's office. Thus the patient can perform the simple screen at home and then contact the practitioner for further diagnostic workup. Patients at highest risk for a UTI include individuals with a history of frequent UTIs, pregnant women, patients with diabetes, men older than 50 years of age, and patients with catheters.

The home kit tests do not always test for UTIs in the same fashion. Some kits test for bacterial reduction of urinary nitrate to nitrite associated with a UTI. Others test for a catalase activity that occurs within white blood cells (WBC) and bacteria. Normally, the urine does not contain WBCs or bacteria, so it should have no catalase activity. If a UTI exists, then catalase levels will rise and can be used for testing purposes.

Tips Worth Tweeting

- Some UTIs caused by enterococci and streptococci do not cause nitrate to nitrite reduction; thus some kits may not detect these organisms or the UTIs with which they are associated.
- Color vision is necessary for the kits that show the nitrate to nitrite reduction.
- Color changes need to be read within 2 minutes of exposure to urine.
- Urine can be stored in the refrigerator if not tested immediately, but must be brought back to room temperature before the test is performed.
- Some kits may contain ingredients that irritate the skin.
- To improve sensitivity of the test, it should be repeated on three consecutive morning samples.
- The first morning urine is the best sample for both types of tests.
- False-positive tests can occur with the nitrate to nitrite tests when the patient has taken drugs that dye the urine, such as phenazopyridine.
- Vitamin C (more than 250 mg/day) may block the test reaction, causing a false-negative result.
- Antibiotic usage may also cause a false-negative result.
- The catalase kit requires you to add four drops of activator to the tube of urine. White foam on top of blue liquid is a positive result.

TOPIC: DIABETES HOME TESTING

Diabetes mellitus is a disease state for which substantial evidence shows that tight glucose control can help patients achieve a better quality of life. Self-monitoring is a critical component of diabetes control. Pharmacists can take a leading role in educating patients about the importance of self-monitoring. Many times patients rely on their pharmacists when they have questions about their meters, their strips, or their medications because pharmacists are the most accessible healthcare professionals.

Home testing for diabetes involves blood glucose monitoring (most frequent), measurement of urine ketones (rarely done except with brittle diabetics or when blood sugars exceed 300 mg/dL), and the newest device for measuring hemoglobin A_{1c}. Self-monitoring and making appropriate changes in lifestyle and therapy are great ways for patients to participate in their care. Additionally, self-monitoring results provide valuable information that assist healthcare providers to adjust drug therapy.

The most critical issue is the initial selection of the meter. Many different meters are available, and they each have some advantages. Some are smaller, whereas others are larger (good choices for patients with arthritis). With some meters, smaller amounts of blood are necessary. Other units offer audio alerts for users with vision impairments. Some devices offer alternative site testing when patients develop an aversion to the constant finger sticking. This consideration also comes into play with the various lancet devices.

Tips Worth Tweeting

- Interview the patient and match a meter to his or her needs.
- Alternative site testing requires a different head for the lancet—one that creates a vacuum.
- Remember to test sugars on sick days and days with emotional stress.
- Monitor sugars with pregnancy when indicated or when exercising.
- Check the expiration dates on test strips.
- Keep logs of your measurements.
- Store meters and test strips at room temperature.

TOPIC: HEMOGLOBIN A_{1C} HOME TEST

Hemoglobin A_{1c} (or A_{1C}) tests measure the percentage of glycated hemoglobin levels in the blood, which is an indicator of blood sugar levels or control of glucose levels over about a 120-day span of time. Thus A_{1C} is a better reflection of long-term control of blood sugar levels in patients. Most evidence-based guidelines suggest A_{1C} levels should be between 6.5 and 7.0% for good control. Current recommendations also suggest that A_{1C} can be used as a screening tool for diabetes or prediabetes.

Tips Worth Tweeting

- The American Diabetes Association (ADA) recommends checking an A_{1C} level at least every 6 months.
- Use only finger stick blood, which is added to the tube first; it does not go directly into the meter.
- No dietary restrictions are necessary for use of such tests, and you can test anytime during the day.
- The result takes approximately 5 minutes to appear.

ANNOTATED BIBLIOGRAPHY

Home diagnostics/devices. In: *Nonprescription Drug Therapy™: Guiding Patient Self-Care,* 6th ed. St. Louis: Wolters Kluwer Health; 2007.

Home testing medical devices. In: *Handbook of Nonprescription Drugs: An Interactive Approach to Self-Care,* 16th ed. Washington, DC: American Pharmacists Association: 2011.

Drug Information, Research Design, and Statistics

CHAPTER

28

TOPIC: DRUG INFORMATION RESOURCES

Section Coordinator: Jean E.Cunningham
Contributor: Terri L. Levien

Introduction

Pharmacists are the drug experts. Regardless of the setting in which they practice, all pharmacists are called upon to provide drug information to patients or other healthcare professionals. Pharmacists are not expected to know everything about all drugs, but they should have a method they use to research and respond to requests for information.

Modified Systematic Approach

A popular approach to research and responding to drug information requests is the modified systematic approach. This method, originally developed by Watanabe, is now commonly taught in pharmacy schools and can be applied to any pharmacy setting. The steps included in a modified systematic approach are as follows:

1. Receive the request for information.
2. Determine and categorize the ultimate question.
3. Research the question.
4. Perform evaluation, analysis, and synthesis.
5. Formulate and provide the response.
6. Complete follow-up and documentation.

Receive the Request for Information

The first step is to receive the question or request for information, whether as a telephone call, fax, email, or a question posed at the pharmacy counter or in the hospital corridor. The pharmacist must secure requestor demographics, including the person's name and contact information, and determine the urgency and mode of delivery for the response. Often it is useful to obtain background information to determine what has prompted the question. If it is patient specific, patient information such as age, gender, renal function, current disease states and medications, and drug allergies should be obtained. Information about a patient's medical coverage may also be useful in making certain treatment recommendations. Finally, the pharmacist may want to ask which references have already been consulted, if any.

Determine and Categorize the Ultimate Question

The next step is to determine the real question being asked and to categorize the question by type. This becomes easier with practice and experience. It is important to determine the real question being asked to ensure that the pharmacist gathers appropriate information and formulates an appropriate response, and also to anticipate subsequent questions that may arise. By categorizing the question, the pharmacist can identify the best resource to use to research the question.

Consider the following example of the need to determine the real question. A nurse asks, "Can isotretinoin cause hair loss?" A simple reply, which would be technically correct, is "yes." However, it is important to get to the real question. Is the question patient specific? Is it suspected that the patient may be experiencing hair loss associated with his or her therapy? Is the nurse wondering if hair loss is likely being caused by the drug and whether it is reversible? Is the nurse wondering if there is a treatment? Or has the nurse heard that hair loss is a potential side effect and before starting therapy wants to know how common it is? At this point the question may be categorized as an adverse reaction question, which would help to narrow the list of references used to research the question.

The pharmacist may need to gather additional patient-specific information once the real question is identified. If the preceding case was patient specific, for example, it would be important to know how long the person had been on isotretinoin therapy and which other medications he or she taking.

Research the Question

Once the real question has been determined and categorized, the pharmacist can develop a strategy for researching the question. Appropriate references can be selected and searches conducted. The types of resources used will be influenced by the type of question and the intended audience for the response.

Tertiary Literature

Tertiary literature, such as textbooks, compendia, review articles, and drug information databases such as Clinical Pharmacy, Facts and Comparisons eAnswers, Lexi-Comp Online, and Micromedex, are often used first when researching a question. These resources are often sufficient for locating information used to respond to questions from patients and many healthcare providers. Secondary resources, which include references that index or abstract the primary literature, may be consulted if the answer cannot be located in a tertiary reference.

Pharmacists should be familiar with the tertiary references available in their work setting. A variety of references may be necessary depending on the types of questions received. Table 28-1 lists common tertiary references that may be used to research specific types of questions.

Drug information databases for handheld digital devices and smart phones are increasingly available and expand the availability of tertiary references. As the speed and memory of these devices improve, the content and capabilities of these databases are becoming ever more comprehensive. Table 28-2 lists several examples of widely used mobile databases.

Table 28-1 Examples of Tertiary Resources for Pharmacists

Question Type	Example Resources
Adult dosing and administration	AHFS Drug Information Clinical Pharmacology Facts and Comparisons eAnswers Micromedex DRUGDEX Lexi-Comp's *Drug Information Handbook*/Lexi-Drugs Online Package inserts
Adverse reactions	AHFS Drug Information Clinical Pharmacology Facts and Comparisons eAnswers Lexi-Comp's *Drug Information Handbook*/Lexi-Drugs Online Meyler's *Side Effects of Drugs* Micromedex DRUGDEX Package inserts
Bioequivalence	*Approved Drug Products with Therapeutic Equivalence Evaluations* (FDA's Orange Book)
Chemical data	*Merck Index* *Remington: The Science and Practice of Pharmacy*
Compatibility/ stability	AHFS Drug Information Clinical Pharmacology *Extended Stability for Parenteral Drugs* *Handbook on Injectable Drugs* *King Guide to Parenteral Admixtures* Micromedex DRUGDEX Trissel's *Stability of Compounded Formulations* *Remington: The Science and Practice of Pharmacy*
Compounding	Allen's *Compounded Formulations* *Extemporaneous Formulations* Micromedex DRUGDEX *Remington: The Science and Practice of Pharmacy* Trissel's *Stability of Compounded Formulations* USP Pharmacists' Pharmacopeia
Drug interactions	AHFS Drug Information Clinical Pharmacology Hansten and Horn's *Drug Interactions Analysis and Management* Drug Interaction Facts/Facts and Comparisons eAnswers Lexi-Comp Online/Lexi-Interact Micromedex DRUGDEX
Drug–laboratory interference	*Basic Skills in Interpreting Laboratory Data* *Laboratory Test Handbook* Lexi Lab Tests and Diagnostic Procedures

Table 28-1 (*continued*)

Question Type	Example Resources
Drug pricing	*Redbook: Pharmacy's Fundamental Reference*
Drugs in pregnancy and lactation	*Drugs in Pregnancy and Lactation: A Reference Guide to Fetal and Neonatal Risk* Micromedex REPRORISK National Library of Medicine LactMed *Neonatal Risk*
FDA-approved indications	AHFS Drug Information Clinical Pharmacology Facts and Comparisons eAnswers Micromedex DRUGDEX Package inserts
Foreign drug identification	European Drug Index Index Nominum Lexi-Drugs International Online *Martindale: The Complete Drug Reference* Micromedex DRUGDEX
Geriatric drug dosing	Lexi-Comp's *Geriatric Dosing Handbook*/ Geriatric Lexi-Drugs Online *The Merck Manual of Geriatrics* Package inserts
Hepatic drug dosing	AHFS Drug Information Lexi-Drugs Online Micromedex DRUGDEX
Manufacturer information	Clinical Pharmacology Facts and Comparisons eAnswers *Physician's Desk Reference* *Redbook: Pharmacy's Fundamental Reference* Package inserts
Natural products/ dietary supplements	Lexi-Natural Products Micromedex AltMedDex Natural Medicines Comprehensive Database *Natural Standard* *PDR for Herbal Medicine* *The Review of Natural Products*
Off-label uses	AHFS Drug Information Micromedex DRUGDEX Off-Label Drug Facts/Facts and Comparisons eAnswers
Over-the-counter medications	Facts and Comparisons eAnswers *Handbook of Nonprescription Drugs: An Interactive Approach to Self-Care*
Patient counseling	Clinical Pharmacology MedCounselor Facts and Comparisons eAnswers Lexi-Comp Online Patient Education Micromedex Drug Information for the Consumer

Table 28-1 (*continued*)

Question Type	Example Resources
Pediatric dosage recommendations	AHFS Drug Information *Harriet Lane Handbook* Lexi-Comp's *Pediatric Dosing Handbook*/ Pediatric Lexi-Drugs Online Micromedex DRUGDEX *Pediatric Injectable Drugs (The Teddy Bear Book)* Neofax
Pharmacokinetics	Applied Pharmacokinetics and Pharmacodynamics Basic Clinical Pharmacokinetics Clinical Pharmacokinetics
Pharmacology	Goodman and Gilman's *The Pharmacological Basis of Therapeutics* *Basic and Clinical Pharmacology*
Renal drug dosing	AHFS Drug Information Drug Prescribing in Renal Failure Micromedex DRUGDEX
Tablet/capsule identification	Micromedex IDENTIDEX Ident-A-Drug Facts and Comparisons eAnswers Lexi-Comp Online Lexi-DrugID Clinical Pharmacology Drug Identifier
Therapeutics/ drugs of choice	*Applied Therapeutics: The Clinical Use of Drugs* Cecil's *Textbook of Medicine* Conn's *Current Therapy* Harrison's *Principles of Internal Medicine* *Pharmacotherapy: A Pathophysiologic Approach* *Sanford Guide to Antimicrobial Therapy* *Textbook of Therapeutics: Drug and Disease Management* *The Medical Letter* Up-to-Date
Toxicology/ poisonings	Lexi-Comp's *Poisoning and Toxicology Handbook*/Lexi-Tox Online Micromedex POISINDEX National Library of Medicine TOXNET *Poisoning and Drug Overdose*
Veterinary pharmacy	CVP Compendium of Veterinary Products Plumb's *Veterinary Drug Handbook* *The Merck Veterinary Manual* Veterinary Pharmacy

Table 28-2 Examples of Mobile Database Drug References

Clinical Pharmacology Onhand
DrDrugs
Epocrates Rx
iFacts
Lexi-Drugs/Lexi-COMPLETE
mobileMicromedex
Mosby Drugs
PEPID Portable Drug Companion
Tarascon Pocket Pharmacopoeia

Internet Resources

Increasingly, Internet resources are being used by both patients and pharmacists to gather information about drugs and diseases. Pharmacists must be able to assess a website to determine whether the information is reliable before making recommendations using that information. They must also be able to assess sites that patients have used as a source of their information and to recommend sites appropriate for patient use. In evaluating a website, pharmacists should ask themselves several questions:

- Is the organization or individual responsible for the content of the site identifiable, and is contact information provided?
- Are funding sources reported and advertising clearly identified?
- Is the individual author of the information identified, and are the author's credentials appropriate for the type of information?
- Is the information accurate, current, and unbiased?
- Is the information appropriately detailed and referenced?

Table 28-3 Reliable Online Resources for Consumers

Centers for Disease Control and Prevention: www.cdc.gov
ClinicalTrials.gov: www.clinicaltrials.gov
Consumer Reports Health: www.consumerreports.org/health/
Drugs.com Drug Information Online: www.drugs.com
Mayo Clinic: www.mayoclinic.com
MedlinePlus: www.medlineplus.gov
The Merck Manual Home Health Handbook Online Edition: www.merckhomeedition.com
National Cancer Institute: www.cancer.gov
U.S. Food and Drug Administration: www.fda.gov/ForConsumers
WebMD: www.webmd.com

Some examples of websites that provide reliable patient information are list in Table 28-3.

Secondary Resources

Secondary resources are used to identify primary literature. Most secondary resources are accessed electronically, although some are still available in print. Examples of secondary resources include PubMed, International Pharmaceutical Abstracts, EMBASE, and Web of Science. Table 28-4 lists several databases commonly used to identify primary literature, along with their scope of coverage.

Most secondary resources are searched using queries constructed with Boolean operators such as AND, OR, or NOT (Figure 28-1). The operator AND will combine two terms, providing responses that only contain both terms. The operator OR will include all citations where either term is used. The operator NOT will eliminate responses that include the term.

As an example, suppose a pharmacist wanted to find articles that discuss the use of fluoxetine in the

Table 28-4 Examples of Secondary Resources

Database	Scope
BIOSIS	Basic sciences information from multiple sources, including journal articles, conference proceedings, patents, and books
CINAHL	Nursing and allied health literature from more than 2,900 journals
Cochrane Library	More than 4,000 systematic reviews on the effectiveness of healthcare treatments and interventions
EMBASE	Articles in the biomedical field from more than 7,000 peer-reviewed journals
International Pharmaceutical Abstracts (IPA)	Articles on a broad range of pharmacy-related topics from more than 750 pharmaceutical, medical, and health-related journals, plus abstracts of presentations at American Society of Health System Pharmacists meetings
Google Scholar	Multidisciplinary scholarly literature including articles, theses, books, abstracts, and court opinions
Iowa Drug Information Service (IDIS/Web)	Articles about drugs and drug therapy from more than 200 medical and pharmaceutical journals
LexisNexus	Medical, legal, and business news
PubMed/Medline	Articles from 5,400 biomedical journals
Web of Science	Articles from more than 10,000 journals in the sciences, social sciences, and arts and humanities, plus proceedings from more than 120,000 conferences

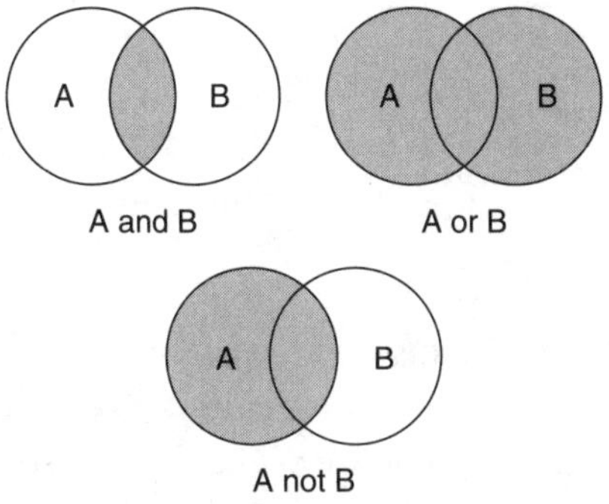

Figure 28-1 Boolean Operators

treatment of anorexia. A PubMed search using the query "fluoxetine AND anorexia" yielded 133 citations. A search using the query "fluoxetine OR anorexia" would not be useful in this situation, as it would not identify articles on the specific topic, but would identify any article that mentioned either search term. If information on either fluoxetine or olanzapine in the treatment of anorexia was desired, the OR term would be useful: "(fluoxetine OR olanzapine) AND anorexia." If the searcher found that many of the results included patients with bulimia and not just anorexia, the search could be further limited with the use of NOT: "(fluoxetine OR olanzapine) AND anorexia NOT bulimia." This query would exclude articles that included mention of bulimia; however, articles that discussed only anorexia would be included. Searches can also be limited by language, study or publication type, subject age or gender, and the year of publication.

Primary Literature

The primary literature, which is often identified in secondary resources, consists of clinical studies such as randomized controlled trials, cohort studies, and even case reports. It includes studies published in journals and unpublished studies. Primary literature is generally the most current information available. The pharmacist must personally assess the applicability and validity of the information.

Perform Evaluation, Analysis, and Synthesis

Information located by searching primary, secondary, or tertiary literature must be assessed to determine its credibility and relevance to the situation. One must consider whether the information located provides an answer to the real question being asked. For a patient-specific question, patient-specific information will help to determine which information gathered is relevant to the situation and must be considered when formulating the response. One must also consider whether the information is current. Finally, one must synthesize all the relevant information.

Formulate and Provide the Response

Considering all the information gathered, evaluated, and synthesized, the next step is to formulate a response. This can be written or verbal, but must be targeted at the appropriate level for the requestor. The target audience will determine the depth of information provided. The responder must clearly distinguish the information identified in the search from the information that consists of personal opinion or interpretation of the information. A verbal response should be clear and concise, and provided using an appropriate tone, confidence, tact, and professionalism. If the message is delivered in person, eye contact and body language appropriate for the target audience are important. If the response is given on the telephone, proper phone manners are critical, including clearly identifying oneself when calling back with the information. Written communication should also be clear and concise, using appropriate terminology for the requester, as well as correct grammar and spelling, and professional style and tone. Regardless of the method of delivery, the response should be timely, current, accurate, complete, concise, well referenced, objective, balanced, and applicable, and should address the real question that was being asked.

Complete Follow-up and Documentation

Depending on the nature of the question and the requestor, the final step may include conducting a follow-up and documenting the question and response.

Summary

Using a modified systematic approach to the drug information question and knowledge of the available resources, pharmacists should be able respond to most questions posed to them.

TOPIC: RESEARCH DESIGN METHODOLOGY

Section Coordinator: Jean E. Cunningham
Contributor: Jean E. Cunningham

Objective

Evaluate the suitability, accuracy, and reliability of information from reference sources by explaining and evaluating the adequacy of experimental design.

Background

In the ideal world, research starts with an idea that develops into a research question, which is then formulated into a research hypothesis. Once the

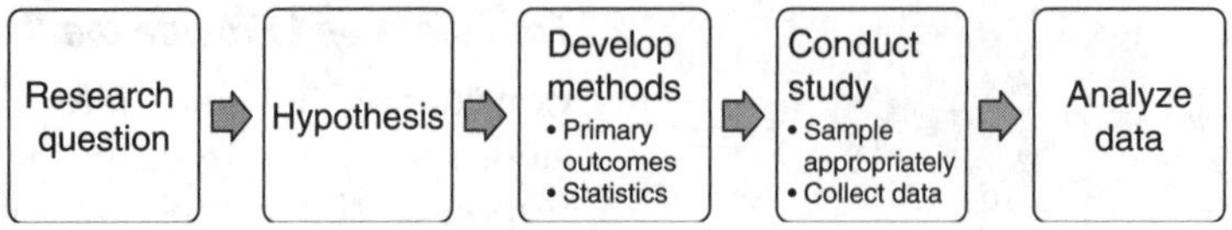

Figure 28-2 General Flow of Research Design

hypothesis is identified, investigators outline the study details, describing these as study methods. The methods should explain in detail which outcomes and objectives will be measured (outcomes should help answer the research question) and which statistical tests will best assess the type of data generated from the outcomes. The investigators then conduct the study as outlined in the methods, gather and analyze the data, and compare findings to the hypothesis. The results should provide some insight into the original research question. In some cases, then a final step is to present or even prepare and write findings in a manuscript that will be submitted for publication.

Practitioners must have some general knowledge about the basics of study design to understand clinical research. Knowing which type of study design should and can be used to address certain types of research questions will help practitioners determine whether a study was designed and performed appropriately. Practitioners who have the ability to evaluate this information will be able to decide on their own if a study was well designed and if the proposed response to the research question is accurate, objective, and valid.

Types of Clinical Research

Clinical research is commonly divided into two types: observational or experimental. Observational research is best defined as research that does not involve an intervention by the investigator. In other words, researchers merely observe a population/sample. In contrast, in experimental research, the investigator intervenes during the study or actually does something (e.g., gives a drug, performs a procedure, provides instruction) to the patient population.

For example, if investigators wanted to study the effects of drinking beer on bone loss, they could do so in one of two ways: observationally or experimentally. In a study with an observational design, an investigator might survey the population and determine whether there is any correlation between beer drinking and the presence or absence of bone loss. In an experimental design, the investigator would have to intervene. For example, the investigator might randomly sample and separate the population into either a control group (who receive a placebo) or an active group (who drink beer), and then compare bone loss between the two groups.

Observational Design

In observational studies, investigators observe and analyze naturally occurring events. The most commonly used types of observational studies in the medical literature are cohort, case-control, and cross-sectional studies.

Cohort Study

The cohort study is designed to determine an association between exposure to various factors and the development of a certain disease or outcome while following a group (or cohort) of patients over time. To determine whether certain factors are associated with developing a disease, the investigator must be able to separate the population into those who are exposed to the risk factor and those who are not exposed to the same risk factor. The investigator follows those patients prospectively and monitors for any signs or symptoms that a patient is developing the disease of interest.

As depicted in Table 28-5, determining who was or was not exposed to the risk factor can affect the results. Thus these patients should be clearly identified in terms of recruitment and all susceptibility to the disease of interest should be as equal as possible so as to focus only on the effect of the exposure of interest. When evaluating the design and methods of cohort studies, the reader should first attempt to ensure that the research question is clearly stated as well as verify that all attempts at measuring the development of the disease state of interest (outcome) are thoroughly performed. A clearly defined research question, similar patients enrolled in the exposure groups, and consistently measured outcomes lead to a better cohort study design.

Outcomes of interest or results from cohort studies are commonly reported as relative risk. Reporting relative risk is appropriate for this study design because it is consistent with the purpose of the study design, which is to demonstrate the likelihood that someone

Table 28-5 Cohort Study Design

Was the patient exposed?	**Present time** (When the investigator begins to test the hypothesis)	Will the patient develop the disease?
+ (yes)		+ (yes)
– (no)		– (no)
Past	**Current**	**Future**

Table 28-6 Cohort Study Design Evaluation Checklist

Clearly defined research question
Similar patients enrolled in different exposure groups
Outcome of interest (disease development) consistently measured and reported
Results reported as relative risk

who has been exposed to a risk factor will develop the outcome as compared to someone who has not been exposed to that risk factor.

Case-Control Study

The case-control study is designed to examine the possible relationship of an exposure or risk factor to a certain disease. Another term for the case-case control study is the trohoc study, as it is very similar to a cohort study, but performed in reverse—that is, the trohoc study starts with the outcome and looks back at the exposure (recall that cohort studies start with the exposure and follow it until the outcome occurs). To determine whether a certain disease is associated with exposure to possible variables, the investigator must be able to separate the population into those who have the outcome of interest versus those who do not have the outcome of interest. The investigator then reviews the patient's history and determine whether the patient was previously exposed to the risk factors of interest.

In examining the case-control study design, one can see that patients who have the disease of interest (cases) are compared to those without the disease of interest (controls). Once cases and controls are identified, investigators will obtain detailed background information about the patient exposure history to compare patients and produce a ratio. This ratio is not a representation of incidence rates, but instead represents the odds of exposure among those with the disease compared to the odds of exposure among those without the disease. This so-called odds ratio is an estimate of relative risk.

When evaluating case-control studies, practitioners should be wary of several limitations that can bias results. Cases should be selected from the same population or a similar population to the controls, as association of disease and risk factors may be affected by unmatched cases and controls. In addition, patients with the disease should be as similar as possible to best represent and limit disease variations that might influence the results. One last area to consider when evaluating case-control studies is the potential for recall bias, as patients with the disease may be more aware of previous exposure compared to those without the disease. This source of bias is best minimized by using data or means of measuring exposure that are as objective as possible.

Table 28-7 Case-Control Study Design

Did the patient have exposure to certain risk factors in the past?	Does the patient currently have the disease of interest?	**Present time** (When the investigator begins to test the hypothesis)
+ (yes)	+ (yes = cases)	
– (no)	– (no = controls)	
Past	**Current**	

Table 28-8 Case-Control Study Design Checklist

Cases and controls as similar as possible
Cases are at the same or similar point in disease progression
Exposure measured objectively
Results reported in odds ratios

Table 28-9 Cross-sectional Study Design Checklist

Clearly defined research question
Sample population is as homogenous as possible
Outliers or potential for inaccurate results are discussed
Timing of survey does not affect results (transient effects)

Cross-sectional Study

The cross-sectional study differs from case-control and cohort studies in that it assesses risk factors and disease development simultaneously. Cross-sectional studies are commonly used to identify the prevalence or characteristics of diseases in populations at one point in time. Because the focus of a cross-sectional study is on the prevalence of a disease, it should not be used to establish causality. When evaluating cross-sectional studies, many of the properties discussed earlier must be considered; however, a few differences do exist.

First, because results are measured at one point in time, it is difficult for investigators to quickly recognize the effects of outliers, inaccurate results, or unidentified sources of bias. In addition, because cross-sectional studies are not longitudinal, populations can provide certain responses based on the time and condition in which they are observed. This is known as a form of transient effects and is best realized and discussed retrospectively.

Experimental Design

Randomized Controlled Trial

Randomized controlled trials (RCTs) are the best way to establish a cause-and-effect relationship between a factor and an outcome of interest. The RCT is considered the gold standard for medical evidence and is a useful tool for addressing many of the limitations associated with observational study design. The basics of RCT study design require investigators to randomly select patients from the general population and assign them to either a treatment or a control/placebo group. Randomization of patients into a clinical trial is important, as it helps to evenly distribute patients between both groups and creates what is hoped to be well-matched study groups based on a variety of baseline characteristics. Several different randomization methods are currently used, but the ultimate goal of an accurate randomization method is to provide groups that are closely matched. Of note, in small sample sizes, full randomization may lead to unequal distribution of patients; thus block randomization may provide some assurance that large imbalances between groups will not exist.

Another important aspect of RCT study design is the elimination of a variety of biases through blinding. In a single-blind study design, patients do not know which type of treatment (active or placebo) is received; in a double-blind study design, neither patients nor investigators know which patients are receiving which therapy.

In addition to assessing whether randomization and blinding are appropriate, practitioners must determine whether the type of patient being recruited is a true representation of the target population. This can be done by closely reviewing the stated inclusion and exclusion criteria. Certain treatments may also be affected by a patient's past medication use, so a wash-out or run-in period may be appropriate depending on the disease state of interest.

After reviewing the initial design and methods of the study, practitioners should focus on the feasibility of the primary and secondary outcomes. It is important to determine whether the outcomes are truly related to the initial research question and hypothesis. The primary outcome should provide results that will prove or disprove the research hypothesis. It is also important to determine how the investigators are measuring the primary outcome (type of data) and whether the appropriate statistical test is being used to measure that data. (This issue will be discussed in more depth later in this chapter.) With regard to the outcomes, clinical endpoints will always be more helpful in providing insights into meaningful cause-and-effect relationships, whereas surrogate measures of clinical endpoints will provide a level of association.

When investigators perform any type of research, some data will not be available at the end of the study. Whether the absence is due to patient dropout, lack of information, or loss to follow-up, the lack of these data can affect the results. One way to limit the impact of missing data is to analyze data using the intent-to-treat (ITT) principle. This analysis requires that data for all patients randomized at the beginning of the study must be reported and accounted for at the end of the trial. Other approaches include analyzing only those patients who follow the study protocol (per-protocol) or even just the as-treated patients. Because the ITT principle maintains the initial randomization of the trial, it is the preferred method.

Table 28-10 Randomized Clinical Trial Study Design Checklist

Type of randomization and blinding are appropriate
Patient population is described in detail and represents the target population
Study design is appropriate, including any necessary wash-out/run-in periods
Primary outcome is representative of the research hypothesis
Clinical endpoints are used over surrogate measures
Type of data analysis used (ITT preferred)
Results can be extrapolated to target population

Finally, when reviewing the results of a RCT, one question a practitioner should ask is whether the results can be extrapolated to similar populations. This question should be carefully considered when evaluating the study as a whole. In addition, it is important to consider whether the appropriate statistical tests were used, and to ask whether statistically significant results are also clinically significant. As practitioners develop their fields of expertise, it becomes easier to apply clinical experience to trial results and to formulate an opinion as to whether the RCT results should be extrapolated to practice.

Objective

Apply and evaluate statistical tests and parameters.

Applied Statistics

The type of statistical test selected completely depends on the type of data generated from the study. To understand whether the test is appropriate, practitioners must first be able to categorize and identify the different types of data. Data are first separated into discrete or continuous categories. Discrete data comprise numerical data with a limited set of values (data that cannot be fractionated), whereas continuous data have an infinite number of evenly spaced potential values between two points (data that can have any value within a defined range).

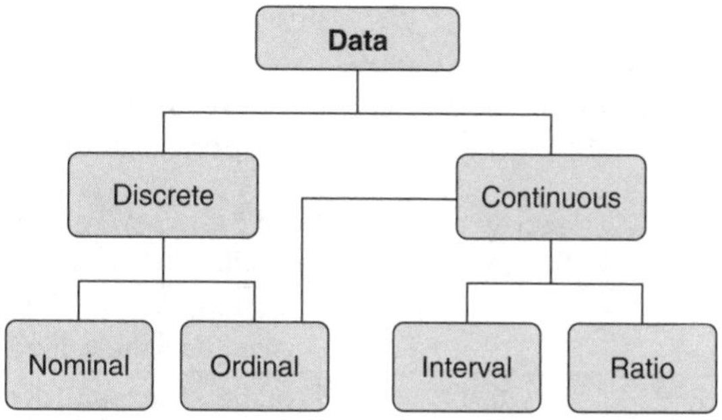

Figure 28-3 Types of Data and Levels of Measurement

Further differentiating types of data requires practitioners to be aware of the different scales of measurement: nominal, ordinal, interval, or ratio data. Nominal data consist of non-numerical data that fit into a category with a finite number of possible values and no implied rank or order. Ordinal data are ranked in order but lack a consistent magnitude of difference between ranks. Interval and ratio data are very similar but with one distinct difference: interval data have an equal distance or interval between values, whereas ratio data also have equal distance or interval between values but with an absolute zero.

Descriptive Statistics

Statistical tests are usually referred to as descriptive or inferential. Descriptive statistics are commonly used to present, organize, and summarize data and serve as a means of basic analysis (i.e., median, mode, standard deviation). Inferential statistics allow for the results from a sample to be generalized to the larger population. Ultimately, inferential statistics make assumptions and consider chance and are commonly used to determine a difference, association, or relationship between variables.

Descriptive statistics are commonly referred to as measures of central tendency, which is represented by the following:

- Mean (average)
- Median (50th percentile)
- Mode (most common value)

Table 28-11 Scales of Measurements and Examples

Scale of Measurement	Example
Nominal	Yes/no, male/female, race, education, blood type, marital status
Ordinal	Severity of disease, pain scales, opinion scores
Interval	Fahrenheit, Celsius
Ratio	Blood glucose, weight, age

Data can also be summarized by measuring the spread of values—for example, through the range, percentiles, and standard deviation (SD). Standard error of the mean (SEM) represents sampling variability.

SD reflects scatter or variation of a series of observational values from the mean and can show how much variation there is from the "average" (mean). *If observational values are "normally" distributed,* then 68.3% of *observational values* are within one SD of the mean, 95.4% are within two SDs of the mean, and 99.7% are within three SDs of the mean.

SEM estimates the true mean of the population from the mean of the sample. It also indicates that separate samples from a population can provide different parameter estimates. The SEM calculation as follows:

$$\text{SEM} = \text{SD}/(\sqrt{\text{N}})$$

If observational values are "normally" distributed, then 68.3% of *observational means* are within one SEM of the mean, 95.4% are within two SEMs of the mean, and 99.7% are within three SEMs of the mean.

Inferential Statistics

Inferential statistics require practitioners to be able to differentiate between a dependent variable and an independent variable. A dependent variable is usually the outcome of interest in a research study (treatment/effect). The independent variable defines the conditions under which the dependent variable is to be examined (cause). It can also be thought of as the variable that influences corresponding measurements of the dependent variable.

Two important areas of inferential statistics are estimation and hypothesis testing. Estimation provides

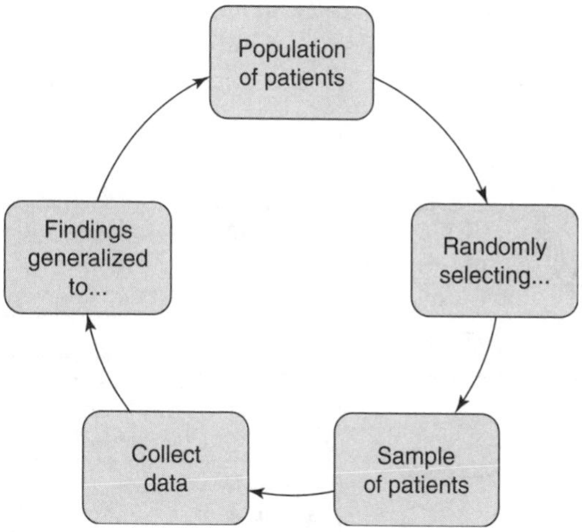

Figure 28-4 Application of Inferential Statistics

estimates of parameters of interest and accounts for uncertainty; uncertainty is commonly represented by reporting confidence intervals. Hypothesis testing recognizes and accounts for the fact that outcomes may occur by chance. Investigators demonstrate hypothesis testing by reporting *p*-values.

Estimation

A 95% confidence interval (CI) is a statistical term that represents the "best guess" or possible values for the true difference between interventions that are supported by the data. Another way to visualize the CI is to note if the same study was performed 100 times, then 95 out of the 100 trials would have a CI that would contain the true mean difference.

Example: A Hypothetical Study of Antihypertensive Drugs

If one drug lowered systolic blood pressure by an average of 5 mm Hg and another drug lowered it by an average of 3 mm Hg, this difference might be reported as a difference of 2 mm Hg with a 95% confidence interval: 95% CI = 0–5.

The results of this trial can be interpreted as a mean difference in antihypertensive drug effect of 2 mm Hg, and a CI showing that the true difference between these drugs could be as small as 0 mm Hg (no difference) or as large as 5 mm Hg.

One benefit of reporting CIs is that the range alone can show whether the results are significant without the need to report *p*-values. A 95% CI is the general standard to determine statistical significance; however, it is possible to have higher CI levels (e.g., 99%). The numbers encompassed by the CI are all possible values for the real difference between groups; a CI that includes a value consistent with no difference cannot represent a statistically significant finding (correlates with a *p*-value > 0.05). To determine if the difference in two means is statistically significant, the CI between the means cannot cross "0". As an example, take a look at the following table, which represents the CI reported as means:

Example Study	Incidence of Adverse Outcome	Absolute Difference (95% CI)	Is It Statistically Significant?
Drug A	27.6%	–	–
Drug B	24.9%	–2.7% (–7.6% to +2.2%)	No, because the CI contains the value "0"
Drug C	20.3%	–7.3% (–12.2% to –2.5%)	Yes, because the CI does not cross the value "0"

To determine if the difference in two treatments, expressed as a ratio, is statistically significant, the CI cannot include or cross "1". As an example, the following table represents the CI reported as ratios:

Study	Hazard Ratio (95% CI)	Is It Statistically Significant?
Study X	0.81 (0.73 to 0.90)	Yes, because the CI does not contain the value "1"
Study Y	1.395 (0.9097 to 2.1398)	No, because the CI does contain the value "1"

Hypotheses

The hypothesis is the researcher's assumption regarding probable study results; it must contain both a null hypothesis and an alternative hypothesis. The alternative hypothesis (H_A) represents expectations in terms of study results. The null hypothesis (H_0) is the "no difference" hypothesis and assumes equality amongst study groups. The null hypothesis serves as the basis for all statistical tests and must be rejected to support the researcher's assumptions.

Type I and Type II Error

Alpha (α) error (Type I) can be thought of as the error that results if a true null hypothesis is rejected. Other ways to remember Type I error are:

- Investigators conclude that there is a difference when no difference actually exists.
- Investigators state a difference was measured even though there really is no difference.
- Investigators state that Drug A was better than placebo, but in truth Drug A was no different from placebo.

Type I error can only occur for *one* reason: chance. To control for this possibility, an acceptable level of risk for Type I error is generally set at 5%. Because patients are at risk, the medical community in general accepts a 5% probability that chance was the reason a difference in effect was measured between the intervention group and the control group. The process of setting the probability of Type I error (false-positive result) as no greater than 5% is known as setting the α value. Many times clinical trials will refer to this step in a variety of ways:

- Setting the statistical significance to 0.05
- Significance level of 0.05
- *p*-values < 0.05 are statistically significant

Investigators should keep in mind that a 5% chance indicates that in 1 of 20 trials, a difference in effect being measured between the groups can be due to chance.

Beta (β) error (Type II) is the error that results if a false null hypothesis is not rejected or if a difference is not detected when a difference exists. Other ways to describe Type II error are:

- Investigators state that no difference exists when a difference actually does exist.
- Investigators state that Drug A was no different from placebo, but in truth Drug A was better than placebo.

Unlike Type I error, Type II error can occur for *two* reasons: chance and sample size. Again, an acceptable level of risk for Type II error has been set. Because it can be said that in Type II error industry is at risk (i.e., a potentially useful therapy may not be used), the medical community is more lax regarding Type II error than Type I error, and generally accepts a 20% probability that chance or sample size (too small) was the reason no difference in effect was measured between the intervention group and the control group.

The process of setting the probability of Type II error (false-negative result) as no greater than 20% is directly related to the study's power. A study's power is represented by the following equation:

$$\text{Power} = 1 - \beta$$

Because the generally accepted level of Type II error is 20%, this translates into a power of 80%. The power equation is also referred to as the β error rate. Some important considerations regarding power include the following:

- If a study lowers the β error rate, the power will be increased.
- An increase in the sample size will reduce the β error rate and increase the study power.

In general, β is calculated by using the number of subjects (*N*) and the difference that the investigators are trying to detect. These parameters must be established before the study begins (a priori) to improve the quality and validity of the study design. A power of less than 80% (or 0.80) suggests that the study may not have enrolled enough subjects to detect a difference between groups. Ultimately, smaller differences in effect between intervention and control groups can be detected with larger sample sizes.

Trial Results	Truth	
	Truly ineffective	Truly effective
Apparently ineffective	Correct (Probability = 1 − α)	Type II error (Probability = β)
Apparently effective	Type 1 error (Probability = α)	Correct (Probability = 1 − β)

Here is another way to look at the situation:

Trial Results	Truth	
	Truly ineffective	Truly effective
Apparently ineffective	Correct: 95%	Pharmaceutical company's risk: 20%
Apparently effective	Patient's risk: 5%	Correct: 80%

Methods to Evaluate the Appropriateness of Statistical Tests Used

The following process is intended to guide students and practitioners through a basic process to determine whether investigators appropriately utilized statistical techniques in a clinical trial.

Step 1: Identify the type of variable (nominal, ordinal, or continuous [interval or ratio]).
Step 2: Determine whether the researcher has control over that specific variable (independent or dependent variable).
Step 3: Determine the number of groups measured (two or more than two?).
Step 4: Use the following simplified chart to determine if the appropriate statistical test was used.

Type of Variable	Independent or Dependent	Number of Groups	Recommended Statistical Test
Nominal	Independent	Two	Chi-squared
	Dependent (paired)	Two	McNemar
		Three or more	Chi-squared
Ordinal	Independent	Two	Mann-Whitney U
		Three or more	Kruskal-Wallis
	Dependent (paired)	Two	Wilcoxon signed ranks
		Three or more	Friedman
Continuous		Two	Student *t*-test
		Three or more	Analysis of variance (ANOVA)
			Analysis of covariance (ANCOVA)

Relative Risk and Additional Calculations

Risk and ratios were discussed earlier in the observational study section. It is important to remember that relative risk (RR) is a measure of disease frequency when a specific factor is present or absent. RR is calculated using the following equation:

$$RR = \frac{\text{Incidence rate among those exposed to a particular factor}}{\text{Incidence rate among those not exposed to the same factor}}$$

- RR = 1.0 means no difference.
- RR > 1.0 means a positive association between the treatment or factor and the outcome.
- RR < 1.0 means a negative association between the treatment or factor and the outcome.

Once relative risk has been ascertained, a few more calculations can be performed:

- Relative risk reduction (RRR) is calculated by subtracting the relative risk from 1 (i.e., 1 − RR = RRR).
- Absolute risk reduction (ARR) is calculated by determining the absolute difference in rates of an outcome (or absolute difference in RR) between two different treatment groups.
- Number needed to treat (NNT) describes the number of patients who need to be treated with a specified therapy for one patient to benefit from treatment; it is sometimes a useful estimate of clinical significance. The calculation is as follows:

$$NNT = \frac{1}{ARR}$$

Survival Analysis

Survival analysis allows for investigators to study the time between patient entry into the trial and the event of interest. It places each subject at time zero and follows the patient until the designated outcome occurs or the study ends, whichever comes first. For survival analysis, there are four general requirements:

- The subject must have identified starting point and must be as consistent as possible.
- The trial must have a clearly defined outcome or endpoint.
- Dropout rates must be independent of the outcome.
- Diagnostic and therapeutic practices must be consistent during observational periods.

The Kaplan-Meier method is commonly used to perform survival analysis. This method utilizes survival times to represent the probability of not experiencing the event over time. It is commonly used for estimating the effect of a variable on survival beyond a certain time point (usually in the form of life tables and survival curves). The outcome measured does not have to be survival, however; it can be any dichotomous (yes or no) outcome measured over a period of time. Nevertheless, if subject differences at baseline are noted during a survival analysis, they should be adjusted based on the type of variable. For differences relating to dichotomous variables (i.e., gender), the Mantel-Haenszel test would be appropriate. For differences relating to continuous variables at baseline, Cox's proportional hazard adjusts for differences and controls for confounding variables.

ANNOTATED BIBLIOGRAPHY

Bryant PJ, Norris KP, McQueen CE, et al. Literature evaluation II: beyond the basics. In: Malone PM, Kier KL, Stanovich JE, eds. *Drug Information: A Guide for Pharmacists.* 4th ed. New York: McGraw-Hill; 2012. Chapter 5. Available at: http://www.accesspharmacy.com.libpublic3.library.isu.edu/content.aspx?aID=55671574. Accessed October 29, 2012.

De Muth JE. Overview of biostatistics used in clinical research. *Am J Health-Syst Pharm* 2009;66:70–81.

DeYoung GR. Biostatistics: a refresher. In: Bressler L, DeYoung GR, El-Ibiary S, et al. *Updates in Therapeutics: The Pharmacotherapy Preparatory Course.* Lenexa, KS: American College of Clinical Pharmacy; 2010.

Hartung DM, Touchette DR. An overview of clinical research design. *Am J Health-Syst Pharm* 2009;66:398–408.

Promoting Wellness

CHAPTER

29

TOPIC: DIETARY SUPPLEMENTS

Section Coordinator: Barb Mason
Contributor: M. Chandra Sekar

Tips Worth Tweeting

- The levo isomer of arginine is one of the amino acids that makes up a protein molecule.
- Astragalus contains a number of active components, which include glycosides, flavonoids, amino acids, and minerals.
- Black cohosh exerts estrogen-like effects.
- Choline is part of phosphatidylcholine, an essential phospholipid in both the plasma membrane and the neurotransmitter acetylcholine.
- Another name for coenzyme Q10 is ubiquinone.
- Bromelin from pineapple and papain from unripe papaya constitute the major proteolytic enzymes in digestive supplements.
- The active ingredient of feverfew is parthenolide (sesquiterpene lactones).
- Garlic's pharmacological activity is due to allicin, a sulfhydral compound.
- *Acidophilus* keeps the intestine more acidic and produces natural antibiotics called bacteriocins.
- Flavonoids are present in milk thistle (*Silybum marianum*).
- Red yeast rice mediates its effect by inhibition of HMG-CoA reductase.

Patient Care Scenario: Community Pharmacy

M. C., 55 y/o, customer for more than a decade, 5'4", 137 lbs, 130/82, pulse 66.
C/o mood swings and headaches and decreased interest in sex with her husband, who recently started taking Viagra.

Date	Physician	Drug	Quantity	Sig	Refills
6/1	Steen	Alendronate 70 mg	#4	One tablet once weekly	6
3/1	Steen	Verapamil XR 60 mg	#30	One tablet daily	6
3/1	Steen	Digoxin 0.125 mg	#30	One tablet daily	6
4/15	Jade	Calcium citrate/ vitamin D 500 mg	#60	One tablet bid	4

1.1.0 Patient Information

Over the last 2 decades, sales of dietary supplements—which include herbs, minerals, and vitamins—have grown exponentially. Some of the factors responsible for this growth are (1) increased consumer involvement in personal health, (2) over-the-counter availability of these products; (3) general belief that as these products are "natural" and therefore safe, and (4) an overall disillusionment with the medical and pharmaceutical establishment. Choosing the "right" herbal product or an appropriate alternative therapeutic regimen for one's patient is more of an art than a science. When judging the effectiveness of a supplement to treat a condition, it may be prudent to use a sliding scale of evidence as suggested by the director of the Arizona Center for Integrative Medicine at the University of Arizona, Dr. Weill—that is, requiring greater rigor of proven effectiveness from products capable of causing greater harm.

Arginine

The levo isomer of arginine is one of the amino acids that makes up a protein molecule.

Mechanism of Action: Arginine releases nitric oxide, a key signal-transducing molecule in the cell capable of causing vasodilation.
Common Uses: Arginine is beneficial in diseases of the vasculature such as coronary artery disease, peripheral artery disease, and erectile dysfunction.
Efficacy Data: Some studies have shown arginine's usefulness in boosting immune system.
Doses: Typical doses of arginine ranges from 5–9 g daily. Arginine is generally safe, but at higher doses its use may be accompanied by diarrhea, nausea, and dizziness.
Drug Interactions: Patients using drugs such as nitroglycerin, Viagra (PDE5 inhibitors), ACE inhibitors, and diuretics should consult their doctors before taking arginine.

Astragalus

Name: Astragalus (*Astragalus membranaceus*) is native to northern China and Tibet.
Plant Part: Its root has been used in medicine for centuries.
Common Uses: In the United States, this herb, in combination with echinacea, has been often used in to treat common respiratory infections such as colds, flu, and bronchitis.
Efficacy Data: Astragalus is considered to be more effective for flu prophylaxis than as an actual treatment for flu. Recently, a website claimed that a product containing astragalus was capable of preventing and treating H1N1 virus, the most famous flu virus of this decade. The FDA forced the company to take down the site, as there is no scientific evidence to support this claim. While manufacturers and promoters of herbs can make general claims, such as that their products "strengthen the immune system," they cannot make any specific claim that these drugs can treat or cure a disease. Protective effects of astragalus have been reported in patients receiving immunosuppression therapy for transplant or cancer. In small clinical trials, protective effects of astragalus in coxsackie B virus–induced myocarditis have been reported.
Active Constituent: Astragalus contains a number of active components, including glycosides, flavonoids, amino acids, and minerals.
Mechanism of Action: Although the exact mechanism of action is unknown, both in vitro and in vivo studies have shown positive effects of astragalus on various biochemical components of the immune response as reflected by increased amounts of lymphocytes and cytokines.
Dose: The usual dose is 9–15 g of dried root daily as tea in divided doses or 250–500 mg of solid extract three times daily.
Adverse Effects: At higher doses, astragalus use is accompanied by few mild side effects such as gastrointestinal upset and diarrhea.

Black Cohosh

Name: *Cimicifuga racemosa.*
Plant Part: Roots of black cohosh were used by Cherokee and the Iroquois Native American tribes.
Common Uses: Black cohosh tea is used to alleviate rheumatic pain, to promote lactation and menses, and for various other gynecological problems. Black cohosh is mainly used to treat "women's health" problems. It is more popular in Europe than in the United States, and it has been approved by the German Commission E for use in easing menstrual discomfort, mood swings, and headaches. The recent gain in popularity of black cohosh accompanied the finding that long-term use of conjugated estrogens is associated with increased incidence of cancer and cardiovascular complications.
Mechanism of Action: While the exact chemical constituent is not identified, black cohosh exerts estrogen-like effects in certain parts of the body. In addition to dried root, black cohosh is available in capsule, tablet, and elixir form.
Dose: The typical recommended dosage is 40 mg of standardized extract three times a day.
Precautions: While black cohosh can be used safely in adults, it should not be used during pregnancy because of its estrogen-like effects.
Drug Interactions: Physician consultation is suggested when black cohosh is used in combination with estrogen replacement therapy, as side effects have been observed with this combination.

Calcium

National Institutes of Health studies have clearly demonstrated that a large population across the United States is "calcium deficient."

Common Uses: While calcium's role in maintaining healthy teeth and bone is well established, new studies indicate increased calcium intake is associated with lower body fat and body weight, decreased risk of colon cancer, alleviation of unpleasant premenstrual syndromes, and beneficial effects on blood pressure.
Dose: The minimum daily requirement for adults is 1,000 mg calcium, with an increased requirement of 1,200 mg in persons older than 51 years of age, as well as higher requirements for teenagers and pregnant women.
Drug Interactions: Calcium supplements should be taken with vitamin D for better absorption, and calcium in the form of calcium citrate is most rapidly absorbed. Calcium deficiency is further enhanced by an increased consumption of soft drinks containing phosphates, which are capable of chelating calcium.

Chamomile

Name: *Matricaria recutita*. The German chamomile is mainly used in United States as tea.
Plant Part: Active ingredients of chamomile are present in the blue oil extracted from this plant's flowers.
Common Uses: When taken internally, chamomile is used to treat insomnia as well as gastrointestinal problems including peptic ulcer, gastritis, gastrointestinal discomfort, indigestion, and diarrhea. It may also be used externally for inflammatory skin conditions and canker sores and irritation of the gums and mouth
Efficacy Data: German Commission E has approved the use of this product for the previously mentioned conditions. There is some evidence to suggest that chamomile possesses both anti-inflammatory and antibacterial properties.
Dose: The usual dose is 2–4 g of dried flower as tea or infusion, three times daily. When taken as capsules, the usually recommended dose is two capsules, each containing 300–400 mg of standardized chamomile extract, three times a day
Drug Interactions: While chamomile is generally safe, caution should be exercised by patients who are also using warfarin, heparin, clopidogrel, ticlopidine, and pentoxifylline.

Choline

The Food and Nutrition Board of the U.S. National Academy of Science has recognized choline as an essential nutrient, whose RDI of 125–550 mg (depending on the patient's age, and other factors) needs to be obtained through diet or supplements.

Mechanism of Action: Choline is part of both phosphatidylcholine, an essential phospholipid in the plasma membrane, and acetylcholine, an important neurotransmitter.
Efficacy Data: Human and animal studies have shown the positive effects of choline supplementation in producing improvement in mild to moderate Alzheimer's disease, healthy brain development in fetuses, enhanced effect of interferon (an immune-stimulating cytokine), and protection in hepatitis B and hepatitis C.
Adverse Effects: Choline supplements up to 3 g have no side effects; occasionally, nausea or diarrhea may be seen at higher doses.

Chondroitin

Common Uses: Osteoarthritis is accompanied by cartilage loss. An important component of cartilage is chondroitin, so it appears logical that supplying the body with chondroitin supplements should be helpful. Chondroitin is a large molecule, and it is not understood how it is absorbed; nevertheless, several clinical trials have demonstrated positive results with chondroitin in osteoarthritis. This supplement is also often recommended for other ailments, such as tendonitis, as well as sprains and strains because of its ability to heal tissue and reduce pain and swelling.

Chondroitin is often combined with glucosamine for increased absorption. It is essential to recommend that the patient choose a product that has been independently verified.
Dose: The typical recommended dose is 1,200 mg/day with meals. Chondroitin has no serious side effects.
Adverse Effects: Minor side effects include gastrointestinal discomfort, heartburn, and nausea.

Chromium

Dose: Chromium is a heavy metal, and the daily RDI for this agent ranges from 11 to 44 mcg, depending on the patient's age, sex, and other factors.
Efficacy Data: Several studies have shown chromium's ability to enhance insulin action, though the exact mechanism is unknown. Chromium's ability to "burn fat" is unsubstantiated, but some evidence suggests chromium can improve cholesterol levels and increase the effectiveness of antidepressants.
Adverse Effects: While the chromium found in food and supplements is nontoxic (industrial chromium is highly toxic and is capable of causing cancer), in large amounts there is a distinct possibility that chromium may cause kidney or liver damage.

Drug Interactions: As chromium can enhance the effectiveness of certain antidiabetic drugs, its dosage may need adjustments with chromium use. Aspirin and NSAIDs may increase the absorption of chromium, while antacids may decrease its absorption.

Coenzyme Q10

Name: Also known as ubiquinone.

Common Uses: Aging as well as certain pathological conditions cause decreased production of this cofactor. CoQ10 supplementation has been found to be beneficial in many cardiovascular conditions, including heart failure, high blood pressure, angina, coronary artery disease, and stroke. Other conditions where there is some evidence of CoQ10's benefits include macular degeneration, migraines, Parkinson's disease, diabetes, and emphysema.

Mechanism of Action: CoQ10 produces its positive effects by improving energy production in cells as well as through its antioxidant activity. To obtain the most benefit, it is recommended to take CoQ10 along with the patient's standard prescription medications.

Dose: CoQ10 is available in capsule, wafer, and tablet forms. The usual dose is 30–300 mg, although some people consume as much as 1,200 mg/day.

Adverse Effects: No serious side effects are observed at smaller doses, but higher doses (more than 200 mg) may result in some gastrointestinal discomfort, as well as nausea and dizziness.

Dihydroepiandrosterone

Name: DHEA (dihydroepiandrosterone) is a male hormone produced by the adrenal glands, gonads, and brain. The maximum level of this hormone in humans is seen around age 25, after which its level decreases.

Common Uses: It is hypothesized that supplementation with DHEA will "reverse aging" and restore youthfulness.

Efficacy Data: There is very little scientific evidence to support this hypothesized effect. Isolated studies have reported that DHEA supplementation leads to increased muscle mass, increased libido in both men and women, decreased symptoms of lupus in women, and improved effectiveness of certain medications treating schizophrenia.

Adverse Effects: DHEA supplements contain variable amounts of this product. As it is an androgen, use of DHEA supplementation by women may lead to "increased masculinization," which may include growth of facial hair, hair loss, and increased sweating; in men, surprisingly, DHEA may promote breast development and tenderness.

Precautions: People with many types of cancers, as well as pregnant and nursing women, should not take DHEA.

Digestive Enzymes

Complete digestive enzyme supplements contain enzymes capable of digesting proteins, carbohydrates, and fats.

Active Constituent: Bromelin from pineapple and papain from unripe papaya constitute the major proteolytic enzymes in digestive supplements.

Common Uses: Beside improving digestion and decreasing heartburn, some studies have shown these enzymes' usefulness as anti-inflammatory agents in patients with low back pain, neck pain, and some other inflammatory conditions.

Dose: For pancreatic insufficiency, 3–4 g of 4× pancreatin is taken with each meal to improve digestion.

Precautions: Patients with cystic fibrosis should not take this medication, and bromelin should not be given to patients taking sedative or antibiotic medications.

Fenugreek

Name: Fenugreek (*Trigonella foenumgraecum*) has been used both for culinary and medicinal purposes for more than a thousand years by people in India, North Africa, and the Middle East.

Common Uses: German Commission E has approved fenugreek as an appetite stimulant and for decreasing skin inflammation.

Efficacy Data: Like many herbs, fenugreek has had a multitude of uses in the past. While some of its uses have no scientific basis, others, such as its effectiveness in reducing blood sugar and cholesterol, have experimental support. Soluble fiber (mucilage), like that present in fenugreek, may slow digestion of food and thereby decrease blood glucose increase. One lipid-lowering effect of fenugreek is due to the presence of saponins.

Dose: As a supplement, fenugreek is available in tablet, capsule, and powder forms. The recommended dose is 6 g daily.

Precautions: Pregnant or nursing mothers should avoid fenugreek.

Adverse Effects: Side effects of fenugreek include minor gastrointestinal discomfort.

Feverfew

Name: Feverfew (*Tanacetum partheniu*) is native to most of Europe and has been used in the past to alleviate symptoms of fever, arthritis, gastrointestinal discomfort, and asthma.

Common Uses: Currently, feverfew is mainly used to treat migraine and inflammatory joint diseases.

Efficacy Data: There is more scientific evidence to support this supplement's use in migraine than in arthritis.

Active Constituent: Its active ingredient, to which feverfew extract is standardized and which is considered to be responsible for many of its therapeutic effects, is parthenolide (sesquiterpene lactones).

Dose: In the form of fresh or powdered leaves, 380 mg of feverfew can be taken, as often as three times daily. When given as a capsule containing 250 mg parthenolide, feverfew is given once daily.

Mechanism of Action: Like NSAIDs, feverfew decreases prostaglandin formation. This effect is not due to inhibition of cyclooxygenase, but rather to phospholipase inhibition that prevents arachidonic acid release.

Adverse Effects: Chewing of feverfew leaves may result in mouth ulcers and loss of taste.

Precautions: Pregnant and nursing women should not take feverfew.

Drug Interactions: Patients taking warfarin, Plavix, aspirin, and other NSAIDs should consult their doctor before starting feverfew.

Garlic

Name: Garlic (*Allium sativum*) has been used for its medicinal value since ancient times.

Active Constituent: Many of its effects are attributed to allicin, a sulfahydral compound responsible for both garlic's odor and its pharmacological activity.

Common Uses: Garlic also possesses antibacterial, antiviral, antifungal, and antiparasitic activity. It is considered "heart healthy" because of its ability to reduce platelet adhesion. German Commission E recommends taking 4 g (1 clove) of garlic daily for its lipid-lowering effect.

Dose: Garlic is available in several formulations. For best results, choose a formulation that contains 1.3% allicin or 5,000–6,000 mg of "allicin potential."

Adverse Effects: Minor gastrointestinal side effects may accompany garlic use. Garlic should not be taken before surgery or with anticoagulants, as it can cause bleeding.

Ginseng

Ginseng is considered an adoptogen by herbalists, which means that it has nonspecific action and can create balance in the entire body.

Common Uses: Ginseng has been used in Chinese medicine for more than 5,000 years. Currently, it is used for relieving stress and fatigue, increasing endurance, strengthening immune system, and counteracting hyperglycemia.

Active Constituent: Three major types of ginseng are available—American, Asian, and Siberian. In chemical content, American and Asian ginseng are similar; each contains the active constituent ginsenoside. Siberian ginseng contains eleutheroside, which is completely different.

Plant Part: In all three types of ginseng, roots are used in the medicine.

Efficacy Data: Compared to Asian and American ginseng, Siberian ginseng is less expensive. While biochemical evidence supports the contention that ginseng administration causes increases in the levels of adrenocorticotropic hormone and corticosteroids, there is little clinical evidence to indicate it is really effective in treating any of the conditions for which it is used.

Doses: As an "adoptogen," different doses of ginseng are considered to produce "clinically" different effects. The same doses given to different patients with differing physiological states can have different actions.

Drug Interactions: Ginseng is relatively safe to use, but should be used with caution in patients taking blood-thinning agents, monoamine oxidase inhibitors, and antidepressants.

Green Tea

Name: Green tea (*Camellia sinensis*). When tea is obtained from unfermented leaves, it is referred to as green tea.

Active Constituent: Polyphenols, the major active ingredient in green tea, are considered to be more potent antioxidants than vitamin C.

Common Uses: Based on its ability to neutralize free radicals, beneficial effects of green tea are observed in certain types of cancer. This supplement has been shown to decrease side effects in patients undergoing chemotherapy or radiation and can boost the immune system. Another characteristic of green tea is its ability to cause prolonged thermogenesis, which has resulted in incorporation of this product in weight-loss products.

Dose: Many people do take this supplement as tea, although extract of green tea is also available in capsule form. The typical extract dosage is 100 mg containing 70% of tea catechins as epigallocatechin.
Adverse Effects: At normal doses, green tea has no side effects.
Drug Interactions: Patients taking prescription medications should consult their doctor before taking large quantities of green tea.

Hawthorn

Name: Hawthorn (*Crategus monogyna*) is currently used for cardiovascular disorders.
Mechanism of Action: Flavonoids from this plant have vasodilatory properties.
Common Uses: Coronary artery disease, atherosclerosis, hypertension, and hypercholesterolemia. The antioxidant properties of this herb have led to its use in decreasing inflammation in tissues damaged by sprains and strains.
Dose: Hawthorn is available in capsule, tincture, liquid, and solid extract form. The usual dosage is 300–600 mg/day in divided doses.
Adverse Effects: Its use is relatively safe except for some minor gastrointestinal discomfort.
Drug Interactions: Caution should be exercised when hawthorn is used in combination with prescription cardiovascular drugs such as digoxin, vasodilators, and alpha-agonists, among others.

Iron

Mechanism of Action: Iron is an essential supplement that plays an important role in the oxygen-carrying capacity of blood. Presently, iron deficiency is one of the most widespread nutritional deficiencies in the world and is accompanied by anemia (decreased number of red blood cells in blood).
Dose: The RDI for iron ranges from 0.27–27 mg depending on the age of the person and his or her physiological status. People who have healthy diets can meet most of their daily requirement for iron through food consumption. Iron can be classified into heme and non-heme iron. Heme iron is obtained from beef, egg yolk, fish, and other sources; non-heme iron is obtained from fruits, vegetables, and grains.
Drug Interactions: Absorption of non-heme iron can be enhanced by ascorbic acid. Although iron is essential for maintaining the body's health children can be poisoned through ingestion of an excessive amount of iron.
Besides tetracycline, ACE inhibitors, histamine blockers, proton pump inhibitors, and a few other drugs are capable of inhibiting iron absorption, as are zinc, calcium, soy, copper, and manganese supplements. Therefore, it is usually recommended that iron supplements be taken 2 hours before these drugs.

Kava Kava

Name: Kava kava (*Piper methysticum*) is used in Western countries to relieve anxiety and provide relaxation.
Active Constituent: Kavalactones present in kava has been shown to possess relaxant and anti-anxiety property.
Common Uses: Kava kava is often used to combat insomnia, stress, and restlessness.
Adverse Effects: While this supplement does not have many of the side effects associated with prescription medications used to treat anxiety and depression (i.e., nonaddictive, nondevelopment of tolerance), several cases of severe liver damage associated with its use have been reported. Although kava kava is a legal supplement in the United States (it is banned in Canada), patients should be encouraged to use it only under the supervision of physicians.
Dose: The usual dose is a 100 mg standardized extract of 70% kavalactones twice or thrice daily.
Adverse Effects: The most common side effect associated with kava kava is stomachache. Prolonged use may cause itching, scaling, and yellowing of skin.
Drug Interactions: Caution should be exercised when kava kava is used in combination with medications to treat seizures, sleep disturbances, anxiety, schizophrenia, or Parkinson's disease.

Lactobacillus Acidophilus

Lactobacillus *acidophilus* is a wonderful example of a "good bacterium" that has a symbiotic relationship with human beings. Yogurt contains lactobacillus *thermophilus* and lactobacillus *bulgaricus* but may or may not contain the *acidophilus* strain.

Name: *Acidophilus* is also referred to as "probiotic."
Common Uses: *Acidophilus* not only helps with digestion, but is also beneficial in treating vaginal yeast infections, ulcers, and urinary tract infections. Increased use of proton pump inhibitors (e.g., pantoprozole, omeprazole), by altering the bacterial culture of the gastrointestinal tract, have increased the need for lactobacillus supplementation. Indirectly, *acidophilus* supplementation helps the immune system.
Mechanism of Action: *Acidophilus* keeps the intestine more acidic and produces natural antibiotics called bacteriocins.

Dose: *Acidophilus* can be taken as a capsule, tablet, or powder; in liquid form; or as yogurt. It needs to be refrigerated. The usual dosage is 1–2 billion living organism daily, but it can sometimes be as high as 10 billion organisms given for a short period.

Adverse Effects: This supplement is usually safe, but minor discomfort such as gas may be experienced by some people.

Milk Thistle

Name: *Silybum marianum*.

Common Uses: The flavonoids present in milk thistle have been shown to possess both liver-protecting and liver-regenerating activity and, therefore, are useful in cirrhosis and infectious hepatitis.

Mechanism of Action: Milk thistle protects the depletion of glutathione, such as that caused by acetaminophen toxicity, and it protects the liver.

Dose: Crushed or powdered seeds of milk thistle are available as capsules, tablets, liquid extracts, and tinctures. The dose range is from 140–280 mg of products containing 70–80% silymarin, taken three times daily.

Adverse Effects: Milk thistle is a safe supplement with very few side effects.

Drug Interactions: Patients taking prescription medications that are metabolized through cytochrome P450 pathway should consult their physician. Milk thistle will reduce the effectiveness of oral contraceptives.

Niacin

Niacin is both a supplement and a prescription drug.

Name: A form of vitamin B_3.

Common Uses: Niacin is currently used for decreasing levels of low-density lipoproteins and triglycerides while increasing high-density lipoprotein levels. The RDI for niacin ranges from 2–18 mg, with requirements increasing with age.

Mechanism of Action: Niacin plays an important role in various physiological processes, including the production of hormones, the production of blood cells, and fat, carbohydrate, and protein metabolism.

Dose: The medicinal dose of niacin is much higher than the suggested RDI. Niacin supplements are available in regular and slow-release formulations.

Adverse Effects: Some of the side effects of niacin include flushing, headaches, and hypotension. At higher doses, regular blood tests should be carried out to monitor for liver damage.

Precautions: Pregnant and nursing women should not take high doses of niacin.

Omega-3 Fatty Acids

Omega-3 fatty acids are unsaturated fatty acids. Abundant consumption of such unsaturated fatty acids by the Japanese population is considered to be responsible for that group's overall good health and longevity.

Common Uses: Supplementation with omega-3 fatty acids, which cannot be synthesized by humans, has been found useful in conditions including heart disease, rheumatism, asthma, and depression, among others.

Mechanism of Action: While the exact mechanism of action for their numerous effects are unknown (as is the case for arachidonic acid), omega-3 fatty acids are considered to be converted to prostaglandins and eicosanoids.

Dose: The most common recommended dose is 3 g of omega-3 fatty acids present in 10 g of fish oil per day.

Precautions: Omega-3 fatty acids are considered generally safe, but people who have a tendency to bleed as well as women who are pregnant or nursing should consult their doctor before starting them. For people who do not want to take fish oil, an alternative source of omega-3 fatty acids is flax seed oil.

Red Yeast Rice

Name: Red yeast rice contains an agent called monacolins—the same agent present in the prescription medicine, lovastatin.

Mechanism of Action: Red yeast rice mediates its effect by inhibition of HMG-CoA reductase.

Common Uses: Used for centuries in China as a food staple, red yeast rice is currently used in the United States as an aid to lower cholesterol.

Dose: Red yeast rice is usually taken as capsule, and the typical dosage is 1,200 mg twice daily. It is advisable to take this drug under the supervision of a doctor, and supplementation with CoQ10 is recommended when a person is taking this supplement.

Adverse Effects: Minor side effects are gastrointestinal in nature. Discontinue the medication and seek medical advice if muscle weakness or myopathy occurs.

Saw Palmetto

Name: Saw palmetto (*Serenoa repens*).

Common Uses: Saw palmetto is currently mainly used for male genitourinary problems, such as prostate enlargement and erectile dysfunction.

Efficacy Data: There is a greater degree of scientific evidence to support its effectiveness in prostate enlargement than in erectile dysfunction.

Mechanism of Action: While the actual mechanism of action is unknown, polysaccharides present in saw palmetto berries may have an anti-inflammatory and immune-stimulating activity that may help with enlarged prostate. Patients on prescription medications for prostate enlargement should seek a doctor's advice before starting saw palmetto.

Dose: Different formulations of saw palmetto are available. The usual total daily dose is 320 mg containing at least 85–95% fatty acid and sterols. Take this supplement with meals if stomach upset occurs.

St. John's Wort

Name: SJW, *Hypericum perforatum*.

Common Uses: While the ancient Greeks were the first to use St. John's wort, by mid-19th century this herb was used to treat "nervous disposition" and "hysteria." SJW is currently one of the top 10 selling herbs in the United States. Its flower tops and petals are used as medicines. Currently, SJW is mostly used by patients to self-treat depression, and secondarily as an antiviral agent to treat the common cold, herpes, and human immunodeficiency virus. Less commonly, infused oil from SJW is used topically to treat muscle aches.

Efficacy Data: Some clinical studies suggest that SJW is as effective as selective serotonin reuptake inhibitors (SSRIs) and tricyclic antidepressants. However, there is no information on the active ingredients responsible for these antidepressant effects and the effects of long-term SJW use.

Dose: Recommended products should contain at least 0.3% hypericin or 3–5% hyperforin. The typical dose is 300 mg three times daily of standardized extract or 2–4 g three times daily of dried herb.

Drug Interactions: Two major concerns with SJW use by patients are interaction with the cytochrome P450 pathway (CYP3A4) and the induction of the multidrug-resistance gene product P-glycoprotein. Reports have shown that concomitant use with SJW have resulted in decreased levels of ethinyl estradiol, indinavir, and cyclosporine—all of which use the cytochrome P450 pathway for metabolism. Reduced digoxin levels have been attributed to the induction of P-glycoprotein by SJW. Patients taking warfarin, a drug with low therapeutic index for their cardiovascular problem, or prescription SSRIs should be extremely cautious using SJW.

ANNOTATED BIBLIOGRAPHY

Schulman RA. *Solve It with Supplements*. Emmaus, PA: Rodale; 2007.

White L, Foster S. *The Herbal Drugstore*. Emmaus, PA: Rodale; 2000.

TOPIC: IMMUNIZATIONS

Section Coordinator: *Michael Klepser*

Contributors: *Katherine A. Campbell-Petkewicz, Scott J. Bergman, and Emily H. Collins-Lucey*

Tips Worth Tweeting

- There are two types of immunity: innate and active.
- Live vaccines may be contraindicated in immunocompromised individuals because of the potential for uncontrolled virus replication.
- An advantage of live vaccines is that they do not require booster doses.
- Any number of live and inactive vaccines can be administered simultaneously on the same date.
- Rotavirus vaccines are administered orally as a liquid suspension.
- Pneumovax is not effective in preventing all pneumococcal pneumonia.
- No person should receive more than two doses of PPSV in a lifetime.
- IM PPSV may be less painful than subcutaneous injection.
- Two Tdap products are available: Boostrix and Adacel.
- A booster shot is needed at 12–15 months for Hib vaccination, regardless of which vaccine is used.
- All varicella-containing vaccines should be frozen at a temperature of 5°F.

Patient Care Scenario: Ambulatory Setting

D. M., 4 y/o, 66 lbs, enrolled in kindergarten to begin next fall. He is up-to-date on all of his immunizations and had all of his last primary doses before 3 years of age.

Immunology Foundation

An antigen can be described as any foreign substance or product that can provoke an immune response. For example, both influenza viruses and the influenza vaccine are considered antigens. Antibodies are molecules produced by B cells that are part of the body's immune system. They recognize specific antigens and induce a cellular response that leads to destruction of the antigen. The ability of the human body to respond to a foreign substance and protect the body from adverse consequences induced by any such foreign substance is known as immunity.

There are two main types of immunity: innate and active. Innate immunity, also known as passive immunity, is immunologic protection an individual achieves temporarily by receiving antibodies against a pathogen. The protection is immediate, such that the body does not have to mount a cellular response to the specific antigen that needs to be accounted for. Antibodies provided to an infant via a mother's breastmilk are an example of innate immunity. Sometimes antibodies are utilized to protect persons exposed to an antigen when immediate protection is desired. For example, hepatitis B immunoglobulin is administered to persons who have been exposed to the hepatitis B virus, but who have not received previous immunization to such a virus. Innate immunity protects an individual for only a limited amount of time.

In contrast, active immunity requires a cellular response by the immune system's B cells so that T cells and memory cells are produced in a series of events that result in the recruitment of various cells to destroy and eliminate the antigens. Memory cells then provide antibodies for protection against future exposure to the same antigen. Protection acquired through receiving a vaccine is an example of active immunity. Active immunity tends to provide much longer, even lifelong protection in comparison to innate immunity.

Vaccines are described as either live (attenuated) or inactive. Live vaccines contain virus that is technically alive, but the viruses' virulent properties that can produce disease are significantly reduced. Thus the body mounts an active immune response as the live virus replicates, but the virus is not capable of causing severe disease. Live vaccines must replicate in the body to provoke an immune response, so anything that may prevent this replication process—such as a recent blood transfusion, which may provide temporary immunity—can cause the vaccine to be ineffective. Live vaccines are often contraindicated in severely immunocompromised individuals because of the potential for uncontrolled replication of the virus. In addition, live vaccines are not recommended for pregnant females. One advantage of live vaccines is that most offer prolonged protection and do not require booster doses.

In contrast, inactive vaccines are chemically altered such that they do not replicate in the body but still stimulate an immune response. Inactive vaccines are generally considered safe for use in immunosuppressed individuals and may also be utilized in pregnant females. Inactive vaccines often require several doses for optimal protection as well as booster doses for prolonged protection.

Immunization Resources and Schedules

Knowing where to find current evidence-based recommendations regarding immunizations is necessary for pharmacists who incorporate immunization services into their practice. The leading entity that publishes immunization recommendations is the Advisory Committee on Immunization Practices (ACIP). The role of the ACIP is to provide advice that will lead to a reduction in the incidence of vaccine-preventable diseases in the United States and an increase in the safe use of vaccines and related biological products.

Recommendations include the age for vaccine administration, number of doses and dosing interval, and precautions and contraindications. Childhood, adolescent, adult, and catch-up immunization schedules are published yearly by the ACIP and can be found at www.cdc.gov/vaccines. This website, which is maintained by the Centers for Disease Control and Prevention, is arguably the best resource for immunization information, as its content is updated daily.

Vaccine Timing, Safety, and Storage

It is not uncommon for a patient to need both a live vaccine and an inactive vaccine at the same health visit. Any number of live and inactive vaccines can be administered simultaneously on the same date. However, additional live vaccines of a different type or antibodies cannot be administered for at least 4 weeks thereafter, because there will likely be a reduced immune response. Most vaccines are very safe, but unique side effects are listed for each product. Local injection-site reactions, including pain, swelling, and erythema, are the most common adverse reactions for intramuscular (IM) and subcutaneous injections. Vaccination is contraindicated in any person with a severe allergic reaction to a vaccine component. Unless noted, vaccines should be stored in the refrigerator at temperatures of 35–46°F (2–8°C) and never frozen.

Vaccine-Preventable Diseases

Rotavirus

1.1.0 Patient Information

Signs and Symptoms

Rotavirus infection is a common disease among infants and children. It causes gastroenteritis, characterized by severe diarrhea, nausea and vomiting, abdominal pain, and fever.

Diseases and Medical Conditions

This highly contagious virus is most commonly transmitted via person-to-person contact, by fecal–oral spread. Children between 3 and 35 months of age have the highest risk of contracting this virus. In particular, children who attend daycare programs, are admitted to a hospital setting, or are immunocompromised are at great risk.

1.2.0 Pharmacotherapy

Indication

All children should receive the rotavirus vaccine unless it is contraindicated.

Two rotavirus vaccines are licensed for use in the United States. The first approved, called RotaTeq (Merck & Co., Whitehouse Station, New Jersey), contains five different types of rotavirus (RV5) that are a combination of human and bovine strains. The second, called Rotarix (GlaxoSmithKline, Research Triangle, North Carolina), contains only one type of rotavirus (RV1), but it is fully human. Both vaccines are live-attenuated viruses that are administered orally as liquid suspensions. Starting at 2 months of age, the first dose of two for RV1 or three for RV5 should be administered, and the next doses given approximately 2 months after the previous dose. The maximum age for any dose is 28 weeks, according to the ACIP.

Package, Storage, Handling, and Disposal

Both rotavirus vaccines need to be stored in the refrigerator and should never be frozen.

Pneumococcal Disease

1.1.0 Patient Information

Signs and Symptoms

Pneumococcal disease, caused by the bacterium *Streptococcus pneumoniae*, accounts for many known diseases, including bacteremia, meningitis, pneumonia, and otitis media. The last of these is the most common among children. Although it can spread throughout the year, pneumococcal disease is usually transmitted from person to person through respiratory droplets during the winter and early spring.

1.2.0 Pharmacotherapy

The childhood pneumococcal vaccine (Prevnar, Wyeth/Pfizer Pharmaceuticals, Philadelphia, Pennsylvania) contains the serotypes of *S. pneumoniae* responsible for most disease among children, and is administered IM. This pneumococcal conjugate vaccine (PCV) originally had seven serotypes; the updated version contains 13 serotypes to protect against strains not included in the first version of PCV. All infants should be immunized with PCV in a four-dose series at 2, 4, and 6 months, with a booster dose at 12–15 months of age. PCV is not routinely recommended for children older than 59 months of age.

Pneumonia is the most common pneumococcal disease among adults and is a common complication resulting from influenza. Pneumovax (Merck & Co., Whitehouse Station, New Jersey) is a 23-valent polysaccharide vaccine (PPSV23) for adults that contains purified capsular polysaccharide antigens from pneumococcal bacteria that are responsible for nearly 88% of disease. The vaccine is 60–70% effective in preventing invasive disease, but it has not been shown to be effective in preventing all pneumococcal pneumonia and should not be referred to as the "pneumonia vaccine." Nevertheless, PPSV can benefit patients who do develop pneumococcal pneumonia, as these patients often have less severe symptoms, a shorter duration of disease, and a reduced death rate.

Table 29-1 Indications for Pneumococcal Vaccine

- All children younger than 24 months of age (PCV series)
- Children 24–59 months of age with an incomplete pneumococcal vaccine schedule
  - PPSV
- Patients 65 years of age or older
- Patients 19–64 years of age who smoke
- Patients 2–64 years of age with chronic illnesses

PPSV should be routinely administered either IM or subcutaneously to all adults age 65 years and older, and to persons 2 years of age and older with certain risk factors, including asplenia and a compromised immune system (Table 29-1). Routine revaccination with the polysaccharide vaccine is not necessary, but certain groups are candidates for a second dose: those 2 years of age or older with certain risk factors (refer to Table 29-1) or anyone age 65 and older who was vaccinated before age 65 *and* for whom 5 years have passed since the original vaccination. No person should receive more than two doses total of PPSV in a lifetime. The intramuscular route of administration seems to be associated with less pain in comparison to subcutaneous injection.

Diphtheria, Tetanus, and Pertussis

1.1.0 Patient Information

Signs and Symptoms

Diphtheria is a toxin-mediated disease caused by the bacterium *Corynebacterium diphtheriae*; it is most often spread from person to person via respiratory droplets. Tetanus is caused by the anaerobic bacterium *Clostridium tetani* and is distinguished by rigidity and convulsive spasms of the skeletal muscles. The bacterium most commonly enters the body through contaminated wounds. Pertussis is a highly contagious disease caused by the bacterium *Bordetella pertussis* that produces an acute cough, otherwise known as whooping cough. It is transmitted from person to person via respiratory droplets.

1.2.0 Pharmacotherapy

Indications

Due to the severity of these diseases, all children should be routinely vaccinated against them. DTaP, an inactivated vaccine combination of diphtheria, tetanus toxoids, and acellular pertussis, comes in three different brands, but the recommendations for each are the same. DTaP is the preferred vaccine for children 6 weeks through 6 years of age. The primary series consists of four doses at 2, 4, 6, and 15–18 months of age. A booster dose is recommended between 4 and 6 years of age if the last primary dose was given before the child turned 4 years of age.

Young children have the highest risk of complications from pertussis, but adolescents and adults can be infected with pertussis and serve as the source of infection for children. A tetanus, diphtheria, and pertussis combination vaccine exists for adults and adolescents (Tdap) that includes a smaller amount of diphtheria than the childhood vaccine to avoid excessive injection-site swelling. Tdap should be administered starting at age 10 to those persons who have completed the primary DTaP series, and followed by a tetanus/diphtheria (Td) booster every 10 years to decrease the risk of these infections. Two Tdap products are available: Boostrix (GlaxoSmithKline, Research Triangle Park, North Carolina), and Adacel (Sanofi Pasteur, Swiftwater, Pennsylvania)

Haemophilus influenzae Type b

1.1.0 Patient Information

Signs and Symptoms

Haemophilus influenzae type b (Hib) is a gram-negative coccobacillus mainly associated with bacterial meningitis. This disease usually affects persons younger than the age of 5 years; it is not a disease often encountered in adults. The Hib bacterium is transmitted from person to person via respiratory droplets and then percolates to the cerebral spinal fluid, blood, pleural fluid, or joint fluid, which can result in osteomyelitis, arthritis, cellulitis, pneumonia, and bacteremia.

1.2.0 Pharmacotherapy

Indication

This invasive disease most commonly affects children between 6 and 11 months, which is why all infants more than 6 weeks old should receive this vaccination. Two Hib conjugate vaccines are available: ActHIB (Sanofi Pasteur, Swiftwater, Pennsylvania) and PedvaxHIB (Merck & Co., Whitehouse Station, New Jersey). ActHIB is a three-dose primary series given at 2, 4, and 6 months, whereas PedvaxHIB only requires a two-dose primary series at 2 and 4 months. Regardless of which brand is used, a booster shot needs to be given between 12 and 15 months. The Hib vaccines are interchangeable, but if even one dose of ActHIB is used, then a third dose will be needed before the booster. Some other vaccines contain Hib vaccine as part of a combination vaccine package, but those should be used only for booster doses after the primary Hib series has been completed using one of the noncombination products.

Hepatitis A

Hepatitis A virus (HAV) is transmitted primarily through fecal–oral spread from contaminated food or water, or from personal contact with an infected person.

1.1.0 Patient Information

Signs and Symptoms

Hepatitis A is highly contagious and replicates in the liver to result in jaundice. Symptoms of acute HAV infection are typically abrupt in onset and consist of fever, malaise, anorexia, nausea, and jaundice.

1.2.0 Pharmacotherapy

Indication

All children should be routinely vaccinated with the hepatitis A vaccine. Two HAV vaccines are available, each in both pediatric and adult formulations. Havrix (GlaxoSmithKline, Research Triangle Park, North Carolina) and Vaqta (Merck & Co., Whitehouse Station, New Jersey) are inactivated whole-virus vaccines and should be administered IM to all children older than 12 months of age, with a booster dose at least 6 months after the first injection.

Hepatitis B

Hepatitis B virus (HBV) is transmitted through bodily fluids from an infected person.

1.1.0 Patient Information

Signs and Symptoms

The effects of this infection can be catastrophic, causing jaundice, cirrhosis, and even hepatocellular carcinoma.

1.2.0 Pharmacotherapy

Indication

All infants should receive one of the two brands of hepatitis B vaccine—Recombivax HB (Merck & Co., Whitehouse Station, New Jersey) or Engerix-B (GlaxoSmithKline, Research Triangle Park, North Carolina)—in a three-dose series. The injection is given IM, using the deltoid muscle in adults and children, and the anterolateral thigh in infants and neonates. The usual schedule is at birth (to protect against perinatal transmission), 1–2 months later, and again at 6–18 months. If not done at birth, then adolescents should be routinely vaccinated with a three-dose schedule of 0, 1 month, and 4–6 months. Catch-up vaccination of adults can be considered for certain high-risk groups, including, but not limited to, those at risk for sexually transmitted HBV, intravenous drug users, healthcare and public safety workers, international travelers, or those who share a household with a person with HBV.

A combination hepatitis A and B vaccine, Twinrix, (GlaxoSmithKline, Research Triangle Park, North Carolina) is approved for persons age 18 years and older with indications for both vaccines. It is administered in a three-dose series at 0, 1, and 6 months. The HAV component in Twinrix is only half the normal adult dose, so the combination vaccine should be used for the entire series. This product should not be confused with other multicomponent vaccines, such as Comvax (Merck & Co., Whitehouse Station, New Jersey), which is a combination vaccine that contains HBV and Hib and is given in a three-dose series at 2, 4, and 12–15 months of age.

Varicella

The varicella zoster virus (VZV) causes two forms of disease: primary infection, known as chickenpox, and reactivation, commonly called shingles. Because VZV is part of the herpesvirus class, shingles is sometimes referred to as herpes zoster. This highly contagious virus is transmitted through respiratory droplets and direct contact with lesions of an infected person.

1.1.0 Patient Information

Signs and Symptoms

Chickenpox usually presents with numerous fluid-filled vesicles in nearly any area of the body. The vesicles cause pruritus, burst, and then dry to become scab-like. The most common secondary complication associated with chickenpox is bacterial skin infection, although it can cause much more serious disease. Recurrent infection occurs when the virus, which remains dormant in sensory nerve ganglia after primary infection, becomes reactivated. Factors associated with reactivation include increasing age, intrauterine exposure, immunosuppression, and primary disease at age younger than 18 months. With shingles, the varicella vesicles erupt along the distribution of a sensory nerve. The patient may experience pain and tingling for several days prior in the area where the vesicles will erupt. The most common complication associated with the shingles is postherpetic neuralgia (PHN). PHN causes pain that may persist for years, and can severely reduce a patient's quality of life.

1.2.0 Pharmacotherapy

The childhood varicella vaccine (Varivax, Merck & Co., Inc., Whitehouse Station, New Jersey), is a live-attenuated virus given by subcutaneous administration.

Indication

All children should receive the varicella vaccine, except for children with certain contraindications such as immunosuppressive disease. The first dose should be given between 12 and 15 months of age, and a second dose should be administered between ages 4 and 6 years.

The adult herpes zoster vaccine (Zostavax, Merck & Co., Whitehouse Station, New Jersey) used to prevent shingles is approved for use in persons aged 60 years and older. It contains a much higher amount of the same live-attenuated varicella virus as the childhood and vaccines. The vaccine efficacy declines with age, but when vaccinated patients do develop shingles, it is less severe and associated with less postherpetic neuralgia. ACIP recommends that persons aged 60 and older be given a one-time dose of the vaccine, regardless of prior varicella vaccination and disease history.

Contraindications, Warnings, and Precautions

Pregnancy, pregnancy planned within 4 weeks of vaccine administration, leukemia, lymphoma, and other immunosuppressive conditions are contraindications to the VZV vaccine. Caution should be used when deciding to vaccinate a patient with acute illness and current treatment with a drug with activity against herpesviruses (such as acyclovir).

Package, Storage, Handling, and Disposal

It is imperative that all varicella-containing vaccines be frozen at a temperature of 5°F (–15°C). However, the vaccine diluent may be stored separately at room temperature or in the refrigerator. If the vaccine is not given within 30 minutes of reconstitution, it should be disposed of and a new vaccine dose should be prepared.

Measles, Mumps, and Rubella

1.1.0 Patient Information

Signs and Symptoms

Measles is a highly contagious virus. The clinical features of this infection consist of a maculopapular rash that begins at the hairline and then spreads downward toward the extremities. Similar to measles, mumps is also a highly contagious virus whose clinical features include symptoms of parotitis and aseptic meningitis. The rubella virus presents with a maculopapular rash similar to mumps, except fainter. Measles, mumps, and rubella (MMR) are all transmitted from person to person via respiratory droplets.

1.2.0 Pharmacotherapy

Indication

A live combination vaccine simply called MMR II (Merck & Co., Whitehouse Station, New Jersey) is approved for children older than 1 year of age. The primary series consists of two doses; the first dose given between 12 and 15 months of age, and the second dose is recommended before the child enters kindergarten, usually between 4 and 6 years of age. A combination measles–mumps–rubella–varicella (MMRV) vaccine (ProQuad, Merck & Co., Whitehouse Station, New Jersey) is approved for children aged 12 months to 12 years. MMRV may be used for both the first and second doses of MMR *and* varicella in children. If the varicella vaccine is not administered at the same time as other vaccines, it needs to be separated by at least 28 days due to the live nature of the vaccine.

Contraindications, Warnings, and Precautions

All children should receive the MMR vaccine except those with certain contraindications to live vaccines (i.e., those with severe immunosuppression).

Adverse Effects

The most common adverse effect associated with MMR vaccine is fever. It is important to note that MMR and MMRV contain gelatin and neomycin.

Package, Storage, Handling, and Disposal

The MMR diluent can be stored either in the refrigerator with the vaccine or at room temperature. Reconstituted vaccine should be used immediately; it must be discarded if not used within 8 hours.

Polio and Childhood Vaccine Combinations

Polio is a disease caused by a highly contagious virus most commonly transmitted through the mouth, by fecal–oral spread.

1.1.0 Patient Information

Signs and Symptoms

Once poliovirus enters the body through the gastrointestinal tract, it travels to the spinal cord and ultimately causes paralysis. In developing countries, where the risk of disease is still quite high, oral polio vaccine is used because it is the most effective version.

1.2.0 Pharmacotherapy

Indication

Inactivated polio vaccine (IPV) is given in areas where disease is uncommon because side effects are rare. All children in the United States should receive a three-dose primary series of IPV at ages 2, 4, and 12–18 months. Children who receive three doses as scheduled before they turn 4 years old should also receive a booster injection between 4 to 6 years of age.

Kinrix (GlaxoSmithKline, Research Triangle Park, North Carolina) is a combination vaccine that contains DTaP and IPV. Kinrix is approved specifically for the fifth dose of DTaP and fourth dose of IPV that children receive at 4–6 years of age.

Pentacel (Sanofi Pasteur, Swiftwater, Pennsylvania), a combination vaccine containing DTaP, Hib, and IPV, is approved for the primary doses of each vaccine. Given to children 6 weeks through 4 years of age, Pentacel should typically be administered at the ages of 2, 4, 6, and 15–18 months. Pentacel is not approved for children older than 5 years of age. Note that IPV contains streptomycin, polymyxin B, and neomycin, which may trigger a reaction in patients allergic to these antibiotics.

Pediarix (GlaxoSmithKline, Research Triangle Park, North Carolina) is approved for use up to 7 years of age and contains diphtheria, tetanus, acellular pertussis (DTaP), IPV, and hepatitis B vaccines. It is given as three-dose primary series at 2, 4, and 6 months of age and is not approved for booster doses.

Contraindications, Warnings, and Precautions

Combination vaccines should never be used for the birth dose of hepatitis B vaccine (single-entity hepatitis B vaccines are the only vaccines approved for infants less than 6 weeks old), but can be used in the second and third doses of the hepatitis B vaccine series.

Human Papillomavirus

Human papillomavirus (HPV) is the most common sexually transmitted infection in the United States.

1.1.0 Patient Information

Signs and Symptoms

There are more than 100 types of HPV, which affect the skin and cause common warts; approximately 40 types can affect mucosal epithelium. Infections range from benign to severe with complications such as anogenital warts and cervical cancers. High-risk HPV types are found in virtually all cervical cancers: types 16 and 18 together account for 70% of all cervical cancers. Types 6 and 11 account for a large proportion of anogenital warts (condyloma acuminata).

1.2.0 Pharmacotherapy

Indication

A quadrivalent HPV vaccine (HPV4) called Gardasil (Merck & Co., Whitehouse Station, New Jersey), containing noninfectious virus-like particles, confers immunity to HPV types 6, 11, 16, and 18. Gardasil is approved for use in females and males between 9 and 26 years of age. Cervarix (GlaxoSmithKline, Research Triangle Park, North Carolina) is a bivalent recombinant vaccine (HPV2) indicated for the prevention of disease caused by HPV types 16 and 18 only; it is approved for use in females age 10 through 25 years of age.

HPV vaccine is recommended by ACIP for routine IM administration to adolescents 11–12 years old. HPV4 is a three-dose series at 0, 2, and 6 months for both girls and boys, whereas HPV2 is administered to girls only at 0, 1, and 6 months. Booster doses are not indicated at this time.

Contraindications, Warnings, and Precautions

An increased occurrence of syncope after injection of Gardasil in adolescent girls has been documented. Given this finding, it is important to administer HPV vaccines to patients in a sitting or supine position instead of standing. Some syncope episodes have been accompanied by tonic–clonic-like activity. This activity usually resolves quickly and is improved by placing the patient in the Trendelenburg position.

Meningococcal Disease

Neisseria meningitidis is an encapsulated gram-negative diplococcus responsible for meningococcal diseases such as meningitis, bacteremia, and focal infections. Five serotypes are responsible for most invasive disease: A, B, C, Y, and W-135. Meningococcal meningitis is the most common form of invasive disease, and results from exposure to the droplets or secretions of an infected person or carrier.

1.1.0 Patient Information

Signs and Symptoms

Meningococcal sepsis can occur with or without meningitis and is characterized by a petechial rash. Disease incidence peaks in infants younger than 12 months of age, then increases among adolescents and young adults, especially those in close contact with one another.

1.2.0 Pharmacotherapy

Indication

Three quadrivalent vaccines are available for protection against meningococcal disease due to serotypes A, C, Y, and W-135, but none protects against serotype B. Menomune (Sanofi Pasteur, Swiftwater, Pennsylvania) is a polysaccharide vaccine (MPSV4); Menactra (Sanofi Pasteur) is a conjugated polysaccharide vaccine (MCV4); and Menveo (Novartis, Cambridge, Massachusetts) is a conjugated oligosaccharide vaccine. Immunity wanes among recipients of Menomune, even with repeated dosing. With Menactra and Menveo, the polysaccharide antigens are conjugated to diphtheria toxoid protein, which the body recognizes from previous immunizations and, therefore, can produce longer-acting immunity. Hence Menactra is preferred over Menomune in those 2–55 years old who are candidates for its administration. Menveo was recently approved for prevention of meningitis and other invasive meningococcal disease in persons ages 11–55 and will likely also be a preferred agent, as it provides longer-acting immunity relative to Menomune. Thus, when either Menactra or Menveo is available, use of Menomune is recommended to be limited to persons older than age 55. Menactra is recommended for all children at 11 or 12 years of age, with catch-up immunization recommended up to age 18. In addition, all college freshmen who live in a dormitory and persons aged 2–55 years who are at increased risk of disease should be vaccinated. The most important of these additional risk factors for pharmacists to recognize is functional or anatomic asplenia. Because the immune system of patients without a spleen cannot recognize encapsulated bacteria, meningococcal, streptococcal, and *Haemophilus influenzae* type B vaccines should all be given to these individuals.

Contraindications, Warnings, and Precautions

Menomune contains lactose, so it should not be used in patients who are allergic to this substance. A small number of cases of Guillain-Barré syndrome (GBS) have been reported after receipt of MCV4, but data are insufficient to determine whether this vaccine truly increases the risk of GBS.

Package, Storage, Handling, and Disposal

Menomune is administered subcutaneously and must be used within 30 minutes of reconstitution. In contrast, Menactra is given IM and should not be drawn into a syringe until immediately before use.

Influenza

Influenza is an RNA virus and occurs as type A, B, or C. Subtypes of A are determined by two surface antigens, hemaglutinin (H1, H2, or H3) and neuraminidase (N1 or N2).

1.1.0 Patient Information

Signs and Symptoms

It is spread through droplet inhalation, and illness is characterized by the abrupt onset of fever, myalgia, fatigue, sore throat, headache, and nonproductive cough. The most frequent complication is bacterial pneumonia.

1.2.0 Pharmacotherapy

Indication

Yearly influenza epidemics account for a large worldwide disease burden. Infants, pregnant women, and persons older than age 65 are at high risk for hospitalization

Table 29-2 Indications for Influenza Vaccination

Recommendations for annual TIV administration:
• Age ≥ 50 years
• All children 6 months to 18 years*
• Long-term care facility residents
• Pregnant women
• Children 6 months to 18 years receiving aspirin therapy*
• Age ≥ 6 months with chronic illnesses†

*Children 6 months to 8 years of age require two doses, 4 weeks apart, for the first year of immunization.

†Pulmonary disease, cardiovascular illness, metabolic disease, renal dysfunction, immunosuppression, or any disease that would compromise respiratory function.

and death. Two versions of influenza vaccine are available, both of which contain the same two types of A virus and one B virus each year. The most widely produced is trivalent inactivated influenza vaccine (TIV), which is administered IM. It is available as Fluzone (Sanofi Pasteur, Swiftwater, Pennsylvania), Fluvirin (Novartis, Cambridge, Massachusetts), Fluarix and FluLaval (both GlaxoSmithKline, Research Triangle Park, North Carolina), and AFLURIA (CSL Biotherapies, King of Prussia, Pennsylvania). Of these products, Fluzone is the only one approved for use in children younger than 48 months. Other persons who may consider vaccination are those who provide essential community services, those traveling outside the United States, and those desiring a reduced chance of infection.

The other available vaccine is a live-attenuated influenza vaccine (LAIV). Known as FluMist (MedImmune, Gaithersburg, Maryland), this vaccine is administered intranasally by spraying 0.1 mL into each nostril. The dose does not need to be repeated if the patient sneezes after administration. This vaccine is approved only for healthy, nonpregnant persons aged 2 through 49 years. Children 2–8 years should still receive two doses, 4 weeks apart. Other inactivated vaccines may be administered at any time before or after the LAIV. Other live vaccines may be administered on the same day, or else must be separated by 4 weeks from the date of LAIV administration.

Persons in close contact with high-risk groups should also be vaccinated with TIV or LAIV vaccine (as long as they meet the LAIV criteria). Exception include persons in close contact with severely immunocompromised, hospitalized patients, who should not receive LAIV because of theoretical concern for transmission. For example, a healthcare worker who is caring for a recent bone marrow transplant recipient in isolation should not receive the LAIV vaccine.

Contraindications, Warnings, and Precautions

Severe allergic reactions to eggs and egg proteins, as well as a previous serious allergic reaction to any vaccine component, are contraindications for any influenza vaccine. Allergies to gentamicin, neomycin, and polymyxin are possible contraindications, depending on the formulation. Children and adolescents receiving aspirin therapy, pregnant women, immunosuppressed patients, and those with chronic disease states should *not* be given LAIV. Persons with a history of developing GBS within 6 weeks of previous influenza vaccination should avoid further influenza immunization.

Package, Storage, Handling, and Disposal

Multidose vials of TIV may be used after opening until the manufacturer's expiration date, as long as there is no visible contamination.

Vaccines for International Travelers

Depending on their itinerary, international travelers may need additional vaccines to protect themselves from infectious diseases not present in the United States. Yellow fever, typhoid, and Japanese encephalitis are examples of these diseases, although there are many other infections that are not vaccine preventable. For travel to most developing countries, it is also important to receive hepatitis A, hepatitis B, polio, and MMR vaccines. For travel to the "meningitis belt" of sub-Saharan African or pilgrimage to Hajj in Saudi Arabia, meningococcal vaccine is also recommended.

Yellow fever occurs only in sub-Saharan Africa and tropical South America, where it is transmitted by mosquitoes. This infection causes a yellowing of the skin and can be fatal. Entry into many of these countries is restricted to visitors who have an International Certificate of Vaccination for yellow fever signed and validated with a stamp from a clinic certified to administer it. The vaccine must be given every 10 years for reentry into endemic areas. A medical exemption waiver is also acceptable, as this vaccine has a few severe side effects. Yellow fever vaccine is made from live virus and, therefore, is contraindicated in patients with immunocompromising conditions such as thymus disease or AIDS with a CD4+ count less than 200 cells/mL. Pregnancy and breastfeeding are relative contraindications depending on the risk of actual infection as weighed against the theoretical risk of vaccine virus transmission. Persons younger than age 6 months or older than age 60 years may also be contraindicated for the vaccine because of increased risk of side effects in these patients. These adverse reactions include potentially life-threatening yellow fever vaccine-associated neurologic and viscerotropic disease.

Typhoid fever is a risk to travelers to parts of the world that have poor sanitation, including unclean drinking water and food. This disease occurs when the bacterium Salmonella *enteriditis* subtype *typhi* enters the gastrointestinal tract and leads to a life-threatening systemic illness. Two vaccines are available for prevention of typhoid fever, although neither is 100% effective. The live-attenuated, oral vaccine (Vivotif, Berna Products, Coral Gables, Florida) provides protection for 5 years if given 4 times every other day for 1 week prior to travel. It should not be taken with hot beverages or antibacterial agents, as these can inhibit the bacterial replication. The IM vaccine (Typhim Vi, Sanofi Pasteur, Swiftwater, Pennsylvania) is protective for 2 years.

Japanese encephalitis is a mosquito-borne viral illness present in much of west and southern Asia (similar to the West Nile virus found in the United States). Travelers visiting rural areas for more than 1 month or planning to participate in outdoor activities especially during the evening may wish to be protected where it is endemic. The current inactivated Japanese encephalitis vaccine (IXIARO, Intercell/Novartis, Cambridge, Massachusetts), which was approved by the FDA in 2009, is given IM in two doses 28 days apart. The product that it replaced was a mouse-brain–derived inactivated vaccine that was discontinued in 2006. This vaccine occasionally caused serious hypersensitivity reactions and rare neurologic symptoms, but experience with the new vaccine is limited. The duration of protection is unknown, but circulating antibodies were detected 2–3 years of initial vaccination with the older product.

Other persons who may consider vaccination are those who provide essential community services, those traveling outside the United States, and those desiring a reduced chance of infection.

ANNOTATED BIBLIOGRAPHY

Atkinson W, Hamborsky J, McIntyre L, Wolfe S, eds. Centers for Disease Control and Prevention *Epidemiology and Prevention of Vaccine-Preventable Diseases*. 11th ed. Washington, DC: Public Health Foundation; 2009.

Brunette GW, ed. Centers for Disease Control and Prevention. *CDC Health Information for International Travel 2010: The Yellow Book*. Atlanta: U.S. Department of Health and Human Services, Public Health Service; 2009.

Centers for Disease Control and Prevention (CDC). General recommendations on immunizations: recommendations of the Advisory Committee on Immunization Practices (ACIP). *MMWR* 2006;55: 3–42.

Centers for Disease Control and Prevention (CDC). Preventing tetanus, diphtheria, and pertussis among adults: use of tetanus toxoid, reduced diphtheria toxoid and acellular pertussis vaccines: recommendations of the Advisory Committee on Immunization Practices (ACIP). *MMWR* 2006;55(RR-17): 1–50.

Pharmacy Law

SECTION

5

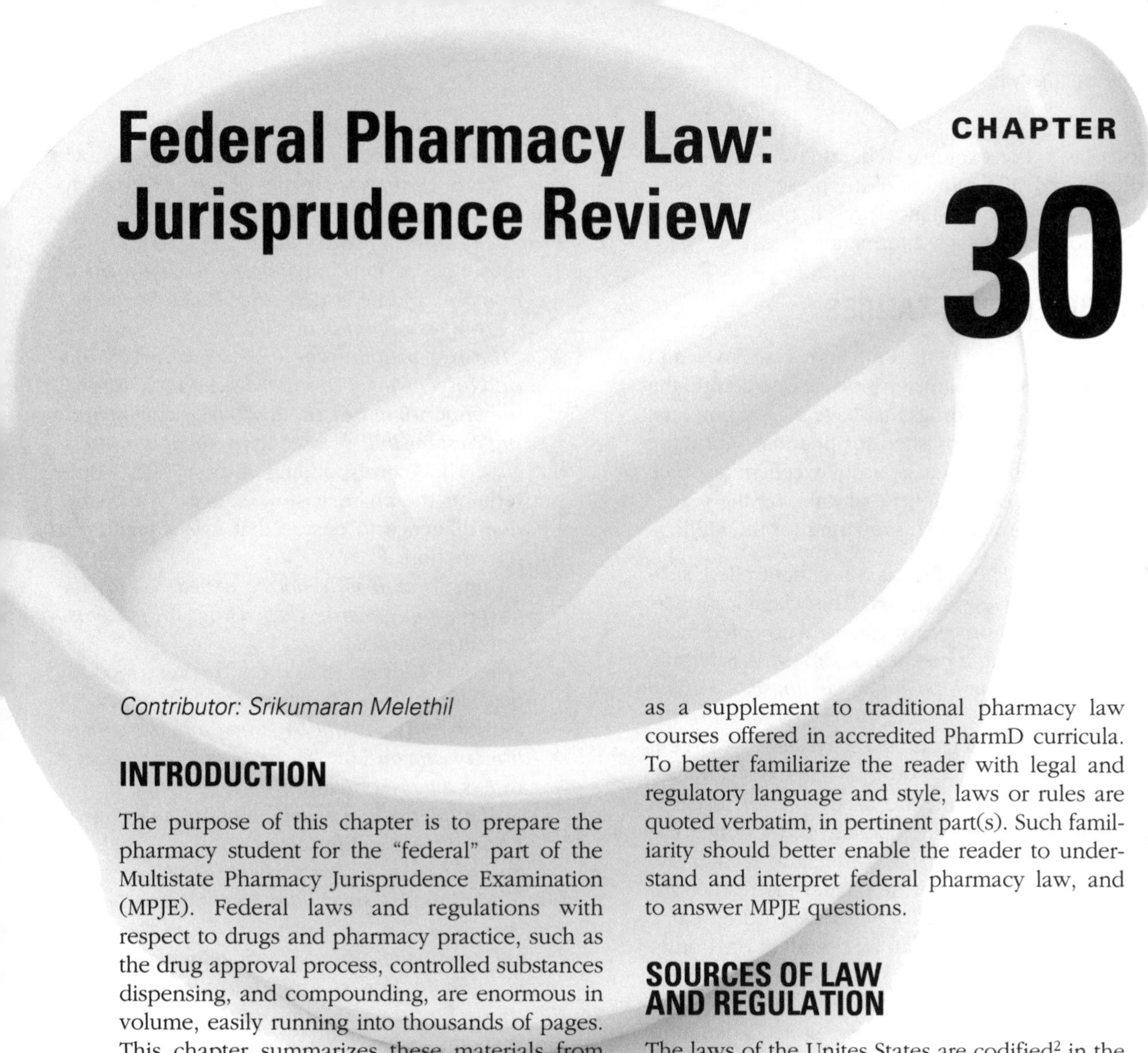

Federal Pharmacy Law: Jurisprudence Review

CHAPTER 30

Contributor: Srikumaran Melethil

INTRODUCTION

The purpose of this chapter is to prepare the pharmacy student for the "federal" part of the Multistate Pharmacy Jurisprudence Examination (MPJE). Federal laws and regulations with respect to drugs and pharmacy practice, such as the drug approval process, controlled substances dispensing, and compounding, are enormous in volume, easily running into thousands of pages. This chapter summarizes these materials from the "MPJE perspective." A significant portion (approximately 78%) of MPJE questions cover "Pharmacy Practice"; approximately 17% of the questions are from the area designated as "Licensure, Registration, Certification and Operational Requirements"; and approximately 5% of MPJE questions come from an area designated as "Regulatory Structure and Terms."[1] Specifically, topics included in this discussion are pertinent sections of the Federal Drug and Cosmetic Act (FDCA), Controlled Substances Act (CSA), and the Omnibus Budget Reconciliation Act of 1990 (OBRA-90), as well as regulations relating to compounding and retail sale of methamphetamine precursors—namely, phenylpropanolamine, ephedrine, and pseudoephedrine. Limited efforts are also made to provide legal insights.

It is important to emphasize that this chapter does not include *everything* one needs to know to pass the MPJE. Instead, it serves as a supplement to traditional pharmacy law courses offered in accredited PharmD curricula. To better familiarize the reader with legal and regulatory language and style, laws or rules are quoted verbatim, in pertinent part(s). Such familiarity should better enable the reader to understand and interpret federal pharmacy law, and to answer MPJE questions.

SOURCES OF LAW AND REGULATION

The laws of the Unites States are codified[2] in the United States Code (USC). Agencies (e.g., FDA, DEA) responsible for implementation of these laws develop rules consistent with the mandate of these laws; these rules are found in the Code of Federal Regulations (CFR). From a practical standpoint, rules have the same force as laws. Major federal sources of drug law can be found in (1) Title 21, Foods and Drugs, Chapter 9.[3] Title 21 of the CFR (which has the same title as the USC) provides the rules.[4]

Pharmacy practice is governed by both state and federal law. Therefore, a pharmacist must comply with both sets of regulations. Practically, this means the strictest law "trumps" the

[1] http://www.nabp.net/programs/assets/NAPLEXMPJEBulletin.pdf, pp. 23–24.

[2] Codification is the "process of collecting and arranging systematically, usually by subject, the laws of a state or country, or the rules and regulations covering a particular area or subject of law or practice" (*Black's Law Dictionary*, 6th ed., p. 258).

[3] http://www.law.cornell.edu/uscode/html/uscode21/usc_sup_01_21_10_9.html

[4] http://www.access.gpo.gov/nara/cfr/waisidx_04/21cfrv1_04.html

less strict laws. For example, federal law requires that the address and DEA number of the prescriber be written on a controlled substance prescription; California law does not require such information.[5]

CONTROLLED SUBSTANCES

The primary purpose of federal and state laws and regulations related to pharmacy practice is to control the distribution and use of drugs that have a great potential for abuse. A manual published for pharmacists by the DEA, written in plain language, is an excellent resource on the regulation of controlled substances;[6] the reader must read this manual when preparing for the MPJE.

a. **Schedules[7]:** The DEA classifies controlled substances into five categories. This classification is primarily based on each substance's accepted medical use, safety, and potential for abuse. A Schedule I drug[8] *"has a high potential for abuse," "has no currently accepted medical use in treatment in the United States,"* and lacks *"accepted safety . . . [even] under medical supervision"* (emphasis added). Drugs in this schedule are used only for research purposes. Starting with Schedule II, the lower the schedule classification of a drug, the greater the potential for abuse and the greater the restrictions on its use. For example, a Schedule III drug has a lesser abuse potential than a Schedule I or II drug. Specific drugs belonging to these five schedules are listed in the CFR.[9] In terms of notation, the abbreviation CII or C-II may be used to denote a Schedule II drug; similar notations can be used for other scheduled drugs.
b. **Prescriptions for controlled substances:** Each state has its own laws and regulations regarding the use of these substances in medical practice. Thus a pharmacist must be familiar with both sets of laws—federal and state. A new development is the proposal to allow electronic prescribing of scheduled drugs. On March 31, 2010, the DEA published interim final rules[10] relating to electronic prescribing of Schedule II through V drugs. Federal laws and regulations regarding "issuance, filling, and filing" of prescriptions can be found in the CFR[11]; key provisions are listed here (*in italics*) and are self-explanatory.

[5] Abood RR. *Pharmacy Practice and the Law*. 5th ed. Sudbury, MA: Jones and Bartlett; 2008:166).

[6] http://www.deadiversion.usdoj.gov/pubs/manuals/pharm2/2pharm_manual.pdf

[7] 21 USC § 812.

[8] The term "drug" is used to refer to a drug or any chemical.

[9] 21 CFR §1306.08.

[10] http://www.deadiversion.usdoj.gov/fed_regs/rules/2010/fr0331.pdf

[11] 21 CFR §1306

i. *Persons entitled to issue prescriptions.*[12] As is obvious, *"Only authorized persons"* are allowed to prescribe.

ii. *Purpose of issue of prescription*[13]
   1. Prescriptions must have a *"legitimate medical purpose"* and be issued *"in the usual course of . . . professional practice."*
   2. *"The responsibility for the proper prescribing and dispensing of controlled substances is upon the prescribing practitioner, but a corresponding responsibility rests with the pharmacist . . . .* The "corresponding responsibility" duty requires the pharmacist to exercise reasonable due diligence to ensure that it is a legitimate prescription.
   3. *"A prescription may not be issued . . . for the purpose of general dispensing to patients"* (emphasis added).
   4. Schedule II drugs should not be prescribed for detoxification or maintenance treatments. *"A prescription may not be issued for "detoxification treatment" or "maintenance treatment," unless the prescription is for a Schedule III, IV, or V narcotic drug [specifically] approved by the Food and Drug Administration. . . ."*

iii. *Manner of issuance of prescriptions*[14]*: All prescriptions for controlled substances shall be dated as of, and signed on, the day when issued and shall bear the full name and address of the patient, the drug name, strength, dosage form, quantity prescribed, directions for use, and the name, address, and registration number of the practitioner.*
   1. *Where a prescription is for gamma-hydroxybutyric acid, the practitioner shall note on the face of the prescription the medical need of the patient for the prescription.* Note that gamma-hydroxybutyric acid—also known as the "date rape drug"—is a Schedule I drug. Again, given the potential for abuse, there is a duty of "corresponding responsibility" for the pharmacist.

iv. *Persons entitled to fill prescriptions*[15]
   1. *"A prescription . . . may only be filled by a pharmacist . . ."* (emphasis added).

v. *Requirement of prescription*[16]: Regulations for Schedule II drugs are more restrictive than for the other scheduled drugs.
   1. *"A pharmacist may dispense . . . a controlled substance listed in Schedule II . . . only pursuant to a written prescription signed by the practitioner. . ."* (emphasis added). Note: See

[12] 21CFR §1306.03

[13] 21 CFR 1306.04

[14] 21 CFR §1306.05

[15] 21 CFR §1306.06

[16] 21 CFR § 1306.11

the emergency, compounding, long-term care facility (LTCF), and hospice exceptions later in this section.

2. Emergency exception[17]: *"In the case of an emergency situation, . . . a pharmacist may dispense a controlled substance listed in Schedule II upon receiving oral authorization of a prescribing individual practitioner, provided that:*
   i. *"The quantity prescribed and dispensed is limited to the amount adequate to treat the patient during the emergency period . . . .*
   ii. *"The prescription shall be immediately reduced to writing by the pharmacist and shall contain all [required] information . . . except for the signature of the prescribing individual practitioner;*
   iii. *"If the prescribing individual practitioner is not known to the pharmacist, he must make a reasonable effort to determine that the oral authorization came from a registered individual practitioner, which may include a call back to the prescribing individual practitioner using his phone number as listed in the telephone directory and/or other good faith efforts to ensure his identity* (emphasis added)*; and*
   iv. *"Within 7 days after authorizing an emergency oral prescription, the prescribing individual practitioner shall cause a written prescription for the emergency quantity prescribed to be delivered to the dispensing pharmacist.*
   v. *"The pharmacist shall notify the nearest office of the Administration if the prescribing individual practitioner fails to deliver a written prescription to him; failure of the pharmacist to do so shall void the authority conferred by this paragraph to dispense without a written prescription of a prescribing individual practitioner.*
   vi. *"Central fill pharmacies shall not be authorized under this paragraph to prepare prescriptions for a controlled substance listed in Schedule II upon receiving an oral authorization from a retail pharmacist or an individual practitioner."*

[17] The term "emergency situation" (21 CFR 290.10) means *"those situations in which the prescribing practitioner determines that immediate administration of the controlled substance is necessary, for proper treatment of the intended ultimate user; and that no appropriate alternative treatment is available, including administration of a drug which is not a controlled substance under Schedule II of the Act; and that it is not reasonably possible for the prescribing practitioner to provide a written prescription to be presented to the person dispensing the substance, prior to the dispensing."*

3. Compounding exception: *"A prescription . . . written for a Schedule II narcotic substance to be compounded for the direct administration to a patient by parenteral, intravenous, intramuscular, subcutaneous, or intraspinal infusion may be transmitted by the practitioner . . . by facsimile. The facsimile serves as the original written prescription . . ."* Note: The oral route is not included.
4. Long-term care exception (LTCF) exception: *"A prescription . . . written for a Schedule II substance for a resident of a long-term care facility may be transmitted by the practitioner . . . to the dispensing pharmacy by facsimile. The facsimile serves as the original written prescription . . . ."*
5. Hospice exception: *"A prescription . . . written for a Schedule II narcotic substance for a patient enrolled in a hospice care program . . . may be transmitted by the practitioner . . . to the dispensing pharmacy by facsimile. The practitioner or the practitioner's agent will note on the prescription that the patient is a hospice patient. The facsimile serves as the original written prescription . . . ."*

vi. *Refilling prescriptions* (§ 1306.12—Schedule II and § 1306.22—Schedules III and IV)

1. Schedule II drugs:
   i. *"The refilling of a prescription for a controlled substance listed in Schedule II is prohibited"* (emphasis added).
   ii. *"An individual practitioner may issue multiple prescriptions authorizing the patient to receive a total of up to a 90-day supply of a Schedule II controlled substance provided the following conditions are met:*
   iii. *"Each separate prescription is issued for a legitimate medical purpose by an individual practitioner acting in the usual course of professional practice.*
   iv. *"The individual practitioner provides written instructions on each prescription (other than the first prescription, if the prescribing practitioner intends for that prescription to be filled immediately) indicating the earliest date on which a pharmacy may fill each prescription."*
   v. *"The issuance of multiple prescriptions as described in this section is permissible under the applicable state laws"* (emphasis added).
2. Schedule III or IV drugs: The "6 months, 5 times rule"

"No prescription for a controlled substance listed in Schedule III or IV shall be filled or refilled

more than six months after the date on which such prescription was issued and no such prescription authorized to be refilled may be refilled more than five times" (emphasis added).

vii. *Partial filling of prescriptions* (§ 1306.13—Schedule II and § 1306.23—Schedules III and V)

1. Schedule II
   i. *"The partial filling of a prescription for a controlled substance listed in Schedule II is permissible, if the pharmacist is unable to supply the full quantity called for in a written or emergency oral prescription. . . . The remaining portion of the prescription may be filled within 72 hours of the first partial filling; however, if the remaining portion is not or cannot be filled within the 72-hour period, the pharmacist shall so notify the prescribing individual practitioner. No further quantity may be supplied beyond 72 hours without a new prescription.*
   ii. *"A prescription for a Schedule II controlled substance written for a patient in a long-term care facility (LTCF) or for a patient with a medical diagnosis documenting a terminal illness may be filled in partial quantities to include individual dosage units.*
   iii. *"If there is any question whether a patient may be classified as having a terminal illness, the pharmacist must contact the practitioner prior to partially filling the prescription. Both the pharmacist and the prescribing practitioner have a corresponding responsibility to assure that the controlled substance is for a terminally ill patient. The pharmacist must record on the prescription whether the patient is "terminally ill" or an "LTCF patient. . . . Schedule II prescriptions for patients in a LTCF or patients with a medical diagnosis documenting a terminal illness shall be valid for a period not to exceed 60 days from the issue date unless sooner terminated by the discontinuance of medication"* (emphasis added).
2. Schedule III, IV, or V drugs
   i. *"The partial filling of a prescription for a controlled substance listed in Schedule III, IV, or V is permissible, provided that:*
      a. *Each partial filling is recorded in the same manner as a refilling,*
      b. *The total quantity dispensed in all partial fillings does not exceed the total quantity prescribed, and*
      c. *No dispensing occurs after 6 months after the date on which the prescription was issued.*

viii. *Dispensing without prescription*[18]

1. *"A controlled substance listed in Schedules II, III, IV, or V which is not a prescription drug . . . may be dispensed by a pharmacist without a prescription to a purchaser at retail, provided that:*
   i. *Such dispensing is made only by a pharmacist . . .;*
   ii. *Not more than 240 cc (8 ounces) of any such controlled substance containing opium, nor more than 120 cc (4 ounces) of any other such controlled substance nor more than 48 dosage units of any such controlled substance containing opium, nor more than 24 dosage units of any other such controlled substance may be dispensed at retail to the same purchaser in any given 48-hour period;*
   iii. *The purchaser is at least 18 years of age;*
   iv. *The pharmacist requires every purchaser of a controlled substance under this section not known to him to furnish suitable identification (including proof of age where appropriate);*
   v. *A bound record book for dispensing of controlled substances under this section is maintained by the pharmacist, which book shall contain the name and address of the purchaser, the name and quantity of controlled substance purchased, the date of each purchase, and the name or initials of the pharmacist who dispensed the substance to the purchaser."*

ix. Maintenance of records and inventories[19]

1. 2-year rule: *"[Records relating to the purchase, receipt, distribution, and disposition of controlled substances] . . . must be kept by the registrant and be available, for at least 2 years from the date of such inventory or records, for inspection and copying . . ."*
2. Schedule I and II drug records and inventories must be separately maintained from records and inventories of the other scheduled drugs.
3. *"Each registered pharmacy shall maintain the inventories and records of controlled substances as follows:*
   i. *"Inventories and records [for drugs] listed in Schedules I and II shall be maintained separately from all other records of the pharmacy, and prescriptions for such substances shall be maintained in a separate prescription file; and*

[18] 21 CFR§1306.26

[19] 21 CFR 1304.04 and 1304.11

ii. *Inventories and records [for drugs] listed in Schedules III, IV, and V shall be maintained either separately from all other records of the pharmacy or in such form that the information required is readily retrievable from ordinary business records of the pharmacy, and prescriptions for such substances shall be maintained either in a separate prescription file for controlled substances listed in Schedules III, IV, and V only or in such form that they are readily retrievable from the other prescription records of the pharmacy.".*

iii. *2-year inventory rule: ". . . the registrant shall take a new inventory of all stocks of controlled substances on hand at least every two years."*

iv. *Inventories of dispensers*[20]. . .

a. *If the substance is listed in Schedule I or II, make an exact count or measure of the contents, or*

b. *If the substance is listed in Schedule III, IV or V, make an estimated count or measure of the contents, unless the container holds more than 1,000 tablets or capsules in which case he/she must make an exact count of the contents (emphasis added).*

COMPOUNDING

Federal (FDA) guidelines can be found at the agency website.[21] According to FDCA, "manufactured" drugs and drug products require premarket approval by the FDA. Compounded drug products do not need such approval. There are instances, however, where a manufactured marketed product is not suitable for a patient. Some examples of unsuitability are when patients have allergies to inert excipients contained in such marketed products or, as with pediatric patients, when palatability issues need to be resolved. In such cases, pharmacists are allowed to compound "limited" quantities of drug products, similar to marketed products, for individual patients. The FDA is concerned that "an increasing number of retail pharmac[ies] are engaged in manufacturing and distributing new drugs for human use in a manner that is clearly outside the bounds of traditional pharmacy practice and that violates the Act."[22]

Compounding of drug products is exempted from this requirement if the compounded product is not commercially available and the amount compounded is not "excessive." A pharmacy or pharmacist may not *"compound regularly or in inordinate amounts (as defined by the Secretary [of Health and Human Services]) any drug products that are essentially copies of a commercially available drug product."* In practice, amounts compounded during the normal course of business are in compliance with the law. Compounding is allowed if *"the drug product is compounded for an identified individual patient based on the unsolicited receipt of a valid prescription . . . if the compounding is by a licensed pharmacist . . ."* (emphasis added). A pharmacist may prepare a compounded product in *"limited quantities before the receipt of a valid prescription order for such individual patient; . . . based on a history of the licensed pharmacist receiving valid prescription orders for the compounding of the drug product . . ."* (emphasis added). General advertising and promotion activities are allowed. *"The pharmacy [or] licensed pharmacist, . . . may advertise and promote the compounding service[s] provided by the pharmacist"* (emphasis added). Advertising or promotion of *"the compounding of any particular drug, class of drug, [or] type of drug"* is *not permitted* (emphasis added). These rules do not apply to *"compounded positron emission tomography drugs . . . or radiopharmaceuticals."*

The following is a nonexhaustive list of prohibited acts as per the FDA compounding rules:

1. *"Compounding of drugs in anticipation of receiving prescriptions, except in very limited quantities in relation to amounts of drugs compounded after receiving valid prescriptions."*
2. *"Compounding drugs that were withdrawn or removed from the market for safety reasons."*
3. *"Compounding finished drugs from bulk active ingredients that are not components of FDA-approved drugs without an FDA-sanctioned investigational new drug application (IND) . . ."*
4. *"Receiving, storing, or using drug substances without first obtaining written assurance from the supplier that each drug substance has been made in an FDA-registered facility."*
5. *"Receiving, storing, or using drug components not guaranteed or otherwise determined to meet official compendia requirements."*
6. *"Using commercial-scale manufacturing or testing equipment."*
7. *"Compounding drugs for third parties who resell to individual patients or offering compounded drug products at wholesale to other state-licensed persons or commercial entities for sale."*
8. *"Compounding drug products that are commercially available . . . or that are essentially copies of commercially available FDA-approved drug products."* Exception: Sometimes compounding of *"a small quantity*

[20] 21 CFR 1304.11

[21] § 503A. [21 USC §353a] Pharmacy Compounding

[22] http://www.fda.gov/ICECI/ComplianceManuals/CompliancePolicyGuidanceManual/ucm074398.htm

of a drug that is only slightly different than an FDA-approved drug is allowed with documented medical need" for *"the particular variation of the compound for the particular patient."*

9. Failing to comply with state law.

METHAMPHETAMINE PRECURSORS: "BEHIND-THE-COUNTER DRUGS"[23]

Methamphetamine has become a major drug of abuse in our society. It can be easily synthesized from three precursor drugs contained in over-the-counter (OTC) cough and cold products: phenylpropanolamine, pseudoephedrine, and ephedrine (abbreviated PSE for convenience). The Combat Methamphetamine Epidemic Act 2005 was enacted[24] to restrict the availability of such drugs to the public. This law created a new class of controlled substances known as "scheduled listed chemical products." All products containing one or more of these drugs are subject to this law. Under this law:

a. The *"daily sales limit of ephedrine base, pseudoephedrine base or phenylpropanolamine base is [set] at 3.6 grams, per purchaser, regardless of the number of transactions."* Because the law is written in free base amounts, the DEA provides "equivalency charts" for converting salt forms to free base equivalents.
b. *"It is unlawful for any person to knowingly or intentionally purchase at retail more than 9 grams during a 30-day period."* Note that the 9-gram limit is for all three drugs. The limit is 7.5 grams for mail-order purchases.
c. The *"seller must place product such that customers do not have direct access before the sale is made ("behind the counter" placement) or in a locked cabinet that is located in an area of the facility to which customers do have direct access. Regulated seller must deliver product directly into the custody of the purchaser. In addition, the seller must*
   i. *"Maintain a written or electronic list (logbook) of sales that identifies:*
      1. *Products by name;*
      2. *Quantity sold;*
      3. *Names and addresses of purchasers; and*
      4. *Date and time of the sales.*
   ii. *"The logbook requirement does not apply to any purchase by an individual of a single sales package that contains not more than 60 mg of pseudoephedrine.*
d. *"Seller may not sell the product unless prospective purchaser presents a photographic identification card issued by a State or the Federal Government . . .*
e. *"Purchaser must sign the logbook and enter his or her name, address, and date and time of sale.*
f. *"Seller must determine that the name entered into the logbook corresponds to the name provided on such identification and that the date and time entered are correct.*
g. *"The logbook must contain a notice to purchasers that entering false statements or misrepresentations in the logbook may subject the purchaser to criminal penalties. . . . such notice must specify the maximum fine ($250,000.00) and term of imprisonment (5 years).*
h. *"Seller must maintain each entry in the logbook for not fewer than two years after the date on which the entry is made* (emphasis added).
i. *"Seller must self-certify to the Attorney General that each individual who is responsible for delivering such products into the custody of purchasers, or who deals directly with purchasers by obtaining payment for the products, has undergone training provided by the seller to ensure that the individual understands the requirements that apply to the sale of these products.*
j. *"Accessing, using, or sharing the logbook information for any purpose other than to comply with the Controlled Substances Act or to facilitate a product recall to protect public health and safety [is] prohibited."*

THE OMNIBUS BUDGET RECONCILIATION ACT OF 1990[25]

The major purpose of OBRA-90 was to reduce healthcare costs. To accomplish this goal, one aspect of the law requires pharmacists to be actively involved in patient drug therapy. It requires the education of pharmacists (and physicians) to make patient drug therapy safer and more effective. Key aspects of the law, which include prospective and retrospective drug review, are highlighted here:

[23] http://www.deadiversion.usdoj.gov/meth/cma2005.htm

[24] http://www.deadiversion.usdoj.gov/meth/q_a.htm

[25] Drug Use Review (under OBRA 90) 42 U.S.C. §1396r-8(g).

a. **Drug use review**

i. *"[A] State shall provide . . . for a drug use review program . . . for . . . drugs in order to assure that prescriptions are appropriate, are medically necessary, and are not likely to result in adverse medical results"* (emphasis added). *Among other issues, such as minimizing fraud, the program is required to educate pharmacists (and physicians) to "identify and reduce the frequency of patterns of . . . abuse, gross overuse, or inappropriate or medically unnecessary care . . . associated with specific drugs or groups of drugs, as well as potential and actual severe adverse reactions to drugs including education on therapeutic appropriateness, overutilization and underutilization, appropriate use of generic products, therapeutic duplication, drug–disease contraindications, drug–drug interactions, incorrect drug dosage or duration of drug treatment, drug–allergy interactions, and clinical abuse/misuse."*

ii. Key practice of aspects of OBRA-90, as provided under the "Prospective drug review" section, are listed here:

1. *"Before each prescription is filled or delivered to an individual receiving benefits under [Medicare], a pharmacist is required to screen for:*
   i. *Potential drug therapy problems due to therapeutic duplication,*
   ii. *Drug–disease contraindications,*
   iii. *Drug–drug interactions (including serious interactions with nonprescription or over-the-counter drugs),*
   iv. *"Incorrect drug dosage or duration of drug treatment,"*
   v. *"Drug–allergy interactions," and*
   vi. *"Clinical abuse/misuse."*

2. *"The pharmacist must offer to discuss with each individual . . . or caregiver . . . who presents a prescription, matters which in the exercise of the pharmacist's professional judgment . . . the pharmacist deems significant," including the following:*
   i. *The name and description of the medication.*
   ii. *The route, dosage form, dosage, route of administration, and duration of drug therapy.*
   iii. *Special directions and precautions for preparation, administration, and use by the patient.*
   iv. *Common severe side or adverse effects or interactions and therapeutic contraindications that may be encountered, including their avoidance, and the action required if they occur.*
   v. *Techniques for self-monitoring drug therapy.*
   vi. *Proper storage.*
   vii. *Prescription refill information.*
   viii. *Action to be taken in the event of a missed dose.*
   ix. *"A reasonable effort must be made by the pharmacist to obtain, record, and maintain at least the following information regarding individuals . . .":*
      a. *Name, address, telephone number, date of birth (or age), and gender.*
      b. *Individual history where significant, including disease state or states, known allergies and drug reactions, and a comprehensive list of medications and relevant devices.*
      c. *Pharmacist comments relevant to the individual's drug therapy.*
      d. *This law does not require "a pharmacist to provide consultation when a [patient] . . . refuses such consultation. . . ."*

SELECT SECTIONS OF THE FOOD, DRUG AND COSMETIC ACT (FDCA)

The Durham-Humphrey Amendment of 1951[26] to FDCA distinguished for the first time prescription and nonprescription drugs. Pertinent parts of this amendment are reproduced here:

iii. *Prescription by physician; exemption from labeling and prescription requirements; misbranded drugs; compliance with narcotic and marijuana laws*

1. *A drug intended for use by man which —because of its toxicity or other potentiality for harmful effect, or the method of its use, or the collateral measures necessary to its use—is not safe for use except under the supervision of a practitioner licensed by law to administer such drug; or*
2. *is limited . . . to use under the professional supervision of a practitioner licensed by law to administer such drug;*
   shall be dispensed only
   (i) upon a written prescription of a practitioner licensed by law to administer such drug, or (ii) upon an oral prescription of such practitioner . . . , or (iii) by refilling any such written or oral prescription . . .
3. *A drug that is subject to paragraph (i) shall be deemed to be misbranded if at any time prior to dispensing the label of the drug fails to bear, at a minimum, the symbol "Rx only."*

[26] 21 USC §353

The Kefauver-Harris Act of 1962,[27] also called the Drug Efficacy Amendment of 1962, was enacted after the discovery of the fetal toxicity of thalidomide, mostly in European patients. This drug was not approved for use in the United States. Drug approval requires submission of a new drug application (NDA), and requires the manufacturer to provide data relating to the safety and efficacy of the drug. The Kefauver-Harris Act also gave the FDA more jurisdiction over prescription drugs. It instituted measures for protection of patients, such as informed consent, Good Manufacturing Practices, inspection of manufacturing facilities every 2 years, and reporting of adverse drug reactions to the FDA.

[27] 21 CFR 312

Top 101 Over-the-Counter Medications

APPENDIX

A

Shannon Hartke and Jennifer Hawkey

	Brand Name	Generic Name	Therapeutic Class	Use
1	Abreva	Docosanol	Antiviral agent	Treats herpes simplex labialis (HSL).
2	Advil	Ibuprofen	NSAID	Reduces fever and inflammation/pain caused by conditions such as headache, toothache, back pain, arthritis, menstrual cramps, or minor injury.
3	Advil Cold & Sinus	Ibuprofen and pseudoephedrine	NSAID and decongestant	Treats stuffy nose, sinus congestion, cough, and pain or fever caused by the common cold or flu.
4	Afrin	Oxymetazoline nasal	Decongestant	Treats congestion associated with allergies, hay fever, sinus irritation, and the common cold.
5	Aleve	Naproxen	NSAID	Treats pain or inflammation caused by conditions such as arthritis, ankylosing spondylitis, tendinitis, bursitis, gout, and menstrual cramps.
6	Anbesol	Benzocaine	Anesthetic, local	Relieves pain and irritation caused by sore throat, sore mouth, or canker sores.
7	Azo Standard	Phenazopyridine	Urinary analgesic	Treats pain, burning, and discomfort caused by infection/irritation of the urinary tract.
8	Bayer Aspirin	Aspirin	Salicylate, antiplatelet agent	Treats mild to moderate pain, fever, and inflammation; sometimes used to treat or prevent heart attacks, strokes, and chest pain.
9	Benadryl Oral	Diphenhydramine	Antihistamine, antitussive, antiemetic, antivertigo agent, antidyskinetic	Treats sneezing, runny nose, itching, watery eyes, hives, rashes, itching, and other symptoms of allergies and the common cold.
10	BENGAY	Methyl salicylate topical	Analgesic, local	Treats minor aches and pains of the muscles and joints.
11	Bonine	Meclizine	Antihistamine	Treats and prevents nausea, vomiting, and dizziness caused by motion sickness, along with other symptoms associated with vertigo.
12	Bufferin	Aspirin	Salicylate, antiplatelet agent	Treats mild to moderate pain, fever, and inflammation; sometimes used to treat or prevent heart attacks, strokes, and chest pain.

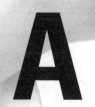

	Brand Name	Generic Name	Therapeutic Class	Use
13	Caladryl	Calamine, pramoxine	Topical analgesic and skin protectant	Temporarily relieves pain and itching associated with conditions such as rashes, insect bites, and minor skin irritations or cuts. Dries oozing and seeping associated with poison ivy, oak, and sumac contact.
14	Capzasin-P	Capsaicin topical	Analgesic	Relieves muscle and joint pain.
15	Carmex	Ammonium alum, salicylic acid, menthol, camphor	Lip balm	Relieves and prevents dry, chapped, and irritated lips; protects lips from sun or wind chaffing.
16	Cêpastat	Phenol	Anesthetic	Relieves sore throat, mouth, gum, and throat irritations.
17	Chloraseptic	Benzocaine topical	Antipruritic and local anesthetic	Reduces pain and discomfort caused by minor skin irritations, sore throat, sunburn, insect bites, teething pain, vaginal or rectal irritation, ingrown toenails, hemorrhoids, and other causes of minor pain; numbs skin or surfaces inside the mouth, nose, throat, vagina, or rectum.
18	Chlor-Tri-meton	Chlorpheniramine	Antihistamine; histamine H1 antagonist	Relieves sinus congestion and pressure, runny nose, watery eyes, itching of the nose and throat, and sneezing caused by respiratory infections, allergies, and hay fever.
19	Citracal	Calcium citrate	Calcium salt	Treats and prevents calcium deficiency or hyperosphatemia; used as an antacid.
20	Claritin	Loratadine	Histamine H1 antagonist	Treats sneezing, watery eyes, runny nose, and itching of the nose and throat caused by seasonal allergies; treats skin hives and itching due to chronic skin reactions.
21	Claritin-D	Loratadine and pseudoephedrine	Alpha/beta agonist; histamine H1 antagonist	Treats sneezing, cough, runny/stuffy nose, itchy/watery eyes, hives, skin rash, itching, and other symptoms of allergies and the common cold.
22	Colace	Docusate	Stool softener	Relieves constipation; prevents hard, dry stool.
23	COLD-EEZE	Zinc supplement	Antidote, mineral	Treats and prevents zinc deficiencies.
24	Compound W	Salicylic acid topical	Keratolytic agent; topical skin product	Treats corns, calluses, and warts.
25	Cortaid	Hydrocortisone	Corticosteroid	Reduces inflammation, redness, and swelling.
26	DayQuil	Acetaminophen, dextromethorphan, and pseudoephedrine	Analgesic, antitussive, and decongestant	Treats stuffy nose, sinus congestion, cough, pain, and fever caused by the common cold and flu.
27	Debrox	Carbamide peroxide	Anti-inflammatory; otic agent	Softens and loosens ear wax.
28	Delsym	Dextromethorphan	Antitussive	Treats cough caused by the common cold.
29	Desitin	Zinc oxide	Topical skin product	Prevents and treats diaper rash, skin irritation, and abrasions.
30	Dimetapp	Brompheniramine and pseudoephedrine	Alpha/beta agonist; histamine H1 antagonist	Treats nasal and sinus congestion caused by allergies, hay fever, and the common cold.
31	Dramamine	Dimenhydrinate	Histamine H1 antagonist	Prevents and treats nausea, vomiting, and dizziness caused by motion sickness.
32	Dulcolax	Bisacodyl	Laxative, stimulant	Relieves constipation and irregularity.
33	Ecotrin	Aspirin	Salicylate, antiplatelet agent	Treats mild to moderate pain, fever, and inflammation; sometimes used to treat/prevent heart attacks, strokes, and chest pain.
34	Emetrol	Dextrose, fructose, and phosphoric acid	Antiemetic	Treats nausea and vomiting.
35	Estroven	Folic acid	Vitamin B complex	Treats anemia; dietary supplement; prevents neural tube defects; reduces risk of vascular disorders
36	Eucerin	Water, petrolatum, mineral oil, ceresin	Emollient cream	Treats dry skin conditions such as cracking skin, eczema, psoriasis, and atopic dermatitis.

	Brand Name	Generic Name	Therapeutic Class	Use
37	Excedrin	Acetaminophen, aspirin, and caffeine	Analgesic	Treats pain from headaches, migraines, muscle aches, menstrual cramps, arthritis, toothaches, the common cold, and nasal congestion.
38	FiberCon	Polycarbophil	Antidiarrheal	Treats constipation and diarrhea; helps to maintain regular bowel movements.
39	First Response	N/A	Home diagnostic aid	Product line includes home pregnancy (measures hCG), ovulation (measures LH), and fertility tests (FSH).
40	Fungi-Nail	Salicylic acid topical	Topical skin product	Treats fungal nail infections.
41	Gas-X	Simethicone	Antiflatulent	Relieves pressure pain, discomfort, and bloating caused by excess gas in the stomach and intestines.
42	Imodium A-D	Loperamide	Antidiarrheal	Treats diarrhea; reduces the amount of stool; slows the rhythm of digestion for the small intestines to have more time to absorb fluid and nutrients.
43	Ivy Dry	Benzyl alcohol and zinc acetate	Antiseptic and astringent	Treats itching, skin rash, oozing, and other irritation caused by insect bites, poison ivy, poison oak, or poison sumac.
44	Lactaid	Lactase	Enzyme	Helps an individual consume dairy foods without experiencing gas, cramps, bloating, or diarrhea.
45	Lamisil AT	Terbinafine	Antifungal agent	Treats fungal infections of the fingernails and toenails.
46	Lotrimin AF	Miconazole	Antifungal agent	Relieves itching, scaling, burning, and discomfort caused by athlete's foot, jock itch, or ringworm.
47	Maalox and Maalox Plus	Aluminum, magnesium, and simethicone	Antacid, antiflatulent	Relieves symptoms of acid indigestion, heartburn, gas, or sour stomach.
48	Metamucil	Psyllium	Antidiarrheal, laxative	Treats occasional constipation; helps restore regulation; reduces risk of coronary heart disease.
49	Midol and Midol PMS	Acetaminophen, pamabrom, and pyrilamine	Analgesic, diuretic	Treats muscles aches, cramps, bloating, headache, fatigue, breast tenderness, and water weight gain due to menstrual periods.
50	Miralax	Polyethylene glycol 3350	Laxative	Treats constipation and irregular bowel movements.
51	Monistat Vaginal	Miconazole nitrate	Antifungal	Treats vulvovaginal candidiasis.
52	Motrin IB	Ibuprofen	Non-steroidal anti-inflammatory drug (NSAID)	Reduces fever; treats minor aches and pains caused by the common cold, toothaches, back/muscle aches, menstrual cramps, and arthritis.
53	Mucinex	Guafenesin	Expectorant	Loosens phlegm and thins bronchial secretions to make coughs more productive.
54	Mylanta	Calcium carbonate and magnesium carbonate	Antacid	Treats indigestion, heartburn, and sour stomach.
55	Mylicon Drops	Simethicone	Antiflatulent	Relieves pressure pain due to excess gas in the stomach and intestines; allows for easier passage of gas.
56	Myoflex	Trolamine salicylate	Analgesic, salicylate, topical skin product	Relieves minor pain and inflammation.
57	Naphcon A	Naphazoline, pheniramine	Histamine H1 antagonist, ophthalmic agent	Relieves itchy, red, watery eyes caused by allergies from pollen, ragweed, grass, or animal hair or dander.
58	Nasalcrom	Cromolyn sodium	Anti-inflammatory, mast cell stabilizer	Prevents and relieves symptoms of hay fever and allergies, including runny/itchy nose, sneezing, and nasal congestion.
59	Neosporin	Neomycin sulfate, polymyxin B sulfate, and bacitracin zinc	Antibiotic combination	Treats and prevents infection due to minor cuts, scrapes, and burns.
60	Nicoderm CQ	Nicotine	Smoking deterrent	Aids in smoking cessation (patch).

	Brand Name	Generic Name	Therapeutic Class	Use
61	Nicorette	Nicotine	Smoking deterrent	Aids in smoking cessation (gum).
62	Nix	Permethrin	Pediculicide	Treats head lice.
63	Nizoral Shampoo	Ketoconazole	Antifungal	Treats tinea (pityriasis) versicolor, a sensitive fungus.
64	NoDoz	Caffeine	Central nervous system stimulant	Restores mental alertness or wakefulness.
65	NyQuil	Acetaminophen, dextromethorphan, doxylamine, and pseudoephedrine	Decongestant, antihistamine, antitussive, and analgesic combination	Relieves symptoms of colds, upper respiratory tract infections, and allergies, including runny nose, sinus congestion, sneezing, and cough.
66	Ocean Nasal	Water, sodium chloride	Decongestant	Treats nasal congestion, including chronic nasal and sinus congestion, dry nose, and irritated nasal passages.
67	Orabase	Benzocaine	Local analgesic	Reduces pain associated with sources of the surface of the body. Examples: sore throat, sunburn, teething pain, vaginal or rectal irritation, ingrown toenails, and hemorrhoids.
68	OralBalance	Lactoperoxidase, lysozyme, glucose oxidase, lactoferrin	Line of products for dry mouth, including moisturizing gel, toothpastes, mouth spray, liquid, oral rinse, and gum	Saliva substitute for dry mouth relief.
69	Os-Cal	Calcium carbonate	Mineral supplement	Treats and prevents calcium deficiencies.
70	PediaCare	Dextromethorphan	Antitussive	Treats cough; will not treat cough associated with smoking, asthma. or emphysema.
71	Pepcid-AC	Famotidine	Histamine H2 blocker	Prevents and relieves heartburn associated with upset stomach and indigestion; can also be used for short-term treatment of gastric and duodenal ulcers and gastroesophageal reflux disease (GERD).
72	Pepcid Complete	Famotidine, calcium carbonate, and magnesium hydroxide	Histamine H2 blocker and antacid combination	Treats heartburn associated with upset stomach and indigestion (not for the prevention of these symptoms).
73	Pepto Bismol	Bismuth subsalicylate	Salicylate	Treats indigestion, upset stomach, nausea, heartburn, and other symptoms associated with eating or drinking too much.
74	Peri-Colace	Docusate and senna	Stool softener and laxative	Treats occasional constipation.
75	Phillips' MOM	Magnesium hydroxide	Laxative/antacid	Relieves occasional constipation and indigestion, stomach ache, and heartburn.
76	Pin-X	Pyrantel	Antihelmintic (antiworm)	Treats infections caused by worms such as roundworm and pinworm.
77	Preparation H	Pramoxine, phenylephrine, glycerin, and petrolatum	Topical analgesic, vasoconstrictor, and skin protectant	Relieves pain, burning, soreness, and irritation of the anal area associated with hemorrhoids.
78	Prilosec OTC	Omeprazole	Proton pump inhibitor	Treats GERD and other conditions associated with excess stomach acid.
79	RID	Permethrin topical	Antiparasite	Treats head lice and scabies.
80	Robitussin	Guaifenesin	Expectorant	Reduces chest congestion caused by the common cold, allergies, or infection.
81	Rogaine	Minoxidil topical	Vasodilator	Treats male pattern baldness; dilates vessels in the scalp, which is thought to stimulate hair follicle function and hair growth.
82	Salivart	Artificial saliva	Artificial saliva	Moistens and lubricates the mouth and throat.

	Brand Name	Generic Name	Therapeutic Class	Use
83	Senokot	Sennosides	Laxative	Irritates bowel tissues to result in bowel movements.
84	Similasan Earache Relief	Chamomilla calmative, mercurius solubilis, and sulfur	Homeopathic earache remedy	Treats discomfort associated with earache in adults and children.
85	Slow-Mag	Magnesium chloride	Mineral supplement	Prevents and treats magnesium deficiencies.
86	Solarcaine	Benzocaine	Topical analgesic	Relieves pain and itching caused by insect bites or stings, poison ivy, poison oak, sunburn, and other minor cuts, scratches, and burns.
87	Sudafed	Pseudoephedrine	Decongestant	Treats nasal, sinus, and Eustachian tube congestion caused by dilated blood vessels in the nasal passages; constricts blood vessels in the nasal passages.
88	Tears Naturale	Ocular lubricant, ophthalmic	Ocular lubricant	Relieves burning, irritation, and discomfort caused by dry eyes; moisturizes the eye.
89	Tums	Calcium carbonate	Antacid	Treats heartburn, stomach ache, acid indigestion.
90	Tylenol	Acetaminophen	Pain reliever/fever reducer	Treats mild pain associated with backache, toothache, headache, arthritis and colds, along with reducing fever.
91	Tylenol Allergy & Sinus	Acetaminophen, chlorpheniramine, and pseudoephedrine	Pain reliever/fever reducer, antihistamine, and decongestant	Treats runny/stuffy nose, sinus congestion, sneezing, and pain/fever caused by allergies or the common cold.
92	Tylenol Cold & Flu	Acetaminophen, dextromethorphan, and pseudoephedrine	Pain reliever/fever reducer, antitussive and decongestant	Treats sinus congestion, stuffy nose, cough, and pain/fever caused by the common cold or flu.
93	Tylenol PM	Acetaminophen and diphenhydramine	Pain reliever/ fever reducer and antihistamine	Treats watery eyes, runny nose, sneezing, and other symptoms of the common cold and flu; treats nighttime pain and induces drowsiness.
94	Unisom	Doxylamine	Antihistamine	Depresses the central nervous system to induce drowsiness.
95	Visine	Tetrahydrozoline ophthalmic	Vasoconstrictor	Relieves burning, redness, dryness, and irritation of the eyes.
96	Zaditor	Ketotifen	Antihistamine and mast cell stabilizer	Prevents itching of the eye due to allergic reactions; blocks the release of chemicals from cells involved in allergic reactions.
97	Zantac OTC	Ranitidine	H2 blocker	Reduces acid production in the stomach; treats and prevents ulcers of the stomach and intestines.
98	Zicam Cold Remedy	Zincum gluconicum	Homeopathic cold remedy	Claimed to shorten the duration and severity of cold symptoms. The nasal spray and gel swabs were recalled in 2009 due to reports of associated loss of sense of smell.
99	Zilactin and Zilactin-B	Benzocaine	Oral analgesic	Relieves pain associated with irritation or minor injury to the mouth, including cold sores, canker sores, fever blisters, and toothaches.
100	Zyrtec	Cetirizine	Antihistamine	Prevents and treats symptoms of hay fever and symptoms of colds and allergies, including sneezing, itching, watery eyes, and runny nose.
101	Zyrtec-D	Cetirizine and pseudoephedrine	Antihistamine and decongestant	Prevents and treats symptoms of hay fever and symptoms of colds and allergies, including sneezing, itching, watery eyes, and runny nose; relieves nasal congestion and shrinks swollen nasal passages.

Courtesy of: Shannon Hartke, PharmD Candidate, The University of Findlay, Class of 2013 and Jennifer Hawkey, PharmD Candidate, The University of Findlay, Class of 2013; Data from: Bernardi RR, Kroon LA, McDermott JH, Newton GD, Oszko MA, Popovich NG, et al, eds. *Handbook of Nonprescription Drugs*, 15th ed. Washington, DC: American Pharmacists Association; 2006; Data from: Drug Topics. *Pharmacy Today Survey Recommends Top OTC Products.* North Olmsted, OH: Advanstar Communications; 2012. Available at: www.drugtopics.modernmedicine.com. Accessed July 23, 2012; Data from: *Clinical Pharmacology,* Tampa, FL: Elsevier/Gold Standard; 2012. Available at: www.clinicalpharmacology.com. Accessed July 23, 2012; Data from: Lexicom. Hudson, OH: Lexicom; 2012. Available at: www.lexi.com. Accessed July 23, 2012. Data from: Micromedex. New York, NY: Thomson Reuters; 2012. Available at: www.micromedex.com. Accessed July 23, 2012.

Top 200 Prescription Drugs

APPENDIX

B

Suzanne Lifer

	Generic Name	Brand Name	Therapeutic Class	Function	Strengths and Formulations
1	Hydrocodone bitartrate with acetaminophen	Lortab	Analgesic combination (opioid)	Hydrocodone: opioid receptor agonist Acetaminophen: centrally acting prostaglandin inhibitor	2.5 mg/500 mg, 5 mg/500 mg, 7.5 mg/500 mg, 10 mg/500 mg; tablets. 7.5 mg/500 mg, 10 mg/500 mg per 15 mL; elixir.
2	Levothyroxine sodium	Synthroid	Thyroid product	Synthetic thyroid hormone supplement	25 mcg, 50 mcg, 75 mcg, 88 mcg, 100 mcg, 112 mcg, 125 mcg, 137 mcg, 150 mcg, 175 mcg, 200 mcg, 300 mcg; tablets. 200 mcg, 500 mcg; powder for IV or IM injection.
3	Lisinopril	Prinivil, Zestril	Angiotensin-converting enzyme (ACE) inhibitor	Angiotensin-converting enzyme inhibitor (ACE-I)	2.5 mg, 5 mg, 10 mg, 20 mg, 40 mg; tablets.
4	Simvastatin	Zocor	Antilipemic agent, HMG-CoA reductase inhibitor	Inhibits HMG coenzyme A and up-regulates hepatic LDL receptors	5 mg,10 mg, 20 mg, 40 mg, 80 mg; tablets.
5	Amoxicillin trihydrate	Amoxil	Antibiotic, penicillin	Inhibits cell-wall synthesis of mucopeptide	250 mg, 500 mg; capsules. 125 mg/5 mL, 250 mg/5 mL, 400 mg/5 mL; suspension. 50 mg/ mL; drops.
6	Azithromycin dihydrate	Zithromax and Zmax	Antibiotic, macrolide; antibiotic, ophthalmic	Inhibits microbial protein synthesis	Zithromax: 250 mg, 500 mg, 600 mg; tablets. 100 mg/5 mL, 200 mg/5 mL; oral suspension. 500 mg/vial; IV infusion. Zmax: 2 g; powder for oral suspension.

	Generic Name	Brand Name	Therapeutic Class	Function	Strengths and Formulations
7	Atorvastatin calcium	Lipitor	Antilipemic agent, HMG-CoA reductase inhibitor	Inhibits HMG coenzyme A and up-regulates hepatic LDL receptors	10 mg, 20 mg, 40 mg, 80 mg; tablets.
8	Metformin hydrochloride	Glucophage	Antidiabetic agent, biguanide	Multiple MOAs suspected. Main effect believed to be inhibition of hepatic gluconeogenesis	Glucophage: 500 mg, 850 mg, 1g; tablets. Glucophage XR: 500 mg, 750 mg; tablets.
9	Hydrochlorothi-azide	Hydrochlorothi-azide	Diuretic, thiazide	Diuretic effect: blocks reabsorption of sodium and chloride from renal tubules. Antihypertensive effect: unknown.	25 mg, 50 mg; tablets.
10	Alprazolam	Xanax	Benzodiazepine	Benzodiazepine: binds to receptors in the central nervous system	0.25 mg, 0.5 mg, 1 mg, 2 mg; tablets.
11	Albuterol sulfate (salbutamol)	Proventil HFA, Proair HFA, Ventolin HFA	$Beta_2$ agonist	$Beta_2$ receptor agonist	90 mcg/inhalation; metered-dose aerosol.
12	Metoprolol succinate	Toprol-XL	Beta blocker, $beta_1$ selective	$Beta_1$ receptor blocker	25 mg, 50 mg, 100 mg, 200 mg; tablets.
13	Atenolol	Tenormin	Beta blocker, $beta_1$ selective	$Beta_1$ receptor blocker	25 mg, 50 mg, 100 mg; tablets.
14	Furosemide	Lasix	Diuretic, loop	"Loop diuretic": blocks sodium and chloride reabsorption from kidney tubules	20 mg, 40 mg, 80 mg; tablets.
15	Amlodipine besylate	Norvasc	Calcium-channel blocker	Dihydropyridine calcium-channel blocker	2.5 mg, 5 mg, 10 mg; tablets.
16	Zolpidem tartrate	Ambien and Ambien CR	Hypnotic, nonbenzodiazepine	Agonist of benzodiazepine GABA-A subunit	Ambien: 5 mg, 10 mg; tablets. Ambien CR: 6.25 mg, 12.5 mg; tablets.
17	Potassium chloride	Potassium chloride	Electrolyte supplement, oral; electrolyte supplement, parenteral	Potassium supplement	8 mEq, 10 mEq, 15 mEq, 20 mEq, 25 mEq; tablets.
18	Metoprolol tartrate	Lopressor	Beta blocker, $beta_1$ selective	$Beta_1$ receptor blocker	50 mg, 100 mg; tablets.

	Generic Name	Brand Name	Therapeutic Class	Function	Strengths and Formulations
19	Oxycodone hydrochloride with acetaminophen	Percocet	Analgesic, opioid	Oxycodone: opioid receptor agonist. Acetaminophen: centrally acting prostaglandin inhibitor	2.5 mg/325 mg, 5 mg/325 mg, 7.5 mg/325 mg, 7.5 mg/500 mg, 10 mg/325 mg, 10 mg/650 mg tablets.
20	Sertraline hydrochloride	Zoloft	Antidepressant, selective serotonin reuptake inhibitor (SSRI)	SSRI	25 mg, 50 mg, 100 mg; tablets. 20 mg/ mL; oral solution.
21	Omeprazole	Prilosec	Proton pump inhibitor (PPI)	PPI	10 mg, 20 mg, 40 mg; capsules.
22	Esomeprazole magnesium	Nexium	Proton pump inhibitor	PPI	20 mg, 40 mg; capsules. 20 mg/ vial, 40 mg/vial; powder for IV injection.
23	Prednisone	Prednisone	Corticosteroid, systemic	Inhibits phospholipase, prostaglandins and leukotrienes (mediators of inflammation)	1 mg, 2.5 mg, 5 mg, 10 mg, 20 mg, 50 mg; tablets.
24	Escitalopram oxalate	Lexapro	Antidepressant, selective serotonin reuptake inhibitor	SSRI	5 mg, 10 mg, 20 mg; tablets. 1 mg/ mL; oral solution.
25	Warfarin sodium (crystalline)	Coumadin	Anticoagulant, coumarin derivative; vitamin K antagonist	Inhibits vitamin K–dependent clotting factors II, VII, IX, and X	1 mg, 2 mg, 2.5 mg, 3 mg, 4 mg, 5 mg, 6 mg, 7.5 mg, 10 mg; tablets. 2 mg/mL; powder for IV injection.
26	Montelukast sodium	Singulair	Leukotriene receptor antagonist	Leukotriene receptor antagonist	10 mg, tablets. 4 mg, 5 mg; chewable tablets.
27	Ciprofloxacin hydrochloride	Cipro (XR)	Antibiotic, ophthalmic; antibiotic, quinolone	Inhibits bacterial DNA synthesis, quinolone antibiotic	Cipro: 250 mg, 500 mg, 750 mg; tablets. 250 mg/5 mL, 500 mg/ 5 mL; suspension. 10 mg/ mL; solution for IV infusion after dilution. 2 mg/mL; solution for IV infusion. Cipro XR: 500 mg, 1,000 mg; tablets.
28	Ibuprofen	Motrin	Nonsteroidal anti-inflammatory drug (NSAID), oral; NSAID, parenteral	NSAID; inhibits prostaglandin synthesis	400 mg, 600 mg, 800 mg; tablets. Motrin IB (OTC): 200 mg; gelcaps, capsules, tablets. 100 mg; caplets. 50 mg, 100 mg; chewable tablets. 100 mg/5 mL; suspension. 40 mg/ mL; drops.
29	Clopidogrel bisulfate	Plavix	Antiplatelet agent	Platelet adenosine diphosphate (ADP) receptor antagonist	75 mg, 300 mg; tablets.

	Generic Name	Brand Name	Therapeutic Class	Function	Strengths and Formulations
30	Fluoxetine hydrochloride	Prozac	Antidepressant, selective serotonin reuptake inhibitor	SSRI	10 mg, 20 mg, 40 mg; capsules. 20 mg/5 mL; oral solution.
31	Tramadol hydrochloride	Ultram	Analgesic, opioid	Binds to opioid receptor, and also inhibits reuptake of norepinephrine (NE) and 5-HT.	50 mg, 100 mg, 200 mg, 300 mg; tablets.
32	Cephalexin	Keflex	Antibiotic, cephalosporin (first generation)	Cephalosporin: inhibits bacterial cell-wall synthesis	250 mg, 333 mg, 500 mg, 750 mg; capsules.
33	Lorazepam	Ativan	Benzodiazepine	Benzodiazepine: binds to receptors in the CNS	0.5 mg, 1 mg, 2 mg; tablets.
34	Clonazepam	Klonopin	Benzodiazepine	Benzodiazepine; believed to enhance GABA activity	0.5 mg, 1 mg, 2 mg; tablets.
35	Citalopram hydrobromide	Celexa	Antidepressant, selective serotonin reuptake inhibitor	SSRI	10 mg, 20 mg, 40 mg; tablets. 2 mg/ mL; oral solution.
36	Bupropion hydrochloride	Wellbutrin (SR, XL)	Antidepressant, dopamine-reuptake inhibitor; smoking cessation aid	Inhibits dopamine (DA) and norepinephrine (NE) uptake	Wellbutrin: 75 mg, 100 mg; tablets. Wellbutrin SR: 100 mg, 150 mg, 200 mg; tablets. Wellbutrin XL: 150 mg, 300 mg; tablets.
37	Gabapentin	Neurontin	Antiepileptic medication; treatment for neuropathic pain	Unknown. May bind to $alpha_2$ -delta receptors in the CNS.	100 mg, 300 mg, 400 mg; capsules. 600 mg, 800 mg; tablets. 250 mg/5 mL; oral solution.
38	Propoxyphene napsylate with acetaminophen	Darvocet	Analgesic combination (opioid)	Acetaminophen: centrally acting prostaglandin inhibitor Propoxyphene: binds to opioid receptor (like codeine, hydrocodone).	50 mg/325 mg, 100 mg/650 mg, 100 mg/500 mg; tablets. Withdrawn from the U.S. market in 2010.
39	Lisinopril with hydrochlorothi-azide	Zestoretic, Prinzide	Angiotensin-converting enzyme (ACE) inhibitor; diuretic, thiazide	ACE-I	10 mg/12.5 mg, 20 mg/12.5 mg, 20 mg/25 mg; tablets.
40	Triamterene with hydrochlorothi-azide	Dyazide	Diuretic, potassium sparing; diuretic, thiazide	Triamterene: inhibits the reabsorption of sodium in exchange for potassium and hydrogen ions in the renal tubule. HCTZ: inhibits sodium and chloride reabsorption at the distal renal tubule.	37.5 mg/25 mg; capsules.

	Generic Name	Brand Name	Therapeutic Class	Function	Strengths and Formulations
41	Amoxicillin trihydrate with clavulanate potassium	Augmentin (XR)	Antibiotic, penicillin	Amoxicillin: beta-lactam antibiotic; inhibits cell-wall synthesis of mucopeptide. Clavulanic acid: beta-lactamase inhibitor, which increases the antibacterial activity of beta-lactam antibiotics.	250 mg/125 mg, 500 mg/125 mg, 875 mg/125 mg, 1,000 mg/62.5 mg; tablets. 125 mg/31.25 mg per 5 mL, 200 mg/28.5 mg per 5 mL, 250 mg/62.5 mg per 5 mL, 400 mg/57 mg per 5 mL; suspensions and chewable tablets. ES: 600 mg/42.9 mg per 5 mL; suspension.
42	Cyclobenzaprine hydrochloride	Flexeril	Skeletal muscle relaxant	Reduces motor activity in brain stem; used as a muscle relaxant	5 mg, 10 mg; tablets.
43	Sulfametho-xazole with trimethoprim	Bactrim	Antibiotic, miscellaneous; antibiotic, sulfonamide derivative	Sulfamethoxazole: inhibits production of dihydrofolic acid, which kills bacteria. Trimethoprim: interferes with the production of folic acid. Bacteriocidal.	400 mg/80 mg, 800 mg/160 mg; tablets.
44	Venlafaxine hydrochloride	Effexor (XR)	Antidepressant, serotonin/ norepinephrine reuptake inhibitor	Potentiates activity of serotonin, norepinephrine, and dopamine	Effexor: 25 mg, 37.5 mg, 50 mg, 75 mg, 100 mg; tablets. Effexor XR: 37.5 mg, 75 mg, 150 mg; capsules.
45	Lansoprazole	Prevacid	Proton pump inhibitor	PPI	15 mg, 30 mg; capsules, solutabs, or oral suspension. 30 mg/vial; powder for IV infusion.
46	Fluticasone propionate with salmeterol xinafoate	Advair	Beta$_2$ agonist; beta$_2$-adrenergic agonist, long-acting; corticosteroid, inhalant (oral)	Fluticasone: inhibits phospholipase, prostaglandins and leukotrienes (mediators of inflammation). Salmeterol: beta$_2$ receptor agonist.	100 mcg/50 mcg, 500 mcg/50 mcg, 250 mcg/ 50 mcg; dry powder for inhaler.
47	Trazodone hydrochloride	Desyrel	Antidepressant, serotonin reuptake inhibitor/antagonist	Unknown. Believed to increase serotonin levels.	50 mg, 100 mg, 150 mg, 300 mg; tablets.
48	Paroxetine hydrochloride	Paxil (CR)	Antidepressant, selective serotonin reuptake inhibitor	SSRI	Paxil: 10 mg, 20 mg, 30 mg, 40 mg; tablets. 10 mg/5 mL; suspension. Paxil CR: 12.5 mg, 25 mg, 37.5 mg; tablets.
49	Fexofenadine hydrochloride	Allegra	Histamine H1 antagonist; histamine H1 antagonist, second generation	Fexofenadine: H1 receptor blocker/antagonist	30 mg, 60 mg, 180 mg; tablets. 30 mg; ODT. 6 mg/mL; suspension.

	Generic Name	Brand Name	Therapeutic Class	Function	Strengths and Formulations
50	Fluticasone propionate (nasal)	Flonase	Corticosteroid, inhalant (oral); corticosteroid, nasal; corticosteroid, topical	Glucocorticoid receptor agonist	50 mcg/spray; aqueous nasal spray.
51	Alendronate sodium	Fosamax	Bisphosphonate derivative	Osteoclast inhibitor	5 mg, 10 mg, 35 mg, 40 mg, 70 mg; tablets. 70 mg/75 mL; oral solution. Plus D: 70 mg; tablets.
52	Valsartan	Diovan	Angiotensin II receptor blocker	Angiotensin receptor blocker (ARB)	40 mg, 80 mg, 160 mg, 320 mg; tablets.
53	Glipizide	Glucotrol	Antidiabetic agent, sulfonylurea	Sulfonylurea: increases pancreatic insulin secretion	Glucotrol: 5 mg, 10 mg; tablets. Glucotrol XL: 2.5 mg, 5 mg, 10 mg; tablets.
54	Lovastatin	Mevacor	Antilipemic agent, HMG-CoA reductase inhibitor	Statin	10 mg, 20 mg, 40 mg; tablets.
55	Rosuvastatin calcium	Crestor	Antilipemic agent, HMG-CoA reductase inhibitor	Statin	5 mg, 10 mg, 20 mg, 40 mg; tablets.
56	Carvedilol	Coreg and Coreg CR	Beta blocker with alpha-blocking activity	Nonselective beta recepter blocker; blocks activity at both $beta_1$ and $beta_2$ receptors	Coreg: 3.125 mg, 6.25 mg, 12.5 mg, 25 mg; tablets. Coreg CR: 10 mg, 20 mg, 40 mg, 80 mg; capsules.
57	Amphetamine and dextroamphet-amine salts	Adderall (XR)	Stimulant	Sympathetic amine with effects similar to epinephrine	Adderall: 7.5 mg, 10 mg, 12.5 mg, 15 mg, 20 mg, 30 mg; tablets. Adderall XR: 5 mg, 10 mg, 15 mg, 20 mg, 25 mg, 30 mg; capsules.
58	Ezetimibe with simvastatin	Vytorin	Antilipemic agent, 2-azetidinone; antilipemic agent, HMG-CoA reductase inhibitor	Cholesterol absorption inhibitor and HMG-CoA reductase inhibitor and cholesterol absorption inhibitor, respectively	10 mg/10 mg, 10 mg/20 mg, 10 mg/40 mg, 10 mg/80 mg; tablets.
59	Duloxetine hydrochloride	Cymbalta	Antidepressant, serotonin/ norepinephrine reuptake inhibitor	Selective serotonin and norepinephrine reuptake inhibitor (SSNRI)	20 mg, 30 mg, 60 mg; capsules.
60	Diazepam	Valium	Benzodiazepine (BZD)	BZD. Binds to receptors in the CNS.	2 mg, 5 mg, 10 mg; tablets. 5 mg/mL; injection.
61	Pravastatin sodium	Pravachol	Antilipemic agent, HMG-CoA reductase inhibitor	Statin	10 mg, 20 mg, 40 mg, 80 mg; tablets.

	Generic Name	Brand Name	Therapeutic Class	Function	Strengths and Formulations
62	Acetaminophen with codeine phosphate	Acetaminophen with codeine	Analgesic, opioid	Acetaminophen: centrally acting prostaglandin inhibitor. Codeine: opioid receptor agonist.	300 mg/30 mg, 300 mg/60 mg; tablets.
63	Amitriptyline hydrochloride	Elavil	Antidepressant, tricyclic (tertiary amine)	Increases 5-HT and NE levels (prevents reuptake). Known as a tricyclic antidepressant (TCA).	10 mg, 25 mg, 50 mg, 75 mg, 100 mg, 150 mg; tablets.
64	Valsartan with hydrochlorothi-azide	Diovan-HCT	Angiotensin II receptor blocker; diuretic, thiazide	Valsartan: ARB. Hydrochlorothiazide (HCTZ): inhibits sodium and chloride reabsorption at the distal renal tubule	80 mg/12.5 mg, 160 mg/12.5 mg,160 mg/25 mg, 320 mg/12.5 mg, 320 mg/25 mg; tablets.
65	Naproxen	Naprosyn	NSAID, oral	NSAID	250 mg, 375 mg, 500 mg; tablets. 125 mg/5 mL; suspension.
66	Fluconazole	Diflucan	Antifungal agent, oral; antifungal agent, parenteral	Inhibits fungal steroid production	50 mg, 100 mg, 200 mg; tablets. 10 mg/mL, 40 mg/mL; powder for oral suspension. 2 mg/mL; IV infusion.
67	Levofloxacin	Levaquin	Antibiotic, quinolone; respiratory fluoroquinolone	Quinolone antibiotic: inhibits bacterial DNA synthesis	250 mg, 500 mg, 750 mg; tablets. 25 mg/mL; oral solution and solution for slow IV infusion after dilution. 5 mg/mL; solution for slow IV infusion.
68	Enalapril maleate	Vasotec	Angiotensin-converting enzyme (ACE) inhibitor	ACE-I	2.5 mg, 5 mg, 10 mg, 20 mg; tablets.
69	Ranitidine hydrochloride	Zantac	Histamine H2 antagonist	Histamine 2 (H2) receptor antagonist	75 mg, 150 mg, 300 mg; tablets. 25 mg; effervescent tablets. 15 mg/mL; syrup. 25 mg/mL; IM or IV injection. 1 mg/mL; IV infusion.
70	Doxycycline hyclate	Vibramycin	Antibiotic, tetracycline derivative	Inhibits bacterial protein synthesis	50 mg, 100 mg; capsules. 50 mg/5 mL; syrup. 25 mg/5 mL; suspension. 100 mg; tablets.
71	Pioglitazone hydrochloride	Actos	Antidiabetic agent, thiazolidinedione	Peroxisome proliferator-activated receptor (PPAR) gamma agonist	15 mg, 30 mg, 45 mg; tablets.
72	Pantoprazole sodium	Protonix	Proton pump inhibitor, substituted benzimidazole	PPI	20 mg, 40 mg; tablets. 40 mg/packet; oral suspension. 40 mg/vial; powder for IV infusion.
73	Carisoprodol	Soma	Skeletal muscle relaxant	Unknown. Works centrally to produce muscle relaxation.	250 mg, 350 mg; tablets.

	Generic Name	Brand Name	Therapeutic Class	Function	Strengths and Formulations
74	Digoxin	Lanoxin	Antiarrhythmic agent, class IV; cardiac glycoside	Inhibits sodium-potassium ATPase	0.125 mg, 0.25 mg; tablets. 0.25 mg/mL, solution for IV or IM injection.
75	Allopurinol	Zyloprim	Xanthine oxidase inhibitor	Xanthine oxidase inhibitor, which decreases uric acid production	100 mg, 300 mg; tablets.
76	Methylprednis-olone	Medrol	Corticosteroid, systemic	Inhibits phospholipase, prostaglandins, and leukotrienes (mediators of inflammation)	2 mg, 8 mg, 16 mg, 32 mg; tablets. Dosepak: 4 mg; tablets. Depo-Medrol: 20 mg/mL, 40 mg/mL, 80 mg/mL; suspension for IM injection. Solu-Medrol: 40 mg, 125 mg, 500 mg, 1 g, 2 g; powder for IV or IM injection.
77	Meloxicam	Mobic	NSAID, oral	NSAID	7.5 mg, 15 mg; tablets. 7.5 mg/5 mL; oral suspension.
78	Insulin glargine (RDNA origin)	Lantus	Insulin, long-acting	Synthetic insulin	100 IU/mL; injection.
79	Amlodipine besylate with benazepril hydrochloride	Lotrel	Angiotensin-converting enzyme (ACE) inhibitor; calcium-channel blocker	Amlodipine: dihydropyridine calcium-channel blocker (DHP CCB). Benazepril: ACE-I.	2.5 mg/10 mg, 5 mg/10 mg, 5 mg/20 mg, 10 mg/20 mg, 5 mg/40 mg, 10 mg/40 mg; capsules.
80	Tamsulosin hydrochloride	Flomax	$Alpha_1$ blocker	$Alpha_1$ receptor antagonist. BPH: "maximum urine flow."	0.4 mg; capsules.
81	Quetiapine fumarate	Seroquel	Antipsychotic agent, atypical	Serotonin (5-HT), dopamine (DA), histamine, and alpha receptor blockers	Seroquel: 25 mg, 50 mg, 100 mg, 200 mg, 300 mg, 400 mg; tablets. Seroquel XR: 50 mg, 150 mg, 200 mg,300 mg, 400 mg; tablets.
82	Clonidine hydrochloride	Catapres	$Alpha_2$-adranergic agonist	$Alpha_2$ receptor agonist	0.1 mg, 0.2 mg, 0.3 mg; tablets.
83	Ezetimibe	Zetia	Antilipemic agent, 2-azetidinone	Cholesterol absorption inhibitor (CAI)	10 mg; tablets.
84	Diltiazem hydrochloride	Cardizem (CD)	Antiarrhythmic agent, class IV; calcium-channel blocker	Non-DHP CCB	Cardizem: 30 mg, 60 mg, 90 mg, 120 mg; tablets. Cardizem LA: 120 mg, 180 mg, 240 mg, 300 mg, 360 mg, 420 mg; tablets. Cardizem CD: 120 mg, 180 mg, 240 mg, 300 mg, 360 mg; capsules.
85	Fenofibrate	TriCor	Antilipemic agent, fibric acid	PPAR alpha agonist	48 mg, 145 mg; tablets.

	Generic Name	Brand Name	Therapeutic Class	Function	Strengths and Formulations
86	Celecoxib	Celebrex	NSAID, COX-2 selective	Cyclooxygenase 2 (COX-2) inhibitor	50 mg, 100 mg, 200 mg, 400 mg; capsules.
87	Norgestimate with ethinyl estradiol	Ortho Tri-Cyclen	Contraceptive, estrogen and progestin combination	Progesterone and estrogen receptor agonists, respectively	0.18 mg/35 mcg, 0.215 mg/35 mcg, 0.25 mg/35 mcg; tablets.
88	Mometasone furoate monohydrate (intranasal)	Nasonex	Corticosteroid, inhalant (oral); corticosteroid, nasal; corticosteroid, topical	Inhibits phospholipase, prostaglandins, and leukotrienes (mediators of inflammation)	50 mcg/spray; aqueous nasal spray.
89	Estrogens (conjugated)	Premarin	Estrogen derivative	Estrogen receptor agonist; (derived from a pregnant mare's urine)	0.3 mg, 0.45 mg, 0.625 mg, 0.9 mg, and 1.25 mg, 2.5 mg; tablets. 0.625 mg/g; cream.
90	Promethazine hydrochloride	Phenergan	Antiemetic; histamine H1 antagonist; histamine H1 antagonist, first generation	H1 receptor blocker	12.5 mg, 25 mg, 50 mg; tablets or suppositories.
91	Sildenafil citrate	Viagra	Phosphodiester-ase-5 enzyme inhibitor	Phosphodiesterase-5 (PDE-5) inhibitor	25 mg, 50 mg, 100 mg; tablets.
92	Drospirenone with ethinyl estradiol (24)	Yaz	Contraceptive, estrogen and progestin combination	Ethinyl estradiol: estrogen receptor agonist. Drospirenone: progesterone receptor agonist.	3 mg/20 mcg; tablets.
93	Pregabalin	Lyrica	Analgesic, miscellaneous; anticonvulsant, miscellaneous	Unknown. May bind to alpha$_2$ -delta receptors in the CNS.	25 mg, 50 mg, 75 mg, 100 mg, 150 mg, 200 mg, 225 mg, 300 mg; capsules.
94	Ramipril	Altace	Angiotensin-converting enzyme (ACE) inhibitor	ACE-I	1.25 mg, 2.5 mg, 5 mg, 10 mg; capsules or tablets.
95	Isosorbide mononitrate	Imdur	Vasodilator	Organic nitrate, which causes arterial and venous dilation	30 mg, 60 mg, 120 mg; tablets.
96	Folic acid	Folic acid	Vitamin, water-soluble	Folic acid supplement	1 mg; tablets. 5 mg/mL; liquid.
97	Spironolactone	Aldactone	Diuretic, potassium sparing; selective aldosterone blocker	Aldosterone antagonist at the distal convoluted renal tubule	25 mg, 50 mg, 100 mg; tablets.

	Generic Name	Brand Name	Therapeutic Class	Function	Strengths and Formulations
98	Glimepiride	Amaryl	Antidiabetic agent, sulfonylurea	Sulfonylurea. Increases pancreatic insulin release	1 mg, 2 mg, 4 mg; tablets.
99	Valacyclovir	Valtrex	Antiviral agent; antiviral agent, oral	Inhibits viral DNA replication	500 mg, 1 g; caplets.
100	Losartan potassium	Cozaar	Angiotensin II receptor blocker	ARB	25 mg, 50 mg, 100 mg; tablets.
101	Glyburide	Micronase and DiaBeta	Antidiabetic agent, sulfonylurea	Sulfonylurea: Increases pancreatic insulin release.	1.25 mg, 2.5 mg, 5 mg; tablets.
102	Drospirenone with ethinyl estradiol (21)	Yasmin	Contraceptive; estrogen and progestin combination	Ethinyl estradiol: estrogen receptor agonist. Drospirenone: progesterone receptor agonist.	3 mg/30 mcg; tablets.
103	Lamotrigine	Lamictal	Anticonvulsant, miscellaneous	Unknown. May block neuronal sodium channels.	25 mg, 100 mg, 150 mg, 200 mg; tablets. 2 mg, 5 mg, 25 mg; chewable tablets. 25 mg, 50 mg, 100 mg, 200 mg; ODT.
104	Verapamil hydrochloride	Isoptin and Calan	Antiarrhythmic agent, class IV; calcium-channel blocker	Non-dihydropyridine (non-DHP) calcium-channel blocker (CCB).	Isoptin SR: 120 mg, 180 mg, 240 mg; tablets. Calan: 40 mg, 80 mg, 120 mg; tablets.
105	Cefdinir	Omnicef	Antibiotic, cephalosporin (third generation)	Inhibits bacterial cell-wall synthesis	300 mg; capsules. 125 mg/5 mL, 250 mg/5 mL; oral suspension.
106	Temazepam	Restoril	Benzodiazepine	Benzodiazepine (BZD). Binds to receptors in the CNS.	7.5 mg, 15 mg, 22.5 mg, 30 mg; capsules.
107	Topiramate	Topamax	Anticonvulsant, miscellaneous	Unknown. Believed to potentiate effects of GABA. Also used to treat essential tremor and migraines.	25 mg, 50 mg, 100 mg, 200 mg; tablets.
108	Triamcinolone acetonide (topical)	Kenalog	Corticosteroid, inhalant (oral); corticosteroid, nasal; corticosteroid, ophthalmic; corticosteroid, systemic; corticosteroid, topical	Inhibits phospholipase, prostaglandins, and leukotrienes (mediators of inflammation)	0.025%, 0.1%, 0.5%; ointment. 0.025%, 0.1%; lotion. 0.025%, 0.1%, 0.5%; cream. 0.147 mg/g; spray. 10 mg/mL; injection.

	Generic Name	Brand Name	Therapeutic Class	Function	Strengths and Formulations
109	Penicillin V potassium	Penicillin V Potassium	Antibiotic, penicillin	Inhibits cell-wall mucopeptide synthesis	250 mg, 500 mg; tablets. 125 mg/5 mL, 250 mg/5 mL; oral suspension.
110	Methylphenidate hydrochloride	Concerta	Central nervous system stimulant	Activates brain cortex and brain stem arousal system.	18 mg, 27 mg, 36 mg, 54 mg; tablets.
111	Oxycodone hydrochloride (IR)	OxyIR	Analgesic, opioid	Opioid receptor agonist	5 mg; capsules.
112	Risperidone	Risperdal	Antimanic agent; antipsychotic agent, atypical	Unknown. Affects serotonin (5-HT) and dopamine (DA) receptors.	0.25 mg, 0.5 mg, 1 mg, 2 mg, 3 mg, 4 mg; tablets. 1 mg/mL; oral solution.
113	Nitrofurantoin	Macrodantin and Macrobid	Antibiotic, miscellaneous	Inhibits bacterial carbohydrate metabolism	Macrodantin: 25 mg, 50 mg, 100 mg; capsules. Macrobid: 100 mg; capsules.
114	Oxycodone hydrochloride (ER)	OxyContin	Analgesic, opioid	Opioid receptor agonist	10 mg, 15 mg, 20 mg, 30 mg, 40 mg, 60 mg, 80 mg; tablets.
115	Benazepril hydrochloride	Lotensin	Angiotensin-converting enzyme (ACE) inhibitor	ACE-I	5 mg, 10 mg, 20 mg, 40 mg; tablets.
116	Risedronate sodium	Actonel	Bisphosphonate derivative	Osteoclast inhibitor	5 mg, 30 mg, 35 mg, 75 mg, 150 mg; tablets.
117	Tiotropium bromide	Spiriva	Anticholinergic agent	Anticholinergic, causing airway smooth muscle relaxation	18 mcg/inhaler; oral inhalation handihaler.
118	Clindamycin hydrochloride (oral)	Cleocin	Antibiotic, lincosamide; topical skin product, acne	Suppresses bacterial protein synthesis.	75 mg, 150 mg, 300 mg; capsules. 75 mg/5 mL; oral solution. 150 mg/mL; injection.
119	Olmesartan medoxomil	Benicar	Angiotensin II receptor blocker	ARB	5 mg, 20 mg, 40 mg; tablets.
120	Metronidazole	Flagyl	Amebicide; antibiotic, miscellaneous; antibiotic, topical; antiprotozoal, nitroimidazole	Causes bacterial DNA strand breakage	250 mg, 500 mg; tablets. 375 mg; capsules. 500 mg/vial, 500 mg/100 mL; IV injection.
121	Diclofenac sodium (oral)	Voltaren	NSAID, ophthalmic; NSAID, oral; NSAID, topical	NSAID	Voltaren: 25 mg, 50 mg, 75 mg; tablets. Voltaren-XR: 100 mg; tablets.

	Generic Name	Brand Name	Therapeutic Class	Function	Strengths and Formulations
122	Metoclopramide hydrochloride	Reglan	Antiemetic; gastrointestinal agent, prokinetic	Antiemetic: inhibits DA (dopamine) receptors, which increases vomiting threshold. GI motility stimulant: cholinergic activity becomes greater than that of dopamine, which increases smooth muscle response to acetylcholine and causes GI motility.	5 mg, 10 mg; tablets.
123	Divalproex sodium	Depakote (ER)	Anticonvulsant, miscellaneous; antimanic agent; histone deacetylase inhibitor	Unknown. May increase brain GABA levels.	Depakote: 125 mg, 250 mg, 500 mg; tablets. Depakote ER: 250 mg, 500 mg; tablets.
124	Nifedipine	Procardia	Calcium-channel blocker	DHP CCB	30 mg, 60 mg, 90 mg; tablets.
125	Latanoprost	Xalatan	Ophthalmic agent, antiglaucoma; prostaglandin, ophthalmic	Prostaglandin analogue (for glaucoma)	0.005%; ophthalmic solution.
126	Olmesartan medoxomil with hydrochlorothi-azide	Benicar-HCT	Angiotensin II receptor blocker; diuretic, thiazide	Olmesartan: ARB. HCTZ: HCTZ: inhibits sodium and chloride reabsorption at the distal renal tubule..	20 mg/12.5 mg, 40 mg/12.5 mg, 40 mg/25 mg; tablets.
127	Donepezil hydrochloride	Aricept	Acetylcholinester-ase inhibitor (ACh-I; central)	ACh-I	5 mg, 10 mg; tablets and ODT.
128	Norgestimate with ethinyl estradiol (triphasic)	Tri-Cyclen Lo	Contraceptive; estrogen and progestin combination	Progesterone and estrogen receptor agonists, respectively	0.18 mg/25 mcg, 0.215 mg/25 mcg, 0.25 mg/25 mcg; tablets.
129	Losartan potassium with hydrochlorothi-azide	Hyzaar	Angiotensin II receptor blocker; diuretic, thiazide	Losartan: ARB. HCTZ: HCTZ: inhibits sodium and chloride reabsorption at the distal renal tubule.	50 mg/12.5 mg, 100 mg/12.5 mg, 100 mg/25 mg; tablets.
130	Estradiol	Estrace	Estrogen derivative	Estrogen receptor agonist	0.5 mg, 1 mg, 2 mg; tablets.
131	Hydroxyzine hydrochloride	Atarax	Antiemetic; histamine H1 antagonist; histamine H1 antagonist, first generation	H1 receptor blocker. You *do* need to remember the salt, as hydroxyzine *pamoate* is Vistaril, a different drug.	10 mg, 25 mg, 50 mg, 100 mg; tablets. 10 mg/5 mL; syrup.
132	Gemfibrozil	Lopid	Antilipemic agent, fibric acid	Increases activity of lipoprotein lipase	600 mg; tablets.

	Generic Name	Brand Name	Therapeutic Class	Function	Strengths and Formulations
133	Nitroglycerin	Nitrostat	Vasodilator	Increases release of nitric oxide, resulting in vasodilation/relaxation of vascular smooth muscle	0.3 mg, 0.4 mg, 0.6 mg; sublingual tablets.
134	Propranolol hydrochloride	Inderal (LA)	Antiarrhythmic agent, class II; beta blocker, nonselective	Beta blocker (beta receptor antagonist)	Inderal: 10 mg, 20 mg, 40 mg, 60 mg, 80 mg; tablets. Inderal LA: 60 mg, 80 mg, 120 mg, 160 mg; capsules.
135	Vitamin D, ergocalciferol	Drisdol	Vitamin D analog	Synthetic vitamin D supplement	50,000 IU or 1.25 mg; capsules. 8,000 IU/mL; solution.
136	Tadalafil	Cialis	Phosphodiesterase-5 enzyme inhibitor	PDE-5 inhibitor; causes vasodilation	2.5 mg, 5 mg, 10 mg, 20 mg; tablets.
137	Rabeprazole sodium	Aciphex	Proton pump inhibitor; substituted benzimidazole	PPI	20 mg; tablets.
138	Quinapril hydrochloride	Accupril	Angiotensin-converting enzyme (ACE) inhibitor	ACE-I	5 mg, 10 mg, 20 mg, 40 mg; tablets.
139	Mupirocin	Bactroban	Antibiotic, topical	Inhibits bacterial protein synthesis	2%; ointment, cream.
140	Eszopiclone	Lunesta	Hypnotic, nonbenzodiazepine	Agonist at GABA receptors in the CNS	1 mg, 2 mg, 3 mg; tablets.
141	Promethazine HCl with codeine phosphate	Phenergan with Codeine	Antiemetic; histamine H1 antagonist; histamine H1 antagonist, first generation	H1 receptor blocker (promethazine) and opioid receptor agonist (codeine)	6.25 mg/10 mg per 5 mL; syrup.
142	Doxazosin mesylate	Cardura (XL)	Alpha$_1$ blocker	Alpha$_1$ receptor antagonist	Cardura: 1 mg, 2 mg, 4 mg, 8 mg; tablets. Cardura XL: 4 mg, 8 mg; tablets.
143	Mirtazapine	Remeron	Antidepressant, alpha$_2$ antagonist	Increases central NE and 5-HT (serotonin) activity	15 mg, 30 mg, 45 mg; tablets.
144	Tolterodine tartrate	Detrol (LA)	Anticholinergic agent	Muscarinic receptor antagonist	Detrol: 1 mg, 2 mg; tablets. Detrol LA: 2 mg, 4 mg; capsules.
145	Varenicline tartrate	Chantix	Partial nicotine agonist; smoking cessation aid	Partial agonist at nicotine receptors	Starting month and continuing month packs. 0.5 mg, 1 mg; tablets.

	Generic Name	Brand Name	Therapeutic Class	Function	Strengths and Formulations
146	Irbesartan	Avapro	Angiotensin II receptor blocker	ARB	75 mg, 150 mg, 300 mg; tablets.
147	Phenytoin sodium (extended)	Dilantin	Antiarrhythmic agent, class IB; anticonvulsant, hydantoin	Enhances neuronal sodium efflux	30 mg, 100 mg; capsules. 50 mg; chewable tablets. 125 mg/5 mL; suspension.
148	Phentermine hydrochloride	Adipex-P	Anorexiant; sympathomimetic	Amphetamine that stimulates the hypothalamus to decrease appetite	37.5 mg; tablets or capsules.
149	Aripiprazole	Abilify	Antipsychotic agent, atypical	Partial DA and 5-HT receptor agonist	2 mg, 5 mg, 10 mg, 15 mg, 20 mg, 30 mg; tablets. 1 mg/mL; oral solution. 7.5 mg/mL; solution for IM injection.
150	Acyclovir	Zovirax	Antiviral agent; antiviral agent, topical	Inhibits viral DNA replication	200 mg; capsules. 400 mg, 800 mg; tablets. 200 mg/5 mL; suspension.
151	Meclizine hydrochloride	Antivert	Antiemetic; histamine H1 antagonist; histamine H1 antagonist, first generation	Antihistamine	12.5 mg, 25 mg, 50 mg; tablets.
152	Niacin (extended release)	Niaspan	Antilipemic agent, miscellaneous; vitamin, water soluble	Enhances lipoprotein lipase activity	500 mg, 750 mg, 1 g; tablets.
153	Fentanyl (transdermal)	Duragesic	Analgesic, opioid; anilidopiperidine opioid; general anesthetic	Opioid receptor agonist	12 mcg/hr, 25 mcg/hr, 50 mcg/hr, 75 mcg/hr, 100 mcg/hr; transdermal system.
154	Levalbuterol hydrochloride	Xopenex	Beta$_2$ agonist	Beta$_2$ receptor agonist (results in bronchial smooth muscle relaxation)	45 mcg/inhalation; metered-dose inhaler.
155	Buspirone hydrochloride	BuSpar	Antianxiety agent, miscellaneous	Dopamine and serotonin agonist	5 mg, 10 mg, 15 mg, 30 mg; tablets.
156	Ipratropium bromide with albuterol sulfate MDI	Combivent	Bronchodilator	Ipratropium: anticholinergic (blocks activity at muscarinic smooth muscle receptor). Albuterol: beta$_2$ receptor agonist (results in bronchial smooth muscle relaxation).	10 mcg/90 mcg; metered-dose inhaler.

	Generic Name	Brand Name	Therapeutic Class	Function	Strengths and Formulations
157	Sitagliptin phosphate	Januvia	Antidiabetic agent, dipeptidyl peptidase IV (DPP-IV) inhibitor	DPP-IV inhibitor	25 mg, 50 mg, 100 mg; tablets.
158	Ibandronate sodium	Boniva	Bone resorption inhibitor/ bisphosphonate derivative	Osteoclast inhibitor	2.5 mg, 150 mg; tablets. 3 mg/3 mL; solution for IV injection.
159	Etonogestrel with ethinyl estradiol (vaginal)	NuvaRing	Contraceptive; estrogen and progestin combination	Ethinyl estradiol: estrogen receptor agonist. Etonogestrel: progesterone receptor agonist.	120 mcg/15 mcg per day; vaginal ring.
160	Glyburide with metformin hydrochloride	Glucovance	Antidiabetic agent, biguanide; antidiabetic agent, sulfonylurea	Glyburide: Sulfonylurea: Increases pancreatic insulin release. Metformin: Multiple MOAs suspected. Main effect believed to be inhibition of hepatic gluconeogenesis	1.25 mg/250 mg, 2.5 mg/500 mg, 5 mg/500 mg; tablets.
161	Methotrexate sodium	Methotrexate	Antineoplastic agent, antimetabolite (antifolate); antirheumatic, disease modifying	Dihydrofolate reductase inhibitor (blocks conversion of dihydrofolate to tetrahydrofolate, thereby interfering with DNA synthesis)	2.5 mg, 5 mg, 7.5 mg, 10 mg, 15 mg, 20 mg, 50 mg, 1 g; tablets. 10 mg/mL, 25 mg/mL; injection.
162	Oxybutynin chloride	Ditropan and Ditropan XL	Antispasmodic agent, urinary	Anticholinergic, which causes the smooth muscle of the bladder to relax	Ditropan: 5 mg; tablets. 5 mg/ 5 mL; syrup. Ditropan XL: 5 mg, 10 mg, 15 mg; tablets.
163	Fexofenadine HCl with pseudoephedrine HCl	Allegra-D	Alpha/beta agonist; histamine H1 antagonist; histamine H1 antagonist, second generation	Fexofenadine: H1 receptor blocker/antagonist. Pseudoephedrine: dextro-isomer of ephedrine. Acts as alpha receptor agonist, causing vasoconstriction.	60 mg/120 mg (Allegra-D 12 hour), 180 mg/240 mg (Allegra-D 24 hour); tablets.
164	Codeine phosphate with guaifenesin	Mytussin AC	Antitussive; cough preparation; expectorant	Codeine: opioid receptor agonist. Guaifenesin: mucolytic.	10 mg–100 mg/5 mL; syrup.
165	Clotrimazole with betamethasone dipropionate	Lotrisone	Antifungal agent, topical; corticosteroid, topical	Increases permeability of fungal cell wall	Betamethasone 0.05%, clotrimazole 1%; cream or lotion.
166	Fluticasone propionate MDI	Flovent	Corticosteroid, inhalant (oral); corticosteroid, nasal; corticosteroid, topical	Inhibits phospholipase, prostaglandins. and leukotrienes (mediators of inflammation	44 mcg/inhalation, 110 mcg/ inhalation, 220 mcg/inhalation; metered-dose inhaler.

	Generic Name	Brand Name	Therapeutic Class	Function	Strengths and Formulations
167	Sumatriptan succinate	Imitrex	Antimigraine agent; serotonin 5-HT1b,1d receptor agonist	5-HT1 receptor agonist	25 mg, 50 mg, 100 mg; tablets. 5 mg/20 mg; nasal spray. 4 mg/0.5 mL, 6 mg/0.5 mL; SC injection.
168	Benzonatate	Tessalon	Antitussive	Suppresses cough by anesthetizing the stretch receptors in the respiratory tract	100 mg, 200 mg; capsules.
169	Methadone hydrochloride	Methadone	Analgesic, opioid; narcotic	Opioid receptor agonist	5 mg, 10 mg, 40 mg; tablets. 5 mg/5 mL, 10 mg/5 mL; solution. 10 mg/mL; injection.
170	Raloxifene hydrochloride	Evista	Selective estrogen receptor modulator (SERM)	SERM. Only binds to certain estrogen receptors.	60 mg; tablets.
171	Butalbital, acetaminophen, and caffeine	Fioricet	Barbiturate	Acetaminophen: centrally acting prostaglandin inhibitor. Butalbital: causes sensory depression by inhibiting conduction in areas of the brain. Caffeine: stimulates CNS by increasing levels of cAMP.	Butalbital 50 mg, acetaminophen 325 mg, caffeine 40 mg; tablets.
172	Polyethylene glycol 3350, NF	Miralax	Laxative, osmotic	Osmotic agent. Causes water to be retained in the stool.	PEG 3350; powder for reconstitution.
173	Bisoprolol fumarate with hydrochlor-othiazide	Ziac	Beta blocker, $beta_1$ selective; diuretic, thiazide	Bisoprolol: nonselective beta blocker (blocks $beta_1$ and $beta_2$ receptors). HCTZ: HCTZ: inhibits sodium and chloride reabsorption at the distal renal tubule.	2.5 mg/6.25 mg, 5 mg/6.25 mg, 10 mg/6.25 mg; tablets.
174	Minocycline hydrochloride	Minocin	Antibiotic, tetracycline derivative	Competitively binds to bacterial 30S ribosomal subunit	50 mg, 100 mg; capsules.
175	Terazosin hydrochloride	Hytrin	$Alpha_1$ blocker	$Alpha_1$ receptor antagonist	1 mg, 2 mg, 5 mg, 10 mg; capsules.
176	Moxifloxacin hydrochloride	Avelox	Antibiotic, ophthalmic; antibiotic, quinolone; respiratory fluoroquinolone	Inhibits bacterial synthesis by inhibiting DNA gyrase (topoisomerase II) and topoisomerase IV	400 mg; tablets. 400 mg/250 mL; solution for IV infusion.

	Generic Name	Brand Name	Therapeutic Class	Function	Strengths and Formulations
177	Ropinirole hydrochloride	Requip (XL)	Anti-Parkinson's agent, dopamine agonist	Dopamine agonist	Requip: 0.25 mg, 0.5 mg, 1 mg, 2 mg, 3 mg, 4 mg, 5 mg; tablets. Requip XL: 2 mg, 4 mg, 8 mg, 12 mg; tablets.
178	Irbesartan with hydrochlorothiazide	Avalide	Angiotensin II receptor blocker; diuretic, thiazide	Irbesartan: ARB. HCTZ: HCTZ: inhibits sodium and chloride reabsorption at the distal renal tubule.	150 mg/12.5 mg, 300 mg/12.5 mg, 300 mg/25 mg; tablets.
179	Nabumetone	Relafen	NSAID, oral	NSAID	500 mg, 750 mg; tablets.
180	Insulin	Humulin	Antidote; insulin, short-acting/ antidiabetic agent	Synthetic insulin	70/30, 50/50, R U-100, R U-500, N; injection.
181	Lidocaine transdermal	Lidoderm	Analgesic, topical; antiarrhythmic agent, class IB; local anesthetic; local anesthetic, ophthalmic	Stabilizes neuronal cell membranes by inhibiting fast-sodium channels. Inhibits depolarization.	5%; adhesive patch.
182	Famotidine	Pepcid	Histamine H2 antagonist	H2 receptor antagonist	20 mg, 40 mg; tablets. 40 mg/ 5 mL; suspension. 10 mg/ mL; solution for IV injection or infusion after dilution. 20 mg/ 50 mL; solution for IV infusion.
183	Tizanidine hydrochloride	Zanaflex	Centrally acting skeletal muscle relaxant/alpha$_2$-adrenergic agonist	Alpha$_2$ receptor agonist	4 mg; tablets. 2 mg, 4 mg, 6 mg; capsules.
184	Ferrous sulfate		Iron salt; mineral, oral	Iron supplement	75 mg, 159 mg, 160 mg, 190 mg, 195 mg, 200 mg, 250 mg, 300 mg, 324 mg, 325 mg, 525 mg; tablets. 220 mg/5 mL; elixir. 300 mg/5 mL, 75 mg/ 0.6 mL, 90 mg/5 mL; liquid.
185	Olanzapine	Zyprexa	Antimanic agent; antipsychotic agent, atypical	Unknown. Believed to antagonize effects of DA and 5-HT.	2.5 mg, 5 mg, 7.5 mg, 10 mg, 15 mg, 20 mg; tablets. 10 mg/ vial; IM injection.
186	Memantine hydrochloride	Namenda	Central nervous system agents, miscellaneous/*N*-methyl-D-aspartate (NMDA) receptor antagonist	NMDA receptor antagonist	5 mg, 10 mg; tablets. 2 mg/mL; oral solution.

	Generic Name	Brand Name	Therapeutic Class	Function	Strengths and Formulations
187	Chlorphenir-amine with hydrocodone	Tussionex	Analgesic, opioid; antitussive; histamine H1 antagonist; histamine H1 antagonist, first generation	Chlorpheniramine: H1 receptor antagonist. Hydrocodone: opioid receptor agonist.	10 mg/8 mg per 5 mL; suspension.
188	Thyroid, desiccated	Thyroid, desiccated	Thyroid product	Thyroid hormone replacement	15 mg, 30 mg, 60 mg, 90 mg, 120 mg, 180 mg, 240 mg, 300 mg; tablets.
189	Insulin lispro (RDNA origin)	Humalog	Insulin, rapid-acting (faster than humulin); antidiabetic agent	Synthetic insulin supplement	100 units/mL; solution for SC injection. Mix 75/25, 50/50; SC injection.
190	Methocarbamol	Robaxin	Skeletal muscle relaxant	Central nervous system depressant; blocks pain impulses.	500 mg, 750 mg; tablets.
191	Finasteride	Proscar	5-alpha-reductase inhibitor	5-alpha-reductase inhibitor; prevents conversion of dihydrotestosterone to testosterone	5 mg; tablets.
192	Norgestrel with ethinyl estradiol	Lo/Ovral	Contraceptive; estrogen and progestin combination	Synthestic progresterone and synthetic estrogen, respectively	0.3 mg/30 mcg; tablets.
193	Insulin aspart, (RDNA origin)	Novolog	Insulin, rapid-acting; antidiabetic agent	Synthetic insulin supplement	100 units/mL. Mix 70/30; solution for SC injection.
194	Clobetasol propionate	Temovate	Anti-inflammatory agents (skin and mucous membrane); corticosteroid, topical	Inhibits phospholipase, prostaglandins, and leukotrienes (mediators of inflammation)	0.5%; cream, gel, ointment.
195	Chlorhexidine gluconate	Peridex	Antibiotic, oral rinse; antibiotic, topical	Bacteriostatic activity as a result of altering bacterial cell osmotic equilibrium	0.12%; liquid.
196	Moxifloxacin hydrochloride (ophthalmic)	Vigamox	Antibiotic, ophthalmic	Inhibits bacterial DNA synthesis	0.5%; ophthalmic solution.
197	Clarithromycin	Biaxin (XL)	Antibiotic, macrolide	Inhibits microbial protein synthesis	Biaxin: 250 mg, 500 mg; tablets. Biaxin XL: 500 mg; tablets. 125 mg/5 mL, 250 mg/5 mL; suspension.

	Generic Name	Brand Name	Therapeutic Class	Function	Strengths and Formulations
198	Oseltamivir phosphate	Tamiflu	Antiviral agent, neuraminidase inhibitor	Neuramidase inhibitor	30 mg, 45 mg, 75 mg; capsules. 12 mg/mL; oral suspension.
199	Buprenorphine HCl with naloxone HCl	Suboxone	Analgesic, opioid	Buprenorphine: opioid receptor agonist. Naloxone: opioid receptor antagonist. (Combining these reduces potential for abuse by IV administration.)	2 mg/0.5 mg, 8 mg/2 mg; tablets.
200	Methylphenidate hydrochloride	Ritalin (LA, SR)	Central nervous system stimulant	CNS stimulant	Ritalin: 5 mg, 10 mg, 20 mg; tablets. Ritalin LA: 10 mg, 20 mg, 30 mg, 40 mg; capsules. Ritalin SR: 20 mg; tablets.

Data from: Sigler's Drug Cards, 27th edition. http://siglerdrugcards.com

Index

C